Middleton's Allergy Seventh edition
Principles & Practice

Commissioning Editors: Thu Nguyen, Claire Bonnett
Development Editor: Joanne Scott
Editorial Assistant: Kirsten Lowson
Project Manager: Alan Nicholson
Design: Charles Gray
Illustration Managers: Gillian Richards, Kirsteen Wright
Illustrators: Oxford Illustrators, Chartwell
Marketing Managers (UK/USA): Clara Toombs, William Veltre

Middleton's Allergy Seventh edition
Principles & Practice

N FRANKLIN ADKINSON JR MD

Professor of Medicine
and Training Program Director
Division of Allergy and Clinical Immunology
Johns Hopkins University School of Medicine
Johns Hopkins Asthma and Allergy Center
Baltimore MD
USA

BRUCE S BOCHNER MD

Professor of Medicine
Director, Division of Allergy and Clinical
Immunology
Johns Hopkins University School of Medicine
Johns Hopkins Asthma and Allergy Center
Baltimore MD
USA

WILLIAM W BUSSE MD

Professor of Medicine
Department of Medicine
University of Wisconsin School of Medicine
and Public Health
Madison WI
USA

STEPHEN T HOLGATE MD

MRC Clinical Professor of Immunopharmacology
School of Medicine
Infection, Inflammation and Repair Division
Southampton University and Hospitals Trust
Southampton
UK

ROBERT F LEMANSKE JR MD

Professor of Pediatrics and Medicine
Head, Division of Pediatric Allergy, Immunology and
Rheumatology
University of Wisconsin School of Medicine and
Public Health
Madison WI
USA

F ESTELLE R SIMONS MD

Professor of Pediatrics and Immunology
Faculty of Medicine
University of Manitoba
Winnipeg MB
Canada

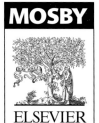

MOSBY
ELSEVIER

An affiliate of Elsevier Inc.

First edition 1978
Second edition 1983
Third edition 1988
Fourth edition 1993
Fifth edition 1998
Sixth edition 2003

ISBN (Premium Edition): 978-0-323-04884-2
ISBN (Basic Edition): 978-0-323-05659-5

British Library Cataloguing in Publication Data
A catalogue record for this book is available from the British Library

Library of Congress Cataloging in Publication Data
A catalog record for this book is available from the Library of Congress

Notice
Medical knowledge is constantly changing. Standard safety precautions must be followed, but as new research and clinical experience broaden our knowledge, changes in treatment and drug therapy may become necessary or appropriate. Readers are advised to check the most current product information provided by the manufacturer of each drug to be administered to verify the recommended dose, the method and duration of administration, and contraindications. It is the responsibility of the practitioner, relying on experience and knowledge of the patient, to determine dosages and the best treatment for each individual patient. Neither the Publisher nor the author assume any liability for any injury and/or damage to persons or property arising from this publication.

The Publisher

Printed in China

Last digit is the print number: 9 8 7 6 5 4 3 2 1

Contents

VOLUME 1

SECTION A IMMUNOLOGY

Contents

Contents

VOLUME 2

SECTION D CLINICAL SCIENCE

Contents

Preface

Over thirty years ago, Elliott Middleton, Jr., Charles E. Reed, and Elliot F. Ellis conceived of the idea for a new comprehensive textbook of asthma and allergic disorders, and they set about to publish the first edition of *Allergy: Principles and Practice*. The seventh edition of the now classic *Middleton's Allergy: Principles and Practice* is an ongoing tribute to the original editors' foresight in bringing their innovative vision to fruition, subsequent wide acceptance, and preeminence. As stated in their original preface, which is traditionally reprinted in each edition, 'it is our opinion that some chapters in this book represent the most comprehensive summaries of the subject material found in print. Thus, *Allergy: Principles and Practice* serves as not only a textbook, but as a reference book.' Moreover, it was their goal that 'the final product … turns out to be a book we hope will be useful to all students of allergy, practitioners, clinical investigators, other researchers, allergy trainees, and medical students.' Each subsequent edition has also achieved this goal. It is the design and hope of the current editors that our efforts have produced a worthy sequel that provides updated and new authoritative information on every important aspect of allergic inflammation, and associated allergic disorders.

To accomplish this, we have adhered to the successful strategy developed by our original forebears to provide information on the basic science underpinnings of allergy (principles) and integrate this information into clinical applications (practice). Our approach follows current efforts in 'translational' research to follow findings or knowledge in basic science discoveries through to their applications in clinical medicine. Fundamental 'principles' of allergic inflammation and its origins is addressed in Volume 1 with sections for immunology (including the cellular biology of immunology, as it relates to allergic processes), aerobiology and allergens; and then physiology, which reflects the functional interactions of the sensitized host with its environment. Volume 2 presents the 'practice' implications of these basic sciences as they are translated to clinical sciences, the diagnostic approach to the patient, and finally therapeutics. Within this structure, we have attempted to infuse the clinical sciences with evidence-based medicine for best practices in the specialty of allergy and clinical immunology.

The achievement of these ambitious goals was a collaborative venture undertaken with our knowledgeable and dedicated authors of the various chapters. As in the past, authors were chosen not only because they are experts in their subject matter, but also because they are able to 'tell the story' in a comprehensive, integrated and understandable manner. We are grateful for the care, dedication and knowledge of the 174 authors and co-authors who contributed to the 97 chapters of this 7th edition. Of these authors 90 are new to the 7th edition and reflect the editors' commitment to find the best contributors within an increasingly global scientific and medical community. Another aspect of this commitment to the inclusion of new and fresh perspectives is our longstanding policy of turning over the authorship of even the most excellent chapters every second or third edition.

The growth of knowledge in biomedical science during the past decade has been nothing short of stupendous, and allergy and clinical immunology have been no exceptions to this. To recognize these advances, 14 new chapters have been added to Middleton's seventh edition. These include the new scientific arenas of innate immunity, stem cells, and dendritic cell biology. A new chapter reviews the factors associated with the increasing prevalence of allergic disorders and asthma. New clinical chapters detail current knowledge of eosinophilic gastroenteropathies, immunologic non-asthmatic lung diseases, oral challenge testing, approach to the patient with chronic cough, and approach to the patient requiring emergency treatment for acute asthma. Other new chapters on therapeutics in the seventh edition include the important topics of environmental controls for allergic diseases, adherence to medical regimens, and pharmacogenomics, as well as the evolving role of anti-IgE therapy. Noteworthy is chapter 27, 'Protease-activated Pathways of Inflammation,' contributed by founding editor Charles Reed along with Hirohito Kita and Catherine Weiler. Although the final application of this new field to allergic diseases and asthma has yet to be fully defined, Charles Reed's vision of new horizons of importance to allergy has always been keen, and we are delighted to include his 'cutting edge' viewpoint.

We think it will not go unnoticed that this edition of *Middleton's Allergy: Principles and Practice* is for the first time printed in full-color format. The design includes color coding and accenting to further enhance organizational structure. And there are more than 400 new illustrations (700 in all) to bring home the message graphically on virtually every page. Appendix A has been thoroughly updated and now covers all 334 CD surface markers and their cellular expression patterns. This seventh edition has also expanded its appendix of Internet Resources useful in the science and practice of allergology. We have also provided in Appendix C summary tables from the new Expert Panel 3 Report outlining US Guidelines for the Diagnosis and Management of Asthma, and the corresponding GINA (Global Initiative for Asthma) guidelines that we hope will be of use and benefit to our readership. We have also added a new feature at the beginning of each chapter: a bulleted list of the salient scientific or clinical principles highlighted in the chapter. These principles should make the text more useful for a wide range of readers seeking information at differing levels of detail. Overall these innovations are intended to make this seventh edition the best yet.

John Yunginger stepped down as an editor with the completion of the sixth edition and his immense contributions have been missed. Dr. Yunginger was a seasoned and savvy member of the editorial team to which he brought understanding and knowledge in insect hypersensitivity, latex allergy, and allergen structure, as well as an important pediatric perspective. Equally important were his uncanny ability to encapsulate key points, and his dogged insistence on clarity and brevity. We thank him for his years of service and leadership. Robert F. Lemanske, Jr., is our new pediatric editor who brings valuable special interests and expertise to this enterprise, particular in the arenas of pediatric asthma and the origins of asthma and allergic diseases.

Lastly, the editors are very grateful for all of the goodwill and patient cooperation that made this collaborative venture possible. In addition to our stalwart authors, there are a few other people without whose skills and persistence this seventh edition would never have been completed. We acknowledge with gratitude the excellent editorial planning and oversight from our three acquisitions editors at Elsevier, Thu Nguyen, Karen Bowler and Claire Bonnett. And we are especially thankful for the indispensable editorial assistance from our Elsevier team who saw us through to completion: Joanne Scott, Kirsten Lowson, John Leonard and Alan Nicholson.

N Franklin Adkinson, Jr
Managing Editor
Bruce S Bochner
William W Busse
Stephen T Holgate
Robert F Lemanske, Jr
F Estelle R Simons

May, 2008

Preface to the first edition

Allergy, once a confusing subject for clinician and researcher alike, has emerged as a medical science in which immunology, physiology, and pharmacology interface uniquely. Our present state of knowledge is the culmination of the efforts of many workers over many decades of research in the clinic and laboratory. We want to acknowledge our incalculable debt to these investigators, both basic scientists and clinicians, who taught us not only fact but more importantly concepts and scientific method.

Several textbooks on allergy are already in existence. Why another one? We pondered this question for some time before embarking on what turned out to be, expectedly, a rather formidable task. It was our opinion that a truly comprehensive book about allergy should focus strongly not only on the exciting developments of the past decade or two in immunology but also provide in-depth coverage of equally pertinent new information on physiology and pharmacology, two areas of critical importance to the student of allergy. We have made no attempt to cover all of the subject matter considered to fall under the general rubric of clinical immunology and so do not include sections dealing with rheumatology, other connective tissue disorders, immunohematology, or tumor immunology, for example, since these subjects are well covered elsewhere.

The chapters dealing with immunology, pharmacology, and physiology appear at the beginning in the basic science section of the book to provide the necessary conceptual framework for the clinical science section, which deals with the variety of clinical states that fall within the purview of allergy and the allergist. The value of the clinical descriptions is vastly enhanced by a careful reading of the earlier chapters.

We were most fortunate in securing a truly outstanding "star-studded" cast of contributors who managed to find time in their already overcrowded schedules to help us write the book. We thank them all for their efforts and are grateful for the patient indulgence of a few who put up with some predictable editorial fussing meant to achieve proper balance and avoid excessive overlap.

Most of the chapters can be read as free-standing articles or monographs on that particular subject. This has led to a certain irreducible amount of duplication. By and large, there is consistency among chapters in which comparable material has been presented by different authors, but the reader will find occasional areas of controversy, a natural state of affairs in a rapidly growing field.

It is our opinion that some chapters in this book represent the most comprehensive summaries of the subject matter to be found in print. Thus Allergy: Principles and Practice serves not only as a textbook but as a reference book. Indeed, this was our intent, but original estimates for the length of the book were necessarily revised upward as it became clear that much excellent material could not properly be left out. The final product then turns out to be a book we hope will be useful to all students of allergy: practitioners, clinical investigators, other researchers, allergy trainees, and medical students.

The generous and unstinting help of many people in addition to the contributors made this book possible. Without the competent and devoted secretarial assistance of Marci Dame, Evelyn Beimers, Bonnie Barcy, Carol Speery, and Candace Anderson, the task could not have been accomplished. We thank our wives and families for their forbearance, while we were sequestered away from home for day and night weekend sessions during the planning and editing phases. From the beginning their support has been essential to the successful completion of our job. A number of colleagues, too numerous to name, provided help in critical reading of manuscripts. To these and others who were helpful in a variety of ways, we offer thanks.

We are saddened that two contributors died during the preparation of the book. Jane Harnett is the senior author of the chapter dealing with aspirin idiosyncrasy. Dr. Harnett compiled much of the information for the chapter and worked on the manuscript under extremely difficult circumstances up to within only a few days of her untimely death. She is remembered fondly and with respect by all those with whom she worked. Robert P. Orange, one of the most brilliant and creative investigators of his generation, died suddenly during the preparation of the book. No one can guess what additional important discoveries Dr. Orange would have made had he not died so prematurely.

We would like to record here our personal sorrow at the loss of these fine physicians. We hope that their representation in this textbook will help keep memories of them alive.

Elliott Middleton, Jr
Charles E Reed
Elliot F Ellis

Contributors

DARRYL J ADAMKO MD FRCPC

Associate Professor, Pulmonary Research Group
Department of Pediatrics
Heritage Medical Research Centre
University of Alberta
Edmonton AB
Canada

N FRANKLIN ADKINSON JR MD

Professor of Medicine
and Training Program Director
Division of Allergy and Clinical Immunology
Johns Hopkins University School of Medicine
Johns Hopkins Asthma and Allergy Center
Baltimore MD
USA

CEZMI A AKDIS MD

Professor of Immunology
Director
Swiss Institute of Allergy and Asthma Research
Davos
Switzerland

YASSINE AMRANI PHD

Reader in Respiratory Immunology
Department of Infection, Immunity and Inflammation
University of Leicester School of Medicine
Leicester
UK

ANDREA J APTER MD MA MSC

Professor of Medicine
Division of Pulmonary, Allergy and Critical Care Medicine
Department of Medicine
School of Medicine
University of Pennsylvania
Philadelphia PA
USA

ERIKA AVILA-TANG MHS PHD

Research Associate
Department of Epidemiology
Johns Hopkins Bloomberg School of Public Health
Baltimore MD
USA

CLAUS BACHERT MD PHD

Professor of Medicine, Chief of Clinics
Head, Upper Airway Research Laboratory
ENT Department
University Hospital Ghent
Ghent
Belgium

KATHERINE J BAINES BBIOMEDSCI (HONS) PHD

Post-Doctoral Fellow
Department of Respiratory Medicine
Center for Asthma and Respiratory Diseases
University of Newcastle
Newcastle NSW
Australia

Contributors

MARK BALLOW MD

Professor of Pediatrics
University of Buffalo School of Medicine and Biomedical Sciences
Division of Allergy and Immunology
Women and Children's Hospital of Buffalo
Buffalo NY
USA

JENNIFER L BANKERS-FULBRIGHT PHD

Assistant Professor of Medicine
Division of Allergy
Mayo Clinic
Rochester MN
USA

PETER J BARNES DM DSC FMEDSCI FRS

Head of Respiratory Medicine
National Heart and Lung Institute
Imperial College London
London
UK

NEAL P BARNEY MD

Associate Professor of Ophthalmology
Department of Ophthalmology and Visual Sciences
University of Wisconsin School of Medicine
Madison WI
USA

LEAH BELLEHSEN PHD

Visiting Professor
Department of Pharmacology and Experimental Therapeutics
School of Pharmacy, Faculty of Medicine
The Hebrew University of Jerusalem
Jerusalem
Israel

BRUCE G BENDER PHD

Professor of Psychiatry
Head, Division of Pediatric Behavioral Health
National Jewish Medical and Research Center
Denver CO
USA

PAUL J BERTICS PHD

Kellett Professor of Biomolecular Chemistry
School of Medicine and Public Health
Department of Biomolecular Chemistry
University of Wisconsin
Madison WI
USA

EUGENE R BLEECKER MD

Professor of Medicine
Co-Director, Center for Human Genomics
Wake Forest University
Winston-Salem NC
USA

BRUCE S BOCHNER MD

Professor of Medicine
Director, Division of Allergy and Clinical Immunology
Johns Hopkins University School of Medicine
Johns Hopkins Asthma and Allergy Center
Baltimore MD
USA

MARK BOGUNIEWICZ MD

Professor of Pediatrics
Division of Allergy-Immunology
National Jewish Medical and Research Center
and University of Colorado School of Medicine
Denver CO
USA

LARRY BORISH MD

Professor of Medicine
Asthma and Allergic Disease Center
University of Virginia Health System
Charlottesville VA
USA

LOUIS-PHILIPPE BOULET MD FRCPC FCCP

Lung Specialist
Institute of Cardiology and Pulmonology of Laval University
Laval Hospital
Quebec QC
Canada

JEAN BOUSQUET MD

Professor of Pulmonology
Department of Allergology
Arnaud de Villeneuve Hospital
University Hospital of Montpellier
Montpellier
France

JOSHUA A BOYCE MD

Co-Director, Inflammation and Allergic Diseases Research Section
Associate Professor of Medicine
Harvard Medical School
Division of Rheumatology, Immunology and Allergy
Brigham and Women's Hospital
Boston MA
USA

DAVID H BROIDE MBCHB

Professor of Medicine
Division of Allergy and Immunology
University of California, San Diego
La Jolla CA
USA

REBECCA H BUCKLEY MD

J Buren Sidbury Professor of Pediatrics
Professor of Immunology
Departments of Pediatrics and Immunology
Duke University Medical Center
Durham NC
USA

A WESLEY BURKS MD

Professor of Pediatrics
Pediatric Allergy and Immunology
Duke University Medical Center
Durham NC
USA

ROBERT K BUSH MD

Professor of Medicine
Department of Medicine
University of Wisconsin School of Medicine and Public Health
Madison WI
USA

PAULA J BUSSE MD

Assistant Professor of Medicine
Department of Internal Medicine
Mount Sinai School of Medicine
New York NY
USA

WILLIAM W BUSSE MD

Professor of Medicine
Department of Medicine
University of Wisconsin School of Medicine and Public Health
Madison WI
USA

WILLIAM J CALHOUN MD

Sealy and Smith Distinguished Professor
Vice Chair for Research
Department of Internal Medicine
University of Texas Medical Branch
Galveston TX
USA

CARLOS A CAMARGO JR MD DRPH

Associate Professor of Medicine
Department of Emergency Medicine
Massachusetts General Hospital
Harvard Medical School
Boston MA
USA

BRENDAN J CANNING PHD

Associate Professor of Medicine
Johns Hopkins University School of Medicine
Johns Hopkins Asthma and Allergy Center
Baltimore MD
USA

THOMAS B CASALE MD

Professor of Medicine
Chief, Division of Allergy/Immunology
Division of Allergy/Immunology
Creighton University School of Medicine
Omaha NE
USA

GÜLFEM ELIF ÇELIK MD

Professor of Chest Disease and Allergy
Department of Allergy
Ankara University School of Medicine
Cebeci Hospital
Ankara
Turkey

CHRISTINA D CHAMBERS PHD MPH

Associate Professor
Department of Pediatrics and Family and Preventative Medicine
University of California San Diego School of Medicine
UCSD Medical Center
San Diego CA
USA

MOIRA CHAN-YEUNG MB FRCPC FRCP

Professor of Medicine
Respiratory Division
Department of Medicine
University of British Columbia
Vancouver BC
Canada

Contributors

JAVIER CHINEN MD PHD

Assistant Professor
Department of Pediatrics
Allergy and Immunology Section
Baylor College of Medicine
Houston TX
USA

DONALD W COCKCROFT MD FRCPC

Professor of Respiratory Medicine
Division of Pulmonary Medicine
University of Saskatchewan
Royal University Hospital
Saskatoon SK
Canada

LAUREN COHN MD

Associate Professor, Pulmonary and Critical Care
Department of Internal Medicine
Yale University School of Medicine
New Haven CT
USA

ELLEN B COOK PHD

Associate Scientist
Department of Medicine
University of Wisconsin Medical School
Madison WI
USA

JONATHAN CORREN MD

Associate Clinical Professor of Medicine
David Geffen School of Medicine
University of California
Los Angeles CA
USA

RONINA COVAR MD

Staff Physician
Department of Pediatrics
National Jewish Medical and Research Center
Denver CO
USA

ADNAN CUSTOVIC MD PHD

Professor of Allergy
North West Lung Centre
University of Manchester
Wythenshawe Hospital
Manchester
UK

TIMOTHY DECAPITE MD

Dermatology Resident
Department of Dermatology
University of Maryland
Baltimore MD
USA

PASCAL DEMOLY MD PHD

Professor of Pulmonology
Department of Allergology
INSERM
Arnaud de Villeneuve Hospital
Montpellier
France

ANNE E DIXON MA BM BCH

Assistant Professor of Medicine
Vermont Lung Center
University of Vermont
Burlington VT
USA

MYRNA B DOLOVICH P.ENG

Associate Clinical Professor Medicine
Faculty of Health Sciences
Head, Firestone Research Aerosol Laboratory
Center for Molecular Imaging of the Lung
St Joseph's Healthcare
Hamilton ON
Canada

STEPHEN R DURHAM MA MD FRCP

Professor of Allergy and Respiratory Medicine
National Heart and Lung Institute
Imperial College School of Medicine
London
UK

RONALD ECCLES DSC

Professor
Common Cold Centre
Cardiff School of Biosciences
Cardiff
UK

ALAN M EDWARDS MBBCHIR

Clinical Assistant (Allergy)
The David Hide Asthma and Allergy Research Centre
St. Mary's Hospital
Newport
Isle of Wight
UK

ROBERT E ESCH PHD

Vice President
Research and Development
Greer Laboratories, Inc.
Lenoir NC
USA

JOHN V FAHY MD

Professor of Medicine
Division of Pulmonary and Critical Care Medicine
University of California, San Francisco
San Francisco CA
USA

REUBEN FALKOFF MD PHD

Clinical Physician
Department of Allergy
Kaiser Permanente Medical Center
San Diego CA
USA

THOMAS A FLEISHER MD

Chief, Department of Laboratory Medicine
NIH Clinical Center
National Institutes of Health
Bethesda MD
USA

SUSAN C FOLEY MD

Postdoctoral Fellow
Meakins-Christie Laboratories
Department of Medicine
McGill University
Montreal QC
Canada

MICHAEL M FRANK MD

Samuel L Katz Professor of Pediatrics, Medicine and Immunology
Department of Pediatrics
Duke University Medical Center
Durham NC
USA

ALLISON D FRYER PHD

Professor of Physiology and Pharmacology
Professor of Pulmonary and Critical Care Medicine
Department of Physiology and Pharmacology
Oregon Health Sciences University
Portland OR
USA

ANTHONY A GASPARI MD

Professor of Dermatology
Department of Dermatology
University of Maryland
Baltimore MD
USA

PHILIPPE GEVAERT MD PHD

Scientific Staff
Department of Otorhinolaryngology
Faculty of Medicine and Health Sciences
University of Ghent
Ghent
Belgium

PETER G GIBSON MBBS FRACP

Clinical Professor of Medicine
Department of Respiratory Medicine
Hunter Medical Research Institute
John Hunter Hospital
New Lambton NSW
Australia

MICHAEL D GOBER MD PHD

Resident Physician
Department of Dermatology
University of Pennsylvania
Philadelphia PA
USA

DAVID B K GOLDEN MD

Associate Professor of Medicine
White Marsh Professional Center
Johns Hopkins University School of Medicine
Baltimore MD
USA

FRANK M GRAZIANO MD PHD

Professor of Medicine
Department of Medicine
University of Wisconsin School of Medicine and Public Health
Madison WI
USA

THERESA GUILBERT MD

Assistant Professor of Pediatrics
Department of Pediatrics
University of Wisconsin
Madison WI
USA

Contributors

SUDHIR GUPTA MD PHD MACP FRCPC

Professor of Medicine, Pathology, and Laboratory Medicine
and Microbiology and Molecular Genetics
Chief, Basic and Clinical Immunology
University of California, Irvine
Irvine CA
USA

QUTAYBA HAMID MD PHD

James McGill Professor of Medicine
and Associate Director
Meakins-Christie Laboratories
Department of Medicine
McGill University
Montréal QC
Canada

ROBERT G HAMILTON PHD D.ABMLI

Professor of Medicine and Pathology
Division of Allergy and Clinical Immunology
Johns Hopkins University School of Medicine
Johns Hopkins Asthma and Allergy Center
Baltimore MD
USA

HAMIDA HAMMAD PHD

Assistant Professor of Medicine
Division of Internal Medicine
Laboratory of Immunoregulation and Mucosal Immunology
University Hospital Ghent
Ghent
Belgium

C GARREN HESTER MD

Laboratory Research Analyst
Department of Pediatrics
Duke University Medical Center
Durham NC
USA

STEPHEN T HOLGATE BSC MD DSC FRCP FRCPATH FIBIOL
FMEDSCI

MRC Clinical Professor of Immunopharmacology
School of Medicine
Infection, Inflammation and Repair
Southampton University and Hospitals Trust
Southampton
UK

FLORENCE IDA HSU MD

Instructor in Medicine, Harvard Medical School
Division of Rheumatology, Immunology and Allergy
Brigham and Women's Hospital
Chestnut Hill MA
USA

CHARLES G IRVIN PHD

Professor, Department of Medicine
Director, Vermont Lung Center
Department of Medicine
University of Vermont
Burlington VT
USA

ELLIOT ISRAEL MD

Director, Pulmonary Clinical Research
Associate Professor of Medicine
Harvard Medical School
Brigham and Women's Hospital
Boston MA
USA

DAVID B JACOBY MD

Professor of Physiology and Pharmacology
Professor of Pulmonary and Critical Care Medicine
Department of Physiology and Pharmacology
Oregon Health and Science University
Portland OR
USA

PETER K JEFFERY FRCPATH DSC (MED) PHD MSC BSC

Emeritus Professor of Lung Pathology
Senior Research Investigator
Honorary Consultant Pathologist
Lung Pathology Unit
Royal Brompton Hospital
Imperial College London
London
UK

CHRISTINE COLE JOHNSON PHD MPH

Senior Scientist and Director
Department for Biostatistics and Research Epidemiology
Henry Ford Hospital Center for Allergy, Asthma and Immunology
Research
Detroit MI
USA

RICHARD B JOHNSTON JR MD

Executive Vice President for Academic Affairs
National Jewish Medical and Research Center
Professor of Pediatrics, Associate Dean for Research Development
University of Colorado School of Medicine
Denver CO
USA

SUJANI KAKUMANU MD

Clinical Instructor
Department of Medicine
University of Wisconsin School of Medicine and Public Health
Madison WI
USA

ALLEN P KAPLAN MD

Professor of Medicine
Division of Pulmonary and Critical Medicine and Allergy
and Clinical Immunology
Department of Medicine
Medical University of South Carolina
Charleston SC
USA

ARTHUR KAVANAUGH MD

Professor of Medicine
Division of Rheumatology, Allergy and Immunology
University of California San Diego
La Jolla CA
USA

PRAMOD KELKAR MD

Partner
Allergy and Asthma Care, PA
Maple Grove MN
USA

H WILLIAM KELLY BS PHARMD

Professor Emeritus
Departments of Pediatrics and Pharmacy
University of New Mexico Health Sciences Center
Albuquerque NM
USA

JOHN M KELSO MD

Clinical Professor of Pediatrics and Medicine
University of California, San Diego
Division of Allergy, Asthma and Immunology
Scripps Clinic
La Jolla CA
USA

HIROHITO KITA MD

Professor of Medicine
Departments of Allergy and Immunology, Otorhinolaryngology
and Immunology
Mayo Clinic
Rochester MN
USA

CYNTHIA J KOZIOL PHD

Research Fellow
Department of Biomoloecular Chemistry
University of Wisconsin
Madison WI
USA

PAIGE LACY PHD

Associate Professor of Medicine
Pulmonary Research Group
Department of Medicine
Heritage Medical Research Centre
University of Alberta
Edmonton AB
Canada

BART N LAMBRECHT MD PHD

Professor of Medicine
Division of Internal Medicine
Laboratory of Immunoregulation and Mucosal Immunology
University Hospital Ghent
Ghent
Belgium

ROBERT F LEMANSKE JR MD

Professor of Pediatrics and Medicine
Head, Division of Pediatric Allergy, Immunology and
Rheumatology
University of Wisconsin School of Medicine and Public Health
Madison WI
USA

DONALD Y M LEUNG MD PHD

Professor of Pediatrics
University of Colorado Health Sciences Center
Head, Division of Pediatric Allergy/Immunology
National Jewish Medical and Research Center
Denver CO
USA

Contributors

FRANCESCA LEVI-SCHAFFER PHD

Isaac and Myrna Kaye Chair in Immunopharmacology
Professor of Immunopharmacology
Department of Pharmacology and Experimental Therapeutics
School of Pharmacy, Faculty of Medicine
The Hebrew University of Jerusalem
Jerusalem
Israel

IAN P LEWKOWICH PHD

Post-doctoral Fellow
Division of Immunobiology
Cincinnati Children's Hospital
Cincinnati OH
USA

JAMES T LI MD

Professor of Medicine
Division of Allergic Diseases
Mayo Clinic
Rochester MN
USA

PHILLIP L LIEBERMAN MD

Clinical Professor of Medicine and Pediatrics
Division of Allergy and Immunology
University of Tennessee College of Medicine
Germantown TN
USA

ANDREW H LIU MD

Associate Professor
Allergy and Clinical Immunonlogy
Department of Pediatrics
National Jewish Medical and Research Center
University of Colorado School of Medicine
Denver CO
USA

RICHARD F LOCKEY MD

Distinguished University Health Professor
Professor of Medicine, Pediatrics and Public Health
Director, Division of Allergy and Immunology
Joy McCann Culverhouse Chair in Allergy and Immunology
University of South Florida College of Medicine
and James A Haley Veterans' Hospital
Tampa FL
USA

ANDREW D LUSTER MD PHD

Professor of Medicine
Harvard Medical School
Chief, Division of Rheumatology, Allergy and Immunology
Massachusetts General Hospital
Boston MA
USA

DONALD W MacGLASHAN JR MD PHD

Professor of Medicine
Division of Allergy and Clinical Immunology
Johns Hopkins University School of Medicine
Johns Hopkins Asthma and Allergy Center
Baltimore MD
USA

ERIC MACY MD FAAAAI

Assistant Clinical Professor of Medicine
University of California, San Diego
Department of Allergy
Kaiser Permanente Medical Center
San Diego CA
USA

JEAN-LUC MALO MD

Professor and Chest Physician
Department of Chest Medicine
Sacré Coeur Hospital
and University of Montréal
Montréal QC
Canada

ELIZABETH MATSUI MD MHS

Assistant Professor of Pediatrics
Division of Pediatric Allergy and Immunology
Johns Hopkins Hospital
Baltimore MD
USA

E R McFADDEN JR MD

Argyl J Beams Professor of Medicine
Director, Center for Academic Clinical Research
Case Western Reserve University School of Medicine
Division of Pulmonary, Critical Care and Sleep Medicine
MetroHealth Medical Center
University Hospital Cleveland
Cleveland OH
USA

MICHAEL H MELLON MD

Associate Clinical Professor of Pediatrics
University of California San Diego
Department of Allergy
Kaiser Permanente Medical Center
San Diego CA
USA

DEAN D METCALFE MD

Laboratory Chief
Laboratory of Allergic Diseases
National Institute of Allergy and Infectious Diseases
National Institutes of Health
Bethesda MD
USA

DEBORAH A MEYERS PHD

Co-Director
Center for Human Genetics
Wake Forest University
Winston-Salem NC
USA

ZAMANEH MIKHAK MD

Instructor in Medicine
Harvard Medical School
Center for Immunology and Inflammatory Diseases
Division of Rheumatology, Allergy and Immunology
Massachusetts General Hospital
Boston MA
USA

REDWAN MOQBEL PHD FRCPATH

Professor and Director, Pumonary Research Group
Department of Medicine
Heritage Medical Research Centre
University of Alberta
Edmonton AB
Canada

MARK H MOSS MD

Associate Professor
Department of Medicine
Section of Allergy, Pulmonary and Critical Care Medicine
University of Wisconsin School of Medicine
Madison WI
USA

HEDWIG S MURPHY MD PHD

Assistant Professor
Department of Pathology
University of Michigan
Ann Arbor MI
USA

ARNON NAGLER MD MSC

Professor of Medicine
Director, Division of Hematology
Chaim Sheba Medical Center
Tel Hashomer
Israel

HAROLD S NELSON MD

Professor of Medicine
Department of Medicine
National Jewish Medical and Research Center
and University of Colorado Health Sciences
Denver CO
USA

EWA NIŻANKOWSKA-MOGILNICKA MD

Professor
Centrum Innowacji
Jagiellonian University
Krakow
Poland

PAUL M O'BYRNE MB FRCPI FRCP(C) FRCPE FRCP(GLAS)

E J Moran Campbell Professor
Chair, Department of Medicine
Michaekl G DeGroote School of Medicine
Faculty of Health Sciences
McMaster University
Hamilton ON
Canada

SOLOMON O (WOLE) ODEMUYIWA DVM PHD

Research Fellow in Pulmonary Medicine
Pulmonary Research Group
Department of Medicine
University of Alberta
Edmonton AB
Canada

NARA T ORBAN MRCS(ENG) DLO

Clinical Research Fellow in Rhinology
Department of Allergy and Clinical Immunology
Imperial College London
Royal Brompton Hospital
London
UK

DENNIS R OWNBY MD

Betty B Wray Professor of Pediatrics
Professor of Medicine
Head, Section of Allergy and Immunology
Medical College of Georgia
Augusta GA
USA

REYNOLD A PANETTIERI JR MD

Adjunct Professor, Wistar Institute
and Professor of Medicine
Pulmonary, Allergy and Critical Care Division
Airways Biology Initiative
University of Pennsylvania School of Medicine
Philadelphia PA
USA

MARY E PAUL MD

Associate Professor of Pediatrics
Allergy and Immunology Center
Texas Children's Hospital
Houston TX
USA

DAVID B PEDEN MD MS

Professor of Pediatrics, Medicine and Microbiology/Immunology
Director, Center for Environmental Medicine, Asthma and Lung
Biology
University of North Carolina at Chapel Hill
Chapel Hill NC
USA

R STOKES PEEBLES JR MD

Associate Professor of Medicine
Division of Allergy, Pulmonary and Critical Care Medicine
Vanderbilt University Medical Center
Nashville TN
USA

WERNER J PICHLER MD

Head of Allergology
Department for Rheumatology and Clinical Immunology/
Allergology
Inselspital, University of Bern
Bern
Switzerland

MARK R PITTELKOW MD

Consultant
Department of Dermatology, Biochemistry and Molecular Biology
The Mayo Clinic
Rochester MN
USA

DOUGLAS A PLAGER PHD

Assistant Professor of Dermatology
Department of Dermatology
Mayo Clinic
Rochester MN
USA

THOMAS A E PLATTS-MILLS MD PHD

Professor and Division Chief
Department of Internal Medicine
University of Virginia Health Science Center
Charlottesville VA
USA

DAVID PROUD PHD

Professor
Department of Physiology and Biophysics
University of Calgary Faculty of Medicine
Calgary AB
Canada

HENGAMEH HEIDARIAN RAISSY PHARMD

Research Assistant Professor of Pediatrics
Department of Pediatrics
University of New Mexico
Albuquerque NM
USA

CYNTHIA S RAND PHD

Professor of Medicine
Department of Pulmonary and Critical Care Medicine
Johns Hopkins University School of Medicine
Baltimore MD
USA

ANURADHA RAY PHD

Professor of Medicine and Immunology
Departments of Medicine and Immunology
University of Pittsburgh School of Medicine
Pittsburgh PA
USA

CHARLES E REED MD

Professor of Medicine, Emeritus
Department of Internal Medicine
Mayo Medical School
Rochester MN
USA

CLIVE ROBINSON PHD FHEA

Reader in Respiratory Cell Science
Ion Channels and Cell Signalling Centre
Division of Basic Medical Sciences
St George's, University of London
London
UK

ANTONINO ROMANO MD

Associate Professor of Internal Medicine
Department of Internal Medicine and Geriatrics
Universita Cattolica del Sacro Cuore
Allergology Section
Rome
Italy

LANNY J ROSENWASSER MD

Dee Lyons/Missouri Endowed Chair in Pediatric Immunology
Research
Professor of Pediatrics
Allergy-Immunology Division
Children's Mercy Hospital and Clinics
and Professor of Pediatrics, Medicine and Basic Science
University of Missouri-Kansas City School of Medicine
Kansas City MO
USA

MARC E ROTHENBERG MD PHD

Director and Endowed Chair, Division of Allergy and Immunology
Professor of Pediatrics
Cincinnati Children's Hospital Medical Center
University of Cincinnati College of Medicine
Cincinnati OH
USA

BRIAN H ROWE MD MSC

Professor and Research Director
Department of Emergency Medicine
University of Alberta
Edmonton AB
Canada

MICHAEL C SAAVEDRA MD MS

Chief Fellow
Division of Allergy, Pulmonary, Immunology, Critical Care and
Sleep
University of Texas Medical Branch
Galveston TX
USA

ALIREZA SADEGHNEJAD MD PHD

Research Assistant Professor
Center for Human Genetics
Wake Forest University School of Medicine
Winston-Salem NC
USA

HESHAM SALEH MBBCH FRCS FRCS (ORL-HNS)

Consultant Rhinologist/Facial Plastic Surgeon and Honorary
Senior Lecturer
ENT Department
Charing Cross Hospital
London
UK

JONATHAN M SAMET MD MS

Professor and Chair
Department of Epidemiology
Johns Hopkins Bloomberg School of Public Health
Baltimore MD
USA

HUGH A SAMPSON MD

Kurt Hirschhorn Professor of Pediatrics
Dean for Translational Biomedical Sciences
Chief, Department of Pediatric Allergy and Immunology
Director, Jaffe Food Allergy Institute
Department of Pediatrics
Mount Sinai School of Medicine
New York NY
USA

Contributors

MAREK SANAK MD PHD

Head, Division of Molecular Biology and Clinical Genetics
Department of Medicine
Faculty of Medicine
Jagiellonian University
Krakow
Poland

MICHAEL SCHATZ MD MS

Clinical Professor of Medicine
University of California, San Diego
Chief, Department of Allergy
Kaiser Permanente Medical Center
San Diego CA
USA

R ROBERT SCHELLENBERG MD FRCPC

Professor
Department of Medicine
James Hogg iCAPTURE Centre for Cardiovascular
and Pulmonary Research
Vancouver BC
Canada

ROBERT P SCHLEIMER PHD

Professor of Medicine
Chief, Division of Allergy-Immunology
Northwestern University
Feinberg School of Medicine
Chicago IL
USA

JOHN T SCHROEDER PHD

Associate Professor of Medicine
Division of Allergy and Clinical Immunology
Johns Hopkins University School of Medicine
Johns Hopkins Asthma and Allergy Center
Baltimore MD
USA

CHUN Y SEOW PHD

Associate Professor
Department of Pathology and Laboratory Medicine
University of British Columbia
James Hogg iCAPTURE Centre for Cardiovascular
and Pulmonary Research
St Paul's Hospital
Vancouver BC
Canada

WILLIAM T SHEARER MD PHD

Professor of Pediatrics and Immunology
and Chief, Allergy and Immunology
Texas Children's Hospital
Department of Pediatrics
Baylor College of Medicine
Houston TX
USA

JAMES H SHELHAMER MD

Deputy Chief, Senior Investigator
Critical Care Medicine Department
Clinical Center
National Institutes of Health
Bethesda MD
USA

HANS-UWE SIMON MD PHD

Professor of Pharmacology
Chairman of the Department of Pharmacology
University of Bern
Bern
Switzerland

F ESTELLE R SIMONS MD FRCPC

Professor of Pediatrics and Immunology
Faculty of Medicine
University of Manitoba
Winnipeg MB
Canada

JODIE L SIMPSON PHD

Research Fellow
Department of Respiratory Medicine
John Hunter Hospital
New Lambton NSW
Australia

JAY E SLATER MD

Laboratory of Immunobiochemistry
Division of Bacterial, Parasitic and Allergenic Products
Office of Vaccine Research and Review
Center for Biologics Evaluation and Research
US Food and Drug Administration
Rockville MD
USA

PHILIP H SMITH MD

Associate Professor of Medicine
Allergy–Immunology Section
Medical College of Georgia
Augusta GA
USA

MICHAEL C SNELLER MD

Medical Officer
Clinical and Molecular Retrovirology Section
Laboratory of Immunoregulation
National Institute of Allergy and Infectious Disease
National Institutes of Health
Bethesda MD
USA

CHRISTINE A SORKNESS PHARMD

Professor of Pharmacy and Medicine
Pharmacy Practice Division
School of Pharmacy
University of Wisconsin
Madison WI
USA

JOSEPH D SPAHN MD

Director on Immunopharmacology Laboratory
Associate Professor of Pediatrics
Division of Clinical Pharmacology
University of Colorado School of Medicine
Denver CO
USA

P SRIRAMARAO PHD

Associate Dean for Research
Professor of Medicine
Department of Vet and Biomedical Sciences
University of Minnesota
St Paul MN
USA

JAMES L STAHL PHD

Associate Scientist
Department of Medicine
University of Wisconsin Medical School
Madison WI
USA

GEOFFREY A STEWART BSC PHD(BIRM)

Professor of Microbiology and Immunology
Head of the School of Biomedical, Biomolecular
and Chemical Sciences
The University of Western Australia
Crawley WA
Australia

JEFFREY R STOKES MD

Associate Professor of Medicine
Department of Medicine
Program Director, Allergy/Immunology
Creighton University Medical Center
Omaha NE
USA

KATHLEEN E SULLIVAN MD PHD

Professor of Pediatrics
University of Pennsylvania School of Medicine
Chief, Division of Allergy and Immunology
Children's Hospital of Philadelphia
Philadelphia PA
USA

ANDRZEJ SZCZEKLIK MD PHD

Professor and Chairman
Department of Medicine
Collegium Medicum
Jagiellonian University
Krakow
Poland

STANLEY J SZEFLER MD

Helen Wohlberg & Herman Lambert Chair in Pharmacokinetics
Head, Pediatric Clinical Pharmacology
Director, Weinberg Clinical Research Unit–Pediatrics Section
National Jewish Health
and Professor of Pediatrics and Pharmacology
University of Colorado at Denver Health Sciences Center
Denver CO
USA

STEPHEN L TAYLOR PHD

Professor of Food Science and Technology
Institute of Agriculture and Natural Resources
University of Nebraska
Lincoln NE
USA

Contributors

ABBA I TERR MD

Clinical Professor of Medicine
Department of Allergy
University of California, San Francisco Medical Center
San Francisco CA
USA

SHIBU THOMAS MD

Fellow
Division of Pulmonary and Critical Care Medicine
University of Texas Medical Branch
Galveston TX
USA

OMAR TLIBA DVM PHD

Research Assistant Professor of Medicine
Airways Biology Initiative
Pulmonary, Allergy and Critical Care Division
University of Pennsylvania Medical Center
Philadelphia PA
USA

ALKIS TOGIAS MD

Chief, Asthma and Inflammation Section
Division of Allergy, Immunology and Transplantation
National Institute of Allergy and Infectious Diseases
National Institutes of Health
Bethesda MD
USA

BRADLEY J UNDEM PHD

Professor of Medicine
Division of Allergy and Clinical Immunology
Johns Hopkins University School of Medicine
Johns Hopkins Asthma and Allergy Center
Baltimore MD
USA

PAUL VAN CAUWENBERGE MD PHD

Head of Department
Department of Otorhinolaryngology
Faculty of Medicine and Health Sciences
University of Ghent
Ghent
Belgium

JAMES VARANI PHD

Professor of Microbiology and Immunology
Department of Pathology
University of Michigan Medical School
Ann Arbor MI
USA

DONATA VERCELLI MD

Professor of Cell Biology
University of Arizona College of Medicine
Arizona Respiratory Center
Tuscon AZ
USA

STEPHAN VON GUNTEN MD PHD MME

Postdoctoral Fellow
Division of Allergy and Clinical Immunology
Johns Hopkins University School of Medicine
Johns Hopkins Asthma and Allergy Center
Baltimore MD
USA

MARTIN WAGENMANN MD

Associate Professor of Otorhinolaryngology
Head of Rhinology, Allergy, and Endoscopic skull base surgery
Department of Otorhinolaryngology, Head and Neck Surgery
University Clinic, Düsseldorf
Düsseldorf
Germany

ULRICH WAHN MD

Professor of Pediatrics, Allergology
Department of Pediatric Pneumology and Immunology
Charité Universitätsmedizin Berlin
Berlin
Germany

PETER A WARD MD

Godfrey Dr Stobbe Professor of Pathology
Department of Pathology
The University of Michigan Medical School
Ann Arbor MI
USA

MICHAEL E WECHSLER MD MMSC

Assistant Professor of Medicine
Harvard Medical School
Associate Director
Brigham and Women's Hospital Asthma Research Center
Brigham and Women's Hospital
Boston MA
USA

CATHERINE R WEILER MD PHD

Assistant Professor of Medicine
Division of Allergy and Immunology
Mayo Clinic
Rochester MN
USA

DAVID WELDON MD FACAAI FAAAAI

Associate Professor of Internal Medicine
Director, Allergy and Pulmonary Lab Services for College Station
Texas A&M University Health Sciences Center
College Station TX
USA

PETER F WELLER MD FACP

Professor of Medicine, Harvard Medical School
Chief, Allergy and Inflammation Division
Department of Medicine
Beth Israel Deaconess Medical Center
Boston MA
USA

SALLY E WENZEL MD

Professor of Pulmonary Medicine
Division of Pulmonary, Allergy and Critical Care Medicine
University of Pittsburgh Medical Center
Pittsburgh PA
USA

GREGORY J WIEPZ PHD

Senior Scientist
Department of Biomolecular Chemistry
University of Wisconsin
Madison WI
USA

DENISE G WIESCH PHD

Scientific Review Administrator
Epidemiology of Cancer Study Section
Health of the Population Integrated Review Group
Center for Scientific Review
National Institutes of Health
Bethesda MD
USA

MARSHA WILLS-KARP PHD

Professor of Pediatrics
Director, Division of Immunobiology
Cincinnati Children's Hospital Medical Center
Cincinnati OH
USA

ROBERT A WOOD MD

Professor of Pediatrics
Director, Pediatric Allergy and Immunology
Johns Hopkins University School of Medicine
Johns Hopkins Hospital
Baltimore MD
USA

LEMAN YEL MD FAAP FAAAAI

Assistant Professor of Clinical Medicine
Division of Basic and Clinical Immunology
Department of Medicine
University of California, Irvine
Irvine CA
USA

JOHN W YUNGINGER MD

Emeritus Professor of Pediatrics and Medicine
Department of Pediatric and Adolescent Medicine,
and Department of Internal Medicine
Mayo Clinic College of Medicine
Rochester MN
USA

MICHAEL A ZASLOFF MD PHD

Professor, Departments of Surgery and Pediatrics
Director of Surgical Immunology
Department of Surgery
Georgetown University Medical Center
Washington DC
USA

ROBERT S ZEIGER MD PHD

Clinical Professor of Pediatrics
University of California, San Diego
and Senior Physician Investigator
Kaiser Permanente San Diego
San Diego CA
USA

JIHUI ZHANG PHD

Drug Discovery Programme Manager
Ion Channels and Cell Signalling Centre
Division of Basic Medical Sciences
St George's, University of London
London
UK

section A

IMMUNOLOGY

The Immune System: an Overview

Javier Chinen, Thomas A Fleisher, and William T Shearer

CONTENTS

- Introduction 3
- Components of the immune system 4
- The immune response 11
- Immunopathology – mechanisms of immune-mediated diseases 13
- Conclusion 16

SUMMARY OF IMPORTANT CONCEPTS

>> Immune responses involve the interplay of innate and adaptive immune mechanisms, complementing each other with their different onset of action and capacity of memory

>> Three types of inflammatory responses are defined: Th1, induced by IL-12 and responsible for T cell-mediated cytotoxicity; Th2, induced by IL-4 and responsible for the development of IgE-mediated allergic disease; and Th17, which leads to a characteristic neutrophilic inflammation and is pathogenic in some experimental models of autoimmunity. IL-23, TGF-β, and IL-6 are essential cytokines to develop the Th17 response

>> Regulatory T cells, together with central and peripheral tolerance processes, ensure that the immune system is not activated against host tissues

>> Distinct mechanisms of immune-mediated diseases are: IgE-mediated hypersensitivity, antibody-mediated cytotoxicity, immune complex reaction, delayed hypersensitivity response, antibody-mediated activation/inactivation of biological function, cell-mediated cytotoxicity, and granuloma reaction

INTRODUCTION

The modern practice of allergy is based on the understanding of the pathogenesis of allergic disorders. This body of knowledge is growing exponentially with the ongoing expansion in our understanding of the immune system. This system is focused on host defense and is composed of specific cellular and protein components that develop and function in a highly complex manner, in order to neutralize or destroy dangerous non-self while preserving self. However, as part of, or as a consequence of the development of this defense system, some types of immune responses may prove inadequate or detrimental in certain circumstances, leading to human illnesses.

Allergic responses are clear examples of the detrimental side of the immune system, because they represent immunological reactions to innocuous environmental elements, resulting in annoying and sometimes debilitating effects in the affected individuals. The allergic response involves hypersensitivity reactions directed at allergens; in contrast to similar hypersensitivity mechanisms that provide host protection to parasitic infections. Thus, allergy is an integral part of the manifestations of immunity, and physicians who treat allergic disease must understand the scope and breadth of immunology. The modern allergist, armed with the knowledge of the underlying pathogenesis of allergic diseases, is better prepared to effectively manage patient symptoms employing scientifically based therapeutic measures.

This chapter summarizes current knowledge of the immune system, the interactions among the constituent parts of the immune network, and the immunopathological mechanisms of the hypersensitivity responses. As such, it serves as a reference point for all subsequent chapters, which discuss the clinical presentations, specific treatments, and management strategies of allergic disease.

THE IMMUNOLOGICAL BASIS OF ALLERGIC DISEASE

The basic foundation of the immune system is the capacity to distinguish *non-self* molecules, with potential to cause harm, from *self* molecules, a characteristic that exists in a delicate balance between tolerance to self and response/rejection of non-self. Autoimmunity and allergy are disorders in which this balance is disrupted.

Autoimmunity defines a state in which tolerance to self is lost and the immune response is activated against host tissues, such as the pancreatic beta cells in insulin-dependent diabetes mellitus. Allergic and hypersensitivity reactions are the result of immune responses to innocuous non-self molecules that are called allergens. This response is mediated by immunoglobulin (Ig) E antibody specific to the allergen. Mast cells and basophils are activated after IgE binding, starting a series of cellular and molecular events that results in the clinical manifestations of allergic disease. IgE-mediated immunity is critical for our defense against parasites; however, the low prevalence of parasitic infections in modern societies has made the role of IgE in allergic disorders of more importance in medical care. Other immune mechanisms producing hypersensitivity reactions include antigen-antibody immune complexes and delayed hypersensitivity (DTH), which are briefly described later in this Chapter.

ENVIRONMENTAL AND GENETIC FACTORS AFFECT THE ALLERGIC IMMUNE RESPONSE

The increasing prevalence of allergic disorders in urban communities is being intensively studied.[1,2] Some of the possible causes accounting for this observation are related to the environment, such as ambient pollution,[3] increased concentration of indoor allergens, diet, and the decrease of childhood infections. The 'hygiene hypothesis', which attempts to explain this increasing prevalence of allergy, is based on the possible immunomodulation induced by bacterial and viral infections early in infancy, modifying the chances of developing an allergic response. However, environmental factors do not fully explain the increase of allergic disease.[4,5] Genetic predisposition to allergic disorders has also been extensively explored recently, as allergists have known for decades that children of allergic parents are more likely to develop allergic disease (see also Chapter 4). Genetic studies, including linkage analysis of large families, have identified several possible loci containing candidate genes that may confer increased susceptibility to allergic disease.[6–8] For example, susceptibility to allergic rhinitis and atopy has been linked to a single nucleotide polymorphism that substitutes an arginine for a glutamine in the exon 4 of the IL-13 gene on chromosome 5q31; also elevated serum IgE levels have been significantly linked to the 3017 G/T polymorphism in intron 2 of the IL-4 gene.[9] It is not unexpected that allergic disorders, with their variety of presentations, may result from a complex interplay between a genetic predisposition of particular populations and specific environmental factors.

INNATE IMMUNITY VS ADAPTIVE IMMUNITY

The immune system involves two complementary sets of defense mechanisms against potentially pathogenic microorganisms: one to provide an immediate, quick response called innate immunity, and a second set to develop a long lasting and highly specific protection, known as adaptive immunity. Innate immunity responses are discussed in more detail in Chapter 2. Components of the innate immunity include the epithelial barriers (skin and mucosa) with the surface antimicrobial substances produced by the epithelial cells; the unique group of proteins that circulate in the blood called the complement system; and diverse blood cells that, upon contact with a pathogen or an infected cell, either directly induce cytotoxicity or initiate a phagocytosis process and intracellular killing. Innate immunity mechanisms present the first line of host defense. The specificity of innate immunity is based on pattern recognition, involving molecules that are shared by multiple microbes, however not present in the host.

In contrast, adaptive immunity mechanisms are designed to specifically recognize and distinguish a large number of molecules, together with an ability to amplify the response with repeated exposures to the same pathogen or molecule. Both innate and adaptive immunity have the capacity to activate each other. Thus, recognition of a particular pathogen by the adaptive immunity may result in enhanced killing by phagocytes. Conversely, activation of complement proteins facilitates chemotaxis and migration of lymphocytes, which develop the adaptive response. A remarkable aspect of the adaptive immune system is its property of memory, which provides effective protection against a repeat exposure to harmful microbial agents even if the events are separated by prolonged periods, even decades. Immunologic memory is made possible by the clonal expansion of lymphocytes in response to antigen (or allergen) stimulation. From the time the human immune system first begins to differentiate in fetal life, uniquely reacting lymphocytes are created by the recombination of genes encoding antigen receptors expressed on the lymphocyte cell membrane. Through the expression of these receptors, each lymphocyte has the ability to bind to and become activated by a specific antigen, either natural or artificial. Interaction with antigen not only activates the lymphocytes but also results in the generation of long-lived antigen-specific memory cell clones. Thus, when the same antigen enters the body, there is immediate recognition by these memory cells. Both cellular and humoral responses to the antigen are produced more rapidly than in the first encounter, and more memory cells are generated. This process of expansion of clonal populations of uniquely reacting lymphocytes first explained the B cell origin of antibody diversity and applies to cellular (T cell) immune responses as well.[10,11]

■ COMPONENTS OF THE IMMUNE SYSTEM ■

All the cells of the immune system derive from the pluripotent hematopoietic stem cell found in the bone marrow (Fig. 1.1). This pluripotential stem cell gives rise to lymphoid stem cells and myeloid stem cells. The lymphoid stem cell differentiates into three types of cells – the T cell, the B cell, and the natural killer (NK) cell progenitors – and contributes to the development of subsets of dendritic cells. The myeloid stem cell gives rise to dendritic cells, mast cells, basophils, neutrophils, eosinophils, monocytes, and macrophages, as well as megakaryocytes and erythrocytes. Differentiation of these committed stem cells is critically dependent on an array of cytokine and cell-cell interactions. An ever-increasing number of biologically important surface membrane proteins are being characterized on cells of the immune system. Many of these molecules have been assigned a sequential number based on the cluster of differentiation (CD) nomenclature and are useful to identify cells and their developmental stage; for example, $CD3^+$ and $CD8^+$ markers define a particular subset of T cells with a role in cytotoxicity.

T CELLS

T cell progenitors derived from the common lymphoid progenitor cells leave the bone marrow through the bloodstream and enter the thymus gland, likely based on the expression of particular adhesion proteins. These cells remain in the thymus gland, where precursor cells ultimately develop into mature T cells, emerging with distinct, surface antigens and functional

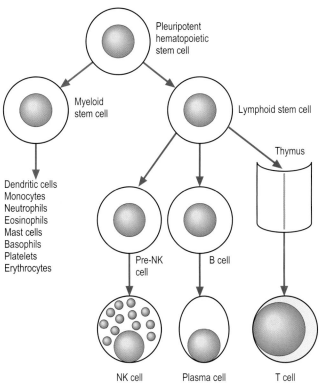

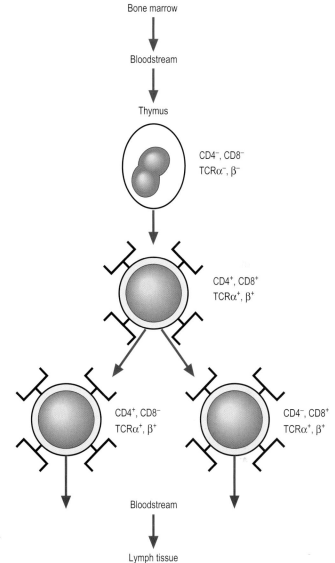

Fig. 1.1. Maturation of the cells of the immune system and hematopoietic system. Pluripotent stem cells are derived from the yolk sac and ultimately reside in the bone marrow. All lymphocytes are derived from the lymphoid stem cell and differentiate into three types of lymphocytes: (1) mature T cells after passage through the thymus gland, (2) large granular lymphocyte cells that possess natural killer (NK) function, and (3) B cells that can differentiate into plasma cells capable of secreting antibodies. Monocytes and macrophages are derived from myeloid stem cells; in addition, neutrophils, eosinophils, erythrocytes, megakaryocytes, mast cells, basophils, and dendritic cells are also derived from this stem cell. The differentiation of stem cells into mature specialized cells is under the control of numerous cytokines and cell-secreted factors.

characteristics (Fig. 1.2).[12,13] T cell progenitors entering the thymus lack surface antigens, including the T cell antigen receptor (TCR) complex and mature T cell markers (e.g., CD4, CD8) that are associated with specific effector functions. These 'double-negative' thymocytes (CD4−/CD8−) are induced to express CD1, CD2, CD5, CD6, CD7, and interleukin-2 receptor (IL-2R) molecules, which serve as critical receptor-ligand functions during early ontogeny. Subsequently, these progenitor T cells undergo rearrangement of the alpha (α) and beta (β) (or gamma (γ) and delta (δ)) genes of the TCR, generating immature T cells.

The genes that encode the variable and constant regions of the TCR α- and β-chains are rearranged for transcription of a complete ribonucleic acid (RNA) message. The coding sequence of the variable (V) region of the α-chain gene is formed by rearrangement of a V gene segment with a joining (J) gene segment, whereas V, diversity (D), and J gene segments of DNA rearrange to produce β-chain variable region coding sequences. The V region sequences are next joined to the constant (C) region sequences. The net result of these DNA rearrangements and subsequent

Fig. 1.2. Ontogeny and lineage relationships of maturing T cells expressing TCR. Most thymocytes express both CD4 and CD8. T cell antigen receptor (TCR) expression commences in this double-positive stage, beginning with low numbers of receptors on each cell and increasing as maturation proceeds. Single-positive, that is CD4+ or CD8+ TCRαβ-expressing, mature cells are selected from this population. A small population of double-negative T cells bearing TCRγδ also leaves the thymus (not shown).

messenger RNA (mRNA) splicing during T cell development in the thymic cortex is to provide for an enormous diversity of TCR antigen specificity.[14] Cell surface expression of the TCR depends on coexpression of the CD3 complex, which is a cluster of gamma (γ), delta (δ), epsilon (ε), and zeta (ζ) chains (see below).[15] Together, the TCR and CD3 molecules form the TCR complex.

5

T cell development within the thymus involves positive and negative selection based on TCR affinity for antigens that ultimately results in the release of mature T cells with the capacity to distinguish between self and non-self antigens presented in the context of self-MHC molecules. This 'education' process is under the control of specialized cortical cells of the thymus, dependent on cell–cell contact and the secretion of cytokines, with subsequent elimination of most precursors that enter the thymus. There are primarily two types of T cells that leave the thymus to circulate in the peripheral blood, lymphatic system, and tissues: TCR-$\alpha\beta^+$/CD4$^+$ T cells and TCR-$\alpha\beta^+$/CD8$^+$ T cells. Fewer than 10% of mature T cells emerge from the thymus as TCR-$\gamma\delta^+$ T cells, which are predominantly CD4$^-$/CD8$^-$. All peripheral T cells bear the TCR complex, and thus CD3 represents a pan-T cell marker. T cell activation occurs when the TCR binds to immunogenic epitopes displayed on a cell (see below). CD8$^+$ T cells recognize antigenic peptides displayed in the context of class I MHC molecules, which are displayed on virtually all nucleated cells, whereas CD4$^+$ T cells recognize antigens peptides presented in the context of class II MHC molecules, which are found on a limited range of cells referred to as antigen-presenting cells (APCs): monocytes, macrophages, B cells, dendritic cells.

Although CD4$^+$ T cells are sometimes functionally referred to as helper T cells and CD8$^+$ T cells as cytotoxic T cells, CD4$^+$ T cells and CD8$^+$ T cells can have diverse functions. Thus, these phenotypes should be recognized for their capacity to respond to antigen in the context of MHC. Upon antigen recognition, the CD3 complex of proteins transduces the signal through the cell membrane lipid bilayer to the cell interior and nucleus (see below). Essential to the proliferation of antigen-activated T cells is their expression of the CD25 (IL-2R α-chain, p55) which combines with the β-chain (p75, CD122) and γ-chain (CD132) to form the high-affinity IL-2R. Signaling through this receptor initiates the production of IL-2, resulting in autocrine cell activation and proliferation. A number of accessory glycoprotein adhesion molecules stabilize the binding of T cells to the APC during the recognition phase or to the target cell in the effector phase, as well as providing for a co-stimulatory signal required for T cell activation (Table 1.1).

When TCR-$\alpha\beta$ binds to a specific peptide presented in the context of an appropriate MHC molecule in the presence of an effective co-stimulatory signal, a signal is imparted to the T cell that results in the following activation events: (1) hydrolysis of the phospholipid component of the lipid bilayer, phosphatidyl inositol bisphosphate, into inositol trisphosphate (IP$_3$) and diacylglycerol (DAG); (2) elevation of intracellular calcium levels produced partly by IP$_3$; (3) activation of protein kinase C (PKC) by interaction with DAG; and (4) phosphorylation and activation of tyrosine kinase (Fig. 1.3).[16,17] All these activation events convey messages to the cell nucleus and appropriate target genes for the nuclear factor of activated T cells (NFAT) and the proto-oncogene c-fos, or transcriptional regulator proteins, such as activator protein-1 (AP-1), that together regulate cell activity. These activated genes in turn code for proteins that commit the T cell to a subsequent specific function. Thus, there is an orderly appearance of proteins produced by the activated cell that are important in subsequent cell function or that interact with other immune cells.

These intricate cell activation events are of considerable importance to the clinical practice of allergy and immunology because their discovery and elucidation explain mechanisms underlying efficacious treatments given to patients for decades. Glucocorticoids, for example, inhibit early T cell gene activation events by the induction of proteins that bind to DNA sequences in the region of promoter response elements, whereas cyclosporin A and tacrolimus inhibit a serine/threonine-specific protein phosphatase called calcineurin that blocks specific gene transcription.

Table 1.1 Molecules (receptor-ligand pairs) that participate in the binding of T cells to antigen-presenting cells (APCs)

T cell	APC
T cell receptor	HLA and peptide
CD4	HLA-DR, HLA-DQ, HLA-DP (Class II MHC)
CD8	HLA-A, HLA-B, HLA-C (Class I MHC)
CD11a (LFA-1α), CD18	CD54 (ICAM-1), ICAM-2, ICAM-3
CD2 (LFA-2)	CD58 (LFA-3)
CD40L	CD40
CD28	CD80 (B7-1), CD86 (B7-2)
CD152 (CTLA-4)	CD80 (B7-1), CD86 (B7-2)

LFA, leukocyte function-associated antigen; ICAM, intercellular adhesion molecule.

B CELLS

The B cell matures in the bone marrow, but during fetal life, their maturation occurs in the liver. During differentiation of the B cell, a series of DNA rearrangements of immunoglobulin heavy-chain genes and light-chain genes occurs for production of membrane-bound and secreted immunoglobulin molecules (Table 1.2). As the pre-B cell matures, it undergoes μ-chain gene rearrangement together with a surrogate invariant light heavy chain (λ-5 and V pre-B) necessary for effective transport of the μ-chain to the cell surface expressed as the pre-B cell receptor. Association of the pre-B cell receptor with the Igα and Igβ proteins provides the means for signal transduction that facilitates further maturation of the pre-B cell, associated with kappa (κ) or lambda (λ) gene rearrangements. These events ultimately result in the expression of an IgM molecule on the cell surface. Mature B cells co-express surface IgM and IgD as a result of heavy-chain mRNA splicing. The B cell maturation process up to this stage is antigen independent, while subsequent differentiation of the IgM$^+$/IgD$^+$ mature B cells released into the periphery is antigen driven. Thus, activation of mature B cells into immunoglobulin-secreting B cells or long-lived memory B cells and final differentiation into plasma cells depend on antigen interaction. Isotype switching involves the further rearrangement of immunoglobulin heavy-chain genes and DNA splicing and is a process under T cell control.[18] The switching mechanisms involve at least two factors: (1) T cell to B cell contact (T cell receptor/B cell antigen presentation and B cell CD40/activated T cell CD40L) and (2) secretion of interleukin molecules, which are thought to make accessible the nine switch regions of the heavy-chain DNA sequence enabling transcription of all subclasses genes, and leading to production of IgG, IgA, or IgE. These immunoglobulins express the same heavy-chain variable regional sequences and light-chain sequences, thus maintaining antigen specificity. Recently, it has been determined that both class switch and somatic hypermutation are driven by the activity of the enzyme activation-induced cytidine deaminase. When this enzyme activity is absent, patients develop an autosomal recessive form of hyper IgM syndrome.[19]

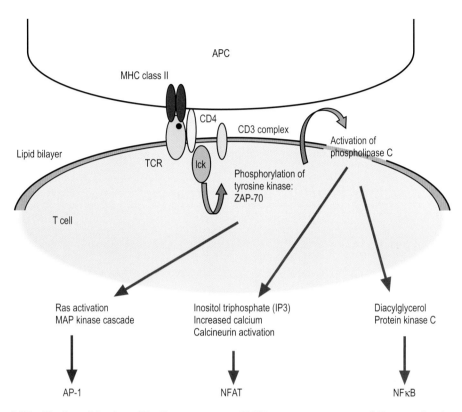

Fig. 1.3. Activation of CD4+ T cells, with binding of T cell antigen receptor (TCR) to antigen-presenting cell (first signal) and accessory molecules (second signal). Cross-linking of TCR causes aggregation with the CD3 complex containing ζ, δ, and ε chains. AP-1, NFAT and NFκB are transcription factors that will activate genes necessary for cell proliferation and differentiation. APC, antigen-presenting cell; ZAP-70, Zeta-associated protein-70; MHC, major histocompatibility complex; MAP, mitogenic-associated proliferation; NFκB, nuclear factor κ of B cells, NFAT, nuclear factor of activated T cells; AP-1, activator protein-1; lck, tyrosine kinase.

Concomitant with the immunoglobulin gene rearrangements and expression of surface immunoglobulin by developing B cells is the appearance of certain B cell markers that are useful in identifying stages of maturation and differentiation. B cell markers include the variable expression of terminal deoxynucleotidyl transferase (TdT); class II antigens; common acute lymphoblastic leukemia antigen (CALLA or CD10); the B cell-specific molecules CD19 and CD20; various membrane immunoglobulin isotypes, such as IgM; CD21, the complement receptor 2 (CR-2), which specifically binds the C3d fragment of complement component 3; CD23, the low-affinity Fc receptor for IgE; CD25, the IL-2 receptor α-chain, and CD27, the antigen that distinguishes memory B cells. Thus the phenotypic expression of markers can distinguish the stage of B cell differentiation (Table 1.2). Similar to events in the thymus with the maturation and differentiation of T cells, the maturation and differentiation of B cells is thought to be under the control of cytokines. For example, interleukin-1 (IL-1) and IL-2 promote B cell activation and growth; IL-4 induces IgE isotype switch; IL-5 enhances eosinophils and B cell growth and terminal differentiation; IL-6 increases the rate of secretion of immunoglobulin by B cells; and IL-7 promotes proliferation of pre-B cells. The cytokine interferon gamma (IFN-γ) can exert a positive or negative influence on the effects of IL-6 on B cells.

Antibody diversity results from the recombination of immunoglobulin genes, generating millions of different immunoglobulin molecules. Heavy-chain genes, located on chromosome 14, and light-chain genes, located on either chromosome 2 (κ light chains) or on chromosome 22 (λ light chains), must rearrange for the production of immunoglobulin molecules using intracellular processes that are similar to those for TCR. The heavy-chain variable region is encoded by VDJ gene segments, which are then juxtaposed to specific C regions for transcription of a complete RNA message. The light-chain variable region is encoded by VJ gene segments, which are juxtaposed to their respective C segment (see Chapter 5). Antigen activation of B cells is initiated by ligation of membrane-bound immunoglobulin, which has cytoplasmic tails consisting of only three amino acids, inadequate for signal transduction. A complex of molecules non-covalently associated with membrane immunoglobulin has cytoplasmic tails sufficient to be phosphorylated and initiate signal transduction.[20,21] These molecules include an IgM-specific 32-kDa μ-chain and an IgD-specific 33-kDa δ-chain, each of which is disulfide linked with a 37-kDa α and a 34-kDa β-chain. This membrane immunoglobulin-associated complex is considered to be analogous to the CD3 molecule of the TCR complex.

B cell activation events occur by many of the same signal transduction pathways described for T cells.[22] Binding of the B cell antigen receptor by anti-IgM induces the rapid hydrolysis of phosphatidylinositol

Table 1.2 Characteristics of B cell differentiation stages

Characteristic	Stem cell	Pre-B cell	Immature B cell	Mature naïve B cell	Activated memory B cell	Antibody-secreting B (plasma) cell
Antigen dependency	–	–	–	–	+	+
Compartment	BM	BM	BM + PB	PB	PB	PB
Intracellular proteins		RAG-1 RAG-2 μ				
Heavy-chain genes	Germline	VDJ	VDJ	VDJ	Isotype switch	Isotype switch
Light-chain genes	Germline	Germline	VJ	VJ	VJ	VJ
Surface markers	CD45 CD34	CD45R MHC-II CD10 CD19 CD20 CD38 CD40	CD45R MHC-II IgM CD19 CD20 CD40	CD45R MHC-II IgM, IgD CD19 CD20 CD21 CD40	CD45R MHC-II IgM CD19 CD20 CD21 CD40 CD27	PC-1 CD20 CD38 CD135
Immunoglobulin (Ig) production	None	Cytoplasm μ-chain	Membrane IgM	Membrane IgD, IgM	Low-rate Ig (G, A, M, D, E)	High-rate Ig (G, A, M, D, E)

Modified from Janeway CA Jr, Travers P. Immunobiology, 6th edn. New York: Garland Science; 2005:310. (Only representative stages are described). BM, bone marrow; PB, peripheral blood; TdT, terminal deoxynucleotidyl transferase; RAG, recombinase activating gene; V, variable; J, joining; D, diversity (gene segments); MHC-II, major histocompatibility complex class II. PC-1, plasma cell antigen-1.

bisphosphate, production of IP_3 and DG, activation of PKC, and eventual production of immunoglobulin. The intervening gene activation events are beginning to be explored, and findings similar to those seen in activated T cells are being discovered. In studies involving human B cell lines stimulated by the binding of platelet-activating factor (PAF) to B cell membrane receptors, in addition to the release of IP_3 and DG from the lipid bilayer, arachidonic acid is released from phospholipids by phospholipase A_2 or DG lipase and is subsequently converted to 5-hydroxyeicosatetraenoic acid (5-HETE) by activated 5-lipoxygenase. These secondary messengers are associated with the activation of the proto-oncogenes c-fos and c-jun.[23,24] In activated human peripheral blood B cells, stimulated by antigens such as HIV gp120, cyclic adenosine monophosphate (cAMP) metabolism was stimulated, cell growth occurred, the B cell receptor was downregulated, and immunoglobulin production was increased.[25] Thus, justification can be made for B cell activation events that link cell membrane receptor binding, signal transduction pathways, intracellular cyclic nucleotide metabolism, secondary fatty acid metabolite production, activation of proto-oncogenes, and immunoglobulin secretion.

ANTIGEN-PRESENTING CELLS: MONOCYTES AND MACROPHAGES

Differentiation of myeloid stem cell lineage leukocytes occurs under the influence of stromal cells and cytokines with both pleiotrophic and lineage-specific effects (Fig. 1.1). The pleiotrophic cytokines include granulocyte-macrophage colony-stimulating factor (GM-CSF) and several interleukins, especially IL-3. Lineage-specific cytokines include a growth factor for terminal differentiation of granulocytes (G-CSF) and for monocytes and macrophages (GM-CSF) (see also Chapter 22). IL-5 is a specific terminal growth factor for eosinophils. GM-CSF plus IL-3 supports the differentiation of basophils; and stem cell factor, which binds to c-kit (CD 117), can induce mast cell differentiation from multipotent hematopoietic stem cells.[26]

Although not programmed with immune memory, the circulating peripheral blood monocyte, tissue macrophage, and dendritic cell are essential components of specific immune responses because they process and present antigens in a highly structured fashion to T cells. These cells contain a number of important receptors that facilitate their interactions with antigens. These receptors are specific for the Fc region of IgG molecules and the third complement component. Monocytes and macrophages can express both class I and class II MHC molecules and thus present antigenic epitopes to TCR on either $CD8^+$ or $CD4^+$ T cells during antigen recognition. The contributions of the monocyte/macrophage system to the general inflammatory response and the specific immune response are diverse, including functioning as phagocytic cells for intracellular pathways and as cytotoxic effector cells, particularly as effectors of ADCC. In addition, these cells produce multiple cytokines, including IL-1, IL-12, and tumor necrosis factor (TNF), that are central to inflammatory immune responses and that induce an extraordinary diversity of effects on hematopoietic and non-hematopoietic cells and tissues.

NK CELLS

NK cells are a non-T, non-B cell lineage of lymphocytes which is defined both phenotypically and functionally.[27] Lacking rearranged immunoglobulin or TCR genes, these cells do not express surface immunoglobulin or the TCR complex. Functionally, they may possess natural cytotoxic activity against tumor cells (NK activity), can mediate antibody-dependent cell-mediated cytotoxicity (ADCC) by activation through their IgG Fc receptors and release of cytolysins, or participate in T cell-mediated responses. NK cells have the morphologic appearance of large granular lymphocytes (LGLs) and phenotypically are CD3-/TCR-, CD16+, CD56+, and CD57+. Uniquely among lymphocytes, NK cells also express the IL-2R β-chain (p75, CD122) and γ-chain (CD132) in a resting state.[28] Because this heterodimer has an intermediate affinity for IL-2 and a cytoplasmic extension capable of participating in signal transduction, resting LGL can be activated directly by IL-2 derived from antigen-activated T cells. The differentiation of NK cells depend entirely on the signal provided by IL-15 stimulation.[29]

NK cell recognition of target cells has become more clear with the identification of a specific class of receptors, the killer immunoglobulin-like receptors (KIRs). The outcome of this signal can be inhibitory or activating and this is linked to MHC class-I molecules. The actual inhibitory versus activating signal is dependent on the internal signaling motif (ITIM or ITAM) utilized.[30] KIRs provide an inhibitory signal in response to cells expressing selected (less polymorphic MHC), explaining the failure to respond to host MHC molecules.

NEUTROPHILS

These are the most numerous leukocytes present in peripheral blood, and are also called polymorphonuclear cells, because their nuclei have irregular shape (see also Chapter 17). They circulate in the blood and migrate to tissues in response to cytokines, chemokines, and other proteins present in areas of inflammation. Neutrophils present with cell surface receptors for the Fc portion of IgG, toll-like receptor ligands and for complement products, which facilitate their function of phagocytosing and killing microorganisms present in the phagosomes and in the spaces called neutrophils extracellular traps (NET). Thus, they are part of the innate immunity, as they are the first responder when tissue invasion occurs.[31]

EOSINOPHILS

The eosinophils (see also Chapter 18) are thought to have evolved as a critical component in the host defense against parasitic infections, because of their increase in number associated with these infections. Their granules, containing lysozymes, peroxidases, and cationic proteins specific to the eosinophil, are cytotoxic to parasites and are released by activation of their Fc epsilon RI receptor. They are also increased in inflammatory processes secondary to allergic reactions: for example, in the respiratory tract of patients with allergic asthma. Their contribution to tissue damage and remodeling is mediated by growth factors such as TGF-β.[32]

BASOPHILS AND MAST CELLS

Basophils are present in the blood in very small numbers, and are similar to eosinophils in that they are recruited to sites of allergic inflammation and are activated after IgE binding to their high-affinity IgE receptors.

However, basophils have cytoplasmic granules containing substances that stain with basophilic dyes and are also present in mast cells (see also Chapters 19, 20).[33] Mast cells are present primarily in skin and mucosal tissues, with increased abundance when there is a parasitic infection or an atopic process. Mast cells release preformed inflammatory mediators upon binding and cross-linking of their Fc epsilon RI receptors, by IgE. These mediators, including proteases, hydrolases, and peptidases, appear to be important in the elimination of parasites. They also release histamine, which is preformed and stored intracellularly for immediate release upon cell activation. Histamine plays a central role in triggering the clinical manifestations of anaphylactic reactions. De novo synthesis of inflammatory lipid mediators and Th2 cytokines also occurs upon activation, contributing to the clinical signs of late-phase hypersensitivity reactions.[34]

THE COMPLEMENT SYSTEM

Serum complement (see also Chapter 6) was first described more than 125 years ago as the fraction of serum that could be inactivated by heat.[35] Even today, after the description of more than 25 of its component proteins, the complexity of nomenclature often obscures the vital role complement plays in innate immunity (Fig. 1.4). Most complement factors are produced in the liver, with smaller contributions made by monocytes and fibroblasts. Complement is a distinct humoral immune system that contributes to host protection against infection. It acts in concert with antibodies, promoting both physical clearance of pathogens and non-specific inflammation. Coating a foreign body surface membrane with complement proteins (opsonization) facilitates phagocytosis of the foreign particle. Anaphylatoxins and chemotactic factors, derived from complement proteins (e.g., C5a), contribute to non-specific inflammation. Anaphylatoxins promote the release of histamine from basophils, promoting easy entry of inflammatory cells from the blood stream to the tissue compartment. Chemotactic factors attract inflammatory cells to sites of complement activation and form part of the biologic amplification system.

Three discrete pathways are known to mediate complement activation. The classic pathway requires existing antibody, notably IgM and most subclasses of IgG (IgG1, IgG2, IgG3). The alternative pathway directs complement function in the absence of existing antibody, thus providing early immune protection for the naive host. The lectin activation pathway depends on a protein, mannan-binding lectin, to initiate the complement cascade. Although these pathways differ in their use of C3 and production of C5 convertase, they converge at the level of generation of opsonins and chemotactic factors, as well as in the formation of the membrane attack complex (MAC).[36]

The Fc portion of the antigen-bound immunoglobulin molecule provides the link between the antibodies and the classic complement pathway.[37] The C1 complex becomes activated when one of its components, C1q, binds to the Fc components of antibody bound to antigen. Activated C1 leads to sequential activation of C4 and C2 to produce the enzyme complex C4b2a, acting as a C3 convertase on the antigen-expressing cell surface. Hydrolysis of C3 results in C3a, a potent anaphylatoxin and chemotactic factor, and C3b, an important opsonin when bound to the target cell surface. Opsonic C3b enhances the involvement of phagocytes in the killing process. C3b interacts with C4b2a to form a C5 convertase that can produce C5a and

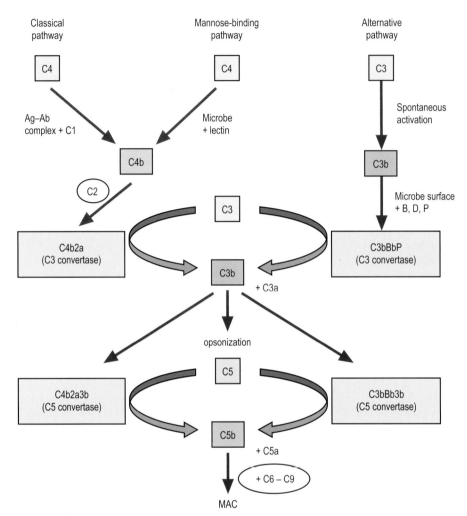

Fig. 1.4. Comparison of classical, mannose-binding lectin, and alternative pathways of complement. All pathways generate C3b, an important opsonin, and result in the formation of the membrane attack complex (MAC). The alternative pathway is initiated by any mechanism that increases the rate of C3b production or reduces the rate of C3b breakdown, such as the presence of microorganisms. The mannose-binding pathway is activated by serum mannose-binding lectins attaching to microbes with mannose residues on cell walls. The classic pathway initiates with the interaction of preexisting antibody (Ab) and C1q to facilitate the subsequent cleavage of C4. The alternative pathway C3 convertase forms through the interaction of C3b, factor B (B), and factor D (D). The resulting C3bBb, stabilized by properdin (P), converts C3 to C3b, which can act as an opsonin or contribute to the C5 convertase (C3bBb3b). The classical pathway uses C4b2a to convert C3 to C3b, which subsequently participates in the C5 convertase (C4b2a3b). Production of C5b by either C5 convertase allows progression to the lytic pathway, where C6, C7, C8, and C9 participate in the generation of the MAC, which would lead to cell lysis. In the course of both pathways, cleavage of C3 and C5 generates C3a and C5a, which possess anaphylatoxin activity.

C5b. C5a is released into the fluid phase to also act as an anaphylatoxin and chemotactic factor. C5b remains on the membrane surface, where it recruits C6, C7, C8, and C9 in forming the MAC, which has lytic capability. It is important to note that C3b is generated in much greater quantity than the other complement products.

In addition, complement component C3 plays a critical role in the alternative pathway and is joined by factor B, factor D, and properdin. Even in the absence of specific antibodies, foreign membranes can be coated with C3b, although the source of the initial C3b is unclear, perhaps being generated at a continuous low level. Serum factors B and D attach near C3b on the surface membrane and are stabilized by the properdin factor. The resulting molecule, C3bBb, acts as a C3 convertase in a manner similar to that of C4b2a in the classic pathway. Activation of the alternative pathway can lead to production of opsonins, anaphylatoxins, and chemotactic factors, including C3b, C3a, and C5a, as well as generation of the lytic MAC. Several complement receptors (CRs) bind to peptide fragments of complement activation. CR1 (CD3b) is a high-affinity receptor for specific fragments of C3 and C4 (e.g., C3b, C4b). CR2 (CD21) is the major receptor for C3d and is also a receptor on B cells for Epstein–Barr virus and for CD23 a low-affinity receptor for IgE. CR3 (CD11b/CD18) bonds to C3 fragments (C3b1, C3b, C3d). CR4 (CD11c/CD18) binds to C3b1 and C3b.[38]

CYTOKINES AND CHEMOKINES

The influences of cytokines (see also Chapters 10, 11) on T cell stimulation have been examined in great detail (see inside cover).[39] On the binding of APCs to resting (G_0) T cells, several interleukins (IL-1, IL-4, IL-6) and TNF-α facilitate the transformation to activated T cells (G_1), which secrete IL-2 and up-regulate their own IL-2R. IL-2 produced now by G_1-phase T cells autostimulates cells to express additional IL-2 receptors on T cell surfaces, thus enhancing their ability to become further activated. G_1-phase T cells under the continuing stimulation by IL-2 become actively replicating cells that begin to secrete additional cytokines, which themselves modulate immune and inflammatory responses.

Several of these T cell-derived cytokines (IL-3, IL-4, and IL-5) have profound effects on immediate hypersensitivity reactions and IgE-derived reactions (Table 1.3, Box 1.1).[40,41] IL-4 is important during B cell activation and induces switching of immunoglobulin production to IgE. IL-3 stimulates the proliferation of basophils. IL-3, GM-CSF, and IL-5 stimulate the growth of eosinophils. Moreover, IL-6 acts as a stimulant to the polyclonal production of immunoglobulin by B cells and may enhance IL-4-induced IgE production.

Because the immune system has such a powerful capacity to stimulate itself, it is appropriate that a counter-regulatory side exists to dampen or turn off immune responses.[42] The immune circuits that inhibit excessive stimulation use cytokines (e.g., TGF-β, IL-10), as well as regulatory T cells (see below). These circuits allow for managing the magnitude and duration of an immune response and appear to depend, at least in part, on a process referred to as 'programmed cell death' (apoptosis). The two general pathways of apoptosis at play in the immune system are a passive process of cell death initiated by the removal of artificial growth factors and an active pathway that involves the interaction between specialized receptors and their specific ligands. Apoptosis is a mechanism for controlling a specific immune response, and it also is a central process in the elimination of autoreactive lymphocytes. Recent evidence suggests that complex regulatory processes are involved in apoptosis that differ between activated and non-activated cells.[43] In addition, apoptosis appears to be a mechanism for controlling other inflammatory cells involved in the immune response and an effector pathway for cytolytic lymphocytes.[44]

Chemokines are generally small-molecular-weight polypeptides that are capable of regulation of numerous cell functions (e.g., chemotaxis, adhesion, degranulation), except proliferation. At a functional level, chemokines are classified as being proinflammatory (e.g., IL-8, MIP-1α, eotaxin, MIP-1β) or developmental/homeostatic (e.g., SDF-1, α-defensins, lymphotactin).[45,46] The chemokines are further classified with regard to the pairs of cysteine amino acids that bind their molecules internally to maintain their folded structure, such as CC (double-cysteine molecules), CXC (cysteine residues separated by a single amino acid), C (single-cysteine molecule), and CX3C (cysteine residues separated by three amino acids). All chemokine receptors share a 7-transmembrane structure, a feature shared with G-protein type receptors. Chemokines signal through their corresponding chemokine receptors (e.g., CC) and produce changes in target cell response, either initiating new biologic responses in the case of the proinflammatory chemokines or maintaining an ongoing response in the case of developmental/homeostatic chemokines (see Appendix A).

One unexpected discovery was that certain microbial organisms utilize chemokine receptors to enter target cells and carry out their life cycles.

The best known of these is human immunodeficiency virus type 1 (HIV-1), which enters monocytes and macrophages by the cognate recognition of the CCR5 receptor and enters CD4 T helper cells by a similar mechanism involving the SDF-1 receptor CXCR4 and CD4.[47,48] The specificity of these chemokine receptor entry systems was established when it was demonstrated that the soluble chemokines macrophage inflammatory protein-1a (MIP-1α), MIP-1β, and RANTES (regulated on activation, normal T cells expressed and secreted) inhibited the binding of the HIV virion to target monocytes. Also, SDF-1 inhibited HIV binding to CD4 T cells.

The extraordinary importance of the role of chemokine receptors in human disease was further demonstrated when studies showed that gene deletions or mutations either rendered humans resistant to HIV infection or altered the course of HIV disease progression. Moreover, some viruses have incorporated the genetic code for chemokine receptors into their own genome to facilitate cell entry. These interesting findings raise the possibility that designer chemokine or soluble chemokine receptor molecules may be capable of being employed as specific immunotherapy for viral infections.

THE IMMUNE RESPONSE

ANTIGEN PRESENTATION

The cellular components of the specific adaptive immune response are T cells, B cells, and monocytes/macrophages. Antigen-presenting cells (APCs) (dendritic cells, monocytes, macrophages) process and present antigen within an antigen-binding cleft of MHC molecules. CD4$^+$ T cells recognize the antigen when presented in the context of a class II MHC molecule (Fig. 1.5) together with the appropriate co-stimulatory signal or signals; and become activated to secrete IL-2, in response to monocyte-derived IL-1 and other cytokines, including autocrine stimulation by IL-2 itself. The activated CD4$^+$ T cell affects additional CD4$^+$ or CD8$^+$ T cells through the secretion of IL-2 and activates B cells by secreting B cell growth and differentiation factors (IL-2, IL-4, IL-6, and IFN-γ). Thus, CD4$^+$ T cells augment immune responses by stimulating B cells activated by antigen and by stimulating CD8$^+$ T cells sensitized by binding of specific antigen in the context of class I MHC molecules. Cell-to-cell contact is important in transmission of messages between cells, and soluble interleukins and other cytokines also play a critical role in the communication between cells.

ANTIGEN RECOGNITION

The biologic basis for antigen recognition in the context of MHC molecules is to allow distinction between self and non-self. In humans the MHC gene complex is located on chromosome 6 and comprises genes that code for human leukocyte antigens (HLA).[49] Class I MHC molecules (HLA-A, HLA-B, HLA-C) are composed of a 44-kDa variant chain that is non-covalently associated with the 12-kDa non-MHC invariant chain, β_2-microglobulin. Class II MHC molecules (HLA-DR, DP, DQ) are composed of two, non-covalently linked variant chains, a 34-kDa protein and a 29-kDa protein. The biologic role of the MHC molecules is to display antigenic peptides to interact with appropriate TCRs. In general, class I MHC molecules present endogenously derived antigenic peptides after antigen processing, such as viral epitopes,

Table 1.3 Effects of cytokines on precursor cells involved in immediate hypersensitivity (IgE-induced) reactions

Activity		IL-3	IL-4	IL-5	IL-9	IL-13	SCF
1.	B cell proliferation	−	+	+	+	+	−
2.	IgE production	−	+	−	+	+	−
3.	MHC class II	−	+	−	+	+	−
4.	CD23 (FcεRII)	−	+	−	+	+	−
5.	B cell differentiation	+	+	−	+	+	−
6.	Mast cell maturation	+	+	−	+	+	+
7.	Eosinophil maturation	+	+	+	+	+	−
8.	Basophil maturation	+	+	+	+	+	+

IgE, immunoglobulin E; IL, interleukin; SCF, stem cell factor; MHC, major histocompatibility complex.

to $CD8^+$ T cells,[50] whereas class II MHC molecules present exogenously derived antigenic peptide, such as soluble bacterial protein-derived antigenic peptide, to $CD4^+$ T cells.[51] Both class I and class II MHC gene products exhibit simple Mendelian inheritance with co-dominant expression. Thus, single cells from any individual typically express pairs of the MHC gene products corresponding to the maternal and paternal alleles.

Class I MHC molecules have three external domains, and their crystalline structure has been resolved.[52] The antigen-binding site resides within a groove formed by the first and second (α_1 and α_2) external domains of the class I MHC molecule, and the appropriate TCR on $CD8^+$ T cells recognizes the antigen in association with these epitopes; the α_3 domain has been implicated in the interaction with CD8 (Fig. 1.5). The class II MHC α- and β-chains each have two immunoglobulin-like external domains. The crystalline structure of class II molecules also has been determined, demonstrating a putative antigen-binding cleft on the distal face of the molecule.[53] The appropriate TCR on $CD4^+$ T cells recognizes the antigenic peptide in this binding cleft, whereas the CD4 molecule binds to a non-polymorphic epitope or epitopes on the class II MHC molecule.[54] Unlike antigenic peptides, certain microbial antigens referred to as superantigens can activate large numbers of T cells by direct interaction with class II MHC and the ζ-chain of the TCR. Antigen-induced activation of T cells requires a combination of two different signals. The first is provided by a TCR-based interaction between the receptor and the appropriate MHC-antigenic peptide. A second or co-stimulatory signal is required for antigen-induced T cell activation, for example, the interaction between CD28 on the T cell and CD80 on the APC.

Because generation of an effector immune response depends on helper T cell function, usually mediated by $CD4^+$ T cell TCR recognition of an antigenic peptide presented in the groove of a class II MHC molecule, these molecules are referred to as the products of immune response genes. Thus, the potential to mount an immune response depends on the class II MHC gene repertoire, as well as an appropriate T cell receptor gene repertoire. Changes as subtle as a single amino acid difference at a critical site within the class II MHC molecule can alter its capacity to present an immunogenic peptide sequence derived from the intact antigen. These changes within class II MHC molecules occur within the amino terminal domain and can be associated with a responder or non-responder state, and may also translate into disease resistance or susceptibility. For example, disease resistance for juvenile-onset diabetes can be conferred by having aspartate encoded at position 57 of a DQ α chain; this alters the salt bridge in the antigen-binding cleft of the DQ molecule.[55] Likewise, susceptibility for development of rheumatoid arthritis and other autoimmune diseases is strongly associated with particular class II MHC amino acid residues.[56] Efforts to identify HLA susceptibility genes for allergic disorders have had mixed results, with associations found for hypersensitivity to drugs such as the HIV inhibitor nevirapine,[57] but not for peanut allergy.[58]

TH1 VS TH2 RESPONSES

The link of the immune response and immune regulation to allergic processes, such as immediate hypersensitivity, includes the recruitment of cells involved in their pathogenesis, eosinophils and mast cells and the regulation of IgE production. This is exquisitely dependent on T cell control, as observed in the initial descriptions of human T cell deficiency diseases, where IgE levels in patients were extremely elevated and returned to normal after T cell reconstitution following bone marrow transplantation. Because a significant portion of the clinical practice of allergists actually deals with the exaggeration of IgE responses, it is appropriate for allergists to understand the fundamental pathways of IgE biosynthesis.

Evidence has accumulated showing that T helper (Th) cell subsets play a role in the cytokine regulation of immune responses.[59] At a conceptual level, the T helper 1 (Th1) cells are associated with cytotoxic or delayed-type hypersensitivity (DTH) immune responses mediated by IFN-γ and IL-12, whereas Th2 inflammatory immune responses involve IgE and eosinophils with production of IL-4 and IL-5. Th1 cells generate an immunologic response that provides an effective defense against viral infections and other intracellular pathogens and depends on T cell-monocyte/dendritic cell interactions. Th2 cells exert their effect on immunologic responses to parasites with augmentation of inflammation from IgE production and eosinophilic infiltration. In one study of the immunoregulation of allergic responses, $CD4^+$ T cell clones specific for dust mite allergens were isolated from atopic and non-atopic individuals. Clones from the atopic persons secreted IL-2 and IL-4, but not IFN-γ and supported in vitro production of IgE. Clones from non-atopic persons secreted IL-2 and IFN-γ but little IL-4 and suppressed in vitro IgE production. It has been suggested that the susceptibility to develop allergic disease is determined by the Th1/Th2 balance established during infancy.[60] Thus a functional compartmentalization of T cells seemed to produce varied proportions of IL-4 vs IFN-γ production, which has a profound effect on IgE production by B cells.

Immunotherapy of allergic disease has been shown to induce T cells capable of turning off allergen-specific IgE responses that likely involves a switch from Th2 to Th1 allergen-specific T cells.[61] Undoubtedly, all the steps of immune sensitization described previously, beginning with presentation of antigen to T cells by APCs and ending with plasma cell secretion of antibody, apply to the IgE response to allergens. Moreover, the demonstration that IL-4 drives IgE switch provides the impetus to search for antagonist cytokines or molecules capable of downregulating IL-4 secretion or the expression of IL-4 receptors.

IMMUNE TOLERANCE AND REGULATORY T CELLS

The defensive capacity of the immune system needs a mechanism to counterbalance its power and minimize unnecessary tissue damage. Several processes ensure that the different immune effector cells are not activated against host tissues, innocuous substance or for prolonged periods of time, after the threat is resolved. Together, these processes constitute immune tolerance, and could be classified as central, if occurring in primary lymphoid organs, or peripheral, if occurring in other tissues.[61,62] An example of central tolerance is the deletion of T cells in the thymus, or B cells in the bone marrow, if these cells express antigen receptors with specificity for self-antigens. The protein AutoImmune REgulator, or AIRE, is a transcription factor that promotes in the thymus the expression of genes which are characteristically expressed in other organs, presumably to present self-antigens to newly formed T cells, and facilitates the elimination of self-reactive T cells, as part of the immune tolerance process. AIRE-deficient patients develop severe autoimmunity, involving multiple endocrine organs, in a syndrome named Autoimmune PolyEndocrinopathy Candidiasis, Ectodermal Dystrophy (APECED). Because not all self-antigens are expressed during the central induction of tolerance, other self-reactive T cells may need to be inactivated in the periphery. In lymphoid organs, lymphocytes with high affinity are deleted upon encounter with self-antigens. In other peripheral tissues, immune tolerance occurs by the induction of anergy. It was observed in experimental models that a T cell subset with the capacity of inhibiting autoimmune responses emerged during tolerance induction. In addition, it was noted that IL-2 knockout mice developed significant autoimmunity. Recent studies have provided evidence of a subset of T cells characterized by high levels of CD25 expression (IL-2R-α-chain), named regulatory T cells or 'Tregs', which suppress the function of other T cells when present in the same site (Fig. 1.6).[63] The modulatory function of these cells appears to require the expression of the forkhead protein FoxP3. T cell proliferation and cytokine responses are blunted in the presence of Tregs. In experimental models, Tregs can function through cell–cell contact and in other models through the secretion of IL-10 and/or TGF-β, inducing activation-induced cell death or anergy. A rare human disorder caused by mutations in the FoxP3 gene, the Immunodeficiency PolyEndocrinopathy, Enteropathy X-linked (IPEX), is characterized by a deficiency of CD4+CD25+ T regulatory cells, and subsequent development of severe autoimmunity, including insulin-dependent diabetes mellitus and inflammatory colitis, as well as

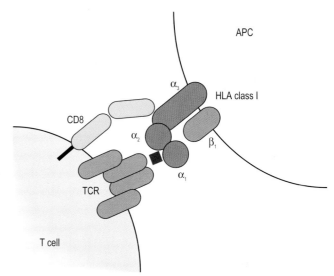

Fig. 1.5. Interaction of a HLA class I molecule (blue) on antigen-presenting cell (APC) with a CD8+ T cell. The antigen receptor (TCR) complex (purple) recognizes a complex of an antigen peptide (red) and an HLA molecule (brown and orange). The CD8 molecule in the T cells interacts with the α_3 domain of the HLA molecule. HLA class II molecules present antigen peptides to CD4+ of T cells in a similar manner, interacting with both the TCR and the CD4 molecules.

atopic dermatitis and asthma.[64] Other types of regulatory T cells have been described that are not CD25+. T_h3 cells produce IL-4, IL-10 and TGF-β and are predominantly located in the mucosa. Tr1 are cells that produce TGF-β only, and are induced by high concentrations of IL-10.

■ IMMUNOPATHOLOGY – MECHANISMS OF IMMUNE-MEDIATED DISEASES ■

Immunopathology is the study of untoward reactions produced by immune mechanisms that primarily exist for protection. For many years, the classification system of Gell and Coombs enjoyed wide acceptance as a guide to understanding complex immunologic reactions that regularly produce clinical illness. The allergist and clinical immunologist caring for patients with these hypersensitivity diseases are, in fact, observing and treating the results of the unexpected excesses of the immune response, some of which are autoimmune in nature. The original Gell and Coombs classification lists four types of hypersensitivity (immunopathologic) reactions: I, immediate (IgE mediated); II, cytotoxic (IgG/IgM mediated); III, immune (IgG/IgM immune complex mediated); and IV, delayed type hypersensitivity (T cell mediated). We endorse an alternate classification system based on one proposed by Sell that categorizes immunopathologic reactions on the basis of seven mechanisms (Box 1.1).[65] In attempting to classify the type of immunopathologic reactions that some patients experience, several of these mechanisms may be applied. For example, patients who are allergic to drugs (e.g., penicillin) may display symptoms compatible with several of these mechanisms, such as those caused by anaphylaxis and immune complexes.

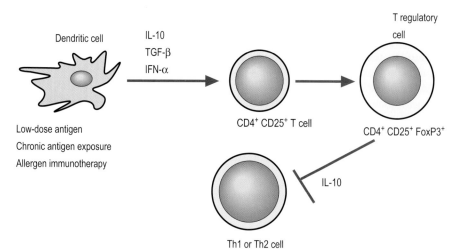

Fig. 1.6.   Regulatory T cells are generated by the interaction of antigen-presenting cells and T cells, mediated by the cytokines IL-10, TGF-β, and IFN-α. These cytokines are secreted when the antigen is presented under certain conditions, such as when administering allergen immunotherapy at very low concentration. Regulatory T cells secrete IL-10 and inhibit effector T cells that share similar antigen specificity.

> **BOX 1.1 PATHOGENIC MECHANISMS OF IMMUNE REACTIONS[65]**
>
> 1. Allergic reactions – IgE mediated
> 2. Cytotoxic or cytolytic antibody reactions
> 3. Immune complex reactions
> 4. Delayed hypersensitivity reactions
> 5. Inactivation/activation antibody reactions
> 6. T cell cytotoxic reactions
> 7. Granulomatous reactions

Over the years, the word 'allergy' has been used to describe many of these reactions. The division of untoward immunologic reactions into specific categories, although having merit for purposes of classification, has led many clinicians into explaining allergic reactions by oversimplified mechanisms. In reality, allergic reactions typically involve components of the immune and inflammatory responses that are common to all immune reactions. A brief consideration of each of the seven general types of immunologic reactions illustrates the integration of immunology in the expression of allergic reactions.

IgE-MEDIATED REACTIONS (GELL AND COOMBS TYPE I) – ANAPHYLAXIS

The immediate hypersensitivity reaction with release of mast cell or basophil mediators creating immediate and delayed (4–8 h) responses to sensitizing allergens appears to be the result of host defense mechanisms to parasites. Anaphylactic responses require allergen-specific IgE antibody to attach to high-affinity IgE receptors on mast cell or basophil surfaces, providing the means for triggering the cascade of cellular events after allergen binding, as with anaphylaxis to penicillins or with allergic rhinitis to ragweed pollen. Anaphylactoid responses are caused by

IgE-independent mechanisms of mast cell or basophil degranulation, such as those associated with high-osmolar radiocontrast material or exposure to morphine derivatives.

Although not directly involved in the immediate reaction, eosinophils are drawn to the site of the reaction by specific chemotactic factors. Eosinophils contain cationic proteins, the best characterized being major basic protein, which have the potential to contribute to ongoing inflammatory reactions by producing cellular injury[66] (see Chapter 19). In addition to eosinophils, it is likely that neutrophils are drawn to the site of an immediate hypersensitivity reaction by chemotactic factors.

Therefore, at least four cell types (mast cell, basophil, eosinophil, neutrophil) may participate in the full expression of anaphylactic reactions. Each of these cells is programmed to secrete significant quantities of mediators, which contributes to the general state of inflammation. These mediators include histamine, prostaglandins, leukotrienes, and PAF. In the case of chronic allergic reactions such as asthma, mononuclear cell infiltrates containing T cells are prominently found at the site of inflammation, such as the lung (see Chapter 30).[67]

Investigators have described that the early-phase, late-phase, and chronic manifestations of asthma involve a stepwise participation of many, if not all, components of the immune and inflammatory responses. T cells, monocytes, eosinophils, cytokines, chemokines, and arachidonic acid metabolites all contribute to the clinical expressions of asthma. In addition, the expression of adhesive glycoproteins on bronchial endothelial cells are upregulated by cytokines and play a role in late-phase allergic reactions in model lung systems.[68] IL-1 and TNF-α upregulate the expression of intercellular adhesion molecule-1 (ICAM-1; Table 1.1), endothelial-leukocyte adhesion molecule-1 (ELAM-1), and vascular cell adhesion molecule-1 (VCAM-1) in the endothelial cell surfaces, which in turn recruit and produce adherence of neutrophils, eosinophils, and basophils.[69,70] Monoclonal antibodies to ICAM-1 and ELAM-1 reduced the adhesiveness of all cell types to IL-1 upregulated adhesion molecules, and anti-VCAM-1 antibody reduced adherence of basophils and eosinophils.

These new facts have changed the clinical management of allergic disease, with a progressive increase in the use of drugs that modify inflammatory responses. Drugs such as corticosteroids are now being used to blunt the excesses of the inflammatory responses underlying all forms of asthma. Therapies focused on the use of antagonists of cytokines, chemokines, and their receptors important in both IgE production and eosinophil, basophil, and mast cell growth are currently under study.

The sum total of immune events that characterize the immediate hypersensitivity reactions describe a multicomponent response, with allergen activated IgE-sensitized mast cells or basophils by allergen binding playing the leading role. Undoubtedly, most if not all components of the immediate hypersensitivity reaction are important in host defense.

ANTIBODY-MEDIATED CYTOLYTIC REACTIONS (GELL AND COOMBS TYPE II)

These immune reactions involve IgG and IgM and to a lesser extent IgA, directed to cell surface antigens on erythrocytes, neutrophils, platelets, and epithelial cells of glandular or mucosal surfaces or to antigens on tissues (e.g., basement membranes). The sensitizing antigens in these cases can be natural cell surface antigens, modified cell surface antigens, or haptens attached to cell surfaces. There are three categories of mechanism II immunopathologic reactions. The first occurs by opsonization, which is facilitated by complement activation; the second induces complement-mediated lysis; the third is cytotoxicity mediated by ADCC. These mechanisms are well known to afford protection against infections and eradication of malignant cells but can also result in damage to self-antigens in various tissues.

An example of the first category is the phagocytic cell destruction of antibody-coated platelets (opsonization) leading to thrombocytopenia. The platelet antigens to which autoantibodies bind are glycoprotein IIb (CD41) and glycoprotein IIIa (CD42). The second-category reaction is illustrated when penicillin binds to the surfaces of erythrocytes, creating a non-self antigen composed of penicillin-modified erythrocyte cell surfaces.[71] These new antigens elicit an immune response. Antipenicilloyl antibodies, initially IgM and later IgG, fix to erythrocyte surfaces and concomitantly activate complement, leading to the lysis of the cell with penetration of the terminal hydrophobic complement MAC (C5–9). Clinically, this condition is known as penicillin-induced autoimmune hemolytic anemia. Other clinical examples of this reaction include quinidine-induced autoimmune thrombocytopenia and methyldopa-induced autoimmune hemolytic anemia. Because of the biologic amplification mechanism inherent in the activation process of complement, the thousands of activated complement components generated from a few target cells under immune attack by antibody can damage non-antibody-bound target cells, the 'innocent bystander effect.'

Several other classic forms of autoimmunity involve these immunopathologic reactions.[72] Certain forms of thyroiditis involve both antibody and complement-mediated cytotoxic reactions and ADCC (third category) attack of antithyroid antibody-coated thyroid glandular cells. The stimulus of this form of autoimmunity is not known but is thought to result from viral infections that alter the state of tolerance defined early in life when T cells are programmed in the thymus gland not to react to self-antigens. Another example is the ADCC reaction produced when eosinophils bind through FcαR receptors to IgA-bound helminths and release cytolytic major basic protein.

IMMUNE COMPLEX REACTIONS (GELL AND COOMBS TYPE III)

IgG and IgM antibodies, activated complement, and neutrophils are participants in immune complex-mediated reactions, again as the result of vigorous immune responses in genetically predisposed individuals on exposure to certain antigens, with a resultant immune injury. Knowledge of this immunologic disease became widespread in the early 1900s, when physicians began using hyperimmune animal sera, usually equine derived, to treat bacterial infections.[73,74] As many as 25% of patients treated with animal sera become seriously ill or even died. Even with the rudimentary understanding of the immune system at that time, physicians ascribed the clinical findings of inflammation of the reticuloendothelial system, skin, kidneys, and joints to an antibody process. With succeeding decades, it became clear that immune complexes of antibody and antigen, activated complement components, and chemotaxis of neutrophils were important participants in this hypersensitivity reaction. Clinical investigators described the appearance of dual sensitization, whereby the IgG (and/or IgM) and IgE immune responses were stimulated. Highly sensitized patients would sustain the immune complex-mediated reaction 10–14 days after exposure to antigen, and this delayed reaction would have been heralded by a classic immediate allergic reaction.

DELAYED HYPERSENSITIVITY REACTIONS (GELL AND COOMBS TYPE IV)

The typical cellular immune response is the delayed hypersensitivity reaction, known to be caused by sensitized T cells, in particular the $CD4^+$ (helper) cell population (see also Chapter 27). A representative clinical example of reaction is contact dermatitis resulting from poison ivy Rhus antigen. This form of hypersensitivity reaction is typically considered an allergic reaction that is actually a $CD4^+$ T cell-mediated Th1 type of response (rather than a Th2 response). Although the most apparent focus is on delayed hypersensitivity reactions involving the skin and sensitizing antigens, reactions involving other organ systems and target antigens are known.

There is also an increasing awareness of the participation of other immune and inflammatory cells and cytokines in delayed hypersensitivity reactions. In the skin, for example, the $HLA-DR^+$ Langerhans' cell presents antigen to T cells, and IFN-γ, IL-1, and TNF-α all modulate the intensity of the immune response. This type of immune response appears to play a central role in certain autoimmune diseases, such as rheumatoid arthritis, and serves as the theoretic basis for new therapeutic approaches directed at blocking inflammatory cytokines.

ANTIBODY-MEDIATED INACTIVATION/ACTIVATION OF BIOLOGICAL FUNCTION

Antibodies to a hormone, hormone receptor, blood-clotting factor, growth factor, enzyme, or drug may cause disease or treatment failure by inactivating the vital biologic function of these molecules. In addition, antibodies to receptors on cells may activate the secretory function of the cell. The disease caused by activation or inactivation depends on the function of the biologically active molecule or cell involved.

Two non-destructive and paradoxical antibody-mediated reactions are characterized by either (1) target cell stimulation or (2) negative signaling or ligand blockade. Antibody to the thyrotropin receptor on thyroid epithelial cells is an example of an autoantibody that can act equivalent to the ligand for the hormone receptor, yielding a positive signal to the cell.[75] Autoantibodies to the insulin receptor in type IIB insulin-resistant diabetes mellitus can cause opposite effects on blood glucose levels over time in the same individual, depending on the relative levels of insulin receptor-stimulating or insulin receptor-blocking antibodies.

CELL-MEDIATED CYTOTOXICITY

T cells or NK cells cause this category of immunopathogenic reactions. An example of such reactions is the T cell infiltration of blood vessels and alveoli in chronic asthma. Components of the immune system involved are $CD4^+$ T cells, $CD8^+$ T cells, and NK cells. $CD8^+$ T cell cytolytic responses to viruses and alloantigens are clinical examples of such immune reactions in which tissue damage is observed. NK cells play an important role in immune surveillance against certain viruses and tumor cells.

GRANULOMATOUS REACTIONS

Granulomas are focal collections of inflammatory cells in tissues, including macrophages, histiocytes, epithelioid cells, and giant cells, as well as lymphocytes and plasma cells surrounded by varying amounts of fibrous tissue.[65] The characteristic epithelioid cell is derived from a macrophage and has a prominent eosinophilic amorphous cytoplasm and a large, oval, pale-staining nucleus with a sharp, thin nuclear membrane and large nuclei. This characteristic pathologic appearance has been recognized for more than 150 years. These cells have been called epithelioid because of their resemblance to epithelial cells. Granulomas may progress from high cellular reactions to fibrous scars. Granulomatous reactions are cellular responses to irritating, persistent, and poorly soluble substances. These reactions are characteristically initiated by sensitized lymphocytes reacting with antigen but may also occur in response to antigen-antibody complexes that persist locally.

Not all granulomas have their origin in an immune response. Common granulomatous reactions are those surrounding insoluble suture material or around urate deposits in gouty lesions. Similar lesions may be induced by other foreign bodies. Antibody-antigen complexes may provide a stimulus for granuloma formation and inflammation if the complex is insoluble and poorly digestible. Clinical conditions involving granulomatous reactions include tuberculosis, leprosy, parasitic diseases, berylliosis, and asbestosis.

■ CONCLUSION ■

The inflammatory response includes elements comprising non-specific and specific cellular and humoral immunity and a network of interacting soluble mediators, cytokines, and chemokines. The 'classic' allergic diseases use selected components of the inflammatory response against innocuous substances resulting in clinical symptoms of varying severity. The various chapters of this textbook are directed at the understanding of these inflammatory responses and corresponding clinical conditions. For example, chapters on allergic rhinitis, asthma, allergic bronchopulmonary aspergillosis, hypersensitivity pneumonitis, sinusitis/otitis/recurrent infections, anaphylaxis, urticaria, atopic dermatitis, and food allergy all attempt to convey information on clinically diagnosed conditions and describe how specific immune responses are excessive, misguided, or deficient in producing clinical illness.

Systems that once were thought to operate only within the context of classic allergy have now been shown to exert effects in many effector systems. For example, major basic protein is thought to produce significant inflammatory effects in atopic eczema, chronic asthma, graft-versus-host disease, and immune surveillance against tumors. The interleukin family of peptide regulators exerts effects on mast cells, IgE production, T cells, and B cells. The integrin supergene family of surface accessory glycoproteins transcends cell type and displays an economy of DNA inheritance in molecular recognition, cellular adhesion, signal transduction, and cell activation. Also increasingly evident is the interaction between innate and adaptive immune responses; and the role of regulatory T cell to control the extent of the immune responses.

This overview provides a sampling of the new areas of research in allergy and clinical immunology that are covered in detail in subsequent chapters. With these advances come unprecedented opportunities to develop and apply new approaches to the diagnosis and management of allergic and immunologic disorders.

References

Introduction

1. Selnes A, Nystad W, Bolle R, et al. Diverging prevalence trends of atopic disease in Norwegian children. Results from three cross-sectional studies. Allergy 2005; 60:894–899.
2. Romagnani S. The increasing prevalence of allergy and the hygiene hypothesis: missing immune deviation, reduced immune suppression, or both? Immunology 2004; 112:352–363.
3. Heinrich J, Wichmann HE. Traffic related pollutants in Europe and their effect on allergic disease. Curr Opin Allergy Clin Immunol 2004; 4:341–348.
4. Platts-Mills TA, Erwin E, Heymann P, et al. Is the hygiene hypothesis still a viable explanation for the increased prevalence of asthma? Allergy 2005; 60(suppl 79):25–31.
5. Riedler J, Braun-Fhralander C, Eder W, et al. Exposure to farming early in life and development of asthma and allergy: a cross sectional survey. Lancet 2001; 116:675–682.
6. Ober C. Asthma genetics 2006; the long and winding road to gene discovery. Genes Immunol 2006; 7:95–100
7. Kurz T, Hoffjan S, Hayes MG, et al. Final mapping and positional candidate studies on chromosome 5p13 identify multiple asthma susceptibility loci. J Allergy Clin Immunol 2006; 118:396–402.
8. Heinzmann A, Jerkic SP, Ganter K, et al. Association study of the IL-13 variant Arg110Gln in atopic diseases and juvenile idiopathic arthritis. J Allergy Clin Immunol 2003; 112:735–739.
9. Basehore MJ, Howard TD, Lange LA, et al. A comprehensive evaluation of IL-4 variants in ethnically diverse populations: association of total serum IgE levels and asthma in white subjects. J Allergy Clin Immunol 2004; 114:80–87.
10. Delves PJ, Roitt IM. The immune system (in two parts). N Engl J Med 2000; 343:37–49, 108–117.
11. Parkin J, Cohen B. An overview of the immune system. Lancet 2001; 357:1777–1789.

Components of the immune system

12. Kruisbeek AM. Introduction: regulation of T cell development by the thymic microenvironment. Semin Immunol 1999; 11:1–2.
13. Jamieson BD, Douek DC, Killian S, et al. Generation of functional thymocytes in the human adult. Immunity 1999; 10:569–575.
14. Arstila TP, Casrouge A, Baron V, et al. A direct estimate of the human alpha/beta T cell receptor diversity. Science 1999; 286:958–961.
15. Garcia KC, Teyton L, Wilson IA. Structural basis of T cell recognition. Ann Rev Immunol 1999; 17:369–397.
16. DeFranco AL, Weiss A. Lymphocyte activation and effector function. Curr Opin Immunol 1998; 10:243–367.
17. Healy JI, Goodnow CC. Positive versus negative signaling by lymphocyte antigen receptors. Annu Rev Immunol 1998; 16:645–670.
18. Kenter AL. Class switch recombination: an emerging mechanism. Curr Top Microbiol Immunol 2005; 290:171–199.
19. Honjo T, Nagaoka H, Shinkura R, et al. AID to overcome the limitations of genomic information. Nat Immunol 2005; 6:655–661.
20. Kurosaki T. Genetic analysis of B cell antigen receptor signaling. Annu Rev Immunol 1999; 17:555–592.
21. Scharenberg AM, Kinet JP. The emerging field of receptor-mediated inhibitory signaling: SHP or SHIP. Cell 1996; 87:961–964.
22. Ruland J, Mak TW. Transducing signals from antigen receptors to nuclear factor kappaB. Immunol Rev 2003; 193:93–100.

23. Schulam PG, Kuruvilla A, Putcha G, et al. Platelet activating factor induces phospholipid turnover, calcium flux, arachidonic acid liberation, eicosanoid generation, and oncogene expression in a human B cell line. J Immunol 1991; 146:1642–1648.

24. Kuruvilla A, Pielop C, Shearer WT. Platelet-activating factor induces the tyrosine phosphorylation and activation of phospholipase C-gamma 1, Fyn and Lyn kinases, and phosphatidylinositol 3-kinase in a human B cell line. J Immunol 1994; 153(12):5433–5442.

25. Patke C, Shearer WT. gp120- and TNF-alpha-induced modulation of human B cell function: proliferation, cyclic AMP generation, Ig production, and B cell receptor expression. J Allergy Clin Immunol 2000; 105:975–982.

26. Mekori YA, Oh CK, Metcalfe DD. IL-3-dependent murine mast cells undergo apoptosis on removal of IL-3. J Immunol 1993; 151:3775.

27. Biron CA, Nguyen KB, Pien GC, et al. Natural killer cells in antiviral defense: function and regulation by innate cytokines. Annu Rev Immunol 1999; 17:189–220.

28. Raulet DH, Held W. Natural killer cell receptors: the offs and ons of NK cell recognition. Cell 1995; 82:697–700.

29. Becknell B, Caligiuri MA. Interleukin-2, interleukin-15 and their roles in the human natural killer cells. Adv Immunol 2005; 86:209–239.

30. Moretta L, Bottino C, Pende D, et al. Surface NK receptors and their ligands on tumor cells. Semin Immunol 2006; 18:151–8.

31. Cho JH, Fraser IP, Fukase K, et al. Human peptidoglycan recognition protein S is an effector of neutrophils-mediated innate immunity. Blood 2005; 106:2551–2558.

32. Williams TJ. The eosinophil enigma. J Clin Invest 2004; 113:507–509.

33. Falcone FH, Hass H, Gibbs BF. The human basophil: a new appreciation of its role in the immune responses. Blood 2000; 96:4028–4038.

34. Rivera J, Gilfillam AM. Molecular regulation of mast cell activation. J Allergy Clin Immunol 2006; 117:1214–1225.

35. Holers VM.Complement. In: Rich RR, Fleisher TA, Shearer WT, et al., eds, Clinical immunology: principles and practice. 2nd edn. St Louis: Mosby; 2001:1–18.

36. Walport M. Complement (in two parts). N Engl J Med 2001; 344: 1058–1066. 1140–1144.

37. Hawlisch H, Kohl J. Complement and toll-like receptors: key regulators of adaptive immune responses. Mol Immunol 2006; 43:13–21.

38. Thurman JM, Holers VM. The central role of the alternative complement pathway in human disease. J Immunol 2006; 176:1305–1310.

39. Oppenheim JJ, Feldman M, eds. Cytokine reference: a compendium of cytokines and other mediators of host defense, London: Academic Press; 2000.

40. McKenzie GJ, Fallon PG, Emson CL, et al. Simultaneous disruption of interleukin (IL)-4 and IL-13 defines individual roles in T helper cell type 2-mediated responses. J Exp Med 1999; 189: 1565–1572.

41. Nelms K, Keegan AD, Zamorano J, et al. The IL-4 receptor: signaling mechanisms and biologic functions. Annu Rev Immunol 1999; 17:701–738.

42. Fitch FW, McKisic MD, Lancki DW, et al. Differential regulation of murine T lymphocyte subsets. Annu Rev Immunol 1993; 11:29.

43. Wickremasinghe RG, Hoffbrand AV. Biochemical and genetic control of apoptosis: relevance to normal hematopoiesis and hematological malignancies. Blood 1999; 93:3587–3600.

44. Scaffidi C, Kirchhoff S, Krammer PH, et al. Apoptosis signaling in lymphocytes. Curr Opin Immunol 1999; 11:277–285.

45. Zlotnik A, Yoshie O. Chemokines: a new classification system and their role in immunity. Immunity 2000; 12:121–127.

46. Von Andrian UH, Mackay CR. T cell function and migration: two sides of the same coin. N Engl J Med 2000; 343:1020–1034.

47. Lusso P. HIV and the chemokine system: 10 years later. EMBO J 2006; 25:447–456.

48. Lederman MM, Penn-Nicholson A, Cho M, et al. Biology of CCR5 and its role in HIV infection and treatment. JAMA 2006; 296:815–826.

The immune response

49. Klein J, Sato A. The HLA system (in two parts). N Engl J Med 2000; 343:702–709, 782–786.

50. Salter RD, Benjamin RJ, Wesley PK, et al. A binding site for the T-cell co-receptor CD8 on the alpha 3 domain of HLA-A2. Nature 1990; 345:41.

51. Chapman HA. Endosomal proteolysis and MHC class II function. Curr Opin Immunol 1998; 10:93–102.

52. Bjorkman PJ, Saper MA, Samraoui B, et al. Structure of the human class I histocompatibility antigen, HLA-A2. Nature 1987; 329:506–512.

53. Brown JH, Jardetzky TS, Gorga JC, et al. Three-dimensional structure of the human class II histocompatibility antigen HLA-DR1. Nature 1993; 364:33.

54. Stern LJ, Brown JH, Jardetzky TS, et al. Crystal structure of the human class II MHC protein HLA-DR1 complexed with an influenza virus peptide. Nature 1994; 368:215–221.

55. Khalil I, d'Auriol L, Gobet M, et al. A combination of HLA-DQ beta Asp57-negative and HLA-DQ alpha Arg 52 confers susceptibility to insulin-dependent diabetes mellitus. J Clin Invest 1990; 85:1315–1319.

56. Thorsby E, Lie BA. HLA-associated genetic predisposition to autoimmune diseases: genes involved and possible mechanisms. Transpl Immunol 2005; 14:175–182.

57. Littera R, Carcassi C, Masala A, et al. HLA-dependent hypersensitivity to nevirapine in Sardinian HIV patients. AIDS 2006; 20:1621–1626.

58. Shrefler WG, Charlop-Powers Z, Sicherer SH. Lack of association of HLA Class II alleles with peanut allergy. Ann Allergy Asthma Immunol 2006; 96:766–768.

59. Renz H, Mutius H, Illi S, et al. T(H)1/T(H)2 immune response profiles differ between atopic children in eastern and western Germany. J Allergy Clin Immunol 2002; 109:338–342.

60. Romagnani S. Immunologic influences on allergy and the TH1/TH2 balance. J Allergy Clin Immunol 2004; 113:395–400.

61. Frew AJ. Immunotherapy for allergic disease. In: Rich RR, Fleisher TA, Shearer WT, et al., eds. Clinical immunology: principles and practice. 2nd edn. St Louis: Mosby; 2001:1–10.

62. Goodnow CC, Adelstein S, Basten A. The need for central and peripheral tolerance in the B cell repertoire. Science 1990; 248:1373–1379.

63. Sakaguchi S. Regulatory T cells: key controllers of immunological self-tolerance. Cell 2000; 101:455–458.

64. Verhagen J, Blaser K, Akdis CA, et al. Mechanisms of allergen-specific immuno-therapy: T-regulatory cells and more. Immunol Allergy Clin North Am 2006; 26:207–231.

Immunopathology - mechanisms of immune-mediated diseases

65. Sell S. Immunopathology. In: Rich RR, Fleisher TA, Schwartz BD, et al., eds. Clinical immunology: principles and practice. St Louis: Mosby, 1996:449–477.

66. Gleich GJ, Adolphson CR, Leiferman KM. The biology of the eosinophilic leukocyte. Annu Rev Med 1993; 44:85.

67. Busse W, Lemanske RF Jr. Asthma. N Engl J Med 2001; 344:350–362.

68. Leung DYM, Pober JS, Cotran RS. Expression of endothelial-leukocyte adhesion molecule-1 in elicited late-phase allergic reactions. J Clin Invest 1991; 87:1805–1809.

69. Bochner BS. Cellular adhesion and its antagonism. J Allergy Clin Immunol 1997;100:581–585.

70. Wardlaw AJ. Molecular basis for selective eosinophil trafficking in asthma: a multistep paradigm. J Allergy Clin Immunol 1999; 104:917–926.

71. Smith LA. Autoimmune hemolytic anemias: characteristics and classification. Clin Lab Sci 1999; 12:110–114.

72. McIntosh RS, Asghar MS, Weetman AP. The antibody response in human autoimmune thyroid disease. Clin Sci 1997; 92:529–541.

73. Kojis FG. Serum sickness and anaphylaxis: analysis of 6,211 patients treated with horse serum for various infections. Am J Dis Child 1942; 64:93–143.

74. Lawley TJ, Bielory L, Gascon P, et al. A prospective clinical and immunologic analysis of patients with serum sickness. N Engl J Med 1984; 311:1407–1413.

75. Devendra D, Eisenbarth GS. Immunologic endocrine disorders. J Allergy Clin Immunol 2003; 111:S624–S636.

Innate Immunity

Andrew H Liu, Michael A Zasloff, and Richard B Johnston Jr

2

CONTENTS

- Introduction 19
- Microbial pattern recognition by the innate immune system 20
- Pattern recognition receptors 20
- Resident cellular responses of innate immunity 25
- Infiltrative cellular responses of innate immunity 26
- Innate instruction of adaptive immune responses 27
- Homeostasis in the innate immune system 27
- Innate immunity and allergy 30

SUMMARY OF IMPORTANT CONCEPTS

>> The innate immune system distinguishes molecular components of microorganisms that are not made by the host. These pathogen-associated molecular patterns (PAMPs) are recognized by pattern recognition receptors (PRRs) on cells and in serum

>> Antimicrobial peptides and proteins secreted in the skin and mucous membranes control the body's relationship with commensal microbes and protect against invasion by pathogens

>> Innate immune activation leads to multifaceted antimicrobial responses by resident cells (macrophages, dendritic cells, epithelial cells, mast cells) and infiltrating cells (neutrophils, NK cells, dendritic cells, monocytes)

>> The innate immune system activates and instructs the adaptive immune system for antigen-specific T- and B-lymphocyte responses and the development of immunological memory

>> Innate immune defenses are highly efficient and include homeostatic mechanisms that downregulate inflammation to optimize the health of the host

>> Like antimicrobial immunity, allergic sensitization and atopic immune responses appear to originate in the innate immune system

INTRODUCTION

This integrated overview of innate immunity reviews its roles in host defense and in orchestrating optimal immune responses and immune development in man. How innate immune responses might lead to allergic responses and disorders are also considered. The innate immune system has a long evolutionary heritage with elements shared by most vertebrates and even with plants and insects. All of these organisms require an innate immune system in order to exist in a microbe-laden environment. Seemingly, evolution has worked elegance into the protective and homeostatic mechanisms provided by innate immunity.

Innate immune responses can be characterized as receptor-guided responses that are specific for molecular components of microorganisms that are not made by the host. These so-called pattern recognition receptors (PRRs) are innate or inborn; they are not adapted, tailored, or expanded by clonal selection as are the recognition receptors of T and B lymphocytes in acquired immunity. Early in the life of an organism, innate immunity is ready to respond immediately to and provide host defenses against microorganisms. Innate immunity has

sensitive detection systems that rapidly amplify other innate immune components when needed. Innate immune responses bridge the gap to adaptive immune responses that require days to amplify to become effective. In addition to its sentinel detection and first-responder roles, the innate immune system activates and instructs adaptive immunity, regulates inflammation, and maintains an efficient homeostasis to allow the organism to develop, grow, and thrive in its environment. Immunological homeostasis, which drives towards physiologic stability, depends on a sentinel function that continuously samples the environment and communicates with all components of the immune response. Adaptive immunity is complementary to and evolutionarily superimposed on a foundation of innate immunity.

MICROBIAL PATTERN RECOGNITION BY THE INNATE IMMUNE SYSTEM

Microbial recognition by the innate immune system is mediated by germline-encoded receptors with genetically predetermined specificities for microbes. Natural selection has formed and refined the repertoire of innate immune receptors to recognize highly conserved molecular structures that distinguish large groups of microorganisms from the host. These microbe-specific molecular structures are generally referred to as 'pathogen-associated molecular patterns (PAMPs)' and the receptors of the innate immune system that recognize them are called 'pattern recognition receptors (PRRs)' (Table 2.1). Although PAMP structures are biochemically distinct, they share common features:

- PAMPs are produced only by microbes, not by their hosts
- PAMP structures recognized by the innate immune system are usually fundamental to the integrity, survival, and pathogenicity of the microorganisms
- PAMPs are typically invariant structures shared by entire classes of pathogens.

For example, bacterial endotoxin is a lipopolysaccharide PAMP that makes up most of the outer layer of the outer membrane of all Gram-negative bacteria. Toll-like receptor 4 (TLR4) is a PRR that specifically interacts with the lipid A component of endotoxin (Fig. 2.1).[1,2] Lipid A is a highly conserved structure of the lipid bilayer of the outer bacterial cell membrane that confers much of endotoxin's biological activities.[3] Other PAMP examples are other membrane components common to large categories of bacteria (e.g., peptidoglycan, mannans), unmethylated microbial DNA, double-stranded RNA, glucans, and polysaccharide or protein moieties that are common to microbes but not to animals or man.

This approach to microbial recognition by PRRs in innate immunity is fundamentally different from the development of microbial recognition in the adaptive immune system by T and B lymphocytes. Each T and B lymphocyte acquires a structurally unique receptor during developmental processes of somatic recombination. This process generates a very diverse, nearly limitless repertoire of antigen specificities, from which the useful receptors (i.e., those specific for microbial pathogens and not self) are selected for clonal expansion and, in antibody recognition, further diversification and specificity refinement by somatic hypermutation and affinity maturation. Useful receptors of adaptive immunity are identified and 'learned' in the individual organism over time and cannot be passed onto progeny.

Thus, the innate immune system relies on PRRs, each distinguishing large classes of microbes from self via shared, conserved PAMPs. Their usefulness has been determined through eons of natural selection. PRRs are germline-encoded and passed onto progeny. In comparison, the adaptive immune system relies on somatic mechanisms that generate great antigen receptor diversity (approximately 10^{14} different immunoglobulin receptors and 10^{18} different T-cell receptors), paired with instructive, selective processes that are individualized for each host.

PATTERN RECOGNITION RECEPTORS

Pattern recognition receptors (PRRs) of the innate immune system can be divided into two groups: secreted receptors and transmembrane signal-transducing receptors (Table 2.1). *Secreted PRRs* typically have multiple effects in innate immunity and host defense, ranging from direct microbial killing, helper proteins for transmembrane receptors (e.g., CD14 and LPS binding protein for TLR4), opsonization for phagocytosis, and chemoattraction of innate and adaptive immune effector cells. The diversity and innate functionality of secreted PRRs are well demonstrated by two main categories in humans: antimicrobial peptides and collectins. *Transmembrane signaling PRRs* are expressed on many innate immune cell types, and importantly on macrophages, dendritic cells, monocytes, and B lymphocytes – the professional antigen-presenting cells. These PRRs are well exemplified by the toll-like receptors and their associated detection-enhancing proteins: MD-2, LPS binding protein, and CD14. Innate immune efficiency is achieved in part by the constitutive expression of some of these receptors as sentinels, with rapid upregulation of other PRRs with innate immune activation.

ANTIMICROBIAL PEPTIDES

Antimicrobial peptides (AMPs) are secreted PRRs that are microbicidal and rapidly acting. When secreted onto epithelial surfaces, they create a microbicidal shield against microbes prior to their attachment and invasion. As components of the antimicrobial repertoire of phagocytic cells, they complement oxidative microbicidal activities within phagolysosomes. AMPs have antimicrobial activity against a broad range of bacteria, fungi, chlamydiae, and enveloped viruses.[4]

AMPs target the membranes of microorganisms for their toxic activity. While there is a great diversity of AMPs between and within species, they share a fundamental feature in their molecular structures of clustering hydrophobic, cationic amino acids to carry out their microbicidal function (Fig. 2.2).[5,6] This molecular feature exploits a distinct feature and vulnerability in the structure of bacterial and other microbial membranes: the outer bilayer of bacterial membranes is largely populated by negatively charged phospholipids, an attractive surface for the cationic and hydrophobic domains of AMPs to bind. In contrast, the outer cell membranes of plants and animals are composed of lipids with no net charge. AMPs integrate into the microbial outer membrane and form pores and cracks, thereby disrupting cell membrane integrity and function.

There are two main categories of AMPs in humans: defensins and the cathelicidin LL-37 (Table 2.1). Two types of defensins are present in humans, the alpha (α) and beta (β) classes. α-defensins in humans are granule proteins of neutrophils (e.g., human neutrophil peptides 1 through 4) and are also synthesized by Paneth cells at the base of small intestinal crypts (α-defensins 5 and 6).[7] β-defensins are expressed on all epithelial surfaces, including those of the airways, urinary and gastrointestinal tracts, and skin. Their production by epithelial cells can be constitutive (as for HBD-1) or inducible (HBD-2, HBD-3, HBD-4). HBD-2 expression is induced in epithelial cells by bacterial PAMPs via TLR2 or TLR4.[8,9] Stimulation of epithelium by innate inflammatory cytokines, including IL-1β and TNF-α, also induces defensin production.[10]

Cathelicidin LL-37 is released from both neutrophils and epithelial cells, and exhibits a broad range of antimicrobial activities.[11] LL-37 is also

Table 2.1 Pattern recognition receptors in humans*

	Recognize	Functions
Secreted		
Antimicrobial peptides	Microbial membranes	Opsonization
Defensins		Microbial cell lysis
Cathelicidin		Chemoattractant
Collectins		
Mannose-binding lectin	Microbial mannose	Complement activation
Surfactant proteins A & D	Bacterial cell wall lipids; viral coat proteins	Opsonization, killing, pro- and antiinflammatory mediator
C-reactive protein	Bacterial phospholipids	Complement activation; opsonization
Membrane-bound		
Toll-like receptors	Microbial PAMPs	Immune cell activation
MD-2	Endotoxin	TLR4 co-receptor
Macrophage mannose receptor	Microbial mannose	Phagocytosis
Macrophage scavenger receptor	Bacterial cell walls	Phagocytosis
N-formylmethionine receptor	Bacterial N-formylmethionine	Phagocytosis
Secreted and membrane-bound		
CD14	Endotoxin	TLR4 signaling
LPS binding protein	Endotoxin	TLR4 signaling
Cytosolic		
Nod 1 and 2	Bacterial peptidoglycans	Immune cell activation
RIG-1 and Mda-5	Viral double-stranded RNA	Immune cell activation

*Principal examples are shown.

induced by vitamin D. The gene encoding LL-37 has a vitamin D receptor binding site.[12,13] In both keratinocytes and macrophages, stimulation of TLR2 results in the induction of CYP27B1, the cytochrome P450 enzyme that converts $25(OH) D_3$ to the active form of vitamin D, $1,25 (OH)_2D_3$, which in turn induces the expression of the antimicrobial peptide LL-37. By this route, vitamin D can influence microbicidal defenses of both skin and circulating phagocytic cells.[14] It has been proposed that certain human infections, such as by *Mycobacterium tuberculosis*, might be more prevalent among populations with inadequate plasma levels of vitamin D.[15]

AMPs generally work in concert with larger secreted antibacterial proteins such as lysozyme, bacterial permeability increasing protein (BPI), lactoferrin, and lipocalin, and are often synthesized by the same cells. Lysozyme, for example, is produced by epithelial cells, such as Paneth cells, and is found in neutrophil granules; lysozyme degrades the bacterial peptidoglycan cell wall of bacteria killed by AMPs.[16] A genomic search for defensin sequence homology in humans revealed five β-defensin gene clusters with as many as 25 additional defensins.[17] Other types of AMPs have been described, e.g., dermicidin in sweat.[18]

This suggests that what is currently known about human AMPs may only be a sampling of what is available and utilized.

Epithelial and innate immune cells express multiple AMPs from several different structural classes. The expression of a diverse, germline-encoded repertoire of AMPs would seem to subvert the development of AMP resistance; the development of AMP resistance is indeed uncommon. An interesting twist to bacterial AMP resistance occurs in the GI tract. The GI tracts of healthy humans are colonized by commensal bacteria that are relatively resistant to AMPs. These commensals provide continuous stimulation of gut epithelial cells to produce AMPs that are toxic to gut pathogens, thereby giving commensals a survival advantage.[19]

AMPs also serve as chemoattractants for innate and adaptive immune cells. Human α-defensin attracts immature dendritic cells and peripheral blood T cells, enhancing antigen-specific adaptive immune responses.[20] For chemoattraction, some AMPs bind to receptors that also bind PAMPs or chemokines. For example, cathelicidin LL-37 attracts neutrophils, monocytes, mast cells, and T lymphocytes via formyl peptide-like receptor 1 – a PRR that also binds bacterial formyl peptides.[21]

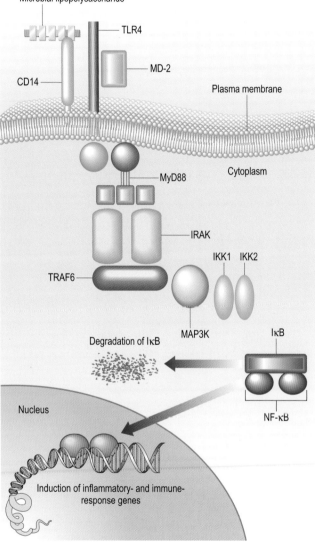

Fig. 2.1. Endotoxin recognition and cell activation via toll-like receptor 4. Lipopolysaccharide from the outer cell wall of Gram-negative bacteria (i.e., endotoxin) is a prototypical microbial pathogen-associated molecular pattern (PAMP) that is recognized by toll-like receptor (TLR) 4. Endotoxin recognition includes two other molecules: MD-2 is a membrane co-receptor of endotoxin, while CD14 binds and enhances endotoxin's interaction with TLR4. Binding of most TLRs, including TLR4, activates the nuclear factor-κB (NF-κB) signaling pathway by recruiting the adaptor protein MyD88. MyD88 is associated with a series of signal transduction intermediates: IL-1 receptor-associated kinases (IRAK) 1–4 and, after IRAK phosphorylation, the adaptor protein TNF receptor-associated factor (TRAF) 6. TRAF-6 oligomerization activates mitogen-activated protein kinase (MAP3K), leading to the activation of IκB kinase 1 (IKK1) and IκB kinase 2 (IKK2). These kinases phosphorylate IκB, which is then degraded, thereby releasing NF-κB, which moves into the nucleus and induces the transcriptional activation of a wide variety of inflammatory- and immune-response genes. TLR4 engagement also induces IRAK phosphorylation and NF-κB translocation through a MyD88-independent pathway mediated by the TIR domain-containing adaptor protein inducing IFN-β (TRIF). (Adapted from Medzhitov R, Janeway C Jr. Innate immunity. N Engl J Med 2000; 343:338–344, Figure 2. © 2000 Massachusetts Medical Society. All rights reserved.)

COLLECTINS

Secreted PRRs can serve as opsonins by binding to microbial cell walls and flagging them for phagocytosis and recognition by the complement system. *Mannose-binding lectin (MBL)* is a secreted PRR that is structurally similar to the complement component C1q and, like C1q, can opsonize microbes for phagocytosis via the C1q receptor. MBL is an acute phase reactant produced by the liver that recognizes terminal mannose residues of carbohydrates on Gram-positive and Gram-negative bacteria, fungi yeast, and some viruses and parasites.[24] MBL and surfactant proteins form a structurally related family of collectins, so named because they contain a collagenous domain.[25] MBL can activate the complement pathway via MBL-associated serine proteases that are related to C1r and C1s, the serine proteases of the classical, antibody-dependent complement pathway. Like C1r and C1s, MBL-associated proteases cleave C4 and C2; activated C2 then cleaves the central protein of the complement cascade, C3. The larger C3b fragment deposits in the microbial membrane and serves as an opsonin for recognition by the CR1 and CR3 receptors on phagocytes. C3b deposition in combination with factor B cleaves C5, which becomes the nidus for localization of other complement components that complex to form membrane pores and lyse cells. Fragments of these complement proteins that are generated during these processes, C3a and C5a, are chemoattractants for neutrophils. Thus, this MBL-triggered complement cascade leads to several immediate antimicrobial effects: microbial cell lysis, chemoattraction of neutrophils, and phagocytosis.

Two of the four pulmonary surfactant proteins, SP-A and SP-D, are collectins with similar structures and multiple innate immune functions. Structurally, they share carbohydrate domains that bind oligosaccharides specific for a variety of microbes (Gram-positive and Gram-negative bacteria, viruses, fungi). They recognize PAMPs such as bacterial LPS, tubercle lipoarabinomannan, a variety of other bacterial lipids, and common viral proteins (e.g., influenza hemagglutinin and neuraminidase envelope glycoproteins, RSV G- and F-fusion proteins).[26] SP-A and SP-D mediate multiple antimicrobial functions. They aggregate and opsonize microbes for phagocytosis by a variety of immune cells, including alveolar macrophages, monocytes, neutrophils, and dendritic cells.

HBD-2 and HBD-3 are inducible and chemoattractive for immature dendritic cells and memory T lymphocytes via the chemokine receptor CCR6.[20] Recruitment of dendritic cells by AMPs induces their maturation. The β-defensins and LL-37 are also chemoattractive for mast cells and can induce their degranulation.[22,23]

To summarize, when AMPs are induced at a site of injury, they act directly to destroy microbial invaders and to attract an array of defensive cells to provide potential 'back-up' support to defend the breached barrier. In states of health, the defenses provided by AMPs are by and large clinically silent. Inflammation is clinically recognized when the AMP-based defenses have proved inadequate and a robust secondary defensive response involving the adaptive immune system is mobilized.

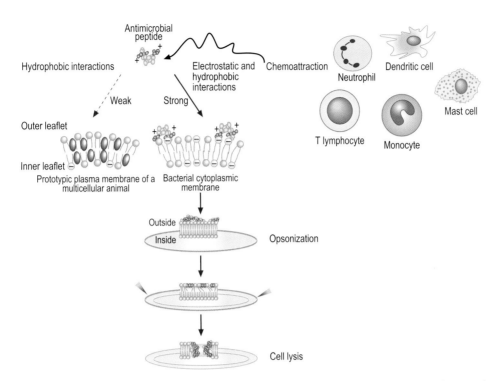

Fig. 2.2. Antimicrobial peptide mechanisms. Antimicrobial peptides (AMPs), cationic and hydrophobic in nature, target the exposed outer membrane of bacteria that is dense with negatively charged phospholipid headgroups. This differs from the cell membranes of plants and animals that are spared of AMP binding because their outer cell membrane lipids have no net charge. AMPs integrate into bacterial membranes and form holes that physically disrupt membrane integrity and lyse target cells. AMPs are also chemoattractive for a variety of immune cells, while carpeting and opsonizing bacterial targets for recognition and uptake by phagocytes bearing AMP receptors. (Adapted from Zasloff M. Antimicrobial peptides of multicellular organisms. Nature 2002; 415:389–395, Figures 2 and 3).[5]

They also mediate nuclear factor-κB (NF-κB) activation and cytokine production via TLR4 and TLR2. SP-A induces the expression of scavenger and mannose receptors on phagocytes, thereby improving phagocytosis. SP-A and SP-D also induce both inflammatory and regulatory responses. SP-A and SP-D have direct bactericidal[27] and fungicidal[28] properties, and also help to dampen inflammatory responses by enhancing the uptake of pro-inflammatory apoptotic cells by macrophages.[29]

Another example of a secreted PRR is C-reactive protein (CRP), a plasma acute phase reactant that is produced by the liver and specifically binds bacterial phospholipids such as phosphorylcholine. CRP opsonizes bacteria by binding the complement factor C1q that can subsequently bind C1q receptors on phagocytes. CRP also directly binds Fc-γ receptors on phagocytes, promoting phagocytosis.

TOLL-LIKE RECEPTORS AND ASSOCIATED PRRs

The immediate cellular responders of the innate immune system (e.g., monocytes, macrophages, dendritic cells, epithelial cells, neutrophils) and many other cell types express a family of transmembrane PRRs with functional roots to the toll receptor of Drosophila.[30] These toll-like receptors (TLR) are structurally similar, with large leucine-rich extracellular domains and cytoplasmic domains that are notably similar to that of the mammalian IL-1 receptor (Table 2.2).[31] Accordingly, the IL-1 receptor and TLRs share a MyD88-dependent signaling pathway that leads to NF-κB activation.

TLR4 was the first human TLR identified and is specific for bacterial endotoxin (Fig. 2.1). Endotoxin, a prototypical PAMP, is a lipopolysaccharide (LPS) that comprises most of the outer bilayer of the outer cell membrane of all Gram-negative bacteria. Its immune stimulatory capacity is largely attributed to the lipid A moiety of endotoxin, which is specifically recognized by TLR4 and is highly conserved across different bacterial species.[1] Very small amounts of endotoxin (i.e., picogram amounts, estimated to equal ~10 LPS molecules/cell) are immune stimulatory.[32]

This very high sensitivity for endotoxin-mediated cell activation is in part attributable to the TLR4-related enhancer proteins, lipopolysaccharide binding protein (LPS BP) and CD14, and on the TLR4 recognition co-receptor, MD-2 (Fig. 2.1). LPS BP is a soluble protein that is produced by the liver, binds endogenous and exogenous LPS, and shuttles to TLR4.[33] CD14 is a soluble and cell surface receptor that binds LPS and improves TLR4 sensitivity and detection of endotoxin.[34] LPS BP and CD14 are not classical PRRs in that their binding specificity is not limited to PAMPs. In comparison, MD-2 is an extracellular adaptor protein that binds both the hydrophobic portion of LPS and the extracellular domain of TLR4.[35] MD-2 is constitutively associated with TLR4 and is required for TLR4 recognition of endotoxin. Thus, the variability of TLR4 sensitivity to endotoxin is in part attributable to whether or not there are detection-dependent (MD-2) and/or detection-enhancing proteins (LPS BP, CD14) in sufficient quantities.

Other factors that heighten immune cellular sensitivity to endotoxin include the constitutive expression of TLR4 on cell surfaces versus other

Table 2.2 Toll-like receptors in humans

	Ligands	Microbial sources
TLR1	Lipoproteins, lipoteichoic acid	Gram-positive bacteria, mycoplasma
TLR2	Lipoproteins	Bacterial cell walls, mycoplasma
	Peptidoglycan, lipoteichoic acid	Gram-positive bacteria cell walls
	Zymosan	Fungi
	Lipoarabinomannan	Mycobacteria cell walls
TLR3	Double-stranded RNA	Viral RNA
TLR4	Endotoxin	Gram-negative bacteria cell walls
	Viral coat proteins	Respiratory syncytial virus
TLR5	Flagellin	Bacteria
TLR6	Lipoproteins, lipoteichoic acid	Gram-positive bacteria, mycoplasma
TLR7	Single-stranded RNA	Viral RNA
TLR8	Single-stranded RNA	Viral RNA
TLR9	Unmethylated CpG DNA	Bacterial and viral DNA
TLR10	Not reported	

TLRs that are inducibly and internally expressed. TLR4-mediated activation is primed by innate immune cytokines (e.g., IFNs), low-level endotoxin exposure, or other PAMP exposures.[32,36–38] Conversely, high endotoxin exposure suppresses TLR4-mediated activation.[38]

Ten human TLRs have been identified and collectively recognize a broad array of microbes (Table 2.2). The different TLRs recognize a remarkably diverse range of microbial cell wall components, proteins, and nucleic acids, all classic PAMPs that distinguish microbes from their mammalian hosts. In comparison to Gram-negative bacteria, Gram-positive bacterial cell walls do not contain endotoxin, but contain peptidoglycan and lipoproteins that are recognized by TLR2.[39] Similarly, mycoplasma does not have a cell wall, but its cell membrane has lipoproteins recognized by TLR2, TLR1, and TLR6.[39] TLR5 recognizes bacterial flagellin.[40] The CpG sequences throughout bacterial and viral DNA are unmethylated, distinguishing microbial DNA from mammalian DNA; microbial unmethylated CpG is recognized by TLR9.[41] TLR7 and TLR8 are closely related to TLR9 and recognize virus-derived single-stranded RNA.[42] Double-stranded RNA, unique to certain viruses, is recognized by TLR3.[43]

Nod1 and Nod2 are cytosolic PRRs with leucine-rich repeat regions that recognize bacterial peptidoglycans.[44] They are the best characterized of a large family of Nod proteins with structural similarities. Nod1 is expressed primarily in GI tract epithelial cells and is specific for peptidoglycans of Gram-negative, but not Gram-positive, bacteria.[45,46] In comparison, Nod2 is produced in macrophages, dendritic cells, and Paneth cells under resting conditions, and is induced by TNF-α and IFN-γ in GI epithelial cells.[47] Nod2 detects the peptidoglycan muramyl dipeptide in both Gram-positive and Gram-negative bacteria.[48,49] Nod2 has been of particular interest in Crohn's disease because, in humans, mutations in the Nod2 gene are strongly associated with increased risk of this disorder.[50] Other known cytoplasmic PRRs are helicases RIG-1 and Mda-5 that recognize double-stranded RNA and mediate antiviral immune responses to different double-stranded RNA viruses.[51]

Activation through TLRs primarily occurs through MyD88 (except TLR3), an intracellular signal-transducing adaptor molecule, leading to intracellular association with multiple IL-1 receptor-associated kinases (IRAK-1 through IRAK-4), activation of TNF receptor-associated factor 6 (TRAF6), and NF-κB translocation (Fig. 2.1).[52] NF-κB translocation results in the expression of co-stimulatory molecules (e.g., CD80) and inflammatory cytokines, including TNF-α, IL-1, IL-6, and IL-8, that are central to innate and adaptive immune responses. While TLRs share the MyD88-dependent activation pathway, they also have differing alternative signaling pathways. For example, TLR4 also activates NF-κB through a MyD88-independent pathway that is relatively insensitive to endotoxin stimulation, and with delayed kinetics.[52] This MyD88-independent pathway, mediated by the 'TIR domain-containing adaptor protein inducing IFN-β' (TRIF), mediates TLR3 as well as TLR4 activation of NF-κB.[53] TLR2 also has a MyD88-independent pathway that differs from that of TLR4 and is mediated via an extracellular signaling pathway that modulates the activity of the transcription factor *c-fos*.[54]

PRRs LINKED TO PHAGOCYTOSIS

In addition to the secreted PRRs that bind PAMPs and opsonize pathogens for phagocytosis, some membrane-bound PRRs on the surface of phagocytes identify microbes for phagocytosis. Upon recognizing PAMPs on a microbial cell, these receptors mediate the phagocytosis-associated release of toxic oxidants and uptake and delivery of pathogens to lysosomes filled with microbicidal products. In macrophages, pathogen-derived proteins are processed into peptides and presented by major histocompatibility complex (MHC) molecules on the surface of the macrophages to engage and instruct antigen-specific T lymphocytes. The *macrophage mannose receptor*, a member of the calcium-dependent lectin family, specifically recognizes carbohydrates with terminal mannan that are characteristic of a variety of microbes, especially fungi, and mediates their phagocytosis

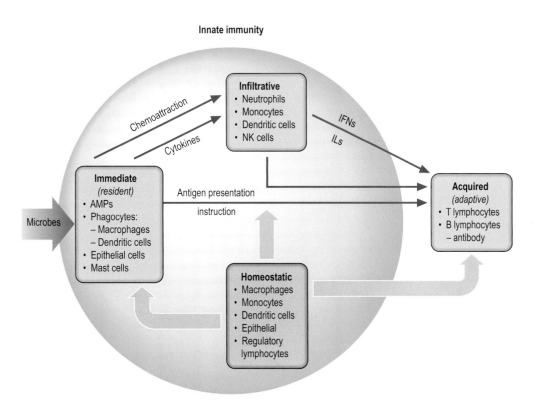

Innate immunity

Fig. 2.3. Spectrum of innate immune responses. Innate immune responses to microbes can be broadly characterized as antimicrobial or homeostatic. Antimicrobial responses begin with protective layers of antimicrobial peptides and detection by immune cells residing at the epithelial interface. Often, these immediate responses sufficiently protect the host. If this first layer of host defense is inadequate, then the front-line responders attract infiltrative innate immune cells that are activated as they approach the source of inflammation. Both immediate and infiltrating immune cells stimulate adaptive immune responses and educate lymphocytes via antigen presentation and co-stimulation. Homeostatic responses by innate immune cells downregulate inflammatory and antimicrobial immune responses when they are no longer needed in order to optimize the utilization of resources and well-being of the host.

by macrophages.[24,55] Macrophages also bind fungal mannan through TLR2 and TLR4.[55] *Macrophage scavenger receptors* are another family of phagocytic PRRs that bind to bacterial cell walls and play a part in the clearance of bacteria.[56]

Another example of a membrane-bound PRR that promotes phagocytosis is the *N-formylmethionine receptor*. The sequence *N*-formylmethionine initiates all bacterial proteins, but only mitochondrial proteins in mammalian cells.[57] Their engagement by the *N*-formylmethionine receptor recruits phagocytes that express this receptor and activates them for phagocytosis and killing. The MHC class I-b molecule of mice is a specific binding receptor for microbial *N*-formyl peptides, thereby forming an intriguing link between MHC class I and microbial PRR-type recognition.[58]

RESIDENT CELLULAR RESPONSES OF INNATE IMMUNITY

Microbial detection via cell surface PRRs leads to the activation of cells that express them. Those in front-line positions for detection are the first responders of the innate immune system: macrophages, dendritic cells, epithelial cells, and mast cells (Fig. 2.3).

Myeloid dendritic cells (mDC) are emerging as key sentinels of the innate immune system and exemplify its immediate cellular response. mDCs are constantly produced in the bone marrow and recruited from the blood into histologic sites with high antigen exposure (e.g., skin, mucosal surfaces, lymph nodes, spleen).[59] With their long dendrites and their PRR-rich cell surfaces, mDCs form a subepithelial web that is sensitive to microbes, inflammation, and cellular stress. In the airways, antigens are captured by mucosal mDCs immediately across epithelial tight junction barriers.[60] In the gastrointestinal tract, mucosal mDCs extend dendrites in between epithelial cells into the gut lumen for antigen sampling.[61] Once activated, mDCs respond quickly in order to alert and instruct the immune system by secreting activating cytokines such as interferons and migrating to draining lymph nodes for T lymphocyte instruction.

mDCs are also among the first immune cells to respond to environmental microbial exposures or cellular stress. For example, in rats, the inhalation of bacteria or viral particles induced a very rapid influx of mDCs into their airway mucosal surfaces, apparent in minutes and peaking 2 h after challenge.[62] This mDC recruitment occurred prior to neutrophil, macrophage, or lymphocyte influx. A wide array of stimuli are chemoattractive for mDCs, including chemokines, complement split products, and bacterial peptides.[63]

mDCs express a discrete division of cellular functions that is developmentally related.[63,64] mDCs migrate from the bone marrow to peripheral tissues in a so-called 'immature' form when their role is primarily sentinel detection. They have a high capacity to sense, sample, and process incoming antigen via dense PRR expression (e.g., TLRs), but a poor ability to stimulate T lymphocytes. Once sensing environmental microbial PAMPs or inflammatory stress, mDCs become activated scavengers of antigen, and subsequently head back to draining lymph nodes. During migration, they 'mature' such that, as mature mDCs, their antigen uptake and processing functions are shut down while large amounts of processed antigen are displayed on cell surface MHC molecules with a battery of T-cell co-stimulatory factors for T lymphocyte education.

mDCs are further characterized by different subtypes, including Langerhans cells in epithelial surfaces of skin and mucosa, subepithelial/interstitial DCs, plasmacytoid DCs, and monocyte-derived DCs, which are derived from circulating monocyte precursors.[64] Different mDC subtypes express different TLRs that recognize different PAMPs, and TLR-mediated activation results in some differences in expressed cytokines.[65] Plasmacytoid DCs express TLR7 and TLR9 for recognizing viral infections and, upon simulation, release large amounts of IFN-α to limit viral replication.[66] Other mDCs express TLR 1–6 for recognizing bacterial infections and are superior stimulators of NK and NKT cells by virtue of their robust IL-12 production.[64] DC-stimulated NK and NKT cells produce much IFN-γ, which in turn promotes both clonal expansion of Th1 cells, maturation of resident DCs, and priming of macrophages and monocytes.

Macrophages are similar to DCs in their histologic location in areas of high environmental antigen exposure, cell surface expression of PRRs, capacity to be immediate cellular responders, and ability to phagocytose organisms, digest them, and present antigens to lymphocytes. In addition, macrophages are distributed throughout all central organs where they protect tissues through phagocytic killing, removed dead tissue and apoptotic cells, and secrete over 100 proteins that mediate host defense and inflammation. Tissue macrophages are derived from blood monocytes, which leave the circulation and migrate into organs and tissues where they differentiate into the macrophage characteristic of that tissue (e.g., Kupffer cells of the liver). Functionally, macrophages are a central keeper of immunological homeostasis and well-being, as discussed later in this chapter.

In addition to these traditional antigen-presenting cells of innate immunity, *epithelial cells and mast cells* are also resident sentinel cells of immediate innate immune responses. These cells are in anatomic positions of high antigenic exposure, express PRRs that allow them to recognize and respond to PAMPs, and respond immediately. The continuous physical barrier and clearance mechanisms (e.g., mucociliary system) that epithelial cells provide between the external environment and the host are often considered to be part of the innate immune system, although this aspect of their protective function does not involve microbial pattern recognition. Human airway epithelial cells express multiple TLRs and, when PAMP stimulated, produce pro-inflammatory cytokines, including IL-8.[67] Human keratinocytes express a mannose-binding receptor that mediates killing of candida.[68] In the GI tract, TLR-mediated epithelial responses to commensal bacteria PAMPs (i.e., TLR4 and TLR2 ligands) mediate epithelial integrity and resilience to injury.[69]

Mast cells live in large numbers in the interstitium of peripheral tissues. They express TLR1, TLR2, TLR4, and TLR6,[70] complement receptors for C3a and C5a,[71] and mannose-binding lectin receptors. Upon PRR activation, mast cells synthesize numerous cytokines and mediators that characterize innate immune responses. In particular, they are key sources

of immediate release of TNF-α and IL-8, which are uniquely preformed in mast cells; their immediate TNF-α release may have a central role in effective antimicrobial responses to infections.[72,73] Mast cells also make classic inflammatory mediators (histamine, heparin, leukotrienes, platelet-activating factor), proteases (e.g., tryptase, chymase), and antimicrobial peptides (cathelicidin LL-37,[74] defensins[75]). Mast cells are poised to be among the immediate responders to microbial exposures.

INFILTRATIVE CELLULAR RESPONSES OF INNATE IMMUNITY

Infiltrative cellular responses are potent antimicrobial effectors that are generally recruited by an innate immune intermediary to induce the full weight of their response, but can respond directly to microbial stimuli via their own surface-expressed PRRs (Fig. 2.3).

Neutrophils, the most abundant circulating phagocytes in the human host, are recruited into sites of infection and inflammation via a variety of chemotactic signals. Large numbers of circulating neutrophils are short-lived, approximately 24 h, such that ~10^{11} die each day.[76] This constant stream of neutrophil death would be potently inflammatory without the extraordinarily efficient uptake and processing of apoptotic neutrophils by macrophages and dendritic cells to prevent release of toxic constituents, a process termed efferocytosis (discussed later in this chapter).[77]

In response to infection, circulating neutrophils adhere to adjacent vascular endothelium, migrate to the site of infection, and ingest and kill the invaders. Neutrophils have PRRs for different types of chemoattractants, including N-formyl bacterial oligopeptide, complement-derived C5a, and leukotriene B4 secreted by numerous immune cells upon activation. Activated innate immune cells and epithelial cells secrete the neutrophil chemokine IL-8. These neutrophil chemoattractants diffuse from the site of infection to provide a chemotactic gradient for neutrophil migration and to further activate neutrophils as they transmigrate.[78,79]

Upon reaching the infected site, neutrophils phagocytose invading microorganisms that are opsonized by innate and acquired immune processes, such as fixation of complement C3 fragments (e.g., C3b, iC3b[80]) and IgG.[81] Following phagocytosis, microbicidal mechanisms kill the ingested microbes almost immediately by internally merging the microbe-containing phagosome with intracellular granules containing microbicidal products such as α-defensins (HNPs 1–4) and highly reactive oxidizing agents generated by membrane NADPH oxidase and myeloperoxidase (e.g., O_2^-, H_2O_2, hypochlorous acid).[82] The phagocyte NADPH oxidase has an essential role in killing and preventing infection with certain common organisms (e.g., *S. aureus, Serratia, enteric bacteria, Aspergillus*).[83] Recently, an increased role for neutrophil granule proteases (neutrophil elastase and cathepsin G) has been recognized. These cationic proteases, usually bound and rendered inactive by proteoglycans, are released and activated with alkalinization and K^+ ion fluxes into phagocytic vacuoles.[84] These pH and potassium requirements for protease solubilization and activity restrict their toxicity to phagocytic vacuoles and limit damage to host tissues.[82]

Natural killer (NK) cells are an innate immune cell type with unique features. They are lymphoid cells that do not express antigen-specific receptors derived from recombination and clonal selection, such as T-cell receptors or surface immunoglobulin.[85] Although NK cells express PRRs such as TLRs 2–5, TLR7, and TLR8, and recognize and respond to the respective TLR ligands directly,[86,87] they are best known for responding in an antigen-independent manner to help contain viral infections (especially herpes infections) and malignant tumors by recognizing aberrant host cells for elimination. NK cells distinguish healthy host cells through *inhibitory receptors* such as the 'killer cell immunoglobulin-like receptor' (KIR) and CD94/NKG2A receptors that recognize MHC class I molecules expressed on healthy cells (Fig. 2.4).[88,89] Binding of these receptors inhibits NK cell-mediated lysis and cytokine secretion. Virus-infected and malignant cells often downregulate MHC class I molecules, rendering them susceptible to attack by NK cells.[90] These inhibitory receptors on NK cells are counterbalanced by *activating receptors*, such as the NKG2D receptor that recognizes 'stress' ligands expressed on cell surfaces in response to intracellular DNA damage.[91]

Recruited and activated NK cells mediate antimicrobial activities via the induction of apoptosis of cell targets and cytokine secretion that is believed to promote innate immune functions and contribute to adaptive immune responses. Target cell apoptosis results from granule exocytosis and death receptor engagement. NK cells have granules with perforins and granzymes that, upon activation, are released into the synapse between target and effector cell, disrupting target cell membranes and inducing apoptosis (Fig. 2.4).[92] NK cells also mediate apoptosis by expressing Fas ligand and 'TNF-related apoptosis-inducing ligand' (TRAIL) that bind Fas and TRAIL-R on target cells, respectively.[93]

Activated NK cells are known for their secretion of IFN-γ in particular, but also secrete TNF-α, growth factors, IL-5, IL-10, IL-13, and chemokines.[94] Dendritic cells recruit, interact with, and activate NK cells through cytokines (e.g., type I IFNs, IL-12, IL-18) and cell-to-cell surface interactions.[94] NK cells can activate bystander immature dendritic cells by producing TNF-α and IFN-γ along with cell–cell contact.[95] Reciprocal NK-dendritic cell interactions occur in secondary lymphoid organs, where NK cells respond to IL-12 produced by mature DCs by producing IFN-γ and promoting the development of Th1 and cytotoxic T lymphocytes.[96–98]

INNATE INSTRUCTION OF ADAPTIVE IMMUNE RESPONSES

The immediate and infiltrative responses of innate immunity set the stage for their instruction of adaptive immunity and the maintenance of immunologic memory. Because the adaptive immune system essentially has a limitless antigen receptor repertoire, instruction is necessary to guide adaptive antimicrobial immune responses toward pathogens, and not self-antigens or harmless environmental antigens. Microbial pattern recognition by innate immune cells controls the activation of adaptive immune responses by directing microbial antigens linked to TLRs through the cellular processes leading to antigen presentation[99] and the expression of co-stimulatory molecules (e.g., CD80 and CD86).

A legacy of research on the prototypical PAMP endotoxin is helpful in understanding PAMP control of adaptive immunity. It has long been known that endotoxin can be used as an essential adjuvant in the induction of antigen-specific T cell memory.[100,101] Although T cells will mount a short-lived proliferative response to protein antigens alone, classic memory immunity – the generation of long-lived memory/effector T lymphocytes and a persistent antibody response – is dependent on immunization with an adjuvant such as endotoxin.[102,103] Endotoxin potently induces

IL-12 and IFN-γ secretion, which are key regulators of memory Th1-type immune development.[104] LPS-generated, antigen-specific memory T lymphocytes have been shown to be IFN-γ-producing effector T cells.[105] LPS strongly influences innate antigen-presenting cells, and especially dendritic cells, to produce IL-12 and to co-stimulate naive T lymphocytes to become effector T lymphocytes that primarily secrete IFN-γ.[106–108] In a reciprocating manner, IFN-γ primes innate immune cells to produce greater amounts of IL-12 in response to stimulation,[107,109–111] fostering a positive feedback relationship between the innate and adaptive immune compartments for Th1-type immune development.

Among antigen-presenting cells, dendritic cells are perhaps the most efficient educators of T lymphocytes. Immature DCs in the periphery are activated via PRRs. Myeloid DCs express TLRs 1–6, while plasmacytoid DCs express TLR7 and TLR9,[112] illustrating DC subtype differences in PAMP recognition. Once activated, DCs scavenge antigen and migrate to T-cell areas of draining lymph nodes, guided by TLR-mediated expression of the chemokine receptor CCR7 (Fig. 2.5). During their migration, they mature to redirect their cellular energy to the processes of antigen presentation in MHC class II molecules and the expression of stimulatory cytokines and cell surface molecules.

In draining LNs, mature DCs attract antigen-specific T cells (Fig. 2.5). Classical activation of naive T lymphocytes requires at least two concurrent receptor interactions: T-cell receptor recognition of peptide-MHC class II complex, and co-stimulation by CD80 or CD86. On the first day, activated T cells receive intense stimulation from DCs via prolonged cell surface receptor interactions, followed on the second day by T lymphocyte proliferation after dissociation from the DCs.[113] These activated T lymphocytes subsequently migrate to other lymph nodes and back to the mucosa, where they again interact with and are sustained by mature DCs in the subepithelial periphery. This peripheral tissue-specific interaction between mature DCs and progeny effector T cells may underlie the persistence of organ-specific immune memory.[114]

HOMEOSTASIS IN THE INNATE IMMUNE SYSTEM

The breadth and depth of innate immune activities to defend the host in its microbe-laden environment are silent from a clinical perspective. Inflammation seems to be the exception rather than the norm. This immune tranquility of the well-defended host is testament to the seamless efficiency of front-line defenses (e.g., antimicrobial peptides) combined with active homeostatic processes that regulate inflammatory responses within the innate immune system.

Homeostatic processes of innate immunity can be viewed as inducible or constitutive in nature. Inducible homeostatic mechanisms re-establish equilibrium after innate immune activation, limiting host bystander cellular injury from inflammation and conserving host resources. In comparison, constitutive homeostatic mechanisms are independent of microbe-induced activation and recycle host resources without compromising host defense.

Macrophages are believed to have an essential role in maintaining immune homeostasis (Fig. 2.6). Airway macrophages well exemplify this antiinflammatory role that is revealed when they are depleted from the airways.[115,116] Pulmonary alveolar macrophages appear to actively suppress DC maturation, antigen presentation, and function in mouse

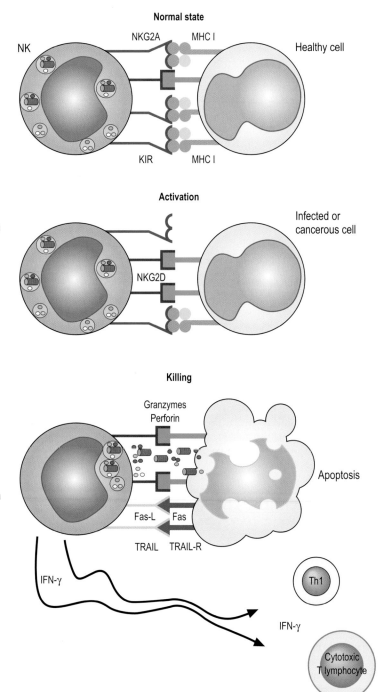

Fig. 2.4. Natural killer cell mechanisms. Natural killer (NK) cells recognize and target infected or malignant cells in an antigen-independent manner. NK cells distinguish healthy host cells by receptors on NK cells (e.g., KIR, NKG2A/CD94) that interact with MHC class I molecules on host cells to inhibit NK cell activation. Pathogen-infected or malignant cells typically downregulate MHC class I expression while concurrently expressing stress ligands that are recognized by activating receptors on NK cells (e.g., NKG2D). Such changes in the balance of activation-to-inhibition receptor engagement lead to NK cell activation and targeting for killing. NK cells induce target cell apoptosis by the release of toxic granules containing granzymes and perforins that disrupt cell membranes. NK cells also express apoptosis-inducing Fas ligand (Fas-L) and TRAIL that interact with their counterparts on target cells (Fas and TRAIL-R, respectively). Activated NK cells produce stimulatory cytokines and chemokines, and are a rich source of IFN-γ that augment innate and adaptive cytotoxic T lymphocyte and T-helper lymphocyte, type 1 immune responses. (Adapted from Jordan JS, Ballas ZK. Clin Immunol 2006; 118:1–10, Figure 2.)

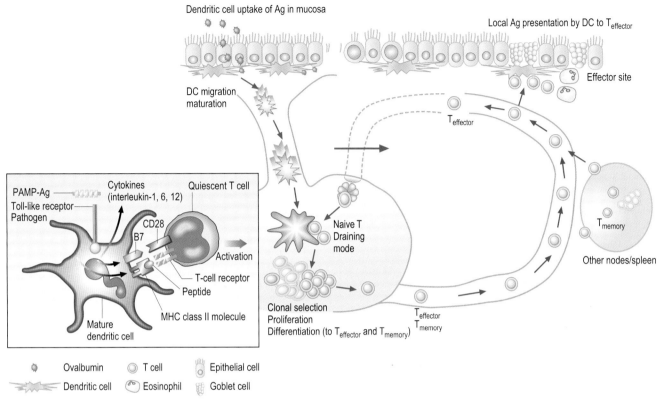

Fig. 2.5. Innate immune instruction of adaptive immunity, exemplified by dendritic cells (DCs) in the lung. Microbial stimuli activate immature dendritic cells DCs in the periphery to take up antigen and migrate to draining lymph nodes. DC migration is linked to antigen processing and DC maturation. Upon reaching lymph nodes, DCs secrete chemokines that attract T lymphocytes. The activities of mature DCs – presenting processed antigen, secreting cytokines, and expressing co-stimulatory molecules – induce antigen-specific T lymphocyte activation, proliferation, and differentiation. While memory T lymphocytes migrate to other lymph nodes and effector T lymphocytes migrate to peripheral tissues, mature DCs also migrate back to peripheral tissues, where their interactions with effector T lymphocytes are thought to underlie tissue-specific immune memory. (Adapted from Lambrecht BN. Dendritic cells and the regulation of the allergic immune response. Allergy 2005; 60:271–282.[114] Inset from: Medzhitov R, Janeway C Jr. Innate immunity. N Engl J Med 2000; 343:338–344, Figure 3. © 2000 Massuchusetts Medical Society. All rights reserved.)

airways.[116] PAMP/PRR activation temporarily diverts alveolar macrophages from their antiinflammatory mode and primes them for antimicrobial functions.[117,118] Classical activation of macrophages induces not only pro-inflammatory responses, but also antiinflammatory mediators: IL-10, TGF-β, and PGE$_2$, that downregulate macrophage and DC functions (Fig. 2.6). In this regard, microbe-induced activation of the innate immune system is tightly linked to the concurrent induction of down-regulatory mechanisms to regain immune homeostasis. An 'alternative' pathway of macrophage activation, via IL-4 and IL-13, has also been proposed based on studies in mice. This modified response modestly downregulates macrophage and DC function and induces antiinflammatory IL-10, IL-1 receptor antagonist and 'decoy' non-signaling IL-1 receptor II, while promoting MHC class II antigen presentation and antibody production.[119]

Macrophages also control inflammation through their constitutive ability to rapidly ingest and clear apoptotic cells, recently termed *efferocytosis* (Fig. 2.6).[77,120] The efficiency of this process is illustrated by the observation that more than 10[11] circulating neutrophils are eliminated each day without a trace of inflammation.[77] Apoptotic neutrophils inevitably release cytotoxic, pro-inflammatory constituents

into their environment without this constitutive antiinflammatory process of apoptotic cell recognition and ingestion. Macrophages recognize apoptotic cells via molecular pattern recognition reminiscent of microbial recognition by innate immune cells. The plasma membrane of viable cells actively maintains an asymmetric phospholipid distribution such that phosphatidylserine is kept on the inner side of the membrane bilayer. Apoptosis perturbs this asymmetry and exposes phosphatidylserine on the cell's outer surface, leading to their recognition by macrophages bearing phosphatidylserine receptors.[121–123] Upon recognition of apoptotic cells, macrophages release antiinflammatory IL-10, PGE$_2$, and TGF-β to complete the task of maintaining immune homeostasis.

The complement component C1q and the collectins, mannose-binding lectin and surfactant proteins A and D, also bind to apoptotic cells and can mediate their clearance.[29] This exemplifies multifunctional components in the innate immune system for both microbial and apoptotic cell clearance. The innate immune system relies on PRRs to recognize both microbes and distinct 'apoptotic cell associated molecular patterns (ACAMPs)'.[124] Although macrophages have received most of the attention in mediating efferocytosis in the immune system, other cell types

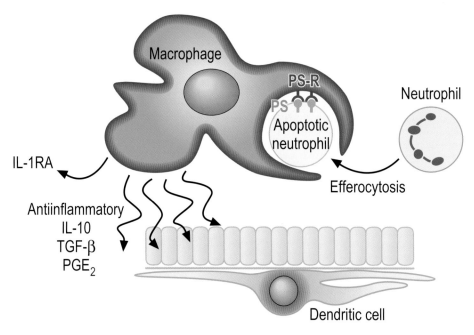

Fig. 2.6. Homeostasis in innate immunity. Macrophages have specialized regulatory functions that prevent inflammatory responses. Activation of macrophages induces antiinflammatory mediators such as IL 1 receptor antagonist, IL-10, PGE_2, and TGF-β that are thought to downregulate dendritic cell maturation and function. Macrophages also control inflammation by rapidly ingesting apoptotic cells in order to prevent their inflammatory rupture in the microenvironment, a process known as 'efferocytosis'. The cell membranes of apoptotic cells have externalized phosphatidylserine (PS) that is actively maintained by healthy cells on the inner side of cell membranes. Macrophages have PS receptors (PS-R) that recognize apoptotic cells, triggering their ingestion and the release of antiinflammatory cytokines.

can efferocytose, including epithelial cells, endothelial cells, fibroblasts, and stromal cells; the relative contribution of these different cell types to handle the efferocytosis workload is not clear.

These macrophage functions exemplify the inducible and constitutive homeostatic processes that are essential to optimal, efficient innate immune function. The innate immune system adjusts its cellular and molecular responses depending on the microbial burden of exposure, in order to optimize host defense while maintaining homeostasis.

INNATE IMMUNITY AND ALLERGY

The innate immune system, the gateway for environmental pathogen recognition for host defense, may also mediate immune responses to nonpathogenic allergens. Like microbial antigens, allergens can engage innate PRRs, are processed through innate immune cells, and can lead to pathogenic, allergic immune responses. Although the circumstances leading to allergic immunity in humans are not clear, existing evidence suggests that allergic susceptibilities can originate in the innate immune system.

INNATE IMMUNE ACTIVATION BY ALLERGENS

A variety of innate PRRs play a role in the uptake of allergens by innate immune cells. Fungal, grass pollen, and dust mite allergens have protease activity that is recognized by protease-activated receptors (PARs)

expressed by epithelial cells, macrophages, monocytes, mast cells, and inflammatory cells.[125] House-dust mite proteases *Derp1*, *Derp3*, and *Derp9* stimulate pro-inflammatory cytokine release by airway epithelial cells via PAR-2.[126,127] In other examples, the uptake and presentation of *Derp1* by mDCs is mannose receptor-dependent.[128] Grass pollen allergen is naturally contained in starch granules that are phagocytosed by alveolar macrophages, but not mDCs, in a C-type lectin binding-dependent manner.[129]

Many naturally occurring allergens and allergenic extracts are associated with a variety of TLR ligands. Commercial cockroach, dust mite, house-dust, and cat allergen extracts are high in endotoxin content; grass and ragweed pollen also have measurable endotoxin.[130] Grass and ragweed pollen and cat allergen extracts are also high in β-glucan content; there is no significant correlation between endotoxin and β-glucan content.[131] TLR ligands of such allergens could come from associated or contaminating microbes (e.g., bacteria, fungi), or inherent qualities of the allergens themselves; they might be covalently linked to the allergens. In the case of dust mites, the notably higher levels of endotoxin in *D. farinae* versus *D. pteronyssinus* cultures might be attributable to Gram-negative bacteria (i.e., *Bartonella* species) in the microflora of *D. farinae*.[132]

INNATE TLR ACTIVATION AND ALLERGY

Since mice with globally impaired TLR responses (i.e., MyD88-deficient mice) are skewed to IgE/Th2 immune responses, one might suspect that TLR ligand exposure protects against allergies.[133] This is the immunological basis for the 'hygiene hypothesis' for allergic diseases, that a greater microbial burden of exposure has a protective influence on the development of allergic sensitization and diseases. Recent research has revealed that the relationship between TLR ligand exposure and allergy is more complex than a unimodal protective effect. Key determinants of healthful or harmful outcomes from TLR ligand exposure have been elucidated and include: (1) dosage, (2) timing, and (3) genetic variation altering responses to TLR ligands.

Endotoxin has been a prototypical TLR ligand for understanding the influence of such microbial exposures on allergy and asthma outcomes in laboratory and clinical settings. In rodent models of allergic sensitization and asthma, the dosage and timing of endotoxin exposure alters disease outcomes. Experimental allergen without concurrent TLR stimulation (i.e., ovalbumin stripped of endotoxin) does not induce a persistent immune response; however, ovalbumin with low-level endotoxin induces IgE-mediated allergic sensitization and a Th2-type allergic inflammatory response.[134] TLR4 stimulation of dendritic cells is necessary for pathogenic Th2 inflammatory responses in the airways.[135,136] In contrast, higher levels of endotoxin with allergen lead to non-pathogenic IgG and Th1-type immune responses specific to the allergen.[134] Endotoxin in higher concentrations induces innate antigen-presenting cells, and especially dendritic cells, to produce IL-12 and to co-stimulate T cells to become effector T cells that primarily secrete IFN-γ.[106,107,137] The timing of endotoxin exposure relative to allergen exposure also alters allergy and asthma outcomes. Endotoxin prior to or within the first few days of allergen exposure induces a non-pathogenic IgG-specific response.[138] In contrast, endotoxin exposure in the later stages of the response amplifies the pathogenic allergic immune response upon re-exposure to allergen.

These experiments exemplify the influence of dosage and timing on TLR-mediated allergic outcomes. In rodent models, it may be a key stimulus to a pathogenic allergic immune response by breaking the tolerogenic state that is the usual outcome of chronic inhaled exposure to allergen.[139–141] Yet, greater TLR stimulation, if early in the development of an allergen-specific immune response, leads to a non-pathogenic one. Later in a developing allergic response, TLR stimulation amplifies allergic inflammation.

TLR stimulation may also have an important role in modifying allergic responses to foods. The natural source of TLR ligands in this circumstance is the natural bacterial microflora of the GI tract. In murine studies of peanut allergy, intragastric administration of peanut allergen and a mucosal adjuvant (cholera toxin) induced allergen-specific IgE and peanut anaphylaxis in three strains of TLR4-deficient mice, but not in six TLR-sufficient mouse strains.[142] TLR4-sufficient mice were rendered susceptible to peanut allergy by administering antibiotics in early life to greatly reduce commensal bacteria in the GI tract. In comparison, TLR4-deficient mice were protected against the development of peanut allergy by co-administration of CpG DNA (TLR9 ligand) with sensitizing peanut. The immunologic hallmark of the TLR4-sufficient mice and the TLR9 co-stimulated mice that were protected from developing peanut allergy was an IFN-γ (i.e., Th1), but not a Th2 cytokine response of CD4+ T cells to peanut allergen stimulation in vitro. In this model of peanut allergy, TLR signaling in the gut via commensal bacteria or CpG DNA converted an intragastric stimulus capable of inducing a Th2 immune response and peanut allergy into a Th1 immune response without peanut allergy.

EPIDEMIOLOGICAL EVIDENCE OF ENDOTOXIN/TLR LIGAND EXPOSURE AND ALLERGY PREVENTION

Epidemiological studies of the hygiene hypothesis have generally found a lower prevalence of allergic rhinitis, atopic dermatitis, allergic sensitization, and atopy-associated asthma in children with greater microbial burden.[143,144] Naturally occurring endotoxin and other TLR ligand exposures, measured in house dust samples, have been studied relative to the development of allergy and asthma. Again, endotoxin has served a prototypical role in our understanding – human epidemiological studies of endotoxin exposure and allergy generally reveal a picture consistent with the basic science and animal model evidence for an atopy-protective influence, with some important twists. An early study associated higher levels of house-dust endotoxin with lack of allergic sensitization in infants (including food allergen sensitization) and higher proportions of Th1 cells in peripheral blood samples.[145] Since then, higher dust endotoxin levels have been associated with less atopic dermatitis.[146–148] less inhalant allergen sensitization, less allergic rhinitis, and less atopy-associated asthma[149,150] in infancy and childhood. The strength of these associations has been demonstrated in multiple longitudinal birth cohort studies,[146–148,151–153] as well as a large European rural farm/non-farm study where a dose-response relationship between endotoxin exposure and less atopy has been shown.[150]

In contrast to these protective influences, higher endotoxin levels have been associated with more wheezing in infants and in non-atopic children, often in the same studies where a protective effect on atopy was concurrently observed.[146,148,150,153–155] This suggests endotoxin-sensitive wheezing phenotypes or asthma in infants and children, similar to endotoxin-sensitive asthma in many occupational settings.[156] Higher endotoxin levels have also been associated with more infantile atopic dermatitis in a New Zealand cohort,[155] and less infant wheezing in a Cincinnati cohort when at least two dogs were also present in the home.[157] These latter epidemiological findings demonstrate that the relationships between endotoxin exposure and atopic or wheezing outcomes are not absolutely consistent across locales and suggest that deviation from the general trends may be due to endotoxin-associated factors.

Functional polymorphisms in genes important to endotoxin-mediated TLR stimulation can alter the likelihood and/or severity of atopy and allergic disease. For example, a common polymorphism in the promoter region (-260C-to-T) of the CD14 gene alters the transcriptional regulation of CD14,[158] such that the C-allele is associated with lower serum levels of soluble CD14, higher serum IgE levels (in skin test-positive individuals), and more allergic sensitization.[159,160] In infants and young children in a birth cohort study, only the low-responder 'CC' homozygous CD14/-260 subgroup demonstrated strong dose-response relationships between higher house-dust endotoxin levels and less subsequent allergic sensitization to inhalant allergens, as well as less atopic dermatitis and more non-atopic wheeze.[161] Conversely, in a study of adult farmers with presumably greater exposure to endotoxin, those who were high-responder 'TT' homozygous at CD14/-260 had significantly lower lung function and a higher prevalence of wheezing.[162] This endotoxin gene-environmental exposure interaction on allergy and wheezing outcomes provides compelling evidence for the relevance of endotoxin in allergy.

Other naturally occurring PAMP exposures may also protect against the development of allergy. Unmethylated CpG motifs in microbial

DNA are PAMPs that are distinguished from non-microbial DNA, and recognized by TLR9.[163] CpG DNA is a particularly effective activator of dendritic cells to induce T cell proliferation and Th1 development.[164,165] DNA from dust samples from farm homes, farm barns, and rural homes in India (where allergy tends to be less common) was found to have a higher proportion of microbial DNA.[166] When combined with a small amount of endotoxin, DNA extracted from dust from farm barns, but not metropolitan homes, augmented IL-10 and IL-12 production by PBMC in vitro. Synthetic DNA-based TLR9 ligands have been developed as immune adjuvants and therapeutic agents to modify the allergic response to allergens.[167–170] An immunostimulatory DNA conjugate to ragweed allergen administered as allergen immunotherapy induced long-lasting (three seasons) suppression of seasonal increases in allergic rhinitis symptoms and allergen-specific IgE.[171]

This epidemiological evidence in humans supports a role for TLR ligand exposures in altering allergy risk. Determinants of healthful outcomes include early timing, moderate dosing, and genetic influences on the innate response to the exposures. This is complementary to the innate immune paradigm that inadequate activation may not stimulate the full development of effector and homeostatic innate immune responses, resulting in inadequate regulatory cell development, adaptive Th2 responses, and allergic consequences.

Innate cellular responses in allergy pathogenesis

First-responder cells of the innate immune system are believed to have central roles in the development of tolerogenic versus inflammatory responses to allergen.[114] In murine models of lung immunity, immature dendritic cells take up model allergens and induce T-cell proliferation and tolerance.[172,173] Partial activation of dendritic cells may result in deletion of activated T lymphocytes and induction of tolerogenic types of antigen-presenting cells – plasmacytoid dendritic cells (pDCs) and alveolar macrophages. In these models, depletion of pDCs leads to an allergic asthma phenotype when tolerance would be the usual outcome; conversely, adoptive transfer of allergen-pulsed pDCs prevents the induction of asthma.[139] In contrast, eliminating myeloid or airway DCs abrogates allergen-mediated inflammation in the lungs.[174] Allergen-pulsed mature mDCs can sensitize the lungs for an allergic inflammatory response,[175,176] but neither immature mDCs nor pDCs are able to fill this role. Thus, plasmacytoid and myeloid DCs may have competing roles in the development of allergic responses.

Airway macrophages may also have an important role in mediating allergic responses in the airways. In murine models, depletion of alveolar macrophages during exposure to harmless antigens greatly enhances primary and secondary immune responses.[115] Antigen-pulsed alveolar macrophages do not promote a pathogenic Th2-type immune response in the airways, as do mDCs; instead, a protective Th1-type immune response is induced.[176,177] A current paradigm in macrophage biology, derived primarily from mouse studies, distinguishes macrophages that are 'alternatively' activated and promote Th2 immune responses from 'classically' activated, Th1-promoting macrophages.[178] The characterization of macrophages as classically activated, alternatively activated, or regulatory macrophages is paradigmatically appealing, although well recognized as an oversimplification.

These studies exemplify some of the numerous innate immune pathways that have been implicated in the pathogenesis of allergic diseases.

Just as it is to microbes, the innate immune system is the gateway to allergen recognition in health and disease. Whether these pathways distinguish the individual who is likely to develop allergic sensitization from others who will not remains unclear.

References

Microbial pattern recognition by the innate immune system

1. Lien E, Means TK, Heine H, et al. Toll-like receptor 4 imparts ligand-specific recognition of bacterial lipopolysaccharide. J Clin Invest 2000; 105:497–504.
2. Hirschfeld M, Ma Y, Weis JH, et al. Cutting edge: repurification of lipopolysaccharide eliminates signaling through both human and murine toll-like receptor 2. J Immunol 2000; 165:618–622.
3. Rietschel ET, Kirikae T, Schade FU, et al. Bacterial endotoxin: molecular relationships of structure to activity and function. FASEB J 1994; 8:217–225.

Pattern recognition receptors

4. Ganz T. Defensins: antimicrobial peptides of innate immunity. Nat Rev Immunol 2003; 3:710–720.
5. Zasloff M. Antimicrobial peptides of multicellular organisms. Nature 2002; 415:389–395.
6. Maloy WL, Kari UP. Structure-activity studies on magainins and other host defense peptides. Biopolymers 1995; 37:105–122.
7. Szyk A, Wu Z, Tucker K, et al. Crystal structures of human alpha-defensins HNP4, HD5, and HD6. Protein Sci 2006; 15:2749–2760.
8. Vora P, Youdim A, Thomas LS, et al. Beta-defensin-2 expression is regulated by TLR signaling in intestinal epithelial cells. J Immunol 2004; 173:5398–5405.
9. Hertz CJ, Wu Q, Porter EM, et al. Activation of Toll-like receptor 2 on human tracheobronchial epithelial cells induces the antimicrobial peptide human beta defensin-2. J Immunol 2003; 171:6820–6826.
10. Birchler T, Seibl R, Buchner K, et al. Human Toll-like receptor 2 mediates induction of the antimicrobial peptide human beta-defensin 2 in response to bacterial lipoprotein. Eur J Immunol 2001; 31:3131–3137.
11. Zanetti M. Cathelicidins, multifunctional peptides of the innate immunity. J Leukoc Biol 2004; 75:39–48.
12. Wang TT, Nestel FP, Bourdeau V, et al. Cutting edge: 1,25-dihydroxyvitamin D₃ is a direct inducer of antimicrobial peptide gene expression. J Immunol 2004; 173:2909–2912.
13. Gombart AF, Borregaard N, Koeffler HP. Human cathelicidin antimicrobial peptide (CAMP) gene is a direct target of the vitamin D receptor and is strongly up-regulated in myeloid cells by 1,25-dihydroxyvitamin D₃. FASEB J 2005; 19:1067–1077.
14. Schauber J, Dorschner RA, Coda AB, et al. Injury enhances TLR2 function and antimicrobial peptide expression through a vitamin D-dependent mechanism. J Clin Invest 2007; 117: 803–811.
15. Liu PT, Stenger S, Li H, et al. Toll-like receptor triggering of a vitamin D-mediated human antimicrobial response. Science 2006; 311:1770–1773.
16. Palaniyar N, Nadesalingam J, Reid KB. Pulmonary innate immune proteins and receptors that interact with gram-positive bacterial ligands. Immunobiology 2002; 205:575–594.
17. Schutte BC, Mitros JP, Bartlett JA, et al. Discovery of five conserved beta-defensin gene clusters using a computational search strategy. Proc Natl Acad Sci U S A 2002; 99: 2129–2133.
18. Schittek B, Hipfel R, Sauer B, et al. Dermicidin: a novel human antibiotic peptide secreted by sweat glands. Nat Immunol 2001; 2:1133–1137.
19. Krisanaprakornkit S, Kimball JR, Weinberg A, et al. Inducible expression of human beta-defensin 2 by Fusobacterium nucleatum in oral epithelial cells: multiple signaling pathways and role of commensal bacteria in innate immunity and the epithelial barrier. Infect Immun 2000; 68:2907–2915.
20. Chertov O, Yang D, Howard OM, et al. Leukocyte granule proteins mobilize innate host defenses and adaptive immune responses. Immunol Rev 2000; 177:68–78.
21. De Y, Chen Q, Schmidt AP, et al. LL-37, the neutrophil granule- and epithelial cell-derived cathelicidin, utilizes formyl peptide receptor-like 1 (FPRL1) as a receptor to chemoattract human peripheral blood neutrophils, monocytes, and T cells. J Exp Med 2000; 192: 1069–1074.
22. Niyonsaba F, Iwabuchi K, Matsuda H, et al. Epithelial cell-derived human beta-defensin-2 acts as a chemotaxin for mast cells through a pertussis toxin-sensitive and phospholipase C-dependent pathway. Int Immunol 2002; 14:421–426.
23. Niyonsaba F, Iwabuchi K, Someya A, et al. A cathelicidin family of human antibacterial peptide LL-37 induces mast cell chemotaxis. Immunology 2002; 106:20–26.
24. Fraser IP, Koziel H, Ezekowitz RA. The serum mannose-binding protein and the macrophage mannose receptor are pattern recognition molecules that link innate and adaptive immunity. Semin Immunol 1998; 10:363–372.
25. Epstein J, Eichbaum Q, Sheriff S, et al. The collectins in innate immunity. Curr Opin Immunol 1996; 8:29–35.
26. Wright JR. Immunoregulatory functions of surfactant proteins. Nat Rev Immunol 2005; 5:58–68.
27. Wu H, Kuzmenko A, Wan S, et al. Surfactant proteins A and D inhibit the growth of Gram-negative bacteria by increasing membrane permeability. J Clin Invest 2003; 111: 1589–1602.

28. McCormack FX, Gibbons R, Ward SR, et al. Macrophage-independent fungicidal action of the pulmonary collectins. J Biol Chem 2003; 278:36250–36256.
29. Vandivier RW, Ogden CA, Fadok VA, et al. Role of surfactant proteins A, D, and C1q in the clearance of apoptotic cells in vivo and in vitro: calreticulin and CD91 as a common collectin receptor complex. J Immunol 2002; 169:3978–3986.
30. Rock FL, Hardiman G, Timans JC, et al. A family of human receptors structurally related to Drosophila Toll. Proc Natl Acad Sci U S A 1998; 95:588–593.
31. Gay NJ, Keith FJ. Drosophila Toll and IL-1 receptor. Nature 1991; 351:355–356.
32. Pabst MJ, Hedegaard HB, Johnston RB Jr. Cultured human monocytes require exposure to bacterial products to maintain an optimal oxygen radical response. J Immunol 1982; 128:123–128.
33. Wright SD, Tobias PS, Ulevitch RJ, et al. Lipopolysaccharide (LPS) binding protein opsonizes LPS-bearing particles for recognition by a novel receptor on macrophages. J Exp Med 1989; 170:1231–1241.
34. Wright SD, Ramos RA, Tobias PS, et al. CD14, a receptor for complexes of lipopolysaccharide (LPS) and LPS binding protein. Science 1990; 249:1431–1433.
35. Visintin A, Iliev DB, Monks BG, et al. Md-2. Immunobiology 2006; 211:437–447.
36. Pabst MJ, Johnston RB Jr. Increased production of superoxide anion by macrophages exposed in vitro to muramyl dipeptide or lipopolysaccharide. J Exp Med 1980; 151:101–114.
37. Forehand JR, Pabst MJ, Phillips WA, et al. Lipopolysaccharide priming of human neutrophils for an enhanced respiratory burst. Role of intracellular free calcium. J Clin Invest 1989; 83:74–83.
38. Shnyra A, Brewington R, Alipio A, et al. Reprogramming of lipopolysaccharide-primed macrophages is controlled by a counterbalanced production of IL-10 and IL-12. J. Immunol 1998; 160(8):3729–3736.
39. Kaisho T, Akira S. Toll-like receptor function and signaling. J Allergy Clin Immunol 2006; 117:979–987; quiz 88.
40. Hayashi F, Smith KD, Ozinsky A, et al. The innate immune response to bacterial flagellin is mediated by Toll-like receptor 5. Nature 2001; 410:1099–1103.
41. Hemmi H, Takeuchi O, Kawai T, et al. A Toll-like receptor recognizes bacterial DNA. Nature 2000; 408:740–745.
42. Heil F, Hemmi H, Hochrein H, et al. Species-specific recognition of single-stranded RNA via toll-like receptor 7 and 8. Science 2004; 303:1526–1529.
43. Alexopoulou L, Holt AC, Medzhitov R, et al. Recognition of double-stranded RNA and activation of NF-kappaB by Toll-like receptor 3. Nature 2001; 413:732–738.
44. Inohara N, Nunez G. NODs: intracellular proteins involved in inflammation and apoptosis. Nat Rev Immunol 2003; 3:371–382.
45. Girardin SE, Boneca IG, Carneiro LA, et al. Nod1 detects a unique muropeptide from gram-negative bacterial peptidoglycan. Science 2003; 300:1584–1587.
46. Chamaillard M, Hashimoto M, Horie Y, et al. An essential role for NOD1 in host recognition of bacterial peptidoglycan containing diaminopimelic acid. Nat Immunol 2003; 4:702–707.
47. Rosenstiel P, Fantini M, Brautigam K, et al. TNF-alpha and IFN-gamma regulate the expression of the NOD2 (CARD15) gene in human intestinal epithelial cells. Gastroenterology 2003; 124:1001–1009.
48. Inohara N, Ogura Y, Fontalba A, et al. Host recognition of bacterial muramyl dipeptide mediated through NOD2. Implications for Crohn's disease. J Biol Chem 2003; 278:5509–5512.
49. Girardin SE, Boneca IG, Viala J, et al. Nod2 is a general sensor of peptidoglycan through muramyl dipeptide (MDP) detection. J Biol Chem 2003; 278:8869–8872.
50. Bouma G, Strober W. The immunological and genetic basis of inflammatory bowel disease. Nat Rev Immunol 2003; 3:521–533.
51. Kato H, Takeuchi O, Sato S, et al. Differential roles of MDA5 and RIG-I helicases in the recognition of RNA viruses. Nature 2006; 441:101–105.
52. Akira S, Takeda K. Toll-like receptor signalling. Nat Rev Immunol 2004; 4:499–511.
53. Yamamoto M, Sato S, Hemmi H, et al. Role of adaptor TRIF in the MyD88-independent toll-like receptor signaling pathway. Science 2003; 301:640–643.
54. Agrawal S, Agrawal A, Doughty B, et al. Cutting edge: different Toll-like receptor agonists instruct dendritic cells to induce distinct Th responses via differential modulation of extracellular signal-regulated kinase-mitogen-activated protein kinase and c-Fos. J Immunol 2003; 171:4984–4989.
55. Netea MG, Gow NA, Munro CA, et al. Immune sensing of Candida albicans requires cooperative recognition of mannans and glucans by lectin and Toll-like receptors. J Clin Invest 2006; 116:1642–1650.
56. Suzuki H, Kurihara Y, Takeya M, et al. A role for macrophage scavenger receptors in atherosclerosis and susceptibility to infection. Nature 1997; 386:292–296.
57. Le Y, Yang Y, Cui Y, et al. Receptors for chemotactic formyl peptides as pharmacological targets. Int Immunopharmacol 2002; 2:1–13.
58. Doyle CK, Davis BK, Cook RG, et al. Hyperconservation of the N-formyl peptide binding site of M3: evidence that M3 is an old eutherian molecule with conserved recognition of a pathogen-associated molecular pattern. J Immunol 2003; 171:836–844.

Resident cellular responses of innate immunity

59. Holt PG, Haining S, Nelson DJ, et al. Origin and steady-state turnover of class II MHC-bearing dendritic cells in the epithelium of the conducting airways. J Immunol 1994; 153:256–261.
60. Takano K, Kojima T, Go M, et al. HLA-DR- and CD11c-positive dendritic cells penetrate beyond well-developed epithelial tight junctions in human nasal mucosa of allergic rhinitis. J Histochem Cytochem 2005; 53:611–619.
61. Niess JH, Brand S, Gu X, et al. CX3CR1-mediated dendritic cell access to the intestinal lumen and bacterial clearance. Science 2005; 307:254–258.
62. McWilliam AS, Nelson D, Thomas JA, et al. Rapid dendritic cell recruitment is a hallmark of the acute inflammatory response at mucosal surfaces. J Exp Med 1994; 179:1331–1336.
63. McWilliam AS, Napoli S, Marsh AM, et al. Dendritic cells are recruited into the airway epithelium during the inflammatory response to a broad spectrum of stimuli. J Exp Med 1996; 184:2429–2432.
64. Rossi M, Young JW. Human dendritic cells: potent antigen-presenting cells at the crossroads of innate and adaptive immunity. J Immunol 2005; 175:1373–1381.
65. Kadowaki N, Ho S, Antonenko S, et al. Subsets of human dendritic cell precursors express different toll-like receptors and respond to different microbial antigens. J Exp Med 2001; 194(6):863–869.
66. Lund JM, Linehan MM, Iijima N, et al. Cutting edge: plasmacytoid dendritic cells provide innate immune protection against mucosal viral infection in situ. J Immunol 2006; 177:7510–7514.
67. Nakanaga T, Nadel JA, Ueki IF, et al. Regulation of interleukin-8 via an airway epithelial signaling cascade. Am J Physiol Lung Cell Mol Physiol 2007; 292:L1289–1296.
68. Szolnoky G, Bata-Csorgo Z, Kenderessy AS, et al. A mannose-binding receptor is expressed on human keratinocytes and mediates killing of Candida albicans. J Invest Dermatol 2001; 117:205–213.
69. Rakoff-Nahoum S, Paglino J, Eslami-Varzaneh F, et al. Recognition of commensal microflora by toll-like receptors is required for intestinal homeostasis. Cell 2004; 118:229–241.
70. Varadaradjalou S, Feger F, Thieblemont N, et al. Toll-like receptor 2 (TLR2) and TLR4 differentially activate human mast cells. Eur J Immunol 2003; 33:899–906.
71. Schulman ES, Post TJ, Henson PM, et al. Differential effects of the complement peptides, C5a and C5a des Arg on human basophil and lung mast cell histamine release. J Clin Invest 1988; 81:918–923.
72. Malaviya R, Ikeda T, Ross E, et al. Mast cell modulation of neutrophil influx and bacterial clearance at sites of infection through TNF-alpha. Nature 1996; 381:77–80.
73. Echtenacher B, Mannel DN, Hultner L. Critical protective role of mast cells in a model of acute septic peritonitis. Nature 1996; 381:75–77.
74. Di Nardo A, Vitiello A, Gallo RL. Cutting edge: mast cell antimicrobial activity is mediated by expression of cathelicidin antimicrobial peptide. J Immunol 2003; 170:2274–2278.
75. Niyonsaba F, Someya A, Hirata M, et al. Evaluation of the effects of peptide antibiotics human beta-defensins-1/-2 and LL-37 on histamine release and prostaglandin D(2) production from mast cells. Eur J Immunol 2001; 31:1066–1075.

Infiltrative cellular responses of innate immunity

76. Walker RI, Willemze R. Neutrophil kinetics and the regulation of granulopoiesis. Rev Infect Dis 1980; 2:282–292.
77. Vandivier RW, Henson PM, Douglas IS. Burying the dead: the impact of failed apoptotic cell removal (efferocytosis) on chronic inflammatory lung disease. Chest 2006; 129:1673–1682.
78. Seo SM, McIntire LV, Smith CW. Effects of IL-8, Gro-alpha, and LTB(4) on the adhesive kinetics of LFA-1 and Mac-1 on human neutrophils. Am J Physiol Cell Physiol 2001; 281:C1568–C1578.
79. Gerard C, Gerard NP. C5A anaphylatoxin and its seven transmembrane-segment receptor. Annu Rev Immunol 1994; 12:775–808.
80. Berger M, O'Shea J, Cross AS, et al. Human neutrophils increase expression of C3bi as well as C3b receptors upon activation. J Clin Invest 1984; 74:1566–1571.
81. Joiner KA, Brown EJ, Frank MM. Complement and bacteria: chemistry and biology in host defense. Annu Rev Immunol 1984; 2:461–491.
82. Segal AW. How neutrophils kill microbes. Annu Rev Immunol 2005; 23:197–223.
83. Winkelstein JA, Marino MC, Johnston RB Jr, et al. Chronic granulomatous disease. Report on a national registry of 368 patients. Medicine (Baltimore) 2000; 79:155–169.
84. Reeves EP, Lu H, Jacobs HL, et al. Killing activity of neutrophils is mediated through activation of proteases by K+ flux. Nature 2002; 416:291–297.
85. Smyth MJ, Cretney E, Kelly JM, et al. Activation of NK cell cytotoxicity. Mol Immunol 2005; 42:501–510.
86. Lauzon NM, Mian F, MacKenzie R, et al. The direct effects of Toll-like receptor ligands on human NK cell cytokine production and cytotoxicity. Cell Immunol 2006; 241:102–112.
87. Hart OM, Athie-Morales V, O'Connor GM, et al. TLR7/8-mediated activation of human NK cells results in accessory cell-dependent IFN-gamma production. J Immunol 2005; 175:1636–1642.
88. Wagtmann N, Rajagopalan S, Winter CC, et al. Killer cell inhibitory receptors specific for HLA-C and HLA-B identified by direct binding and by functional transfer. Immunity 1995; 3:801–809.
89. Lazetic S, Chang C, Houchins JP, et al. Human natural killer cell receptors involved in MHC class I recognition are disulfide-linked heterodimers of CD94 and NKG2 subunits. J Immunol 1996; 157:4741–4745.
90. Cerwenka A, Lanier LL. Natural killer cells, viruses and cancer. Nat Rev Immunol 2001; 1:41–49.
91. Gasser S, Raulet DH. Activation and self-tolerance of natural killer cells. Immunol Rev 2006; 214:130–142.
92. Trapani JA, Smyth MJ. Functional significance of the perforin/granzyme cell death pathway. Nat Rev Immunol 2002; 2:735–747.
93. Sato K, Hida S, Takayanagi H, et al. Antiviral response by natural killer cells through TRAIL gene induction by IFN-alpha/beta. Eur J Immunol 2001; 31:3138–3146.
94. Andoniou CE, Andrews DM, Degli-Esposti MA. Natural killer cells in viral infection: more than just killers. Immunol Rev 2006; 214:239–250.
95. Gerosa F, Baldani-Guerra B, Nisii C, et al. Reciprocal activating interaction between natural killer cells and dendritic cells. J Exp Med 2002; 195:327–333.
96. Ferlazzo G, Pack M, Thomas D, et al. Distinct roles of IL-12 and IL-15 in human natural killer cell activation by dendritic cells from secondary lymphoid organs. Proc Natl Acad Sci U S A 2004; 101:16606–16611.

REFERENCES

Innate instruction of adaptive immune responses

97. Martin-Fontecha A, Thomsen LL, Brett S, et al. Induced recruitment of NK cells to lymph nodes provides IFN-gamma for T(H)1 priming. Nat Immunol 2004; 5:1260–1265.
98. Mailliard RB, Son YI, Redlinger R, et al. Dendritic cells mediate NK cell help for Th1 and CTL responses: two-signal requirement for the induction of NK cell helper function. J Immunol 2003; 171:2366–2373.

Innate instruction of adaptive immune responses

99. Blander JM, Medzhitov R. Toll-dependent selection of microbial antigens for presentation by dendritic cells. Nature 2006; 440:808–812.
100. Dresser DW. Effectiveness of lipid and lipidophilic substances as adjuvants. Nature 1961; 191:1169–1171.
101. Louis JA, Chiller JM, Weigle WO. The ability of bacterial lipopolysaccharide to modulate the induction of unresponsiveness to a state of immunity. Cellular parameters. J Exp Med 1973; 138:1481–1495.
102. Vella AT, McCormack JE, Linsley PS, et al. Lipopolysaccharide interferes with the induction of peripheral T cell death. Immunity 1995; 2:261–270.
103. Pape KA, Khoruts A, Mondino A, et al. Inflammatory cytokines enhance the in vivo clonal expansion and differentiation of antigen-activated CD4+ T cells. J Immunol 1997; 159:591–598.
104. Le J, Lin JX, Henriksen-DeStefano D, et al. Bacterial lipopolysaccharide-induced interferon-gamma production: roles of interleukin 1 and interleukin 2. J Immunol 1986; 136:4525–4530.
105. Reinhardt RL, Khoruts A, Merica R, et al. Visualizing the generation of memory CD4 T cells in the whole body. Nature 2001; 410(6824):101–105.
106. Macatonia SE, Hosken NA, Litton M, et al. Dendritic cells produce IL-12 and direct the development of Th1 cells from naive CD4+ T cells. J Immunol 1995; 154:5071–5079.
107. Hilkens CM, Kalinski P, de Boer M, et al. Human dendritic cells require exogenous interleukin-12-inducing factors to direct the development of naive T-helper cells toward the Th1 phenotype. Blood 1997; 90:1920–1926.
108. Manetti R, Parronchi P, Giudizi MG, et al. Natural killer cell stimulatory factor (interleukin 12 [IL-12]) induces T helper type 1 (Th1)-specific immune responses and inhibits the development of IL-4-producing Th cells. J Exp Med 1993; 177:1199–1204.
109. Snijders A, Kalinski P, Hilkens CM, et al. High-level IL-12 production by human dendritic cells requires two signals. Int Immunol 1998; 10:1593–1598.
110. Ma X, Chow JM, Gri G, et al. The interleukin 12 p40 gene promoter is primed by interferon gamma in monocytic cells. J Exp Med 1996; 183:147–157.
111. Hayes MP, Wang J, Norcross MA. Regulation of interleukin-12 expression in human monocytes: selective priming by interferon-gamma of lipopolysaccharide-inducible p35 and p40 genes. Blood 1995; 86:646–650.
112. Jarrossay D, Napolitani G, Colonna M, et al. Specialization and complementarity in microbial molecule recognition by human myeloid and plasmacytoid dendritic cells. Eur J Immunol 2001; 31:3388–3393.
113. Miller MJ, Safrina O, Parker I, et al. Imaging the single cell dynamics of CD4+ T cell activation by dendritic cells in lymph nodes. J Exp Med 2004; 200:847–856.
114. Lambrecht BN. Dendritic cells and the regulation of the allergic immune response. Allergy 2005; 60:271–282.

Homeostasis in the innate immune system

115. Thepen T, Van Rooijen N, Kraal G. Alveolar macrophage elimination in vivo is associated with an increase in pulmonary immune response in mice. J Exp Med 1989; 170:499–509.
116. Holt PG, Oliver J, Bilyk N, et al. Downregulation of the antigen presenting cell function(s) of pulmonary dendritic cells in vivo by resident alveolar macrophages. J Exp Med 1993; 177:397–407.
117. Lambrecht BN. Alveolar macrophage in the driver's seat. Immunity 2006; 24:366–368.
118. Takabayshi K, Corr M, Hayashi T, et al. Induction of a homeostatic circuit in lung tissue by microbial compounds. Immunity 2006; 24:475–487.
119. Gordon S. Alternative activation of macrophages. Nat Rev Immunol 2003; 3:23–35.
120. Gardai SJ, McPhillips KA, Frasch SC, et al. Cell-surface calreticulin initiates clearance of viable or apoptotic cells through trans-activation of LRP on the phagocyte. Cell 2005; 123:321–334.
121. Bratton DL, Fadok VA, Richter DA, et al. Appearance of phosphatidylserine on apoptotic cells requires calcium-mediated nonspecific flip-flop and is enhanced by loss of the aminophospholipid translocase. J Biol Chem 1997; 272:26159–26165.
122. Fadok VA, Voelker DR, Campbell PA, et al. Exposure of phosphatidylserine on the surface of apoptotic lymphocytes triggers specific recognition and removal by macrophages. J Immunol 1992; 148:2207–2216.
123. Fadok VA, Bratton DL, Rose DM, et al. A receptor for phosphatidylserine-specific clearance of apoptotic cells. Nature 2000; 405:85–90.
124. Gregory CD. CD14-dependent clearance of apoptotic cells: relevance to the immune system. Curr Opin Immunol 2000; 12:27–34.

Innate immunity and allergy

125. Reed CE, Kita H. The role of protease activation of inflammation in allergic respiratory diseases. J Allergy Clin Immunol 2004; 114:997–1008; quiz 9.
126. Asokananthan N, Graham PT, Stewart DJ, et al. House dust mite allergens induce proinflammatory cytokines from respiratory epithelial cells: the cysteine protease allergen, Der p 1, activates protease-activated receptor (PAR)-2 and inactivates PAR-1. J Immunol 2002; 169:4572–4578.

127. Sun G, Stacey MA, Schmidt M, et al. Interaction of mite allergens Der p3 and Der p9 with protease-activated receptor-2 expressed by lung epithelial cells. J Immunol 2001; 167:1014–1021.
128. Deslee G, Charbonnier AS, Hammad H, et al. Involvement of the mannose receptor in the uptake of Der p 1, a major mite allergen, by human dendritic cells. J Allergy Clin Immunol 2002; 110:763–770.
129. Currie AJ, Stewart GA, McWilliam AS. Alveolar macrophages bind and phagocytose allergen-containing pollen starch granules via C-type lectin and integrin receptors: implications for airway inflammatory disease. J Immunol 2000; 164:3878–3886.
130. Trivedi B, Valerio C, Slater JE. Endotoxin content of standardized allergen vaccines. J Allergy Clin Immunol 2003; 111:777–783.
131. Finkelman MA, Lempitski SJ, Slater JE. beta-Glucans in standardized allergen extracts. J Endotoxin Res 2006; 12:241–245.
132. Valerio CR, Murray P, Arlian LG, et al. Bacterial 16S ribosomal DNA in house dust mite cultures. J Allergy Clin Immunol 2005; 116:1296–1300.
133. Schnare M, Barton GM, Holt AC, et al. Toll-like receptors control activation of adaptive immune responses. Nat Immunol 2001; 2:947–950.
134. Eisenbarth SC, Piggott DA, Huleatt JW, et al. Lipopolysaccharide-enhanced, toll-like receptor 4-dependent T helper cell type 2 responses to inhaled antigen. J Exp Med 2002; 196:1645–1651.
135. Dabbagh K, Dahl ME, Stepick-Biek P, et al. Toll-like receptor 4 is required for optimal development of Th2 immune responses: role of dendritic cells. J Immunol 2002; 168:4524–4530.
136. Piggott DA, Eisenbarth SC, Xu L, et al. MyD88-dependent induction of allergic Th2 responses to intranasal antigen. J Clin Invest 2005; 115:459–467.
137. Reis e Sousa C, Hieny S, Scharton-Kersten T, et al. In vivo microbial stimulation induces rapid CD40 ligand-independent production of interleukin 12 by dendritic cells and their redistribution to T cell areas. J Exp Med 1997; 186:1819–1829.
138. Tulic MK, Wale JL, Holt PG, et al. Modification of the inflammatory response to allergen challenge after exposure to bacterial lipopolysaccharide. Am J Respir Cell Mol Biol 2000; 22:604–612.
139. de Heer HJ, Hammad H, Soullie T, et al. Essential role of lung plasmacytoid dendritic cells in preventing asthmatic reactions to harmless inhaled antigen. J Exp Med 2004; 200:89–98.
140. Ostroukhova M, Seguin-Devaux C, Oriss TB, et al. Tolerance induced by inhaled antigen involves CD4(+) T cells expressing membrane-bound TGF-beta and FOXP3. J Clin Invest 2004; 114:28–38.
141. Van Hove CL, Maes T, Joos GF, et al. Prolonged inhaled allergen exposure can induce persistent tolerance. Am J Respir Cell Mol Biol 2007; 36:573–584.
142. Bashir ME, Louie S, Shi HN, et al. Toll-like receptor 4 signaling by intestinal microbes influences susceptibility to food allergy. J Immunol 2004; 172:6978–6987.
143. Liu AH. Endotoxin exposure in allergy and asthma: reconciling a paradox. J Allergy Clin Immunol 2002; 109:379–392.
144. Liu AH, Murphy JR. Hygiene hypothesis: fact or fiction? J Allergy Clin Immunol 2003; 111:471–478.
145. Gereda JE, Leung DY, Thatayatikom A, et al. Relation between house-dust endotoxin exposure, type 1 T-cell development, and allergen sensitisation in infants at high risk of asthma. Lancet 2000; 355:1680–1683.
146. Gehring U, Bolte G, Borte M, et al. Exposure to endotoxin decreases the risk of atopic eczema in infancy: a cohort study. J Allergy Clin Immunol 2001; 108:847–854.
147. Phipatanakul W, Celedon JC, Raby BA, et al. Endotoxin exposure and eczema in the first year of life. Pediatrics 2004; 114:13–18.
148. Perzanowski MS, Miller RL, Thorne PS, et al. Endotoxin in inner-city homes: associations with wheeze and eczema in early childhood. J Allergy Clin Immunol 2006; 117:1082–1089.
149. Gehring U, Bischof W, Fahlbusch B, et al. House dust endotoxin and allergic sensitization in children. Am J Respir Crit Care Med 2002; 166:939–944.
150. Braun-Fahrlander C, Riedler J, Herz U, et al. Environmental exposure to endotoxin and its relation to asthma in school-age children. N Engl J Med 2002; 347:869–877.
151. Gehring U, Bischof W, Fahlbusch B, et al. House dust endotoxin and allergic sensitization in children. Am J Resp Crit Care Med 2002; 166(7):939–944.
152. Gehring U, Heinrich J, Hoek G, et al. Bacteria and mould components in house dust and children's allergic sensitisation. Eur Respir J 2007; 29:1144–1153.
153. Celedon JC, Milton DK, Ramsey CD, et al. Exposure to dust mite allergen and endotoxin in early life and asthma and atopy in childhood. J Allergy Clin Immunol 2007; 120:144–149.
154. Park JH, Gold DR, Spiegelman DL, et al. House dust endotoxin and wheeze in the first year of life. Am J Respir Crit Care Med 2001; 163:322–328.
155. Gillespie J, Wickens K, Siebers R, et al. Endotoxin exposure, wheezing, and rash in infancy in a New Zealand birth cohort. J Allergy Clin Immunol 2006; 118:1265–1270.
156. Rylander R. Endotoxin and occupational airway disease. Curr Opin Allergy Clin Immunol 2006; 6:62–66.
157. Campo P, Kalra HK, Levin L, et al. Influence of dog ownership and high endotoxin on wheezing and atopy during infancy. J Allergy Clin Immunol 2006; 118:1271–1278.
158. LeVan TD, Bloom JW, Bailey TJ, et al. A common single nucleotide polymorphism in the CD14 promoter decreases the affinity of Sp protein binding and enhances transcriptional activity. J Immunol 2001; 167:5838–5844.
159. Baldini M, Lohman IC, Halonen M, et al. A polymorphism in the 5' flanking region of the CD14 gene is associated with circulating soluble CD14 levels and with total serum immunoglobulin E. Am J Respir Cell Mol Biol 1999; 20:976–983.
160. Koppelman GH, Reijmerink NE, Colin Stine O, et al. Association of a promoter polymorphism of the CD14 gene and atopy. Am J Respir Crit Care Med 2001; 163:965–969.
161. Simpson A, John SL, Jury F, et al. Endotoxin exposure, CD14, and allergic disease: an interaction between genes and the environment. Am J Respir Crit Care Med 2006; 174:386–392.
162. LeVan TD, Von Essen S, Romberger DJ, et al. Polymorphisms in the CD14 gene associated with pulmonary function in farmers. Am J Respir Crit Care Med 2005; 171:773–779.

163. Krieg AM. CpG motifs in bacterial DNA and their immune effects. Annu Rev Immunol 2002; 20:709–760.
164. Boonstra A, Asselin-Paturel C, Gilliet M, et al. Flexibility of mouse classical and plasmacytoid-derived dendritic cells in directing T helper type 1 and 2 cell development: dependency on antigen dose and differential toll-like receptor ligation. J Exp Med 2003; 197:101–109.
165. Krug A, Towarowski A, Britsch S, et al. Toll-like receptor expression reveals CpG DNA as a unique microbial stimulus for plasmacytoid dendritic cells which synergizes with CD40 ligand to induce high amounts of IL-12. Eur J Immunol 2001; 31:3026–3037.
166. Roy SR, Schiltz AM, Marotta A, et al. Bacterial DNA in house and farm barn dust. J Allergy Clin Immunol 2003; 112:571–578.
167. Raz E, Tighe H, Sato Y, et al. Preferential induction of a Th1 immune response and inhibition of specific IgE antibody formation by plasmid DNA immunization. Proc Natl Acad Sci U S A 1996; 93:5141–5145.
168. Kline JN, Waldschmidt TJ, Businga TR, et al. Modulation of airway inflammation by CpG oligodeoxynucleotides in a murine model of asthma. J Immunol 1998; 160:2555–2559.
169. Tighe H, Takabayashi K, Schwartz D, et al. Conjugation of immunostimulatory DNA to the short ragweed allergen amb a 1 enhances its immunogenicity and reduces its allergenicity. J Allergy Clin Immunol 2000; 106:124–134.
170. Fanucchi MV, Schelegle ES, Baker GL, et al. Immunostimulatory oligonucleotides attenuate airways remodeling in allergic monkeys. Am J Respir Crit Care Med 2004; 170:1153–1157.

171. Creticos PS, Schroeder JT, Hamilton RG, et al. Immunotherapy with a ragweed-toll-like receptor 9 agonist vaccine for allergic rhinitis. N Engl J Med 2006; 355:1445–1455.
172. Holt PG, Stumbles PA. Regulation of immunologic homeostasis in peripheral tissues by dendritic cells: the respiratory tract as a paradigm. J Allergy Clin Immunol 2000; 105: 421–429.
173. Lambrecht BN, Pauwels RA, Fazekas De St Groth B. Induction of rapid T cell activation, division, and recirculation by intratracheal injection of dendritic cells in a TCR transgenic model. J Immunol 2000; 164:2937–2946.
174. Lambrecht BN, Salomon B, Klatzmann D, et al. Dendritic cells are required for the development of chronic eosinophilic airway inflammation in response to inhaled antigen in sensitized mice. J Immunol 1998; 160:4090–4097.
175. Lambrecht BN, De Veerman M, Coyle AJ, et al. Myeloid dendritic cells induce Th2 responses to inhaled antigen, leading to eosinophilic airway inflammation. J Clin Invest 2000; 106: 551–559.
176. Lambrecht BN, Peleman RA, Bullock GR, et al. Sensitization to inhaled antigen by intratracheal instillation of dendritic cells. Clin Exp Allergy 2000; 30:214–224.
177. Tang C, Inman MD, van Rooijen N, et al. Th type 1-stimulating activity of lung macrophages inhibits Th2-mediated allergic airway inflammation by an IFN-gamma-dependent mechanism. J Immunol 2001; 166:1471–1481.
178. Mantovani A, Sica A, Sozzani S, et al. The chemokine system in diverse forms of macrophage activation and polarization. Trends Immunol 2004; 25:677–686.

REFERENCES

Molecular Biology and Genetic Engineering

Sudhir Gupta and Leman Yel

3

CONTENTS

SUMMARY OF IMPORTANT CONCEPTS

>> The Human Genome Project has been a recent hallmark in human biology with an impact on disease diagnosis, genetic predisposition, pharmacogenetics, and gene therapy

>> Genomics and proteomics, by means of microarray technology, help to translate the human genetic blueprint into knowledge of gene location, expression profiling, and function

>> Pharmacogenetics, the study of interindividual genomic variations related to the effect of drugs, is a rapidly developing area of research to personalize pharmacological treatment

>> RNA interference/RNA silencing, a Nobel Prize winning discovery, is a powerful reverse genetics tool to clarify gene function and to modify expression of the gene of interest

>> DNA methylation and histone modification are two prominent epigenetic mechanisms for formation and storage of cellular information in response to transient environmental signals

It has been just over a half century since the double helix structure of the DNA was described. This landmark in biology has led to a series of accelerating advances in genetics. Classically, the function of a gene was studied by examining the effect of its mutation in the whole organism or in cultured cells. The technology of gene cloning, in vitro mutagenesis, gene expression in heterologous cells, development of transgenic and knockout animals, genomics, and proteomics have revolutionized genetic analysis. The Human Genome Project (HGP), an international research effort to sequence and map all of the genes of our species, *Homo sapiens*, has emerged as one of the great achievements in human biology.

Completed in April 2003, the HGP has started the 'biology century' with a potential impact on numerous areas of molecular medicine including disease diagnosis, genetic predispositions, pharmacogenetics, and gene therapy.

ANATOMY OF THE GENE

The gene, the basic unit of heredity, is carried by the chromosome and stored in the nucleus. Genes are made up of deoxyribonucleic acid (DNA), which is the genetic material for all cellular organisms. DNA contains three main components: the phosphate (PO_4) groups, five-carbon sugars, and nitrogen-containing bases called purines, comprising adenine (A) and guanine (G), and pyrimidines, comprising thymine (T) and cytosine (C). These basic subunits are called nucleotides. Nucleic acids are polymers of repeating subunits of nucleotides. The carbon atoms are numbered 1′ to 5′ proceeding clockwise from the oxygen atom (Fig. 3.1).

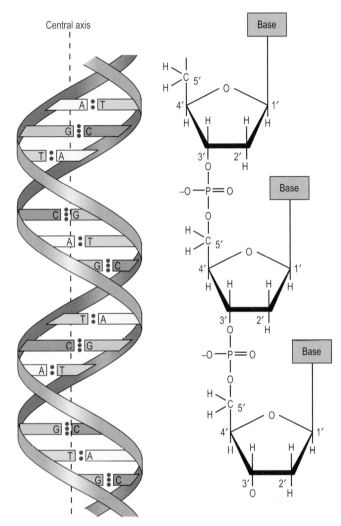

Fig. 3.1. Structure of DNA. (Left) Model of Watson–Crick DNA double helix. A, adenine; T, thymine; G, guanine; C, cytosine. (Right) Chain-linked deoxyribose and phosphate residues forming the sugar–phosphate bond. (Courtesy Baback Roshanravan.)

The phosphate group is attached to the 5′ carbon atom of the sugar, and the base is attached to the 1′ carbon atom. There is an additional free hydroxyl group (–OH) attached to the 3′ carbon atom. The presence of 5′ phosphate and 3′ hydroxyl groups allows DNA and ribonucleic acid (RNA) to form long chains of nucleotides. The 5′ phosphate of one nucleotide interacts with the 3′ hydroxyl group of another nucleotide, and a covalent bond (phosphodiester bond) is formed between the two molecules. This two-unit nucleotide still has a free 5′ phosphate at one end and a 3′ hydroxyl group at the other so that it can interact with other nucleotides at each end. In this manner, a long chain of nucleotides can be joined together to form a DNA or RNA molecule. All four nucleotides are not in equal amounts, but the amount of adenine present in a DNA molecule is always equal to the amount of thymine, and the amount of guanine always equals the amount of cytosine (A = T and G = C).

The three-dimensional structure was not known until early in the 1950s, when British chemist Rosalind Franklin, working in the laboratory of Maurice Wilkins, performed X-ray crystallography of DNA fibers. The diffractional pattern suggested that the DNA molecule had the shape of a helix or corkscrew, with a diameter of 2 nm and a complete helical turn every 3.4 nm. James Watson and Francis Crick[1] built models of nucleotides and tried to assemble the nucleotides into a molecule. After exploring various possibilities, they proposed a 'double helix' structure of the DNA molecule, in which the bases of two strands pointed inward toward one another (base pairing). They proposed that the base pairing was always between purines (large) pointing toward pyrimidines (small), thus keeping the diameter of the molecule at a constant 2 nm. The double helix is stabilized by a hydrogen bond between the bases in a base pair; adenine makes double hydrogen bonds with thymine, and guanine will form three hydrogen bonds with cytosine (Fig. 3.1).

■ RNA AND PROTEIN SYNTHESIS ■

All eukaryotic cells use DNA to direct protein synthesis. Proteins are made in the cytoplasm on the ribosome. These polypeptide-making factories contain more than 50 different proteins, as well as RNA. RNA is similar to DNA, and its presence in ribosomes suggests its important role in protein synthesis (Fig. 3.2). RNA differs from DNA in two ways: RNA contains ribose as sugar rather than the deoxyribose in DNA, and RNA contains the pyrimidine uracil (U) instead of thymine (T).[2] In addition, RNA does not have a regular helical structure. The class of RNA present in ribosomes is called ribosomal RNA (rRNA).[3] rRNA and ribosomal proteins provide sites where polypeptides are assembled. Transfer RNA (tRNA) transports the amino acids to the ribosome for the synthesis of polypeptide.[4,5] There are >40 different tRNA molecules in human cells. tRNA is smaller than rRNA and is present in free form in the cytoplasm. Messenger RNA (mRNA) comprises long strands of RNA molecules that are copied from DNA. mRNA travels to the ribosome to direct the assembly of polypeptides.

RNA is synthesized on a DNA template by a process of DNA transcription in which RNA polymerase enzymes make an RNA copy of a DNA sequence. RNA polymerases are formed from multiple polypeptide chains with a molecular weight of 500 000 Da.[6,7] In eukaryotic cells, there are three different types of RNA polymerases. RNA polymerase II transcribes the gene whose RNAs will be translated into proteins. RNA polymerase I makes the large rRNA precursor (45S rRNA) containing the major rRNAs. RNA polymerase III makes very small, stable RNAs, including tRNA and the small 5S rRNA. In mammalian cells there are approximately 20 000–40 000 molecules of each of the RNA polymerases.

TRANSCRIPTION

The first phase of gene expression is the production of an mRNA copy of the gene. As in all other RNAs, mRNA is formed on a DNA template by a process of transcription.[6–9] Transcription is initiated when RNA polymerase binds to a specific DNA sequence, called the promoter, located at the 5′ end of the DNA, which contains the start site for RNA synthesis and signals where RNA synthesis should start. After binding to the promoter, the RNA polymerase opens up an adjacent area of the double helix to expose the nucleotides on a small stretch of DNA on each strand. One of the two exposed DNA strands serves as a template

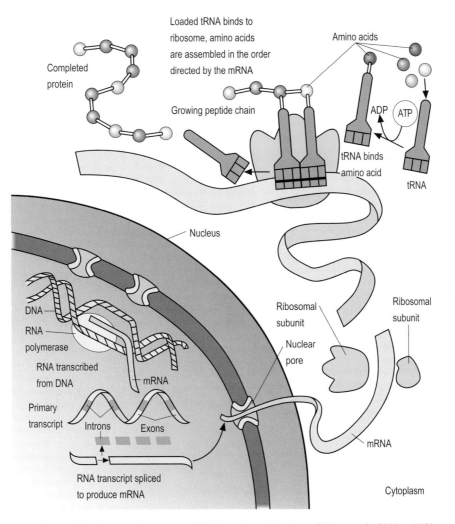

Fig. 3.2. Steps in protein synthesis. ADP, adenosine diphosphate; ATP, adenosine triphosphate; tRNA, transfer RNA; mRNA, messenger RNA. (Courtesy Baback Roshanravan.)

for complementary base pairing with RNA nucleotide. Therefore, G, C, T, and A in the DNA would signal the addition of C, G, A, and U, respectively, to the RNA. The RNA polymerase then moves stepwise along the DNA helix, exposing the next region of DNA for complementary base pairing (from the 5′ to the 3′ end) until the polymerase encounters another area of special sequences in the DNA, the stop (terminal) signal, where polymerase disengages from the DNA and releases the newly assembled single-stranded RNA chain and both the DNA templates. The RNA chain that is complementary to the DNA from which it was copied is called the primary RNA transcript. The primary RNA transcript is approximately 70–10000 nucleotides long because only a selected portion of a DNA is used to produce an RNA molecule.

Primary RNA transcripts (originally called 'heterogenous nuclear RNA') vary greatly in size because of the presence of long non-coding intron sequences. This is in contrast to mature, more uniform, small-size RNA sequences that are needed for encoding proteins. The primary

RNA transcript is then capped by the addition of a methylated G nucleotide to its 5′ end (5′ cap). The 5′ cap plays an important role in protecting growing RNA transcript from degradation and later in the initiation of protein synthesis. The 3′ end of primary RNA transcript is cleaved at a specific site, and a poly-A tail (100–200 residues of adenylic acid) is added by poly-A polymerase. The poly-A tail facilitates the export of mature mRNA from the nucleus, influences the stability of some mRNAs in the cytoplasm, and serves as a recognition signal for the ribosome, which is required for translation of mRNA.

For mRNA to move out of the nucleus, primary modified RNA transcripts undergo one or more RNA splicing events. The non-coding sequences (introns) are removed by ribonucleoprotein complex (the spliceosome), and the coding sequences (exons) on either side of the introns are joined together. These events result in a small, relatively stable, mature mRNA, which represents approximately 3% of the quantity of cellular RNA.

Table 3.1 The genetic code, with 20 specified amino acids[a]

First position (5' end)	Second position				Third position (3' end)
	U	**C**	**A**	**G**	
U	Phe	Ser	Tyr	Cys	U
	Phe	Ser	Tyr	Cys	C
	Leu	Ser	Stop	Stop	A
	Leu	Ser	Stop	Trp	G
C	Leu	Pro	His	Arg	U
	Leu	Pro	His	Arg	C
	Leu	Pro	Gln	Arg	A
	Leu	Pro	Gln	Arg	G
A	Ile	Thr	Asn	Ser	U
	Ile	Thr	Asn	Ser	C
	Ile	Thr	Lys	Arg	A
	Met	Thr	Lys	Arg	G
G	Val	Ala	Asp	Gly	U
	Val	Ala	Asp	Gly	C
	Val	Ala	Glu	Gly	A
	Val	Ala	Glu	Gly	G

[a]Codons are given as they appear in messenger RNA (mRNA).

U, Uracil; C, cytosine; A, adenine; G, guanine; Phe, phenylalanine; Ser, serine; Tyr, tyrosine; Cys, cysteine; Leu, leucine; Stop, stop codon; Trp, tryptophan; Pro, proline; His, histidine; Arg, arginine; Gln, glutamine; Ile, isoleucine; Thr, threonine; Asn, asparagine; Lys, lysine; Met, methionine; Val, valine; Ala, alanine; Asp, aspartic acid; Gly, glycine; Glu, glutamic acid.

TRANSLATION

In the second phase of gene expression the information contained in mRNA is used for the synthesis of polypeptides by a process of translation. During the course of protein synthesis the translational machinery moves from the 5′ to the 3′ direction along an mRNA, and the mRNA sequence is read as a block of three nucleotides at a time, termed a codon (Table 3.1).[10] Because RNA is made up of four types of nucleotides, there are 64 possible sequences composed of three nucleotides. Three of the 64 sequences do not code for amino acids but instead signal the termination of the polypeptide chain. These non-coding sequences are called stop codons. The remaining 61 codons specify only 20 amino acids; therefore most of the amino acids (with the exception of methionine and tryptophan, which have only one codon each) are represented by multiple codons, and the genetic code is considered to be degenerate.

Translation is mediated by tRNA, also termed adapter molecule, which has two important properties.[11–15] First, tRNA is able to represent only one amino acid to which it is covalently bound. Second, tRNA contains a trinucleotide sequence, the anticodon, which is complementary to the codon in mRNA representing its amino acid. The anticodon enables the tRNA to recognize the codon through complementary base pairing. The events in protein synthesis are catalyzed on the ribosome, which consists of two subunits; each subunit consists of several proteins associated with a long RNA (rRNA). A ribosome contains three binding sites for RNA molecules: one for mRNA and two for tRNAs. The site for tRNA

that holds the growing end of the polypeptide chain is called the P-site (peptidyl-tRNA-binding site), whereas the site that holds the incoming tRNA molecules charged with an amino acid is termed the A-site (aminoacyl-tRNA-binding site). To accomplish the sequential synthesis of a protein, the ribosome moves along the mRNA one codon at a time. A ribosome attaches to mRNA at or near the 5′ end of a coding region; moving along the RNA toward the 3′ end, it translates each triplet codon into an amino acid en route. The process of polypeptide chain elongation on a ribosome is a repeat of cycles with three distinct steps. During step 1, an aminoacyl-tRNA molecule binds to a ribosomal A-site by base pairing with the codon on mRNA exposed on A-site. In step 2, the carboxyl end of the polypeptide chain is uncoupled from the tRNA molecule bound to the P-site and joined by a peptide bond to the amino acid linked to the tRNA at the A-site. This reaction is catalyzed by peptidyl transferase. During final step 3, as the ribosome moves along the mRNA, the new peptidyl-tRNA in the A-site is translocated to the P-site. At the same time, the free tRNA molecule that was generated in the P-site in step 2 is released from the ribosome to reenter the pool of cytoplasmic tRNA. After completion of step 3, the unoccupied A-site on the ribosome is ready to take another tRNA linked to the next amino acid, which starts the cycle again. The stop codons (UAA, UAG, and UGA) are responsible for the termination of the translational process. Cytoplasmic proteins, the eukaryotic releasing factor (eRF), bind directly to any stop codon that reaches the A-site on the ribosome, resulting in the alteration of the activity of peptidyl transferase. This results in the addition of a water molecule instead of an amino acid to the peptidyl-tRNA. This frees the –COOH end of the growing polypeptide chain from its attachment to a tRNA molecule. Because only this attachment holds the growing polypeptide to the ribosome, the completed protein is released into the cytoplasm. The ribosome releases mRNA and dissociates into its two subunits, which are ready to assemble on another mRNA to begin the synthesis of a new protein. In summary, the termination reaction involves (1) release of the completed polypeptide from the last tRNA, (2) expulsion of the tRNA from the ribosome, and (3) dissociation of the ribosome from mRNA.

Additional factors are required at each stage of protein synthesis,[11,12] characterized by their cyclic association with, and dissociation from, the ribosome. During the initiation phase of protein synthesis, the two subunits of ribosomes are brought together at the precise location on the mRNA where the polypeptide chain is to begin. An RNA sequence can be translated in any one of three reading frames, each specifying a completely different polypeptide chain. The sequence of the mRNA determines which of the three reading frames are read, which determines how the ribosome assembles. The initiation process involves a number of steps catalyzed by a set of proteins, the initiation factors (IFs). To start a new protein chain, the ribosome must bind an aminoacyl-tRNA molecule in its P-site (normally occupied by peptidyl-tRNA molecule), a special step performed by initiator tRNA, which provides the amino acid methionine that starts a protein chain. The initiator tRNA must be loaded onto a small ribosomal unit, with the help of eukaryotic initiation factor-2 (eIF-2), before this subunit can bind to an mRNA molecule. This process allows the subunit to find the start codon (AUG), as well as allowing the small ribosomal subunit to bind to its larger subunit.

■ DNA REPAIR ■

Individual survival depends on genetic stability. Thousands of random changes are created in human cell DNA every day by heat energy and metabolic accidents; however, most of these spontaneous changes are temporary because they are immediately corrected by a mechanism termed DNA repair.[16,17] Only rarely are these changes in the DNA permanent, termed mutation. The process of DNA repair depends on the presence of a separate copy of the genetic information in each strand of the double helix of the DNA. The DNA repair process takes place in three steps. In step 1, the damaged portion of the DNA strand is recognized and removed by DNA repair nucleases, leaving a small gap in the DNA helix. In step 2, another DNA polymerase makes a complementary copy from the undamaged strand of the double helix, binds to the 3′ –OH end of the cut DNA, and fills in the gap. In step 3, the break or 'nick' that is left in the damaged strand when the DNA polymerase has filled the gap is finally sealed by DNA ligase.

DNA polymerase and DNA ligase are also important in DNA replication. In addition to maintaining the integrity of DNA sequences by DNA repair, an accurate duplication of DNA is a prerequisite for all cell divisions.

■ DNA REPLICATION ■

DNA replication is semiconservative because the original DNA duplex is not conserved after one round of replication; instead, each strand of the duplex becomes part of another duplex. DNA replication in mammalian

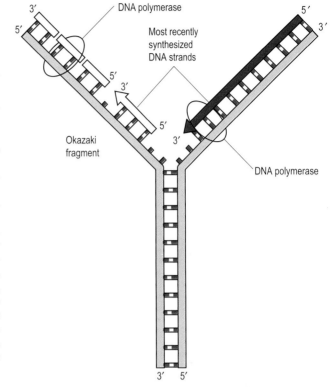

Fig. 3.3. Structure of DNA replication fork. (Courtesy Baback Roshanravan.)

cells occurs at a polymerization rate of about 50 nucleotides/s. The speed and accuracy with which the replication process takes place is regulated by a group of enzymes constituting a 'replication machine.' The basis for the great accuracy of DNA replication is complementarity.[18]

DNA templating is a process in which the nucleotide sequence of a DNA strand or a segment of DNA strand is copied by complementary base pairing in complementary nucleic acid sequence.[19,20] During this process, two strands of DNA helix are separated so that the hydrogen bond donor and acceptor groups on each base become exposed for base pairing. The DNA double helix is opened and untwisted ahead of the replication fork, by DNA helicase and single-stranded DNA-binding proteins.[21,22] This results in the separation of the template strand from its complementary strand, which is a requirement for DNA polymerases to copy the DNA. DNA helicases, when bound to single strands of DNA, hydrolyze adenosine triphosphate (ATP). Using the principle that hydrolysis of ATP can change the shape of a protein, DNA helicases move rapidly along the DNA single strand; where they encounter a region of double helix, they continue to move along their strand, thereby prying the helix apart. Single-strand DNA-binding proteins (helix-destabilizing proteins) bind to exposed DNA strands without covering the bases, allowing them to remain available for templating. These proteins also help open the DNA helix by stabilizing the unwound, single-stranded confirmation. Several classes of eukaryotic DNA polymerase have been identified. DNA polymerase α is a nuclear replicase; however, it synthesizes only one of the daughter strands. DNA polymerase

δ is also involved in replication and probably synthesizes the other daughter strand. DNA polymerases β and ϵ are probably involved in DNA repair reactions, and DNA polymerase γ is responsible for replication of mitochondrial DNA.

The actual process of replication occurs at the DNA replication fork,[23–25] which is asymmetric (Fig. 3.3). The replication of DNA always proceeds in the $5'\rightarrow3'$ direction on a growing DNA strand. Because the two parent strands are antiparallel, new strands are synthesized in opposite directions along the parent templates at each replication fork. Therefore, the new strand must be elongated by different mechanisms. Two DNA polymerases molecules work at the DNA fork, one (polymerase δ) on the leading strand (a strand that elongates toward the replication fork) and the other (polymerase α) on the lagging strand (a strand that is elongated away from the fork). Once the replication fork is established, the DNA polymerase at the leading strand is continuously presented with a base-pair chain onto which it adds a new nucleotide at the $3'$ end in a continuous manner; therefore the DNA daughter strand is synthesized continuously. In contrast, the lagging strand is synthesized discontinuously in a series of short segments called Okazaki fragments, which in eukaryotic cells are about 100–200 nucleotides long. Each Okazaki fragment is synthesized by DNA polymerase at the lagging strand in the $5'-3'$ direction beginning at the replication fork and moving away from it. DNA polymerase requires only approximately 4s to complete each short DNA fragment, after which it starts synthesizing a completely new DNA fragment at a site distant from the template strand. To achieve this, DNA primase, using ribonucleoside triphosphates, synthesizes short RNA primers (approximately 10 nucleotides long). RNA primers are made at intervals on the lagging strand, where they are elongated by DNA polymerase to synthesize Okazaki fragments. Synthesis of each Okazaki fragment ends when the DNA polymerase reaches the RNA primer attached to the $5'$ end of the previous fragment. To produce a continuous chain of DNA from the many DNA fragments made on the lagging strand, old RNA primers are removed and replaced with DNA. The $3'$ end of the new fragment is joined to the $5'$ end of the previous DNA fragment by DNA ligase, completing DNA replication. Because the synthesis of the leading strand is continuous, whereas that of the lagging strand is discontinuous, DNA replication is semicontinuous.

How does the newly synthesized DNA strand become a double helix without tangling? It is estimated that every 10 base pairs replicated at the DNA replication fork correspond to one complete turn about the axis of the parental double helix. For a replication fork to move along the entire length of a chromosome, the fork must rotate rapidly, requiring a large amount of energy. Instead, a swivel is formed in the DNA helix by a group of proteins, the DNA topoisomerases, covalently binding to a DNA phosphate, thereby breaking a phosphodiester bond in a DNA strand.[26,27] Topoisomerase I causes a single-strand break ('nick'). The phosphodiester bond in the strand acts as a swivel point around which two sections of DNA helix on either side of the nick can rotate. Consequently, DNA replication can occur with the rotation of only a short length of helix. Topoisomerase II forms a covalent bond to both strands of the DNA helix at the same time, resulting in a transient double-strand break in the DNA helix. Topoisomerase II enzymes are activated where two double helixes cross over each other. When topoisomerase binds to such a crossing site, (1) breakage of one double helix creates a DNA 'gate,' (2) the second nearby double helix passes through the gate, and (3) the break reseals and dissociates from the DNA, thus preventing potential tangling that would otherwise occur during DNA replication.

CONTROL OF GENE EXPRESSION

Control of gene expression is essential for directing development and maintaining homeostasis and can be regulated at several levels: transcriptional, RNA processing, RNA transport, mRNA degradation, translational, and post-translation by protein phosphorylation.[28–32] The most common and important gene regulation is at the transcription level, which is affected by binding of proteins to regulatory sequences within the DNA.

TRANSCRIPTIONAL CONTROL

To transcribe a gene, RNA polymerase binds to the promoter region, a specific sequence of nucleotides on the gene that informs the RNA polymerase where to begin transcribing. Other protein-binding nucleotide sequences on DNA regulate transcription by affecting the binding of RNA polymerase to the promoter. The interaction of proteins to the regulatory sequence either inhibits transcription by interfering with RNA polymerase binding to the promoter region or stimulates it by facilitating polymerase binding to the promoter.

To initiate transcription, an assembly of a set of proteins, the transcriptional factors, on the promoter is required for the stabilization of binding of RNA polymerase to the promoter. The assembly begins some 25 nucleotides upstream from the transcription start site, where a transcription factor (basal factor) composed of several subunits binds to a short TATA sequence (Fig. 3.4). Other transcriptional factors (coactivators) link the basal transcriptional factors with the regulatory proteins, the activators. This completes the formation of a full transcription complex that is able to engage RNA polymerase. The transcription complex then phosphorylates the bound RNA polymerase, disengaging it from the complex so that it is free to start transcription. Any factor that reduces the availability of a particular transcriptional factor, or blocks its assembly into the transcription complex, will likely inhibit transcription.

Regulatory proteins bind to the edges of base pairs exposed in the major grooves of DNA. Most of these regulatory proteins contain structural motifs, such as zinc finger or leucine zipper. The regulatory proteins are composed of two distinct domains, the DNA-binding domain and the regulatory domain. The DNA-binding domain physically attaches the protein to DNA at a specific site, using one of the structural motifs. The regulatory domain interacts with other regulatory proteins. These two domains of regulatory proteins provide them with an advantage, allowing a regulatory protein to bind to a specific DNA sequence on one site of a chromosome and to exert its regulatory effect over a promoter at another site. The distant sites to which regulatory proteins bind are termed enhancers. The activator regulatory proteins bind to DNA through specific enhancer sequences. Interaction of specific basal transcriptional factors with particular activator proteins is necessary for the proper positioning of RNA polymerase. The rate of transcription is regulated by the availability of these activator regulatory proteins. The repressor regulatory protein, through its regulatory domain, binds to a 'silencer' sequence, located adjacent to or overlapping an enhancing sequence. As a result, the corresponding activator protein will no longer be able to bind to the enhancer sequences and will be unavailable to interact with the transcription complex, repressing transcription.

One question remaining unanswered is how a regulatory protein can affect a promoter when these proteins bind to DNA at enhancer/repressor sites located far from the promoter. The current hypothesis is that the DNA loops around so that the enhancer is positioned near the

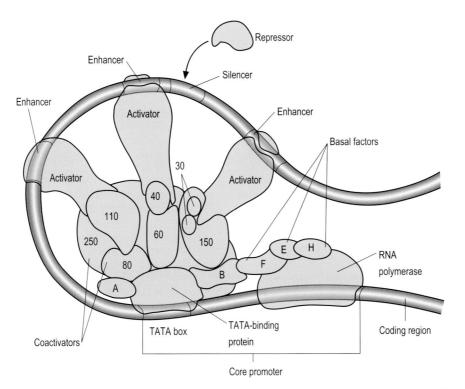

Fig. 3.4. Structure of human transcription complex, consisting of four types of proteins: basal factors, coactivators, activators, and repressors. (Courtesy Baback Roshanravan.)

promoter. This brings the regulatory domain of the protein attached to the enhancer into direct contact with the transcription factor associated with the RNA polymerase attached to the promoter.

POST-TRANSCRIPTIONAL CONTROL

Although gene regulation typically occurs at the level of transcription, there are several post-transcriptional steps at which gene expression can be regulated, including RNA splicing, translational repressor proteins, and selective degradation of mRNA transcripts. Most eukaryotic genes comprise short coding sequences (exons) embedded within long stretches of non-coding sequences (introns). The initial mRNA copied from a gene by RNA polymerase, the primary transcript, is a copy of the entire gene including introns and exons. Before the primary transcript is translated, the introns (composed of approximately 90% of the primary transcript) are removed by enzymes in a process of RNA splicing or RNA processing. This is a point where gene expression can be controlled because the exon can be spliced in different ways to allow different polypeptides to be assembled from the same gene.

Another step in post-transcriptional regulation of gene expression is the level of transport of processed mRNA script from the nucleus to the cytoplasm. The processed mRNA script is transported across the nuclear membrane through a nuclear pore. This active process of transport requires recognition of poly-A tail (a chain of adenine residues at the 3′ end) of processed transcript by receptors lining the interior of the nuclear pore. Although no direct evidence indicates that the gene expression is regulated at this point, it remains a possibility.

Because the translation of processed mRNA in the ribosome involves transcription factors, gene expression can be regulated by modification of one or more of these transcriptional factors. Translation repressor proteins shut down translation by binding to the beginning of the transcript so that it cannot be attached to the ribosome.

Different mRNA transcripts have different half-lives. Transcripts contain sequences near their 3′ end that make them subject to enzymatic degradation. A sequence of A and U nucleotides near the 3′ end of poly-A tail of transcript promotes removal of the tail, destabilizing the mRNA. Other mRNA transcripts contain sequences near their 3′ end that are recognition sites for endonucleases, causing these transcripts to be digested quickly.

■ DNA REARRANGEMENT (GENETIC RECOMBINATION) ■

To adapt to an ever-changing environment, DNA undergoes rearrangement, which is caused by genetic recombination.[33-40] The mechanisms of genetic recombination allow large sections of DNA helix to move from one chromosome to another. There are two classes of genetic recombinations: general, or homologous, and site specific.

In homologous recombination an exchange of genetic material takes place between two pairs of homologous DNA sequences located on two copies of the same chromosome.[36,37] This exchange involves breaking of two homologous DNA double helices and joining of the two broken

43

ends, by base pairing, to their opposite partners (crossover) to create two intact DNA molecules, each composed of parts of the original DNA molecule. The exchange of genetic material can occur anywhere in the homologous DNA sequences of two DNA helixes; however, the mechanism of homologous recombination ensures that two regions of DNA double helix undergo an exchange reaction provided they have extensive sequence homology. The homologous recombination does not normally change the rearrangement of the genes in a chromosome.

In contrast, site-specific recombination alters the relative positions of the nucleotide sequence in a chromosome because DNA homology between the recombining DNA molecule is not required, and the pairing reaction depends on a recombination enzyme-mediated recognition of specific nucleotide sequences present on one or both recombining DNA molecules.[33,38–40] There are two types of site-specific recombinations, conservative and transpositional. The conservative site-specific recombination was first demonstrated in bacteriophage λ.[38] This applies to many viruses. DNA sequences in the virus encode for integrase; in bacteriophage λ it is termed λ integrase. When a virus (in this case, bacteriophage λ) enters a cell, λ integrase is synthesized. Several molecules of integrase protein bind to a specific DNA sequence of the circular bacteriophage chromosome (mobile genetic element). This DNA-integrase complex binds to a related but different specific sequence on the bacterial chromosome (target chromosome), bringing the bacterial and bacteriophage chromosomes close together. Integrase then cuts the DNA section in both the bacteria and the bacteriophage and, by using a short region of sequence homology, reseals the reaction. The integrase then dissociates from the DNA and is ready to be used for the next recombination reaction. In transpositional site-specific recombination, mobile DNA sequences encode integrases that insert their DNA into target chromosome by a mechanism different from that described for bacteriophage λ. Similar to λ integrase, each of these integrases recognizes a specific DNA sequence in the mobile genetic element that must be integrated into the target chromosome. However, these integrases do not require specific DNA sequences in the target chromosome. Instead, both cut ends of the linear DNA sequence of mobile genetic element catalyze a direct attack on the target DNA, leaving two short single-stranded gaps in the recombinant DNA molecule, one at the 3′ end and the other at the 5′ end of the mobile genetic element. These gaps are then filled by DNA polymerase, and thus the entire process of recombination is completed. In summary, in conservative site-specific DNA recombination, integrase encoded by viral DNA (mobile genetic element) is involved in the entire process of recombination, that is, cutting of specific DNA sequences of both the mobile genetic material and the target DNA (cell) and resealing them. On the other hand, in transpositional site-specific recombination, integrase is involved in cutting of the specific DNA sequences of the mobile genetic element only.

■ RECOMBINANT DNA TECHNOLOGY ■

Recombinant DNA technology has revolutionized the field of cell biology and led to the discovery of a large number of new genes and proteins. By allowing the study of the regulatory regions of genes, this technique has provided an important tool to understand and decipher various complex mechanisms of gene regulation in eukaryotic cells. In addition, recombinant DNA technology has been instrumental in the study of conservation of many proteins during evolution and in the determination of the functions of proteins and of individual domains within proteins. Recombinant DNA technology comprises a number of techniques, of which the most significant are the following:

- Fragmentation, separation, sequencing, and recognition of DNA molecules
- Nucleic acid hybridization
- Gene cloning
- Gene isolation
- Gene mapping
- DNA engineering
- Genomics and proteomics
- RNA interference/RNA silencing

■ FRAGMENTATION, SEPARATION, SEQUENCING, AND IDENTIFICATION OF DNA ■

DNA FRAGMENTATION

Cell DNA can be cleaved at specific sites by restriction nucleases to yield DNA fragments that are separated by gel electrophoresis and can be subsequently sequenced.[41,42] The restriction nucleases are bacterial enzymes that protect bacteria from viruses by degrading viral DNA. Each restriction nuclease cuts the double-helical DNA into fragments of DNA (restriction fragments) that are strictly defined by their property of recognizing a specific sequence of four to eight nucleotides. More than 100 restriction nucleases have been purified from various bacteria, most of which recognize different nucleotide sequences. Most of these restriction nucleases are now commercially available (Table 3.2). Certain restriction nucleases produce staggered cuts, leaving short single-stranded tails at the two ends (cohesive ends) of each DNA fragment (Fig. 3.5). Any two DNA fragments can be joined together, provided both DNA fragments have the same cohesive ends (either generated by the same restriction nuclease or with another restriction nuclease, provided the DNA fragment has the same cohesive ends). DNA molecules produced in this manner by splicing together two or more DNA fragments are known as recombinant DNA molecules.

As mentioned, each restriction nuclease yields a series of restriction fragments. A restriction map of a particular region of the gene can be generated by comparing the sizes of restriction fragments obtained by the treatment of DNA from a particular genetic region with a combination of restriction nucleases. Because different short DNA sequences are recognized by different restriction nucleases, these sequences serve as markers, and the restriction map reveals their arrangement in the region of the gene. By using a restriction map, it is possible to study the conservation of a region of chromosome that codes for a particular gene during evolution, that is, whether the coding region has remained unchanged during evolution. Restriction maps are also used in DNA cloning and DNA engineering by identifying the gene of interest on a restriction fragment and therefore facilitating its isolation for DNA cloning and DNA engineering.

Table 3.2 Selected restriction endonucleases and their recognition sequences and cleavage sites (*)

Enzymes	Cleavage sites						
	5'					3'	
Tetranucleotides							
Taql	T	*	C	G	A		
Msp1	C	*	C	G	G		
Pentanucleotides							
EcoRll	*	C	C	T (A)	G	G	
Hinfl	G	*	A	N	T	C	
Hexanucleotides							
BamH1	G	*	G	A	T	C	C
EcoRl	G	*	A	A	T	T	C
HindIll	A	*	A	G	C	T	T
Pstl	C	T	G	C	A	*	G
Smal	C	C	C	*	G	G	G
Sphl	G	C	A	T	G	*	C
Heptanucleotides							
Mstll	C	C	*	T	N	A	G	G

T, Thymine; C, cytosine; G, guanine; A, adenine; N, any base.

SEPARATION OF DNA

Gel electrophoresis techniques separate DNA molecules by size.[43–45] Polyacrylamide gel with a small pore size is used to separate single-stranded DNA fragments less than 500 nucleotides long (size range 10–500 nucleotides) that differ in size by as little as a single nucleotide. Agarose gel with a medium pore size is used to fractionate the double-stranded DNA molecule (size range 300–10000 nucleotide pairs). The DNA bands in polyacrylamide gel and agarose gel electrophoresis are invisible, unless DNA is stained with ethidium bromide or labeled with radioisotope ^{32}P before performing electrophoresis. A variation of agarose gel electrophoresis, the pulse-field agarose gel electrophoresis, separates extremely long DNA molecules. This technique has been used to separate 16 different *Saccharomyces cerevisiae* chromosomes that range in size from 220000 to 2.5 million nucleotide pairs.

LABELING OF PURIFIED DNA MOLECULES

Isolated DNA molecules can be labeled by two methods.[46] In one method, DNA is copied by *Escherichia coli* DNA polymerase I in the presence of nucleotides that have either been labeled with ^{32}P or chemically labeled. These labeled nucleotides are then used as 'DNA probes' for nucleic acid hybridization. In the second method, bacteriophage polynucleotide kinase is used to transfer a single ^{32}P-labeled phosphate from ATP to the 5′ end of each chain of DNA. This method has both advantages

and disadvantages. DNA molecules labeled by this technique have low radioactivity and therefore cannot be used as DNA probes; however, they are extremely useful for DNA sequencing and DNA footprinting.

SEQUENCING OF DNA FRAGMENTS

It is now possible to determine the complete DNA sequence of genes by a chemical or an enzymatic method.[47–50] In the chemical method a set of identical end-labeled double-stranded DNA molecules are dissociated and exposed to a chemical that destroys one of the four bases (e.g., C residue) in the DNA. This generates a family of DNA fragments of different lengths. To determine the full sequence, a similar procedure can be done on four separate samples of identical end-labeled double-stranded DNA, using four different chemicals that cleave DNA preferentially at T, C, G, or A residues. The fragments of DNA produced by mild chemical treatments are then separated on gel and detected by autoradiography. Because the chemical method is less specific than the enzymatic method, it is no longer used.

The enzymatic method is the standard procedure currently used for DNA sequencing. In this procedure, in vitro DNA synthesis is carried out in the presence of chain-terminating nucleoside triphosphate. The DNA to be sequenced is used as a template to synthesize in vitro a set of replicas, using DNA polymerase. All replicas begin at the same place but terminate at different points along the DNA. The most important

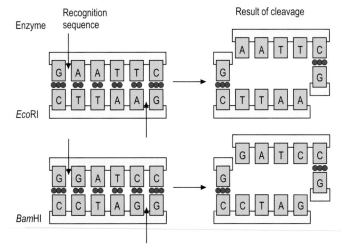

Fig. 3.5. Cleavage sites for commonly used restriction nucleases. (Courtesy Baback Roshanravan.)

step of this method is the use of the dideoxynucleoside dideoxyadenosine triphosphate (ddATP), in which the deoxyribose 3′–OH group present in normal nucleotides is missing. Therefore, when incorporated into a DNA chain, ddATP blocks the addition of the next nucleotide. This reaction generates a ladder of DNA fragments, which can be detected by a chemical or radioactive label that is incorporated either into oligonucleotide primers or into one of the deoxyribonucleoside triphosphates. To determine the full sequence of the desired DNA, four different chain-terminating nucleoside triphosphates are used in separate DNA synthesis reactions on the same primed single-stranded DNA template. Products of these reactions are analyzed in polyacrylamide gel electrophoresis.

RECOGNIZING DNA

DNA recognition is one of the central control points in the regulation of cellular processes. The nuclear proteins scan the surface of DNA molecules with extraordinary sensitivity and specificity, using them as a map to find the correct position for assembling the transcriptional apparatus. The ability of these regulatory factors to recognize specific DNA sequences underlies the selective expression of genes in a particular cell type. Important sequences in a regulatory region are identified by directly examining an interaction between protein and DNA. Several methods have been used to identify such protein-DNA interactions.[51]

Electrophoretic mobility-shift assay

The electrophoretic mobility-shift assay, or gel-shift assay or retardation assay, relies on gel electrophoresis to determine if a radioactive DNA fragment binds nuclear protein and to what extent the binding is sequence specific.[52] The radiolabeled DNA fragment that contains a protein-binding site runs through the gel more slowly than the DNA fragment alone, and therefore the band corresponding to protein-DNA complex shifts upward relative to the band corresponding to DNA alone. To distinguish sequence-specific from sequence-non-specific interactions

between protein and DNA, competitive assays are performed with two competitor DNA, one non-specific competitor (unrelated sequence) and one specific competitor (an exact sequence of the probe). The unlabeled specific competitor competes with the labeled DNA fragment for nuclear protein binding, resulting in the disappearance of the shifted band. A further variation of the gel-shift assay uses antibodies against specific nuclear proteins to confirm that the shifted protein-DNA complexes contain the corresponding protein factor. The antibody binds to the protein, forming a supercomplex of protein-DNA complex, and on autoradiograph is visualized as a 'supershifted' band.

The gel-shift assay cannot identify the position at which the protein binds along the DNA. Furthermore, this assay cannot be used to determine whether the shifted band is caused by two proteins binding to two different sites on the same DNA fragment. The DNA footprinting technique addresses these limitations of gel-shift assay.

DNA footprinting

Some proteins play a crucial role in determining which genes in a particular cell type are active by binding to regulatory DNA sequences that are located outside the coding region of a particular gene.[53,54] To determine the function of a protein, it is important to identify the specific sequences to which it binds. DNA footprinting reveals the site where proteins bind on a DNA molecule. In this technique, first a pure DNA fragment that is labeled at one end with ^{32}P is isolated, then a trace amount of a DNA endonuclease is added to the mixture of nuclear protein and radiolabeled DNA. The endonuclease cuts double-stranded DNA at various sites, except where a protein is bound to the DNA (protein prevents endonuclease cleavage). The DNA fragments are electrophoresed on a gel containing denaturing agents. Only the protein-labeled DNA complex is visualized on autoradiograph. The labeled fragments that terminate with binding sites are missing, leaving a gap in the gel pattern called a 'footprint.'

Binding-site selection assay

In this assay, specificity of DNA-protein interaction is complemented with the amplification capacity of the polymerase chain reaction (PCR) to identify a protein's DNA-binding site without prior knowledge of the gene it may control.[55] A set of synthetic potential DNA binding sites are required for this assay. Nuclear protein is incubated with DNA fragments that allow protein to bind to its preferred binding site among the random collection of DNA. The protein-DNA complexes are separated from unbound DNA fragments by gel-shift or an antibody to protein. The protein is then removed from the DNA by heating, and the selected DNA fragments are amplified by PCR, using primers complementary to the sequences flanking the random oligonucleotides. It is possible to obtain a homogenous DNA sequence containing the preferred DNA binding site by repeating the process of protein binding, purification, and amplification.

■ NUCLEIC ACID HYBRIDIZATION ■

Two strands of the double-helix DNA dissociate when an aqueous solution of DNA is exposed to very high pH (=13) or heated at 100°C, a process called DNA denaturation. However, if the solution is kept at

65°C for a prolonged period, the complementary single strands of DNA will re-form double helixes, a process called DNA hybridization. Similar hybridization will occur between single strands of DNA/DNA, RNA/RNA, or RNA/DNA, provided they have complementary nucleotide sequences.[56,57] The rate of nucleic acid hybridization depends on the rate at which two complementary nucleic acid chains collide, which in turn is proportional to the concentration of the chains. Therefore, the rate of hybridization may represent the concentration of any desired DNA or RNA sequence in a mixture of other sequences. Nucleic hybridization assay requires a pure single-stranded DNA fragment that is complementary in sequence to the desired DNA or RNA. Such a single-stranded DNA fragment can be obtained by cloning or can be chemically synthesized if its sequence is short. The DNA fragment is labeled either with radioisotope or with a chemical and used as an indicator to follow its incorporation during hybridization. Such an indicator DNA is called a DNA probe. Nucleic acid hybridization reactions using DNA probes are so sensitive and selective that one molecule of complementary sequence present in one cell can be detected. Therefore, it is possible to determine the number of copies of a particular DNA sequence in a cell's genome.

DNA probes can also be used to hybridize with RNA rather than DNA to determine whether a particular gene is expressed in a cell. In this case, DNA probe is hybridized with purified cellular RNA to determine whether the RNA includes molecules matching the probe DNA. In more extensive analysis, DNA probe, after hybridization has completed, is treated with specific nucleases to determine the exact region of DNA probe that has hybridized with cellular RNA. The start and stop sites for RNA transcription can thus be determined. The hybridization of DNA probes to cellular RNA also allows determination of whether change in gene expression is caused by controls that act on the transcription of DNA, splicing of the RNA of the gene, or translation of mature mRNA into protein.

NORTHERN AND SOUTHERN BLOTTING

Northern and Southern blotting are gel transfer hybridization techniques to analyze RNA and DNA, respectively.[58,59] In Southern blotting (named for the inventor of the procedure), isolated genomic DNA is cut into fragments of manageable size (which can be readily separated) with usually more than one restriction endonuclease.[43] In general, maximum lengths of DNA that can be directly manipulated are 15–20 kilobases (kb). The double-stranded DNA fragments are then separated according to their size by gel electrophoresis. Double-stranded DNA molecules are separated into single-stranded DNA by alkaline denaturation after the gel has been run. To identify DNA fragments, DNA is transferred from agarose gel to a nitrocellulose filter paper (nylon), on which they become immobilized. This process of DNA transfer from agarose gel to nitrocellulose paper is similar to blotting, therefore the term blotting. DNA fragments on nitrocellulose paper now can be hybridized with radiolabeled DNA probe. Those fragments that are complementary to DNA probe will be hybridized and can be visualized by autoradiography. The size of the DNA molecule in each band that binds to the probe can be determined by reference to bands of DNA standard that are electrophoresed side-by-side with the experimental samples. The usefulness of this technique depends on the specificity of the available probes. In Northern blotting, instead of DNA, RNA encoding gene of interest is analyzed with DNA probe.

Analogous to Southern blotting, in Northern blotting, purified RNA is separated by agarose gel electrophoresis, transferred to nitrocellulose membrane, hybridized with labeled DNA probe, and visualized by autoradiography.

POLYMERASE CHAIN REACTION

PCR is an extremely sensitive and rapid technique to detect the presence of a specific gene and is extremely useful as a diagnostic tool for detecting a large number of disease-causing or associated genes.[60–62] However, the most significant contribution of PCR technology has been in gene cloning. It is possible to isolate a gene from a single cell. This procedure involves in vitro amplification of specific pieces of DNA (Fig. 3.6). Two oligonucleotide primers, which are homologous to some part of the gene of interest, are synthesized. One of the primers is complementary to the sense strand, and the other is complementary to the antisense strand. The primers are mixed with genomic DNA or complementary DNA. The mixture is heated to 95°C to denature the double-stranded DNA and allowed to cool, during which oligonucleotide primers anneal to their complementary sequences. Then a special DNA polymerase (Taq) derived from a bacterium (*Thermus aquaticus*) is added to the mixture, and the temperature is raised to 72°C. The advantage of Taq is that it is not denatured at 95°C and is active at 72°C. During this reaction, DNA replicates with oligonucleotides as primers. This process of denaturing the DNA, reannealing the oligonucleotide primers, and replicating the DNA is repeated 30 times, using an automated thermal cycler, resulting in an exponential amplification of the gene. The DNA product of the PCR reaction can be inserted into a vector, cloned, and sequenced.

Quantitative real-time PCR

The amount of specific DNA product at the end of the PCR run does not correlate with the number of target copies present in the original specimen. However, some applications in medicine and research require quantification of the number of specific targets in the specimen. This has led to development of quantitative PCR techniques. Recent advances in technology allow detection of the increment per cycle of a specifically generated PCR product in 'real-time mode.' Quantitative real-time PCR is based on detection of a fluorescent signal produced proportionally during the amplification of a PCR product.[63–65] A probe (e.g., Taq) is designed to anneal to the target sequence between the traditional forward and reverse primers. The probe is labeled at the 5′ end with a reporter fluorochrome (usually 6-carboxyfluorescein [6-FAM]), and a quencher fluorochrome (6-carboxy-tetramethyl-rhodamine [TAMRA]) is added at the 3′ end. As long as both fluorochromes are on the probe, the quencher molecule stops all fluorescence by the reporter. As Taq polymerase extends the primer, the intrinsic 5′→3′ nuclease activity of Taq degrades the probe, releasing the reporter fluorochrome. The amount of fluorescence released during the amplification cycle is proportional to the amount of product generated in each cycle (Fig. 3.7). Compared to other quantitative PCR methods, the real-time PCR technique is more accurate and sensitive, less labor intensive, does not require post-PCR sample handling, and allows a faster and higher throughput. Therefore, real-time PCR can be performed on very small samples, for example, to quantify cytokine profiles in cells of the immune system.

■ IMMUNOLOGY

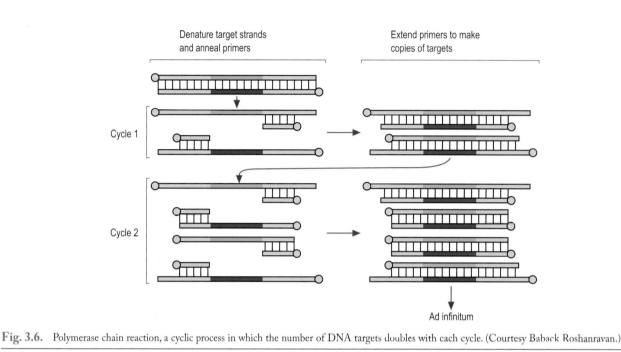

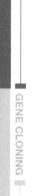

Fig. 3.6. Polymerase chain reaction, a cyclic process in which the number of DNA targets doubles with each cycle. (Courtesy Baback Roshanravan.)

T cell receptor rearrangement excision circle (TREC) measurement is another application of real-time PCR in immunology. TREC offers a novel tool to identify recent thymic emigrants in peripheral blood and T cell production by the thymus.

FLUORESCENCE IN SITU HYBRIDIZATION

Fluorescence in situ hybridization (FISH) is a non-radioactive technique used by cytogeneticists and molecular biologists to identify chromosomal aberrations and gene mapping. Chromosomal aberrations indicate clinical abnormalities and therefore are important in prenatal diagnosis of several diseases. In this technique, DNA probes detect segments of the human genome by DNA-DNA hybridization of samples of lysed metaphase cells prepared under conditions that preserve the morphology of condensed human chromosomes.[66,67] Attachment of the fluorescent molecule to the DNA probe allows the visualization, by light microscope, of the position on a chromosome. FISH is an improvement of in situ hybridization methods that depend on labeling of probes with radioactive isotopes. FISH has played an important role in the Human Genome Project.

■ GENE CLONING ■

One of the most important developments in the field of recombinant DNA technology has been the technique of gene cloning. The first step in the cloning of a specific gene is the construction of a comprehensive collection of cloned DNA fragments, the DNA library or gene library, which includes at least a fragment that contains a gene of interest (see below). The cloning of genetic material begins with the insertion of a DNA fragment that contains a gene of interest into the purified DNA genome of a self-replicating element, generally a virus or a plasmid, and

the propagation of this chimeric DNA molecule in a host organism. The process of gene cloning leads to the amplification of specific DNA fragments more than 10^{12}-fold. This allows the isolation and chemical characterization of specific DNA sequences. A virus or plasmid used in this way is known as a cloning vector. A cloning vector is a DNA molecule that has the following characteristics: (1) it is capable of replicating independently of the host chromosome, (2) an organism containing the vector can be grown preferentially, and (3) additional DNA can be inserted into the vector. There are two classes of vectors: the plasmid vectors and the phage vectors.

PLASMID VECTORS

Plasmids are small, circular molecules of double-stranded DNA derived from larger plasmids that occur naturally in bacteria.[68] Most plasmid-cloning vectors are designed to replicate in *E. coli*.[69] All the enzymes required for replication of the plasmid DNA are produced by a host bacterium. The classic example of plasmid vector is pBR322, which was one of the first plasmids that was recognized. The three important features of plasmid vectors are as follows:

1. Origin of replication. This origin permits the efficient replication of plasmid to a large number of copies of cells, by the plasmids replicon, a region of approximately 1000 base pairs encoding the site at which DNA replication is initiated.
2. Presence of selectable marker. Most plasmid vectors encode a gene that confers bacterial resistance to antibiotic. This allows selection of clones carrying the plasmid in the medium containing antibiotic.
3. Cloning, or restriction enzyme, cleavage site. All cloning vectors must have at least one cloning site (a specific DNA sequence that is recognized and cut by a restriction endonuclease), where the foreign DNA is inserted.

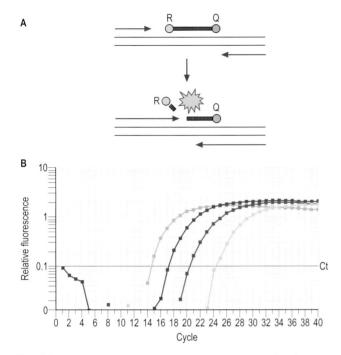

Fig. 3.7. Quantitative real-time polymerase chain reaction (PCR). (A) Primers are extended as in traditional PCR reaction. Probe labeled with reporter fluorochrome (R) and quencher fluorochrome (Q) anneals to the complementary gene sequence between the two primers. Fluorescent signal is generated when R is cleaved from the probe by Taq polymerase on extension of the primer. (B) Amplification window showing the fluorescence obtained in each amplification cycle for each reaction. Threshold cycle (Ct) shows the cycle number at which fluorescence intensities are above background noise.

Three classes of restriction enzymes bind to DNA at the recognition sequence and hydrolyze the phosphodiester bond on both strands of DNA. Such restriction sites usually have twofold symmetry, that is, the restriction sites are palindromic. Class II restriction endonucleases, which recognize a DNA sequence of four to eight nucleotides, are preferred for DNA technology. The restriction enzyme EcoRI, isolated from *E. coli*, cleaves DNA at the sequence 5′-GAATTC.[69] The EcoRI scans the plasmid until it finds the GAATTC sequence, where it hydrolyzes the phosphodiester bond between deoxyguanosine and deoxyadenosine on both strands of the DNA, creating a four-base pair (AATT) single-stranded overhang. Because EcoRI is palindromic, the overhanging single-stranded ends (sticky ends) are complementary to each other and can hybridize or anneal to each other by base pairing. Now the DNA to be cloned (cleaved from its source by EcoRI) is inserted into a plasmid vector whose DNA sequence has been cut by restriction endonuclease. The DNA fragment anneals to the vector through DNA ligase, which catalyzes the covalent joining of the vector DNA to the new piece of DNA (chimeric DNA). The gene (DNA fragment to be cloned) now becomes a passenger on the vector molecule, ready to be introduced into bacteria (DNA transformation).

Electroporation is the most efficient of the several techniques used to achieve DNA transformation.[71] The chimeric DNA is mixed with bacteria in a cuvette, and an electric potential is created across the wall of the container, allowing the DNA to enter the bacteria (transfection). The bacteria are then grown in the presence of antibiotic (e.g., ampicillin, neomycin) for which the resistant gene is present in the chimeric DNA.[70] This will allow the bacteria with recombinant plasmid to proliferate, whereas any bacteria that were not transformed with the recombinant plasmid will die. The clones or colonies of bacteria containing cloning vector can be isolated for further characterization. There are several ways to characterize clones, but the most common technique is to culture individual bacterial clones, isolate their DNA, and analyze the clones. Once the plasmid DNA has been purified, its structure can be analyzed by digesting the DNA with restriction endonuclease (e.g., EcoRI) and then subjecting it to agarose gel electrophoresis. DNA is visualized by staining the gel with ethidium bromide.

PHAGE VECTORS

Practically all phage vectors are based on bacteriophage lambda (λ), a bacterial virus that infects *Escherichia coli*.[72] Phage vectors have several advantages over plasmid vectors. First, phage vectors induce their genes into bacteria with high efficiency. Second, they can be exploited to clone larger pieces of DNA because many phages have large genomes. The bacteriophage λ DNA (approximately 50 kb) encodes approximately 60 genes that are arranged in three groups: the immediate early genes, the delayed early genes, and the late genes. After entry of λ phage DNA into a bacterium, its 12-base cohesive ends (cos) are joined by DNA ligase, resulting in the formation of a circular molecule. The virus then follows a lysogenic (dormant) or lytic pathway, depending on a balance between host and the viral factors. If immediate early genes are not expressed, the viral genome integrates into bacterial chromosome; however, transcription of almost all viral genes is suppressed, and therefore virus is maintained in a dormant or lysogenic state. In contrast, if the immediate early genes are transcribed, their proteins, through gene transcription, lead to expression of delayed early genes. The delayed early genes are responsible for the induction of lytic pathway through their involvement in replication of viral DNA. The late genes, whose expression follows the expression of delayed early genes, encode proteins that are involved in the synthesis of viral capsid, packaging of the viral RNA into the capsid, and lysis of the infected bacterium. The middle third genome of the phage vector, which is critical for the lysogenic pathway, is not critical for the lytic pathway. Therefore, this segment can be replaced with a new piece of DNA. In summary, phage λ cloning vector can be considered as having two pieces of DNA. One piece (≈20 kb) encodes the late genes that are involved in capsid assembly. The other piece (≈10 kb) encodes delayed early genes required for replication of phage DNA and late genes, which regulate the lysis of bacterium. The terminal portions of both pieces are cos sites, which signal the packaging of the viral DNA into capsid. One of the most versatile phage λ vectors is λ zeta-associated protein (λZAP), which has several important features. First, λZAP has a polyclonal site that has multiple restriction enzyme recognition sequences that are large (six to eight bases). The enzymes cut λZAP only in the polyclonal site. Second, λZAP can make fusion proteins that are useful in purifying the protein encoded by the cloned gene. The fusion proteins can also be used to raise antibodies to a cloned gene's product by injecting them in the animal. Third, the promoters of two specific RNA polymerases flank λZAP's polyclonal site. One side has a promoter that is recognized by the RNA polymerase of bacteriophage T3, and on the other side is a promoter that is recognized by the RNA polymerase

GENE CLONING

49

of bacteriophage 7. These RNA polymerases transcribe complementary strands of the cloned insert. The synthetic RNA can be translated in vitro or in vivo to make the protein so that the structure and function of the encoded protein can be studied. Fourth, λZAP encodes a phagemid vector that can be excised in vivo from the λ vector. This is helpful to prepare large amounts of cloned DNA fragments from phagemid vector rather than from a λ vector.

The process of ligating a DNA insert into a λ phage vector is the same as with a plasmid vector. However, a DNA insert must have terminal ends that are compatible with ligation into the λ cloning site. After ligation, the DNA is packaged into phage λ in vitro as protein capsid, using a mixture of structural proteins and enzymes. The recombinant bacteriophages are then allowed to infect the bacterium. The infected bacteria are mixed with agarose and plated. In about 5 h the recombinant bacteriophage undergoes many rounds of replication and lyses bacteria within a 1-mm diameter. As a result, a clear area, the plaque, develops that corresponds to a clone generated by phage λ vector. Each plaque contains 1 million copies of a single viral clone. Individual plaques can be purified, and the phages from the plaque can be grown in large quantities to isolate the DNA. Some phage particles stick to a piece of nitrocellulose paper when it is placed over a plaque. The phage particles can be disrupted and the DNA irreversibly attached to nitrocellulose membrane. This DNA can be screened by hybridization with a radiolabeled nucleic acid probe. Labeled probes are then visualized by radiography. In this way, labeled nucleic acid probes can be used to identify a gene within a λ gene library.

COSMID VECTORS

These are hybrids between plasmid and phage λ vectors. The classic example of cosmid vector is c2RB, which carries an origin of replication and a cloning site and has antibiotic-resistant genes. As with the phage λ vector, the cosmid vector encodes the cos sequences required for packaging of DNA into λ capsid. Cosmid vectors are designed to clone large fragments of DNA and to grow their DNA as a virus or as a plasmid. Cosmid vectors are used in homologous recombination between two different plasmids in the same cell and grown in both bacteria and animal cells. Cosmid vectors, along with λ vectors, are used as standard vectors for the cloning of genomic DNA.[73]

PHAGEMID VECTORS

These are hybrids between plasmids and a gene from a filamentous DNA bacteriophage M13 that infects but does not lyse *E. coli*. These vectors can convert a double-stranded plasmid into a single-stranded plasmid; the latter is useful for DNA sequencing, site-directed mutagenesis, and subtraction hybridization.[74,75]

YEAST PLASMID VECTORS

Although bacterial plasmid vectors are used most often, yeast plasmid vectors are preferred in special circumstances,[76] most notably the development of artificial chromosomes for gene mapping. Yeast plasmid vectors can carry DNA fragments that are 20 times (10^6 bases) as great as the DNA that even the cosmid vectors can propagate. Yeast artificial chromosomes (YACs), the most efficient vectors for cloning large pieces of DNA, encode a bacterial and yeast origin of replication, an antibiotic-resistant gene, a cloning site, a yeast centromere, two telomerases, and a selectable gene for growth in yeast. Because these vectors clone large fragments of DNA, yeast plasmid vectors are particularly useful in demonstrating linkage between two genes that may be >50 kb apart; other cloning techniques will not be able to show such physical linkage. This technique has already resulted in the isolation of several disease-causing genes, including genes for neurofibromatosis type 1, cystic fibrosis, and Duchenne's muscular dystrophy.

EUKARYOTIC PLASMID VECTORS

Eukaryotic plasmid vectors, also known as shuttle vectors, can express genes in both bacteria and eukaryotic cells.[77] These vectors carry a bacterial origin of replication (replicon) and an antibiotic-resistant gene, which allow them to grow in bacteria. In addition, shuttle vectors carry a eukaryotic enhancer and a promoter at 5′ to the coding sequence of a gene and poly-A site located at 3′ to the gene. Furthermore, many of the eukaryotic vectors also have introns, either before or after the coding sequence. Plasmid pSV2gpt was one of the first eukaryotic vectors described. A number of genes have been used as selectable markers in animal cells, including gpt (expressed by pSV2gpt), which encodes for xanthine-guanine phosphoribosyl transferase; apt, encoding for aminoglycoside phosphotransferase; tk, encoding for thymidine kinase; gdfr gene, encoding for dihydrofolate reductase; hpt, encoding for hygromycin B phosphotransferase; and adenosine deaminase gene, the ad gene. Eukaryotic vectors have been used to isolate genes on the basis of their function. Complementary DNA (cDNA) is inserted into the vector between the promoter and the poly-A site. The pCD vector was the first eukaryotic vector designed to express cDNA library in human cells.[78] The function of a eukaryotic gene can be evaluated by introducing the plasmid DNA into eukaryotic cells by electroporation, transfection of precipitable DNA, or microinjection. Eukaryotic expression vectors can also be used to make a transgenic animal that carries a new artificially introduced gene in the embryo.[79,80] A cloned gene in a eukaryotic expression vector is introduced into the female pronucleus of a single-cell embryo by microinjection. This cloned DNA integrates into the host chromosome and becomes a part of the host genome. Transgenic animals have been extensively used to study the effects of mutation and aberrant expression of a gene. Genes can also be introduced into the embryo with eukaryotic viral vectors.

EUKARYOTIC VIRAL VECTORS

Viruses that infect eukaryotic cells can be used to introduce DNA into animal cells not as a primary vector for cloning a gene, but to demonstrate the expression of a cloned gene in eukaryotic cells. First, eukaryotic viral vectors were based on the SV40 papovavirus, which is a double-stranded DNA virus of 5400 base pairs (bp) that carries only a small amount (2000 bp) of new DNA.[81] Two types of eukaryotic viral vector systems have been used: retroviral vectors and herpesvirus vectors.[82,83] The advantage of retroviral vectors is that all genes can be replaced with new DNA. Retroviruses contain a single-stranded RNA genome that is converted into double-stranded DNA by reverse transcriptase (RT) inside the infected cell.[84] The double-stranded DNA integrates into the chromosome of host cells. This provirus transcribes its entire genome, which encodes all the proteins that are required for the synthesis of new virions. Most retroviruses do not kill the cells they infect. Therefore, infected cells continue to make new viruses. In the retroviral genome, tandem long terminal repeats (LTRs) flank the coding sequences of the virus at either end. LTRs play an important role in the integration of provirus into the infected host cell chromosome and in regulating transcription. The sequences just internal to LTRs are involved in replication of viral genome and packaging of viral RNA (packaging sequences, or psi) into the virus. Most of the retroviral genome is composed of three structural genes: gag, pol, and env. The gag gene encodes for several core proteins, the pol gene encodes RT and integrase, and the env gene codes for viral envelope glycoprotein, which is required for viral entry into host cell.

The essential elements of retroviral vectors are a cloning site between two LTRs, the packaging signal, and the sequence necessary for DNA replication. After insertion and ligation of a gene into the cloning site, the vector is grown in bacteria to produce large amounts of DNA. The DNA is purified and introduced into an animal cell line.[85] The recombinant RNA is integrated into a host chromosome and transcribed into recombinant DNA, which carries the packaging signal. The RNA transcript is then packaged into capsid. In addition to its use in making transgenic mice,[86–89] eukaryotic retroviral vectors have been used in gene therapy.[90,91] However, retroviral vectors require cell division, and thus efficient transduction of quiescent stem cells has been difficult to achieve. Currently, more efficient vector systems such as lentiviral vectors are being developed to transduce non-dividing cells (e.g., quiescent hematopoietic stem cells).

GENE LIBRARIES

To clone a specific gene by plasmid or viral vector, one must construct a DNA library, which is a collection of cloned DNA fragments that includes the gene of interest. A DNA library is generally stored in a population of bacterial cells. There are two types of DNA libraries: genomic and complementary DNA. A genomic library is a collection of DNA fragments contained within self-replicating vectors that represent the entire genome of the individual from which the DNA was made. The cDNA library represents a collection of only those DNA fragments that were transcribed into mRNA in the cell from which the mRNA was isolated.[92,93]

A genomic library is constructed from chromosomal DNA. The DNA of the cell is digested with a specific restriction nuclease (e.g., EcoRI) into a large number of DNA fragments. The digestion reaction can be controlled so that the average size of the DNA fragments is approximately 20000 bp (DNA is partially digested). The advantage of the partial-digest library is that it contains a series of overlapping DNA fragments (approximately 18–20 kb) covering the genome. The DNA is then fractionated by size. Because the size of genomic DNA fragments tends to be relatively large (>10000 bases), phage or cosmid vectors (more often phage vectors) are used to generate genomic DNA clones. The bacteriophage λ DNA is cleaved with the same restriction nuclease that is used to cleave genomic DNA, and the two are then mixed; DNA ligase is added, and the chimeric DNA is packaged into phage capsids. The phage capsid is allowed to infect bacteria (e.g., *E. coli*). The recombinant phage multiplies as the bacteria multiply, generating millions of genomic DNA clones. The phage can be purified, and the collection of virions is called a phage genomic library. Genomic libraries are usually stored as phage particles in solution.

A genomic library can be prepared in cosmid vectors provided the partially digested DNA fragments are adjusted to approximately 40–45 kb. A cosmid library has the advantage of a larger insert size; however, rearrangements may occur. More recently, YAC libraries have been constructed for mapping large regions of human genome. Yeasts have advantages over bacteria because they are eukaryotes and therefore more like animal and human cells.

cDNA libraries can be prepared from selected populations of mRNA molecules.[94,95] When the gene of interest is expressed at high levels, most cDNA clones are likely to contain the gene sequence, and therefore cDNAs can be selected from these cells with minimal efforts. However, various methods can be used to enrich particular mRNAs before making the cDNA library from cells in which genes of interest are less abundantly transcribed. One example is the use of antibody against the protein to precipitate selectively those polyribosomes to which the mRNA coding for the protein is attached. The precipitate may enrich the desired mRNA by as much as 1000-fold. mRNA from the cells is isolated by dissolving the cells in a solution that inactivates ribonucleases, and RNA is then separated by cesium chloride density-gradient centrifugation. mRNA (contains poly-A tail) is separated from rRNA and tRNA by passing through chromatographic column containing cellulose to which short polymer of thymidine (oligodeoxythymidine [dT], or poly-dT) are covalently attached. Because of the adenines at the 3′ end of mRNA, mRNA hybridizes to oligo-dT and is retained by the column, whereas the poly-A RNA (e.g., rRNA and tRNA) pass through the column. The pure poly-A plus mRNA is eluted from the column by washing the column with water. mRNA is now converted into double-stranded DNA by means of a series of enzymatic reactions. A double-stranded hybrid molecule containing one strand of RNA and one strand of DNA is made with the help of RT. The RNA strand is then converted into DNA by DNA polymerase, DNA ligase, and RNase H, resulting in a cDNA molecule. The cDNA molecule is ligated into one of several cloning vectors (e.g., phagemid, eukaryotic vector, λ phage). Then DNA is introduced into bacteria to create the cDNA library.

■ ISOLATION OF GENE ■

Once a gene library has been generated, the gene of interest is isolated from millions of clones in the library by a number of screening methods, based on the particular properties of the genes and the proteins they encode. In general, these methods can be categorized into (1) screening by homology to nucleic acid probes, (2) screening for an immunoreactive product with antibodies to the gene's product, (3) screening with a functional assay for the gene product, (4) differential screening, (5) subtraction hybridization, and (6) PCR.

HOMOLOGY TO NUCLEIC ACID PROBES

Many genes have homologies to other genes that have been previously cloned. In this method, one constructs an oligonucleotide probe based on the structure of the known gene, which is suspected to have homology to the gene in question, and then probes to detect a cDNA clone within a cDNA library. For example, to isolate immunoglobulin-G subclass 1 (IgG1) gene expressed by cloned B cells, one makes a cDNA library from the B cells' mRNA and screens the library with a probe homologous to a highly conserved domain in all IgG genes, the IgG constant region domain.[96]

SCREENING WITH ANTIBODIES TO GENE PRODUCT

In this screening technique, antibodies against a particular protein encoded by the gene of interest are used to screen cDNA libraries for a particular gene cloned in an expression vector. The antibody binds to the replica of phage plaques containing the protein encoded by the gene of interest and detected by one of several methods already described. The recombinant phage that bound the antibody is purified and can be sequenced and functionally assayed to confirm that it encodes the gene of interest.[97]

EXPRESSION SYSTEMS TO SCREEN FUNCTIONAL GENE PRODUCT

To verify that the isolated gene encodes for a protein that has a functional role, in vitro and in vivo expression systems are used. One of the methods for analyzing the function of a cloned gene is the oocyte expression system. In this in vitro expression assay, synthetic mRNA made from the cloned cDNA is injected into *Xenopus oocyte* and then translates the transcript in vitro.[98] After translation the presence of the desired protein can be assayed by a number of methods. For example, if an antibody to a protein is available, the protein can be immunoprecipitated, purified, and characterized for its function, or if the gene encodes an enzyme, the enzyme activity can be measured. In the in vivo expression system, the cloned gene is expressed in cells, as in the oocyte expression system. Additional in vivo expression assays depend on eukaryotic expression vector pCD and eukaryotic viral vector systems.

Expression systems have been used to isolate a gene. The expression of a cDNA library in tissue culture cells has been used to isolate cDNA clones encoding lymphokines[99,100] and CD28, a T cell receptor cell surface protein.[101]

DIFFERENTIAL AND SUBTRACTION HYBRIDIZATION

The differential and subtraction hybridization methods are used to identify genes that are expressed in one type of cell but not in another, for example, a gene expressed in terminally differentiated cells but not in undifferentiated precursor cells, or genes encoding for cell surface proteins present in T cells but absent in B cells.

In differential hybridization, mRNA is extracted from two cell types from the same organism, and a cDNA library of a large number of recombinant clones is made from the target tissue from which the gene of interest is to be isolated.[102] Next, a selected library is grown on agar plates as discrete colonies. Bacterial colonies are picked individually and replated in a matrix. Two replicas of the matrix are made on nitrocellulose paper; bacteria on the filter paper are chemically lysed, and their DNA is fixed. The mRNAs from both cell types or tissues are converted into cDNAs, which are now radiolabeled. Two separate hybridizations are performed on two nitrocellulose filters carrying the target bacterial matrix. Each filter is probed with cDNA made from

each cell type or tissue. In this reaction, bacterial colonies that contain cDNA homologous to the probe mRNA will hybridize to the radiolabeled probe, which then can be identified by autoradiography. The differential hybridization is a simple procedure; however, it is less sensitive than subtraction hybridization because it requires abundant mRNA molecule (>0.1%).

Subtraction hybridization is a powerful tool for enriching particular nucleotide sequences before cDNA cloning.[103–105] This procedure can be used to identify any differentially expressed gene. Subtraction hybridization was first used to isolate cDNA encoding for the T cell antigen receptor (TCR),[106] a gene that is expressed only in T cells and is lacking in B cells. In the case of lymphocytes (or in any other cell type), poly-A plus RNA is prepared from both T and B lymphocytes. Then cDNA strands from T cells are synthesized, using oligo-dT primers. The RNA is removed from DNA-RNA hybrids by alkaline hydrolysis. These cDNAs are then hybridized with a large excess of mRNA from B cells. All T cell cDNAs for genes that are also expressed in B cells hybridize to B cell RNA, and the T cell-specific cDNAs remain single stranded and are further purified by passing the mixture on a hydroxyapatite column, which retains double-stranded hybridized molecules and allows the single-stranded T cell-specific cDNA to pass through. These single-stranded cDNAs are converted into double-stranded cDNAs and cloned. The library is screened with a subtracted ^{32}P-labeled cDNA probe.

POLYMERASE CHAIN REACTION

PCR can clone selected DNA fragments. The availability of purified DNA polymerases and chemically synthesized DNA oligonucleotides has made it possible to clone specific DNA sequences rapidly without the need for living cells. PCR cloning technique is rapidly replacing Southern blotting for the diagnosis of genetic disease and for the detection of low levels of viral infection, including human immunodeficiency virus (HIV) infection.

■ GENE MAPPING ■

The power of gene mapping for the study of human diseases is extraordinary. Restriction fragment length polymorphism (RFLP) has been successful in pinpointing the chromosomal location of a number of genes for different diseases, the cause of which is unknown. More than 100 human diseases have been mapped to both X-loci and autosomal loci using RFLP.[107–109]

RESTRICTION FRAGMENT LENGTH POLYMORPHISM

Gene mapping, or restriction endonuclease mapping, has become an important technique to analyze a large number of genetic disorders; large genomes can be mapped by either physical or genetic technique. Physical mapping, which includes restriction maps and a library of genomic clones, directly analyzes the DNA molecules that constitute each chromosome. A restriction map identifies a linear series of sites in the DNA that are separated from one another by actual distance along the nucleic acid. A genetic map is based on the frequency of co-inheritance of two or more features of an organism that serve as a genetic marker. If the difference in DNA sequence in a given population is rare, it is termed mutation; if it is common, it is called polymorphism.

RFLP is a difference in the size of DNA restriction fragment (restriction map) between individuals. It can serve as a useful genetic marker for the analysis and mapping of a large genome. RFLP is based on the principle that small differences in the DNA sequence can alter restriction enzyme cutting patterns. For example, a single base-pair difference in a particular chromosome, or short deletions or insertions of a base pair, may eliminate a site for restriction enzyme action, resulting in a large size difference in DNA restriction fragments. The inherited difference in the size of RFLPs provides a large number of linkage markers for following mutant genes through families.

■ DNA ENGINEERING ■

To determine the role of genes, RNA molecules, and proteins in an intact organism, scientists have relied on naturally occurring mutations and on a number of techniques to generate mutations. DNA engineering has transformed this area of investigation. A specific mutation now can be generated in selected genes, and stable strains of mutants can be produced in cells or mice to study the function of a desired gene.

STUDY OF THE GENE'S FUNCTION

In vitro a mutation in a gene of interest can be produced by two different techniques. In the first, or classic technique, cells in which the gene is known to be expressed are treated with mutagen, and mutant cells are isolated by selecting against expression of gene product. This approach has not been very successful because the mutations can only be detected if both copies of a gene in the diploid cell are mutated, which occurs rarely when using conventional mutagenesis. Therefore the more reliable technique of homologous recombination (discussed previously) is used. Cloned copies of the desired gene are altered to render them non-functional and then introduced into the cell's chromosome, replacing the normal gene with a non-functional copy. Because of the high frequency of homologous recombination, both copies of the gene in a diploid cell can be mutated, resulting in homozygous mutant cells. A defect then can be ascribed to the mutated gene if the mutant phenotype is reverted by a copy of the wild type of gene transferred into the mutant cell by transfection.

Several approaches have been used to study the function of an isolated gene by inserting it in 'foreign' cells. First, using transient expression systems, it is possible to insert genes into cells and study both the quantity and the structure of their transcript. Second, genes can be introduced into established cultures of cells of the appropriate lineage. Third, it is possible to insert chromosomes containing the gene of interest into a foreign cell. Fourth, genes can be introduced into fertilized eggs and their patterns of integration and expression studied over the next several generations; several variations on this approach have developed. For example, the application of homologous recombination to embryonic stem (ES) cells has allowed the manipulation of mouse genome. ES cells are derived from the inner cell mass of a blastocyst and can be kept indefinitely in culture without affecting their totipotent characteristics. New genes can be inserted into the mouse genome by transgenesis, creating transgenic mice.[110] In transgenesis, the desired DNA is injected into the male pronucleus of a fertilized ovum, which is then implanted into the uterus of a pseudopregnant female mouse. The injected DNA is randomly integrated into the genome of some of the eggs. This results in a mouse that has extra genetic material of a known structure (transgene). Therefore, it is possible to study the effect of a transgene on

development, to localize the region of the gene required for its expression in normal tissues, and to study the effect of overexpression and mutation on gene function. Transgenic mice have been especially useful in studying the role of T cell and B cell receptors in lymphocyte development.

In contrast to transgenic animals, in certain circumstances, the function of a particular gene can be understood if a mutant animal that does not express the gene of interest can be obtained, using a technique of gene knockout by homologous recombination. Such mice are called knockout mice.[111] A common approach to disrupt gene function by homologous recombination in ES cells is to construct a target or knockout vector. A standard knockout vector contains a positive selection marker (neomycin gene) within the coding sequence of a genomic DNA fragment that leads to disruption of the target gene. However, to improve the recombination events, a knockout vector containing a positive selection marker that lacks either its own promoter or poly-A site and knockout vectors that contain a negative selection gene in addition to a positive marker have been developed. Furthermore, the frequency of homologous recombination has been increased by using a syngeneic DNA. These approaches have been used to generate a large number of null mutant mice strains, including major histocompatibility complex (MHC) class I-deficient[112] and MHC class II-deficient mice.[113]

The two techniques for generating transgenic mice and knockout mice are now well established. These animals have been instrumental in the in vivo study of the effect of point mutation. As a result, functions of various molecules and the molecular basis of various genetic diseases have been delineated.

■ GENOMICS AND PROTEOMICS ■

GENE ARRAYS

The Human Genome Project, started in 1990 and officially completed in 2003, has initiated a new era in genetics.[114–117] At present, a huge amount of DNA sequence data that make up the entire human genetic blueprint is available. The challenge is to translate the genome into knowledge, making the focus of research to analyze the interaction and regulation of the identified genes. Advances in functional genomic technology help to determine the location, function, and the orchestrated expression of these genes. DNA array technology has become a powerful, high-throughput, versatile tool that can be applied to the study of functional genomics. DNA arrays are collections of large sets of DNA sequences immobilized onto solid substrates as individual spots. The principle of DNA array technology is based on the highly sensitive and specific hybridization of complementary strands of nucleic acids. cDNA is tagged with a radioactive or fluorescent label during reverse transcription from sample RNA and hybridized to an array. This single-stranded tagged cDNA, or probe, binds to corresponding DNA immobilized to an array. Excess and non-specific tagged cDNA is washed away, and the pattern of tagged cDNA binding is imaged and analyzed for the intensity of hybridization to each spot. The intensity of the signal is proportional to the quantity of the hybridized cDNA. The level of expression relative to another cDNA or another DNA sequence spot on the array is calculated (Fig. 3.8). The data processing enables analysis of thousands of transcripts at the same time and profiling of the relationship between the many genes in the arrays, termed expression profiling. The substrates used to immobilize the target DNA can be either porous, such as nylon membrane, or non-porous, such as glass slides. When

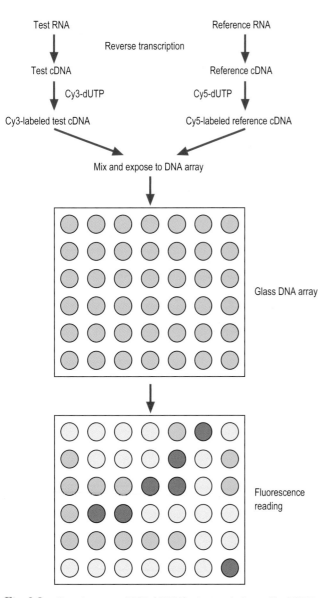

Fig. 3.8. Complementary DNA (cDNA) microarray schema. Total RNA from both the test and reference sample is fluorescently labeled with Cy3- or Cy5-dUTP using reverse transcription. Fluorescent targets are pooled and hybridized to the clones on the array. Fluorescence is measured and data are calculated from a single experiment as a normalized ratio of Cy3/Cy5 in which significant deviations from 1 show increased (>1) or decreased (<1) levels of gene expression relative to the reference sample. dUTP, deoxyuridine triphosphate.

DNAs are dotted onto nylon membranes, the gene arrays are referred as macroarrays. In this case, the detection is based on radioactivity of ^{32}P or ^{33}P and does not rely on competition between an experimental and control set of cDNAs. On the other hand, in glass arrays, i.e. microarrays, also called 'chips,' the detection depends on fluorescence labeling of the probe, which is less sensitive than radioactive system. However, glass has many advantages over nylon as a support. Because of its low autofluorescence, glass does not contribute significantly to background 'noise,' which can mask data in nylon arrays. More importantly, two different probes can be labeled with different fluorochromes and simultaneously incubated with one glass array. The DNA sequences immobilized onto substrate can be either full-length or short oligonucleotides of 10–50 bp. Short oligonucleotides may be more efficient in hybridization.[118,119] Recently, the microarrays have been designed using oligonucleotide probes synthesized in situ by using a resequencing array tiling strategy in order to achieve a high throughput sequencing that allows for the detection of both known and novel single-nucleotide polymorphisms (SNPs).[120] These resequencing arrays can also be used for comprehensive sequence analysis of small genomes of pathogens or mitochondria.

PROTEIN ARRAYS

Proteomics is described as 'the systematic analysis of proteins for their identity, quantity, and function.' It is different from Western blotting, a standard method of identifying the proteins in a tissue sample. With proteomics it is possible to investigate protein populations simultaneously, called multiplexing, unlike with Western blotting, which allows investigation of only one protein at a time. In addition, quantification of proteins of interest is more accurate with proteomics because quantities of sample proteins run in different gel lanes, or because different gels may not be identical in Western blotting. Proteomics is complementary to the area of genomics because (1) the proteins, rather than nucleic acids, maintain the cellular functions, and (2) proteins can be regulated by post-transcriptional mechanisms. Antibody microarrays comprising a large number of antibodies immobilized as individual spots onto solid substrate can be used for analysis of protein expression.[121,122] In this method, lysine moieties in two protein samples are labeled with two different fluorescent dyes, Cy3 and Cy5. The samples are mixed and exposed to a microarray containing antibodies spotted onto glass slides. The fluorescence signals are quantified using a microarray reader, and the relative quantities of the two samples for each of the proteins on the array are calculated (Fig. 3.9). Instead of fluorescence labeling, biotin labeling followed by streptavidin-horseradish peroxidase coupling of the bound proteins can be used. In this case, signals are detected by chemiluminescence, and resultant array images are compared electronically to determine the differential expression of proteins. Hypothetically, antibody arrays are similar to DNA arrays. However, technically, it is more difficult to include the proteasomes extensively because of the abundance of proteins due to multiple protein modifications.

Although the array technology is a powerful tool, the reliability in reproducibility, interpretation, and comparison from one study to another have been a concern.[123] Therefore, there is a great effort to achieve technological improvement to overcome these issues. A recent study on microarray quality control has demonstrated a high level of reproducibility.[124]

PHARMACOGENETICS

Pharmacogenetics is described as the study of interindividual variations in the DNA sequence related to drug absorption, disposition, and action.[125–127] Variations in critical genes that encode the functions of transporters, metabolizing enzymes, receptors, and their proteins can result in individual differences in response to therapeutic agents. SNPs in

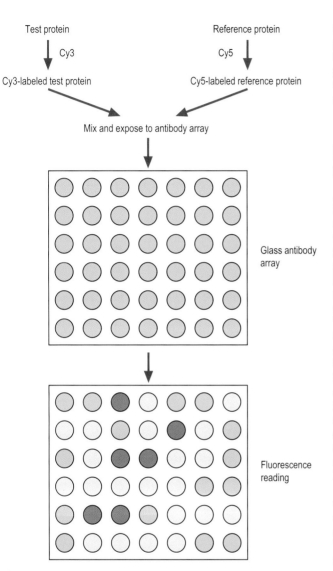

Test protein

↓ Cy3

Cy3-labeled test protein

Reference protein

Cy5 ↓

Cy5-labeled reference protein

Mix and expose to antibody array

Glass antibody array

Fluorescence reading

Fig. 3.9. Antibody microarray schema. Total protein from the test and reference sample is fluorescently labeled with Cy3 or Cy5. Mixed samples are exposed to antibodies on the array. Array images are quantified using the same algorithms used for cDNA microarrays.

these genes may cause an alteration in protein structure and function at the protein expression level. SNPs may also affect the RNA transcript through alternative splicing, and thereby influence the protein synthesis. In allergic diseases, SNPs that alter the drug target have been of major interest. Clinical studies to identify the asthma susceptibility genes have shown that β_2-adrenoreceptor SNPs affect the response to bronchodilator treatment. Asthmatic patients who have Arg16 are more responsive to bronchodilator treatment compared to individuals who carry Gly16. SNPs in other asthma susceptibility genes, identified by positional cloning, e.g., ADAM33, PHF11, DPP10, and GPRA, have the potential to

influence the response to treatment. With the availability of candidate gene and whole-genome SNP maps, and high-throughput resequencing microarray technology, it now appears that we are not far away from personalizing treatment by creating SNP profiles for patients to identify the individuals who are likely to respond favorably to a particular drug, or who are prone to have side effects.

■ RNA INTERFERENCE/RNA SILENCING ■

As this chapter is being written, the Nobel Prize in Physiology and Medicine (2006) has been awarded for the discovery of RNA interference – gene silencing by double-stranded RNA.[128] RNA interference (RNAi) technology is a powerful reverse genetics tool to clarify gene function in a variety of model organisms (e.g., *C. elegans, Drosophila*, plants). RNAi is a highly conserved molecular mechanism used by eukaryotic organisms to control gene expression during development and to defend their genomes against attackers such as RNA viruses. It is a mechanism for 'silencing' the transcript of an active gene, mRNA.[128,129] This process of post-transcriptional gene silencing is initiated by short (small) interfering RNA (siRNA), a double-stranded form of RNA that contains 21–23 bp and is highly specific for the nucleotide sequence of its target in mRNA. In plants and *Drosophila*, siRNAs are generated by an endonuclease called 'dicer.' These siRNAs associate with helicase and nuclease molecules to form a large complex, RNA-induced silencing complex (RISC), which leads to sequence-specific degradation of mRNA (Fig. 3.10). Dicer is not found in differentiated mammalian cells, although transfection of such cells with synthetic siRNA has resulted in highly sequence-specific RNAi. Therefore, it seems that dicer-mediated mechanisms are not required by mammalian cells to form RISCs.

RNAi also has therapeutic implications, such as in inhibition of the viral replication of HIV, poliovirus, and respiratory syncytial virus. Potentially, mutant oncogene mRNA in cancer cells can be targeted while mRNA expressed from the corresponding normal allele is protected. This is one of the most promising technologies to modify expression of the gene of interest.

■ EPIGENETICS ■

In the nucleus, DNA exists as a highly compressed structure, consisting of DNA and chromatin. The epigenome[130] is the sum of both the chromatin and the pattern of DNA methylation, which is the result of interaction of environment with the genome. The epigenetics can be defined as a study of heritable changes in gene functions that occur without a change in the sequence of the DNA, and includes the process of DNA methylation and chromatin remodeling, and the study of certain processes that occur in embryonic development (e.g., inactivation of one X chromosome in females and the phenomenon of gene silencing). Epigenetic mechanisms are widely used for the formation and storage of cellular information in response to transient environmental signals. In recent years, increasing evidence has emerged for a prominent role of epigenetic regulation, including DNA methylation and modification of histones, of immune system genes. This chapter will now discuss DNA methylation and histone modification.

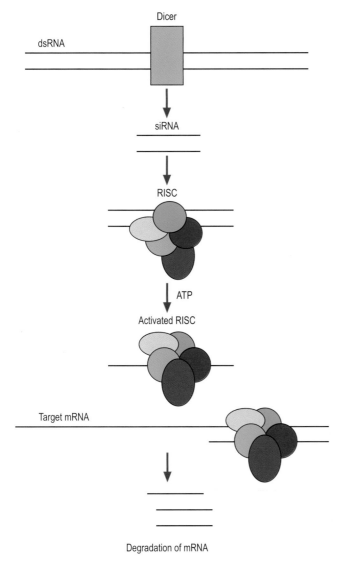

Fig. 3.10. Mechanism of RNA interference. Double-stranded RNA (dsRNA) is cleaved by 'dicer' enzyme into short interfering RNA (siRNA). The siRNA is assembled in a protein complex, called RNA-induced silencing complex (RISC), which is activated by adenosine triphosphate (ATP). Unwound siRNA in the complex guides target mRNA degradation by a ribonuclease.

DNA METHYLATION

Methylation[131,132] is a process of addition of methyl group or groups to a molecule, amino acid, or a nucleotide. At the level of protein, methylation is an addition of a methyl group or groups to the amino acid arginine or lysine, whereas on the DNA level, addition of a methyl group to a cytosine residue to convert it to 5-methylcytosine. When DNA is analyzed for CG dinucleotide pairs, the regions with higher proportions of CG sequences than would be expected by chance are termed as CpG islands. The CpG sites are in regions near the promoter of a gene. CpG islands constitute approximately 1–2% of the total genome, but account for most of the non-methylated CG dinucleotides. The remaining CG dinucleotides occur outside of CpG islands and are highly methylated. The state of methylation of CpG islands is critical to both gene activity and gene expression. Methylation of DNA cytosine bases leads to the inaccessibility of DNA regulatory elements to their transcription factors by a number of mechanisms. A large number of novel proteins involved in DNA methylation have been identified including methylcytosine-binding proteins and members of the DNA methyltransferase family. DNA methylation may suppress gene transcription by two mechanisms: (1) methylated CG dinucleotide may directly interfere with the binding of transcription factors to their recognition sequences, and (2) inhibition of binding of transcription factors to their promoter sequences by methylcytosine-binding proteins (MBPs). MBPs bound to CpG in the promoter region form complexes with histone deacetylases, leading to histone deacetylation, chromatin condensation, and a transcriptionally inactive chromatin. Hypomethylation of CpG dinucleotides within a promoter region allows transcription factors to bind and transcription to occur. A large number of genetic disorders have been linked to congenital deficiencies of a number of proteins involved in DNA methylation. These include the immunodeficiency, centromere instability, and facial anomalies (mutation in DnMt3b) syndrome, Rett syndrome (mutation in methylcytosine-binding protein MeCP2), and ATR-X syndrome, characterized by severe, X-linked mental retardation, facial dysmorphism, urogenital abnormalities, and α-thalassemia (mutation of ATR gene).

HISTONE MODIFICATION[132,133]

Histones are highly basic proteins that function to compress DNA within the nucleus to form chromatin, which provides a platform for regulating gene transcription. Therefore, histone modification, which can occur as a consequence of DNA methylation (see above) or independent of DNA methylation, provides mechanisms for epigenetic tagging of the genome and gene transcription. The interaction between histone and DNA is mediated by the amino(N)-terminal tail of histone proteins, which serve as a platform for 'histone code', a specific pattern of post-translational modification of histone octamer in chromatin. There are number of post-translational modification sites within the N-terminal tails of histone proteins. Post-translational modification of histone tails occurs by acetylation, methylation, ubiquitylation, and phosphorylation. Acetylation of histone tails correlates with transcriptional activity in many genes. *Acetylation* of lysine residues is catalyzed by histone acetyltransferases, resulting in neutralization of their positive charge, which transfer an acetyl group from acetyl-coenzyme A to the ε-NH+ group of a lys residue within a histone. Histone acetylation is a reversible processes, which is catalyzed by histone deacetylases. Histone deacetylation is associated with repression of gene expression. *Histone methylation* also occurs on the ε-NH+ group of a lysine residue and is mediated by histone methyltransferases. However, methylation of lys residues preserves their positive charge. *Ubiquitylation* of histones, similar to other proteins, occurs through the attachment of ubiquitin (76 amino acid protein) to the ε-NH+ group of a lysine residue; most histones are monoubiquitylated. *Phosphorylation* of histones H1 and H3 was discovered in context of chromosome condensation during meiosis. Phosphorylation of Ser10 on H3 is mediated by ribosomal protein S6kinase 2, which is downstream of extracellular signal-regulated kinase, and phosphorylation of Ser28 in H3 is mediated by aurora kinases.

▦ SUMMARY ▦

Molecular biology is a rapidly evolving discipline. The tools of molecular biology have been instrumental in the isolation and characterization of many genes that, when mutated, cause diseases in humans. The molecular nature of genetic defects in many human diseases has been defined. Several approaches relying on recombinant technology have been applied to understand the regulation of genes, functions of proteins, and the production of molecules in quantities large enough to treat a variety of human diseases. Progress in the field of molecular biology will lead to gene-directed therapeutic approaches in many genetically determined human disorders.

References

Anatomy of the gene

1. Watson J, Crick FH. Molecular structure of nucleic acids: a structure for deoxyribose nucleic acid. Nature 1953; 171:737.

RNA and protein synthesis

2. Holley RW, Apgar J, Everett GA, et al. Structure of a ribonucleic acid. Science 1965; 147:1462.
3. Noller HF. Structure of ribosomal RNA. Annu Rev Biochem 1984; 53:119.
4. Rich A, Kim SH. The three-dimensional structure of transfer RNA. Sci Am 1978; 238:52.
5. McClain WH. Transfer RNA identity. FASEB J 1993; 7:72.
6. Kerppola TK, Kane CM. RNA polymerase: regulation of transcript elongation and termination. FASEB J 1991; 5:2833.
7. Sentenac A. Eukaryotic RNA polymerases. CRC Crit Rev Biochem 1985; 18:31.
8. Murphy S, Moorefield B, Pieler T. Common mechanisms of promoter recognition by RNA polymerases II and III. Trends Genet 1989; 5:122.
9. Watson JD. The involvement of RNA in the synthesis of proteins. Science 1963; 140: 17.
10. Crick FH. The genetic code III. Sci Am 1966; 215:55.
11. Hunt T. The initiation of protein synthesis. Trends Biochem Sci 1980; 5:178.
12. Merrick WC. Overview: mechanism of translation initiation in eukaryotes. Enzyme 1990; 44:7.
13. Cavarelli J, Moras D. Recognition of tRNAs by aminoacyl-tRNA synthetases. FASEB J 1993; 7:79.
14. Stern S, Powers T, Changchien L-M, et al. RNA-protein interactions in 30S ribosomal subunits: folding and function of 16S rRNA. Science 1989; 244:783.
15. Kozak M. Structural features in eukaryotic mRNAs that modulate the initiation of translation. J Biol Chem 1991; 266:9867.

DNA repair

16. Barnes DE, Lindahl T, Sedgwick B. DNA repair. Curr Opin Cell Biol 1993; 5:424.
17. Wevrick R, Buchwald M. Mammalian DNA-repair genes. Curr Opin Genet Dev 1993; 3:470.

DNA replication

18. So AG, Downey KM. Eukaryotic DNA replication. Crit Rev Biochem Mol Biol 1992; 27:129.
19. Meselson M, Stahl FW. The replication of DNA in Escherichia coli. Proc Natl Acad Sci U S A 1958; 44:671.
20. Linn S. How many pols does it take to replicate nuclear DNA? Cell 1991; 66:185.
21. Lohman TM. Helicase-catalyzed DNA unwinding. J Biol Chem 1993; 268:2269.
22. Thommes P, Hubscher U. Eukaryotic DNA helicases: essential enzymes for DNA transaction. Chromosoma 1992; 101:467.
23. Ogawa T, Okazaki T. Discontinuous DNA replication. Ann Rev Biochem 1980; 49:421.
24. Thommes P, Hubscher U. Eukaryotic DNA replication: enzymes and proteins acting at the fork. Eur J Biochem 1990; 194:699.
25. Kaguni LS, Lehman IR. Eukaryotic DNA polymerase-primase: structure, mechanism and function. Biochim Biophys Acta 1988; 950:87.
26. Sternglanz R. DNA topoisomerases. Curr Opin Cell Biol 1989; 1:533.
27. Wang JC. DNA topoisomerases: why so many? J Biol Chem 1991; 266:6659.

Control of gene expression

28. Darnell JE Jr. Variety in the level of gene control in production of liver-specific mRNA. Nature 1982; 297:365.
29. Merrick WC. Mechanism and regulation of eukaryotic protein synthesis. Microbiol Rev 1992; 56:219.
30. Mitchell PJ, Tijan R. Transcriptional regulation in mammalian cells by sequence-specific DNA-binding proteins. Science 1989; 245:371.
31. Pabo CO, Sauer RT. Transcription factors: structural families and principles of DNA recognition. Annu Rev Biochem 1992; 61:1053.
32. Hershey JWB. Overview: phosphorylation and translational control. Enzyme 1990; 44:17.

DNA rearrangement (genetic recombination)

33. Sadowski PD. Site-specific genetic recombination: hop, flip and flops. FASEB J 1993; 7:760.
34. West SC. Enzymes and molecular mechanisms of genetic recombination. Annu Rev Biochem 1992; 61:603.
35. Lloyd RG, Sharpless GJ. Genetic analysis of recombination in prokaryotes. Curr Opin Genet Dev 1992; 2:683.
36. Eggleston AK, Kowalczykowski SC. An overview of homologous pairing and DNA strand exchange proteins. Biochimie 1991; 73:163.
37. Kobayashi I. Mechanisms for gene conversion and homologous recombination: the double-strand break repair model and successive half crossing-over model. Adv Biophys 1992; 28:81.
38. Landy A. Dynamic, structure, and regulatory aspects of lambda site-specific recombination. Annu Rev Biochem 1989; 58:913.
39. Stark WM, Boocock MR, Sherratt DJ. Catalysis by site-specific recombinases. Trends Genet 1992; 8:432.
40. Mizuuchi K. Transpositional recombination: mechanistic insights from studies of mu and other elements. Annu Rev Biochem 1992; 61:1011.

Fragmentation, separation, sequencing, and identification of DNA

41. Danna KJ. Determination of fragment order through partial digests and multiple enzyme digests. Methods Enzymol 1980; 65:449.
42. Nathans D, Smith HO. Restriction endonucleases in the analysis and restructuring of DNA molecules. Annu Rev Biochem 1975; 44:273.
43. Southern EM. Detection of specific sequences among DNA fragments separated by gel electrophoresis. J Mol Biol 1975; 98:503.
44. Evans GA. Physical mapping of the human genome by pulsed field gel analysis. Curr Opin Genet Dev 1991; 1:75.
45. Andrews AT. Electrophoresis. 2nd edn. Oxford: Clarendon Press; 1986.
46. Rigby PW, Dieckmann M, Rhodes C, et al. Labeling deoxyribonucleic acid to high specific activity in vitro by nick translation with DNA polymerase I. J Mol Biol 1977; 113:237.
47. Maxam AM, Gilbert W. A new method for sequencing DNA. Proc Natl Acad Sci U S A 1979; 74:560.
48. Sanger F, Nicklen S, Coulson AR. DNA sequencing with chain-terminating inhibitors. Proc Natl Acad Sci U S A 1977; 74:5463.
49. Prober JM, Trainor GL, Dam RJ, et al. A system for rapid DNA sequencing with fluorescent chain-terminating dideoxynucleotides. Science 1987; 336.
50. Griffin HG, Griffin AM. DNA sequencing: recent innovations and future trends. Appl Biochem Biotech 1993; 38:147.
51. Rosenthal N. Recognizing DNA. N Engl J Med 1995; 333:925.
52. Garner MM, Revzin A. A gel electrophoresis method for quantifying the binding of proteins to specific DNA regions: application to components of Escherichia coli lactose operon regulatory system. Nucleic Acids Res 1981; 9:3047.
53. Tullius TD. Physical studies of protein-DNA complex by footprinting. Annu Rev Biophys Chem 1989; 18:213.
54. Cartwright IL, Kelly SE. Probing the nature of chromosomal DNA-protein contacts by in vivo footprinting. Biotechniques 1991; 11:188.
55. Blackwell TK, Weintraub H. Differences and similarities in DNA-binding preferences of MyoD and E2A protein complexes revealed by binding site-selection. Science 1990; 250:1104.

Nucleic acid hybridization

56. Wetmur JG. DNA probes: applications of the principles of nucleic acid hybridization. Crit Rev Biochem Mol Biol 1991; 26:227.
57. Gerhard DS, Kawasaki ES, Bancroft FC, et al. Localization of a unique gene by direct hybridization in situ. Proc Natl Acad Sci U S A 1981; 78:3755.
58. Alwine JC, Kemp DJ, Stark GR. Method for detection of specific RNAs in agarose gels by transfer to diabenzyloxymethyl-paper and hybridization with DNA probes. Proc Natl Acad Sci U S A 1977; 74:5350.
59. Thomas PS. Hybridization of denatured RNA and small DNA fragments transferred to nitrocellulose. Proc Natl Acad Sci U S A 1980; 77:5201.
60. Higuch R. Simple and rapid preparation of samples for PCR. In: Erlich HA, ed. PCR technology: principles and applications for DNA amplification. New York: Stockton; 1989:31.
61. Erlich HA, ed. PCR technology: principles and application for DNA amplification. New York: Stockton; 1989.
62. White TJ, Arnheim N, Erlich HA. The polymerase chain reaction. Trends Genet 1989; 5:185.
63. Gibson UE, Heid CA, Williams PM. A novel method for real-time quantitative RT-PCR. Genome Res 1996; 6:995.
64. Heid CA, Stevens J, Livak KJ, et al. Real-time quantitative PCR. Genome Res 1996; 6:986.
65. McFarland RD, Picker LJ, Koup RA, et al. Recently identified measures of human thymic function. Clin Appl Immunol Rev 2001; 2:65.

66. Landegent JE, Jansen in de Wal N, van Ommen GJ, et al. Chromosomal localization of a unique gene by nonautoradiographic in situ hybridization. Nature 1985; 317:175.
67. Landegent JE, Jansen in de Wal N, Dirk RW, et al. Use of whole cosmid cloned genomic sequences for chromosomal localization by non-radioactive in situ hybridization. Hum Genet 1987; 77:366.

Gene cloning

68. Novick RP. Plasmids. Sci Am 1980; 243:102.
69. Hanahan D. Studies on transformation of Escherichia coli with plasmids. J Mol Biol 1983; 166:557.
70. Foster TJ. Plasmid-determined resistance to antimicrobial drugs and toxic metal ions in bacteria. Microbiol Rev 1983; 47:361.
71. Dower WJ, Miller JF, Ragsdale CW. High efficiency transformation of E. coli by high voltage electroporation. Nucleic Acids Res 1988; 16:6127.
72. Short JM, Fernandez JM, Sorge JA. Lambda ZAP: a bacteriophage lambda expression vector with in vivo expression properties. Nucleic Acids Res 1988; 16:7583.
73. Bates PF, Swift RA. Double cos site vectors: simplified cosmic cloning. Gene 1983; 26:137.
74. Vieira J, Messing J. Production of single-stranded plasmid DNA. Methods Enzymol 1987; 153:3.
75. Meade DA, Kemper B. Chimeric single-stranded DNA phage-plasmid clonic vectors. In: Rodriguez RL, Denhardt DT, eds. Vectors: a survey of molecular cloning vectors and their uses. Boston: Butterworth-Heinemann; 1988:85.
76. Burke DT. The role of yeast artificial chromosome in generating genome maps. Curr Opin Genet Dev 1991; 1:69.
77. Mulligan RC, Berg P. Expression of a bacterial gene in mammalian cells. Science 1980; 209:1422.
78. Okayama H, Berg P. A cDNA cloning vector that permits expression of cDNA inserts in mammalian cells. Mol Cell Biol 1983; 3:280.
79. Jaenisch R. Transgenic animals. Science 1988; 240:1468.
80. Palmiter RD, Brinster RL. Transgenic mice. Cell 1985; 41:343.
81. Hamer DH. DNA cloning in mammalian cells with SV40 vectors. In: Setlow JK, Hillaender A, eds. Genetic engineering: principles and methods. Vol. 2. New York: Plenum; 1980:83.
82. Nicolas JF, Rubenstein JL. Retroviral vectors. In: Rodriguez RL, Denhardt DT, eds. Vectors: a survey of molecular cloning vectors and their uses. Boston: Butterworth-Heinemann; 1988:493.
83. Elroy-Stein O, Fuerst TR, Moss B. Cap-independent translation of mRNA conferred by encephalomyocarditis virus 5′ sequence improves the performance of the vaccinia virus/ bacteriophage T7 hybrid expression system. Proc Natl Acad Sci U S A 1989; 86:126.
84. Varmus H. Retroviruses. Science 1988; 240:1427.
85. Cone RD, Mulligan RC. High efficiency gene transfer into mammalian cells: generation of helper free recombinant retrovirus with broad mammalian host range. Proc Natl Acad Sci U S A 1984; 81:6349.
86. Van der Putten H, Botteri FM, Miller AD, et al. Efficient insertion of genes into the mouse germ line via retroviral vectors. Proc Natl Acad Sci U S A 1985; 82:6148.
87. Huszar D, Balling R, Kothary R, et al. Insertion of a bacterial gene into the mouse germ line using an infectious retrovirus vector. Proc Natl Acad Sci U S A 1985; 82:8587.
88. Stuhlmann H, Cone R, Mulligan RC, et al. Introduction of a selectable gene into different animal tissue by a retrovirus recombinant vector. Proc Natl Acad Sci U S A 1984; 81:7151.
89. Rubenstein JL, Nicolas JF, Jacob F. Introduction of genes into preimplantation mouse embryo by use of a defective recombinant retrovirus. Proc Natl Acad Sci U S A 1986; 83:366.
90. Verma IM. Gene therapy. Sci Am 1990; 263:68.
91. Brenner MK. Gene transfer to hematopoietic cells. N Engl J Med 1996; 335:337.
92. Lenon GG, Lehrach H. Hybridization analyses of array cDNA libraries. Trends Genet 1991; 7:314.
93. Maniatis T, Hardison RC, Lacy E, et al. The isolation of structural genes from libraries of eukaryotic DNA. Cell 1978; 15:687.
94. Okayama H, Berg P. High efficiency cloning of full length cDNA. Mol Cell Biol 1982; 2:161.
95. Calvet JP. Molecular approaches for analyzing differential gene expression: differential cDNA library construction and screening. Pediatr Nephrol 1991; 5:751.

Isolation of gene

96. Shambrook J, Fritsch F, Maniatis T. Molecular cloning: a laboratory manual. 2nd edn. New York: Cold Spring Harbor Laboratory; 1989.
97. Young RA, Davis RW. Efficient isolation of genes by using antibody probes. Proc Natl Acad Sci U S A 1983; 80:1194.
98. Rubenstein JL, Chappell TG. Construction of a synthetic messenger RNA encoding a membrane protein. J Cell Biol 1983; 96:1464.
99. Yokota T, Otsuka T, Mosmann T, et al. Isolation and characterization of a human interleukin cDNA clone, homologous to mouse B-cell stimulatory factor 1, that expresses B-cell and T-cell-stimulating activities. Proc Natl Acad Sci U S A 1985; 82:5894.
100. Lee F, Yokota T, Otsuka T, et al. Isolation and characterization of a mouse interleukin cDNA clone that expresses B-cell stimulatory factor 1 activities and T-cell- and mast-cell-stimulatory activities. Proc Natl Acad Sci U S A 1986; 83:2061.
101. Aruffo A, Seed B. Molecular cloning of a CD28 cDNA by a high-efficiency COS cell expression system. Proc Natl Acad Sci U S A 1987; 84:8573.
102. Cochran BH, Zumstein O, Zullo J, et al. Differential colony hybridization: molecular cloning from zero data base. Methods Enzymol 1987; 147:64.
103. Rubenstein JL, Brice AE, Ciaranello RD, et al. Subtractive hybridization system using single-stranded phagemids with directional inserts. Nucleic Acids Res 1990; 18:4833.
104. Duguid JR, Rohwer RG, Seed B. Isolation of cDNAs of scrapie-modulated RNAs by subtraction hybridization of a cDNA library. Proc Natl Acad Sci U S A 1988; 85:5738.
105. Kowalski J, Smith JH, Ng N, et al. Vectors for the direct selection of cDNA clones corresponding to mammalian cell mRNA of low abundance. Gene 1985; 35:45.
106. Hedrick SM, Cohen DI, Nielsen EA, et al. Isolation of cDNA clones encoding T cell-specific membrane-associated protein. Nature 1984; 308:149.

Gene mapping

107. Kidd KK. Progress towards completing the human linkage map. Curr Opin Genet Dev 1991; 1:99.
108. Pourzand C, Cerutti P. Genotypic mutation analysis by RFLP/PCR. Mutat Res 1993; 288:113.
109. Weatherall DJ, ed. The new genetics and clinical practice. 3rd edn. Oxford: OUP; 1991:103.

DNA engineering

110. Shuldiner AR. Transgenic animals. N Engl J Med 1996; 334:653.
111. Majzoub JA, Muglia LJ. Knock out mice. N Engl J Med 1996; 344:904.
112. Zijtstra M, Li E, Sajjadi E, et al. Germ-line transmission of a disrupted β_2-microglobulin gene produced by homologous recombination in embryonic stem cells. Nature 1989; 342:435.
113. Cosgrove D, Gray D, Dierich A, et al. Mice lacking MHC class II molecules. Cell 1991; 66:1051.

Genomics and proteomics

114. International Human Genome Sequencing Consortium. Initial sequencing and analysis of the human genome. Nature 2001; 409:860.
115. Venter JC, Adams MD, Myers EW, et al. The sequence of the human genome. Science 2001; 291:1304.
116. Collins FS, Morgan M, Patrinos A. The Human Genome Project: Lessons from large-scale biology. Science 2003; 300:286.
117. Collins FS, Green ED, Guttmacher AE, et al. A vision for the future of genomics research. Nature 2003; 422:835.
118. Duggan DJ, Bittner M, Chen Y, et al. Expression profiling using DNA microarrays. Nat Genet 1999; 21:S10.
119. Lockhart DJ, Winzeler EA. Genomic, gene expression and DNA arrays. Nature 2000; 405:827.
120. Cutler DJ, Zwick ME, Carrasguillo MM, et al. High-throughput variation detection and genotyping using microarrays. Genome Res 2001; 11:1913.
121. Haab BB, Dunham MJ, Brown PO. Protein microarrays for highly parallel detection and quantitation of specific proteins and antibodies in complex solutions. Genome Biol 2: 4.1:2001.
122. Jenkins RE, Pennington SR. Arrays for protein expression profiling: towards a viable alternative to two-dimensional gel electrophoresis? Proteomics 2001; 1:13.
123. Knight J. When the chips are down. Nature 2001; 410:860.
124. Shi L, Reid LH, Jones WD, et al. The MicroArray Quality Control (MAQC) project shows inter- and intraplatform reproducibility of geneexpression and measurements. Nat Biotechnol 2006; 24:1151.
125. Roses AD. Pharmacogenetics and the practice of medicine. Nature 2000; 405:857.
126. Lesko LJ, Salerno RA, Spear BB, et al. Pharmacogenetics and pharmacogenomics in drug development and regulatory decision making: Report of the first FDA-PWG-PhRMA-DruSafe workshop. J Clin Pharmacol 2003; 43:342.
127. Holgate ST. Pharmacogenetics: the new science of personalizing treatment. Curr Opin Allergy Clin Immunol 2004; 4:37.

RNA interference/RNA silencing

128. Fire A, Xu SQ, Montgomery MK, et al. Potent and specific genetic interference by double-stranded RNA in Caenorhabditis elegans. Nature 1998; 391:806.
129. Hannon GJ. RNA interference. Nature 2002; 418:244.

Epigenetics

130. Pray L. Epigenetics: genome, meet your environment. Scientist 2004; 18:14.
131. Ng HH, Bird A. DNA methylation and chromatin modification. Curr Opin Genet Dev 1999; 9:158.
132. Attwood JT, Yung RL, Richardson BC. DNA methylation and the regulation of gene transcription. Cell Mol Life Sci 2002; 59:241.
133. Grunstein M. Histone acetylation and chromatin structure and transcription. Nature 1997; 93:349.

Principles of Genetics in Allergic Diseases and Asthma

Alireza Sadeghnejad, Eugene Bleecker, and Deborah A Meyers

4

SUMMARY OF IMPORTANT CONCEPTS

>> There is genetic susceptibility to the development and probably severity of asthma and allergy

>> Multiple genes each with a modest effect are involved as well as environment influences

>> Replication is important in genetic studies in common diseases, such as allergy and asthma

>> Appropriate large population samples of different ethnic groups need to be studied. The degree of genetic variation often differs between races

>> Whole gene wide association studies with hundreds of thousands of genetic variants will provide additional insight

>> Pharmacogenetic analysis of genes in pathways relevant to a given therapy are important to design personalized approaches to treatmonts

INTRODUCTION

It is now well accepted that there is a genetic basis to susceptibility to most common diseases, although environment has an important role. In addition, it is widely recognized that individual response to therapy including adverse reactions probably has a genetic basis. There have been significant advances in genetic studies of allergy and asthma which will be reviewed and discussed in this chapter. Classically, allergy has been defined as the result of immune reaction to antigens known as allergens. Atopy, the genetically mediated predisposition to produce specific IgE following exposure to allergens, is clinically defined as having evidence of allergic sensitization to at least one allergen.[1] Atopy is fundamental to the pathogenesis of allergic disorders, which manifest as any combination of conjunctivitis, food intolerance, asthma, rhinitis, and eczema (atopic dermatitis). However, these clinical presentations can also appear in the absence of atopy.[2] The current definition of asthma describes its pathophysiologic basis, emphasizing the importance of inflammatory mechanisms (Box 4.1).[3] Subjects with asthma have variable airway obstruction and enhanced bronchial responsiveness and are often allergic.[3] Asthma and other allergic diseases are major public health problems.[4] Asthma, in particular, is a disease that places a huge burden on society. Asthma is the most common chronic illness in childhood. It is estimated that asthma affects more than 300 million people worldwide, 15 million in the USA, leading to more than 500000 hospitalizations and over 5000 deaths annually.[5] Therefore, from the public health point of view, asthma is probably the most important allergy-related disease.

The main focus of this chapter is to present the principles and current understanding of genetics in asthma, and its related phenotypes including allergy and atopy. However, most progress towards defining the genetic basis has been seen from studies on asthma; therefore, we will concentrate on genetic studies for asthma. Of course, the methods and principles discussed are applicable to other common disorders. We start with phenotype definition for asthma and proceed with current

BOX 4.1 ASTHMA

Definition. A chronic inflammatory disorder of the airways in which many cells and cellular elements play a role. The chronic inflammation is associated with airway hyperresponsiveness that leads to recurrent episodes of wheezing, breathlessness, chest tightness, and coughing, particularly at night or in the early morning. These episodes are usually associated with widespread, but variable, airflow obstruction within the lung that is often reversible either spontaneously or with treatment.

Clinical spectrum is highly variable, and different cellular patterns have been observed, but the presence of airway inflammation remains a consistent feature.

Risk factors can be divided into host factors (primarily genetic) and environmental factors.

Host factors:
>> Genes predisposing to atopy
>> Genes predisposing to airway hyperresponsiveness
>> Obesity
>> Sex

Environmental factors:
>> Allergens
  – Indoor: domestic mites, furred animals (dogs, cats, mice), cockroach allergen, fungi, molds, yeasts
  – Outdoor: pollens, fungi, molds, yeasts
>> Infections (predominantly viral)
>> Occupational sensitizers
>> Tobacco smoke
  – Passive smoking
  – Active smoking
>> Outdoor/indoor air pollution
>> Diet

BOX 4.2 ASTHMA-RELATED PHENOTYPES

Atopic sensitization: Characterized by high levels of immunoglobulin E (IgE) antibodies or skin-test responsiveness to common allergens.

Wheeze: Noisy, labored breathing due to air moving through narrowed tracheobronchial airways.

Bronchial hyperresponsiveness is the state where bronchi constrict easily and excessively, on exposure to specific (allergen) and non-specific (chemical and physical) stimuli.

Other allergic disorders: Characterized by an immunologically mediated adverse reaction to a foreign substance.

children.[6] Because many asthmatic patients are atopic, it is appropriate to study measures of the allergic phenotype, such as total serum eosinophil counts, skin test responses to common allergens, and specific IgE measures in addition to total serum IgE levels.

Clinical asthma is characterized with prominent activity of mast cells, eosinophils, and lymphocytes, as well as T-helper cell type 2 (Th2) immune cytokines such as interleukin-13 (IL-13).[3] These same cellular and immune components are also prominent in non-atopic asthma and animal models for asthma.[7] Th2 immune activity (Fig. 4.1), which is prominent in atopy and asthma and a key component of natural defenses against certain parasitic helminths, involves the actions of the cytokines IL-3, IL-4, IL-5, IL-9, and IL-13.[8] Two of these cytokines, IL-4 and IL-13, share a receptor subunit (IL-4Ra) and the same signal transducer and activator of transmission, STAT-6. IL-4 is the principal cytokine in inducing Th2 cell growth and IgE synthesis, typical of atopy, whereas IL-13 can also induce IgE synthesis but plays a central role in inducing mucosal changes typical of asthma: bronchial eosinophilic infiltration, mucus hypersecretion, and bronchial smooth muscle hypertrophy.[9] Studying the genes in this pathway is an example of a candidate gene approach which will be discussed later in this chapter.

Investigators have used various approaches, including a reported physician's diagnosis of asthma, questionnaire data on relevant symptoms, objective measures as discussed above, or combinations to define asthma in genetic studies. Reliance on only historical information, such as a prior physician's diagnosis of asthma appears to underestimate the prevalence of asthma and allergy in family and epidemiologic studies.[6] In evaluating genetic studies and comparing results, it is important to be aware of differences in disease definition. While performing well-standardized laboratory testing is time consuming and expensive, it is important to very carefully characterize individuals in genetic studies to avoid biases introduced by inconsistent or not-well defined disease status.

knowledge on asthma genetics, followed by topics on new approaches in asthma and allergy genetics. The newer approaches include gene–gene and gene–environment interactions as well as pharmacogenetics in asthma, comparative genomics and genome-wide association studies.

PHENOTYPE DEFINITION

Because multiple genes are involved in its pathogenesis, asthma is considered a common and complex genetic disease. Clearly defining the disease phenotype is a central issue in genetic studies. There is no uniform phenotypic definition for asthma for research purposes. However, to investigate the genetic basis of asthma, it is useful to evaluate phenotypes associated with the disease, such as bronchial hyperresponsiveness (BHR), bronchodilator reversibility, and pulmonary function, and measures of atopy such as total serum immunoglobulin E levels (IgE) and skin-test reactivity to common allergens. These are objective phenotypes that may be measured in asthma studies using standard methodologies (Box 4.2).[3] BHR is a marker of asthma and associated with atopy, as observed by the close association of serum IgE levels, BHR, and asthma in asymptomatic

EVIDENCE FOR A GENETIC COMPONENT IN ASTHMA

Like other complex genetic diseases, evidence for a genetic component in asthma has been confirmed by several types of genetic studies. From familial aggregation and twin studies, a significant familial aggregation of asthma and associated phenotypes such as BHR and total serum IgE

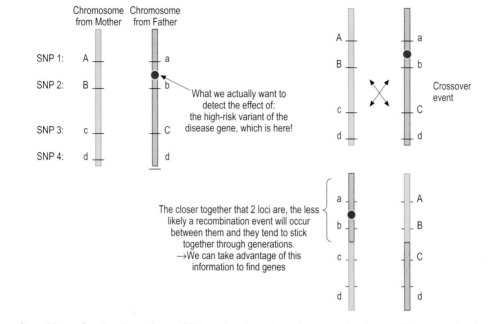

Chromosome from Mother Chromosome from Father

SNP 1: A — a
SNP 2: B — b
What we actually want to detect the effect of: the high-risk variant of the disease gene, which is here!
SNP 3: c — C
SNP 4: d — d

A — a
B — b ● Crossover event
c — C
d — d

The closer together that 2 loci are, the less likely a recombination event will occur between them and they tend to stick together through generations. →We can take advantage of this information to find genes

a — A
b — B
c — C
d — d

Fig. 4.1. Linkage disequilibrium describes the tendency of alleles to be inherited together more often than would be expected under random segregation.

levels has been described in numerous studies.[10–13] The presence of familial aggregation for asthma has been supported by studies reporting that an asthma phenotype is present in approximately 25% of the offspring of a parent with asthma.[10] Higher concordance rates for a disease phenotype in monozygotic twins (who share 100% of their genes) compared with dizygotic twins (who share 50% of their genes identical by descent) also provides important evidence of a genetic component. An increased correlation of total serum IgE levels and a higher concordance of asthma were seen in monozygotic twins compared with dizygotic twins.[11–13]

Although it may be difficult at times to distinguish between a genetic component and shared environment, it is well accepted that there is a significant genetic component to both asthma and allergy. It is also clear that multiple genes with environmental effects, not a few major genes, are responsible for the asthmatic phenotypes.

CURRENT KNOWLEDGE ON GENES ASSOCIATED WITH ASTHMA

Two general approaches have been widely used to study the genetics of asthma: family studies using genome-wide linkage approaches followed by positional cloning and candidate gene association studies usually performed in unrelated asthmatics and controls. The first approach searches for disease susceptibility genes based on their chromosomal location and inheritance of shared chromosomal regions among asthmatics within a given family. This approach uses data from families to identify chromosomal regions that harbor disease-susceptibility genes. Therefore, using this approach, one may find novel genes or pathways regardless of their known physiologic effects as well as known genes with biologic function, possibly, related to asthma.

Candidate gene association studies, on the other hand, evaluate genes that are physiologically suggested (candidates) to be involved in disease pathogenesis. The data for this type of study are usually obtained from unrelated individuals (cases and controls), although family-based methods are also available, such as the 'trio' design, where DNA (without phenotypic information) is obtained from the parents of an asthmatic

A main advantage to case-control candidate studies is the relative ease of obtaining data from well-characterized unrelated asthmatics compared with the difficulties often encountered in recruiting and testing whole family units. In general for most common diseases, investigators have moved towards performing case-control studies instead of family studies, although both approaches have been successful in genetic studies of common diseases such as asthma and allergy.

GENOME-WIDE LINKAGE STUDIES

Genome-wide linkage studies use phenotypic data from all available members of a family (affected and unaffected) and DNA markers to examine whether the markers co-segregate with phenotypes of interest (Fig. 4.1). This approach identifies chromosomal regions that are consistently shared between affected siblings or inherited by affected offspring. The major advantage of linkage studies is that there is no a priori hypothesis of disease pathogenesis. Therefore novel genes or genetic pathways may be identified in regions that have been linked to phenotypes. Positional cloning, which is the identification of a gene from a linkage study, has the advantage of identifying a novel gene, including genes that would not be currently considered a candidate gene based on known biologic processes.

GENOME-WIDE LINKAGE STUDIES

The first step in positional cloning, genome-wide linkage analysis is to genotype family members for a set of highly polymorphic DNA markers, usually tandem repeats and often now SNPs, evenly spread over the whole genome. It is not necessary that these be polymorphisms within genes but simply highly variant markers so that determination of shared chromosomal regions among affected family members is possible. It is important to note that careful and consistent phenotyping is important in family members since the degree of evidence for a shared chromosomal region (containing a susceptibility gene) would be greatly decreased if non-asthmatics are labeled as asthmatics in the data analysis.

By conducting linkage studies, for each marker the analysis will provide a likelihood score (logarithm of odds ratio, LOD) which is a measure of the evidence for linkage between the marker locus and the phenotype of interest. When LOD is between 1.9 and 3.3, it is considered suggestive of linkage while a LOD >3.3 is considered significant evidence for linkage.[14]

The next step, fine mapping, is to include additional markers in regions that are likely to harbor important genes and finally localize the genes involved in pathogenesis. This is an extremely difficult step since the chromosomal region usually detected by family studies is very large and may contain hundreds of genes.

Although positional cloning has been more effective in discovering causal genes for monogenic disorders, there are success stories with regard to asthma genetics. In one of the first linkage study for asthma phenotypes, Daniels et al recruited families from Western Australia and included phenotypic data on asthma, BHR, total serum IgE, and serum eosinophil counts.[15] Except for the study by Daniels et al, which used a 20 cM interval in screening, maps at approximately 10 cM were used in the other linkage studies on asthma-related phenotypes. From these studies there is evidence for linkage to many different chromosomal regions. Perhaps most interesting are those regions showing evidence for linkage in different populations ('replicated' regions), which include chromosomes 1p, 2q, 3q, 4q, 5q, 6p, 11q, 13q, 19p, and 20q.[15–27] However, there are other regions that have been reported in two populations (1q, 2p, 3p, 4p, 7p, 11p, 12q, and 17q).[21,22,26,28–31] Describing all the previous linkage studies is not informative; instead we will concentrate on the linkage studies (Table 4.1) that resulted in six positionally cloned genes, *ADAM33*, *CYFIP2*, *DPP10*, *HLA-G*, *GRPA*, and *PHF11*, for asthma-related phenotypes.[32–37]

ADAM33

Van Eerdewegh et al identified a locus on chromosome 20p13 that was linked to asthma, LOD = 2.94 and bronchial hyperresponsiveness, LOD = 3.93. After genotyping additional markers, they observed evidence that the *ADAM33* gene was significantly associated with asthma using case-control, transmission disequilibrium and haplotype analyses. ADAM proteins are membrane-anchored metalloproteases with diverse functions, which include the shedding of cell-surface proteins such as cytokines and cytokine receptors.[32] We will discuss this gene in more detail in the section on genetic association studies.

CYFIP2

There is strong evidence for linkage between asthma and markers on chromosome 5q33. Noguchi et al performed mutation screening and association analyses of genes in the 9.4-Mb human linkage region.

Linkage analysis revealed that six polymorphisms in cytoplasmic fragile X mental retardation protein (FMRP)-interacting protein 2 gene (*CYFIP2*) were associated significantly with the development of asthma. In real-time quantitative polymerase chain reaction analysis, subjects homozygous for the haplotype overtransmitted to asthma-affected offspring showed a significantly increased level of cytoplasmic FMRP interacting protein 2 gene expression in lymphocytes compared with ones heterozygous for the haplotype.[33]

DPP10

Several reports have linked asthma and related phenotypes to a wide interval between 2q14 and 2q32.[15,23,38,39] Allen et al sequenced the region surrounding their linkage peak and constructed a comprehensive, high-density, single-nucleotide polymorphism (SNP) linkage disequilibrium map. SNP association was limited to the initial exons of a solitary gene of 3.6 kb *(DPP10)*, which extends over 1 Mb of genomic DNA. *DPP10* encodes a homolog of dipeptidyl peptidases (DPPs) that cleave terminal dipeptides from cytokines and chemokines.[34]

HLA-G

Many studies reported linkage of asthma and related phenotypes, especially allergic phenotypes, to chromosome 6p21, making it one of the most replicated region of the genome. As many genes with individually small effects are likely to contribute to risk, identification of susceptibility loci has been challenging. Using four independent samples, Nicholae et al showed evidence in support of *HLA-G* as a novel asthma and bronchial hyperresponsiveness susceptibility gene in the human leukocyte antigen region on chromosome 6p21.[35]

GRPA

Laitinen et al reported a locus for asthma-related traits on chromosome 7p15-p14.[31] *GRPA*, a gene in this region, belongs to the G protein-coupled receptor family. In functional studies, they demonstrated that isoform specific activation of GPRA-A with its agonist, neuropeptide S (NPS), resulted in significant inhibition of cell growth. To clarify disease mechanism, they studied co-expression of the variants without finding any indication that truncated variants would inhibit the receptor transport into the plasma membrane. Furthermore, they detected ubiquitous expression of GPRA-B, and frequent expression of GPRA-A in the epithelia of several organs, including bronchi and gastrointestinal tract. Additionally, they observed aberrant mRNA and protein expression levels of GPRA in the asthmatic bronchi. Finally, they demonstrate that GPRA and NPS are co-expressed in bronchial epithelium. This study provides evidence that GPRA might have functional relevance in modulating asthma by increased expression levels in the relevant tissues under diseased state and by potential inhibitory effect of GPRA-A activation on cell growth.[36]

PHF11

Chromosome 13q14 has showed consistent linkage to atopy and the total serum IgE concentration.[15,22,25] Zhang et al identified association between total serum IgE levels and a novel 13q14 microsatellite and have now localized the underlying quantitative-trait locus (QTL) in a comprehensive single-nucleotide polymorphism (SNP) map. They

Table 4.1 Studies that identified genes for asthma-related phenotypes by positional cloning

Gene	Location	Reference	Function	Phenotype
ADAM33	Chromosome 20	Van Eerdewegh et al 2002[32]	Transmembrane proteins with several distinct domains Involved in cell migration, cell adhesion, cell–cell interactions, and signal transduction	BHR and severity of asthma
CYFIP2	Chromosome 5	Noguchi et al 2005[33]	May be involved in differentiation of T cells	Asthma
DPP10	Chromosome 2	Allen et al 2003[34]	DPP10 encodes a homolog of dipeptidyl peptidases (DPPs) that cleave terminal dipeptides from cytokines and chemokines	Asthma – severe asthma
GRPA	Chromosome 7	Laitinen et al 2001[31]	G protein-coupled receptor for asthma susceptibility	Asthma and high total serum IgE levels
HLA-G	Chromosome 6	Nicolae et al 2005[35]	May inhibit Th-1-mediated inflammation	Asthma, BHR
PHF11	Chromosome 13	Zhang et al 2003[37]	PDH Finger Protein 11 includes two zinc finger motifs in the translated protein which suggests a role in transcriptional regulation	Asthma, serum IgE levels

BHR, Bronchial hyperresponsiveness; IgE, immunoglobulin E.

found evidence for association to IgE levels and severe clinical asthma that were attributed to several alleles in a single gene, *PHF11*. The gene product (PHF11) contains two PHD zinc fingers and may regulate transcription.[37]

CANDIDATE GENE APPROACH

BASIC PRINCIPLES AND POTENTIAL PROBLEMS

The selection of a gene as candidate is based either on its biological function in asthma pathogenesis or evidence of linkage to asthma-related phenotypes. Examples for the first set of genes are those encoding cytokines, chemokines, and their receptors as well as transcription factors, IgE receptor, etc. Using data, usually from unrelated individuals, candidate gene association studies investigate whether allele or genotype frequencies are different in cases with asthma-related phenotypes than unaffected controls. The markers that are usually used to conduct association studies are single nucleotide polymorphisms (SNPs). These are the most common type of polymorphism and it has been estimated that the human genome contains about 10 million SNPs. For a SNP to be useful for association studies, it should have a frequency of at least 10% in the population. Compared with linkage studies, one advantage of association studies with candidate genes is their ability to identify genetic variations that have relatively small effects on susceptibility. Also, association

studies are more efficient in terms of recruiting subjects and financial burden. However, the choice of controls could be difficult because ideally the subjects need to be matched for variables that may confound the results, for example, age, sex, and ethnic background. The other problem is interpretation of the results from association studies may be complicated and there have been some efforts to implement stringent criteria for legitimacy of a candidate gene association study.[40]

One of the main problems of association studies is inflated type I error or false-positive results. Using a p-value of 0.05 as the threshold for significance is equivalent to 5% type I error rate and means that for every 20 tests one 'finding by chance' is expected. The main source for type I error is multiple comparisons because of having multiple polymorphisms in the same gene, polymorphisms in multiple genes, or multiple phenotypes. In these cases, $p < 0.05$ (5% tolerance as the false-positive findings rate when the null hypothesis is not accepted) is no longer applicable because there is a 5% type I error rate expected with each independent comparison (e.g., with polymorphisms in different genes).

Another source of type I error is the large number of negative association studies with candidate genes that are never reported. Because the reported p-values are rarely adjusted for the total number of studies performed (both reported and unreported), the type I error rate in the reported studies is actually higher than the true level. Type I errors can also result from genotyping errors, particularly if there is a systematic error such as overcalling one genotype over another. Lastly, type I errors can result from population substructure, or sampling cases and controls that differ with respect to ethnic background. Because allele frequencies vary among ethnic groups, great care must be taken to assure that case and control subjects have similar ethnic compositions. If they differ, an allele may be significantly more frequent in the cases compared with controls due to differences in ethnicity, but this may be misinterpreted as an association with the disease.

There are several methods to modify inflated type I error in genetic association studies. A simple way of correction for multiple comparisons is known as a Bonferroni correction. In this method, the threshold p-value (usually 0.05) is divided by the number of comparisons. For example, in a study of 10 variants, one would need to obtain a p-value of 0.005 to have the equivalent of a 5% type I error rate. However, the Bonferroni correction can be overly conservative if the multiple tests correspond to correlated variables. For example, phenotypes are often correlated (e.g., asthma and IgE levels), as are the genotypes of SNPs that are in linkage disequilibrium (LD, Fig. 4.2). Thus, these comparisons do not represent independent tests and the Bonferroni correction can be excessive.[41] Because there is no simple correction for multiple correlated comparisons, alternative methods to correct for the error rates are used. Permutation tests are useful because they preserve the correlation structure of the data and provide accurate p-values. They can be used to control the probability of committing any type I error and this can lead to stringent thresholds in studies with a large number of candidate genes. An alternative approach is to control the False Discovery Rate (FDR), which is the proportion of false positives in the set of rejected hypotheses.[42] FDR is a more liberal rate to control, so it is more powerful. With regard to false-positive results due to genotype errors, one approach is to test for Hardy–Weinberg proportions for the genotypes especially in control subjects.

Systematic errors in genotyping will often yield genotype frequencies that are not in Hardy–Weinberg proportions. Markers showing departure from Hardy–Weinberg equilibrium should not be automatically discarded because deviation from Hardy–Weinberg equilibrium among cases is expected for variants close to a susceptibility locus.[43] Nevertheless, markers that show deviations from expectations should be carefully monitored and retyped to ensure that they are correctly genotyped. Finally, for population stratification, there are methods to directly test for stratification and to correct for any imbalances by genotyping the case and control samples for loci that discriminate between pairs of racial or ethnic groups.[44]

The gold standard to handle type I error is the replication of findings in other populations. However, not all associations that are not replicated are false-positive results. An association may not be replicated because of different patterns of LD in different populations. Differences in LD patterns can be caused by differences in allele frequencies and/or the presence of more than one causal variant. This can be addressed by examining haplotypes instead of single SNPs. Some studies have shown that examining multiple SNPs as haplotypes is preferable to single SNP analysis.[45] A haplotype is composed of alleles at different loci that are inherited together on the same chromosome. Thus, even if the disease-causing variant itself is not identified, a shared haplotype that contains the disease variant will be more common in cases than in controls. In addition, this could help to identify the true susceptibility variant.

Another reason for non-replication could be different phenotype definition between studies. For example, the phenotype 'atopy' has been defined as a positive skin prick test (SPT), a positive RAST test, high total serum IgE, or a combination of these tests. Although these phenotypes are clearly related, it is likely that some genes that influence total IgE levels do not influence specific IgE response to allergens, and vice versa. Lastly, positive associations may not be replicated because the true model of genetic susceptibility for diseases such as asthma and atopy is complex. It is highly possible that any particular susceptibility variant has a relatively minor effect on the phenotype and that the magnitude of its effect will be influenced by genes at other loci (gene–gene interactions, epistasis) and by the environmental factors (gene–environment interactions).[46,47] Because background genes and environmental factors differ between populations, it would not be surprising if associations with single SNPs or haplotypes differed between populations.

A statistically significant association between a variant in a candidate gene and a disease phenotype can have three possible explanations.[3] The marker allele truly affects gene function by altering the amino acid sequence or by modifying splicing, transcriptional properties, or mRNA stability, and thereby directly affects disease risk.[1] The marker allele is in linkage disequilibrium (LD) with the true disease-causing variant. LD or allelic association is the non-random association of alleles at linked loci in populations, and will usually only be detected over small distances (= 60 approximated kb), although LD over longer distances has been observed. Thus, the marker allele must be located in relatively close proximity to the disease-causing variant (Fig. 4.1).[2] The association is a false-positive result (type I error).

CANDIDATE GENE ASSOCIATION STUDIES FOR ASTHMA-RELATED PHENOTYPES

There are more than 120 genes that have been reported to be associated with an asthma- or atopy-related phenotype. About half of these have been replicated in independent samples. The 10 highly replicated genes are interleukin-4 (*IL4*), IL-4 receptor (*IL4RA*), interleukin-13 (*IL13*), β_2-adrenergic receptor (*ADRβ2*), human leukocyte antigen DRB1 (*HLA-DRB1*), human leukocyte antigen DQB1 (*HLA-DQB1*), tumor necrosis factor (*TNF*), lymphotoxin-α (*LTA*), high-affinity IgE receptor (*FCER1B*), and *ADAM33*. From these genes we will use examples to illustrate the principles of association studies, including *IL13* because of its well known role in the pathogenesis of asthma, *ADRβ2* because of its implication in asthma therapy and pharmacogenetics, and *ADAM33* because it has found by positional cloning and also studied in association studies for both asthma susceptibility and severity.

IL-13

IL-13 is a Th2 cytokine that has been identified as a critical regulator of the allergic response. Studies in animal models of asthma suggest that IL-13 is necessary and sufficient to induce many pathophysiologic features of allergic asthma.[48] The importance of IL-13 in humans became more significant as strong associations between IL-13 levels and functional polymorphisms were observed.[49,50]

IL13 maps to a genomic region, 5q31, frequently linked to asthma,[51,52] total serum IgE,[53,54] airway responsiveness,[54] and other asthma-related phenotypes.[55] Two well-characterized single nucleotide polymorphisms (SNPs) in *IL13* are a promoter SNP (-1112C/T) and a coding SNP in exon 4 ($Arg_{130}Gln$). These two variants may be functionally important. For example in CD4+ T_H2 lymphocytes, enhanced *IL13* promoter activity was detected for -1112T allele compared with -1112C allele.[56] Also studies showed that the 130Gln substitution results in signal transduction and activation of transcription 6 (STAT6) phosphorylation in monocytes, decreased affinity of IL-13 for IL-13 receptor α-2, and increased expression of IL-13 in patients with asthma.[49,57] These polymorphisms have been associated with asthma and related phenotypes in some studies[58,59] but not in others.[60,61] The most consistent association has been with total serum IgE.[62–66]

ADRβ2

Agonists of β_2-adrenergic receptor are the most commonly used class of medication in the treatment of asthma worldwide and β_2-adrenergic receptor gene (*ADRβ2*) may affect asthma severity.[67] Two common functional variants in *ADRβ2* have been well characterized.[68] Individuals who are homozygous for glycine at position 16 may have more severe asthma and less response to bronchodilator therapy compared to arginine homozygotes.[68,69] However, new studies suggest that it is controversial and is described further in the section on pharmacogenetics. To understand the function of *ADRβ2* in asthma, a comprehensive evaluation of gene variation, haplotype structure, and linkage disequilibrium is critical. In a recent report on *ADRβ2* sequence in several ethnic groups, 49 polymorphisms were identified. In addition to a previously reported coding variant, $Gly_{16}Arg$, 21 novel SNPs and a poly C repeat in the 3' untranslated region were observed. These data suggest that the length of the poly-C repeat may influence lung function and may be important in understanding why individuals respond differently to β-agonist.[70]

ADAM33

The *ADAM33* gene is associated with asthma and airway hyperresponsiveness and is postulated to represent a gene that is involved in regulating structural components of the airways, 'airway remodeling' in asthma. In the first replication study after cloning of *ADAM33*, Howard et al evaluated eight SNPs in the 3' portion of this gene in four asthma populations (African-American, US non-Hispanic white, US Hispanic, and Dutch), and observed significant associations with at least one SNP with asthma in each population ($p=0.0009–0.04$). For asthma susceptibility, significant associations were observed for at least one of the eight SNPs within each population, but no single SNP was consistently associated within all groups. This replication study in four ethnic groups is important; however, *ADAM33* is a large gene (>20 kb) and further evaluation of additional SNPs is needed. A number of studies have replicated these findings, showing that *ADAM33* is a susceptibility gene for asthma in different populations,[71–73] but some studies have not been able to replicate these findings.[74,75] In a cohort of 200 Dutch asthma patients followed for over 20 years, eight single nucleotide polymorphisms were genotyped within the *ADAM33* gene. The S2 polymorphism was significantly associated with an excess decline in FEV_1 after correction for multiple testing.[72] These findings suggest that a variant in *ADAM33* is not only important in the development of asthma but also in disease progression, possibly related to enhanced airway remodeling. In a birth cohort study, children were genotyped for 17 SNPs in *ADAM33* to test for association with early measures of lung function at age 3 ($n=285$) and 5 years ($n=470$). This report concluded that polymorphisms in *ADAM33* predict impaired early-life lung function and suggested that

the functionally relevant polymorphism is likely to be at the 5' end of the gene.[76] Thus, this is an example of a gene that is relevant to both disease susceptibility and disease progression.

GENE BY GENE INTERACTION

Similar to other complex genetic diseases, it has been shown that genes involved in the pathogenesis of asthma interplay with each other (Fig. 4.2). An example of gene–gene interaction in asthma includes *IL13* and *IL4* genes. Binding of IL-13 and IL-4 to their common receptor (IL-4 receptor α, IL-4Rα) induces the initial response for Th2 lymphocyte polarization. Both IL-13 and IL-4 are produced by Th2 cells and are capable of inducing isotype class-switching of B cells to produce IgE after allergen exposure. In a case-control study design in a Dutch population, a significant gene–gene interaction between the SNP S478P in *IL4RA* and the -1112C/T promoter polymorphism in *IL13* was detected. Individuals with the risk genotype for both genes were at almost five times greater risk for the development of asthma compared to individuals with both non-risk genotypes ($p=0.0004$). These data suggest that an interaction between *IL4Rα* and *IL13* markedly increases an individual's susceptibility to asthma.[46] Another study on a large cross-sectional population of 1120 children aged 9–11 years indicated that the combinations of genetic variations in the *IL4/IL13* pathway are significantly related to the development of atopy and childhood asthma.[65]

GENE–ENVIRONMENT INTERACTION IN ASTHMA

The evidence for the increased prevalence of asthma in the last decades is strongly suggestive of an important environmental component to the pathogenesis of asthma, and potential for gene–environment interaction. A dominant opinion of asthma pathogenesis is that onset of the disease and its clinical course are determined by gene–environment interactions, suggesting that individuals who develop asthma are both genetically susceptible and are exposed to a triggering environmental stimulus. Among asthmatics in the population, the relative influence of genes and environmental factors probably varies and that individuals with different asthma-related genotypes have different sensitivities to environmental exposures. Several possible patterns for gene–environment interaction have been suggested.[6] For example, both the presence of a given asthma susceptibility gene and an environmental exposure may be necessary to produce excess risk of a disease. With regards to asthma, there are extensive data showing that tobacco smoking increases airway responsiveness.[77,78]

There is also evidence suggesting that exposure to tobacco smoke during pregnancy may affect airway responsiveness after birth.[79] Several studies have suggested that genetic predisposition changes the effect of tobacco exposure on asthma-related phenotypes.[24,80,81] Passive smoke, as defined by parental smoking during gestation and early childhood, is a risk factor for the development of atopy and asthma, especially in utero cigarette smoke exposure as well as exposure in the first few months of life.[82] In our Dutch study,[24] an even stronger influence of the effects of passive exposure to cigarette smoke on the genome screen linkage results were observed than found previously in the collaborative study on the genetics of asthma (CSGA).[83] The families in

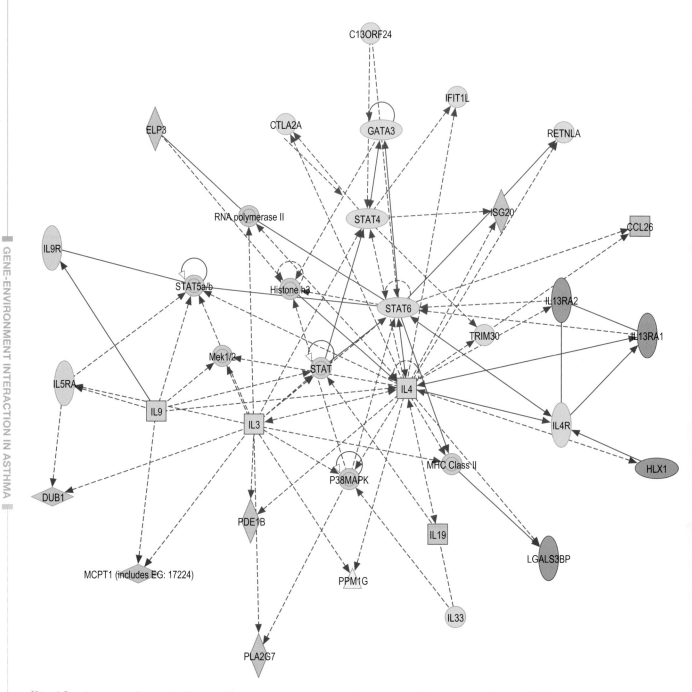

Fig. 4.2. A network of inter-related genes with some members suggested as important candidate genes in asthma and Th2 immune response. (Courtesy of Ingenuity Systems, Inc, Redword City, CA, USA.)

which the children were exposed to passive smoking accounted for all of the evidence for linkage of BHR to 5q. Stronger evidence for linkage to BHR than to asthma was observed in these Dutch families. This is an interesting finding because while all probands with asthma had evidence of BHR, an additional 15% of offspring had asymptomatic BHR. Thus, the linkage on 5q for BHR represents a broader category

that included both family members with diagnosed and symptomatic asthma and those potentially at risk for developing asthma (asymptomatic BHR).

Another example on gene–environment interaction is the opposite effects of *CD14* polymorphism on serum IgE levels in children raised in different environments. CD14 is a pattern recognition receptor for microbial molecules and it was previously reported that a polymorphism in the promoter region of *CD14* (-260 C/T) and serum IgE levels were associated. In 624 children living in two rural communities in Europe, a study compared total and specific serum IgE levels between the genotypes of *CD14/-260* in relation to exposure to animals. The results of this study suggested that the C allele of *CD14/-260* was associated with higher levels of serum IgE to aeroallergens in children with regular contact with pets, whereas in children with regular contact with stable animals, T allele of *CD14/-260* was associated higher levels of serum IgE (associations in opposite directions). These results suggest that the type and concentrations of microbial molecules present in the environment strongly determine the direction of the association between *CD14/-260* and serum markers of atopy.[84]

■ PHARMACOGENOMICS OF ASTHMA ■

Pharmacogenetics refers to the relationship between genotype (genetic variation) and drug response. The term pharmacogenomics is usually used when many genes or the whole genome is analyzed, similar to the genome-wide association studies that are being performed with hundreds of thousands of SNPs for disease susceptibility. It is important to remember that pharmacogenetic studies are still genetic association studies, but only patients with the disease of interest are studied and the outcome is individual response to therapy. The same issues as seen in case-control association studies need to be considered, including sample size and statistical power, population stratification, quality and completeness of phenotyping, and appropriate adjustment for the number of SNPs and genes analyzed. Pharmacogenetics is essentially a gene–environment study where the therapy is the environment.

β_2-receptor agonists, including the short-acting β-agonists (SABAs) and the long-acting β-agonists (LABAs) continue to be widely used in asthma therapy. When analyzing any possible pharmacogenetic response, it is important to consider current guidelines as to the use of a given drug, including dose, therapeutic indications, and whether it is usually used in conjunction with other therapeutic agents. The bronchodilator response obtained from use of a β-agonist may vary between subjects and could be influenced by common factors such as age, sex, and ethnicity, as well as the severity of asthma and airway obstruction, and the concurrent use of medications such as corticosteroids.[85]

The main area of pharmacogenetic research in asthma is the β_2-adrenergic receptor, and the ongoing research will be described as an example of pharmacogenetic studies. The β_2-adrenergic receptor is a G-protein coupled receptor encoded by the gene *ADRβ2*, a single exon gene.[86] Reihsaus et al[68] first described the genetic variation in *ADRβ2*, including two relatively common amino acid changes $Gly_{16}Arg$, and $Gln_{27}Glu$ which are in partial linkage disequilibrium.

In 1997, Martinez et al[69] genotyped the $Gly_{16}Arg$ and $Gln_{27}Glu$ variants in children and tested for association with the change in FEV_1 after administration of the SABA, albuterol. They concluded that there was an effect for the $Gly_{16}Arg$ genotypes but not the $Gln_{27}Glu$ genotypes. The homozygous Arg/Arg children had a great response to albuterol than Arg/Gly or Gly/Gly children.

Two clinical trial studies published in 2000 showed evidence that Arg/Arg subjects did not respond as well to the short-acting β-agonist albuterol based on outcome variables, including changes in peak flow rates and lung function (Table 4.2). These studies were not designed to test pharmacogenetics, so the number of Arg/Arg subjects was small ($n = 17, 16$).[87,88] Therefore, the NHLBI Asthma Clinical Trials Network designed a clinical trial where subjects were genotyped before enrollment in order to have a similar number of Arg/Arg and Gly/Gly subjects. This 'BARGE' study showed evidence that the Arg/Arg subjects do not respond as well to SABA therapy compared to Gly/Gly subjects. Due to sample size restrictions, the heterozygotes were not studied. In general, it is important to analyze all three genotypes and determine whether there is a dominant or recessive effect. A study on the SABA fenoterol did not show evidence for a pharmacogenetic effect although there were only 12 Arg/Arg subjects.[89]

Given the use of LABAs, it is obviously important to determine if there is a pharmacogenetic effect similar to the potential effect described for SABAs. Although Taylor et al observed that Arg/Arg patients had an increase in asthma exacerbations when treated regularly with albuterol, a similar effect was not observed for the LABA salmeterol.[87] However, analysis of data from two ACRN trials provided evidence for an Arg/Arg effect in subjects treated with LABAs. Given the size of the trials and the fact that they were not designed for pharmacogenetic analysis, the number of Arg/Arg subjects is very small ($n = 12$ and 8, see Table 4.2). In a somewhat larger study of 29 Arg/Arg subjects, no effect was observed for treatment with the same LABA, salmeterol.

There are clearly differences besides sample size that may have led to the differing results from the clinical trials described, including the design of the study and the criteria used to select the asthmatic subjects. It is also important to interpret results in terms of current guidelines for asthma therapy which, for example, emphasize the importance of inhaled corticosteroid therapy in conjunction with use of β-agonists.

Due to the pharmacogenetics interest in this gene, Hawkins et al resequenced *ADRβ2* in a large number of subjects, both non-Hispanic whites and African-Americans and found additional genetic variation, both rare and common.[70] The degree of polymorphism and the resulting number of haplotypes differed between the ethnic groups. Although, the rare variants may have a role in a small number of subjects, the key question is whether other relatively common variants in this gene may be associated with response to β-agonist therapy.

The possible relationship between *ADRβ2* genetic variations and β-agonist response is still being debated. In general, there appears to be an affect of the $Gln_{16}Arg$ genotypes when using SABA therapies. However, these studies each contain a small number of subjects with the at-risk genotype (Arg/Arg) and larger studies would be more convincing. Larger studies need to be performed analyzing multiple SNPs in this gene as well as thoroughly genotyping other relevant genes in the pathway. Ideally, this should be performed in multiple ethnic groups since the degree of polymorphism varies between ethnic groups as well as the frequency and severity of asthma. Additional studies of LABAs are especially needed since the current results are inconclusive, although the larger studies do not support a pharmacogenetic effect.

Pharmacogenetics and pharmacogenomics are important areas of research that may lead to individualized therapies for certain diseases. It is most likely that multiple genes, each with a relatively small effect, will be related to drug response, just as variation in multiple genes is associated with susceptibility to many common diseases. In the future, genetic testing may be used to decrease the frequency of adverse effects such as toxicity and to optimize treatment response.

Table 4.2 Clinical trials utilizing pharmacogenetic data on short-(SABA) and long-acting (LABA) β-agonist response

Study	Trial design	β-agonist	Duration (weeks)	Steroid therapy	Arg/Arg studied (n)	Principal outcome	Arg_{16}/Arg_{16} effect
Taylor et al 2000[87]	PC, XO	Albuterol (SABA)	24	Yes	17	AM/PM PEFR, FEV_1, PC_{20}	Yes
Israel et al 2000[88]	PC, PG	Albuterol (SABA)	16	No	16	AM/PM PEFR, albuterol use, FEV_1, symptoms	Yes
Israel et al 2004[88a]	PC, XO	Albuterol (SABA)	16	No	37	AM/PM PEFR, symptoms	Yes
Hancox et al 1998[89]	PC, XO	Fenoterol (SABA)	24	No	12	AM PEFR, exacerbations, FEV_1, PC_{20}	No
Taylor et al 2000[87]	PC, XO	Salmeterol (LABA)	24	Yes	17	AM PEFR, exacerbations	No
Weschler et al 2006[88b]	PG	Salmeterol SOCS (LABA)	28	No	12	AM/PM PEFR, FEV_1, PC_{20}, symptoms	Yes
Weschler et al 2006[88b]	PG	Salmeterol SLIC (LABA)	24	Yes	8	AM/PM PEFR, FEV_1, PC_{20}, symptoms	Yes
Bleecker et al 2006[88c]	PC	Salmeterol (LABA)	12	yes	29	AM PEFR, FEV_1, albuterol use, symptoms	No

All studies were randomized double-blind trials. PC, placebo controlled; XO, crossover; PG, parallel group.

NEW APPROACHES TO ASTHMA GENETICS

FUNCTIONAL GENOMICS

This approach can be a complementary step after positional cloning or association studies for identifying disease genes. It also includes high-throughput techniques such as RNA microarrays, proteomics, metabolomics, and mutation analysis to describe the function of genes. These methods have the potential to identify thousands of genes simultaneously and quantification of specific differential expression under varying physiologic conditions or between cases and controls. One possibility in this approach is to study the physiologic impact of a polymorphism. For example the effect of *IL13+2044Gγα* on the functional properties of IL-13 has been investigated. This SNP changes arginine to glutamine at position 130 in IL-13. The activity of wild-type IL-13 (arginine at position 130) and minor variant of IL-13 (glutamine at position 130) on primary human cells has been studied. The results have shown that minor variant of IL-13 was significantly more active than wild-type IL-13. Also a decreased neutralization of the minor variant was shown to result in an enhanced in vivo activity. Therefore, natural variation in the coding region of *IL13* may be an important genetic determinant of susceptibility to allergy.[49] Multiple association studies have shown evidence for an association of *IL13* polymorphisms and measures of asthma and atopy. The association

results led to the functional studies which are often time consuming and extensive. However, with the advent of new technologies, it may become reasonable to screen a large number of genes for functional relevance and then perform association studies in the relevant populations.

COMPARATIVE GENOMICS

The idea behind this approach is to search for comparable (homologous) genomic regions that affect similar phenotypes in two species. This method is considered a powerful tool in the search for the genes in quantitative trait loci (QTLs) in various ways. Finding a QTL in homologous regions in different species can be interpreted as a replication of that locus and increases the confidence for the presence of a gene in that region. The basic hypothesis is that genes that have survived evolutionary stresses and are present today in multiple species are likely to have important functional roles. Comparative genomics may be useful in narrowing down the QTL regions for both species. For example, when a QTL is found in a region homologous between human and mouse, it is reasonable to consider that a single gene has been responsible for the linkage in both species. It is possible to have a cluster of genes with more than one common gene that are responsible for the phenotypes in the two species. However, the number of genes in common is likely to be much smaller that the number in the linked region in each species; therefore, decreasing the number of genes that need to be studied further.

So far about 340 conserved chromosomal segments between human and mouse have been identified.[90]

GENOME-WIDE ASSOCIATION STUDIES

Although genes have been identified for common diseases such as asthma and allergy from studies of candidate or pathway genes in cases and controls, it would be more powerful if it was possible to scan the whole genome in cases versus controls to identify multiple susceptibility genes, each alone contributing a small effect. This is now possible due to both the HapMap project and the advances in genotyping technology. Chips are now available for genotyping 100 000–1 000 000 SNPs/person. The cost has decreased and the accuracy rates have increased making this a powerful approach for studying the genetics of common diseases. This approach will localize the susceptibility locus to a much smaller region (10–500 kb) than is typically possible in a linkage study and in some situations provide fine mapping markers at the same time. Using SNPs, the first genome-wide studies for complex diseases, case-control designs, were reported in 2005[91] and afterward for other common diseases including asthma.[92] Compared to traditional candidate gene association studies, genome-wide association studies may identify novel genes and pathways. Their advantage over linkage studies in that they can identify genes with small effects. It is expected that genome-wide association studies in large populations of cases and controls will become the next standard approaches to gene discovery.

One of the main problems with genome-wide association studies is the large number of false-positive results given the number of genotypes analyzed. As discussed previously, false-positive results are a major issue in association studies and even more of an issue in genome-wide association studies. Replication in additional populations of positive findings is crucial (Fig. 4.3). In addition, given the large expense and difficulties in performing such large studies in thousands of subjects, it is very important that the subjects are well phenotyped so that disease status and associated phenotypes can be analyzed.

The first genome-wide association study has been published for asthma.[92] In this study, >300 000 SNPs were used to map their association with childhood asthma in 994 patients and 1243 non-asthmatics. The study detected multiple markers on chromosome 17q21 to be strongly associated with childhood-onset asthma (Fig. 4.4). In two independent replication studies the 17q21 locus showed strong association with diagnosis of childhood asthma. In another step, markers of the 17q21

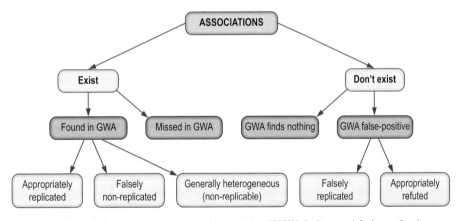

Fig. 4.3. Different possibilities at the level of associations, genome-wide association (GWA) findings, and findings of replication studies. (Reproduced from Ioannidis JP. Non-replication and inconsistency in the genome-wide association setting. Hum Hered 2007; 64:203–213[92b]).

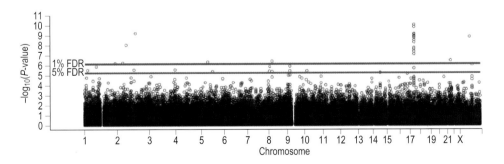

Fig. 4.4. Position in the genome, divided by chromosome, is depicted along the x-axis. Strength of association is shown on the y-axis. The result for each individual marker is depicted as a black circle. The genome-wide thresholds for 1% and 5% false discovery rates (FDR) are shown as horizontal red lines. Numerous markers on chromosome 17q21 show association to asthma above the 1% FDR threshold in the region of maximum association. (Reproduced from Moffatt MF, Kabesch M, Liang L, et al. Genetic variants regulating ORMDL3 expression contribute to the risk of childhood asthma. Nature 2007; 448:470–473.[92])

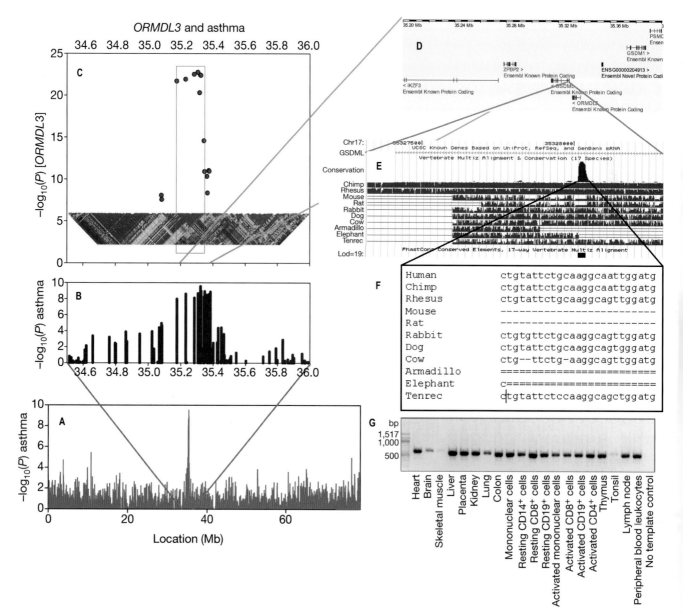

Fig. 4.5. Association to asthma and transcript abundances of *ORMDL3* on chromosome 17q21. (A) Mapping of association to asthma on chromosome 17. (B) Detail of association to SNPs on chromosome 17q21. (C) Association to *ORMDL3* transcript abundance with the same markers. A GOLD plot[93] of linkage disequilibrium between markers is also shown, with red indicating high linkage disequilibrium and blue denoting low. The central island of linkage disequilibrium, which contains maximum association to *ORMDL3* and asthma, is contained within the grey rectangle. (D) Genes contained within the associated interval. (E) Homology plot from the region of maximum association. (F) Sequence homology from intron I of *GSDML*. (G) RT-PCR (34 cycles) of *ORMDL3* cDNA from representative tissues (Clontech). (Reproduced from Moffatt MF, Kabesch M, Liang L, et al Genetic variants regulating ORMDL3 expression contribute to the risk of childhood asthma. Nature 2007; 448: 470–473.[92])

locus and transcript levels of genes in Epstein–Barr virus (EBV)-transformed lymphoblastoid cell lines were evaluated and revealed to be related (Fig. 4.5).[93] This report concluded that *ORMDL3*, a member of a gene family that encodes transmembrane proteins anchored in the endoplasmic reticulum, affects susceptibility to childhood asthma. Strong aspects of this genome-wide association study are the large sample size and use of several independent populations along with the expression experiment. However, it had the limitation of not having a homogeneous characterization for asthma and not using objective asthma-related phenotypes such as BHR in the analysis.[92] This may be the reason for only detecting one major genomic region, since it would be expected to detect multiple regions, including genes previously associated with asthma.

References

Introduction

1. Jarvis D, Burney P. ABC of allergies. The epidemiology of allergic disease. BMJ 1998; 316:607–610.
2. Arshad SH, Tariq SM, Matthews S, et al. Sensitization to common allergens and its association with allergic disorders at age 4 years: a whole population birth cohort study. Pediatrics 2001; 108:E33.
3. National Institutes of Health. National Heart Lung, and Blood Institute Global strategy for asthma management and prevention. Updated 2006. Online. Available: http://www.ginasthma.org.
4. Weiss KB, Sullivan SD. The health economics of asthma and rhinitis. I. Assessing the economic impact. J Allergy Clin Immunol 2001; 107:3–8.
5. Mannino DM, Homa DM, Pertowski CA, et al. Surveillance for asthma – United States, 1960–1995. MMWR CDC Surveill Summ 1998; 47:1–27.

Phenotype definition

6. Wiesch DG, Meyers DA, Bleecker ER. Genetics of asthma. J Allergy Clin Immunol 1999; 104:895–901.
7. Maestrelli P, di Stefano A, Occari P, et al. Cytokines in the airway mucosa of subjects with asthma induced by toluene diisocyanate. Am J Respir Crit Care Med 1995; 151:607–612.
8. Holt PG, Macaubas C, Stumbles PA, et al. The role of allergy in the development of asthma. Nature 1999; 402:B12–17.
9. Zhu Z, Homer RJ, Wang Z, et al. Pulmonary expression of interleukin-13 causes inflammation, mucus hypersecretion, subepithelial fibrosis, physiologic abnormalities, and eotaxin production. J Clin Invest 1999; 103:779–788.

Evidence for a genetic component in asthma

10. Panhuysen CI, Bleecker ER, Koeter GH, et al. Characterization of obstructive airway disease in family members of probands with asthma. An algorithm for the diagnosis of asthma. Am J Resp Crit Care Med 1998; 157:1734–1742.
11. Hopp RJ, Bewtra AK, Watt GD, et al. Genetic analysis of allergic disease in twins. J Allergy Clin Immunol 1984; 73:265–270.
12. Edfors-Lubs ML. Allergy in 7000 twin pairs. Acta Allergol 1971; 26:249–285.
13. Duffy DL, Martin NG, Battistutta D, et al. Genetics of asthma and hay fever in Australian twins. Am Rev Respir Dis 1990; 142:1351–1358.

Genome-wide linkage studies

14. Lander ES, Schork NJ. Genetic dissection of complex traits. Science 1994; 265:2037–2048.
15. Daniels SE, Bhattacharrya S, James A, et al. A genome-wide search for quantitative trait loci underlying asthma. Nature 1996; 383:247–250.
16. Xu J, Meyers DA, Ober C, et al. Genomewide screen and identification of gene-gene interactions for asthma-susceptibility loci in three U.S. populations: collaborative study on the genetics of asthma. Am J Hum Genet 2001; 68:1437–1446.
17. Evans DM, Zhu G, Duffy DL, et al. Major quantitative trait locus for eosinophil count is located on chromosome 2q. J Allergy Clin Immunol 2004; 114:826–830.
18. Huang SK, Mathias RA, Ehrlich E, et al. Evidence for asthma susceptibility genes on chromosome 11 in an African-American population. Hum Genet 2003; 113:71–75.
19. Blumenthal MN, Ober C, Beaty TH, et al. Genome scan for loci linked to mite sensitivity: the collaborative study on the genetics of asthma (CSGA). Genes Immun 2004; 5:226–231.
20. Blumenthal MN, Langefeld CD, Beaty TH, et al. A genome-wide search for allergic response (atopy) genes in three ethnic groups: collaborative study on the genetics of asthma. Hum Genet 2004; 114:157–164.
21. Ober C, Tsalenko A, Parry R, et al. A second-generation genomewide screen for asthma-susceptibility alleles in a founder population. Am J Hum Genet 2000; 67:1154–1162.
22. Xu J, Postma DS, Howard TD, et al. Major genes regulating total serum immunoglobulin E levels in families with asthma. Am J Hum Genet 2000; 67:1163–1173.
23. Koppelman GH, Stine OC, Xu J, et al. Genome-wide search for atopy susceptibility genes in Dutch families with asthma. J Allergy Clin Immunol 2002; 109:498–506.
24. Meyers DA, Postma DS, Stine OC, et al. Genome screen for asthma and bronchial hyperresponsiveness: interactions with passive smoke exposure. J Allergy Clin Immunol 2005; 115:1169–1175.
25. Yokouchi Y, Nukaga Y, Shibasaki M, et al. Significant evidence for linkage to mite-sensitive childhood asthma to chromosome 5q31-q33 near the interleukin 12 B locus by a genome-wide search in Japanese families. Genomics 2000; 66:152–160.
26. Dizier MH, Besse-Schmittler C, Guilloud-Bataille M, et al. Genome screen for asthma and related phenotypes in the French EGEA study. Am J Respir Crit Care Med 2000; 162:1812–1818.
27. Haagerup A, Bjerke T, Schiotz PO, et al. Asthma and atopy – a total genome scan for susceptibility genes. Allergy 2002; 57:680–686.
28. Xu X, Fang Z, Wang B, et al. A genomewide search for quantitative-trait loci underlying asthma. Am J Hum Genet 2001; 69:1271–1277.
29. Ferreira MA, O'Gorman L, Le Souef P, et al. Robust estimation of experiment wise p values applied to a genome scan of multiple asthma traits identifies a new region of significant linkage on chromosome 20q13. Am J Hum Genet 2005; 77:1075–1085.
30. Pillai SG, Chiano MN, White NJ, et al. A genome-wide search for linkage to asthma phenotypes in the genetics of asthma international network families: evidence for a major susceptibility locus on chromosome 2p. Eur J Hum Genet 2006; 14:307–316.

31. Laitinen T, Daly MJ, Rioux JD, et al. A susceptibility locus for asthma-related traits on chromosome 7 revealed by genome-wide scan in a founder population. Nat Genet 2001; 28:87–91.
32. Van Eerdewegh P, Little RD, Dupuis J, et al. Association of the adam33 gene with asthma and bronchial hyperresponsiveness. Nature 2002; 418:426–430.
33. Noguchi E, Yokouchi Y, Zhang J, et al. Positional identification of an asthma susceptibility gene on human chromosome 5q33. Am J Resp Crit Care Med 2005; 172:183–188.
34. Allen M, Heinzmann A, Noguchi E, et al. Positional cloning of a novel gene influencing asthma from chromosome 2q14. Nat Genet 2003; 35:258–263.
35. Nicolae D, Cox NJ, Lester LA, et al. Fine mapping and positional candidate studies identify HLA-G as an asthma susceptibility gene on chromosome 6p21. Am J Hum Genet 2005; 76:349–357.
36. Vendelin J, Pulkkinen V, Rehn M, et al. Characterization of GPRA, a novel G protein-coupled receptor related to asthma. Am J Resp Cell Mol Biol 2005; 33:262–270.
37. Zhang Y, Leaves NI, Anderson GG, et al. Positional cloning of a quantitative trait locus on chromosome 13q14 that influences immunoglobulin E levels and asthma. Nat Genet 2003; 34:181–186.
38. Hizawa N, Freidhoff LR, Chiu YF, et al. Genetic regulation of Dermatophagoides pteronyssinus-specific IgE responsiveness: a genome-wide multipoint linkage analysis in families recruited through 2 asthmatic sibs. Collaborative study on the genetics of asthma (CSGA). J Allergy Clin Immunol 1998; 102:436–442.
39. Wjst M, Fischer G, Immervoll T, et al. A genome-wide search for linkage to asthma. German Asthma Genetics Group. Genomics 1999; 58:1–8.

Candidate gene approach

40. Weiss ST. Association studies in asthma genetics. Am J Respir Crit Care Med 2001; 164:2014–2015.
41. Schwager SJ. Bonferroni sometimes loses. Am Stat 1984; 38:192–197.
42. Benjamini Y, Hochberg Y. Controlling the false discovery rate – a practical and powerful approach to multiple testing. J Roy Stat Soc Series B – Methodological 1995; 57:289–300.
43. Wittke JK, Cox NJ. Departures from Hardy-Weinberg equilibrium for common disease models. Am J Hum Genet 2003; 73:620–620.
44. Pritchard JK, Rosenberg NA. Use of unlinked genetic markers to detect population stratification in association studies. Am J Hum Genet 1999; 65:220–228.
45. Ober C, Leavitt SA, Tsalenko A, et al. Variation in the interleukin 4-receptor alpha gene confers susceptibility to asthma and atopy in ethnically diverse populations. Am J Hum Genet 2000; 66:517–526.
46. Howard TD, Koppelman GH, Xu J, et al. Gene-gene interaction in asthma: Il-4RA and Il-13 in a Dutch population with asthma. Am J Hum Genet 2002; 70:230–236.
47. Baldini M, Vercelli D, Martinez FD. Cd14: An example of gene by environment interaction in allergic disease. Allergy 2002; 57:188–192.

Candidate gene association studies for asthma-related phenotypes

48. Wills-Karp M, Chiaramonte M. Interleukin-13 in asthma. Curr Opin Pulm Med 2003; 9:21–27.
49. Vladich FD, Brazille SM, Stern D, et al. IL13 r130q, a common variant associated with allergy and asthma, enhances effector mechanisms essential for human allergic inflammation. J Clin Invest 2005; 115:747–754.
50. Viale G, Vercelli D. Interleukin-13 regulates the phenotype and function of human monocytes. Int Arch Allergy Immunol 1995; 107:176–178.
51. Postma DS, Bleecker ER, Amelung PJ, et al. Genetic susceptibility to asthma – bronchial hyperresponsiveness co-inherited with a major gene for atopy. N Engl J Med 1995; 333:894–900.
52. A genome-wide search for asthma susceptibility loci in ethnically diverse populations. The collaborative study on the genetics of asthma (CSGA). Nat Genet 1997; 15:389–392.
53. Meyers DA, Postma DS, Panhuysen CI, et al. Evidence for a locus regulating total serum IgE levels mapping to chromosome 5. Genomics 1994; 23:464–470.
54. Bleecker ER, Amelung PJ, Levitt RC, et al. Evidence for linkage of total serum IgE and bronchial hyperresponsiveness to chromosome 5q: a major regulatory locus important in asthma. Clin Exp Allergy 1995; 25 (Suppl 2):84–88; Discussion 95–86.
55. Postma DS, Meyers DA, Jongepier H, et al. Genomewide screen for pulmonary function in 200 families ascertained for asthma. J Allergy Clin Immunol 2005; 172:446–452.
56. Cameron L, Webster RB, Strempel JM, et al. Th2 cell-selective enhancement of human IL13 transcription by IL13–1112C>T, a polymorphism associated with allergic inflammation. J Immunol 2006; 177:8633–8642.
57. Arima K, Umeshita-Suyama R, Sakata Y, et al. Upregulation of IL13 concentration in vivo by the IL-13 variant associated with bronchial asthma. J Allergy Clin Immunol 2002; 109:980–987.
58. Heinzmann A, Mao XQ, Akaiwa M, et al. Genetic variants of IL-13 signalling and human asthma and atopy. Hum Mol Genet 2000; 9:549–559.
59. Howard TD, Whittaker PA, Zaiman AL, et al. Identification and association of polymorphisms in the interleukin-13 gene with asthma and atopy in a Dutch population. Am J Respir Cell Mol Biol 2001; 25:377–384.
60. Hakonarson H, Bjornsdottir US, Ostermann E, et al. Allelic frequencies and patterns of single-nucleotide polymorphisms in candidate genes for asthma and atopy in Iceland. Am J Respir Crit Care Med 2001; 164:2036–2044.
61. Celedon JC, Soto-Quiros ME, Palmer LJ, et al. Lack of association between a polymorphism in the interleukin-13 gene and total serum immunoglobulin E level among nuclear families in Costa Rica. Clin Exp Allergy 2002; 32:387–390.
62. Sadeghnejad A, Karmaus W, Hasan Arshad S, et al. IL13 gene polymorphism association with cord serum immunoglobulin E. Pediatr Allergy Immunol 2007; 18:288–292.

63. Graves PE, Kabesch M, Halonen M, et al. A cluster of seven tightly linked polymorphisms in the IL-13 gene is associated with total serum IgE levels in three populations of white children. J Allergy Clin Immunol 2000; 105:506–513.
64. DeMeo DL, Lange C, Silverman EK, et al. Univariate and multivariate family-based association analysis of the IL-13 arg130gln polymorphism in the childhood asthma management program. Genet Epidemiol 2002; 23:335–348.
65. Kabesch M, Schedel M, Carr D, et al. IL-4/IL-13 pathway genetics strongly influence serum IgE levels and childhood asthma. J Allergy Clin Immunol 2006; 117:269–274.
66. Maier LM, Howson JM, Walker N, et al. Association of IL13 with total IgE: evidence against an inverse association of atopy and diabetes. J Allergy Clin Immunol 2006; 117:1306–1313.
67. Raby BA, Weiss ST. Beta2-adrenergic receptor genetics. Curr Opin Mol Ther 2001; 3:554–566.
68. Reihsaus E, Innis M, MacIntyre N, et al. Mutations in the gene encoding for the beta 2-adrenergic receptor in normal and asthmatic subjects. Am J Respir Cell Mol Biol 1993; 8:334–339.
69. Martinez FD, Graves PE, Baldini M, et al. Association between genetic polymorphisms of the beta2-adrenoceptor and response to albuterol in children with and without a history of wheezing. J Clin Invest 1997; 100:3184–3188.
70. Hawkins GA, Tantisira K, Meyers DA, et al. Sequence, haplotype, and association analysis of ADR beta2 in a multiethnic asthma case-control study. Am J Respir Crit Care Med 2006; 174:1101–1109.
71. Blakey J, Halapi E, Bjornsdottir US, et al. Contribution of ADAM33 polymorphisms to the population risk of asthma. Thorax 2005; 60:274–276.
72. Jongepier H, Boezen HM, Dijkstra A, et al. Polymorphisms of the ADAM33 gene are associated with accelerated lung function decline in asthma. Clin Exp Allergy 2004; 34:757–760.
73. Werner M, Herbon N, Gohlke H, et al. Asthma is associated with single-nucleotide polymorphisms in ADAM33. Clin Exp Allergy 2004; 34:26–31.
74. Lee JH, Park HS, Park SW, et al. ADAM33 polymorphism: Association with bronchial hyper-responsiveness in Korean asthmatics. Clin Exp Allergy 2004; 34:860–865.
75. Lind DL, Choudhry S, Ung N, et al. ADAM33 is not associated with asthma in Puerto Rican or Mexican populations. Am J Respir Crit Care Med 2003; 168:1312–1316.
76. Simpson A, Maniatis N, Jury F, et al. Polymorphisms in a disintegrin and metalloprotease 33 (ADAM33) predict impaired early-life lung function. Am J Respir Criti Care Med 2005; 172:55–60.

Gene–environment interaction in asthma

77. Tashkin DP, Altose MD, Bleecker ER, et al. The lung health study: airway responsiveness to inhaled methacholine in smokers with mild to moderate airflow limitation. The Lung Health Study Research Group. Am Rev Respir Dis 1992; 145:301–310.
78. Kauffmann F, Frette C, Annesi I, et al. Relationships of haptoglobin level to fev1, wheezing, bronchial hyper-responsiveness and allergy. Clin Exp Allergy 1991; 21:669–674.
79. Young S, Le Souef PN, Geelhoed GC, et al. The influence of a family history of asthma and parental smoking on airway responsiveness in early infancy. N Engl J Med 1991; 324:1168–1173.
80. Wang Z, Chen C, Niu T, et al. Association of asthma with beta(2)-adrenergic receptor gene polymorphism and cigarette smoking. Am J Respir Crit Care Med 2001; 163:1404–1409.
81. Kabesch M, Hoefler C, Carr D, et al. Glutathione S transferase deficiency and passive smoking increase childhood asthma. Thorax 2004; 59:569–573.
82. Martinez FD, Antognoni G, Macri F, et al. Parental smoking enhances bronchial responsiveness in nine-year-old children. Am Rev Respir Dis 1988; 138:518–523.
83. Colilla S, Nicolae D, Pluzhnikov A, et al. Evidence for gene–environment interactions in a linkage study of asthma and smoking exposure. J Allergy Clin Immunol 2003; 111:840–846.
84. Eder W, Klimecki W, Yu L, et al. Opposite effects of CD 14/-260 on serum IgE levels in children raised in different environments. J Allergy Clin Immunol 2005; 116:601–607.

Pharmacogenomics of asthma

85. Weiss ST, Litonjua AA, Lange C, et al. Overview of the pharmacogenetics of asthma treatment. Pharmacogenom J 2006; 6:311–326.
86. Hawkins GA, Weiss ST, Bleecker ER. Asthma pharmacogenomics. Immunol Allergy Clin North Am 2005; 25:723–742.
87. Taylor DR, Hancox RJ, McRae W, et al. The influence of polymorphism at position 16 of the beta2-adrenoceptor on the development of tolerance to beta-agonist. J Asthma 2000; 37:691–700.
88. Israel E, Drazen JM, Liggett SB, et al. The effect of polymorphisms of the beta(2)-adrenergic receptor on the response to regular use of albuterol in asthma. Am J Respir Crit Care Med 2000; 162:75–80.
88a. Israel E, Chinchilli VM, Ford JG, et al. Use of regularly scheduled albuterol treatment in asthma: genotype-stratified, randomised, placebo-controlled cross-over trial. Lancet 2004; 364:1505–1512.
88b. Wechsler ME, Lehman F, Lazarus RF Jr, et al. beta-Adrenergic receptor polymorphisms and response to salmeterol. Am J Resp Crit Care Med 2006; 173:519–526.
88c. Bleecker ER, Yancey SW, Baitinger LA, et al. Salmeterol response is not affected by beta2-adrenergic receptor genotype in subjects with persistent asthma. J Allergy Clin Immunol 2006; 118:809–816.
89. Hancox RJ, Sears MR, Taylor DR. Polymorphism of the beta2-adrenoceptor and the response to long-term beta2-agonist therapy in asthma. Eur Respir J 1998; 11:589–593.

New approaches to asthma genetics

90. Pennacchio LA. Insights from human/mouse genome comparisons. Mamm Genome 2003; 14:429–436.

Genome-wide association studies

91. Maraganore DM, de Andrade M, Lesnick TG, et al. High-resolution whole-genome association study of Parkinson disease. Am J Hum Genet 2005; 77:685–693.
92. Moffatt MF, Kabesch M, Liang L, et al. Genetic variants regulating ORMDL3 expression contribute to the risk of childhood asthma. Nature 2007; 448:470–473.
92b. Ionnidis JP, Non-replication and inconsistency in the genome-wide association setting. Hum Hered 2007; 64:203–213.
93. Abecasis GR, Cookson WO. GOLD – graphical overview of linkage disequilibrium. Bioinformatics 2000; 16:182–183.

Immunoglobulin Structure and Function

Jennifer L Bankers-Fulbright and James T Li

5

SUMMARY OF IMPORTANT CONCEPTS

>> Antibodies specific for antigen mediate a variety of biologic effects, including agglutination, precipitation, neutralization, activation of complement, and interaction with specific cell surface Fc receptors

>> To construct functional light and heavy immunoglobulin chain genes, the discontinuous DNA coding sequences must first be rearranged

>> Isotype class switching is highly T cell dependent and is regulated through CD40 and the action of cytokines

>> Monoclonal and polyclonal immunoglobulins are used therapeutically

INTRODUCTION

The central event in the acquired immune response is specific antigen recognition. Only two types of molecules can specifically recognize the diverse antigens humans are exposed to every day: immunoglobulins (Ig) or antibodies and the T cell receptor (TCR). Humans typically generate 10 million antibodies with different antigen-binding specificities, and they have the potential to generate up to 10^{16} different antibodies, each specific for a particular target. The antibody is elegantly constructed in a manner that allows it to serve two primary functions: one region of the molecule confers a capability to recognize and bind an enormous variety of antigenic determinants, and the other region is involved in mediating the biologic effects of the immunoglobulin, such as complement fixation or antibody-dependent cell cytotoxicity.

A key difference between the way the TCR and immunoglobulin recognize antigen is that only the immunoglobulin (secreted or membrane bound) recognizes its native, properly folded form. In contrast, the TCR can only recognize antigens that have been processed and are presented in the context of the major histocompatibility complex (MHC) by an antigen presenting cell. This means that although both a TCR and an immunoglobulin can recognize the same antigen, they are almost surely recognizing different epitopes on that antigen. Thus, knowledge of the structural features and gene organization of the antibody molecule is essential for the understanding of antigen–antibody interactions and immunoregulation. The study of hypersensitivity rightfully includes a review of antibody structural diversity and function.

B LYMPHOCYTES AND THE HUMORAL IMMUNE RESPONSE

B cells are circulating lymphocytes and are ultimately the source of all immunoglobulins. Like other leukocytes, B cells differentiate in the bone marrow from hematopoietic stem cells. However, unlike T cells that mature in the thymus, B cells develop completely in the bone marrow and are released as mature lymphocytes capable of reacting with antigen. Following release from the bone marrow, naïve mature B cells circulate through the blood, lymph, and secondary lymphoid tissues.

Immunoglobulins produced by B lymphocytes are membrane bound or secreted. The only difference between these two forms is an alternative splice of the mRNA coding for the immunoglobulin that results in an added 'tail' on the C-terminal end of the membrane-bound immunoglobulin, which serves as a membrane anchor. Secreted immunoglobulins that lack this tail comprise the bulk of the humoral immune response. Membrane-bound immunoglobulins make up the antigen-recognizing portion of the B cell receptor (BCR). Upon activation,

B cells differentiate into plasma cells that secrete high levels of antibody of the same specificity as the B cell from which they were derived.

B CELL RECEPTOR (BCR) STRUCTURE AND SIGNALING

The BCR is a molecular complex containing membrane immunoglobulin and two polypeptides, Igα (CD79a) and Igβ (CD79b) (Fig. 5.1). Igα and Igβ are glycoproteins that have structural similarity with the components of the TCR-associated CD3. An important structural feature of the Igα and Igβ molecules is the presence of the conserved immunoreceptor tyrosine-based activation motif (ITAM) sequence.

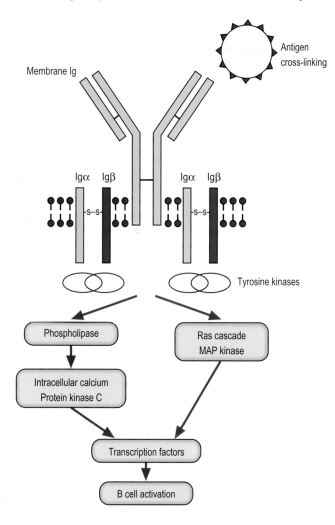

Fig. 5.1. Schematic of B cell activation. The B cell antigen receptor consists of membrane immunoglobulin in non-covalent association with Igα/Igβ heterodimers. Antigen cross-linking of the B cell receptor results in phosphorylation of the ARH1 motifs on Igα and Igβ and subsequent activation of tyrosine kinases. Through a number of intermediary steps not shown here, phospholipases are activated and the Ras cascade initiated, leading to induction of transcription factors and intracellular calcium. MAP, mitogen activated protein.

This 18-amino acid conserved motif is important for signal transduction through tyrosine kinase activation and intracellular calcium mobilization and is found in other receptor systems such as the TCR complex and Fc receptors (Table 5.1).

Igα and Igβ are essential for normal expression and transport of membrane immunoglobulin. All nine isotypes of immunoglobulin bind Igα and Igβ. In the normal pre-B cell, μ heavy chains form intracellular complexes with surrogate light chains and with Igα and Igβ heterodimers. This membrane immunoglobulin-surrogate light chain-Igα/Igβ complex is transiently expressed on the cell surface of the pre-B cell.[1,2] Maturation of the pre-B cell to an immature and then mature B cell involves production of κ or λ light chains that complex with μ heavy chains and the Igα/Igβ heterodimer to form the mature BCR.

Because the cytoplasmic tails of the membrane immunoglobulins are only a few amino acids in length, Igα and Igβ are the key signaling proteins of the BCR.[3-5] Cross-linking of the BCR results in the release of intracellular calcium via activation of phospholipase C and the induction of multiple transcription factors through the activation of tyrosine kinases and the serine-threonine kinase, protein kinase C (PKC.) In resting B cells, the BCR is associated with a variety of tyrosine kinases. Antigen binding to membrane immunoglobulin induces cross-linking of antigen receptors and activation of tyrosine kinases of the *src*, *syk*, and *Janus kinase* (JAK) families, resulting in phosphorylation of the ITAM motifs on Igα and Igβ. Activation of these kinases results in the subsequent activation of other signal transducers, such as PI-3 kinase and phospholipase C (PLC). PLC generates the second messengers inositol triphosphate (IP3) and diacylglycerol (DAG). DAG is required for the activation of classical and novel PKC isoforms and IP3 is involved in the release of calcium from intracellular stores. Additionally, the mitogen activated protein (MAP) kinase pathway is activated following BCR ligation, leading to the production of the transcription factor AP-1.

The importance of tyrosine kinases in BCR signal transduction and B cell development and function is evident by mutations found in certain immunodeficiencies. X-linked agammaglobulinemia is linked to a specific tyrosine kinase expressed in B cells, Bruton's tyrosine kinase (BTK), and JAK-3 deficiency causes combined immunodeficiency characterized by hypogammaglobulinemia.[6,7]

HUMORAL IMMUNE RESPONSE

The cross-linking of membrane-bound immunoglobulins on circulating, naïve B lymphocytes results in their activation and migration to the draining lymph node (or other lymphatic tissue). Depending on the qualities of the antigen, the B cell will follow one of two activation pathways. If the antigen is a thymus-independent (TI) antigen, such as a complex polysaccharide with repeating epitopes, the B cell can become activated in the absence of T cell help, and the secreted immunoglobulins are always of the IgM (or IgG) isotype. Typically, no memory response is observed. Most protein antigens are thymus-dependent (TD) antigens and require T cell help for full B cell activation.[8] Secreted immunoglobulins produced in response to TD antigens follow a typical pattern of primary and secondary serum antibody response (Fig. 5.2). IgM production is characteristic of an early primary immune response, and class switch to IgG occurs soon thereafter. At the end of the primary immune response, both IgM and IgG levels decrease almost to baseline. However, upon subsequent challenge with the same antigen, a secondary response is observed

Table 5.1 Structural overview and cellular expression profiles of Fc receptors.

		Structural overview and cellular expression profiles of Fc receptors		
Receptor	**Structure and apparent M_r**	**Affinity for immunoglobulin**		**Expression**
		Mouse	**Human**	
FcγRIa (CD64)	α 70 kDa γ 9 kDa ITAM	10^7–10^8 M^{-1} to IgG2a>>3, 1, 2b	10^7–10^9 M^{-1} to IgG1$\geq$3>4>>2	Macrophage, monocyte, DC
FcγRIIa (CD32)	40 kDa ITAM-like	NF	<10^7 M^{-1} to IgG3$\geq$1, 2>>4	Macrophage, neutrophil, eosinophil, platelets, DC, LC
FcγRIIb (CD32)	40–60 kDa ITIM-like	<10^7 M^{-1} to IgG1, 2a, 2b>>3 3×10^5 M^{-1} to IgE	<10^7 M^{-1} to IgG3$\geq$1>4>2	B cell, mast cell, basophil, macrophage, eosinophil, neutrophil, DC, LC
FcγRIIIa (CD16)	α human: 60–70 kDa mouse: 40–60 kDa γ (or ζ)	<10^7 M^{-1} to IgG1, 2a, 2b>>3 5×10^5 M^{-1} to IgE	2×10^7 M^{-1} to IgG1, 3>>2, 4	Macrophage, monocyte, NK cell, mast cell, DC, LC, neutrophil (mouse)
FcγRIIIb (CD16)	50 kDa GPI link	NF	<10^7 M^{-1} to IgG1, 3>>2, 4	Neutrophil
FcϵRI	α 46–65 kDa β 32 kDa γ	10^{10} M^{-1} to IgE	>10^{10} M^{-1} to IgE	Mast cell, basophil, LC (human), DC (human)
FcϵRII (CD23)	C-type lectin domain 46 kDa	10^8 M^{-1} to IgE	10^8 M^{-1} to IgE	Ubiquitous, platelets
FcαRI (CD89)	α 55–75 kDa γ	NF	2×10^7 M^{-1} to IgA1, IgA2	Macrophage, neutrophil, eosinophil,
FcRn	α 50 kDa β_2m 12 kDa	10^8 M^{-1} to rat IgG2a>2b, 1, 2c	2×10^8 M^{-1} to IgG	Placenta, small intestine, monocyte, DC
Fcα/μR	α 70 kDa	ND	10^8 M^{-1} to IgM, IgA	B cell, macrophage
Poly-IgR	85 kDa	High, but ND	High, but ND	Epithelium, liver, small intestine, lungs
FcRH1–5*	FcRH2 54 kDa	ND	ND	B cell

β_2m, β_2-microglobulin; DC, dendritic cell; FcRH, Fc-receptor homologue; FcRn, neonatal Fc receptor; GPI, glycosylphosphatidylinositol; Ig, immunoglobulin; LC, Langerhans cell; M_r, relative molecular mass; ND, not determined; NF, not found in mice; NK, natural killer; poly-IgR, polymeric immunoglobulin receptor.
*The complementary DNAs for FcRHs encode type I transmembrane glycoproteins that have 3–6 immunoglobulin-like extracellular domains and a cytoplasmic domain that contains an immunoreceptor tyrosine-based activation motif (ITAM) and/or immunoreceptor tyrosine-based inhibitory motif (ITIM). The protein products have 15–31% identity to their closest FcR relatives. A putative structure of one of the members, FcRH2, is shown. At present, no null alleles for *FcγRIIa or FcγRIIb* are known in humans.
From: Takai T. Roles of Fc receptors in autoimmunity. Nature Rev Immunol 2002; 2:580–592.

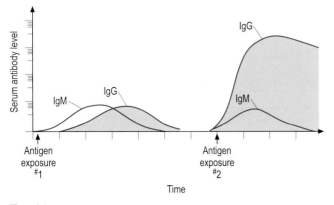

Fig. 5.2. Typical primary and secondary humoral response of serum IgM and IgG levels following the first and second exposures to a given antigen. Units are not shown on the axes because the actual response times and serum antibody levels vary with the antigen, route of immunization, and several other factors. Note that the Y-axis is logarithmic.

that is characterized by much faster and greater production of antigen-specific IgG than was observed in the primary response (Fig. 5.2). In addition, elevated (though not necessarily protective) serum IgG levels are detectable for weeks to years following the elimination of antigen from the host.

Class switch induced by T and B lymphocyte interaction is dependent primarily upon three receptor-ligand interactions, often referred to as the immunological synapse, which take place in the draining lymph node or other lymphatic tissue near the site of antigen exposure. The first interaction is the processing and presentation of an antigen by the B cell in the context of MHC class II for recognition by an appropriate T cell receptor. Second, CD80/CD86 that is expressed on the surface of the B cell binds to CD28, which is expressed on the surface of the T lymphocyte. This interaction induces upregulation of CD40-ligand (CD154) expression on the T cell surface. CD154 can then bind to CD40 expressed by the B cell, which is the third key interaction. These three sequential signals trigger T lymphocyte cytokine secretion, which drives immunoglobulin class switch and also B lymphocyte proliferation and differentiation into short- and long-lived plasma cells. Plasma cells convert to making secreted immunoglobulin and can produce thousands of antibody molecules per second during an active immune response.

Serum antibody levels are tightly regulated by long-lived plasma cells resident primarily in the bone marrow.[9] Antibodies to previously seen antigens are commonly detected in serum decades after the last known exposure and homeostatic production of specific antibody persists even in the apparent absence of the inducing antigen. Although it is clear that long-lived plasma cells can survive quite some time in the bone marrow, it is unknown whether or not an individual plasma cell survives for the life of the host or whether it is continuously replicating at a slow rate. It has been proposed that there is a limited long-lived plasma cell survival niche in humans. Newly formed plasma cells actively compete with those existing plasma cells to reach homeostasis at a finite threshold of long-lived plasma cells per person.[10] Some have suggested that idiotypic-anti-idiotypic antibody immune-complexes may be responsible for immunological humoral memory.[11]

■ IMMUNOGLOBULIN STRUCTURE AND FUNCTION ■

IMMUNOGLOBULIN PROTEIN STRUCTURE

Immunoglobulins are composed of four polypeptides, 2 identical heavy chains and 2 identical light chains (Fig. 5.3). Each light chain is bound to a heavy chain through a covalent disulfide bond, and the heavy chains are linked to each other by a distinct set of disulfide bonds. Each heavy and light chain has two major functional domains: the constant region and the variable region. These are generally denoted as C_L and V_L for the light chains and C_H and V_H for the heavy chains. The variable domains of the light and heavy chains combine to form the antigen-binding site of the antibody. Because there are pairs of heavy and light chains that form each immunoglobulin, each immunoglobulin has two antigen-binding sites, each specific for the same antigen. This is critical to the function of antibodies because it allows for cross-linking of antigen.

The light chain is a polypeptide with an approximate molecular weight of 23 kDa and contains about 220 amino acid residues. Comparison of the amino acid sequences of several light chains reveals that the entire light chain is composed of two similar segments, each of about 110 amino acids. Each segment contains an acidic intrachain disulfide bond formed by cysteine residues approximately 60 amino acids apart. Domains with this general structure are found in many molecules involved in the immune response and are called immunoglobulin-like domains. Molecules with these domains are said to belong to the immunoglobulin superfamily, of which the immunoglobulin molecules are the flagship member. Likewise, the heavy chains have a variable domain (V_H) and three or four constant region domains (C_H1, C_H2, C_H3, and C_H4) depending on the immunoglobulin isotype.

A number of invariant amino acid residues in the heavy- and light-chain sequences are located at contact points between light-chain domains and heavy-chain domains. These invariant residues account for the ability of different light and heavy chains to pair in many combinations. Immunoglobulins are also glycoproteins; however, carbohydrate group attachment is generally limited to the constant regions of the heavy chain. The carbohydrate content of immunoglobulins is variable and appears not to be predetermined. Even monoclonal antibodies exhibit microheterogeneity of carbohydrate content. Furthermore, the carbohydrate groups located on the otherwise identical heavy-chain pair with a single immunoglobulin molecule may be different. Carbohydrate chains are necessary for several effector functions of immunoglobulins. Monoclonal antibodies produced in vitro without carbohydrates demonstrate impaired complement binding, Fc receptor binding, and antibody-dependent cell-mediated cytotoxicity (ADCC) activity.

The constant region of the heavy chain and the combined variable regions of both the heavy and light chains form the two distinct functional regions of immunoglobulins. The antigen-binding fragment (Fab) end is formed by the assembly of heavy and light chain variable regions, recognizes antigen, and contains the immunoglobulin idiotype, the unique protein sequence that identifies each antibody. The crystallizable fragment (Fc) portion is determined by the constant region of the heavy chain only and defines the isotype of the immunoglobulin. The Fc portion binds to Fc receptors and is responsible for all of the functional attributes of an antibody. Limited cleavage of intact immunoglobulin molecules by proteolytic enzymes in vitro yields immunoglobulin fragments that

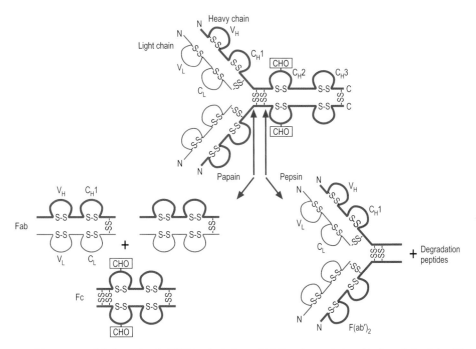

Fig. 5.3. Basic structure of the immunoglobulin molecule. CHO, carbohydrate; thick lines, heavy chains; thin lines, light chains. Note the regularly spaced immunoglobulin domains (half-circles) in both the light and heavy chains. (Reproduced from Spiegelberg HL. Biological activities of immunoglobulins of different classes and subclasses. Adv Immunol 1974; 19:265, with permission)

possess different properties and clearly illustrate the functional properties of the immunoglobulin molecule (Fig. 5.4). Papain cleaves the IgG hinge region at the N-terminal side of the heavy chain disulfide bonds to produce three fragments. Two fragments are identical and are formed by intact light chains bound to the V_H and C_H1 regions of the heavy chains. These fragments bind antigen and are referred to as Fab fragments. They are monovalent and do not exhibit immunoglobulin effector functions (no Fc region). The third fragment is composed of the C-terminal portion of the heavy chains bound to each other. This fragment does not bind antigen but can bind to complement or Fc receptors. The Fc portions of immunoglobulins of a single isotype are identical. Alternatively, the protease pepsin cleaves IgG at the C-terminal side of the heavy chain disulfide bonds, thus releasing a fragment called $F(ab')_2$. This fragment consists of two Fab-like fragments joined by disulfide bond. Because it is bivalent, the $F(ab')_2$ fragment can precipitate and cross-link antigen. Pepsin digestion of an immunoglobulin usually results in substantial degradation of the Fc portion and loss of Fc-mediated biological activities.

X-ray crystallographic studies and electron microscopy of human myeloma proteins and fragments have resulted in elucidation of immunoglobulin structure (Fig. 5.5).[12,13] Immunoglobulin models are typically depicted as a Y- or T-shaped molecule with each globular Fab region linked to the globular Fc regions by the hinge segments. The Fab regions can pivot on the hinge region so that the angle between the two Fab arms can change. Further, the Fab region can rotate alone its long axis. All domains share the same basic secondary structure of two β-pleated sheets, one consisting of four antiparallel strands and the other consisting of three. The two sheets form a sandwich-like structure with the intrachain disulfide bond and hydrophobic amino acid residues between the two layers. The V domains contain an extra loop that contributes directly to the antigen-binding site.

Antibody molecules can be distinguished by antigenic determinants expressed on the variable regions of the molecule. These determinants are referred to as an idiotype. Because the number of variable regions an individual expresses is large, many more idiotypes exist than allotypes or isotypes. Unlike isotypes or allotypes, idiotypes can be expressed on the variable region of the light chain (VL), the variable region of the heavy chain (VH), or on portions of VL and VH combined. Idiotypic determinants often involve the antigen-combining sites of antibody molecules and thus can sometimes serve as clonal markers. However, it is now known that different molecules of similar or even unrelated specificity can share idiotype determinants. Furthermore, some idiotypes may involve only the framework or non-antigen-binding locations on variable regions. Thus although certain idiotypes may be unique to a clone of antibody molecules, other idiotypes may be shared. The study of antiidiotypic antibodies has resulted in a better understanding of immunoregulation. Antiidiotypic antibodies exhibit many immunological functions, including enhancement, suppression, and stimulation.[14] Clinical studies suggest a role for autologous antiidiotypic antibodies in several autoimmune disorders.

The binding of antigenic determinants to the antibody-combining site is similar to other forms of ligand-receptor interaction. However, antibody binding is unique in that a vast number of related molecules have different binding specificities. In their natural environment, antibodies usually bind to complex macromolecules such a proteins, polysaccharides,

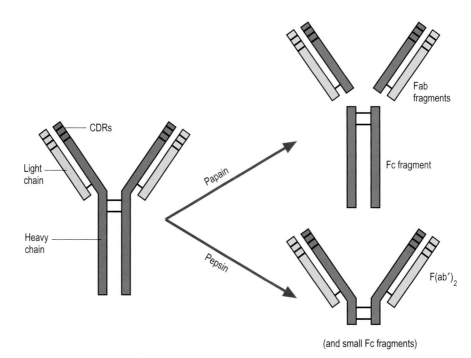

Fig. 5.4. Immunoglobulin fragments generated in vitro with papain and pepsin digestion. Papain cleaves the immunoglobulin molecule into three fragments: 2 Fab fragments, which are each capable of binding a single antigen epitope, and the Fc fragment, which can still bind to Fc receptors. Alternatively, pepsin digestion of immunoglobulins results in a single F(ab')$_2$ fragment, which is still capable of cross-linking and precipitating multivalent antigen. The Fc portion is generally digested into several smaller peptides by pepsin.

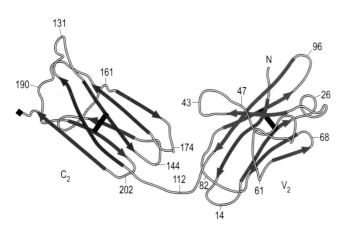

Fig. 5.5. Three-dimensional structure of a Bence-Jones protein (light chain) showing β-pleated sheets (white and cross-hatched arrows) and disulfide bonds (solid bars). C_2, constant domain; V_2, variable domain. (From: Schiffer et al, Structure of lambda-type Bence-Jones protein at 3.5-Å resolution. Biochemistry 1973; 12:4620. Copyright, American Chemical Society)

phospholipids, and nucleic acids. The ability of an antiserum to bind with complex multideterminant macromolecules depends on the number of binding sites in addition to intrinsic equilibrium constants, and immunoglobulins can be generally described in terms of their affinity and their avidity for a particular antigen.

The term affinity reflects antibody binding with a single epitope or binding site. The affinity of an antibody-binding site for an antigenic determinant is determined by the sum of the non-covalent forces between the antigen binding site of the immunoglobulin and the antigen itself. Because the strength of these non-covalent forces is greatly increased at short distances, the strongest binding site/determinant interactions occur when complementarity exists between the two structures. The interaction of oscillating dipoles of adjacent atoms generates van der Waals forces, which result in the atoms' mutual attraction. Because the attractive force is greatest at distances of only 0.18–0.20 nm, the strongest binding of antigen to antibody occurs when complementarity is greatest. The COO$^-$ or NH$_4^+$ side groups on polar amino acids lining the antibody-binding site can interact with oppositely charged moieties on antigenic determinants to form electrostatic bonds. Hydrogen bonds can be involved in antigen binding and are maximal at distances of 0.2–0.3 nm. Thus, both the steric fit of antigen to the combining site and the juxtaposition of attracting chemical groups are essential for efficient antibody-ligand binding. In addition, it may be possible for the VL and VH domains to 'slide' a few nm at the time of antigen binding.[15]

Alternatively, avidity is used in a semiquantitative way to describe the overall binding of antibodies to antigen and is highly dependent upon the valence of the immunoglobulin. Antibody avidity is an average measure of the affinity of the antibodies for a particular antigen in a serum sample and increases in avidity during an immune response are largely a result of somatic hypermutation and subsequent selection of high affinity B cells.[16] When multiple identical sites are present on antigen, the valence of the antibody contributes significantly to the stability of the antigen–antibody complex, such as the binding of pentameric IgM to a multideterminant antigen.

IMMUNOGLOBULIN ISOTYPES AND FUNCTIONS

As mentioned above, the isotype of an immunoglobulin is determined by the Fc portion (or constant region) of the heavy chain (Fig. 5.6). By definition, all isotype genes are expressed in a given individual. These heavy-chain isotypes define the class and subclass of the antibody molecule and are designated $\gamma 1$, $\gamma 2$, $\gamma 3$, $\gamma 4$, μ, $\alpha 1$, $\alpha 2$, δ, and ε. The immunoglobulin isotype is named according to the heavy-chain isotype present. The immunoglobulin isotypes (class or subclass) are IgG1, IgG2, IgG3, IgG4, IgM, IgA1, IgA2, IgD, and IgE.

The four IgG subclasses, IgG1, IgG2, IgG3, and IgG4, are so classified on the basis of shared antigenic determinants and amino acid sequence homology. For example, the γ subclass molecule bears both shared class-specific determinants and individual subclass-specific determinants. The constant regions of the γ subclasses exhibit 90% homology to each other and only 33% homology to the μ constant region. However, because each

IgG subclass constant region is represented by a separate constant region gene segment, the IgG 'subclasses' are in fact simply closely related isotypes. The two α subclasses are similarly related.

Immunoglobulin molecules of certain isotypes can be further classified according to determinants in the constant region that represent allelic variants and therefore segregate in classic Mendelian fashion. These determinants define the allotypes of a heavy or light chain. According to this definition, different individuals may possess different allotypes, and no individual can possess all allotypes. Amino acid sequence studies have shown that most allotypic determinants are defined by a single amino acid substitution in the constant region. Allotypes can be considered polymorphic variants of certain isotypes. The heavy-chain isotypes that exhibit allotypic variants are $\gamma 1$, $\gamma 2$, $\gamma 3$, $\gamma 4$, and $\alpha 2$. The two dozen γ variants are called Gm allotypes. The two known allotypes of the $\alpha 2$ heavy chain are designated A2m(1) and A2m(2).

Light-chain isotypes are known as types and subtypes. The constant regions of the light chains allow for distinction of two types of light chains, κ and λ, which have very limited clinical significance. Comparison of amino acid sequences demonstrates that the two light-chain types

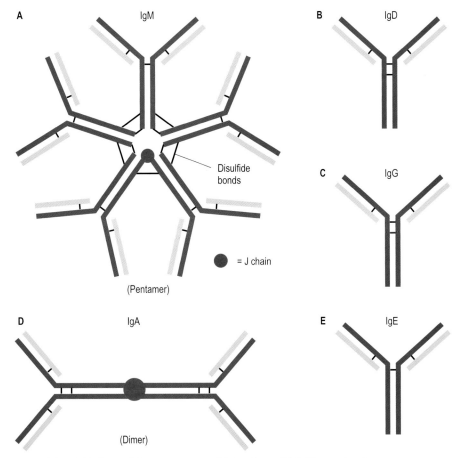

Fig. 5.6. General structures of the soluble forms of the major immunoglobulin classes. (A) IgM is produced as a pentamer, connected by disulfide bonds in the Fc regions as well as a J chain, which is required for mucosal secretion. (B) IgD is rarely if ever present in serum but is present on mature, naïve B cells. (C) IgG is always present in serum as a monomer. (D) IgA can be found as a monomer or as a dimer connected by the same J chain found in the IgM pentameric structure. IgA that is present in secretions and mucosal tissues is dimeric. (E) IgE.

are approximately 40% homologous. There are four isotypic forms of λ chains but only one form of κ chain. The subtypes of λ chains are distinguished by antigenic determinants present in the constant region. Comparison of amino acid sequences among subtypes reveals substitutions in one to four amino acid positions. Of the two light chains expressed in humans, only the κ chain has allotypes, designated Km(1), Km(1,2), and Km(3). Again, although not particularly useful clinically, allotypes can be used to determine whether serum immunoglobulin is of donor or recipient origin in bone marrow transplant recipients, and they can be useful in paternity testing or forensic medicine.

In general, antibodies have three major effector functions following binding of antigen. The first is simple neutralization of the antigen or toxin in soluble complexes by preventing further binding of that antigen to other cells. Second, antibodies can serve to opsonize (promote phagocytosis of) antigens via complement cascade activation or interactions with FcγR. Third, the cross-linking of antibodies bound to Fc receptors on effector immune cells, such as natural killer (NK) cells or macrophages, leads to antibody-dependent cell-mediated cytotoxicity (ADCC). Each antibody isotype and subtype varies in its ability to induce each of these effector functions (Table 5.2).

IgM

Membrane-bound monomeric IgM functions as the earliest BCR on B cells developing in the bone marrow. Antigen binding to mature B cells results in B cell activation and differentiation, leading to pentameric IgM secretion. Indeed, an increase in antigen-specific IgM is generally considered indicative of a primary immune response to that antigen. Pentameric IgM contains the J chain and five IgM monomers linked together via disulfide bonds. The J chain is a 15 kDa glycoprotein rich in cysteine residues and links two of the 5 IgM Fc regions together. IgM is extremely effective at fixing complement and neutralizing antigens and has recently been recognized as being able to bind to effector cells via the Fc receptor Fcα/μR.[17] Because pentameric IgM includes the J chain, it (like dimeric IgA) can bind to the poly-Ig receptor present on the basolateral surface of mucosal epithelial cells. The poly-Ig receptor not only facilitates transport of the

immunoglobulins through the epithelial barrier, but also is ultimately cleaved and remains bound to the mucosal immunoglobulins as the secretory component.[18,19]

IgD

This is present in serum at very low concentrations. The function of IgD is not well understood, but appears to be as a membrane-bound antigen receptor on the B cell surface. During B cell development, IgM and IgD are co-expressed on developing cells. Although some evidence suggests that the presence of surface IgD is correlated with a resistance to the induction of B cell tolerance, the role of IgD in B cell maturation (or any other functions) remains largely unknown.

IgG

IgG is the major immunoglobulin class in serum, comprising approximately 85% of total serum immunoglobulin. An increase in antigen-specific serum IgG is characteristic of a memory response to a given antigen. There are four subtypes of IgG: IgG1, IgG2, IgG3, and IgG4. IgG1 is by far the most prevalent, followed, respectively by IgG2, IgG3, and IgG4. In general, IgG1, IgG2, and IgG3 are considered Th1-type antibodies whereas IgG4 is typically associated with Th2-type responses. Although the IgG subtypes are 90–95% homologous, they have different functional properties as shown in Table 5.3.[20] One key difference is that IgG1, IgG2, and IgG3 (but not IgG4) can activate the complement cascade. A unique role of IgG is providing passive immunity to infants because this is the only immunoglobulin isotype that can cross the placenta. However, IgG2 is relatively inefficient in crossing the placenta. Thus, the other three subclasses make up the majority of passively transferred maternal antibody.

IgA

The major role of IgA is mucosal immunity.[21] There are two subclasses of IgA, IgA1 and IgA2, which can be found in both monomeric and polymeric forms. Although the majority of monomeric serum IgA is

Table 5.2 Select biological properties of human immunoglobulin isotypes

Immunoglobulin	Complement fixation	Placental transfer	SC-dependent transport	ADCC	Immediate hypersensitivity	Half-life (days)
IgG1	++	+	−	+	−	29
IgG2	+	+	−	+	−	27
IgG3	++	+	−	+	−	16
IgG4	−	+	−	±	−	16
IgM	++	−	+	−	−	5
IgA	−	−	+	−	−	6
IgD	−	−	−	−	−	−
IgE	−	−	−	+	+	2

SC, secretory component; ADCC, antibody-dependent cell-mediated cytotoxicity; ±, equivocal.

Table 5.3 Immunoglobulin (Ig) classes

	Class/ subclass	Molecular weight (Da)	Serum concentration (mg/ml)
$\gamma 1$	IgG1	146 000	5–12
$\gamma 2$	IgG2	146 000	2–6
$\gamma 3$	IgG3	165 000	0.5–1.0
$\gamma 4$	IgG4	146 000	0.2–1.0
μ	IgM	970 000[a]	0.5–1.5
$\alpha 1$	IgA1	160 000	0.5–2.0
$\alpha 2$	IgA2	160 000	0–0.2
δ	IgD	170 000	0–0.4
ε	IgE	190 000	0–0.002

From: Spiegelberg 1974.[20]
[a]Pentameric IgM+J chain.

IgA1, secreted IgA is split evenly between the two subtypes. The major polymeric form is the IgA dimer, which contains a single J chain joined to two IgA monomeric subunits (see also IgM above). Like IgM, polymeric IgA can bind to the poly-Ig receptor and be transported across mucosal epithelium and is the primary antibody found in mucosal tissues secretions.

Humans produce more IgA than any other immunoglobulin class, and selective IgA deficiency is the most common primary immunodeficiency. Interestingly, secretory IgA appears to be derived from locally produced IgA and not serum IgA.[22] Studies using radiolabeled polymeric IgA demonstrate that only 2% of the polymeric IgA in saliva is serum derived. Clinically, this finding suggests that intravenous IgA replacement for IgA-deficient patients may not restore IgA mucosal immunity.

IgE

IgE is secreted as a monomer and plays a key role in responses to parasitic infections. Interaction of antigen with IgE bound to Fc receptors on mast cells or basophils is the central event in Type I hypersensitivity (see Chapter 7). Although typically not seen at high circulating levels in 'Westernized' societies, IgE is often elevated in atopic persons.

IMMUNOGLOBULIN Fc RECEPTORS

The major function of immunoglobulins is to render potential pathogens and toxins harmless. Although the immunoglobulin molecule is responsible for recognizing a pathogen or toxin, it alone has a very limited role in their inactivation. However, by binding and aggregating (cross-linking) toxins, viruses, or bacteria via their Fc domains, antibodies can lead directly to neutralization, decreased microbial virulence, or clearance by binding to specific Fc receptors. Activation of complement, neutrophils, monocytes, macrophages, platelets, and lymphocytes is the major mechanism through which specific antibody can clear foreign antigen.

Fc receptors are all members of the immunoglobulin superfamily and are widely distributed.

FcγR

There are four Fc receptors for IgG, FcγRI, FcγRII, FcγRIII,[23,24] and a fourth type of FcγR, called FcγRn, expressed in neonates, where it is responsible for binding maternal IgG for transport across the placenta. FcγRI (CD64) is a 72 kDa glycoprotein and is the only FcγR that binds monomeric IgG with high affinity. Even so, IgG2 does not bind to FcγRI. FcγRI is present on monocytes and macrophages and can be upregulated on neutrophils and eosinophils by IFNγ. FcγRII (CD32) is a 40 kDa glycoprotein present on placental trophoblasts, endothelial cells, and all leukocytes (except NK cells). FcγRII binds monomeric IgG poorly but does bind immune complexes containing IgG1 and IgG3; binding to IgG2 is variable. Expression of FcγRII is upregulated on eosinophils by IFNγ and IL-3. FcRγIII (CD16) is a 50–80 kDa glycoprotein that can be attached to the membrane via a transmembrane tail or it can be GPI linked. FcγRIII binds IgG1, IgG3, and lectins and is highly expressed on neutrophils.

Interestingly, CD32 is expressed both on a human mast cell line, HMC-1,[25] and on human cutaneous mast cells,[26] but not lung or gastrointestinal mast cells.[26,27] Recently it has been shown that only FcγRIIa, but not FcγRIIb is expressed on human skin-derived mast cells.[28] This is key because FcγRIIa and FcγRIIb differ in their signaling response to binding IgG.[29] FcγRIIa is considered an 'activating' receptor - it contains the immunoreceptor tyrosine-based activation motif (ITAM) and cross-linking this receptor on B cells can lead to B cell activation. In contrast, FcγRIIb contains only an immunoreceptor tyrosine-based inhibitor motif (ITIM) associated with downregulation. These recent findings provide evidence that human mast cells can respond not only to cross-linking of Fcε receptors with allergen-specific IgE but also to cross-linking mediated by allergen-specific IgG via FcγRIIa.

FcαR

There are at least three distinct IgA receptors. FcαRI (CD89) is a 55–75 kDa glycoprotein that binds both IgA1 and IgA2 and is expressed on monocytes, macrophages, neutrophils, and eosinophils. FcαR expression on eosinophils is upregulated in atopic individuals and likely plays a key role in eosinophil activation. Interestingly, mice lack this receptor. Although several cells express FcαRI, neutrophils account for the majority of CD89+ cells.[17] IgA can also bind to a relatively recently discovered receptor called Fcα/μR. As its name indicates, this receptor also binds IgM and has been reported to mediate phagocytosis of IgM-coated bacteria. Lastly, the transferrin receptor (CD71) can also bind IgA, although its role in immunity is not well defined.[17]

FcεR

There are two IgE receptors (FcεR). FcεRI (no CD designation) is the high-affinity IgE receptor and is expressed not only by mast cells and basophils but also by dendritic cells and Langerhans cells in the skin. Cross-linking of IgE bound to FcεRI on mast cells and basophils leads to mediator release, resulting in mild to severe allergic reactions. The low-affinity IgE receptor FcεRII (CD23) is expressed on monocytes and B cells.

■ IMMUNOGLOBULIN GENES: GENERATION OF DIVERSITY AND CLASS SWITCH ■

The transcription of immunoglobulins (and T cell receptors) defies many conventions of traditional molecular biology and involves directed DNA breakage, rearrangement, and repair.[30] Although the bulk of the final immunoglobulin protein is encoded in the genomic DNA, each immunoglobulin chain undergoes a specific process of DNA rearrangement to randomly join several DNA 'cassettes' into a newly created coding sequence. In addition to these unique rearrangements, some nucleotides are removed and others are randomly added at the joining ends of each cassette to further enhance the variability of the immunoglobulin library. Finally, following ligation with antigen, the immunoglobulin undergoes somatic hypermutation.[31,32]

In theory, enough diversity must be present so that any potential pathogen can be recognized by a specific antibody. The average human has 10 million unique antibodies. If each of these antibodies were encoded by a unique gene, immunoglobulin genes alone would take up the entire human genome. In reality, the great diversity observed in the immunoglobulin repertoire is not fully dependent upon genomic DNA sequences and is largely formed while the pre-B cell is still developing in the bone marrow, before antigen is ever encountered. Indeed, the stages of B cell development are largely delineated by what is happening with the immunoglobulin genes and proteins (which are functioning as the BCR during development) at each stage.[7] In the pro-B cell stage, signals from the μ heavy chain combined with surrogate light chains and Igα and Igβ shut down further rearrangements of the Ig heavy chain (IgH) at this stage, correlating with the transition to the pre-B cell stage when the light chains rearrange. Interestingly, IgH V(D)J rearrangement appears to be permanently shut down. The recombinases responsible for V(D)J recombination (RAGs) are re-expressed during light-chain rearrangement, but this re-expression does not cause further IgH-chain rearrangement.[33,34]

V(D)J LIGHT- AND HEAVY-CHAIN REARRANGEMENT

To construct functional light- and heavy-chain genes, the discontinuous coding sequences must first be rearranged at the DNA level. This is a process unique to B and T lymphocytes. Both the light chains and the heavy chains undergo recombination at the DNA level during B cell development in the bone marrow. The constant and variable regions of each chain are encoded by separate regions in the germline genome that are recombined at the DNA level during B cell development (Fig. 5.7). A single constant region correlates with a single light- or heavy-chain isotype. The variable regions of the light and heavy chains are encoded by two (light) or three (heavy) exons. Both light and heavy chains have several variable (V) coding regions, one of which attaches to one of several joining segments (J) to create a unique V-J coding sequence in a particular B cell. Heavy chains also include one of approximately 50 additional segments, the diversity (D) segments, between the V and J coding segments to create a V(D)J recombination.

Certain segments of the V regions are highly variable whereas other amino acid residues are relatively constant. The segments that exhibit great sequence variation are called hypervariable regions

or complementarity-determining regions (CDRs). Both human light and heavy chains contain three CDRs referred to as CDR1, CDR2, and CDR3 (Fig. 5.4). The CDRs in the V regions of both the heavy and light chains directly contribute to the diversity of antigen recognition by the immunoglobulin repertoire. The recombination site of the V(D)J segments creates CDR3, the third, most variable CDR and the most critical for determining the idiotype of an immunoglobulin.

The germline configuration of heavy-chain variable genes is composed of a cluster of 51 V_H gene segments located 5′ to a cluster of 27 D (for diversity) gene segments.[35,36] There are seven V_H families with approximately 80% sequence homology within each family. Of these, the V_H 3 family is the largest. Additionally, 6 J_H genes are located 3′ to the D cluster and 5′ to the C_H genes.

Two recombination signal sequences (RSS-12 and RSS-23) are required for V(D)J recombination (Fig. 5.8). All V_H gene segments contain the RSS-12 signal and all J_H segments possess the RSS-23 signal. For heavy chains, the V_H has RSS-23, the D_H has RSS-12 on both ends, and the J region has RSS-23 (thus preventing direct V_H-J_H recombination). Recombination only occurs between dissimilar RSS signals (the 12/23 rule). Thus $V_H J_H$ recombination can take place, whereas $V_H V_H$ or $J_H J_H$ recombination cannot. Without the RSS, RAG is not functional and will not coordinate recombination.

DNA rearrangement results in the creation of a V(D)J segment separated from the C segment by intervening sequence. The V(D)J segment and C segments remain discontinuous and form the final coding sequence for the full heavy or light chain after mRNA processing to yield a function mRNA coding for the mature heavy or light chain (Fig. 5.7).

The exact site of recombination between the V, D, and J segments varies by a few nucleotides which further enhances the diversity of the CDR3 regions. N nucleotides are added at the coding junctions via terminal deoxynucleotidyltransferase. Additionally, palindromic sequences of DNA at the coding ends (P nucleotides) are inserted at the coding ends of the final gene. Because these non-germline encoded additions happen in the CDR3 region, they have a dramatic effect on antigen recognition of the final immunoglobulin molecule.

V(D)J recombination is regulated and mediated by RAG-1 and RAG-2. RAG-1 and RAG-2 have no sequence similarity to each other and are expressed only in B and T lymphocytes. This at least partially explains the limitation of DNA recombination to these cell types. Intriguingly, even though both T and B lymphocytes express RAG-1 and RAG-2 during their development, each rearranges only their unique antigen recognition molecules: the TCR for the T lymphocytes and the immunoglobulin genes for the B lymphocytes. Notably, deficiencies in the RAG genes lead to severe combined immunodeficiency (SCID) syndrome due to the inability of B and T lymphocytes to generate antigen receptors.

The DNA-level recombination of variable region cassettes as well as the 'sloppy' joining of those cassettes means that, by chance, one in three rearrangements will not be functional (will be out of the reading frame) and that autoreactive antibodies may be generated.[37] These autoreactive antibodies are expressed during B cell development in the bone marrow and, if ligated during development by self antigens in the bone marrow, and cause that B cell to be deleted. If B cells expressing autoreactive immunoglobulins on their surface escape this negative selection and are allowed to leave the bone marrow as mature B cells, a second level of regulation must still be overcome. Most B cells are dependent upon

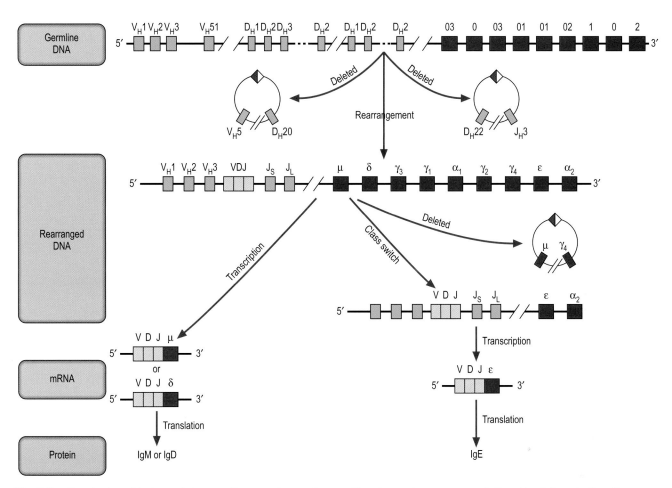

Fig. 5.7. Organization of the heavy-chain genes. Exons are shown as boxes and long intervening sequences are indicated by slash marks. Germline DNA: the human genome consists of 51 distinct V_H genes, 27 distinct D_H genes, and 6 J_H genes. Rearranged DNA: activation of RAG genes initiates the rearrangement of V(D)J regions which results in the excision of and V, D, and J regions ('deleted' circles) from the genomic DNA of maturing B lymphocytes. Once the VDJ regions have recombined, transcription can proceed and the μ exon is brought into proximity to the VDJ exon. If class switch is activated (such as during a secondary response), the DNA undergoes a second recombination which removes the intervening heavy-chain exons ('deleted' circle). mRNA: the recombined VDJ region is joined with the appropriate heavy-chain exon via splicing at the mRNA level (DNA is not affected). Protein: translation of the spliced mRNA results in the production of the immunoglobulin isotype corresponding to the heavy-chain exon transcribed.

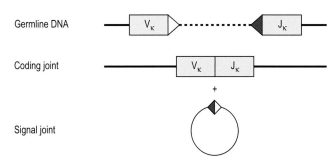

Fig. 5.8. VJ recombination. Each V_κ region is flanked by an RSS-12 signal (open triangle), and each J_κ region is flanked by an RSS-23 signal (closed triangle). Recombination yields a $V_\kappa J_\kappa$ coding joint and an RSS-12/RSS-23 signal joint.

T cells for immunological 'help' to develop into memory and plasma cells. In contrast to B cells, T cells undergo a very extensive process in the thymus to eliminate (or render non-functional) autoreactive T cells. Thus, with no T cells to recognize the same autoantigen, B cells expressing potentially autoreactive immunoglobulin should not be activated. Additionally, autoreactive immunoglobulins expressed on the surface of B cells can also be silenced by receptor editing mediated by RAG-1 and RAG-2.[38–40]

In addition to generated autoreactive immunoglobulins, DNA rearrangements can often produce a non-functional gene. Deletions and recombinations that produce an incorrect reading frame can all result in abortive rearrangements. Study of aberrant rearrangements in B cells reveals that λ-producing B cells usually contain deleted or abortively rearranged κ genes, whereas κ-producing cells contain λ genes in the germline configuration. This suggests that κ genes rearrange first and that

λ genes rearrange only if the κ rearrangement is unsuccessful. Once a successful rearrangement has occurred, the respective allele on the other chromosome is silenced by allelic exclusion to ensure that only one immunoglobulin of one specificity is expressed on any given B cell.

The area around the rearranged variable regions of the heavy and light chains is subject to somatic hypermutation after interaction with antigen.[41] Somatic hypermutation is a random mutation of the DNA sequence that is approximately one million times greater than the spontaneous DNA mutation rate. Although most random mutations result in antibodies with lower specificities for antigen, those that result in higher specificities are selected and ultimately become the antibodies that are most prevalent in the secondary and later responses. This is commonly referred to as affinity maturation. Although somatic hypermutation is frequently observed in most immunoglobulins, it is seldom seen in IgM. Once the VDJ regions of the heavy chain have been rearranged at the DNA level, they represent the permanent idiotype (barring somatic hypermutation) of the immunoglobulin produced by a particular B cell.

CLASS SWITCH RECOMBINATION

Humans have nine distinct heavy-chain genes, all of which are expressed in a given individual and that define the isotype of the antibody (Table 5.3). The genes are named using the Greek letter (e.g., γ) followed by a number (if there is a subclass of the isotype) whereas the proteins (isotypes) are identified using Arabic letters (e.g., IgM). The human immunoglobulin genes are arranged in the following order: μ, δ, $\gamma1$, $\gamma2$, $\gamma3$, $\gamma4$, $\alpha1$, ε, $\alpha2$. The Fc portion of an antibody is completely encoded for by the constant region of the heavy chain genes. All of the genes for the immunoglobulin heavy chains in humans are located on chromosome 14 (band 14q32.33).

The C_H genes are located $3'$ to the V_H, D, and J gene clusters. The exons that code for the μ constant region are located closest to the J cluster (Fig. 5.7). Generation of membrane or secreted immunoglobulins occurs not through DNA rearrangement but through mRNA processing and splicing. Both IgM and IgD are expressed during B cell development and both share the same V regions.

Although the shift from membrane bound to secreted immunoglobulin occurs at the RNA level as a consequence of differential RNA splicing, isotype class switch occurs at the DNA level and involves additional deletion of intervening sequences. In contrast to V(D)J recombination mediated by the RAG enzymes, class switch recombination is mediated by activation-induced deaminase (AID).[42] The usual progression of an antibody immune response involves the production of specific IgM antibodies followed by a switch to IgG (or IgA or IgE) antibodies with the same idiotype. The isotypes share the same recombined V region and, thus, antigen-binding specificity. Class switching occurs in mature B cells during B cell proliferation in the germinal center of the lymph node (or other lymphatic tissue) after antigen exposure. It does not occur in non-dividing plasma cells. The switch in immunoglobulin class is accomplished by translocation of the recombined V(D)J segment to a position immediately $5'$ to one of the constant region exons. Again, this recombination occurs at the DNA level, which means that the order of the heavy-chain genes in the genome is critical. As the immunoglobulins undergo class switch, the heavy-chain genes between the recombined V(D)J segments and the current C_H gene

are deleted, and can never be used again by that B cell. However, sequential isotype switching can occur, meaning that any constant region gene downstream of the gene currently being used is still available for use by that B cell.

Cytokines are primarily responsible for inducing class switch. The Th2-type cytokines, IL-4 and IL-13, can direct class to IgG4 and IgE. IFNγ can inhibit class switch to these two isotypes. Similarly, TGFβ induces class switch to IgA. Isotype switching is highly T cell dependent, although class switch can occur in the absence of T cell help.[43] Not only do T cell-derived cytokines such as IL-4 regulate switching, but direct T and B cell collaboration is also necessary for normal class switching via CD40. The CD40 ligand (CD154) on T cells and other cells is a 33 kDa glycoprotein that provides a mitogenic signal to B cells through the CD40 molecules on the B cell surface. In fact, individuals with hyper-IgM immunodeficiency syndrome lack expression of CD154 and are unable to accomplish normal isotype switching. Not only can isotype switching occur from IgM to other isotypes but also sequential switching can take place, as from IgM to IgG2 to IgE.

THERAPEUTIC APPLICATIONS OF IMMUNOGLOBULINS

Isolated immunoglobulins used for immunotherapy are polyclonal or monoclonal. Polyclonal antibodies generally represent a population of immunoglobulin molecules that are all specific for a particular antigen, but do not have the same idiotypes (or even necessarily the same isotype) and thus do not recognize the same epitope. Replacement intravenous immunoglobulin (IVIG) for certain immunodeficiency diseases is made from the polyclonal immunoglobulins (primarily IgG) of healthy donors because the polyclonal nature of the IVIG is necessary for it to provide passive immunity to the recipient.[44] On the other hand, monoclonal antibodies are generated by cloning individual B cells and expanding one particular (clonal) antibody.[45] All antibodies in a monoclonal antibody culture will be exactly identical, have the same isotype, idiotype, and will recognize the same epitope with the same affinity.

Although potentially a 'magic bullet,' the widespread use of monoclonal antibodies in immunotherapy is just starting to be realized.[46] The initial development of monoclonal antibodies in the 1980s relied on fusing normal mouse B cells with an immortal myeloma cells to create thousands of hybridoma cells. Each hybridoma cell not only retained the immortality of the original myeloma cell but also now expressed the unique immunoglobulin that the normal B cell provided. The hybridoma cells are then serially diluted and cloned so that each monoclonal antibody can be tested for antigen specificity and other desired characteristics before large amounts of antibody are produced.

Therapy with such mouse monoclonal antibodies was severely limited by the rapid production of anti-mouse antibodies by the patient being treated, rendering future treatments with mouse monoclonal antibodies ineffective. This problem was drastically minimized by using genetic engineering techniques to humanize the monoclonal antibodies (Fig. 5.9).[47] A humanized monoclonal antibody has only the CDRs from the original mouse monoclonal antibody, ensuring that the antigen-binding sites are still functional. The rest of the immunoglobulin, including the variable region framework sequences and the constant

Table 5.4 Monoclonal antibodies approved by the FDA for clinical use

Name/trade name	Target	Indication
Transplant rejection		
Muronomab-CD3 Orthoclone OKT3	CD3	Transplant rejection
Daclizumab Zenapax	CD25	Transplant rejection
Basiliximab Simulect	CD25	Transplant rejection
Inflammatory disease		
Abciximab ReoPro	Glycoproteins IIb/IIIa	Cardiovascular disease
Infliximab Remicade	TNFα	Rheumatoid arthritis
Adalimumab Humira	TNFα	Rheumatoid arthritis
Omalizumab Xolair	IgE	Atopic asthma
Efalizumab Raptiva	CD11a	Psoriasis
Natalizumab Tysabri	α4 integrin	Multiple sclerosis
Cancer		
Rituximab Rituxan	CD20	Non-Hodgkin lymphoma
Trastuzumab Herceptin	Her2	Metastatic breast cancer
Gemtuzumab ozogamicin Mylotarg	CD33	Acute myelogenous leukemia
Alemtuzumab Campath 1H	CD52	Chronic lymphocytic leukemia
Ibritumomab tiuxetan Zevalin	CD20	Non-Hodgkin lymphoma
Tositumomab-I^{131} Bexxar	CD20	Non-Hodgkin lymphoma
Cetuximab Erbitux	EGF receptor	Colorectal/head and neck cancers
Bevacizumab Avastin	VEGF	Colorectal cancer
Infectious disease		
Palivizumab Synagis	RSV F protein	Respiratory syncytial virus

Adapted in part from: Reichert JM, Rosensweig CJ, Faden LB et al. Monoclonal antibody successes in the clinic. Nature Biotechnology, 2005; 23:1073–1078, and Waldman TA. Immunotherapy: post, present and future. Nature Medicine 2003; 9:269–277. Copyright Nature Publishing Group.

THERAPEUTIC APPLICATIONS OF IMMUNOGLOBULINS

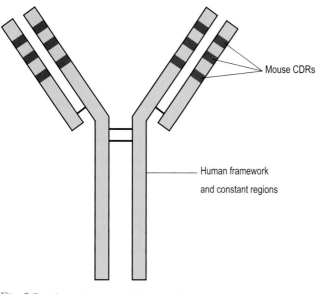

Mouse CDRs

Human framework and constant regions

Fig. 5.9. General structure of humanized monoclonal therapeutic antibodies. All framework and constant regions of the mouse immunoglobulin have been replaced by human immunoglobulin sequences. The only mouse-derived sequences that remain are those in the complimentarity-determining regions (CDRs), which are responsible for the antigen specificity.

BOX 5.1 CLASSIFICATION OF IMMUNOGLOBULINS

Isotype: Defined by heavy-chain constant region genes. All isotypes are present in healthy individuals. Heavy-chain isotypes define immunoglobulin class and subclass.

Allotype: Allelic variants of constant region genes that segregate in classic Mendelian fashion.

Idiotype: Set of determinants expressed on the variable regions of heavy and light chains that generally define the antigen-binding site; often used as a clonal marker.

Sources of antibody diversity
Encoded in genome

1. Several different V, D, and J segments.
2. Sites of hypervariability (CDR1 and CDR2) within V regions of both heavy and light chains.

DNA recombination/mutation

1. Random joining of different V, D, and J segments to form CDR3 domain.
2. N- and P-region nucleotide additions/deletions.
3. Somatic hypermutation following antigen recognition.

Protein assembly

1. Combination of heavy and light chain to make antigen-binding site.

regions are derived from human immunoglobulin sequences using recombinant DNA technology.[48] Additionally, some monoclonal antibodies are made in completely human systems, thus eliminating the possibility of cross-species reaction all together. Information about the source of the antibody can be gleaned from the generic names of the therapeutic monoclonal antibodies listed in Table 5.4.[49] If the generic name ends in '-ximab' or '-zumab' the monoclonal antibody is chimeric or humanized, respectively.[50] An ending of '-omab' indicates it is a mouse antibody, and '-umab' indicates human origins.

■ SUMMARY ■

The dual functions of the antibody molecule – antigen binding and biological effector function – are reflected in antibody structure and genetic organization. The B cell precursor contains immunoglobulin genes inherited from both parents. However, these inherited genes determine only to a limited extent the idiotypic repertoire of the offspring. B cell development is absolutely dependent upon successful rearrangement of immunoglobulin genes and uses membrane-bound immunoglobulins as a key component of the BCR. Diversity of the variable regions of the immunoglobulins is generated by a variety of genetic mechanisms, all of which contribute to the phenomenal variety of idiotypes expressed in the immunoglobulin repertoire (Box 5.1).

Interaction of the IgM cell surface BCR with antigen activates the B cell to produce secreted IgM. With T cell help, immunoglobulin class switching may then occur. The secondary (and subsequent) immune response consists of secreted IgG, IgA, or IgE. Class switching is highly T cell dependent and is regulated through CD40 and the

action of cytokines. Somatic hypermutation can generate additional variability of the antibody idiotype and affinity. Antibodies specific for antigen mediate a variety of biologic effects, including agglutination, precipitation, neutralization, activation of complement, and interaction with specific cell surface Fc receptors. Notably, type I hypersensitivity reactions result when IgE bound to Fcε receptors on mast cells or basophils is cross-linked with antigen. All these functions of antibody ligation are dependent upon the isotype of the antibody.

References

B lymphocytes and the humoral immune response

1. Melchers F. Fit for life in the immune system? Surrogate L chain tests H chains that test L chains. Proc Natl Acad Sci U S A 1999; 96:2571–2573.
2. Vettermann C, Herrmann K, Jack H-M. Powered by pairing: the surrogate light chain amplifies immunoglobulin heavy chain signaling and pre-selects the antibody repertoire. Semin Immunol 2006; 18:44–55.
3. Wang LD, Clark MR. B-cell antigen receptor signaling in lymphocyte development. Immunology 2003; 110:411–420.
4. Geisberger R, Crameri R, Achatz G. Models of signal transduction through the B-cell antigen receptor. Immunology 2003; 104:401–410.
5. Geier JK, Schlissel MS. Pre-BCR signals and the control of Ig gene rearrangements. Semin Immunol 2006; 18:31–39.
6. Tissot JD, Vu DH, Aubert V, et al. The immunoglobulinopathies: from physiopathology to diagnosis. Proteomics 2002; 2:813–824.
7. Weiler CR, Bankers-Fulbright JL. Common variable immunodeficiency: test indications and interpretations. Mayo Clin Proc 2005; 80:1187–1200.
8. McHeyzer-Williams LJ, Malherbe LP, McHeyzer-Williams MG. Helper T cell-regulated B cell immunity. Curr Top Microbiol Immunol 2006; 311:59–83.
9. Manz RA, Hauser AE, Hiepe F, et al. Maintenance of serum antibody levels. Annu Rev Immunol 2005; 23:367–386.
10. Manz RA, Radbruch A. Plasma cells for a lifetime? Eur J Immunol 2002; 32:923–927.
11. Nayak R, Lal G, Shaila MS. Perpetuation of immunological memory: role of serum antibodies and accessory cells. Microbes Infect 2005; 1276–1283.

Immunoglobulin structure and function

12. Roux KH. Immunoglobulin structure and function as revealed by electron microscopy. Int Arch Allerg Immunol 1999; 120:85–99.
13. Schiffer M, Girling RL, Ely KR, et al. Structure of λ-type Bence-Jones protein at 3.5 Å resolution. Biochemistry 1973; 12:4620–4631.
14. Greenspan NS, Bona CA. Idiotypes: structure and immunogenicity. FASEB J 1993; 7:437–444.
15. Pellequer JL, Chen SW, Roberts VA, et al. Unraveling the effect of changes in conformation and compactness at the antibody V(L)-V(H) interface upon antigen binding. J Mol Recognit 1999; 12:267–275.
16. Kelly DF, Pollard AJ, Moxon ER. Immunological memory – the role of B cells in long-term protection against invasive bacteria pathogens. JAMA 2005; 294:3019–3023.
17. Woof JM, Mestecky J. Mucosal immunoglobulins. Immunol Rev 2005; 206:64–82.
18. Kaetzel CS. The polymeric immunoglobulin receptor: bridging innate and adaptive immune responses at mucosal surfaces. Immunol Rev 2005; 206:83–99.
19. Rojas R, Apodaca G. Immunoglobulin transport across polarized epithelial cells. Nat Rev Mol Cell Biol 2002; 3:944–955.
20. Spiegelberg HL. Biological activities of immunoglobulins of different classes and subclasses. Adv Immunol 1974; 19:259–294.
21. Brandtzaeg P. Role of secretory antibodies in the defense against infections. Int J Med Microbiol 2003; 293:3–15.
22. Hahn C-L, Best AM. The pulpal origin of immunoglobulins in dentin beneath caries: an immunohistochemical study. J Endod 2006; 32:178–182.
23. Flesch BK, Neppert J. Functions of the Fc receptors for immunoglobulin G. J Clin Lab Anal 2000; 14:141–156.
24. Radaev S, Sun P. Recognition of immunoglobulins by Fcγ receptors. Mol Immunol 2002; 38:1073–1083.
25. Wedi B, Lewrick H, Butterfield JH, et al. Human HMC-1 mast cells exclusively express the FcγRII subtype of IgG receptor. Arch Dermatol Res 1996; 289:21–27.
26. Ghannadan M, Baghestanian M, Wimazal F, et al. Phenotypic characterization of human skin mast cells by combined staining with toluidine blue and CD antibodies. J Invest Dermatol 1998; 111:689–695.
27. Krauth MT, Majlesi Y, Florian S, et al. Cell surface membrane antigen phenotype of human gastrointestinal mast cells. Int Arch Allergy Immunol 2005; 138:111–120.
28. Zhao W, Kepley CL, Morel PA, et al. FcγRIIa, not FcγRIIb, is constitutively and functionally expressed on skin-derived human mast cells. J Immunol 2006; 177:694–701.
29. Van den Herik-Oudijk IE, Capel PJA, van der Bruggen T, et al. Identification of signaling motifs within human FcγRIIa and FcγRIIb isoforms. Blood 1995; 85:2202–2211.

Immunoglobulin genes: generation of diversity and class switch

30. Schwartz RS. Shattuck Lecture – Diversity of the immune repertoire and immunoregulation. N Engl J Med 2003; 348:1017–1026.
31. Diaz M, Flajnik MF, Klinman N. Evolution and the molecular basis of somatic hypermutation of antigen receptor genes. Philos Trans R Soc Lond B Biol Sci 2001; 356:67–72.

32. Diaz M, Casali P. Somatic immunoglobulin hypermutation. Curr Opin Immunol 2002; 14:235–240.
33. Jung D, Giallourakis C, Mostoslavsky R, et al. Mechanism and control of V(D)J recombination at the immunoglobulin heavy chain locus. Annu Rev Immunol 2006; 24:541–570.
34. Cobb RM, Oestreich KJ, Osipovich OA, et al. Accessibility control of V(D)J recombination. Adv Immunol 2006; 91:45.
35. Giudicelli V, Duroux P, Ginestoux C, et al. IMGT/LIGM-DB, the IMGT comprehensive database of immunoglobulin and T cell receptor nucleotide sequences. Nucleic Acids Res 2006; 34:D781–D784.
36. Pallares N, Lefebre S, Contet V, et al. The human immunoglobulin heavy variable genes. Exp Clin Immunogenet 1999; 16:36–40.
37. Melchers F, Rolink AR. B cell tolerance – how to make it and how to break it. Curr Top Microbiol Immunol 2006; 305:1.
38. Jancovic M, Casellas R, Yannoutsos N, et al. RAGs and regulation of autoantibodies. Annu Rev Immunol 2004; 22:485–501.
39. DeWildt RM, Hoet RMA, van Venrooij, et al. Analysis of heavy and light chain pairings indicates that receptor editing shapes the human antibody repertoire. J Mol Biol 1999; 285:895–901.
40. Seagal J, Melamed D. Role of receptor revision in forming a B cell repertoire. Clin Immunol 2002; 105:1–8.
41. Sale JE, Bemark M, Williams GT, et al. In vivo and in vitro studies of immunoglobulin gene somatic hypermutation. Philos Trans R Soc Lond B Biol Sci 2001; 356:21–28.
42. Stavnezer J, Amemiya CT. Evolution of isotype switching. Semin Immunol 2004; 16: 257–275.
43. He B, Qiao X, Klasse PJ, et al. HIV-1 envelope triggers polyclonal Ig class switch recombination through a CD40-independent mechanism involving BAFF and C-type lectin receptors. J Immunol 2006; 176:3931–3941.

Therapeutic applications of immunoglobulins

44. Grabenstein JD. Somebody else's antibodies: the characteristics and roles of immune globulins. Pharm Pract Manag Q 2001; 20:41–55.
45. Lipman NS, Jackson LR, Trudel LJ, et al. Monoclonal versus polyclonal antibodies: distinguishing characteristics, applications, and information resources. ILAR J 2005; 46:258–268.
46. Schnipper LE, Strom TB. A magic bullet for cancer – how near and how far. N Engl J Med 2001; 345:283–284.
47. Peterson NC. Advances in monoclonal antibody technology: genetic engineering of mice, cells, and immunoglobulins. ILAR J 2005; 46:314–319.
48. Reichert JM, Rosensweig CJ, Faden LB, et al. Monoclonal antibody successes in the clinic. Nat Biotechnol 2005; 23:1073–1078.
49. Waldmann TA. Immunotherapy: past, present and future. Nat Med 2003; 9:269–277.
50. Ballow M. -ximab this and -zumab that! Has the magic bullet arrived in the new millennium of medicine and science? J Allergy Clin Immunol 2005; 116:738.

REFERENCES

The Complement System

Kathleen E Sullivan

6

CONTENTS

SUMMARY OF IMPORTANT CONCEPTS

>> Complement deficiencies are not uncommon. MBL deficiency occurs in approximately 5% of the population and C2 deficiency occurs in 1:10 000 Caucasian individuals

>> Systemic lupus erythematosus and meningococcal disease are the two most common phenotypes associated with complement deficiencies

>> The diagnosis of most complement deficiencies begins with the demonstration of a markedly low CH_{50} or AH_{50}

>> Management of complement deficiencies is not standardized but efforts to minimize infection have been developed

■ OVERVIEW ■

The complement system was first described in the 1880s and 1890s as a system capable of inducing lysis of bacteria and red cells. This is still the most recognized function of the complement cascade, although it is probably not the most important function ascribed to complement. In 1919, the Nobel Prize in Physiology was given to the Belgian microbiologist, Jules Bordet, for his description of the complement system. The term complement was given to the unnamed proteins by Bordet when he fractionated serum from guinea pigs and identified a heat-stable fraction with antibody and a heat-labile fraction which 'complemented' the antibody fraction in a lytic assay.

Today, we understand the complement system as a group of 14 proteins comprising the complement cascade and more than 10 regulatory proteins. In addition, there are at least seven receptors which mediate the biological functions of the complement proteins. A tremendous amount of metabolic energy is expended in the production of the complement proteins, hinting at their importance. Nearly 5% of all serum proteins are complement proteins and this number can rise to 7% of serum proteins in inflammatory states. In addition, the conservation of the complement system across evolution also hints at the importance of these proteins. Lymphocytes and antibody first evolved with cartilaginous fishes and from that point forward in evolution, the complement cascade became more and more intertwined with other elements of host defense. Prior to the evolution of cartilaginous fishes, there existed a simple single C3-like molecule in primitive species such as jawless fishes, sea urchins, and sea squirts. The main function of this simple C3-like molecule was to opsonize pathogens. The term opsonization is derived from the Greek word for condiment or delicacy and refers to the facilitation of phagocytosis by neutrophils. The neutrophils perceive bacteria coated in complement as 'tastier' than bacteria without complement, thus enhancing ingestion. This role of complement as an opsonin is its most important role in host defense.

The majority of serum complement is produced by hepatocytes, although C1q, properdin, and C7 are produced predominantly by myeloid cells and factor D is produced by adipocytes and is also known as adipsin.[1–5] A wide variety of cells produce small amounts of complement

BOX 6.1 DEFINITIONS

Classical pathway: C1, C4, C2, C3 and the terminal components.

Alternative pathway: factor B, factor D, properdin and the terminal components.

Lectin activation pathway: MBL, MASP1, MASP2, C3 and the terminal components.

Anaphylatoxins: C3a, C4a, C5a. These are mediators of smooth muscle contraction, degranulation of mast cells, enhanced neutrophil aggregation, increased vascular permeability.

Opsonization: Renders a particle more easily phagocytosed.

C3 tick-over: This term is occasionally used to describe spontaneous C3 hydrolysis.

Membrane attack complex (terminal components): C5, C6, C7, C8, C9.

CH_{50}: The assay is used to define the dilution of serum capable of lysing 50% of the sensitized sheep red cells. This assay measures the intactness of the classical pathway through the terminal components.

AH_{50}: The assay is used to define the dilution of serum capable of lysing 50% of non-sensitized rabbit red cells. This assay measures the intactness of the alternative pathway through the terminal components.

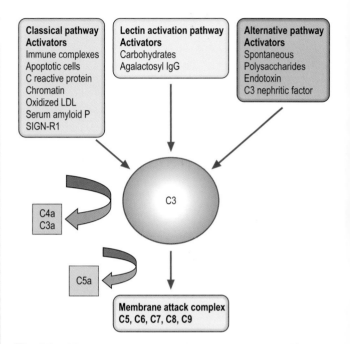

Fig. 6.1. The three activation arms of the complement system. The complement system consists of three activation arms each independently triggered, but all leading to cleavage of C3. Activation of the classical pathway via C1q is driven largely by immune complexes, but many ligands such as amyloid and SIGN-R1, a C-type lectin, can activate the classical pathway under the right circumstances. The lectin activation pathway is driven largely by oligosaccharides present on microbes and the alternative pathway is driven largely by the surface qualities of bacteria. Activation of C3 is important for opsonization, anaphylotoxic activity, and B cell costimulation. Lysis of bacteria is dependent on the membrane attack complex.

components after pro-inflammatory stimuli and this is thought to magnify the local response in times of infection.[6] The regulation of complement component expression is largely transcriptional and is largely induced by inflammatory cytokines although the details vary according to cell type.[7] Thus, interpretation of clinical tests of complement must be placed within the context of the patient. Advanced liver disease compromises the production of complement components and has been shown to render the patient more susceptible to bacterial infections.[8] This decrease in production could be masked by an intercurrent illness, which would induce the expression of complement components from hepatocytes.

This chapter will address the biochemistry of the complement cascade, the biological functions of complement, and disorders related to the complement system. The complement cascade is dedicated to the deposition of C3b on the surface of microbes and the release of small molecule mediators to regulate inflammation.[9,10] Generally, the protein-protein interactions of the complement system involve enzymatic cleavage steps, leading to two or more protein fragments with biological activity. With these tenets in mind, the complement cascade becomes a simple set of protein-protein interactions designed to deposit C3 and cleave complement proteins into smaller fragments with biologicalal activity. While simple in principle, the details are still being investigated in many cases. In addition, the field of complement has daunting nomenclature and, for this reason, a few definitions are given in Box 6.1. The nomenclature follows certain patterns with the classical pathway components generally indicated with an upper case C followed by a number that roughly correlates with the position in the cascade (C4 appears out of order). Alternative pathway members are generally referred to as a 'factor' and are designated with a letter (factor B, factor D, factor H). As protein fragments are cleaved

off, they are given lower case letter identifiers with the 'a' most often designating the smaller fragment (the exception is C2a which is larger than C2b). In some cases, the two fragments can be further cleaved and those smaller fragments are named with additional lower case letters. When a cleavage product is inactive, it is proceeded by the letter 'i.'

■ INTRODUCTION TO THE COMPLEMENT SYSTEM ■

The complement cascade originally evolved to opsonize pathogens and enhance their phagocytosis. As the adaptive immune system evolved, the complement system co-evolved such that it now interfaces with nearly all aspects of host defense. The most important biological functions of the complement system can be divided into those related to innate host defense: opsonization, initiation of an inflammatory response, clearance of apoptotic debris, and direct lysis of gram negative bacteria; and those related to the adaptive responses: B cell activation and T cell priming. In addition, complement regulatory proteins play an important role in endothelial cell homeostasis. Each of these functions will be described as well as disorders associated with loss of one or more of these functions.

A simple model for the organization of the complement cascade has three activation arms: the classical pathway, the lectin activation pathway and the alternative pathway (Fig. 6.1). These three pathways exist to cleave the central protein, C3, and allow it to bind to the nearest surface, usually a pathogen. C3 constitutes a powerful opsonin and markedly enhances phagocytosis of the pathogen. The three activation arms utilize different pathogen recognition strategies and lead to the production of slightly different inflammatory mediators. Once C3 is cleaved, the terminal components proceed to bind to the surface and will ultimately form a pore. Two important functions of the complement cascade, therefore, are related to structural aspects of the complement protein. Opsonization requires the covalent attachment of C3b to the pathogen and direct cell lysis is due to the formation of a membrane-spanning pore. Many of the remainder of the functions of the complement cascade relate to fluid phase mediators. The next three sections discuss the three activation arms and the inflammatory mediators released as a result of their serial cleavage steps.

■ THE CLASSICAL PATHWAY ■

The classical pathway is so named because it was the first pathway to be described and for many years, it was thought to be the only complement activation mechanism. The classical pathway is activated primarily by immune complexes. When antibody binds antigen, a subtle conformational change occurs which renders the antibody molecule capable of interacting with C1.[11,12] Not all antibody is equivalent in terms of its ability to activate complement. Only IgG and IgM activate complement and IgM is much more efficient than IgG. In addition, not all isotypes of IgG are equivalent. IgG3 is the most efficient followed by IgG1 and IgG2. IgG4 is not able to activate complement. A single molecule of IgM is sufficient to activate complement while many molecules of IgG bound to a particle are required to activate complement, presumably because two side-by-side IgG molecules are required for activation and, given a random distribution, a large number would be required on the surface in order to produce two of sufficient proximity.

Immune complexes are not the only molecules capable of activating the classical pathway. C-reactive protein, serum amyloid P, β-amyloid, DNA/chromatin, cytoskeletal filaments, SIGN-R1, and some pathogens can activate the classical pathway although it is not entirely clear how that interaction occurs.[13,14] In addition, C1 can bind apoptotic cells and participates in the removal of apoptotic debris.[15] This function is of critical importance. Many murine models have demonstrated that persistence of apoptotic debris leads to the development of autoantibodies and C1 deficiency in humans is strongly associated with the development of systemic lupus erythematosus (SLE) in humans.[16] The defect in clearance of apoptotic debris probably leads to the exposure of nuclear antigens on the surface of apoptotic cells which then act as a reservoir for immunizing B cells if not properly cleared.

C1 is a large complex of a single C1q (in turn comprised of six polypeptide chains), two C1r and two C1s proteins (Fig. 6.2). The globular head interacts with the Cγ2 domain of IgG or the Cμ3 domain of IgM. Interestingly, other activators of C1 bind to the stalk region rather than the globular head. All protein interactions lead to a conformational change in C1 which allows autoactivation of C1r. The two molecules of active C1r cleave the two molecules of C1s. Once cleaved, the active C1s cleaves C4 into C4a and C4b (not to be confused with the genetically distinct C4A and C4B genes). C4b is a highly reactive molecule which binds to

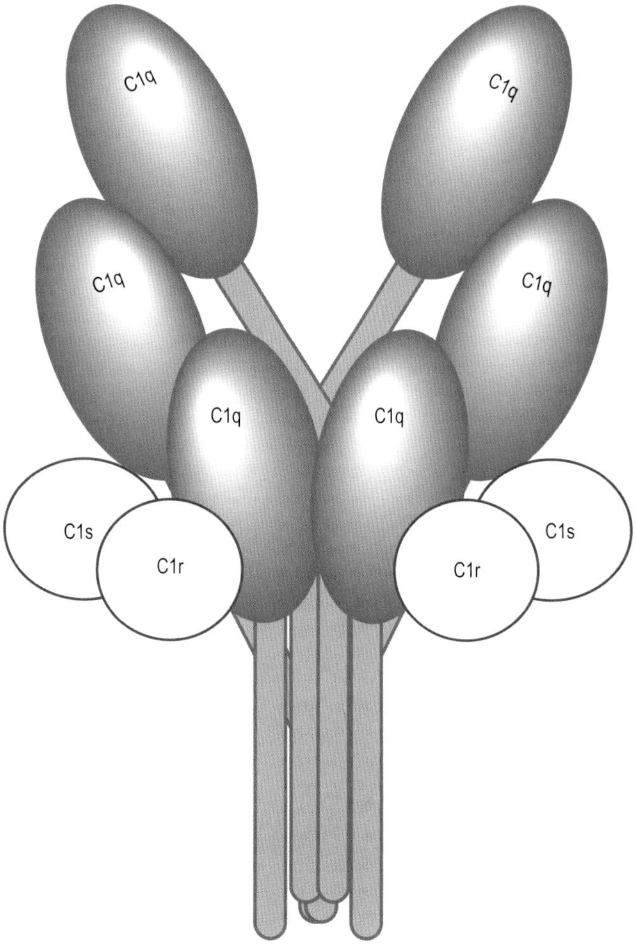

Fig. 6.2. The C1 complex. C1 is a large complex with a configuration resembling a bouquet of tulips. The enzymatically active C1r and C1s are nestled in the stem region. Interaction of C1q with antibody or certain other activators leads to a conformational change which activates C1r and C1s, leading to enzymatic cleavage of C4.

the pathogen surface near the antibody-C1 complex.[17] Binding of C4b to the surface is inefficient and much of the C4b simply diffuses away and is inactivated. Measuring this inactive fragment forms the basis of some complement activation assays. The C4b that becomes attached to the surface of the pathogen serves to nucleate another reaction. The C4b-C1s$_2$ complex with the enzymatically active C1s can cleave C2 into C2a and C2b. The smaller C2b is released and the C2a becomes incorporated into the growing complex. The complement proteins are all physically associated but it is the C4bC2a complex which is referred to as the C3 convertase. In the next stage, C3 binds to this complex and is cleaved by C2a. Once again, two fragments are produced, with C3a being released into the surrounding space and C3b binding to the pathogen surface (Fig. 6.3). C3b securely deposited on the pathogen surface is recognized by specific receptors on neutrophils. The actual deposition is inefficient and the majority of C3 drifts off. This fluid phase C3b is very short lived and is quickly inactivated to become iC3b. At this point, the main focus of

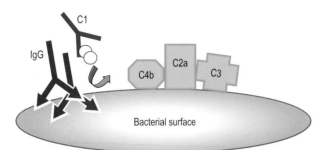

Fig. 6.3. Activation of the classical pathway. The classical pathway C3 convertase consists of C4bC2a. Covalent attachment of C4b to the surface of the antibody-bound pathogen ensures that the opsonization is not misdirected. The attachment of C3b renders the pathogen more easily phagocytosed by neutrophils.

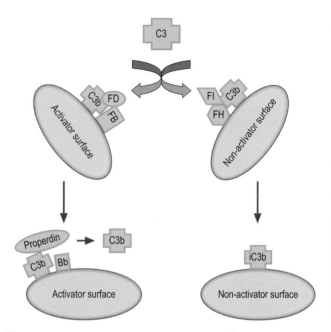

Fig. 6.4. Activation of the alternative pathway. The activation of the alternative pathway relies on distinguishing activator surfaces from non-activator surfaces. This distinction is largely the result of factor H (FH). Factor B (FB) interacts with spontaneously hydrolyzed C3b, is cleaved by factor D (FD), and when stabilized by properdin can continue to cleave additional C3 and ultimately C5 on activator surfaces such as pathogens. On non-activator surfaces, such as host cells, factor H displaces factor B which facilitates an interaction with factor I (FI), which inactivates C3b.

the classical pathway has been achieved: C3b has been deposited on the surface of a pathogen where it can act to enhance phagocytosis.

As a consequence of classical pathway activation, there are a number of small molecule mediators which act to initiate inflammation. C4a, C3a, and C5a are termed anaphylatoxins.[18,19] These fragments are less than 12 kDa and bind specific receptors which lead to mast cell degranulation and neutrophil aggregation. The release of histamine by mast cells and basophils leads to increased vascular permeability and vasodilatation. These anaphylatoxins are not equivalent and C5a is the most potent.[18,20] In addition, C5a acts as a chemotactic factor for neutrophils.[21] Thus, within minutes of an antibody binding to a pathogen, the complement system has ensured that neutrophils are recruited to phagocytose and kill the pathogen and have enhanced the phagocytosis of the pathogen by coating it with C3b. The anaphylatoxins increase blood flow to the site, increase vascular permeability such that additional complement proteins and antibodies can enter into the tissue, and direct neutrophils to the location of the pathogen through the chemotactic activity of C5a. It is therefore no surprise that deficiencies of classical pathway components are associated with an increased predisposition to infection with bacteria.

In summary, the classical pathway is activated by immune complexes, apoptotic debris and a variety of other proteins and nucleic acids. Once activated, C1, C4, and C2 interact to produce a C3 cleaving enzyme: C4bC2a. Cleavage products resulting from this activation pathway lead to inflammation with erythema (vasodilatation) and edema (vascular leak). Neutrophils become activated and are therefore primed to cross the vascular endothelium to enter into tissues to initiate the attack on the pathogen.

■ THE ALTERNATIVE PATHWAY ■

The alternative pathway was discovered and named as the non-classical alternative pathway in the 1950s. This pathway does not require the existence of preformed antibody and it, along with the lectin activation pathway, constitutes the truly innate activation arms of the complement cascade.[22,23] The basis of this pathway is a spontaneous hydrolysis of C3 which occurs in the serum at a rate of 0.2–0.4% per hour.[24] Most of the complement proteins have short half-lives in serum, but C3 has

a particularly high rate of hydrolysis. This spontaneous hydrolysis is often referred to as C3 tick-over because there is always some ongoing complement consumption as a result of this hydrolysis. The hydrolyzed C3 undergoes a conformational change which allows it to interact with factor B. Only when factor B is complexed with hydrolyzed C3 can it be cleaved by the serum protein factor D. The cleaved factor B is termed Bb and there is a small fragment liberated in this enzymatic cleavage known as Ba, which is not thought to be biologically active. C3bBb is the alternative pathway C3 converting enzyme which is stabilized by properdin and cleaves additional C3 into C3b and C3a.[25] As was the case with the classical pathway, the surface is important. In the case of the classical pathway, the surface provides a binding site for antibody and substrate to anchor the accumulated C3 converting enzyme complex. In the case of the alternative pathway, surfaces are either activator surfaces or non-activator surfaces. A non-activator surface (usually our own cells) binds factor H avidly due to rich sialic acid residues.[26–28] Factor H on our own cells displaces factor B from C3b and catabolizes C3b. In contrast, on activator surfaces, factor H cannot displace factor B from C3b and the alternative pathway activation is allowed to proceed (Fig. 6.4). Activator surfaces are often coated with mannose or N-acetylglucosamine. These oligosaccharide moieties are produced primarily by bacteria and yeast. The significance of an activator surface cannot be overstated. Many medical products are activator surfaces and activation of complement via the alternative pathway due to blood flow over membranes is a significant issue for patients on cardiac bypass or undergoing dialysis.

In summary, the alternative pathway can, in some circumstances, be activated directly by immune complexes, but it is generally activated through the recognition of oligosaccharide and charge differences common to pathogens. It is a constituent of the innate immune system. The alternative pathway exploits the instability of the native C3 molecule and, on activator surfaces, nucleates a complex of C3bBb which cleaves additional C3 to fan the flames of inflammation. Note that the classical pathway provides an important substrate for the alternative pathway, C3b.

■ THE LECTIN ACTIVATION PATHWAY ■

The lectin activation pathway also is a part of the innate immune system. In fact, MBL-like proteins have been identified in invertebrates, suggesting that this pathway may be the most evolutionarily ancient. The critical protein, mannose-binding lectin (MBL), recognizes oligosaccharides specific to pathogens in a manner similar to that of factor H discussed above.[29–31] The MBL protein is structurally related to C1q and has the same stalk and globular head arrangement existing as dimers, trimers, tetramers, pentamers, and hexamers. Molecularly, it belongs to the collectin family which includes surfactant proteins and conglutin. Mammalian glycoproteins are generally decorated with galactose and sialic acid, not recognized by MBL. In contrast, MBL avidly binds to oligosaccharides associated with bacteria, yeast, and parasites such as mannose, N-acetylglucosamine, fucose, and glucose.[30] The affinity is highest for mannose.

Upon binding to the carbohydrate ligand, MBL undergoes a conformation change leading to activation of the two associated enzymes, MASP1 and MASP2. The arrangement of these enzymes with MBL is quite similar to the C1q-C1r-C1s arrangement. MASP2 cleaves C4 into the metastable C4b which binds to a nearby surface, and the anaphylatoxin, C4a. MASP1 cleaves C3 and as such, provides substrate for the alternative pathway which can amplify the process. Once C4b is bound to the pathogen surface, the remaining protein-protein interactions are identical to those in the classical pathway (Fig. 6.5). The C3 converting enzyme C4bC2a is formed and C3 is cleaved into C3a which diffuses away and C3b which attaches to the pathogen and both acts as an opsonin and initiates the activation of the terminal components.

The lectin activation pathway is intrinsically an innate immune response; however, MBL binds to α-galactosyl IgG with high affinity.[32] This unusual IgG is produced primarily at times of inflammation and this antibody would therefore amplify the complement response at sites of inflammation by activating both through the classical pathway and the lectin activation pathway.

Given the importance of this molecule in innate defenses, it is predictable that deficiencies of MBL or MASP 1/2 would predispose to infection. Indeed, that appears to be the case.[33–35] Although MBL deficiency is extremely common in the general population, having MBL deficiency does increase the risk of infection. Perhaps less predictable is an increased risk of SLE and enhanced progression of rheumatoid arthritis.[36–39] The mechanism underlying the association with rheumatoid arthritis is not clear; however, the risk of SLE is attributed to the role of MBL in the clearance of apoptotic cells and debris.[40] MBL functions

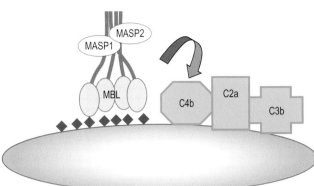

Fig. 6.5. Activation of the lectin pathway. The lectin activation pathway is engaged by pathogen oligosaccharides (black diamonds) and leads to a C3 convertase which is identical to that of the classical pathway. Mannose-binding lectin (MBL) serves as the recognition domain of the complex, while MASP1 and MASP2 are similar in function to C1r and C1s.

much as C1q does and deficiency of MBL would be expected to impair clearance of apoptotic cells. These cells can act to 'immunize' the host to nuclear proteins which are exposed on the surface of apoptotic cells.

In summary, the lectin activation pathway represents an important arm of the innate immune system. This pathway is activated directly by pathogen oligosaccharides and by a specific type of IgG produced in inflammation (α-galactosyl IgG). The C3 convertase produced in the lectin activation pathway is identical to that of the classical pathway and the inflammatory mediators perform the same functions.

■ THE MEMBRANE ATTACK COMPLEX ■

The most important biological activities of the complement system are opsonization, clearance of apoptotic debris, lysis of cells and pathogens, activation of B cells, and activation of T cells. Of these functions, only direct lysis of targets requires the terminal components. Once C3 is cleaved by any of the activation arms described above, it becomes a part of the next enzymatic complex, the C5 convertase. This C5 convertase will either be *C4b2a3b* (classical and lectin activation pathways) or *C3b2Bb* (alternative pathway). The cleavage of C5 follows the typical pattern with the larger fragment becoming attached to a surface and the smaller fragment diffusing into the fluid phase. C5b has a low affinity for lipids but, when bound to C6 and C7, can insert firmly into a lipid membrane.[41,42] C5b, which remains more external than the other components, binds directly to C8 which then becomes incorporated into the complex. This last addition is sufficient to compromise the physical integrity of the membrane and leakage of cytoplasmic proteins and ions begins to occur. The addition of C9 leads to the formation of true pore, as opposed to a leaky patch (Fig. 6.6). Multiple C9 molecules can associate with the C5-C6-C7-C8 complex, although the pore size is remarkably uniform by electron microscopy.[43]

Nucleated cells are resistant to lysis for two reasons. As they are metabolically active, they can repair membrane damage. Additionally, eukaryotic cells are coated with complement regulatory proteins which inhibit completion of the lytic process. In fact, nucleated cells are often stimulated in the presence of sublytic amounts of complement.[44–46] It is not clear why this might be physiologically desirable; however, it may serve to alert the cells of danger. In contrast, many gram negative bacteria and most enveloped viruses are susceptible to complement-mediated lysis. Given the enormous capacity for damage, it is no surprise that there are a large number of regulatory proteins which control this process. These will be discussed in a subsequent section.

It might be imagined that the destructive powers of the terminal components would be essential for host defense. In fact, most people with terminal complement component deficiencies have a limited phenotype or no phenotype. The major susceptibility, as a consequence of a terminal complement component deficiency, is to *Neisseria*. Nevertheless, it would be a mistake to dismiss the terminal components as an afterthought.

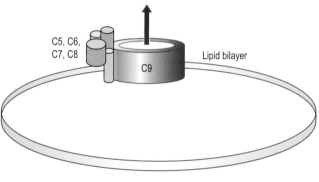

Fig. 6.6. The membrane attack complex or terminal components can form a physical pore in membranes. The terminal components or the membrane attack complex are a carefully ordered set of protein-protein interactions. C5-C6-C7-C8 is sufficient to render the membrane less stable and somewhat leaky; however, the addition of C9 allows a stable pore to be formed. Once formed, if the cell is unable to repair the damage, cell contents leak from the cell.

They play a very important role in tissue damage as a result of autoantibodies.

In summary, the terminal components, also known as the membrane attack complex, serve to induce lysis of a target. They are most efficient at lysing red blood cells which have no capability of repairing membrane damage and gram negative bacteria. In other eukaryotic cells, low levels of membrane attack complex on the surface can be stimulatory.

■ RECEPTORS AND BIOLOGICAL FUNCTIONS ■

Receptors for complement mediate many of the biological functions of complement (Table 6.1). They are often divided into the anaphylatoxin receptors and the receptors recognizing classical pathway components.[47] The anaphylatoxin receptors recognize C3a or C4a and there is a distinct receptor for C5a. Both are G-protein coupled receptors. The same receptor recognizes C3a and C4a; however, the affinity for C3a is approximately 100-fold higher than for C4a.[48–50] The receptors are widely expressed on mast cells, basophils, eosinophils, neutrophils, platelets, endothelial cells, and smooth muscle cells.[51] Through the activation and degranulation of mast cells, histamine-induced vasodilatation occurs, although in some circumstances C3a may be able to induce vasodilatation and gastrointestinal smooth muscle contraction directly. Other biological effects attributed to the C3a/C4a receptor are aggregation of neutrophils, stimulation of mucus release from goblet cells, and activation of macrophages.[52] In the face of an infection, these functions may all be viewed as protective (Fig. 6.7). The vasodilatation acts to deliver additional neutrophils to the site of inflammation, mucus release may facilitate clearance of organisms, activation of macrophages enhances phagocytosis, and aggregation of neutrophils is a surrogate marker for enhanced trans-endothelial migration into the affected tissue.

The C5a receptor provides additional support for an incipient infection.[53] The C5a receptor provides all of the functions of the C3a/C4a

Table 6.1 Complement receptors

Receptor	Ligand	Role	Comments
CR1	C3b, C4b, iC3b	Immune complex clearance, phagocytosis	Four allelic forms differ in size, CD21
CR2	C3d, C3dg, iC3b	B cell activation	CD35
CR3	iC3b, C3d, C3b, ICAM-1	Neutrophil adhesion, phagocytosis	β_2-integrin, 165 kDa α chain, 95 kDa β chain, CD11b/CD18
CR4	iC3b, C3b	Neutrophil adhesion	β_2-integrin, 150 kDa α chain, 95 kDa β chain, CD11c/CD18
CRIg	C3b, iC3b	Intravascular pathogen clearance	
C1qRp	C1q, MBL, surfactant protein A	Phagocytosis	126 kDa, CD93
cC1qR	C1q, MBL, surfactant protein A	Phagocytosis	Recognizes collagen domain
C3aR	C3a >>> C4a	Increases vascular permeability, mast cell degranulation, chemotaxis	48 kDa protein
C5aR	C5a, C5a desArg	Chemotaxis, mast cell degranulation, increases vascular permeability	43 kDa protein, CD88

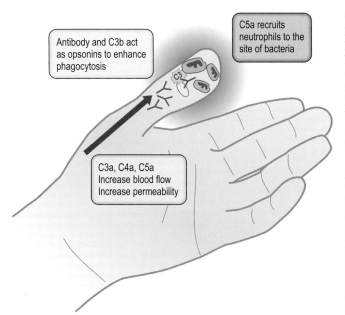

Antibody and C3b act as opsonins to enhance phagocytosis

C5a recruits neutrophils to the site of bacteria

C3a, C4a, C5a
Increase blood flow
Increase permeability

Fig. 6.7. Complement plays an important role in inflammation. The anaphylatoxic activities of the classical pathway are very important in the initiation of the inflammatory process. The purpose of inflammation is to deliver cells and proteins which might participate in host defense to the site. C3a, C4a, C5a enhance blood flow and vascular leak; C3b and/or antibody on the surface of bacteria enhance phagocytosis; C5a plays an important role in the recruitment of neutrophils via its chemotactic effects.

receptor and is even superior in terms of anaphylatoxic activity, although the range of tissue expression is different. In addition to the tissue distribution of the C3a/C4a receptor, the C5a receptor is expressed on hepatocytes, lung endothelium and vascular smooth muscle, umbilical cord endothelium, astrocytes, microglia, and T cells.[54,55] In addition, C5a is the most powerful endogenous chemotactic factor for neutrophils and is a potent chemotactic agent for monocyte/macrophages.[56] Furthermore, C5a induces tissue factor expression on monocytes and endothelial cells as well as IL-8 expression, all of which contributes to fibrin formation. Thus, the early inflammatory response mediated by complement, anaphylatoxins, bradykinin, and other small molecule mediators, serves to deliver increased blood flow to the area, increases extravasation of antibody and complement into the tissues, and then C5a provides directionality for the recruited neutrophils (Fig. 6.7). This is a very efficient system to direct a response to a focal infection.

In overwhelming sepsis, high levels of serum C5a can cause neutrophil aggregation, blockage of pulmonary vessels, and adult respiratory distress syndrome (ARDS). Over-production of C5a in sepsis can also lead to inhibition of neutrophil function, which may partially explain the paradoxical immunocompromise seen in sepsis in the face of high levels of inflammatory mediators.[57] C5a also appears to be one of the major contributors to disseminated intravascular coagulation in sepsis.

The remaining complement receptors recognize either intact complement components or the large cleavage products. There are several poorly defined C1q receptors which have been described. Their function appears to relate to phagocytosis and clearance of apoptotic cell debris.

C1qRp (CD93) is expressed on myeloid cells, endothelium, and platelets and appears capable of also binding MBL,[58] although its function has been called into question recently.[59] There are two proteins which bind C1q which are primarily intracellular but which can appear on the surface after myeloid cell stimulation, CRT (cC1qR/collectin receptor), and a mitochondrial protein, gC1qbp.[60-63] Finally CR1 (discussed below) can bind C1q, although the exact role of the interaction remains to be defined. In general, C1q interactions lead to enhanced phagocytosis, enhanced clearance of apoptotic cells, increased respiratory burst, and improved microbicidal activity.

The CR1 (CD35) receptor has been difficult to study because it is only present in primates. In primates, it is widely expressed and is found on mast cells, basophils, eosinophils, monocytes/macrophages, glomerular cells, B cells, follicular dendritic cells, some T cells, and erythrocytes. The CR1 receptor primarily binds C3b, C4b, and iC3b, although in some systems it may also bind C1q.[64,65] Engagement of the receptor enhances phagocytosis but its most important role appears to be in the clearance of immune complexes. Immune complexes are extremely potent stimuli for inflammation via Fc receptors and complement receptors. In a normal host, immune complexes are maintained in a soluble state by complement through the binding of C3b and it is this C3b that is recognized by the CR1 receptor. Maintaining the immune complexes in a soluble state, prevents their access to the pro-inflammatory Fc receptors and complement receptors. Erythrocytes are extremely numerous and they constitute a non-responsive 'sink' for immune complexes because they are incapable of generating an inflammatory response. The erythrocytes bind the immune complexes and transport them to reticuloendothelial cells of the liver and spleen where they are degraded.[66-68]

Two other functions of the CR1 receptor deserve mention. CR1 has a regulatory role in the inactivation of C3 and the destabilization of the C3 and C5 convertase complexes.[69] It is not clear how important this function is in the regulation of the complement cascade. The other function relates to antigen processing. B cells and other professional antigen-presenting cells may process antigen differently when it is bound by complement and this could theoretically affect antigen presentation. In a more specialized antigen uptake scenario, CR1/CR2 bearing follicular dendritic cells trap antigen, providing a stimulus for B cells.[70-72] A more speculative role for CR1 bearing cells in the bone marrow is that they may become tolerized upon exposure to apoptotic cells bound by complement.[73,74]

The CR2 receptor (CD21) is the receptor for the Epstein–Barr virus and is expressed on B cells, follicular dendritic cells, epithelial cells, and some T cells.[75,76] CR2 binds downstream degradation products of C3 such as C3d. Antigen bound by C3d, as would normally occur on an antigen after complement activation, is far more stimulatory for B cells than antigen which is not bound by C3d. The activation threshold for B cells is dramatically lowered when both the B cell receptor and CR2 are simultaneously engaged.[76-78] Engagement of this receptor seems to be particularly important for the development or survival of B1 B cells.[78] Thus, patients with deficiencies in C3 are compromised in terms of their ability to produce antibody in response to live infections. This is also true for patients with other deficiencies of the classical pathway activation arm; however, because C3 may still be cleaved via the alternative and lectin activation pathways, the compromise in antibody production is less severe.

CR3 and CR4 are both members of the β2 integrin family.[79] These receptors bind iC3b and C3b. The CR3 receptor also binds C3d. While clearly complement receptors, these receptors act primarily as adhesion molecules. CR3 is expressed on monocytes, neutrophils, natural killer cells, and microglia and can mediate phagocytosis of particles opsonized with C3b and adhesion via binding to its ligand, ICAM (intracellular adhesion molecule). The $\beta 2$ integrin family has only three members. Each member utilizes the same β chain, giving the family the name. The second $\beta 2$ integrin is complement receptor CR4. The role of CR4 as a complement receptor is not well understood.

The most recently described complement receptor has been named CRIg and is present on tissue-resident macrophages. It is the primary receptor mediating clearance of complement-tagged bloodborne pathogens. Kupffer cells bearing both CR3 and CRIg appear to have a dominant role in this process and Fc receptors may also play a role in the phagocytic clearance process.[80]

The main roles of complement are opsonization, initiation of inflammation, clearance of apoptotic debris, lysis, and modulation of the adaptive responses. All three activation arms lead to opsonization and the attachment of C3b or iC3b to a particle enhances phagocytosis through an interaction with the CR1, CR3, CR4 or CRIg receptors. Residual C1q may be bound by the CR1 receptor and also contribute to enhanced phagocytosis. The importance of C3 in host defense is clear from the tremendous number of infections seen in patients with C3 deficiency. The infections arise from an inability to opsonize, and an inability to generate the C5a chemotactic factor, and the impaired antibody response due to failure of B cell co-stimulation through the CR2 receptor.

This opsonization most often occurs in tissue space not in the intravascular space. In fact, neutrophils have a safety mechanism such that they are relatively resistant to activation unless bound to a surface. Neutrophils must egress from the vascular space by adhering to the vascular endothelium. Complement plays a role in the early inflammatory response which aids in the recruitment of neutrophils. The release of the anaphylatoxins leads to blood vessel dilatation to deliver more cells to the location, increased leakage of plasma proteins such as antibody and additional complement into the tissue space, and activation of mast cells and platelets initiates the complex adhesion process which directs neutrophils to the site. C5a acts to guide the neutrophils to the pathogen by acting as a chemotactic gradient which the neutrophil senses with its C5a receptor.

The neutrophil rapidly digests the pathogen and for many infections, the arrival of the neutrophil is the end of the threat. While the human body is constantly inundated with bacteria, this early defense system is so effective, the bacteria rarely have an opportunity to proliferate and establish a clinical infection. In certain infections, the neutrophil may not be capable of killing the pathogen or the number of pathogens may overwhelm the system. The CRIg receptor contributes to clearance of intravascular pathogens and bloodstream *S. pneumoniae* can be specifically recognized by SIGN-R1 on marginal zone macrophages leading to SIGN-R1 mediated opsonization of the bacteria and delivery to marginal zone B cells for T-independent antibody production.[81,82] Persistent antigen bound by C3d can stimulate conventional B cells to produce antibody which would aid clearance in subsequent infections. Although the alternative pathway and lectin activation arms are not dependent on antibody, antibody is important for defense against bacteria in two ways. The classical pathway is the most efficient of the activation arms; thus, the presence of antibody to a pathogen maximizes the complement cascade. Secondly, antibody is

itself a powerful opsonin. Most myeloid cells have Fc receptors which also mediate phagocytosis. Dual engagement of Fc receptors and complement receptors by a phagocytic cell results in a synergistic enhancement of phagocytosis.

■ REGULATION OF COMPLEMENT ACTIVATION ■

Unregulated complement activation would lead to host cell lysis, the inappropriate production of inflammatory mediators, and aberrant B cell activation. Nearly as much metabolic energy is spent in the regulation of the complement system as is spent producing the main constituents of the complement cascade. Traditionally, the regulators of complement are divided into fluid phase regulators and membrane-bound regulators; although this is somewhat arbitrary, this is the format used in this chapter (Table 6.2). Another categorization strategy groups the regulators by means of the targeted component. For example, C3 is the most important complement component and the most tightly regulated component. C3 is regulated by factor H, factor I, properdin, C4 binding protein, membrane cofactor protein, CR1, CR2, and decay accelerating factor (DAF, CD55). Several of these molecules have a conserved motif of 60 amino acids, termed the short consensus motif, and belong to the RCA gene cluster on chromosome 1 (Fig. 6.8).

C1 inhibitor is perhaps the most clinically important of the regulatory proteins. Heterozygous deficiencies of C1 inhibitor lead to hereditary angioedema. C1 inhibitor is a serine protease which inhibits the low level autoactivation of C1 and the fluid phase activation of C1 (Fig. 6.9).[83] Immune complex activation of C1 is preserved and is not affected by C1 inhibitor. The mechanism by which C1 inhibitor regulates C1 is by binding to C1s and C1r, leading to dissociation from C1q. It is thought that C1 inhibitor acts on MBL and MASP1/2 through a similar mechanism. C1 inhibitor also has important roles inhibiting factor XII (Hageman factor) and prekallikrein of the contact system of coagulation,[84,85] functions of paramount importance for the clinical features of C1 inhibitor deficiency.

C4 binding protein is another fluid phase regulator of complement and also shares the short consensus motif configuration of many of the complement regulators. It acts to displace C2a and dissociates the classical pathway convertase. In addition, C4 binding protein is a cofactor for factor I cleavage of C4b (Fig. 6.9).[86,87]

Factor I, alongside factor H, regulates the alternative pathway (Fig. 6.10).[88–91] Factor H identifies non-activator surfaces though the recognition of non-pathogen oligosaccharides and displaces Bb from C3b on those surfaces. Factor H can also prevent factor B from ever binding to C3b in the first place. Factor I inactivates C3b by cleaving it to iC3b and its activity is enhanced in the presence of factor H. Together, these two regulators ensure that the spontaneous activation of the alternative pathway remains low level unless an activator surface is available to nucleate a more intensive and sustained activation.

Factor I also acts to inhibit C4b from the classical pathway.[89,92] In this setting, it interacts with C4 binding protein and cleaves C4b into C4c and C4d. C4 binding protein has an interesting structure and regulates the complement cascade as well as the coagulation cascade, as is true for C1 inhibitor. C4 binding protein binds circulating protein S and inhibits it.

Table 6.2 Complement regulatory proteins

Protein	Localization	Function	Comments
C1 inhibitor	Serum	Binds to C1r and C1s and dissociates the C1 complex	105 kDa
C4 binding protein	Serum	Cofactor for factor I cleavage of C4b	550 kDa
Factor I	Serum	Cleaves C3b and C4b	
Factor H	Serum	Defines activator surface	
S-protein	Serum	Inhibits the insertion of the membrane attack complex into the cell membrane	Also known as vitronectin
Decay accelerating factor (DAF)	Ubiquitous/cell membrane	Dissociates both C3 and C5 convertases	GPI-anchored CD55
Membrane cofactor protein	Hematopoietic cells except erythrocytes	Cofactor for C3b cleavage by factor I	CD46
C8 binding protein	Most hematopoietic cells	Binds to C8 and prevents interaction with C9	GPI-anchored; also known as homologous restriction factor
CD59	Hematopoietic cells, endothelial cells, epithelial cells, glomerular cells	Inhibits the membrane attack complex	GPI-anchored; also known as HRF20

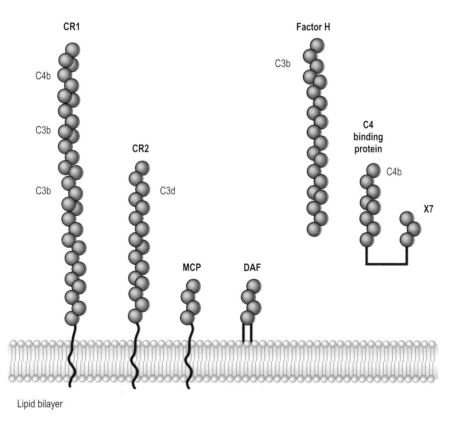

Fig. 6.8. Complement regulatory proteins. The regulators of complement proteins are all composed of short consensus repeats (circles) and are all encoded on chromosome 1q32. The binding sites for various ligands are indicated in the figure. CR1, complement receptor 1; CR2, complement receptor 2; MCP, membrane cofactor protein; DAF, decay accelerating factor.

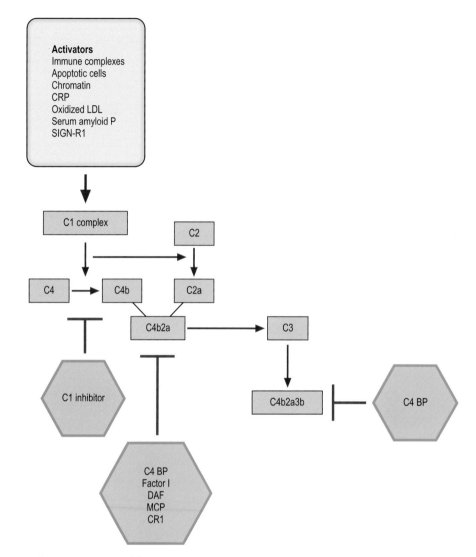

Fig. 6.9. The regulation of the classical pathway. The classical activation pathway is shown with the relevant regulatory proteins shown in the gray hexagons. C4 BP denotes C4 binding protein.

One last fluid phase complement regulatory protein should be mentioned. S-protein (distinct from protein S) is an inhibitor of the membrane attack complex.[93] The majority of terminal complement inhibitors are membrane bound and this soluble inhibitor is thought to act as a back-up strategy to prevent inappropriate lysis of host tissue.

The membrane-bound regulators of complement consist of the ubiquitous 70 kDa molecule termed DAF, membrane cofactor protein (MCP, CD46), C8 binding protein, and CD59.[89,94–99] DAF, C8 binding protein, and CD59 are glycosylinositol phospholipids (GPI) linked proteins and MCP is an integral membrane glycoprotein. DAF is expressed on most cells, C8 binding protein is a 65 kDa protein expressed on all hematopoietic cells, and CD59 is a 20 kDa protein expressed on all cells in contact with blood and certain epithelial cells and brain cells. DAF serves to dissociate the C3 convertase and MCP serves as a cofactor for factor I cleavage of C3b and C4b (Figs 6.9–6.11). CD59 is an important

protein, which, along with S protein, inhibits the membrane attack complex. CD59 accomplishes this by becoming incorporated into the accumulating membrane attack complex and inhibiting C9 binding. C8 binding protein functions similarly, but acts via binding to C8. S protein acts in the fluid phase as an inhibitor of C5b and prevents insertion into the cell membrane.

Several receptors also act as complement regulatory proteins and in these cases, the regulatory activity may be viewed as termination of that specific complement function after the signal has been delivered. CR1 binds C3b and C4b and serves as a cofactor for factor I mediated cleavage. CR1 can further support additional cleavage steps leading to C3dg which can be cleaved by serine proteases to C3d, the fragment capable of co-stimulating B cells.[69] Finally, CR1 accelerates the decay of both C3 convertases. CR2 has a similar role supporting cleavage of C3b.

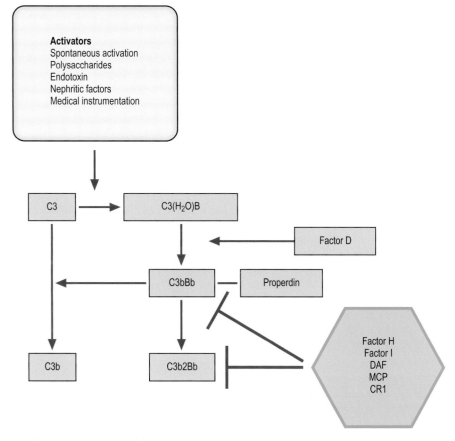

Fig. 6.10. The regulation of the alternative pathway. The alternative activation pathway is shown with the relevant regulatory proteins shown in gray hexagons. C3bBb is stabilized by properdin.

■ DISORDERS ASSOCIATED WITH COMPLEMENT ACTIVATION ■

Complement is easily triggered and, in spite of a broad range of control strategies, can feed back on itself and engender significant harm. The primary examples of wholesale systemic complement activation are post-cardiac bypass syndrome and immune complex diseases. In post-cardiac bypass syndrome, the bypass circuitry is an activator surface and the alternative complement activation pathway is fully activated.[100–102] This leads to activation of the kinin system, fibrinolysis, platelet activation and the release of large amounts of C5a. C5a can directly stimulate TNFα, IL-1, IL-6, and IL-8 release, further fueling the inflammatory process. Neutrophils bind the C5a and become activated and form aggregates. These aggregates interfere with circulation (often in the lung) and can release reactive oxygen species as well as damaging lysosomal enzymes. The systemic consequences of this process are neutropenia due to trapping, thrombocytopenia due to trapping, end organ dysfunction due to impaired circulation, and hypotension due to the action of the anaphylatoxins. In several trials, the use of a C5 inhibitor reduced mortality and morbidity in patients post cardiac bypass.[103,104]

Less dramatically, complement activation contributes to the manifestations of burn injuries, pancreatitis, and crush injuries.[105–107] In these cases, the tissues themselves are altered so as to become activator surfaces. In the case of burns, early colonization of the wound with bacteria also contributes to complement activation. Although most complement components are acute phase reactants and increase in response to TNFα and IL-6, activation of complement necessarily consumes the substrates as each component is cleaved to active fragments. Generally, early after injury, complement levels are low due to consumption; however, later they may be normal or increased in spite of ongoing consumption because the hepatic production of the components has been upregulated.

Serum sickness is uncommon; however, it can occur when soluble antigen is produced at high levels (hepatitis C), when an antigen is administered (OKT3 administration), or when antibodies develop to a medication.[108–110] Immune complexes contribute to the clinical features of a variety of autoimmune disorders where autoantibodies are produced. The classic manifestations of serum sickness relate to the deposition of immune complexes onto vascular beds with either high oncotic pressure or tortuosity. Classic serum sickness consists of a vasculitic rash, glomerulonephritis, and arthritis. Immune complexes are normally maintained in a soluble state by C3. Recognition of C3b by CR1 allows the immune complexes to travel to the Kupffer cells of the liver, where the immune complexes are taken up and degraded.[65–67] Fc receptors in the liver and spleen also contribute to clearance. When the clearance

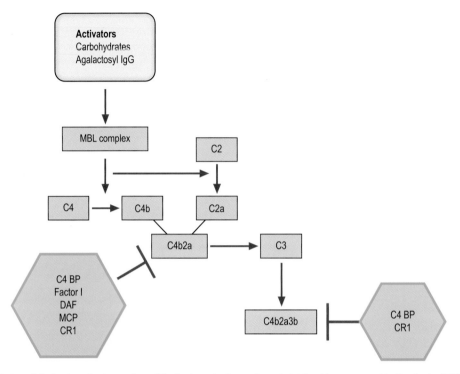

Fig. 6.11. The regulation of the lectin activation pathway. The lectin activation pathway is initiated by mannose-binding lectin (MBL) and utilizes regulatory proteins which are nearly identical to that of the classical pathway. The regulatory proteins are shown in gray hexagons.

pathway is overwhelmed, immune complexes deposit on endothelial cells wherever pressure or tortuosity allows them to do so (usually skin, glomeruli, and synovium). The deposited immune complexes initiate an inflammatory response by interacting with Fc receptors on the endothelial cell. Pre-existing antibody can mediate an immediate response to the antigen with abrupt onset of serum sickness. When a neoantigen is administered, initially there is no response; however, after 10–14 days an antibody response develops and the initial clinical signs of serum sickness ensue. Urticarial or vasculitic rashes are often the first sign, followed by adenopathy, fever, arthritis, and proteinuria.[111,112] Laboratory studies demonstrate hypocomplementemia due to consumption and a leukocytoclastic vasculitis with deposition of C3, IgM, and IgG.

There are four disorders associated with a limited complement activation due to stabilization of complement components by autoantibodies. Nephritic factor is a set of autoantibodies which stabilize C3 convertases.[113] The nephritic factor described initially was an autoantibody directed against C3bBb, the alternative pathway convertase. This nephritic factor stabilizes the active form and resists decay mediated by factors H and I. Thus, the activity of the alternative pathway is prolonged in the presence of nephritic factor. The vast majority of patients with the classic C3bBb nephritic factor have membranoproliferative glomerulonephritis.[114–116] Other types of nephritic factors have been described including antibodies which stabilize the classical pathway convertase. Nephritic factors, in general, are associated with lipodystrophy and membranoproliferative glomerulonephritis. Nearly 80% of patients with dense deposit disease or membranoproliferative glomerulonephritis type II have nephritic factor. Membranoproliferative glomerulonephritis type III disease is

associated with a nephritic factor which stabilizes the alternative pathway convertase and the C5 convertase in 70% of the patients. Type I disease is associated with various nephritic factors in only 15% of cases. The age of onset is typically in late childhood or adolescence. The lipodystrophy is characterized by the progressive loss of subcutaneous tissues, leading to a sunken-eyed appearance.[117] Often the fat below the waist is spared. The renal involvement may precede, or post-date the lipodystrophy by many years. A low C3 is seen with preservation of C4 because the defect is distal to C4. The mechanism of the lipodystrophy is due to the nephritic factor's lysis of factor D producing adipocytes.[118] Why some regions of the body are spared is not understood. The mechanism underlying the membranoproliferative glomerulonephritis is not completely understood. The nephritic factor may act as an immune complex and simply incite inflammation in the glomerulus due to its deposition. The fact that factor H deficiency can be associated with a similar phenotype suggests that there may be something specific about partial activation of the complement cascade and supporting this is the finding that renal podocytes have several complement receptors.

Antibodies to C1q were first described in patients with hypocomplementemic urticarial vasculitis.[119,120] They have since been described in patients with systemic lupus erythematosus. These IgG antibodies are directed against the collagen-like region of C1q. In lupus, the anti-C1q antibodies are preferentially found in renal tissue and the presence of anti-C1q in the serum of patients is a very strong predictor of renal disease.[121–123] The antibody appears to amplify any other injury to the glomerulus. In experimental animal models, antibodies to C1q caused pathology only after pre-existing injury. Given that the antibodies appear to be identical, it is difficult to understand the phenotype of hypocomplementemic urticarial vasculitis. In this disorder, glomerulonephritis is seen; however, cutaneous manifestations such as urticaria and angioedema are the most prominent findings. Ocular inflammation is also common and in patients who smoke, an aggressive obstructive lung disease is seen.[124,125]

Antibodies to factor H and C1 inhibitor, two complement regulatory proteins have been described and cause significant disease. The features of the diseases are comparable to the inherited deficiencies of those proteins and will be covered below.

■ DISORDERS ASSOCIATED WITH COMPLEMENT DEFICIENCY ■

Acquired and inherited deficiencies of complement can have significant biological effects or have very minor consequences. In the following subsections, individual deficiencies will be described (Table 6.3). In most cases, it is possible to predict the effects of a particular deficiency

based on understanding the normal physiological function of that protein. For example, the early classical pathway components function to aid apoptotic cell clearance, to activate C3, and to produce anaphylatoxic activity. The main phenotype associated with defects in C1, C2, and C4 is systemic lupus erythematosus. There is also an increase in the risk of infection. The terminal component deficiencies lead to impaired lysis of gram negative bacteria and the predominant manifestation is an increased risk of neisserial disease.

The vast majority of genetically determined complement deficiencies are inherited in an autosomal recessive fashion. Properdin deficiency is X-linked and C1 inhibitor deficiency is autosomal dominant (hemizygous). Inherited complement component disorders are typically associated with a CH_{50} or AH_{50} of near 0 and can be specifically defined in reference laboratories using a complementation system whereby patients' sera are added to mixes generated with a single missing component. Lysis is achieved except when the component missing in the patients' is identical to the component missing in the lytic mix. Further studies may be done if required to define the mutation; however, this is seldom helpful clinically. Identifying deficiencies of regulatory proteins is much more difficult as mutations must

Table 6.3 Inherited complement deficiencies

Deficiency	Chromosomal location	Number of cases reported	Clinical features, diagnostic strategy
C1q	1p36.12	10–100	SLE, infections, CH_{50} near 0
C1r/s	12p13	10–100	SLE, infections, CH_{50} near 0
C4	6p21.3	10–100	SLE, infections, CH_{50} near 0
C2	6p21.3	Many	SLE, infections, some asymptomatic, CH_{50} near 0
C3	19p13.3-13.2	10–100	Infections frequent and severe, glomerulonephritis, CH_{50} near 0
Factor D	19p13.3	<10	*Neisseria*, AH_{50} near 0
Factor B	6p21.3	<10	*Neisseria*, AH_{50} near 0
Properdin	Xp11.3-11.23	>100	*Neisseria*, AH_{50} diminished
MBL	10q11.2-21	Millions	Most asymptomatic, infections, SLE, CH_{50} normal, MBL assay required
C5	9q33	10–100	*Neisseria*, CH_{50} near 0
C6	5p13	>100	*Neisseria*, CH_{50} near 0
C7	5p13	>100	*Neisseria*, CH_{50} near 0
C8	1p32, 9q34.3	>100	*Neisseria*, CH_{50} near 0
C9		Many	*Neisseria*, CH_{50} diminished
Factor I	4q25	10–100	*Neisseria*, HUS, C3 may be diminished, many require mutation analysis
Factor H	1q32	10–100	*Neisseria*, HUS, C3 may be diminished, many require mutation analysis
MCP	1q32	<10	HUS, mutation analysis required
C1 inhibitor	11q12-13.1	Many	Angioedema, C1 antigen and functional levels
CR3/CR4	16p11.2	>100	Leukocyte adhesion deficiency, very severe systemic infections, lack of pus, flow cytometry
CD59	11p13	<10	Paroxysmal nocturnal hemoglobinuria, flow cytometry

be specifically sought in most cases. C1 inhibitor assays are widely available and are quite reliable, but for other complement regulatory proteins, the assays are infrequently available and often rely on direct mutation detection.

C1q DEFICIENCY

Patients with C1q deficiency present nearly uniformly with early-onset systemic lupus erythematosus (SLE).[126–128] C1q deficiency is the strongest known genetic risk factor for lupus. The manifestations of lupus in these individuals are similar to those seen in non-complement deficient individuals. The autoantibody profile is similar although anti-dsDNA antibodies may be somewhat less common.[129,130] Clinically, the features have more dramatic cutaneous and CNS manifestations than in the typical patient with lupus and the disease may be more severe. Based on a small number of patients, it is also believed that the lupus seen in C1q deficient individuals is less steroid responsive and has an earlier age of onset.[129,130] Patients with C1q deficiency also report an increased rate of infection and this no doubt relates to compromised opsonization and a mild decrease in B cell co-stimulation.

There are a few patients with inherited deficiencies of C1r and C1s.[131–134] It is thought that neither is stable without the other and therefore a mutation in one often leads to diminished levels of both. Glomerulonephritis and lupus have been found in C1r/C1s deficient patients. There are too few patients to define a clear phenotype.

C4 DEFICIENCY

There are two distinct genes for C4, termed C4A and C4B. They are highly homologous although C4A binds more avidly to protein while C4B binds more avidly to carbohydrate. Within each C4 gene, there can be deletions or duplications or simple inactivating mutations.[135,136] Thus, interpretation of a serum level is difficult.[137] A low C4 level may be due to consumption or to the inheritance of an inactive allele. Partial C4 deficiencies are extremely common; 1–2% of the general population and up to 15% of patients with SLE have complete C4A deficiency. While C4A deficiency is a risk factor for SLE, the severity of the disease is often less in patients with C4A deficiency compared to complement sufficient hosts.[138–142] Whereas 1–2% of the population has complete C4B deficiency, up to 15% of patients with invasive bacterial disease are C4B deficient.[143] In contrast to the common partial deficiencies, complete C4 deficiency due to four inactive alleles is quite rare. Well over 50% of the completely C4 deficient individuals have SLE.[142,144,145] Cutaneous manifestations are common and severe and the age of onset is often quite early. The usual array of autoantibodies are found although anti-dsDNA antibodies may be somewhat less frequent in C4 deficient individuals compared to normal hosts. Infection appears to be a significant problem for patients with C4 deficiency and infection is the major cause of death.[146,147] The mechanisms underlying the predisposition to infection are probably related to impaired opsonization and a modestly compromised B cell response to antigen. Each of these defects is partial, because C3 may still be cleaved via the alternative pathway. The association with SLE is due to compromised clearance of apoptotic debris. Persistence of apoptotic cells, with nuclear antigens displayed on the surface, can act as an antigen depot for immunization.

C2 DEFICIENCY

C2 deficiency is the most common of the inherited classical complement component deficiencies in Caucasians. Although rare in some ethnic groups, in Caucasians, it is found with a frequency of 1:10000. Most C2 deficient individuals are asymptomatic in contrast to those patients with C4 and C1 deficiency. Between 20 and 40% of C2 deficient individuals will develop lupus.[146–148] The age of onset is early adulthood, as is true for SLE in the general population, although cerebritis, nephritis, and arthritis are less common in C2 deficient SLE patients compared with the typical SLE patient. Anti-Ro antibodies are extremely common in C2 deficient patients with SLE although anti-dsDNA antibodies are infrequent.[149] Other autoimmune disorders have been described in patients with C2 deficiency although there may be an element of ascertainment bias as CH_{50} assays are commonly run on patients with autoimmune disorders.

Infections are increased in C2 deficient individuals as would be expected, and the most common cause of death among C2 deficient patients is sepsis.[148] Other systemic infections such as meningitis, pneumonia, epiglottitis, and peritonitis have been seen and the most common organisms have been *S. pneumoniae* and *H. influenzae*. With improved vaccination against these organisms, it is possible that the infection pattern will be altered.

C3 DEFICIENCY

The infectious manifestations of C1, C4, and C2 deficiency are not overwhelming and certain patients have no obvious increase in infections. C3 deficiency is the rarest of the four early component deficiencies and it has the most severe phenotype by far.[150–154] Membranoproliferative glomerulonephritis is seen instead of lupus in approximately one-third of the cases of C3 deficiency.[146,147] All patients have a profound predisposition to infection and the infections are sometimes characteristic of neutrophil dysfunction (abscesses), humoral deficiencies (sinopulmonary disease), and complement deficiencies (sepsis, meningitis). These types of infections reflect the various roles of C3. Staphylococcal abscesses probably reflect an inability to opsonize and to generate the C5a chemotactic factor. Recurrent sinopulmonary infections reflect a significant compromise in B cell co-stimulation. Systemic infections are due to a complete failure of C3b opsonization. These multiple defects contribute to the severe infectious manifestations of C3 deficiency.[155]

One other feature of C3 deficiency deserves mention. During infections, a vasculitic rash may appear and symptoms of serum sickness may occasionally be seen. These unusual findings are due to the lack of immune complex solubilization by C3. They are typically transient in nature but can cause confusion with lupus, particularly in the presence of glomerulonephritis.

C3 deficiency is rare, with fewer than 30 cases reported in the literature. There is a founder effect in South Africa among the Afrikaans-speaking population.[156] Slightly more common is a partial deficiency of C3, termed hypomorphic C3.[157,158] This partial deficiency has been seen in a number of autoimmune disorders but is difficult to diagnose and is probably underascertained.

MBL DEFICIENCY

MBL deficiency was originally identified in a cohort of hospitalized patients with a variety of infectious diseases ranging from tuberculosis to sepsis. It is now known that MBL deficiency is quite common with

2–7% of people having MBL deficiency.[159] There are common structural mutations which destabilize the higher-order complexes, leading to accelerated clearance and poor function.[160] There are several promoter mutations which lead to impaired production.[160] Each type of mutation has a characteristic effect on function and serum levels and because each one is relatively common, there are combinations of mild mutations which lead to complete loss of function.

A large number of studies have attempted to characterize the risk of infection in MBL deficient individuals.[159] Studies of children with upper respiratory tract infections have both shown an association with MBL deficiency and have shown no association with MBL deficiency. When sepsis was evaluated, there was clear evidence that MBL deficiency was associated with sepsis.[161,162] Similarly burn patients with MBL deficiency are at markedly increased risk of infection with *Pseudomonas aeruginosa* compared to MBL sufficient burn patients. Studies of patients on chemotherapy and in ICU setting have been inconsistent with respect to the importance of MBL deficiency. In summary, it seems likely that MBL deficiency may modify disease susceptibility but, on its own, contributes minimally to susceptibility to infections.

In addition to the risk of infection, MBL deficiency has been found to double the risk of SLE but to be protective for renal disease.[163] This is similar to what has been seen in C4A deficiency. In rheumatoid arthritis, the presence of MBL deficiency increases radiologic progression of disease.[164] Patients with Crohn's disease are more likely to have MBL deficiency than controls and are more likely to have antibodies to mannan, which is a marker for Crohn's disease.

MASP2 DEFICIENCY

A single patient with mannose-binding protein-associated serine protease 2 (MASP2) deficiency has been described.[165] This patient suffered from ulcerative colitis and SLE. Laboratory evaluations revealed hypocomplementemia, with low levels of C1q. Testing for MASP2 revealed very low levels and a mutation was identified; which interfered with MBL binding.

FACTOR B DEFICIENCY

A single case of factor B deficiency has been reported.[166] The patient was identified after developing meningococcemia and laboratory studies revealed an absent AH_{50}. No mutation was characterized; however, abnormal protein was seen on electrophoresis.

FACTOR D DEFICIENCY

Neisserial infections are the most common manifestation of factor D deficiency.[146,147,167] Systemic streptococcal infections have also been seen. Other complement levels are typically normal in factor D deficiency; however, there is almost no ability to activate the alternative pathway. The phenotype of factor D deficiency confirms the importance of the alternative pathway.

PROPERDIN DEFICIENCY

Properdin deficiency is the only X-linked complement deficiency. It is one of the more common complement deficiencies and occurs largely in Caucasians. Approximately half of the properdin deficient individuals have had one or more episodes of meningococcal disease.[146,147,168–171] Other bacterial infections are also seen, but are much less common. There is a particularly high fatality rate in meningococcal disease in properdin deficient patients in contrast to the protection from mortality seen in patients with terminal complement component deficiencies. There may be a founder effect in Tunisian Jewish people; however, properdin deficiency is seen on all ethnic backgrounds.

The role of properdin is to stabilize C3bBb and, in patients lacking this stabilizing function, activation of the alternative pathway is impaired. It is not completely clear why neisserial species are more subject to complement-mediated lysis than other gram negative species. In vitro, most gram negative organisms are susceptible to complement-mediated lysis and it has been suggested that neisserial species are unusual in that they typically induce colonization of the nasopharynx prior to active infection. It may be that the site of inoculation is important and other gram negative organisms would be encountered predominantly in the gastrointestinal tract where IgA is the dominant antibody and complement is not a prominent form of host defense.

C5 DEFICIENCY

C5 is the major endogenous chemotactic factor for neutrophils; however, C5 deficient patients have the same phenotype as the other terminal component deficiencies: neisserial infections.[146,147,172] Patients have been primarily ascertained through rheumatology clinics, where CH_{50} assays are often run, and after meningococcal disease. C5 deficiency has been detected in patients with SLE and other autoimmune disorders; however, there is little rationale for believing there is a mechanistic relationship and these findings may represent ascertainment bias. C5 does play an important role in the defense against *Neisseria* and the relationship of C5 deficiency to meningococcal and gonococcal disease is more assured. C5 deficiency is found in a number of ethnic and racial backgrounds.

C6 DEFICIENCY

C6 deficiency is one of the more common complement disorders and occurs more frequently in African-Americans and in people of South Africa. As is true for the other terminal component deficiencies, C6 deficiency is associated with meningococcemia, meningococcal meningitis, and disseminated gonococcal disease.[146,147,173,174] There are occasional reports of C6 deficiency associated with autoimmune disease but it is likely that this represents ascertainment bias.

There are two variations on C6 deficiency. In one case, a splice defect leads to a smaller than usual protein, C6SD.[175] This protein functions less efficiently than wild-type C6; however, it is not clear whether bearing C6SD leads to compromised host defense. The other variation is combined C6 and C7 deficiency.[176]

C7 DEFICIENCY

C7 deficiency is not particularly common and of the few patients reported in the literature, they have had varied presentations. The most common presentation was neisserial disease.[146,147,177]

C8 DEFICIENCY

C8 is composed of three chains: α, β, γ. The α and γ chains become covalently attached during synthesis and bind to the β chain. Interestingly, it is the α and β chain genes which are in linkage disequilibrium and map to chromosome 1p32. C8β deficiency is more common in Caucasians while C8α-γ deficiency is more common among African-Americans.[178–181] The majority of the C8β mutations are due to a single base pair transition leading to a premature stop codon. The majority of the C8α-γ mutations are due to a 10bp insertion leading to a stop codon.

Regardless of the genetic basis, all types of C8 deficiency are associated with diminished bactericidal activity in vitro and an in vivo susceptibility to neisserial disease.[146,147] Meningococcal meningitis, meningococcemia, and disseminated gonococcus have been seen. Rarely, C8 deficiency has been identified in a patient with SLE or other autoimmune disorders. The relationship of C8 deficiency to autoimmunity is not certain.

C9 DEFICIENCY

C9 deficiency is seen with high frequency in Japan and Korea.[182–184] Upwards of 0.05% of the population in Japan are C9 deficient. It is less often seen outside of Japan; however, it is more difficult to diagnose than most of the other complement deficiencies described here because the CH_{50} is diminished but not absent.[185] As lytic activity can be generated in the absence of C9, the CH_{50} is typically one-third to one-half of normal in patients with C9 deficiency. This CH_{50} level would not typically lead to further evaluation as mildly diminished levels are commonly seen when the sample is poorly handled or in the presence of active disease leading to complement consumption. As is true for the other terminal complement component deficiencies, C9 deficiency is associated with neisserial disease although the penetrance appears to be less than that seen in other terminal component deficiencies.[186] Rare cases of autoimmune disease have been described.

C1 INHIBITOR DEFICIENCY

Hereditary angioedema is the other clinical designation given to patients with heterozygous deficiencies of C1 inhibitor. No patient with a complete deficiency has been described. Patients with C1 inhibitor deficiency may have a mildly increased susceptibility to infection and have been clearly demonstrated to have an increased risk of SLE, presumably due to chronic consumption of C2 and C4. The most common clinical presentation is angioedema. The angioedema has no distinguishing features. It is not associated with urticaria although there is often a lacey reticular rash that precedes the onset of angioedema.[187] The historical features most helpful in identifying potential C1 inhibitor deficient individuals are recurrent episodes of angioedema, involvement of the airway in the absence of anaphylaxis, abdominal episodes, a positive family history, or angioedema arising after trauma.[187] This section will discuss inherited C1 inhibitor deficiency initially, followed by a brief discussion of acquired C1 inhibitor deficiency.

C1 inhibitor deficiency is often categorized as type I in which there is a concomitant decrease in protein levels and function. Type I deficiency is the most common, occurring in approximately 85% of the inherited cases. Type II deficiency is associated with the production of an antigenically normal but dysfunctional protein. In patients with type II deficiency, the serum levels of C1 inhibitor detected antigenically are normal or elevated, although the function is diminished.[187] It is for this reason that it is recommended that both antigenic and functional levels be obtained when testing for C1 inhibitor deficiency. A typical functional level is approximately 25–40% of normal in both types. As this is a disorder due to heterozygous mutations, a level of 50% would be expected. If the functional allele produced normal amounts of C1 inhibitor, the serum level should be half of what would be expected if two alleles were functional. The explanation appears to be that the C1 inhibitor complexes with its targets and, when one allele is dysfunctional, a greater fraction of the C1 inhibitor is held in protein complexes, thus altering its catabolism.

The main manifestations of C1 inhibitor deficiency are recurrent episodes of submucosal or subcutaneous edema although 5% of people who carry a C1 inhibitor mutation are asymptomatic.[187] Half of patients have had episodes before the age of 10 years. The episodes may be as infrequent as 1/year or as frequent as 1/month and the frequency and the severity of episodes do not correlate with laboratory features and are often inconsistent within a family. The extremities, face, or genitalia are most often involved. Involvement of the gastrointestinal tract can lead to disabling abdominal pain. Abdominal episodes begin with pain and are often accompanied by vomiting, more rarely diarrhea. In one study, one-third of patients with C1 inhibitor deficiency had undergone an appendectomy or exploratory laparotomy for abdominal pain.[187] The most feared type of angioedema is that involving the airway. Although the lungs are not involved, the upper airway can swell, leading to respiratory arrest. This complication can occur in as many as two-thirds of patients with C1 inhibitor deficiency, although improved management has made it somewhat less common. Prior to modern management, slightly over 10% of patients underwent a tracheostomy as a result of airway episodes.

The angioedema typically progresses for 1–2 days and resolves in another 2–3 days. Common precipitants are illness, hormonal fluctuations, trauma, and stress. Although many patients can identify triggers, many episodes have no identifiable trigger which increases anxiety and feelings of loss of control. The C1 inhibitor promoter is androgen responsive which is why men have fewer problems in general than female patients.[188–190] It may also explain the common complaint that symptoms vary with menstruation. It is also the mechanism underlying the main therapeutic modality in the USA, attenuated androgens. The mechanism underlying the angioedema is not completely clear but relates to the role of C1 inhibitor as an inhibitor of both the classical complement pathway activation and as an inhibitor of the kinin pathway (Fig. 6.12).[191] Treatment therefore is directed at correcting either the level of C1 inhibitor through the use of attenuated androgens or direct administration of C1 inhibitor. Other strategies which are under investigation target the kinin system.

Management is typically divided into four categories (Table 6.4).[187,191–193] Ideally, the episodes of angioedema are prevented. The most common strategy for prevention is the use of attenuated androgens. In children, the use of androgens is discouraged due to concerns about closure of the epiphyses and tranexamic acid is often used, although difficult to obtain. Short-term prophylaxis is used for dental procedures, surgical procedures, or other situations where significant trauma may be expected. Attenuated androgens are typically used in these settings and if the risk of angioedema is substantial, then FFP is usually given prior to the event. In Europe and certain other countries, pasteurized C1 inhibitor concentrate is available for both short-term prophylaxis and treatment and is very effective.[193–198] A clinical trial

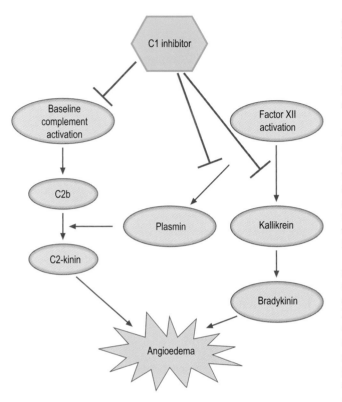

Fig. 6.12. The role of C1 inhibitor. C1 inhibitor deficiency is thought to lead to angioedema through loss of inhibitory activity for the intrinsic coagulation pathway. Factor XII (Hageman factor) is activated by negatively charged molecules and this is most often the case when blood vessels are damaged and collagen exposed. Factor XII activation leads to the activation of bradykinin, which is one of the most potent vasodilators known. In addition, bradykinin leads to vascular leak, and hence, angioedema. This pathway is thought to be the most important for the development of angioedema; however, a cleavage product of C2b, C2-kinin is produced by plasmin. Plasmin is itself activated by factor XII. The C2-kinin has some effect on vasodilation. As activation of factor XII is often due to vascular damage, the role of this mediator may explain why some patients report angioedema after trauma and why surgery represents a significant risk.

in the USA may lead to FDA approval, but as of this printing, C1 inhibitor is available in the USA only under the aegis of a clinical trial. In addition to long-term prophylaxis and short-term prophylaxis, it is often necessary to treat an acute episode. In spite of prophylaxis, breakthrough episodes do occur. Episodes also occur in children, particularly pre-adolescent girls and adolescent girls. These patients may be on an antifibrinolytic agent that is much less effective than an attenuated androgen, and breakthroughs are not uncommon. Finally, acute episodes arise in the undiagnosed patient or in non-compliant patients. In spite of the frequency of acute episodes for all of these reasons, there is little consensus on management. There is general agreement that corticosteroids, epinephrine, and antihistamines have no effect. Beyond that, there is little agreement. Supportive care and close observation are essential as pharyngeal swelling can progress to airway compromise in a few hours. Narcotics are appropriate for abdominal pain episodes. In terms of addressing the angioedema, there are numerous options and almost no

data. C1 inhibitor concentrate is the best option where available. When it is not available, antifibrinolytics are thought to reduce the severity and length of the episode and attenuated androgens may do the same; however, they do not begin to have an effect for 24 h. At various times, FFP and aprotinin have been used for acute episodes; however, the FFP is thought to provide active substrate to enhance further edema and is not routinely used and side effects with aprotinin have limited its use.

The last category of management is fertility and obstetrical management. Polycystic ovary syndrome is seen in approximately one-third of female patients with C1 inhibitor deficiency regardless of prior therapy.[187] The typical endocrine findings of increased luteinizing hormone and testosterone are not seen. Ultrasounds demonstrate polycystic ovaries and the only laboratory feature is often reduced levels of follicle-stimulating hormone. Menstrual irregularities are common and the underlying pathogenesis is the aberrant regulation of complement activation in follicular fluid.[199] Unexpectedly, attenuated androgen therapy improves the polycystic ovaries.

In spite of common menstrual irregularities, fertility is largely preserved and pregnancy poses a particular risk to both the mother and the fetus. The hormonal shifts of pregnancy lead to an increased risk of angioedema although late pregnancy seems to offer some protection. Delivery is itself traumatic and an affected mother has a 50% chance of transmitting the disorder to her offspring. Thus, potentially both mother and child are at risk during delivery. There is no consensus on management. In Europe, C1 inhibitor is given prophylactically or if problems arise. In the USA, low-dose androgens have been utilized although there are risks of androgenization of the baby. In theory, FFP could be administered prophylactically; however, there are no data on this strategy.

Acquired C1 inhibitor deficiency is clinically indistinguishable from inherited C1 inhibitor deficiency except that the age of onset is after 30 years.[187,200,201] A distinction between acquired disease due to lymphoreticular malignancy and acquired disease seen in association with autoimmune disease has not proved practical because anti-C1 inhibitor antibodies have been found in both. The laboratory features are similar to those of hereditary C1 inhibitor deficiency except that C1q levels are diminished in these patients. All patients with acquired C1 inhibitor deficiency require careful surveillance for malignancy. B cell malignancies and monoclonal gammopathies are the most common. Only 14% of patients with acquired C1 inhibitor deficiency had no associated medical condition in one study. Malignancy, infection, and autoimmune disease were most commonly reported. Treatment for acquired C1 inhibitor deficiency is slightly different in that attenuated androgens are seldom helpful. C1 inhibitor has been used successfully although the increased catabolism often mandates that higher doses be used. Antifibrinolytics are as efficacious in acquired disease as in inherited disease and are often used as prophylaxis. There is hope that the new kallikrein inhibitor may bypass the catabolism problem and become an effective therapy for patients with acquired C1 inhibitor deficiency.

C4 BINDING PROTEIN DEFICIENCY

A single kindred with C4 binding protein deficiency has been described.[202] The proband presented with angioedema, vasculitis, and arthritis. The manifestations were thought to relate to uncontrolled activation of the classical pathway and release of anaphylatoxins.

Table 6.4 Therapeutic options for C1 inhibitor deficiency

Treatment	Adult	Pediatric	Comments
Tranexamic acid (Cyklokapron)	1–3 g/day p.o. as divided doses for prophylaxis, 1 g p.o. q. 3–4 h until episode resolves for acute episodes.	25–50 mg/kg b.i.d.–t.i.d. as prophylaxis, 1.5 g/day for acute episodes (available as i.v. form)	Not available in the USA
Epsilon aminocaproic acid (Amicar)	1 g p.o. t.i.d. as prophylaxis, 1 g/h as i.v. therapy for acute attacks	100 mg/kg q.4–6 h not to exceed 30 g/day as therapy. Oral syrup available for prophylaxis but doses not established: 6 g/day for children <11 years and 12 g/day for children >11 years has been used successfully	The only antifibrinolytic available in the USA, has modest efficacy. Cannot be used in neonates. Oral dosing has significant GI side effects
Danazol (Danocrine)	200 mg p.o. q.d. as a starting point for prophylaxis (titrate to effect), 400–600 mg p.o. q.d. for acute episode or short-term prophylaxis	50–200 mg p.o. q.d. as a starting point for prophylaxis (titrate to effect) and consider q.o.d. or q. 3 days in pre-adolescent children; can use up to 400 mg p.o. q.d. as short-term prophylaxis	Concern about androgenization and premature closure of the epiphyses limits the use of attenuated androgens in children. Titration to desired effect is recommended rather than to laboratory criteria
Oxandrolone (Oxandrin)	2.5–20 mg p.o. t.i.d. as prophylaxis (titrate to effect). Not proven as short-term prophylaxis or treatment	0.1 mg/kg per day as prophylaxis. Not proven as short-term prophylaxis or treatment in a formal clinical trial	Has less androgenizing effects than Danazol
Fresh frozen plasma (FFP)	2 U i.v. as short-term prophylaxis. May be required for up to 36 h after surgery	10–15 ml/kg as short-term prophylaxis. May be required for up to 36 h after surgery	Not typically used for acute episodes due to danger of accelerating angioedema; useful for short-term prophylaxis for surgery or dental extractions
C1 inhibitor concentrate	1000 U as treatment	10–30 U/kg as treatment (up to 500–1000 U total)	Very rapid effect, especially useful in pregnancy
DX-88			Kallikrein inhibitor, has shown efficacy in early trials; could be available later in 2007
Icatibant			Bradykinin receptor antagonist; awaiting trial results

Airway protection, fluid replacement, and pain relief are of paramount importance. Some episodes require no intervention. For long-term prophylaxis, consider monitoring the liver by ultrasound and blood studies. Although epinephrine is ineffective systemically, it may provide some benefit when used topically in airway obstruction.

FACTOR I DEFICIENCY

Factor I deficiency has two phenotypes and it is not yet clear whether a genotype–phenotype relationship exists. The first phenotype described relates to the role of factor I as a cofactor for C3bBb dissociation. When factor I is lacking, C3bBb continues to cleave C3 unabated and a secondary deficit in C3 occurs. Both the CH_{50} and AH_{50} are depressed but not absent and C3 antigen levels are low.[203–206] The infectious consequences of low C3 are similar to those seen in true C3 deficiency.[146,147] Neisserial disease has been seen as well as infections with more typical organisms such as *S. pneumoniae* and *H. influenzae*. As is true for inherited C3 deficiency, some patients have developed a serum sickness-like picture.

The second phenotype is atypical hemolytic uremic syndrome (HUS) or membranoproliferative glomerulonephritis II.[207–209] This unusual phenotype has now been described in patients with factor I deficiency, factor H deficiency, and MCP deficiency.[210] HUS is characterized by microangiopathic hemolytic anemia, renal disease, and hypertension. These cases are 'atypical' because they lack the common trigger of infectious diarrhea. Toxins elaborated by certain *E. coli* are typical triggers for HUS. These cases of factor I deficiency are difficult to identify because complement studies are often normal. C3 may be depressed but is not necessarily depressed. The factor I level is typically normal as the mutations are not null, they simply inactivate certain binding sites. It is thought that the mutations in the regulatory proteins adversely affect binding to surface-bound C3b and polyanion surfaces such as endothelium. The fenestrated endothelium of the glomerulus represents a landscape of polyanions where the basement membrane is exposed by the fenestration. Thus, the role of complement regulatory proteins would be greatest on those surfaces. Lack of protection due to lack of complement regulatory proteins or to enhanced activation of C3 by C3 nephritic factor would lead to endothelial damage in the glomerulus.

FACTOR H DEFICIENCY

Infections, atypical HUS, and macular degeneration are the main phenotypes seen in factor H deficiency.[211–214] As is true for factor I deficiency, the first cases described were those with infection. The infections are due to consumption of C3 and a secondary partial C3 deficiency.[155] These can be easily suspected on the basis of diminished C3 levels and low but not absent CH_{50} and AH_{50} and typically the antigenic levels of factor H are low. Factor H deficient pigs were known to develop membranoproliferative glomerulonephritis and next, several kindreds with membranoproliferative glomerulonephritis were identified with factor H deficiency. Finally, factor H was found to be the underlying basis for 15–30% of patients with atypical HUS. Both autosomal recessive and heterozygous mutations have been seen. The age of onset is quite young in most cases and the disease is recurrent.[210] Death is not uncommon. Therapy with FFP may be of benefit. These patients have a diminished C3 level although the antigenic level of factor H is typically normal or elevated. Normal C3 levels are sometimes seen and the only way in which this disorder can be confidently identified is with direct mutation analysis.

The basis for the HUS in factor H deficiency is thought to be due to an inability to protect fenestrated endothelium in the glomerulus from complement-mediated damage.[215] Microtrauma arises frequently due to the high oncotic pressure and the basement membrane is able to support complement activation if not protected. Interestingly, recurrent atypical HUS has been seen in patients with antibodies to factor H suggesting an acquired form as well. This form may be slightly more amenable to therapy.

A common tyrosine-histidine polymorphism of factor H was identified as a significant risk factor for macular degeneration in a genome-wide linkage study.[211,216] Homozygous bearers of this polymorphic variant have a relative risk of 7.4 for the development of macular degeneration. Macular degeneration is the leading cause of blindness in the USA and many other developed countries. The central region of the retina is gradually destroyed by a process that leaves a deposit of protein, termed drusen. These deposits contain factor H and terminal complement components. It has been hypothesized that the abnormal factor H provides less protection to the choroidal vessels, allowing smoldering complement activation and gradual damage to the endothelium.

MEMBRANE COFACTOR PROTEIN (CD46) DEFICIENCY

Deficiencies of membrane cofactor protein (MCP) are associated with a later onset of atypical HUS compared to factor H and factor I deficiencies.[210,217–219] MCP mutations are thought to account for approximately 10% of all atypical HUS. There is no other known phenotype for MCP deficiency. As MCP is a membrane protein, this defect is intrinsic to the kidney. In contrast to factor H and factor I deficiencies, renal transplantation can be successful. Traditional complement analyses are normal although the mechanism is thought to be the same as for factor H and factor I deficiencies.

CD59 DEFICIENCY AND PAROXYSMAL NOCTURNAL HEMOGLOBINURIA

A single patient with CD59 deficiency has been described and the major manifestation was chronic hemolytic anemia and recurrent stroke.[220] CD59 is expressed on most hematopoietic cells and endothelial cells where it confers protection from intravascular complement mediated lysis. This defect in CD59 was suspected because of the phenotypic resemblance to paroxysmal nocturnal hemoglobinuria (PNH).

PNH is characterized by recurrent episodes of hemoglobinuria due to intravascular hemolysis. Thrombosis occurs for unknown reasons and aplastic anemia can both pre-date and post-date the PNH. PNH is typically due to acquired somatic mutations of PIG-A or PIG-M in a clone of bone marrow progenitor cells.[221] These protein products are required for GPI-anchored proteins and C8-binding protein, DAF and CD59 are all GPI-anchored proteins which protect hematopoietic cells from complement-mediated lysis.[222] The red cells are the most vulnerable because they have no ability to repair membrane damage. When the cells develop from the mutation-bearing progenitor, they lack all GPI-anchored membrane proteins although the major features relate to loss of CD59. As DAF deficiency does not have a hemolytic phenotype, it would appear that CD59 is the more important of the two. The diagnosis of PNH is made by flow cytometry for CD59 or CD55 (DAF). Monitoring of the red cell expression is warranted because there have been spontaneous remissions.

DAF DEFICIENCY (CD55)

DAF deficiency is also termed the Inab blood group phenotype.[223–225] The Cromer blood group antigens reside on DAF and the null phenotype is referred to as the Inab phenotype. Certain kindreds with DAF deficiency have had protein-losing enteropathy while others have been completely healthy and have been identified at the time of blood donation or cross matching for a transfusion. None of the patients have had hemolysis, suggesting that CD59 is substantially more important in regulating red cell lysis by complement.

CR1 DEFICIENCY

No known patients with complete inherited CR1 deficiency exist; however, acquired mild C1R deficiency is quite common in immune complex diseases and serum sickness. It appears as though CR1 internalizes immune complexes once bound and a consequence of the internalization leads to a temporary lack of surface expression.[226–228] This appears to be physiologic although it might be imagined that long-term internalization could lead to a secondary inability to clear immune complexes and might further contribute to the inflammatory consequences. A polymorphic variant of CR1 with diminished levels and function exists although it does not appear to be a risk factor for autoimmune disease.[229,230]

CR3/CR4 DEFICIENCY

This disorder is a defect in the three β_2-integrin adhesion molecules. It will be discussed in more detail in the chapter on immunodeficiencies. The more common terminology for this β_2-integrin deficiency is leukocyte adhesion deficiency type I (LAD type I). Mutations in the common β chain (CD18) lead to failure to express adequate α chains: CD11a, CD11b, and CD11c.[231,232] These three proteins are perhaps better known as LFA-1, CR3, and CR4. Most patients with LAD type I do not have complete null mutations and the severity of the disease relates to the residual level of protein expression on the surface.

LAD type I is a very serious disorder with a high mortality rate. Among patients with no residual expression of β_2-integrins, mortality is quite high and bone marrow transplantation is often recommended. These patients have very high resting white blood cell counts, frequent necrotic skin infections without pus formation, a delayed separation of the umbilical cord, and assorted other serious bacterial and fungal infections.[233–235] The infections are characteristic in that necrosis predominates and there is little in the way of neutrophilic infiltrate. In addition, these patients suffer from spontaneous peritonitis which is seldom seen in other immune deficiencies. The patients with some residual β_2-integrin expression may be able to survive without a bone marrow transplant; however, infections are common and the morbidity associated with the infections can compromise the quality of life.

The manifestations of the disorder are due to the combined effects of ineffective opsonization and an inability to traverse the vascular endothelium to phagocytose bacteria. β_2-integrins are essential for the firm adhesion step and diapedesis. Lacking β_2-integrins, the neutrophils remain in the vascular space where they are unable to participate in the defense against bacteria. This also explains the lack of pus at sites of active infection. The high resting white cell count was long thought to be due to an inability of the cells to migrate out of the vasculature. There may be some effect from the abnormal distribution of the cells; however, the major contributor to the elevated absolute neutrophil count is a disruption in the IL-17–IL-23 pathway.[236]

There are two other forms of leukocyte adhesion deficiency. LAD type II is due to a defect in fucosylation of selectin ligands and will not be further discussed in this chapter.[237–239] LAD type III is due to activation defects of integrins. This is probably a heterogeneous group of genetic defects and the major manifestations are the infection pattern described above and a moderate to severe bleeding tendency due to impaired activation of platelet adhesion molecules.[240]

■ MANAGEMENT OF COMPLEMENT DEFICIENCIES ■

The management of complement deficiencies is completely dependent on the type of defect. In some cases, the management is critically dependent on knowing the precise defect present. For example, in inherited forms of atypical HUS, renal transplants are indicated for MCP deficiency but not factor H or factor I deficiency. For this reason, each class of defect will be discussed separately in this section. It is important to realize that with few exceptions there are no trials supporting the management strategies offered here. The management tools offered in this chapter represent possible interventions based on current literature. As this is a rapidly moving field, it is wise to seek out expert advice when confronted with a complement deficient patient.

EARLY CLASSICAL COMPONENT DEFICIENCIES

The major features of early classical component deficiencies are SLE and infection. The therapy which has been used for SLE in complement deficient individuals is no different from that used for other SLE patients. One European study of C2 deficient SLE patients found replacement of C2 to be therapeutically useful; however, this product is not widely available.

Therapy for infection is not standardized, nor have clinical trials demonstrated the benefits of intervention; however, patients are often given vaccines to raise titers of antibodies to encapsulated organisms to high levels. In the case of terminal component deficiencies, high levels of antibody have been shown to partially compensate for the complement deficiency. For early complement component deficiencies the major risks seem to be *S. pneumoniae* and *H. influenzae*.[146–148] Vaccines to these entities exist and there is reason to believe that having high titers of antibody may offer protection. The other strategy often considered is prophylactic antibiotics. In one study, half of the C2 deficient patients had serious infections such as sepsis, and infection was the leading cause of death, accounting for over 10% of the deaths in this cohort.[148] The range of age of deaths was quite broad, suggesting that antibiotic prophylaxis might be required life-long. In addition to death, approximately one-quarter of the patients had meningitis. While not specifically mentioned, it might be expected that neurologic residua compromised the quality of life in some of these patients. Thus, prevention of infection is desirable and vaccination and prophylactic antibiotics should be given consideration. Patients on immunosuppressive medication for rheumatologic disorders may require yet more vigilance.

C3 DEFICIENCY

With very few patients, it is extremely difficult to define optimal therapy for this group of patients. Their infections are the most severe of any of the complement deficiencies and management must address loss of opsonization, loss of B cell co-stimulation, and loss of immune complex solubilization.[155] One could consider the use of IVIG to compensate for the compromised B cell function and prophylactic antibiotic use could ameliorate some of the infections. The membranoproliferative glomerulonephritis seen in C3 deficient patients has no specific intervention. Renal transplantation has been attempted. The recurrence risk has not been characterized; however, one would anticipate some recurrence risk. Nevertheless, as not all C3 deficient patients develop membranoproliferative glomerulonephritis, renal transplantation should be given consideration in patients with end-stage renal disease.

MBL DEFICIENCY

While MBL deficiency is common, infections arising in patients with MBL deficiency are not common.[159,160] Studies implicating MBL deficiency in infection have utilized cohorts of patients with severe infections and have asked whether MBL deficiency is more common than in a control population. Indeed, many associations have been defined in this way although not all have been replicated. No prospective study of MBL deficiency has been performed. Of the many millions of people with MBL deficiency, it is not known what fraction suffer from significant infections although the number is expected to be low. Of those with infection, are there cofactors which synergize with MBL deficiency leading to recurrent infections? If so, management would be best directed at the cofactor. This conundrum is an extremely common one in clinical immunology. At this point, cofactors for infection should be addressed when possible and the consideration for prophylactic antibiotics given.

FACTOR D AND PROPERDIN DEFICIENCY

Patients with factor D and properdin deficiency have manifestations related to secondary consumption of C3. Thus, neisserial disease is common and infections with *S. pneumoniae* and *H. influenzae* are also seen. Vaccination to achieve high titers of antibody to those entities could theoretically provide benefit. Traditionally, prophylactic antibiotics have been used for some patients in an effort to prevent infections.[241–243]

TERMINAL COMPLEMENT COMPONENT DEFICIENCIES

Deficiencies of C5, C6, C7, C8, and C9 are all associated with an increased risk of neisserial disease. Meningococcal disease is by far the most common, but disseminated gonococcal infections have been seen with significant frequency and patients should be warned about the possibility. The prevention of meningococcal disease has been studied thoroughly in Russia and Europe and two things have emerged from these studies. Patients with terminal complement component deficiencies have a rather abrupt onset of meningococcal disease but have a shorter and milder course ultimately.[244] Thus, patients in rural areas may be at increased risk due to potential delay in the initiation of treatment. The other important lesson is that vaccination every 3 years with the meningococcal vaccine decreases the frequency of meningococcal episodes but does not eliminate them.[245–248] The frequency is decreased to 20% of what non-vaccinated individuals experience. No study has examined prophylactic antibiotics and it may be that careful monitoring and hyper-vaccination may be sufficient.

C1 INHIBITOR DEFICIENCY

Management of this regulatory protein defect has been discussed somewhat above. Medical interventions for short-term prophylaxis, long-term prophylaxis, and acute therapy are given in Table 6.4. There are a number of strategies which should be reviewed with each patient.[187] Genetic counseling should be offered to each family. The use of bracelets with medical information is a very individual choice. For patients with anticipated travel or events which might lead to isolation from friends and family familiar with the disorder, bracelets might have some role to inform paramedics and physicians in the event of an emergency. Patients should be counseled to avoid certain medications. ACE inhibitors can induce angioedema as can estrogen-containing birth control pills or post-menopausal hormone replacement. In men, hormonal modulation may also affect their angioedema.

FACTOR H, FACTOR I, AND MCP DEFICIENCY

It is thought that certain mutations in factor II and factor I predispose to meningococcal disease while others predispose to HUS. In kindreds with meningococcal disease, the same strategies utilized for patients with terminal complement component deficiencies would be expected to be of benefit. In kindreds with HUS, the management is less clear. As is done for TTP, some patients receive pheresis and FFP replacement for acute episodes.[217,249] One study evaluating factor H replacement demonstrated benefit, suggesting that FFP alone might be of benefit as prophylaxis. In the case of MCP, where the affected protein is membrane bound, it is less clear that pheresis and FFP would provide benefit, but it could potentially act to clear inciting agents or complement activation products. For patients with end-stage renal disease, the recurrence of disease in patients with factor H or factor I deficiency is unacceptably high and renal transplantation is not recommended. In contrast, renal disease in MCP typically does not recur in the transplanted kidney.

■ LABORATORY ASSESSMENT OF COMPLEMENT ■

There are several themes that arise from discussion of laboratory assessment of complement. The first issue is to define the patient population which would benefit from complement screening analyses. The second issue is to match the appropriate study to the suspected complement deficiency.

EPIDEMIOLOGY

Patients with recurrent sinopulmonary infections are often referred for an immunologic evaluation. Complement deficiencies will be found infrequently in this population. For patients with recurrent sepsis/systemic infection or sepsis on the background of autoimmune disease (or a family history of autoimmune disease), the frequency of identifying a complement defect is probably higher although there are no data to support this approach. A reasonable evaluation would include a CH_{50} and AH_{50} and an assessment of MBL levels for these patients.[250]

Patients with a single meningococcal infection, either meningitis or meningococcemia, probably deserve an evaluation in non-endemic areas.[251–253] The evaluation would include a CH_{50} and AH_{50}. The frequency with which complement deficient individuals are identified in this population is low but not zero. The rationale for evaluating such patients is that identification of a complement deficiency would lead to vaccination and prevention of future episodes; however, there is no consensus that these patients should have an evaluation. There is, however, general consensus that patients with meningococcal disease with an unusual serotype (serotypes X, Y, Z, W135 or 29E), with meningococcal disease on the background of a positive family history, or recurrent meningococcal disease, should have an evaluation with a CH_{50} and AH_{50}. In these patient groups, the frequency of complement deficiency ranges from 10 to 50%.[252,254–257] Chronic meningococcemia appears to be another condition with a high frequency of complement deficiency.[258]

Patients with lupus are often tested for complement deficiency inadvertently. Until recently, it was common to follow patients with serial CH_{50} assays as a measure of complement activation. For this reason, it is known that most Caucasian lupus cohorts have approximately 1–2% of patients with complement deficiency.[259] Most often this is C2 deficiency. Given the high rate of infection, it is important to identify these patients. $CH_{50}s$ are not performed as widely as they once were and it might be reasonable to consider which populations of patients with SLE might benefit from CH_{50} screening for complement deficiency. As patients with C1 and C4 deficiency tend to have severe disease with early presentations, it is possible that testing pediatric-onset severe SLE might be revealing of complement deficiencies. There are no data to support this approach, however. An additional category where a CH_{50} assay might be considered is in the evaluation of patients with clinical symptoms suggestive of SLE but with negative ANA and anti-dsDNA. While often thought of as important indicators of SLE, complement deficient patients have these autoantibodies less frequently and it might support the diagnosis of SLE to know that the patient had a complement deficiency.

Membranoproliferative glomerulonephritis and HUS are more clear-cut patient populations. All patients with atypical HUS should have a complement evaluation.[217,219] An initial screen would include a CH_{50}, an AH_{50}, and a C3 level. In many cases these will be normal and specific studies of factor H, factor I, and MCP mutation analyses should be performed. Patients with membranoproliferative glomerulonephritis type II should also be evaluated when the clinical suspicion of a complement deficiency or nephritic factor exists.

Angioedema presentations have been discussed above. There are several considerations in the evaluation of a patient with angioedema. When it occurs in the setting of a known allergic response, it is much less likely to be due to C1 inhibitor deficiency. Patients with recurrent angioedema in the absence of allergic reactions, patients with a family history of angioedema, patients with angioedema preceded by a reticular rash, and patients with angioedema after trauma should all have an evaluation. A simple but rather insensitive screen is to measure C4 levels. C4 is typically decreased at baseline but is diminished even more during an acute attack due to consumption. A superior strategy is to measure C1 inhibitor antigen and functional levels.

COMPLEMENT LABORATORY ANALYSES

A CH_{50} assay consists of adding dilutions of patient serum to sensitized sheep red cells. The antibody on the sensitized sheep cells initiates complement activation and, when all components are present, leads to lysis. A CH_{50} reports out the dilution of serum capable of lysing 50% of the sheep cells. Similarly, rabbit red cells are used to measure the intactness of the alternative pathway. Note that all components for the activation arm through the terminal components must be intact for a normal CH_{50} or AH_{50}. With the exception of C9 deficiency, deficiencies of all the cascade components lead to a CH_{50} of 0 or near 0. Low levels of CH_{50} or AH_{50} results should be repeated as mishandling of the serum is an extremely common problem leading to diminished complement levels. Other causes of low but not absent CH_{50} results are complement consumption due to active immune complex disease, diminished hepatic production due to liver disease, and immaturity of hepatic production seen in young infants. Less common, but more medically important are the regulatory protein defects leading to consumption of C3 such as factor D, factor H, and factor I deficiency. C9 deficiency also leads to a reduction in both the CH_{50} and AH_{50}.

Once an abnormal CH_{50} or AH_{50} has been confirmed, nephelometry is used to define the serum levels of certain components (C3 and C4 primarily), ELISAs are available for certain other components, and for some components the only strategy is a laborious add-back method. These assays are not widely available but are available through reference laboratories. These assays will lead to the identification of a component which is absent or markedly diminished. Once the specific diagnosis is established, the management path should be clear.

References

Overview

1. Scoazec JY, Delautier D, Moreau A, et al. Expression of complement-regulatory proteins in normal and UW-preserved human liver. Gastroenterology 1994; 107:505–516.
2. Anthony R, el-Omar E, Lappin DF, et al. Regulation of hepatic synthesis of C3 and C4 during the acute-phase response in the rat. Eur J Immunol 1989; 19:1405–1412.
3. Wilkison WO, Min HY, Claffey KP, et al. Control of the adipsin gene in adipocyte differentiation. Identification of distinct nuclear factors binding to single- and double-stranded DNA. J Biol Chem 1990; 265:477–482.
4. Schwaeble W, Huemer HP, Most J, et al. Expression of properdin in human monocytes. Eur J Biochem 1994; 219:759–764.
5. Ziccardi RJ. The first component of human complement (C1): activation and control. Springer Semin Immunopathol 1983; 6:213–230.
6. Passwell J, Schreiner GF, Nonaka M, et al. Local extrahepatic expression of complement genes C3, factor B, C2, and C4 is increased in murine lupus nephritis. J Clin Invest 1988; 82:1676–1684.
7. Lappin DF, Guc D, Hill A, et al. Effect of interferon-gamma on complement gene expression in different cell types. Biochem J 1992; 281:437–442.
8. Homann C, Varming K, Hogasen K, et al. Acquired C3 deficiency in patients with alcoholic cirrhosis predisposes to infection and increased mortality. Gut 1997; 40:544–549.
9. Walport MJ, Complement. Second of two parts. N Engl J Med 2001; 344:1140–1144.
10. Walport MJ, Complement. First of two parts. N Engl J Med 2001; 344:1058–1066.

The classical pathway

11. Gal P, Cseh S, Schumaker VN, et al. The structure and function of the first component of complement: genetic engineering approach (a review). Acta Microbiol Immunol Hung 1994; 41:361–380.
12. Sim RB, Reid KBM. C1: molecular interactions with activating systems. Immunol Today 1991; 12:307–311.
13. Sjoberg AP, Trouw LA, McGrath FD, et al. Regulation of complement activation by C-reactive protein: targeting of the inhibitory activity of C4b-binding protein. J Immunol 2006; 176:7612–7620.
14. Riley-Vargas RC, Lanzendorf S, Atkinson JP. Targeted and restricted complement activation on acrosome-reacted spermatozoa. J Clin Invest 2005; 115:1241–1249.
15. Korb LC, Ahearn JM, C1q binds directly and specifically to surface blebs of apoptotic human keratinocytes. Complement deficiency and systemic lupus erythematosus revisited. J Immunol 1997; 158:4525–4528.
16. Botto M, Dell'agnola C, Bygrave AE, et al. Homozygous C1q deficiency causes glomerulonephritis associated with multiple apoptotic bodies. Nat Genet 1998; 19:56–59.
17. Law SKA, Dodds AW, Porter RR. A comparison of the properties of two classes C4A and C4B of the human complement component C4. EMBO 1984; 3:1819–1823.
18. Weigle WO, Morgan EL, Goodman MG, et al. Modulation of the immune response by anaphylatoxin in the microenvironment of the interacting cells. Fed Proc 1982; 41:3099–3103.
19. Schlaf G, Nitzki F, Heine I, et al. C5a anaphylatoxin as a product of complement activation up-regulates the complement inhibitory factor H in rat Kupffer cells. Eur J Immunol 2004; 34:3257–3266.
20. Hawlisch H, Belkaid Y, Baelder R, et al. C5a negatively regulates toll-like receptor 4-induced immune responses. Immunity 2005; 22:415–426.
21. Robbins RA, Russ WD, Thomas KR, et al. Complement component C5 is required for release of alveolar macrophage-derived neutrophil chemotactic activity. Am Rev Respir Dis 1987; 135:659–664.

The alternative pathway

22. Pangburn MK. Analysis of recognition in the alternative pathway of complement. Effect of polysaccharide size. J Immunol 1989; 142:2766–2770.
23. Pangburn MK. Analysis of the mechanism of recognition in the complement alternative pathway using C3b-bound low molecular weight polysaccharides. J Immunol 1989; 142:2759–2765.
24. Pangburn MK, Muller-Eberhard HJ. Initiation of the alternative complement pathway due to spontaneous hydrolysis of the thioester of C3. Ann N Y Acad Sci 1983; 421:291–298.

25. Nolan KF, Schwaeble W, Kaluz S, et al. Molecular cloning of the cDNA coding for properdin, a positive regulator of the alternative pathway of human complement. Eur J Immunol 1991; 21:771–776.
26. Rodriguez de Cordoba S, Esparza-Gordillo J, Goicoechea de Jorge E, et al. The human complement factor H: functional roles, genetic variations and disease associations. Mol Immunol 2004; 41:355–367.
27. Zipfel PF, Skerka C, Hellwage J, et al. Factor H family proteins: on complement, microbes and human diseases. Biochem Soc Trans 2002; 30:971–978.
28. Zipfel PF. Complement factor H: physiology and pathophysiology. Semin Thromb Hemost 2001; 27:191–199.

The lectin activation pathway

29. Sastry K, Herman GA, Day L, et al. The human mannose binding protein gene. J Exp Med 1989; 170:1175–1189.
30. Childs RA, Drickamer K, Kawasaki T, et al. Neoglycolipids as probes of oligosaccharide recognition by recombinant and natural mannose-binding proteins of rat and man. Biochem J 1989; 262:1018–1022.
31. Matsushita M, Fujita T. Cleavage of the third component of complement (C3) by mannose-binding protein-associated serine protease (MASP) with subsequent complement activation. Immunobiology 1995; 194:443–448.
32. Malhotra R, Wormald MR, Rudd PM, et al. Glycosylation changes of IgG associated with rheumatoid arthritis can activate complement via the mannose-binding protein. Nat Med 1995; 1:237–243.
33. Garred P, Madsen HO, Balslev U, et al. Susceptibility to HIV infection and progression of AIDS in relation to variant alleles of mannose-binding lectin. Lancet 1997; 349:236–240.
34. Kakkanaiah VN, Shen GQ, Ojo-Amaize EA, et al. Association of low concentrations of serum mannose-binding protein with recurrent infections in adults. Clin Diagn Lab Immunol 1998; 5:319–321.
35. Summerfield JA, Ryder S, Sumiya M, et al. Mannose binding protein gene mutations associated with unusual and severe infections in adults. Lancet 1995; 345:886–889.
36. Davies EJ, Snowden N, Hillarby MC, et al. Mannose binding protein gene polymorphism in systemic lupus erythematosus. Arthritis Rheum 1995; 38:110–114.
37. Sullivan KE, Wooten C, Goldman D, et al. Mannose-binding protein genetic polymorphisms in black patients with systemic lupus erythematosus. Arthritis Rheum 1996; 39:2046–2051.
38. Ip WK, Lau YL, Chan SY, et al. Mannose-binding lectin and rheumatoid arthritis in southern Chinese. Arthritis Rheum 2000; 43:1679–1687.
39. Horiuchi T, Tsukamoto H, Morita C, et al. Mannose binding lectin (MBL) gene mutation is not a risk factor for systemic lupus erythematosus (SLE) and rheumatoid arthritis (RA) in Japanese. Genes Immun 2000; 1:464–466.
40. Franz S, Frey B, Sheriff A, et al. Lectins detect changes of the glycosylation status of plasma membrane constituents during late apoptosis. Cytometry A 2006; 69:230–239.

The membrane attack complex

41. Salama A, Bhakdi S, Mueller-Eckhardt C, et al. Deposition of the terminal C5b-9 complement complex on erythrocytes by human red cell autoantibodies. Br J Haematol 1983; 55:161–169.
42. Halperin JA, Taratuska A, Rynkiewicz M, et al. Transient changes in erythrocyte membrane permeability are induced by sublytic amounts of the complement membrane attack complex (C5b-9). Blood 1993; 81:200–205.
43. Bhakdi S, Tranum-Jensen J. C5b-9 assembly: average binding of one C9 molecule to C5b-8 without poly-C9 formation generates a stable transmembrane pore. J Immunol 1986; 136:2999–3005.
44. Gao L, Qiu W, Wang Y, et al. Sublytic complement C5b-9 complexes induce thrombospondin-1 production in rat glomerular mesangial cells via PI3-k/Akt: association with activation of latent transforming growth factor-beta1. Clin Exp Immunol 2006; 144:326–334.
45. Mudge SJ, McRae JL, Auwardt RB, et al. Sublytic complement injury does not activate NF-kappa B, or induce mitogenesis in rat mesangial cells. Exp Nephrol 2000; 8:291–298.
46. Rus HG, Niculescu F, Shin ML. Sublytic complement attack induces cell cycle in oligodendrocytes. J Immunol 1996; 156:4892–4900.

Receptors and biological functions

47. Atkinson JP, Krych M, Nickells M, et al. Complement receptors and regulatory proteins: immune adherence revisited and abuse by microorganisms. Clin Exp Immunol 1994; 97(suppl 2):1–3.
48. Monsinjon T, Gasque P, Ischenko A, et al. C3A binds to the seven transmembrane anaphylatoxin receptor expressed by epithelial cells and triggers the production of IL-8. FEBS Lett 2001; 487:339–346.
49. Humbles AA, Lu B, Nilsson CA, et al. A role for the C3a anaphylatoxin receptor in the effector phase of asthma. Nature 2000; 406:998–1001.
50. Lienenklaus S, Ames RS, Tornetta MA, et al. Human anaphylatoxin C4a is a potent agonist of the guinea pig but not the human C3a receptor. J Immunol 1998; 161:2089–2093.
51. Martin U, Bock D, Arseniev L, et al. The human C3a receptor is expressed on neutrophils and monocytes, but not on B or T lymphocytes. J Exp Med 1997; 186:199–207.
52. Takahashi M, Moriguchi S, Ikeno M, et al. Studies on the ileum-contracting mechanisms and identification as a complement C3a receptor agonist of Oryzatensin, a bioactive peptide derived from rice albumin. Peptides 1996; 17:5–12.
53. Guo RF, Ward PA. Role of C5a in inflammatory responses. Annu Rev Immunol 2005; 23:821–852.

54. Akatsu H, Abe M, Miwa T, et al. Distribution of rat C5a anaphylatoxin receptor. Microbiol Immunol 2002; 46:863–874.
55. Nataf S, Davoust N, Ames RS, et al. Human T cells express the C5a receptor and are chemoattracted to C5a. J Immunol 1999; 162:4018–4023.
56. Hopken UE, Lu B, Gerard NP, et al. The C5a chemoattractant receptor mediates mucosal defence to infection. Nature 1996; 383:86–89.
57. Riedemann NC, Guo RF, Hollmann TJ, et al. Regulatory role of C5a in LPS-induced IL-6 production by neutrophils during sepsis. FASEB J 2004; 18:370–372.
58. Steinberger P, Szekeres A, Wille S, et al. Identification of human CD93 as the phagocytic C1q receptor (C1qRp) by expression cloning. J Leukoc Biol 2002; 71:133–140.
59. McGreal EP, Ikewaki N, Akatsu H, et al. Human C1qRp is identical with CD93 and the mNI-11 antigen but does not bind C1q. J Immunol 2002; 168:5222–5232.
60. Nepomuceno RR, Tenner AJ. C1qRP, the C1q receptor that enhances phagocytosis, is detected specifically in human cells of myeloid lineage, endothelial cells, and platelets. J Immunol 1998; 160:1929–1935.
61. Vegh Z, Kew RR, Gruber BL, et al. Chemotaxis of human monocyte-derived dendritic cells to complement component C1q is mediated by the receptors gC1qR and cC1qR. Mol Immunol 2006; 43:1402–1407.
62. Robles-Flores M, Rendon-Huerta E, Gonzalez-Aguilar H, et al. p32 (gC1qBP) is a general protein kinase C (PKC)-binding protein; interaction and cellular localization of P32-PKC complexes in ray hepatocytes. J Biol Chem 2002; 277:5247–5255.
63. Lim BL, White RA, Hummel GS, et al. Characterization of the murine gene of gC1qBP, a novel cell protein that binds the globular heads of C1q, vitronectin, high molecular weight kininogen and factor XII. Gene 1998; 209:229–237.
64. Weiss L, Fischer E, Haeffner-Cavaillon N, et al. The human C3b receptor (CR1). Adv Nephrol Necker Hosp 1989; 18:249–269.
65. Medof ME, Iida K, Mold C, et al. Unique role of the complement receptor CR1 in the degradation of C3b associated with immune complexes. J Exp Med 1982; 156:1739–1746.
66. Emlen W, Carl V, Burdick G. Mechanism of transfer of immune complexes from red blood cell CR1 to monocytes. Clin Exp Immunol 1992; 89:8–17.
67. Davies KA, Erlendsson K, Beynon HLC, et al. Splenic uptake of immune complexes in man is complement dependent. J Immunol 1993; 151:3866–3873.
68. Cornacoff JB, Hebert LA, Smead WL, et al. Primate erythrocyte immune complex clearing mechanism. J Clin Invest 1983; 71:236–240.
69. Wilson JG, Andriopoulos NA, Fearon DT. CR1 and the cell membrane proteins that bind C3 and C4. A basic and clinical review. Immunol Res 1987; 6:192–209.
70. Ferguson AR, Youd ME, Corley RB. Marginal zone B cells transport and deposit IgM-containing immune complexes onto follicular dendritic cells. Int Immunol 2004; 16:1411–1422.
71. Fang Y, Xu C, Fu YX, et al. Expression of complement receptors 1 and 2 on follicular dendritic cells is necessary for the generation of a strong antigen-specific IgG response. J Immunol 1998; 160:5273–5279.
72. Fischer MB, Goerg S, Shen L, et al. Dependence of germinal center B cells on expression of CD21/CD35 for survival. Science 1998; 280:582–585.
73. Holers VM. Complement receptors and the shaping of the natural antibody repertoire. Springer Semin Immunopathol 2005; 26:405–423.
74. Noorchashm H, Moore DJ, Lieu YK, et al. Contribution of the innate immune system to autoimmune diabetes: a role for the CR1/CR2 complement receptors. Cell Immunol 1999; 195:75–79.
75. Cooper NR, Bradt BM, Rhim JS, et al. CR2 complement receptor. J Invest Dermatol 1990; 94:112S–117S.
76. Marquart HV, Svehag SE, Leslie RG, CR2 is the primary acceptor site for C3 during alternative pathway activation of complement on human peripheral B lymphocytes. J Immunol 1994; 153:307–315.
77. Fischer MB, Ma M, Goerg S, et al. Regulation of the B cell response to T-dependent antigens by classical pathway complement. J Immunol 1996; 157:549–556.
78. Ahearn JM, Fischer MB, Croix D, et al. Disruption of the Cr2 locus results in a reduction in B-1a cells and in an impaired B cell response to T-dependent antigens. Immunity 1996; 4:251–262.
79. Wagner C, Hansch GM, Stegmaier S, et al. The complement receptor 3, CR3 (CD11b/CD18), on T lymphocytes: activation-dependent up-regulation and regulatory function. Eur J Immunol 2001; 31:1173–1180.
80. Helmy KY, Katschke KJ Jr, Gorgani NN, et al. CRIg: a macrophage complement receptor required for phagocytosis of circulating pathogens. Cell 2006; 124:915–927.
81. Roozendaal R, Carroll MC. Emerging patterns in complement-mediated pathogen recognition. Cell 2006; 125:29–32.
82. Kang YS, Do Y, Lee HK, et al. A dominant complement fixation pathway for pneumococcal polysaccharides initiated by SIGN-R1 interacting with C1q. Cell 2006; 125:47–58.

Regulation of complement activation

83. Zahedi K, Prada AE, Davis AE 3rd. Structure and regulation of the C1 inhibitor gene. Behring Inst Mitt 1993; 93:115–119.
84. Cicardi M, Zingale L, Zanichelli A, et al. C1 inhibitor: molecular and clinical aspects. Springer Sem Immunopathol 2005; 27:286–298.
85. Davis AE 3rd. Biological effects of C1 inhibitor. Drug News Perspect 2004; 17:439–446.
86. Gronski P, Bodenbender L, Kanzy EJ, et al. C4-binding protein prevents spontaneous cleavage of C3 in sera of patients with hereditary angioedema. Complement 1988; 5:1–12.
87. Hessing M, van 'T Veer C, Bouma BN. The binding site of human C4b-binding protein on complement C4 is localized in the alpha'-chain. J Immunol 1990; 144:2632–2637.
88. Isenman DE. Conformational changes accompanying proteolytic cleavage of human complement protein C3b by the regulatory enzyme factor I and its cofactor H. Spectroscopic and enzymological studies. J Biol Chem 1983; 258:4238–4244.

89. Masaki T, Matsumoto M, Nakanishi I, et al. Factor I-dependent inactivation of human complement C4b of the classical pathway by C3b/C4b receptor (CR1, CD35) and membrane cofactor protein (MCP, CD46). J Biochem (Tokyo) 1992; 111:573–578.

90. Discipio RG, Hugli TE. Circular dichroism studies of human factor H. A regulatory component of the complement system. Biochim Biophys Acta 1982; 709:58–64.

91. Kinoshita T, Nussenzweig V. Regulatory proteins for the activated third and fourth components of complement (C3b and C4b) in mice. I. Isolation and characterization of factor H: the serum cofactor for the C3b/C4b inactivator (factor I). J Immunol Methods 1984; 71:247–257.

92. Hardig Y, Hillarp A, Dahlback B. The amino-terminal module of the C4b-binding protein alpha-chain is crucial for C4b binding and factor I-cofactor function. Biochem J 1997; 323(Pt 2):469–475.

93. Su HR. S-protein/vitronectin interaction with the C5b and the C8 of the complement membrane attack complex. Int Arch Allergy Immunol 1996; 110:314–317.

94. Lublin DM, Krsek-Staples J, Pangburn MK, et al. Biosynthesis and glycosylation of the human complement regulatory protein decay-accelerating factor. J Immunol 1986; 137:1629–1635.

95. Lublin DM, Lemons RS, Le Beau MM, et al. The gene encoding decay-accelerating factor (DAF) is located in the complement-regulatory locus on the long arm of chromosome 1. J Exp Med 1987; 165:1731–1736.

96. Taguchi R, Funahashi Y, Ikezawa H, et al. Analysis of PI (phosphatidylinositol)-anchoring antigens in a patient of paroxysmal nocturnal hemoglobinuria (PNH) reveals deficiency of 1F5 antigen (CD59), a new complement-regulatory factor. FEBS Lett 1990; 261:142–146.

97. Rollins SA, Zhao J, Ninomiya H, et al. Inhibition of homologous complement by CD59 is mediated by a species-selective recognition conferred through binding to C8 within C5b-8 or C9 within C5b-9. J Immunol 1991; 146:2345–2351.

98. Lublin DM, Liszewski MK, Post TW, et al. Molecular cloning and chromosomal localization of human membrane cofactor protein (MCP). Evidence for inclusion in the multigene family of complement-regulatory proteins. J Exp Med 1988; 168:181–194.

99. Hansch GM, Weller PF, Nicholson-Weller A. Release of C8 binding protein (C8bp) from the cell membrane by phosphatidylinositol-specific phospholipase C. Blood 1988; 72:1089–1092.

Disorders associated with complement activation

100. Tarnok A, Hambsch J, Emmrich F, et al. Complement activation, cytokines, and adhesion molecules in children undergoing cardiac surgery with or without cardiopulmonary bypass. Pediatr Cardiol 1999; 20:113–125.

101. Parry AJ, Petrossian E, McElhinney DB, et al. Neutrophil degranulation and complement activation during fetal cardiac bypass. Ann Thorac Surg 2000; 70:582–589.

102. Donahue MA, Price PM, Aprotinin: antifibrinolytic and anti-inflammatory mechanisms of action in cardiac surgery with cardiopulmonary bypass. Dynamics 2002; 13:16–23.

103. Tofukuji M, Stahl GL, Agah A, et al. Anti-C5a monoclonal antibody reduces cardiopulmonary bypass and cardioplegia-induced coronary endothelial dysfunction. J Thorac Cardiovasc Surg 1998; 116:1060–1068.

104. Shernan SK, Fitch JC, Nussmeier NA, et al. Impact of pexelizumab, an anti-C5 complement antibody, on total mortality and adverse cardiovascular outcomes in cardiac surgical patients undergoing cardiopulmonary bypass. Ann Thorac Surg 2004; 77:942–949; discussion 949–950.

105. Kaneko H, Orii KE, Yamada M, et al. Long-term duration of reduced serum complement level following burn injury. J Investig Allergol Clin Immunol 2001; 11:303–304.

106. Wan KC, Lewis WH, Leung PC, et al. A longitudinal study of C3, C3d and factor Ba in burn patients in Hong Kong Chinese. Burns 1998; 24:241–244.

107. Gloor B, Stahel PF, Muller CA, et al. Predictive value of complement activation fragments C3a and sC5b-9 for development of severe disease in patients with acute pancreatitis. Scand J Gastroenterol 2003; 38:1078–1082.

108. Nielsen H, Sorensen H, Faber V, et al. Circulating immune complexes, complement activation kinetics and serum sickness following treatment with heterologous anti-snake venom globulin. Scand J Immunol 1978; 7:25–33.

109. Bielory L, Gascon P, Lawley TJ, et al. Human serum sickness: a prospective analysis of 35 patients treated with equine anti-thymocyte globulin for bone marrow failure. Medicine (Baltimore) 1988; 67:40–57.

110. Clark BM, Kotti GH, Shah AD, et al. Severe serum sickness reaction to oral and intramuscular penicillin. Pharmacotherapy 2006; 26:705–708.

111. King B, Geelhoed G. Adverse skin and joint reactions associated with oral antibiotics in children: The role of cefaclor in serum sickness-like reactions. J Paediatr Child Health 2003; 39:677–681.

112. Warrington RJ, Martens CJ, Rubin M, et al. Immunologic studies in subjects with a serum sickness-like illness after immunization with human diploid cell rabies vaccine. J Allergy Clin Immunol 1987; 79:605–610.

113. Mold C, Medof ME. C3 nephritic factor protects bound C3bBb from cleavage by factor I and human erythrocytes. Mol Immunol 1985; 22:507–512.

114. West CD, Witte DP, McAdams AJ. Composition of nephritic factor-generated glomerular deposits in membranoproliferative glomerulonephritis type 2. Am J Kidney Dis 2001; 37:1120–1130.

115. Williams DG. C3 nephritic factor and mesangiocapillary glomerulonephritis. Pediatr Nephrol 1997; 11:96–98.

116. Ohi H, Watanabe S, Fujita T, et al. Detection of C3bBb-stabilizing activity (C3 nephritic factor) in the serum from patients with membranoproliferative glomerulonephritis. J Immunol Methods 1990; 131:71–76.

117. Power DA, Ng YC, Simpson JG. Familial incidence of C3 nephritic factor, partial lipodystrophy and membranoproliferative glomerulonephritis. Q J Med 1990; 75:387–398.

118. Mathieson PW, Wurzner R, Oliveria DB, et al. Complement-mediated adipocyte lysis by nephritic factor sera. J Exp Med 1993; 177:1827–1831.

119. Wisnieski JJ. Jones SM. IgG autoantibody to the collagen-like region of C1q in hypocomplementemic urticarial vasculitis syndrome, systemic lupus erythematosus, and 6 other musculoskeletal or rheumatic diseases. J Rheumatol 1992; 19:884–888.

120. Wisnieski JJ, Naff GB. Serum IgG antibodies to C1q in hypocomplementemic urticarial vasculitis syndrome. Arthritis Rheum 1989; 32:1119–1127.

121. Trendelenburg M, Lopez-Trascasa M, Potlukova E, et al. High prevalence of anti-C1q antibodies in biopsy-proven active lupus nephritis. Nephrol Dial Transplant 2006.

122. Jaekell HP, Trabandt A, Grobe N, et al. Anti-dsDNA antibody subtypes and anti-C1q antibodies: toward a more reliable diagnosis and monitoring of systemic lupus erythematosus and lupus nephritis. Lupus 2006; 15:335–345.

123. Marto N, Bertolaccini ML, Calabuig E, et al. Anti-C1q antibodies in nephritis: correlation between titres and renal disease activity and positive predictive value in systemic lupus erythematosus. Ann Rheum Dis 2005; 64:444–448.

124. Wisnieski JJ, Baer AN, Christensen J, et al. Hypocomplementemic urticarial vasculitis syndrome. Clinical and serologic findings in 18 patients. Medicine (Baltimore) 1995; 74:24–41.

125. Wisnieski JJ, Emancipator SN, Korman NJ, et al. Hypocomplementic urticarial vasculitis syndrome in identical twins. Arthritis Rheum 1994; 37:1105–1111.

Disorders associated with complement deficiency

126. Hannema AJ, Kluin-Nelemans JC, Hack CE, et al. SLE syndrome and functional deficiency of C1q in members of a large family. Clin Exp Immunol 1984; 55:106–114.

127. Slingsby JH, Norsworthy P, Pearce G, et al. Homozygous hereditary C1q deficiency and systemic lupus erythematosus. A new family and the molecular basis of C1q deficiency in three families. Arthritis Rheum 1996; 39:663–670.

128. Botto M, Walport MJ. C1q, autoimmunity and apoptosis. Immunobiology 2002; 205:395–406.

129. Bowness P, Davies KA, Norsworthy PJ, et al. Hereditary C1q deficiency and systemic lupus erythematosus. QJM 1994; 87:455–464.

130. Walport MJ, Davies KA. Botto M. C1q and systemic lupus erythematosus. Immunobiology 1998; 199:265–285.

131. Lee SL, Wallace SL, Barone R, et al. Familial deficiency of two subunits of the first component of complement: C1r and C1s associated with a lupus erythematosus-like disease. Arthritis Rheum 1978; 21:958–967.

132. Dragon-Durey MA, Quartier P, Fremeaux-Bacchi V, et al. Molecular basis of a selective C1s deficiency associated with early onset multiple autoimmune diseases. J Immunol 2001; 166:7612–7616.

133. Inoue N, Saito T, Masuda R, et al. Selective complement C1s deficiency caused by homozygous four-base deletion in the C1s gene. Hum Genet 1998; 103:415–418.

134. Rich KC Jr, Hurley J, Gewurz H. Inborn C1r deficiency with a mild lupus-like syndrome. Clin Immunol Immunopathol 1979; 13:77–84.

135. Ballow M, McLean R, Einarson M. Hereditary C4 deficiency – genetic studies and linkage to the HLA. Trans Proc 1979; 11:1710–1712.

136. Fredrikson GN, Truedsson L, Kjellman M. DNA analysis in a MHC heterozygous patients with complete C4 deficiency-homozygosity for C4 gene deletion and C4 pseudogene. Exp Clin Immunogen 1991; 8:29–37.

137. Wilson WA, Armatis PE, Perez MC. C4 concentrations and C4 deficiency alleles in systemic lupus erythematosus. Ann Rheum Dis 1989; 48:600–604.

138. Welch TR, Brickman C, Bishof N, et al. The phenotype of SLE associated with complete deficiency of complement isotype C4A. J Clin Immunol 1998; 18:48–51.

139. Moulds JM, Warner NB, Arnett FC. Complement component C4A and C4B levels in systemic lupus erythematosus: quantitation in relation to C4 null status and disease activity. J Rheumatol 1993; 20:443–447.

140. Howard PF, Hochberg MC, Bias WB, et al. Relationship between C4 null genes, HLA-D region antigens, and genetic susceptibility to systemic lupus erythematosus in Caucasian and black Americans. Am J Med 1986; 81:187–193.

141. Meyer O, Hauptmann G, Tappeiner G, et al. Genetic deficiency of C4, C2 or C1q and lupus syndromes. Association with anti-Ro (SS-A) antibodies. Clin Exp Immunol 1985; 62:678–684.

142. Colten HR. Navigating the maze of complement genetics: a guide for clinicians. Curr Allergy Asthma Rep 2002; 2:379–384.

143. Bishof NA, Welch TR, Beischel LS. C4B deficiency: a risk factor for bacteremia with encapsulated organisms. J Infect Dis 1990; 162:248–250.

144. Mascart-Lemone F, Hauptmann G, Goetz J, et al. Genetic deficiency of C4 presenting with recurrent infections and a SLE-like disease. Genetic and immunologic studies. Am J Med 1983; 75:295–304.

145. Colten HR, Rosen FS. Complement deficiencies. Ann Rev Immunol 1992; 10:809–834.

146. Ross SC, Densen P. Complement deficiency states and infection: epidemiology, pathogenesis and consequences of neisserial and other infections in an immune deficiency. Medicine 1984; 63:243–273.

147. Figueroa JE, Densen P. Infectious diseases associated with complement deficiencies. Clin Microbiol Rev 1991; 4:359–395.

148. Jonsson G, Truedsson L, Sturfelt G, et al. Hereditary C2 deficiency in Sweden: frequent occurrence of invasive infection, atherosclerosis, and rheumatic disease. Medicine (Baltimore) 2005; 84:23–34.

149. Vandersteen PR, Provost TT, Jordan RE, et al. C2 deficient systemic lupus erythematosus. Arch Dermatol 1982; 118:584–587.

150. Peleg D, Harit-Bustan H, Katz Y, et al. Inherited C3 deficiency and meningococcal disease in a teenager. Pediatr Infect Dis J 1992; 11:401–404.

151. Grumach AS, Vilela MM, Gonzalez CH, et al. Inherited C3 deficiency of the complement system. Braz J Med Biol Res 1988; 21:247–257.

152. Botto M, Fong KY, So AK, et al. Molecular basis of hereditary C3 deficiency. J Clin Invest 1990; 86:1158–1163.

153. Botto M, Fong KY, So AK, et al. Homozygous hereditary C3 deficiency due to a partial gene deletion. Proc Natl Acad Sci U S A 1992; 89:4957–4961.

154. Singer L, Whitehead WT, Akama H, et al. Inherited human complement C3 deficiency. An amino acid substitution in the beta-chain (ASP549 to ASN) impairs C3 secretion. J Biol Chem 1994; 269:28494–28499.
155. Reis ES, Falcao DA, Isaac L. Clinical aspects and molecular basis of primary deficiencies of complement component C3 and its regulatory proteins factor I and factor H. Scand J Immunol 2006; 63:155–168.
156. Botto M, Fong KY, So AK, et al. Homozygous hereditary C3 deficiency due to a partial gene deletion. Proc Natl Acad Sci U S A 1992; 89:4957–4961.
157. McLean RH, Bryan RK, Winkelstein J. Hypomorphic variant of the slow allele of C3 associated with hypocomplementemia and hematuria. Am J Med 1985; 78:865–868.
158. McLean RH, Weinstein A, Damjanov I, et al. Hypomorphic variant of C3, arthritis, and chronic glomerulonephritis. J Pediatr 1978; 93:937–943.
159. Thiel S, Frederiksen PD, Jensenius JC. Clinical manifestations of mannan-binding lectin deficiency. Mol Immunol 2006; 43:86–96.
160. Garred P, Larsen F, Seyfarth J, et al. Mannose-binding lectin and its genetic variants. Genes Immun 2006; 7:85–94.
161. Hansen TK, Thiel S, Wouters PJ, et al. Intensive insulin therapy exerts antiinflammatory effects in critically ill patients and counteracts the adverse effect of low mannose-binding lectin levels. J Clin Endocrinol Metab 2003; 88:1082–1088.
162. Sutherland AM, Walley KR, Russell JA. Polymorphisms in CD14, mannose-binding lectin, and Toll-like receptor-2 are associated with increased prevalence of infection in critically ill adults. Crit Care Med 2005; 33:638–644.
163. Garred P, Voss A, Madsen HO, et al. Association of mannose-binding lectin gene variation with disease severity and infections in a population-based cohort of systemic lupus erythematosus patients. Genes Immun 2001; 2:442–450.
164. Graudal N. The natural history and prognosis of rheumatoid arthritis: association of radiographic outcome with process variables, joint motion and immune proteins. Scand J Rheumatol Suppl 2004; 1–38.
165. Stengaard-Pedersen K, Thiel S, Gadjeva M, et al. Inherited deficiency of mannan-binding lectin-associated serine protease 2. N Engl J Med 2003; 349:554–560.
166. Densen P, Weiler J, Ackermann L, et al. Functional and antigenic analysis of human factor B deficiency. Mol Immunol 1996; 33(suppl 1):68.
167. Kluin-Nelemans H, van Velzen-Blad H, van Helden HPT, et al. Functional deficiency of complement factor D in a monozygous twin. Clin Exp Immunol 1984; 58:724–730.
168. Densen P, Weiler J, Griffiss JM, et al. Familial properdin deficiency and fatal meningococcemia. Correction of the bactericidal defect by vaccination. N Engl J Med 1987; 316:922–926.
169. Fredrikson GN, Westburg J, Kuijper EJ, et al. Molecular genetic characterization of properdin deficiency type III: dysfunction due to a single point mutation in exon 9 of the structural gene causing a tyrosine to aspartic acid interchange. Mol Immunol 1996; 33(suppl 1):1.
170. Nielson HE, Kock C. Congenital properdin deficiency and meningococcal infection. Clin Immunol Immunopathol 1987; 44:134–138.
171. Sjoholm AG, Braconier JH, Soderstrom C. Properdin deficiency in a family with fulminant meningococcal infections. Clin Exp Immunol 1982; 50:291–297.
172. Wang X, Fleischer DT, Whitehead WT, et al. Inherited human complement C5 deficiency. Nonsense mutations in exons 1 (Gln1 to Stop) and 36 (Arg1458 to Stop) and compound heterozygosity in three African-American families. J Immunol 1995; 154:5464–5471.
173. Zhu ZB, Totemchokchyakarn K, Atkinson TP, et al. Molecular defects leading to human complement component C6 deficiency. FASEB J 1996; 10:A1446.
174. Nishizaka H, Horiuchi T, Zhu Z-B, et al. Molecular bases for inherited human complement component C6 deficiency in two unrelated individuals. J Immunol 1996; 156:2309–2315.
175. Wurzner R, Hobart MJ, Fernie BA, et al. Molecular basis of subtotal complement C6 deficiency. J Clin Invest 1995; 95:1877–1883.
176. Fernie BA, Wurzner R, Morgan BP, et al. Molecular basis of combined C6 and C7 deficiency. Mol Immunol 1996; 33(suppl 1):59.
177. Nishizaka H, Horiuchi T, Zhu Z-B, et al. Genetic bases of human complement C7 deficiency. J Immunol 1996; 157:4239–4243.
178. Kojima T, Horiuchi T, Nishizaka H, et al. Genetic basis of human complement C8 alpha-gamma deficiency. J Immunol 1998; 161:3762–3766.
179. Kotnik V, Luznik-Bufon T, Schneider PM, et al. Molecular, genetic, and functional analysis of homozygous C8 beta-chain deficiency in two siblings. Immunopharmacology 1997; 38:215–221.
180. Kaufmann T, Hansch G, Rittner C, et al. Genetic basis of human complement C8 beta deficiency. J Immunol 1993; 150:4943–4947.
181. Komatsu M, Yamamoto K, Mikami H, et al. Genetic deficiency of complement component C8 in the rabbit: evidence of a translational defect in expression of the alpha-gamma subunit. Biochem Genet 1991; 29:271–274.
182. Kang HJ, Kim HS, Lee YK, et al. High incidence of complement C9 deficiency in Koreans. Ann Clin Lab Sci 2005; 35:144–148.
183. Kira R, Ihara K, Watanabe K, et al. Molecular epidemiology of C9 deficiency heterozygotes with an Arg95Stop mutation of the C9 gene in Japan. J Hum Genet 1999; 44:109–111.
184. Hayama K, Sugai N, Tanaka S, et al. High-incidence of C9 deficiency throughout Japan: there are no significant differences in incidence among eight areas of Japan. Int Arch Allergy Appl Immunol 1989; 90:400–404.
185. Hobart MJ, Fernie BA, Wurzner R, et al. Difficulties in the ascertainment of C9 deficiency: lessons to be drawn from a compound heterozygote C9-deficient subject. Clin Exp Immunol 1997; 108:500–506.
186. Fukumori Y, Yoshimura K , Ohnoki S, et al. A high incidence of C9 deficiency among healthy blood donors in Osaka, Japan. Int Immunol 1989; 1:85–89.
187. Agostoni A, Aygoren-Pursun E, Binkley KE, et al. Hereditary and acquired angioedema: problems and progress: proceedings of the third C1 esterase inhibitor deficiency workshop and beyond. J Allergy Clin Immunol 2004; 114:S51–S131.
188. Prada AE, Zahedi K, Davis AE 3rd. Regulation of C1 inhibitor synthesis. Immunobiology 1998; 199:377–388.
189. Lener M, Vinci G, Duponchel C, et al. Molecular cloning, gene structure and expression profile of mouse C1 inhibitor. Eur J Biochem 1998; 254:117–122.
190. Falus A, Feher K, Walcz E, et al. Hormonal regulation of complement biosynthesis in human cell lines I. Androgens and gamma interferon stimulate the biosynthesis and gene expression of C1 inhibitor in human cell lines U937 and HepG2. Mol Immunol 1990; 27:191–195.
191. Davis AE 3rd. The pathophysiology of hereditary angioedema. Clin Immunol 2005; 114:3–9.
192. Bowen T, Cicardi M, Farkas H, et al. Canadian 2003 International Consensus Algorithm For the Diagnosis, Therapy, and Management of Hereditary Angioedema. J Allergy Clin Immunol 2004; 114:629–637.
193. Gompels MM, Lock RJ, Abinun M, et al. C1 inhibitor deficiency: consensus document. Clin Exp Immunol 2005; 139:379–394.
194. Levi M, Choi G, Picavet C, et al. Self-administration of C1-inhibitor concentrate in patients with hereditary or acquired angioedema caused by C1-inhibitor deficiency. J Allergy Clin Immunol 2006; 117:904–908.
195. Bork K, Meng G, Staubach P, et al. Treatment with C1 inhibitor concentrate in abdominal pain attacks of patients with hereditary angioedema. Transfusion 2005; 45:1774–1784.
196. De Serres J, Groner A, Lindner J. Safety and efficacy of pasteurized C1 inhibitor concentrate (Berinert P) in hereditary angioedema: a review. Transfus Apher Sci 2003; 29:247–254.
197. Bork K, Barnstedt SE. Treatment of 193 episodes of laryngeal edema with C1 inhibitor concentrate in patients with hereditary angioedema. Arch Intern Med 2001; 161:714–718.
198. Kunschak M, Engl W, Maritsch F, et al. A randomized, controlled trial to study the efficacy and safety of C1 inhibitor concentrate in treating hereditary angioedema. Transfusion 1998; 38:540–549.
199. Perricone R, De Carolis C, Giacomello F, et al. Impaired human ovarian follicular fluid complement function in hereditary angioedema. Scand J Immunol 2000; 51:104–108.
200. Carreer FM, The C1 inhibitor deficiency. A review. Eur J Clin Chem Clin Biochem 1992; 30:793–807.
201. Nusinow SR, Zuraw BL, Curd JG. The hereditary and acquired deficiencies of complement. Med Clin North Am 1985; 69:487–504.
202. Trapp RG, Fletcher M, Forristal J, et al. C4 binding protein deficiency in a patient with atypical Behçet's disease. J Rheumatol 1987; 14:135–138.
203. Bonnin AJ, Zeitz HJ, Gewurz A. Complement factor I deficiency with recurrent aseptic meningitis. Arch Intern Med 1993; 153:1380–1383.
204. Leitao MF, Vilela MM, Rutz R, et al. Complement factor I deficiency in a family with recurrent infections. Immunopharmacology 1997; 38:207–213.
205. Vyse TJ, Morley BJ, Bartok I, et al. The molecular basis of hereditary complement factor I deficiency. J Clin Invest 1996; 97:925–933.
206. Vyse TJ, Spath PJ, Davies KA, et al. Hereditary complement factor I deficiency. Q J Med 1994; 87:385–401.
207. Fremeaux-Bacchi V, Dragon-Durey MA, Blouin J, et al. Complement factor I: a susceptibility gene for atypical haemolytic uraemic syndrome. J Med Genet 2004; 41:e84.
208. Genel F, Sjoholm AG, Skattum L, et al. Complement factor I deficiency associated with recurrent infections, vasculitis and immune complex glomerulonephritis. Scand J Infect Dis 2005; 37:615–618.
209. Kavanagh D, Kemp EJ, Mayland E, et al. Mutations in complement factor I predispose to development of atypical hemolytic uremic syndrome. J Am Soc Nephrol 2005; 16:2150–2155.
210. Caprioli J, Peng L, Remuzzi G. The hemolytic uremic syndromes. Curr Opin Crit Care 2005; 11:487–492.
211. Klein RJ, Zeiss C, Chew EY, et al. Complement factor H polymorphism in age-related macular degeneration. Science 2005; 308:385–389.
212. Sanchez-Corral P, Perez-Caballero D, Huarte O, et al. Structural and functional characterization of factor H mutations associated with atypical hemolytic uremic syndrome. Am J Hum Genet 2002; 71:1285–1295.
213. Nielsen HE, Christensen KC, Koch C, et al. Hereditary, complete deficiency of complement factor H associated with recurrent meningococcal disease. Scand J Immunol 1989; 30:711–718.
214. Dragon-Durey MA, Fremeaux-Bacchi V, Loirat C, et al. Heterozygous and homozygous factor H deficiencies associated with hemolytic uremic syndrome or membranoproliferative glomerulonephritis: report and genetic analysis of 16 cases. J Am Soc Nephrol 2004; 15:787–795.
215. Pangburn MK. Cutting edge: localization of the host recognition functions of complement factor H at the carboxyl-terminal: implications for hemolytic uremic syndrome. J Immunol 2002; 169:4702–4706.
216. Haines JL, Hauser MA, Schmidt S, et al. Complement factor H variant increases the risk of age-related macular degeneration. Science 2005; 308:419–421.
217. Caprioli J, Noris M, Brioschi S, et al. Genetics of HUS: the impact of MCP, CFH, and IF mutations on clinical presentation, response to treatment, and outcome. Blood 2006; 108:1267–1279.
218. Richards A, Kemp EJ, Liszewski MK, et al. Mutations in human complement regulator, membrane cofactor protein (CD46), predispose to development of familial hemolytic uremic syndrome. Proc Natl Acad Sci U S A 2003; 100:12966–12971.
219. Zimmerhackl LB, Besbas N, Jungraithmayr T, et al. Epidemiology, clinical presentation, and pathophysiology of atypical and recurrent hemolytic uremic syndrome. Semin Thromb Hemost 2006; 32:113–120.
220. Yamashina M, Ueda E, Kinoshita T, et al. Inherited complete deficiency of 20-kilodalton homologous restriction factor (CD59) as a cause of paroxysmal nocturnal hemoglobinuria. N Engl J Med 1990; 323:1184–1189.
221. Shichishima T, Noji H. Heterogeneity in the molecular pathogenesis of paroxysmal nocturnal hemoglobinuria (PNH) syndromes and expansion mechanism of a PNH Clone. Int J Hematol 2006; 84:97–103.
222. Shichishima T. Glycosylphosphatidylinositol (GPI)-anchored membrane proteins in clinical pathophysiology of paroxysmal nocturnal hemoglobinuria (PNH). Fukushima J Med Sci 1995; 41:1–13.
223. Reid ME, Cromer-related blood group antigens and the glycosyl phosphatidylinositol-linked protein, decay-accelerating factor DAF (CD55). Immunohematol 1990; 6:27–29.
224. Telen MJ, Green AM. The Inab phenotype: characterization of the membrane protein and complement regulatory defect. Blood 1989; 74:437–441.

225. Hue-Roye K, Powell VI, Patel G, et al. Novel molecular basis of an Inab phenotype. Immunohematol 2005; 21:53–55.
226. Cohen J, Lutz HU, Pennaforte JL, et al. Peripheral catabolism of the CR1(the C3b receptor, CD35) on erythrocytes from healthy individuals and patients with systemic lupus erythematosus. Clin Exp Immunol 1992; 87:422–428.
227. Wakabayashi M, Ohi H, Tamano M, et al. Acquired loss of erythrocyte complement receptor type 1 in patients with diabetic nephropathy undergoing hemodialysis. Nephron Exp Nephrol 2006; 104:e89–e95.
228. Miyaike J, Iwasaki Y, Takahashi A, et al. Regulation of circulating immune complexes by complement receptor type 1 on erythrocytes in chronic viral liver diseases. Gut 2002; 51:591–596.
229. Cohen J, Caudwell V, Levi-Strauss M, et al. Genetic analysis of CR1 expression on erythrocytes of patients with systemic lupus erythematosus. Arthritis Rheum 1989; 32:393–397.
230. Sullivan KE, Jawad AF, Piliero LM, et al. Analysis of polymorphisms affecting immune complex handling in systemic lupus erythematosus. Rheumatology (Oxford) 2003; 42:446–452.
231. Kishimoto TK, Hollander N, Roberts TM, et al. Heterogeneous mutations in the beta subunit common to the LFA-1, Mac-1, and p150,95 glycoproteins cause leukocyte adhesion deficiency. Cell 1987; 50:193–202.
232. Arnaout MA, Dana N, Gupta SK, et al. Point mutations impairing cell surface expression of the common beta subunit (CD18) in a patient with leukocyte adhesion molecule (Leu-CAM) deficiency. J Clin Invest 1990; 85:977–981.
233. Bunting M, Harris ES, McIntyre TM, et al. Leukocyte adhesion deficiency syndromes: adhesion and tethering defects involving beta 2 integrins and selectin ligands. Curr Opin Hematol 2002; 9:30–35.
234. Engel ME, Hickstein DD, Bauer TR Jr, et al. Matched unrelated bone marrow transplantation with reduced-intensity conditioning for leukocyte adhesion deficiency. Bone Marrow Transplant 2006; 37:717–718.
235. Kishimoto TK, Springer TA. Human leukocyte adhesion deficiency: molecular basis for a defective immune response to infections of the skin. Curr Prob Dermatol 1989; 18:106–115.
236. Stark MA, Huo Y, Burcin TL, et al. Phagocytosis of apoptotic neutrophils regulates granulopoiesis via IL-23 and IL-17. Immunity 2005; 22:285–294.
237. Helmus Y, Denecke J, Yakubenia S, et al. Leukocyte adhesion deficiency II patients with a dual defect of the GDP-fucose transporter. Blood 2006; 107:3959–3966.
238. Etzioni A, Tonetti M. Leukocyte adhesion deficiency II – from A to almost Z. Immunol Rev 2000; 178:138–147.
239. Etzioni A, Sturla L, Antonellis A, et al. Leukocyte adhesion deficiency (LAD) type II/carbohydrate deficient glycoprotein (CDG) IIc founder effect and genotype/phenotype correlation. Am J Med Genet 2002; 110:131–135.
240. Etzioni A, Alon R. Leukocyte adhesion deficiency III: a group of integrin activation defects in hematopoietic lineage cells. Curr Opin Allergy Clin Immunol 2004; 4:485–490.

Management of complement deficiencies

241. Biesma DH, Hannema AJ, van Velzen-Blad H, et al. A family with complement factor D deficiency. J Clin Invest 2001; 108:233–240.
242. Hiemstra PS, Langeler E, Compier B, et al. Complete and partial deficiencies of complement factor D in a Dutch family. J Clin Invest 1989; 84:1957–1961.
243. Sjoholm AG, Kuijper EJ, Tijssen CC, et al. Dysfunctional properdin in a Dutch family with meningococcal disease. N Engl J Med 1988; 319:33–40.

244. Platonov AE, Beloborodov VB, Vershinina IV. Meningococcal disease in patients with late complement component deficiency: studies in the U.S.S.R. Medicine 1993; 72:374–392.
245. Fijen CA, Kuijper EJ, Drogari-Apiranthitou M, et al. Protection against meningococcal serogroup ACYW disease in complement-deficient individuals vaccinated with the tetravalent meningococcal capsular polysaccharide vaccine. Clin Exp Immunol 1998; 114:362–369.
246. Schlesinger M, Kayhty H, Levy R, et al. Phagocytic killing and antibody response during the first year after tetravalent meningococcal vaccine in complement-deficient and in normal individuals. J Clin Immunol 2000; 20:46–53.
247. Drogari-Apiranthitou M, Fijen CA, Van De Beek D, et al. Development of antibodies against tetravalent meningococcal polysaccharides in revaccinated complement-deficient patients. Clin Exp Immunol 2000; 119:311–316.
248. Platonov AE, Beloborodov VB, Pavlova LI, et al. Vaccination of patients deficient in a late complement component with tetravalent meningococcal capsular polysaccharide vaccine. Clin Exp Immunol 1995; 100:32–39.
249. Goodship TH. Factor H genotype-phenotype correlations: lessons from aHUS, MPGN II, and AMD. Kidney Int 2006; 70:12–13.

Laboratory assessment of complement

250. Ekdahl K, Truedsson L, Sjoholm AG, et al. Complement analysis in adult patients with a history of bacteremic pneumococcal infections or recurrent pneumonia. Scand J Infect Dis 1995; 27:111–117.
251. Ernst T, Spath PJ, Aebi C, et al. Screening for complement deficiency in bacterial meningitis. Acta Paediatrica 1997; 86:1009–1010.
252. Fijen CA, Kuijper EJ, te Bulte MT, et al. Assessment of complement deficiency in patients with meningococcal disease in The Netherlands. Clin Infect Dis 1999; 28:98–105.
253. Ellison RT, Kohler PH, Curd JG, et al. Prevalence of congenital and acquired complement deficiency in patients with sporadic meningococcal disease. N Engl J Med 1983; 308:913–916.
254. Nielsen HE, Koch C, Magnussesn P, et al. Complement deficiencies in selected groups of patients with meningococcal disease. Scand J Infect Dis 1989; 21:389-344.
255. Fijen CA, Juijper EJ, Hannema AJ, et al. Complement deficiencies in patients over ten years old with meningococcal disease due to uncommon serogroups. Lancet 1989; ii:585–588.
256. Merino J, Rodriguez-Valverde V, Lamelas JA. Prevalence of deficits of complement components in patients with recurrent meningococcal infections. J Infect Dis 1983; 148:331–336.
257. Cremer R, Wahn V. Deficiency of late complement components in patients with severe and recurrent meningococcal infections. Eur J Pediatr 1996; 155:723–724.
258. Nielsen HE, Koch C, Mansa B, et al. Complement and immunoglobulin studies in 15 cases of chronic meningococcemia: properdin deficiency and hypoimmunoglobulinemia. Scand J Infect Dis 1990; 22:31–36.
259. Sullivan KE, Wisnieski JJ, Winkelstein JA, et al. Serum complement determinations in patients with quiescent systemic lupus erythematosus. J Rheumatol 1996; 23:2063–2067.

Immunobiology of IgE

Donata Vercelli

7

CONTENTS

- Induction of IgE synthesis: cell–cell interactions 115
- Molecular events in the induction of IgE synthesis 118
- IgE regulation and the environment 123
- Isotype switching in tissues 124
- IgE regulation: bench to bedside 125
- The genetic regulation of IgE responses 126

SUMMARY OF IMPORTANT CONCEPTS

>> Isotype switching to IgE requires two signals: signal 1 typically depends on Th2 cells and cytokines, results in the activation of transcription at a specific region in the Ig locus, and dictates isotype specificity. Signal 2 is CD40-dependent and results in DNA switch recombination and IgE expression. Circuits involving accessory molecules can amplify the response, leading to high-rate IgE synthesis.

>> The synthesis of IgE and antibody isotype other than IgM requires isotype switching. This process, also known as class switch recombination, consists of an intrachromosomal DNA recombination that involves repetitive switch (S) regions located upstream of each constant heavy chain (CH) gene, except $C\delta$. Switch recombination reflects a 'cut and paste' process in which breaks are introduced into the DNA of two participating S regions, which are subsequently fused. Three successive events are required for isotype switching to occur: transcription of target S region sequences, DNA cleavage, and DNA repair. Class switching can be direct or sequential.

>> Environmental exposures exert strong, allergen-specific influences on IgE regulation. For instance, exposure to a farming environment protects against grass-specific responses at every step along the sequential IgG1/IgG4/IgE switching pathway, but has no significant impact on mite responses. In contrast, protection from responses to cat allergen is concentrated at the IgG1 level.

>> IgE switching occurs not only in lymphoid organs but also in peripheral tissues, as evidenced by molecular analysis.

>> IgE regulation is strongly affected by genes variants arrayed along the main signaling pathways leading to Th2-dependent class switch recombination.

Immunobiology of IgE includes themes as diverse as IgE structure, IgE receptors, and IgE regulation. This chapter will focus on IgE regulation, and will address the basic cell–cell interactions required for class switching to IgE and the molecular events that such interactions induce. IgE modulation by environmental stimuli, potential therapeutic targets, and the effects of genetic variants on IgE responses will then be discussed.

INDUCTION OF IgE SYNTHESIS: CELL–CELL INTERACTIONS

THE TWO-SIGNAL MODEL

During an immune response, a B lymphocyte can express different immunoglobulin (Ig) heavy-chain isotypes sharing the same VDJ region. This process (isotype switching, or class switch recombination) allows a single B cell clone to produce antibodies with the same fine specificity but different effector functions. The functional diversification of the antibody response achieved through class switching is essential for a normal immune response, as eloquently shown by the severe immunodeficiency observed in patents with hyper-IgM syndrome, whose B cells can produce antigen-specific IgM but fail to switch to other isotypes.[1]

Isotype switching to IgE requires two signals: signal 1 is typically T cell- and cytokine-dependent, results in the activation of transcription at a specific region in the Ig locus, and dictates isotype specificity. Signal

2 is CD40-dependent and results in DNA switch recombination and IgE expression. Circuits involving accessory molecules can amplify the response, leading to high-rate IgE synthesis. It should be emphasized the definition of 'signal 1' and 'signal 2' reflects a B cell-centered perspective. However, high-rate cytokine secretion (signal 1) and full B cell activation

via CD40/CD40 ligand (CD154) interactions (signal 2) may enhance one another and involve additional ligand-receptor pairs (Fig. 7.1).

SIGNAL 1 IS DELIVERED BY IL-4 OR IL-13

The interaction between IL-4 and the IL-4 receptor (IL-4R) delivers the first signal for switching to IgE. The most compelling evidence for the central role of IL-4 in IgE induction came from gene targeting experiments. Mice in which the IL-4 gene had been knocked out by homologous recombination (IL-4 KO mice) were unable to mount an antiparasite IgE response; the IgG1 response was also suppressed, although to a lesser extent, whereas the production of other isotypes was unaffected.[2]

More recently it became clear that another cytokine, IL-13, shares many of the functional properties of IL-4, including the ability to induce IgE synthesis by B cells. Although the sequence homology between IL-13 and IL-4 is only $\approx 30\%$, all residues that contribute to the hydrophobic core of IL-4 are conserved or have conservative hydrophobic replacements in IL-13. Furthermore, the IL-4Rα chain is a component of both the IL-4R (IL-4Rα:γc) and the IL-13R (IL-4Rα:IL-13Rα1) (Fig. 7.2). However, IL-4 and IL-13, as well as their receptors, are by no means identical. IL-13 does not bind to cells transfected either with complementary DNA (cDNA) for the IL-4R α chain and/or the γ chain and most importantly, unlike IL-4, it has no effects on human T cells. The biology of IL-4, IL-13, and their receptors has been extensively reviewed.[3,4]

Marked differences exist in the kinetics of IL-4 and IL-13 production after T cell stimulation through the antigen receptor. IL-4 is secreted in low amounts during the first 24h, whereas IL-13 is secreted abundantly for at least 6 days.[5] Furthermore, it has been shown that naive $CD4^+CD45RO^-$ human T cells develop into effector cells that secrete IL-13, IL-5, and interferon-γ (IFN-γ) but not IL-4 upon T cell receptor cross-linking.[6] These cells are able to provide efficient help for IgE production. These findings suggest the intriguing possibility that, at least at certain stages of T helper (Th) differentiation, the production of IL-13 and IL-4 may be independently regulated. Comparison of IL-4 or IL-13 single KO mice to animals carrying a simultaneous disruption in both IL-4 and IL-13 demonstrates that only the double KO mice exhibited no IgE in response to challenge with *Schistosoma mansoni*. Unlike IL-4$^{-/-}$ mice, IL-13 null mice fail to clear helminthes and to recover basal IgE levels after stimulation with IL-4.[7] However, it is not yet clear to what extent interference with *cis* regulatory elements on the linked allele may have contributed to the phenotypes observed in these experiments.

SIGNAL 2 IS DELIVERED BY CD40/CD154 INTERACTIONS

The engagement of CD40 on B cells by CD154 expressed on T cells provides the second signal required for switching to IgE. CD154 can be replaced in vitro by anti-CD40 mAbs. Indeed, this was the first system in which the B cell-activating signal for human IgE synthesis could be delivered in vitro by antibody-induced engagement of a discrete B cell surface antigen.[8] CD40 is a 50 kDa surface glycoprotein that belongs to the tumor necrosis factor receptor (TNFR) superfamily and is expressed on human B lymphocytes, cytokine-activated monocytes, follicular dendritic cells, epithelial cells (including thymic epithelium), but not T cells. CD40 plays a key role in the survival, growth, and differentiation of B cells. Signaling through CD40 rescues B cells from apoptosis induced

by Fas (CD95) or cross-linking of the IgM complex. Selected anti-CD40 mAbs trigger significant proliferation of highly purified resting B cells in the absence of other co-stimuli.[9]

The common structural framework of the CD40 extracellular domain is reflected by the ability of the TNFR family members to interact with a parallel family of TNF-related molecules that includes the ligands for CD40 (CD154), CD27, CD30, OX40, TNF-α, and lymphotoxin. CD154 is a 261 amino acid type 2 membrane glycoprotein transiently expressed on activated, but not resting, Th1 and Th2 cells. Cells transfected with CD154 induced IgE synthesis by both murine and human B cells, in the presence of IL-4, whereas a soluble CD40-Ig fusion protein inhibited IL-4-dependent IgE synthesis in human peripheral blood mononuclear cells. These results clearly indicate that CD40/CD154 interactions are critical for delivering the second signal required for IgE production. The central role of the CD40/CD154 pathway in IgE synthesis, and more generally in isotype switching, was confirmed by the finding that defective switching in patients with X-linked hyper-IgM syndrome is due to mutations in CD154 that result in impaired CD40/CD154 interactions.[10] Furthermore, no IgG, IgA, or IgE response to thymus-dependent antigens was detectable in CD40[11] and CD154[12] KO mice, and no germinal centers were recognizable in lymphoid organs. In contrast, responses to thymus-independent antigens were preserved. Finally, the inability of human newborn B cells to switch, and the consequent transient immunodeficiency observed in human neonates, have been ascribed to a decrease in both CD154 expression and responses to CD40 agonists. Thus data from a number of in vitro and in vivo models consistently point to the crucial role of CD40/CD154 interactions in germinal center formation, B cell activation, isotype switching, and antibody production.[13]

The interactions between CD40 and CD154 are tightly regulated. T cells only become competent to activate B cells via CD40 after they express CD154, and this in turn requires T cell antigen receptor-dependent T cell activation. The latter process seems to be somewhat constrained, since in secondary lymphoid tissues CD154 is only expressed at the site of cognate T/B cell interactions. Interestingly, a subset of $CD4^{+/-}$ memory T cells in germinal centers contains pre-formed CD154 that is rapidly (within minutes) but transiently expressed on the cell surface after T cell receptor-mediated activation. Rapid expression of CD154 on T cells may be crucial in germinal centers because centrocytes either leave the light zone within a few hours of activation or die by apoptosis in situ. On the other hand, the availability of CD154 is drastically limited because the interaction with CD40 induces rapid endocytosis of surface CD154, and release of soluble CD40 by B cells downregulates CD154 mRNA.[13]

INTERACTIONS BETWEEN CO-STIMULATORY MOLECULES AMPLIFY SIGNAL 1 AND SIGNAL 2

Several pairs of co-stimulatory molecules have been shown to participate in T/B cell interactions conducive to IgE synthesis by complementing and/or upregulating the T cell-dependent activation of B cells that follows the engagement of CD40 by CD154 (Fig. 7.1). A major accessory role is likely to be played by the CD28/CD80-CD86 ligand receptor pairs. Both CD28 on T cells and its B cell counter-receptors, CD80 (B7.1) and CD86 (B7.2), are part of a reciprocal amplification mechanism that amplifies T/B cell interactions mediated via CD40/CD154. Engagement of CD40 is known to result in expression of CD80 and CD86 on B cells.

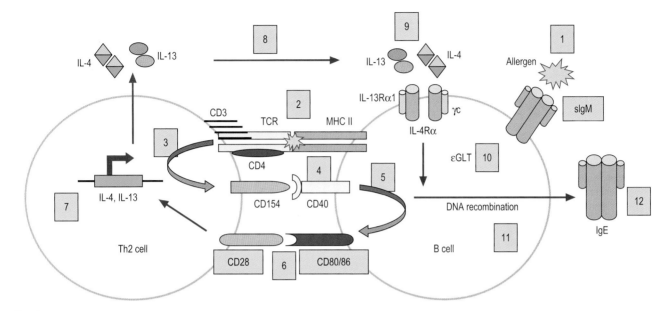

Fig. 7.1. T/B cell interactions leading to IgE isotype switching. The signals required for isotype switching are provided to the B cell through a complex series of interactions with an antigen (allergen)-specific T cell. A B cell that expresses IgM specific for the allergen (1) binds the allergen via surface immunoglobulins (sIgM), processes it, and presents it to an allergen-specific Th2-like T cell, i.e. a T cell programmed to secrete IL-4 but not IFN-γ (2). Engagement of the T cell receptor/CD3 complex by MHC class II molecules results in the rapid expression of CD154 (3), that engages CD40, the counterreceptor constitutively expressed on B cells (4). T/B cell interactions mediated via CD40/CD154 are amplified by interactions between co-stimulatory molecules, particularly the CD28/CD80-CD86 ligand/receptor pair. Engagement of CD40 upregulates CD80-CD86 expression on B cells (5). CD80-CD86 engage CD28 (6), inducing high-rate transcription (7) and secretion (8) of IL-4 and/or IL-13, that will bind their heterodimeric receptors (9). At this stage, the B cell is receiving both signals required for IgE switching: IL-4 triggers ε germline transcription (10), thereby targeting the ε switch region for recombination. Cross-linking of CD40 by CD40L activates DNA recombination to the targeted ε S region (11), leading to IgE isotype switching and IgE secretion (12).

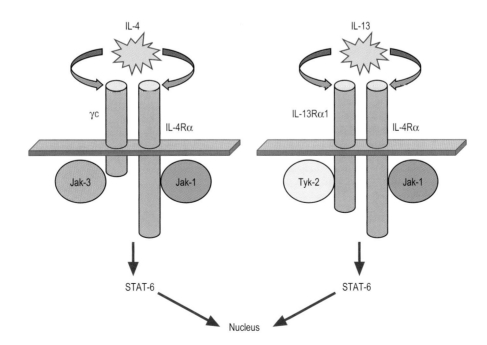

Fig. 7.2. Structure of the receptors for IL-4 and IL-13. The chains that form the heterodimeric IL-4R and IL-13R are shown, together with the associated Jak kinases specific to each receptor complex. Engagement of either receptor results in STAT6 phosphorylation and nuclear translocation.

On the other hand, engagement of CD28 results in increased expression of CD154 on T cells. It appears that CD28 activation is required for strong transcriptional activation of the CD154 promoter in response to T cell receptor ligation. Most importantly, both CD28 and CD80/CD86 KO mice have reduced basal Ig levels. Even more strikingly, mice deficient in both CD80 and CD86 failed to generate antigen-specific antibody responses and lacked germinal centers when immunized by a number of routes, even in the presence of complete Freund's adjuvant. These mice also exhibited an inhibition of IL-4 production accompanied by enhanced IFN-γ production. Thus, CD28/B7 interactions appear to be critical for both IL-4 secretion and CD40-mediated B cell activation and ultimately potentiate both signal 1 and signal 2.[14]

CD86 expression is markedly increased by cross-linking of major histocompatibility complex (MHC) class II molecules on B cells, particularly when ICAM-1 is simultaneously engaged. Thus interactions through MHC class II and ICAM-1 complement T cell help provided via CD40/CD154 interactions.[15] The inducible co-stimulator (ICOS) is the newest member of the CD28/CD152 receptor family involved in regulating T cell activation. It delivers distinct signals to T cells that can be specifically inhibited by ICOSIg.[16] It is upregulated early on all T cells through the CD28/CD80-CD86 pathway and binds specifically to its counter-receptor B7RP-1, but not to CD80 or CD86. In vivo, a lack of ICOS results in severely deficient T cell-dependent B cell responses, impaired germinal center formation, low levels of IL-4, and defective class switching to IgE.[17] As such, it appears that ICOS may be an important component of the cascade of events required for T cell activation.

AMPLIFICATION OF IgE SYNTHESIS BY NON-T CELLS

Human basophils and mast cells have been recently reported to secrete IL-4 and IL-13 and to express CD154. Thus basophils and mast cells may in principle provide both signal 1 and signal 2 for IgE synthesis. However, these non-T cells conceivably play a role in IgE amplification, rather than IgE induction. The optimal physiologic stimulus for secretion of IL-4 and IL-13 seems to be allergen-dependent cross-linking of allergen-specific, receptor-bound IgE. Thus cytokine secretion is predicated on the production of allergen-specific IgE, which in turn requires the signals and cells (primarily, allergen-specific T cells) discussed previously. Once IgE has been produced, it can recruit basophils and mast cells by binding to their IgE receptors, thus inducing IL-4/IL-13 secretion and CD154 expression. Only at this point may non-T cells trigger an IgE response, which would not necessarily be allergen-specific but may be polyclonal as well. Consistent with this scenario, a significant proportion of the IgE response in hyper-IgE states is frequently polyclonal rather than allergen-specific. Furthermore, and most importantly, IgE responses in IL-4-deficient mice were restored by reconstitution with T, but not non-T, cells.[14]

■ MOLECULAR EVENTS IN THE INDUCTION OF IgE SYNTHESIS ■

The synthesis of IgE and antibody isotypes other than IgM requires isotype switching. This process, also known as class switch recombination, consists of an intrachromosomal DNA recombination that involves repetitive switch (S) regions located upstream of each constant heavy-chain (CH) gene, except Cδ, and results in the juxtaposition of different downstream CH genes to the expressed VDJ transcription unit. Since the switching process is highly conserved between mice and humans, much of our current understanding of the mechanisms underlying class switching derives from mouse studies. This work conclusively showed that, mechanistically, switch recombination reflects a 'cut and paste' process, in which breaks are introduced into the DNA of two participating S regions, which are subsequently fused. Three successive events are required for isotype switching to occur: transcription of target S region sequences, DNA cleavage, and DNA repair (Fig. 7.3).[18]

TRANSCRIPTION OF TARGET S REGION SEQUENCES: THE EXPRESSION OF GERMLINE TRANSCRIPTS

S regions include segments of highly repeated tandem arrays of short specific sequence units. For instance, the Sμ region contains a tandem repeat region, $(GAGCT)_3GGGGT$, which recurs approximately 150 times to make up a 3 kb element. Each S region has a distinctive repeat but all exhibit at least some GAGCT and GGGGT sequence motifs. Deletion of most of the Sμ region has been shown to severely impair switching to downstream CH genes, whereas deletion of the entire Sγ1 region essentially blocks switching to IgG1, suggesting that the S regions are specialized targets for the switch recombination process.[19]

Transcription through a particular S region is required for switching to the corresponding CH gene. It has been shown that upstream of each S region are promoters for sterile RNAs, known as germline transcripts. Germline transcripts are transcribed through the S and CH genes, and terminate at the normal termination sites for mature mRNAs. They are also spliced, polyadenylated and exported to the cytoplasm, although they do not appear to be translated. After splicing, germline transcripts contain an I exon encoded upstream of the S region spliced to the normal CH1 splice acceptor for the mature heavy chain mRNA (Fig. 7.4). Although there is no significant sequence similarity between germline transcripts of different isotypes, their overall structure is conserved.[20]

The requirement for transcription and transcription-control elements for isotype switching has been demonstrated directly in gene targeting experiments, in which deletion of I exon promoters or certain 3'IgH enhancer elements abolished or greatly reduced germline transcription of the corresponding CH genes and switching to these genes. Furthermore, constitutively active heterologous promoters inserted in place of endogenous I region promoters can also drive switching.[18,20] Therefore, transcription directly influences class switch recombination.

The choice of the isotype expressed as a result of class switch recombination is mediated by germline transcription and directed by Th cell-derived cytokines in combination with antigen-dependent, CD40-mediated B cell activation. The cytokines IL-4 and IL-13, expressed by allergen-activated Th2 cells, have a unique capacity to induce ε germline transcription and IgE switching, such that IgE expression provides a molecular signature of Th2-dependent activation events in both humans and mice.[2] IL-4-dependent ε germline transcription is strongly upregulated upon CD40 engagement,[21] an effect that is believed to be critical for the efficiency of switching.

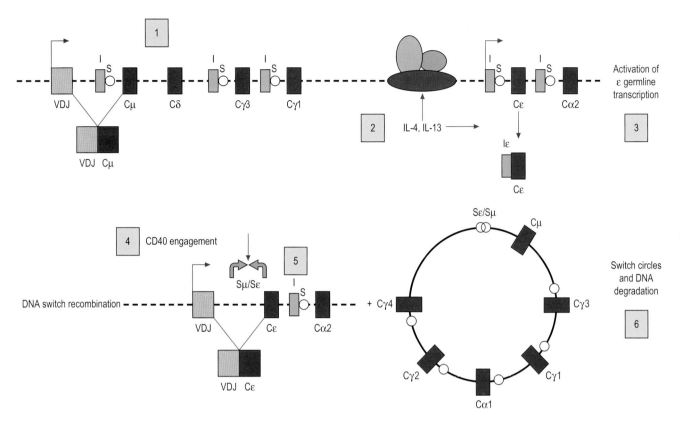

Fig. 7.3. Molecular events in IgE isotype switching. Before switching occurs, the IgE locus is in germline configuration, with all the heavy-chain constant genes still unrearranged. However, VDJ recombination has already occurred, thus determining the antigen specificity of the antibody **(1).** Stimulation with IL-4 or IL-13 **(2)** results in the transcriptional activation of the IgE locus, still in germline configuration **(3).** Induction and correct splicing of germline transcripts is thought to be necessary to target the appropriate switch region for recombination and switching. CD40 engagement **(4)** activates class switch recombination. DNA rearrangement at the targeted S region generates chimeric Sμ/Sε regions composed of the 5′ Sμ joined to the 3′ portion of the targeted Sε region. **(5).** During recombination, the region containing the germline promoter and the I exon is deleted as part of a switch circle and subsequently degraded **(6).**

Full activation of the ε germline promoter in response to IL-4 and CD40 engagement requires a constellation of nuclear factors that are either constitutively expressed or recruited to the promoter by specific activating signals (Fig. 7.2). Among these factors, STAT6 and NF-κB/Rel appear to be most critical for transcriptional activation. Transduction of the IL-4 signal to the nucleus depends on the phosphorylation, dimerization, and activation of STAT6, and STAT6-deficient mice do not express IgE.[22] NF-κB/Rel proteins bind two distinct sites in the ε germline promoter and play an essential role in IL-4-dependent responses, cooperating with STAT6 for the synergistic activation of human ε germline transcription. NF-κB activation mediates the CD40-dependent enhancement of IL-4-induced ε germline transcription. This effect is likely to reflect the physical association between NF-κB/Rel proteins and STAT6. Upon interaction with NF-κB, STAT6 DNA binding affinity is substantially enhanced and transactivating ability is induced. Thus, direct STAT-6/NF-κB interactions appear to be necessary for the synergistic activation of transcription from promoters containing both cognate sites. Notably, activation of neither STAT-6 nor NF-κB requires de novo protein synthesis, allowing for the rapid transmission of the IL-4/CD40 signal to the nucleus.[23]

The role of germline transcription in class switching has long been a subject of speculation. Transcription has been postulated to function at several non-mutually exclusive levels, including rendering S region chromatin structures accessible to the enzymes involved in recombination and generating DNA structures able to act as substrates of a switch recombinase. Support for the DNA structure model arises from the notable feature of all mammalian S regions: that the non-template strand is G-rich. Moreover, when S regions are transcribed in vitro in the normal physiological orientation, the transcripts stably associate with the template strand of the DNA to form RNA-DNA hybrids. These RNA-DNA hybrids were demonstrated to form R loops, in which the displaced non-template strand exists as single-stranded DNA, both in vitro and in vivo (Fig. 7.5).

DNA CLEAVAGE

Although IL-4 (signal 1) is sufficient for the initiation of transcription through the Sε region, switching and expression of mature Cε transcripts (containing the VDJ region spliced to Cε1-4) require signal 2 (engagement of CD40 by CD154). The role of signal 2 in the induction of IgE switching is complex. In addition to triggering DNA recombination,

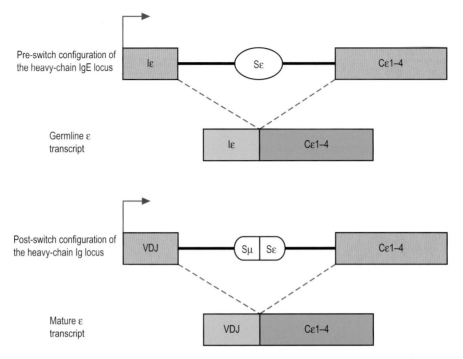

Fig. 7.4. Structure of transcripts expressed during class switch recombination to IgE. Before switching occurs, the IgE locus is in germline, unrearranged configuration. The germline transcripts then expressed in response to Th2 cytokines contain the $C\varepsilon$1-4 heavy-chain exons. Upstream of them is a short I exon ($I\varepsilon$), transcribed off a sequence located a few kb 5' of the ε switch region. The $I\varepsilon$ exon is only present in the genome *before* switching occurs, and is deleted upon recombination. Thus the corresponding transcripts are designated as germline, because they reflect the germline (unrearranged) configuration of the Ig heavy-chain locus. After switching, $I\varepsilon$ is deleted and the 5' portion of the mature IgE transcript is now provided by the assembled VDJ transcription unit, which encodes the variable region of the immunoglobulin molecule. mRNA splicing joins the $C\varepsilon$1-4 heavy-chain exons to the $I\varepsilon$ or VDJ exons (dashed lines).

CD40/CD154 interactions are also critically involved in upregulating IL-4-induced ε germline transcription. Because optimal transcription through the S region is thought to be required for an efficient targeting of recombination,[24] this transcriptional effect of CD40 engagement may be crucial for switching.

Sequencing of chimeric $S\mu/S\varepsilon$ switch fragments composed of the 5' $S\mu$ joined to the 3' portion of the targeted $S\varepsilon$ region, or of switch circles, their reciprocal products, formally proved that switch recombination occurs through deletion of intervening DNA. The same process underlies switching to other isotypes. Deletional switch recombination is preceded by double-stranded breaks in the targeted S regions, a key event the mechanism for which remained long unknown. A major breakthrough came with the discovery of a gene crucial for class switch recombination and formation of DNA breaks. Surprisingly, the same gene turned out to be required for somatic hypermutation. Using a murine lymphoma B cell line (CH12F3-2), transfection of DNA constructs containing $S\mu$ and $S\alpha$ regions constitutively transcribed by separate promoters demonstrated that isotype switching occurred only when the cells were stimulated.[25] Since the transgene was constitutively transcribed and thus accessible for recombination, and switching was inhibited in these cells by treatment with cycloheximide, the stimulation requirement for transgene recombination was linked to the induction of a new protein involved in recombination. Analysis of the clones identified a novel member of the cytidine deaminase family, activation-induced cytidine deaminase

(AID). AID is specifically expressed in germinal center B cells and is induced by in vitro stimulation with IL-4 and LPS or CD154.[26] Overexpression of AID in these cells augmented class switching from IgM to IgA without a need for cytokine stimulation,[27] while AID deficiency abolished isotype switch recombination, even though germline transcription was fully preserved. Furthermore, immunization of AID[-/-] mice failed to induce accumulation of mutations in the antigen-specific variable region gene.[27] These results indicated AID is involved in regulation of the DNA modification step of both isotype switching and somatic hypermutation. Of note, AID[-/-] mice exhibited a hyper-IgM phenotype with enlarged germinal centers containing strongly activated B cells.

Several studies[18,28,29] support the notion that AID is responsible for deoxycytosine deamination to uridine in DNA and leads to DNA repair activities that could result in either somatic hypermutation or isotype switching. The finding that AID deaminates only single-stranded DNA in vitro supports the argument that switching might be enhanced by single-stranded DNA targets, such as those provided by R-loop formation (see above). Indeed, the G-rich DNA that supported isotype switching in vivo was efficiently deaminated by AID in vitro, mainly on the non-template strand (i.e. the single-stranded DNA of the R loop), when the reaction was coupled to transcription. Conversely, C-rich DNA that did not target switch recombination in vivo was a poor AID substrate when transcribed in vitro. According to the current model, transcription through mammalian S regions could generate single-stranded DNA

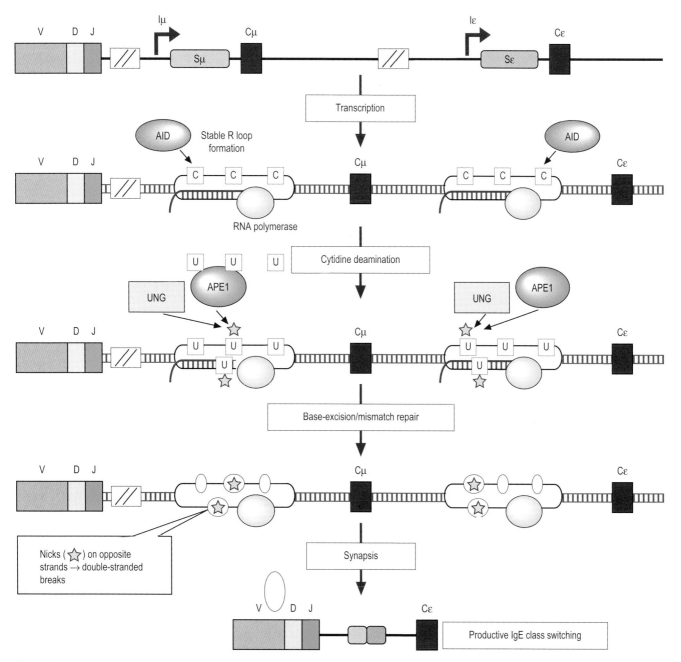

Fig. 7.5. Model for class switch recombination. Transcription through the two participating switch (S) regions generates R loops that provide single-stranded DNA substrates for activation-induced cytidine deaminase (AID). Subsequently, the activities of uracil-DNA glycosylase (UNG) and apurinic/apyrimidinic endonuclease 1 (APE1) can introduce a high density of nicks on the non-template strand, and this, combined with a closely spaced nick on the opposite strand, can generate double-stranded breaks in the S regions. The breaks are synapsed in a process that requires the putative participation of several proteins. Isotype switching is completed by fusion of two S regions double-stranded breaks, possibly by the non-homologous end-joining pathway.

R-loop substrates for the cytidine deaminase activity of AID, thereby generating the initiating DNA lesion that is ultimately processed into a DNA break in the S region (Fig. 7.5).

The generation of an episomal circle in class recombination strongly suggests that switching proceeds through DNA double-stranded break intermediates. Double-stranded breaks have been detected in S regions, and appear to be AID dependent.[30] If double-stranded breaks are essential intermediates in switch recombination, how does AID-mediated DNA deamination lead to such breaks? According to the current model, the AID-introduced deoxyuridine in S region DNA is removed by the base-excision-repair enzyme uracil-DNA glycosylase (UNG) to generate an abasic site, the processing of which, by the apurinic/apyrimidinic endonuclease 1 (APE1), creates a 'nick' (Fig. 7.5).[31] A closely spaced, similarly created nick on the opposite strand could lead to a staggered double-stranded break. In addition, the deoxyuridine-deoxyguanosine mismatch could also be processed by components of the mismatch repair machinery to generate staggered double-stranded breaks. Accordingly, both UNG[32] and MMR[33] deficiencies result in isotype switching defects in both mice and humans.[34] Therefore, deaminated DNA might be processed by several DNA repair pathways, which ultimately lead to the generation of a DNA double-stranded break.

The AID protein has limited sequence specificity, being able to deaminate most deoxycytosine residues. The highest activity of AID is on deoxycytosine residues within WRC motifs (in which W represents A or T and R represents a purine). Switch recombination is found to occur preferentially in sequences that are the best targets for AID deamination. These preferred sequences have been found in all S region tandem repeats, and it seems probable that the tandem repeats reflect evolutionary duplication events selected, at least in part, to provide high concentrations of preferred AID target sites. Interestingly, the roles of AID in somatic hypermutation and class switching appear to be separable, because the C terminal region of AID can be mutated, or the C terminal-most 10 amino acids of AID can be deleted, without interfering with its ability to support somatic hypermutation, although this eliminates its ability to support switch recombination. Conversely, mutations in the N-terminus of AID eliminate somatic hypermutation but have no effect on switching. These data suggest that specific domains of AID may interact with other proteins that allow somatic hypermutation or isotype switching. The fact that different domains of AID may have different functions is especially interesting in light of the fact that somatic hypermutation evolved prior to class switching.[20]

Recent data suggest AID activity is post-translationally regulated. Biochemical assays showed replication protein A (RPA), a single-stranded DNA-binding protein, associates with phosphorylated AID and enhances AID activity on transcribed double-stranded DNA containing switch recombination target sequences.[35] This AID-RPA association, which requires phosphorylation, may provide a mechanism for allowing AID to access double-stranded DNA targets in activated B cells. The same group later showed that AID from B cells is phosphorylated on a consensus protein kinase A (PKA) site, and that PKA is the physiological AID kinase.[36]

Although AID motifs are important in recombination targeting, there are clearly higher levels of regulation that control whether any given AID motif will be accessible for class switching. Analyses of mutant mice that lack the Sμ tandem repeat region show that sequences that flank this region can clearly undergo switch recombination in mutant but not in wild-type mice. Comparisons of mutant and wild-type mice indicate that class switching is constrained to a DNA region that is bounded upstream by the S region transcriptional promoter (Iμ), extends 4–5 kb downstream, and is bounded downstream (in wild-type mice) near the end of the tandem repeat region. The mechanism that establishes this recombination 'domain' is not known. Since different S regions have quite different lengths, isotype-specific factors may provide the different recombination domain lengths. Factors important for switching to specific isotypes have been detected,[37] but the roles of these factors are not yet known. It is also possible that chromatin modifications or structure might define the DNA domain that is accessible to the recombination machinery.[19]

DNA END JOINING

Completion of class switch recombination appears to involve the joining of two broken S regions (Fig. 7.5). The two main pathways that form a synapsis by joining broken DNA ends in mammalian cells are homologous recombination and non-homologous end joining (NHEJ). The limited or complete lack of homology at S region junctions rules out the possibility that the former pathway has a main role, leaving NHEJ as the most probable candidate. A role for NHEJ in class switching was indicated by the observation that isotype switching was severely impaired in Ku70- or Ku80-deficient B cells reconstituted with rearranged IgH and IgL chains.[38,39] However, such an effect could be indirect as Ku-deficient B cells had proliferative defects and died when induced to switch.[39]

Unlike Ku-deficient B cells, B cells from mice with a targeted disruption of DNA-PKcs, which completely eliminates expression of any DNA-PKcs protein, showed no proliferation defects, yet exhibited severely impaired switching to all IgH isotypes except IgG1,[40] strongly indicating a direct role for DNA-PKcs in class switching. The role of DNA-PKcs in isotype switching might be separate from its role in NHEJ, which requires a functional kinase domain, and may reflect the DNA bridging properties of DNA-PKcs, which are independent of its kinase activity.[41] Several other proteins are likely to be involved in double-stranded break joining during switching, but none of these factors have been found to be absolutely required for class switching.[18]

One puzzling feature of the switch recombination process is its ability to join AID-dependent double-stranded breaks within two large IgH locus S regions that lie up to 200 kb apart. Recent experiments tested the postulated roles of S regions and AID in isotype switching by generating mutant B cells in which donor Sμ and acceptor Sγ1 regions were replaced with yeast I-SceI endonuclease sites. Site-specific I-SceI double-stranded breaks mediated recombinational class switching from IgM to IgG1 without S regions or AID.[42] These results suggest that class switching evolved to exploit a general DNA repair process that promotes joining of widely separated double-stranded breaks within a chromosome.

CLASS SWITCH RECOMBINATION DEFECTS

During the last few years, the molecular mechanisms and signals involved in class switch recombination have been further understood through the dissection of a group of disorders (collectively named class switch recombination defects, and previously known as hyper-IgM syndromes) characterized by impaired switching and variably associated with defects in somatic hypermutation. The clinical phenotypes and molecular alterations associated with switching defects were extensively reviewed.[34]

SEQUENTIAL SWITCHING

Sequencing of switch circles generated in B cells triggered to switch to IgE by IL-4 and anti-CD40 mAb revealed μ–γ–ε switching and even more complex sequential events (μ–α1–γ–ε). However, μ–ε circles representing direct switching events were also found at high frequency. Likewise, sequence analysis of Sμ/Sε switch fragments from patients with atopic dermatitis showed a predominance of direct Sμ/Sε joining, indicating sequential and direct switching coexist.[43] Of note, some fragments amplified from B cells stimulated with IL-4 and hydrocortisone contained insertions at the Sμ/Sε junction that were derived from Sγ4,[44] which suggested some B cells had undergone sequential IgM-IgG4-IgE switching. Indeed, IL-4 has been shown to induce isotype switching to IgG4 as well as to IgE, and single B cells can give rise to clones that secrete IgG4 and IgE. Support for sequential μ–γ4–ε switching was also provided by ex vivo and in vivo (see below) studies in humans. Potential implications of sequential switching in humans are discussed below. Here it is important to emphasize that, since class switching entails looping-out and deletion of the DNA located between the S regions involved in recombination, this process is both irreversible and unidirectional, i.e. when occurring sequentially it can only proceed forward along the locus, according to the order in which individual CH genes are arrayed (Cγ3, Cγ1, Cα1, Cγ2, Cγ4, Cε, and Cα2 for the human Ig locus on chromosome 14).

◼ IgE REGULATION AND THE ENVIRONMENT ◼

Invariably a major question about allergy is, why when every individual in the population is exposed to allergens, only some individuals mount a Th2-dependent IgE response to them. A much-needed way out this conundrum is provided by the hygiene hypothesis. The hypothesis was initially formulated to explain the steep increase in the prevalence of allergies in western societies observed over the last few decades, and proposed that reduced exposure to infections in early childhood due to a combination of diminishing family size, improved living standard, and higher personal hygiene may result in increased risk of developing allergic disease.[45] As the integration between epidemiology and immunology intensified, the hypothesis converged with the then dominant Th1/Th2 dichotomy to state that hygienic environments typical of western lifestyles deprive the immune system of stimuli required to boost Th1 responses, leading to a surge in the prevalence of Th2-mediated disease.[46] Once it became clear that the western world is witnessing an increase in both Th2-mediated allergic disorders and Th1-mediated autoimmune diseases,[47] the hygiene hypothesis took on a regulatory twist, stating that evolution endowed our species with immune regulatory mechanisms that are activated by the interaction with the microbial environment and serve to fine tune both Th1 and Th2 antigen-driven effector responses.[48] The innate immune system senses the environment and modulates accordingly the T regulatory arm, which acts as the ultimate keeper of the balance between tolerance and responsiveness. The efficiency of the regulatory interface would be currently jeopardized by a decrease in the microbial burden the immune system evolved to deal with.[49]

The hygiene hypothesis has focused the attention of allergy researchers on the role that exposure to bacterial products, such as endotoxin/lipopolysaccharide (LPS), may have in influencing allergic sensitization. In support of the hypothesis, children raised in rural areas and heavily exposed to animals and LPS have a remarkably lower prevalence of allergy and asthma compared with children living in the same areas but not exposed to animals.[50] Endotoxin concentrations were highest in stables of farming families, but also indoors in dust from kitchen floors and in the children's mattresses, indicating that contact with livestock determines an overall increase in endotoxin exposure.[51] Another recent study found that the homes of allergen-sensitized infants contain significantly lower concentrations of house-dust endotoxin than those of non-sensitized infants. Increased house-dust endotoxin concentrations correlated with increased proportions of IFN-γ-producing CD4 T cells.[52]

In utero exposure to a milieu rich in microbial compounds appears to act as a critical determinant of immune responses occurring later in life. Both atopic sensitization and the expression of major innate immune receptor genes (TLR2, TLR4, CD14) in school-age children were found to be strongly determined by maternal exposure to stables during pregnancy, whereas current exposures had much weaker or no effects.[53] Interestingly, a dose-response relation was found between the extent of upregulation of these genes and the number of different farm animal species the mother had encountered in her pregnancy; that is, each additional farm animal species increased the expression of TLR2, TLR4, and CD14. That time of exposure to bacterial ligands relative to sensitization is critical has been recently reiterated by mouse models showing that mucosal exposure to ovalbumin and/or endotoxin in the neonatal period inhibited allergic responses following subsequent allergen challenge.[54]

Inasmuch as IgE synthesis by human B cells typically results from allergen-dependent, Th2-initiated class switch recombination, the impact of environmental exposures on IgE expression is likely to involve a modulation of isotype switching. Understanding the mechanisms responsible for the protective effect of a farming environment on IgE responses could therefore provide insights into the regulation of isotype switching in vivo and propose a paradigm leading to effective preventive and therapeutic strategies. A recent study assessed the co-expression of allergen-specific serum IgE and IgG subclasses in a large population of farm-exposed or non-exposed children to reconstruct patterns of allergen-induced isotype switching, determine at which steps in the switching process farm exposure exerts its protective effects, and define the correlation between specific IgE switching pathways and prevalence of atopic disease. Farm exposure did not affect allergen-specific IgG2 and IgG3, but had complex, allergen-specific effects on IgG1, IgG4, and IgE. Exposure protected against grass-specific responses at every step along the IgG1/IgG4/IgE switching pathway, but had no significant impact on mite responses. Protection from cat responses was concentrated at the IgG1 level. For all allergens, failure to express IgG1 was associated with low prevalence of IgG4 or IgE responses. Notably, co-expression of IgG1, IgG4, and IgE to grass was associated with increased risk of allergic disease and higher IgE compared to production of IgG1 and IgE without IgG4, suggesting IgG4 co-expression marks stronger activation of Th2-dependent events (Fig. 7.6).[55]

The results of this work revealed novel features of allergen-induced antibody responses, their modulation by exposure, and their relationship with disease. First, for all the allergens examined (timothy grass, mite, cat), virtually no IgE was detected without a concomitant IgG1 (and, less frequently, IgG4) response of the same specificity.

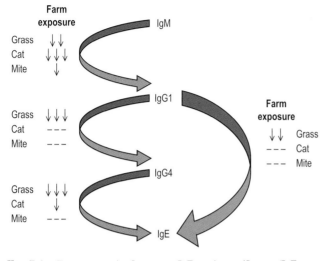

Fig. 7.6. Environmental influences on IgE regulation. (See text 'IgE regulation and the environment'.)

Furthermore, virtually no individual in the population produced allergen-specific IgG4 without IgG1. These findings suggest expression of IgG1 may be a prerequisite for switching to CH genes, such as IgG4 and/or IgE, positioned more downstream in the Ig locus. More generally, the coexistence of IgG1, IgG4, and IgE responses of the same allergen specificity, combined with a prevalence pattern that closely reflects the location of the corresponding CH genes in the Ig locus (IgG1 more prevalent than IgG4, IgG4 more prevalent than IgE), suggests ongoing in vivo expression of Th2-dependent Ig isotypes in response to recurrent or continuous allergen exposure may be regulated coordinately and sequentially.

Farm exposure exerted its effects at discrete stages of Th2-dependent IgG1, IgG4, and IgE switching, indicating that distinct signals regulate the transition from one isotype to the other in vivo. On the other hand, the inability of exposure to affect IgG2 and IgG3 responses implies that the latter are likely controlled by different, so far unknown mechanisms. As importantly, at variance with the common notion that allergens are immunogenic only for selected, genetically predisposed individuals, only a minority of children failed to express IgG1 to grass and mite, and the same was true for anti-cat IgG1, although the non-responsive group was larger. These results suggest that inter-individual (e.g., genetically determined) differences in allergen responsiveness are more likely to affect the profile of antibody responses than the ability to initiate a response.[55]

Analysis of the interaction between isotype switching pathways and exposure to a farming environment also revealed unexpected complexities of the allergen-specific response. Indeed, each allergen-induced pathway was influenced by exposure according to a distinct pattern. Farm exposure protected against grass-specific responses at every step along the IgG1/IgG4/IgE switching pathway, such that the strong global protection against IgE responses detected in the farming population appeared to result from multiple, possibly synergistic effects at distinct steps within the process. In contrast, protection from responses to cat was concentrated mostly at the IgG1 level, whereas farm exposure had no significant impact on antibody responses to mite. Since patterns

of isotype switching to different allergens were assessed within one and the same population, these findings are unlikely to result from inter-individual differences in genetic background and/or allergen exposure conditions. Furthermore, although the contexts of exposure (outdoor versus indoor) were different, all of the test allergens are inhaled, making it unlikely that tissue district-specific differences in dendritic cell function could account for the different patterns of isotype switching we observed. Rather, allergen-specific patterns of antibody responses likely resulted from peculiarities in the biology of allergen/immune system interactions. The unique interactions between farm exposure and antibody responses to specific allergens suggest interventions aimed at arresting the march of allergen-induced class switch recombination towards the IgE isotype may need to be tailored to specific target antigens.[55]

Finally, this work revealed a complex relationship between isotype switching patterns and prevalence of IgE-mediated disease. Risk for allergic disease was substantially increased in individuals co-expressing grass-specific IgG1, IgG4, and IgE compared with those who did not express IgG4. The relationship between presence of grass-specific IgG4 and increased prevalence of disease appeared to be mediated by the expression of markedly higher levels of IgE, such that IgG4 expression in IgE-positive individuals may have signaled a more robust activation of allergen-dependent Th2-mediated events. This enhanced activation, rather than the presence of allergen-specific IgG4 per se, likely contributed to higher disease prevalence in children expressing both IgG4 and IgE.[55]

ISOTYPE SWITCHING IN TISSUES

Classically, isotype switching to IgE was considered to be restricted to lymphoid tissues, such as regional lymph nodes and spleen.[56] IgE+ cells found within peripheral sites of allergic inflammation, such as the respiratory mucosa, were thought to have migrated to the tissue from these centers. In some strong sense, the standard methods for the diagnosis of allergy (skin tests and serum levels of allergen-specific IgE) rely on this view. However, IgE has been detected at sites of allergic inflammation even in the absence of positive skin tests or elevated serum IgE,[57] raising the possibility that B cells residing within tissues may also support IgE production by local isotype switching.

All or most of the main players in class switch recombination are found in the respiratory tract.[43] Populations of IgM+ and IgG4+ B cells have been observed within the nasal mucosa. IgE protein and mRNA have been identified in nasal lavage fluid of patients with symptoms of allergy. IgE-expressing B cells are over 1000-times more frequent among nasal B cells than in peripheral blood. Increased numbers of T cells express IL-4 and IL-13 mRNA. Mast cells, basophils, and eosinophils may express CD154. Within the mucosa of sensitized individuals, these cells are present in ample number and bear IgE in anticipation of allergen exposure. When the latter occurs, allergen cross-linking of surface-bound IgE induces these cells to release IL-4 and engage in IL-13 production. In effect, following initial sensitization, these cells may be an important source of the signals required to induce B cell isotype switching to IgE.

The strongest evidence for IgE switching in the respiratory mucosa was provided by studies that used molecular markers to document the occurrence of defined steps in switch recombination. Nasal challenge with allergen and diesel exhaust particles resulted in nasal lavage B cells that express Sμ-Sε switch circle DNA.[58] Cells undergoing ε germline transcription were demonstrated within the nasal mucosa of allergic rhinitis patients following allergen exposure[59] and in bronchial biopsies from atopic asthmatics.[60] Furthermore, local ε germline transcription as well as class switch recombination were confirmed by the presence of Iε RNA as well as Sμ-Sε and Sε-Sγ switch circle DNA in nasal mucosa exposed to allergen ex vivo.[61] ε germline transcription was inhibited when the tissue was cultured with a combination of allergen and neutralizing Abs against IL-4 and IL-13, suggesting de novo cytokine production mediated isotype switching. The same study showed allergen-induced appearance of Sε-Sγ DNA switch circles and upregulation of Cγ4 mRNA, illustrating that sequential switching to IgE also occurred. More recently, mRNA for AID, multiple germline gene transcripts, and IH-ε circle transcripts were detected in the nasal mucosa of allergic, but not non-allergic control subjects, confirming that local switching occurs in allergic rhinitis. The germline gene transcripts and ε circle transcripts in grass pollen-allergic subjects were upregulated during the season and also when biopsies from allergic subjects were incubated with the allergen ex vivo, demonstrating that allergen stimulates local switching to IgE.[62] The same molecular approach also offered provocative data about the potential role of local IgE switching in asthma pathogenesis. ε germline transcripts and AID mRNA were detectable in bronchial biopsies from atopic patients with asthma, non-atopic patients with asthma, atopic controls without asthma, and non-atopic controls without asthma subjects. In contrast, Iε-Cμ and Iε-Cγ circle transcripts and ε mRNA were detectable in the bronchial mucosa of the majority of both atopic and non-atopic patients with asthma, but rarely in the controls without asthma. These data suggested the bronchial mucosa is a site primed in all individuals for class switching to IgE, because of B cell expression of ε germline transcripts and AID mRNA. However, it is only in patients with asthma, regardless of atopic status, that class switching to IgE occurs.[63]

IgE REGULATION: BENCH TO BEDSIDE

As IgE regulation is understood in more detail, several steps in the induction of IgE synthesis emerge as potential targets for therapeutic strategies. A number of approaches – most of them still at an experimental stage – are currently being devised. Strategies aimed at blocking signal 1 promise to result in an inhibition of switching that should be relatively IgE isotype-specific. In contrast, targeting of signal 2 looks more problematic. A blockade of CD40 signaling would in fact be expected to hamper not only IgE production but also switching to other isotypes. Recent observations, however, suggest that this may not necessarily be the case. Finally, approaches directed at the IgE molecule, either in the membrane-bound or in the secreted form, are actively pursued because of the well-defined specificity of the target. Here the strategies that at this time seem to be most promising in terms of rationale and/or feasibility are briefly discussed.

The synthesis of IL-4 and IL-13, both products of Th2 cells, is dysregulated in atopics.[64] This abnormal commitment to a Th2 response is likely to play a critical role in the pathogenesis of allergic disease. The potential usefulness of soluble cytokine receptors that inactivate naturally occurring cytokine without mediating cellular activation has received some attention of late. Clinical trials show that inhalation of a nebulized soluble recombinant human IL-4R results in significant improvement

of lung function in asthmatics.[65] Soluble IL-13R also appears to abrogate asthma-like symptoms in mice,[66] although this molecule has not yet been studied in humans. Blocking these cytokine pathways may lower IgE levels, which may be responsible for the observed clinical improvement; however, this remains to be determined.

The strong protective effects of traditional farming environments against allergic sensitization and asthma[67] is one of the strongest arguments in favor of the hypothesis and consistently points to bacterial products such as endotoxin and muramic acid. In line with the epidemiologic findings, the search for the molecular mechanisms of the hygiene hypothesis has focused mostly on the interactions between bacterial products and Toll-like receptors (TLR), the main transducers of microbial signals to the immune system and critical regulators of CD4 T cell activation. Several animal models have been developed to define how the administration of bacterial stimuli affects antigen-specific immune responses and the development of allergic inflammation. Unfortunately, the results are confusing because no two models are identical in terms of mouse strain, type and dose of antigen, route of antigen administration, type and dose of TLR ligand, time and route of administration of TLR ligand relative to the antigen. It is fair to say that most groups have reported a protective effect of natural or synthetic TLR2 and/or TLR4 ligands on allergen-induced lung inflammation, but disease-enhancing effects have been observed as well. There is also disagreement as to whether downregulation of Th2-dependent inflammation is or is not accompanied by a concomitant upregulation of Th1 responses. Interestingly, the ability to modulate allergic responses is not unique to TLR2/4 ligands. Early life administration of CpG-containing immunostimulatory DNA sequences, agonists of TLR9, has also been shown to exert a protective effect against allergic inflammation in a murine mode of maternal asthma transmission, and the same TLR9 ligand conferred protection against a classic allergen challenge. However, immunostimulatory oligonucleotides failed to inhibit allergic airway responses in a clinical trial,[68] indicating that further work is required before TLR-mediated manipulation of allergen-induced immune responses can be translated into an effective preventive or therapeutic strategy.[69]

Recently, it became clear the role of glucocorticoids in the treatment of allergic disease may have to be redefined and extended. In vitro, glucocorticoids have complex and paradoxical effects on IgE synthesis because they actually deliver a potent signal 2 to human B cells and thus induce IgE (and IgG4) production in the presence of exogenous IL-4, even though they have no significant direct effect on ε germline transcription.[70] However, the in vivo effect of glucocorticoids seems to be dominated by their ability to induce long-term suppression of IL-4 and IL-13 production, thus blocking the very first step in IgE induction. Local administration of glucocorticoids was recently shown to inhibit ε germline transcription and IgE synthesis in the respiratory mucosa. The use of topical corticosteroids with the ability to block IgE production in the tissue has provided a significant contribution to the efficacy of these agents.[59]

In vitro studies have indicated that cromolyn sodium and nedocromil sodium, drugs often used as prophylactic agents in asthma, block IgE isotype switching by acting directly at the B cell level and targeting deletional switch recombination.[71] Interestingly, these drugs do not seem to interfere with the CD40-delivered signal because they also suppress IgE production by B cells stimulated with hydrocortisone and IL-4. The synthesis of isotypes other than IgE was suppressed as well. In contrast, GL transcription was unaffected. The inhibitory effect on IgE synthesis, combined with the known inhibitory activity on a wide variety of inflammatory cells involved in the allergic response, may further enhance the efficacy of these agents.

A number of studies are currently ongoing to evaluate the therapeutic potential of a variety of anti-IgE antibodies.[72] Two different approaches have been proposed: producing antibodies to the portion of IgE that is part of membrane but not secreted IgE, and targeting the IgE binding site for the high-affinity IgE receptor (FcεR1). Although both approaches target the IgE molecule, their rationales are quite different. The first approach is predicated on the existence of a structurally distinct IgE isoform selectively expressed on B cell membranes and is aimed at the ablation of surface IgE-bearing cells. The other relies on an extensive analysis of IgE/FcεR1 interactions, on the identification of IgE residues involved in FcεR1 binding,[73] and on the generation of high-affinity humanized antibodies capable of preventing IgE binding to the receptor, such as rhuMab-E25. Clinical trials have demonstrated that E25 is effective in suppressing allergen-induced symptoms of allergic asthma, such as FEV_1, and reducing serum IgE levels, possibly through a decrease in the density of IgE receptors on mast cells and basophils.[74,75]

■ THE GENETIC REGULATION OF IgE RESPONSES ■

The search for genetic variants that can modulate IgE responses is intense, and is currently based on both candidate gene approaches and linkage studies followed by positional cloning.[76] If complex diseases result from combinations of, and interactions among, mild defects rather than individual massive genetic disruptions, deciphering the contribution of these defects to the pathogenesis of allergic inflammation may require going beyond a one gene-by-one gene approach, and interrogating multiple genes within a pathway. A roadmap for the analysis of gene-gene interactions relevant to IgE dysregulation is shown in Figure 7.7. The figure shows several sets of molecular and cellular interactions essential for IgE regulation. For some of the genes encoding these molecules, association or linkage studies exist and are referenced. For others, associations were found with phenotypes other than IgE (e.g., asthma), but these genes are included because asthma and increased IgE levels frequently co-occur.[77]

The most upstream events in the map are the interactions occurring at the innate sensing interface which involve allergens, microbial products, and dendritic cells surveying the microenvironment. Dendritic cells, in turn, present antigen to CD4 Th precursors under the influence of T regulatory cells. It is well known that polymorphisms in some of the key genes involved in these interactions (such as TLR2, CD14, IL-10, TGF-β) impact significantly on downstream events, including IgE regulation and allergic inflammation,[78] but the molecular mechanisms underlying these effects remain to be determined. Interestingly, it has been recently proposed that pollen-associated phytoprostanes, bioactive molecules which resemble endogenous prostaglandins E_2 not only structurally but also functionally, may act directly on dendritic cells to decrease IL-12 expression, thus favoring Th2 cell polarization.[79] In this case, receptors for phytoprostanes may represent another important target of genetic variation, which might reset the threshold for allergen-mediated

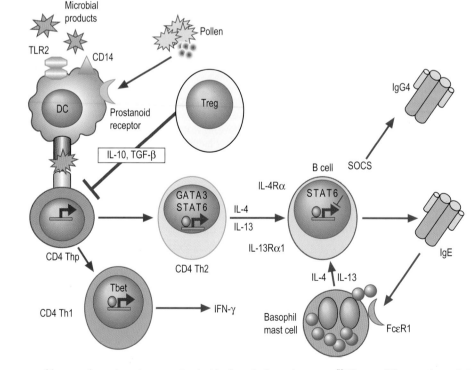

Fig. 7.7. Pathways targeted by natural genetic variants associated with allergy/asthma phenotypes.[78] (See text 'The genetic regulation of IgE responses'.)

induction of Th2 responses. Variation in the prostanoid DP receptor has been recently shown to be associated with increased susceptibility to asthma,[80] reiterating the potential role of prostanoids in the modulation of allergic inflammation.

The differentiation of CD4 Th cell precursors into a Th2, rather than a Th1, polarized effector phenotype is another key process that has implications for IgE regulation. There is good evidence that the process of T cell fate determination is highly plastic, particularly in human T_h cells.[81] Upon encountering antigens presented by professional antigen-presenting cells, T cell receptor signaling rapidly induces modest bursts of GATA3 and T-bet (transcription factors specifically associated with Th2 and Th1 differentiation, respectively). This early transcriptional activity is independent of cytokines and their signaling molecules, but is not sufficient to maintain Th cell differentiation. Full Th2 polarization requires additional IL-4/STAT6 signals, which further induce GATA3. GATA3 then undergoes a STAT6-independent positive feedback process (autoactivation) which enhances its own expression. Interestingly, GATA3 activity is inhibited by T-bet through tyrosine kinase-mediated interactions between the two transcription factors that interfere with the binding of GATA3 to its target DNA.[82] Conversely, GATA3 overexpression inhibits IL-12Rα2 expression and Th1 development even in Th1-inducing conditions. An analogous cascade of events controls Th1 differentiation. In Th1 polarizing conditions, IFN-γ/STAT1 signals increase the initial levels of T-bet expression, which then directly induces IFN-γ and IL12-Rβ2 chain gene transcription. Thus, GATA3 and T-bet appear to act as master switches for Th1 and Th2 differentiation, respectively. Of note, common variants of GATA3,[83] TBX21 (the gene encoding T-bet),[84] and STAT6[85] have been recently found to be associated with allergic inflammation phenotypes, including high serum IgE levels and improved response to corticosteroid treatment in asthma.

The effector phase of allergic inflammation witnesses the involvement of multiple pathways and mechanisms orchestrated by the Th2 cytokines IL-4 and IL-13. Our model focuses on the events leading to the synthesis of IgE, which plays a pivotal effector role in allergy and asthma. Since IL-4 and IL-13 are the only cytokines which instigate IgE synthesis, it is not surprising that polymorphisms in these genes (particularly, two functional ones in IL-13[86,87]) are strongly associated with high serum IgE levels.[88] Th2 cytokines signal to B cells through the IL-4Rα and IL-13Rα1 chains. The interaction between IL-13 and its receptor provides an excellent example of gene-gene interaction, since susceptibility to allergic asthma is strongly increased in individuals who express IL-13 R130Q and the gain-of-function IL4-R V50R551 variant[88] or carry IL-13-1112CT and IL-4RA S478P.[89]

Binding of Th2 cytokines to their receptors activates STAT6 signaling. Further downstream, the signals which determine whether Th2-dependent sequential isotype switching progresses from the IgG4 to the IgE isotype remain unknown, but this choice is likely to be under genetic control, since only a minority of allergen-exposed individuals express IgE, although virtually everyone expresses allergen-specific IgG4[55] (see above). Of note, polymorphisms in IL-13 or IL-4 may influence IgE amplification dependent on Th2 cytokines expressed by basophils and mast cells, as well as T cell-dependent induction of IgE synthesis. In addition, since IgE-mediated FcER1 cross-linking is the main stimulus for Th2 cytokine secretion by mast cells and basophils, and SNPs in the IgE receptor are associated with atopy,[90] polymorphisms in FcER1

may affect not only IgE-dependent release of effector mediators but also the signaling pathways which control Th2 cytokine expression in non-T cells.

References

Induction of IgE synthesis: cell–cell interactions

1. Durandy A, Honjo T. Human genetic defects in class-switch recombination (hyper-IgM syndromes). Curr Opin Immunol 2001; 13:543–548.
2. Geha R, Jabara H, Brodeur S. The regulation of immunoglobulin E class-switch recombination. Nat Rev Immunol 2003; 3:721–732.
3. Nelms K, Keegan AD, Zamorano J, et al. The IL-4 receptor: signaling mechanisms and biological functions. Annu Rev Immunol 1999; 17:701–738.
4. Hershey GK. IL-13 receptors and signaling pathways: an evolving web. J Allergy Clin Immunol 2003; 111:677–690.
5. de Vries J. The role of IL-13 and its receptor in allergy and inflammatory responses. J Allergy Clin Immunol 1998; 102:165–169.
6. Brinkmann V, Kristofic C. TCR-stimulated naive human CD4+45RO- T cells develop into effector cells that secrete IL-13, IL-5, and IFN-γ, but no IL-4, and help efficient IgE production by B cells. J Immunol 1995; 154:3078–3087.
7. McKenzie GJ, Fallon PG, Emson CL, et al. Simultaneous disruption of IL-4 and IL-13 defines individual roles in T helper cell type 2-mediated responses. J Exp Med 1999; 189:1565–1572.
8. Jabara HH, Fu SM, Geha RS, et al. CD40 and IgE: synergism between anti-CD40 mAb and IL-4 in the induction of IgE synthesis by highly purified human B cells. J Exp Med 1990; 172:1861–1864.
9. van Kooten C, Banchereau J. CD40-CD40 ligand. J Leukoc Biol 2000; 67:2–17.
10. Fuleihan R, Ramesh N, Loh R, et al. Defective expression of the CD40 ligand in X-chromosome-linked immunoglobulin deficiency with normal or elevated IgM. Proc Natl Acad Sci U S A 1993; 90:2170–2173.
11. Castigli E, Alt FW, Davidson L, et al. CD40 deficient mice generated by RAG-2 deficient blastocyst complementation. Proc Natl Acad Sci U S A 1994; 91:12135–12139.
12. Xu J, Foy TM, Laman JD, et al. Mice deficient for the CD40 ligand. Immunity 1994; 1:423–431.
13. Quezada SA, Jarvinen LZ, Lind EF, et al. CD40/CD154 interactions at the interface of tolerance and immunity. Annu Rev Immunol 2004; 22:307–328.
14. Oettgen HC, Geha RS. IgE regulation and roles in asthma pathogenesis. J Allergy Clin Immunol 2001; 107:429–440.
15. Poudrier J, Owens T. CD54/intercellular adhesion molecule 1 and major histocompatibility complex II signaling induces B cells to express interleukin 2 receptors and complements help provided through CD40 ligation. J Exp Med 1994; 179:1417–1427.
16. Aicher A, Hayden-Ledbetter M, Brady WA, et al. Characterization of human inducible costimulator ligand expression and function. J Immunol 2000; 164:4689–4696.
17. Tafuri A, Shahinian A, Bladt F, et al. ICOS is essential for effective T-helper-cell responses. Nature 2001; 409:105–109.

Molecular events in the induction of IgE synthesis

18. Chaudhuri J, Alt FW. Class-switch recombination: interplay of transcription, DNA deamination and DNA repair. Nat Rev Immunol 2004; 4:541–552.
19. Selsing E. Ig class switching: targeting the recombinational mechanism. Curr Opin Immunol 2006; 18:249–254.
20. Stavnezer J, Amemiya CT. Evolution of isotype switching. Semin Immunol 2004; 16:257–275.
21. Shapira SK, Vercelli D, Jabara HH, et al. Molecular analysis of the induction of IgE synthesis in human B cells by IL-4 and engagement of CD40 antigen. J Exp Med 1992; 175:289–292.
22. Linehan LA, Warren WD, Thompson PA, et al. STAT6 is required for IL-4-induced germline Ig gene transcription and switch recombination. J Immunol 1998; 161:302–310.
23. Vercelli D. IgE and its regulators. Curr Opin Allergy Clin Immunol 2001; 1:61–65.
24. Lee CG, Kinoshita K, Arudchandran A, et al. Quantitative regulation of class switch recombination by switch region transcription. J Exp Med 2001; 194:365–374.
25. Kinoshita K, Tashiro J, Tomita S, et al. Target specificity of immunoglobulin class switch recombination is not determined by nucleotide sequences of S regions. Immunity 1998; 9:849–858.
26. Muramatsu M, Sankaranand VS, Anant S, et al. Specific expression of activation-induced cytidine deaminase (AID), a novel member of the RNA-editing deaminase family in germinal center B cells. J Biol Chem 1999; 274:18470–18476.
27. Muramatsu M, Kinoshita K, Fagarasan S, et al. Class switch recombination and hypermutation require activation-induced cytidine deaminase (AID), a potential RNA editing enzyme. Cell 2000; 102:553–563.
28. Shinkura R, Tian M, Smith M, et al. The influence of transcriptional orientation on endogenous switch region function. Nat Immunol 2003; 4:435–441.
29. Chaudhuri J, Tian M, Khuong C, et al. Transcription-targeted DNA deamination by the AID antibody diversification enzyme. Nature 2003; 422:726–730.
30. Catalan N, Selz F, Imai K, et al. The block in immunoglobulin class switch recombination caused by activation-induced cytidine deaminase deficiency occurs prior to the generation of DNA double strand breaks in switch mu region. J Immunol 2003; 171:2504–2509.
31. Petersen-Mahrt SK, Harris RS, Neuberger MS. AID mutates E. coli suggesting a DNA deamination mechanism for antibody diversification. Nature 2002; 418:99–103.

IMMUNOLOGY

32. Imai K, Slupphaug G, Lee WI, et al. Human uracil-DNA glycosylase deficiency associated with profoundly impaired immunoglobulin class-switch recombination. Nat Immunol 2003; 4:1023–1028.
33. Ehrenstein MR, Neuberger MS. Deficiency in Msh2 affects the efficiency and local sequence specificity of immunoglobulin class-switch recombination: parallels with somatic hypermutation. EMBO J 1999; 18:3484–3490.
34. Notarangelo LD, Lanzi G, Peron S, et al. Defects of class-switch recombination. J Allergy Clin Immunol 2006; 117:855–864.
35. Chaudhuri J, Khuong C, Alt FW. Replication protein A interacts with AID to promote deamination of somatic hypermutation targets. Nature 2004; 430:992–998.
36. Basu U, Chaudhuri J, Alpert C, et al. The AID antibody diversification enzyme is regulated by protein kinase A phosphorylation. Nature 2005; 438:508–511.
37. Kenter AL. Class switch recombination: an emerging mechanism. Curr Top Microbiol Immunol 2005; 290:171–199.
38. Casellas R, Nussenzweig A, Wuerffel R, et al. Ku80 is required for immunoglobulin isotype switching. EMBO J 1998; 8:2404–2411.
39. Manis JP, Gu Y, Lansford R, et al. Ku70 is required for late B cell development and immunoglobulin heavy chain class switching. J Exp Med 1998; 187:2081–2089.
40. Manis JP, Dudley D, Kaylor L, et al. IgH class switch recombination to IgG1 in DNA-PKcs-deficient B cells. Immunity 2002; 16:607–617.
41. DeFazio LG, Stansel RM, Griffith JD, et al. Synapsis of DNA ends by DNA-dependent protein kinase. EMBO J 2002; 21:3192–3200.
42. Zarrin AA, Del Vecchio C, Tseng E, et al. Antibody class switching mediated by yeast endonuclease-generated DNA breaks. Science 2007; 315:377–381.
43. Gould HJ, Sutton BJ, Beavil AJ, et al. The biology of IgE and the basis of allergic disease. Annu Rev Immunol 2003; 21:579–628.
44. Jabara HH, Loh R, Ramesh N, et al. Sequential switching from μ to ε via γ4 in human B cells stimulated with IL-4 and hydrocortisone. J Immunol 1993; 151:4528–4533.

IgE regulation and the environment

45. Strachan DP. Hay fever, hygiene, and household size. BMJ 1989; 299:1259–1260.
46. Sheikh A, Strachan DP. The hygiene theory: fact or fiction? Curr Opin Otolaryngol Head Neck Surg 2004; 12:232–236.
47. Bach JF. The effect of infections on susceptibility to autoimmune and allergic diseases. N Engl J Med 2002; 347:911–920.
48. Wills-Karp M, Santeliz J, Karp CL. The germless theory of allergic disease: revisiting the hygiene hypothesis. Nat Rev Immunol 2001; 1:69–75.
49. Vercelli D. Innate immunity: sensing the environment and regulating the regulators. Curr Opin Allergy Clin Immunol 2003; 3:343–346.
50. von Mutius E. Influences in allergy: epidemiology and the environment. J Allergy Clin Immunol 2004; 113:373–379.
51. Von Mutius E, Braun-Fahrlander C, Schierl R, et al. Exposure to endotoxin or other bacterial components might protect against the development of atopy. Clin Exp Allergy 2000; 30:1230–1234.
52. Gereda JE, Leung DY, Thatayatikom A, et al. Relation between house-dust endotoxin exposure, type 1 T-cell development, and allergen sensitisation in infants at high risk of asthma. Lancet 2000; 355:1680–1683.
53. Ege MJ, Bieli C, Frei R, et al. Prenatal farm exposure is related to the expression of receptors of the innate immunity and to atopic sensitization in school-age children. J Allergy Clin Immunol 2006; 117:817–823.
54. Wang Y, McCusker C. Neonatal exposure with LPS and/or allergen prevents experimental allergic airways disease: development of tolerance using environmental antigens. J Allergy Clin Immunol 2006; 118:143–151.
55. Stern DA, Riedler J, Nowak D, et al. Exposure to a farming environment has profound, allergen-specific effects on in vivo isotype switching in response to common inhalants. J Allergy Clin Immunol 2007; 119:351–358.

Isotype switching in tissues

56. Ganzer U, Bachert U. Localisation of IgE synthesis in immediate-type allergy to the upper respiratory tract. ORL J Otorhinolaryngol. Relat Spec 1988; 50:257–264.
57. Small P, Barrett D, Frenkiel S, et al. Local specific IgE production in nasal polyps associated with negative skin tests and serum RAST. Ann Allergy 1985; 55:736–739.
58. Fujieda S, Diaz-Sanchez D, Saxon A. Combined nasal challenge with diesel exhaust particles and allergen induces in vivo IgE isotype switching. Am J Respir Cell Mol Biol 1998; 19:507–512.
59. Cameron LA, Durham SR, Jacobson MR, et al. Expression of IL-4, Cε RNA, and Iε RNA in the nasal mucosa of patients with seasonal rhinitis: effect of topical corticosteroids. J Allergy Clin Immunol 1998; 101:330–336.
60. Ying S, Humbert M, Meng Q, et al. Local expression of ε germline gene transcripts and RNA for the ε heavy chain of IgE in the bronchial mucosa in atopic and nonatopic asthma. J Allergy Clin Immunol 2001; 107:686–692.
61. Cameron L, Gounni AS, Frenkiel S, et al. S epsilon S mu and S epsilon S gamma switch circles in human nasal mucosa following ex vivo allergen challenge: evidence for direct as well as sequential class switch recombination. J Immunol 2003; 171:3816–3822.
62. Takhar P, Smurthwaite L, Coker HA, et al. Allergen drives class switching to IgE in the nasal mucosa in allergic rhinitis. J Immunol 2005; 174:5024–5032.
63. Takhar P, Corrigan CJ, Smurthwaite L, et al. Class switch recombination to IgE in the bronchial mucosa of atopic and nonatopic patients with asthma. J Allergy Clin Immunol 2007; 119:213–218.

IgE regulation: bench to bedside

64. Romagnani S. The role of lymphocytes in allergic disease. J Allergy Clin Immunol 2000; 105:399–408.
65. Borish LC, Nelson HS, Corren J, et al. Efficacy of soluble IL-4 receptor for the treatment of adults with asthma. J Allergy Clin Immunol 2001; 107:963–970.
66. Wills-Karp M, Luyimbazi J, Xu X, et al. Interleukin-13: central mediator of allergic asthma. Science 1998; 282:2258–2261.
67. Schaub B, Lauener R, von Mutius E. The many faces of the hygiene hypothesis. J Allergy Clin Immunol 2006; 117:969–977.
68. Gauvreau GM, Hessel EM, Boulet LP, et al. Immunostimulatory sequences regulate interferon-inducible genes but not allergic airway responses. Am J Respir Crit Care Med 2006; 174:15–20.
69. Vercelli D. Mechanisms of the hygiene hypothesis – molecular and otherwise. Curr Opin Immunol 2006; 18:733–737.
70. Jabara HH, Ahern DJ, Vercelli D, et al. Hydrocortisone and IL-4 induce IgE isotype switching in human B cells. J Immunol 1991; 147:1557–1560.
71. Loh RK, Jabara HH, Geha RS. Disodium cromoglycate inhibits Sμ→Sε deletional switch recombination and IgE synthesis in human B cells. J Exp Med 1994; 180:663–671.
72. Jardieu P. Anti-IgE therapy. Curr Opin Immunol 1995; 7:779–782.
73. Presta L, Shields R, O'Connell L, et al. The binding site on human immunoglobulin E for its high affinity receptor. J Biol Chem 1994; 269:26368–26373.
74. Milgrom H, Fick RB Jr, Su JQ, et al. Treatment of allergic asthma with monoclonal anti-IgE antibody. rhuMAb-E25 Study Group. N Engl J Med 1999; 341:1966–1973.
75. Saini SS, MacGlashan DW Jr, Sterbinsky SA, et al. Down-regulation of human basophil IgE and FC epsilon RI alpha surface densities and mediator release by anti-IgE-infusions is reversible in vitro and in vivo. J Immunol 1999; 162:5624–5630.

The genetic regulation of IgE responses

76. Hoffjan S, Nicolae D, Ober C. Association studies for asthma and atopic diseases: a comprehensive review of the literature. Respir Res 2003; 4:14.
77. Burrows B, Martinez FD, Halonen M, et al. Association of asthma with serum IgE levels and skin test reactivity to allergens. N Engl J Med 1989; 320:271–277.
78. Vercelli D. Genetic regulation of IgE responses: Achilles and the tortoise. J Allergy Clin Immunol 2005; 116:60–64.
79. Traidl-Hoffmann C, Mariani V, Hochrein H, et al. Pollen-associated phytoprostanes inhibit dendritic cell interleukin-12 production and augment T helper type 2 cell polarization. J Exp Med 2005; 201:627–636.
80. Oguma T, Palmer LJ, Birben E, et al. Role of prostanoid DP receptor variants in susceptibility to asthma. N Engl J Med 2004; 351:1752–1763.
81. Murphy KM, Reiner SL. The lineage decisions of helper T cells. Nat Rev Immunol 2002; 2:933–944.
82. Hwang ES, Szabo SJ, Schwartzberg PL, et al. T helper cell fate specified by kinase-mediated interaction of T-bet with GATA-3. Science 2005; 307:430–433.
83. Pykalainen M, Kinos R, Valkonen S, et al. Association analysis of common variants of STAT6, GATA3, and STAT4 to asthma and high serum IgE phenotypes. J Allergy Clin Immunol 2005; 115:80–87.
84. Tantisira KG, Hwang ES, Raby BA, et al. TBX21: a functional variant predicts improvement in asthma with the use of inhaled corticosteroids. Proc Natl Acad Sci U S A 2004; 101:18099–18104.
85. Schedel M, Carr D, Klopp N, et al. A signal transducer and activator of transcription 6 haplotype influences the regulation of serum IgE levels. J Allergy Clin Immunol 2004; 114:1100–1105.
86. Vladich FD, Brazille SM, Stern D, et al. IL-13 R130Q, a common variant associated with allergy and asthma, enhances effector mechanisms essential for human allergic inflammation. J Clin Invest 2005; 115:747–754.
87. Cameron L, Webster RB, Strempel JM, et al. Th2-selective enhancement of human IL13 transcription by IL13–1112C>T, a polymorphism associated with allergic inflammation. J Immunol 2006; 177:8633–8642.
88. Vercelli D. Genetics of IL-13 and functional relevance of IL-13 variants. Curr Opin Allergy Clin Immunol 2002; 2:389–398.
89. Howard TD, Whittaker PA, Zaiman AL, et al. Identification and association of polymorphisms in the interleukin-13 gene with asthma and atopy in a Dutch population. Am J Respir Cell Mol Biol 2001; 25:377–384.
90. Shirakawa T, Li A, Dubowitz M, et al. Association between atopy and variants of the β subunit of the high-affinity immunoglobulin E receptor. Nat Genet 1994; 7:125–129.

Signal Transduction

8

Paul J Bertics, Cynthia J Koziol, and Gregory J Wiepz

CONTENTS

- Introduction 129
- General principles 130
- Cell structures 130
- General features of receptors and signaling 130
- Mechanisms mediating intracellular signaling 132
- Selected signaling systems relevant to allergy 143
- Additional therapeutic considerations 146

INTRODUCTION

The processes whereby various external and internal stimuli (signals) serve to modulate cellular behavior are collectively known as signal transduction. These events are critical for the control of cell growth, differentiation, function, and adaptability. The stimuli to which cells can respond are quite diverse and range from small molecules, such as ions and various nutrients, to larger molecules, including hormones, cytokines, growth factors, toxins, and allergens. In addition, processes such cell–cell contact, cell adhesion to matrix components, cell deformation or even cell damage can all elicit specific signal transduction processes, thereby allowing the cell to respond appropriately to differing situations and challenges. Furthermore, although many studies have focused on the capacity of external factors to transduce intracellular signals and alter cell behavior (a process termed outside-in signaling), there is an increasing appreciation for the reverse process (inside-out signaling), wherein intracellular events control how the cell interacts with its external environment. For example, certain intracellular signals can result in the activation/inhibition of cell–cell or cell–matrix adhesion molecules such as the integrins. In general, signal transduction events are tightly regulated and involve the coordinated action of numerous molecules to affect the proper change in cell phenotype and function.

The study of cell signaling is a diverse and rapidly expanding field driven by the observation that an understanding of how cells respond

SUMMARY OF IMPORTANT CONCEPTS

>> The processes whereby various external and internal stimuli (signals) serve to modulate cellular behavior are collectively known as signal transduction

>> The initiation of outside-in signaling begins with a receptor, which is generally a protein(s) that selectively binds the signal-initiating factor (ligand)

>> Receptors exist on the cell surface (plasma membrane) for ligands that cannot readily enter the cell, or at intracellular sites (nucleus) for ligands that are lipophilic/cell permeable

>> Cell-surface receptors often respond to ligand binding by activating enzymes (e.g., protein and lipid kinases), inducing changes in G-protein activity, regulating ion channels, altering gene transcription/mRNA processing, or serving as scaffolding sites for other signaling proteins

>> Intracellular receptors generally act as DNA/chromatin binding molecules that promote or inhibit specific gene transcriptional activities

>> Signal transduction from cell-surface receptors often involves the action of intermediates (second messengers); these processes include the regulated synthesis/turnover of cAMP, the initiation of Ca^{++} fluxes, and the generation of phospholipid metabolites

>> Common signaling events in immune cells also include the regulation of protein kinase cascades (e.g., MAP kinases), the regulation of transcriptional regulators (Jak-STAT and NF-κB), and the involvement of various stimulatory and inhibitory receptor systems containing ITAM and ITIM motifs, respectively (Fc receptors, paired receptors)

>> Receptor activation can regulate multiple cellular activities and functions, including secretion/degranulation, migration, replication, differentiation, and apoptosis

>> Modulation of distinct intracellular pathways offers tremendous possibilities for specific disease management

to various stimuli often results in the development of therapeutics that can selectively target specific cell behaviors. Accordingly, knowledge of the mechanisms by which various hormones, cytokines, chemokines, and allergens can modulate immune cell function is important to the field of allergy. Although research into signal transduction is quite large and cannot be fully covered in one chapter, there are several major themes that can be defined at the general cellular level and with respect to immune cell function.[1] Thus, this chapter will first focus on general principles in cell signaling, such as receptors, relevant cell structures, and common signaling mechanisms. These considerations will then be followed by a discussion of selected systems that are key in immune function and will include a discussion of several families of activating and inhibitory receptors, their downstream signaling cascades and their modulation. Furthermore, throughout the text, therapeutic aspects associated with certain signaling processes will be examined.

GENERAL PRINCIPLES

In this chapter, the discussion will focus on the signal transduction mechanisms initiated at the plasma membrane (outside-in signaling). Because cell signaling involves many effector molecules and cellular structures, it is important to first define several basic concepts (Fig. 8.1). For example, external stimuli that cannot freely enter the cell, such as water-soluble factors (e.g., cytokines, chemokines) or various externally tethered molecules (e.g., cell surface proteins, extracellular matrix components) generally interact with specific cellular recognition molecules ('receptors') that possess an externally facing ligand-binding site. These cell-surface receptors then transduce information into the cell via various conformational/enzymatic activities that allow for signal amplification and the regulation of specific enzyme activities, ion fluxes, cytoskeletal reorganization, and/or secretory events. Also, depending on the receptor, cell-surface-initiated signaling may alter transcriptional activities, chromatin structure, mRNA stability/processing, translational activity, and/or post-translational processing. Furthermore, signaling via cell-surface receptors can result in receptor desensitization, internalization, and/or recycling to achieve feedback control and to prevent excessive stimulation that may lead to pathology. With respect to lipid-soluble factors that can penetrate the membrane, such as steroid hormones, the receptors for these molecules are largely located within the cell, often in the nucleus, wherein ligand–receptor complex formation generally serves to modulate gene transcription. Once again, feedback pathways exist to properly contain the magnitude and duration of signals initiated by intracellular receptor systems. In the following sections, specific cellular structures, receptors, and processes that are common to numerous signal transduction systems associated with allergy will be discussed.

CELL STRUCTURES

PLASMA MEMBRANE

Eukaryotic cells are encapsulated by a plasma membrane that makes the cell selectively permeable to many extracellular factors, including nutrients, lipids, proteins, ions, and pathogens. The plasma membrane is a fluid lipid bilayer containing a complex mixture of phospholipids, glycolipids, sterols, and proteins. This structure serves as an effective barrier to molecules that are poorly lipid soluble and also plays a critical role in the

bidirectional flow of information. This conduction of information includes the recognition of extracellular factors that function to modulate cellular responses. In this regard, cells can selectively recognize and respond to numerous extracellular stimuli, including hormones, toxins, adhesion molecules and pathogens. As noted above, the recognition of these factors at the plasma membrane is mediated by receptors, and receptor engagement elicits changes in cell behavior via the alteration of intracellular processes (signal transduction). These processes entail receptor-initiated changes in the action of various enzymes, structural proteins, adaptor molecules, and transcription factors. In addition, the regulated flow of ions (such as Ca^{++}) across the plasma membrane can modulate various signaling events.

Another important feature of the plasma membrane is the presence of specialized microdomains ('lipid rafts') that consist of a unique composition of sterols, lipids, and proteins. These localized differences in membrane structure promote the recruitment of certain receptors and associated molecules to these regions, thereby facilitating the rapid activation of these signaling complexes in response to appropriate stimuli.

CELLULAR ORGANELLES

Besides the plasma membrane, the endoplasmic reticulum (ER), nucleus, and mitochondria play key roles in cell signaling. The ER is a membranous network of tubules and cisternae that is continuous with the nuclear envelope. This structure participates in many cell functions, including protein synthesis, ion sequestration, and the processing/trafficking of membrane-associated and secreted proteins. The ER, similar to the plasma membrane, contains channels that allow for ions, especially Ca^{++}, to undergo regulated release into the cytoplasm wherein they modulate various signaling processes.

The nucleus is a membrane-enclosed organelle that contains most of the cell's genetic information (chromosomes) and is the major site of gene regulation. Cell responses to external/internal stimuli can lead to changes in gene expression via the alteration of transcription factor activity and chromatin structure. In this regard, DNA is tightly wrapped around proteins called histones, thereby forming higher-order structures known as nucleosomes. Modifications such as acetylation and methylation in response to cellular, environmental, or developmental cues can modulate histone function and affect gene expression. Following gene transcription, the mRNA is processed, transported out of the nucleus, and translated into protein at sites such as the ER. These processes are subject to regulation by distinct signal transduction networks.

Mitochondria are a major site of metabolic function, including lipid/carbohydrate metabolism, oxidative phosphorylation, and ATP synthesis. This organelle participates in the metabolism (e.g., hydroxylation, sulfation) of molecules for excretion and in the destruction of oxidative free radicals. Also, alterations in mitochondrial membrane potential/permeability that occur upon certain signaling events can mediate programmed cell death (apoptosis).

GENERAL FEATURES OF RECEPTORS AND SIGNALING

The initiation of outside-in signaling begins with a receptor, which is generally a protein(s) that selectively binds the signal-initiating factor (e.g., cytokine, hormone). Receptors exist on the cell surface (plasma

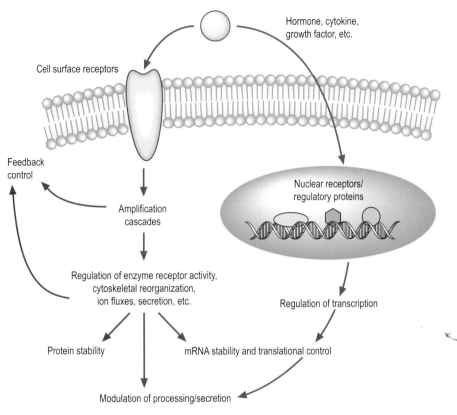

Fig. 8.1. Overview of signal transduction. This model depicts many of the primary pathways that are initiated following ligand binding to its cognate receptor. In general, receptor activation leads to signal amplification and alterations in gene expression (transcription, mRNA stability, protein induction) and/or modification of cellular events, including secretion, cytoskeletal changes, and certain enzymatic activities. These processes exhibit complex feedback controls. An understanding of these signaling systems is valuable in the development of therapeutics for allergic disorders.

membrane) for ligands that cannot readily enter the cell, and/or at intracellular sites (e.g., nucleus) for ligands that are lipophilic/cell permeable. Ligand–Receptor (LR) interaction is selective and is required for initiating the signaling response. The biological response is often proportional to LR complex formation, which can be described by the equilibrium expression:

$$[L] + [R] \rightleftharpoons [LR]$$

where $[L]$, $[R]$, and $[LR]$ are the levels of free ligand, unoccupied receptor, and ligand–receptor complex, respectively. The dissociation constant (Kd) for LR breakdown is:

$$Kd = [L] \times [R] / [LR]$$

In general, ligand–receptor interaction is of high affinity ($Kd < 10^{-9}$ M) and the receptor number/cell is small (saturable), which limits the signal that is produced. Because $[LR]$ is proportional to output, the signal can be regulated by altering ligand or receptor concentration, or by modulating receptor affinity (Kd). In some cases, multiple receptors for the same ligand permit separate signaling behaviors, ligand sensitivities and distinct cell type responses. Receptor affinity and internalization/turnover are often controlled by ligand binding, and these events can regulate or

desensitize LR formation and cell responsiveness. Furthermore, various endpoints may require different degrees of receptor occupancy, e.g., some effects are detected at low receptor occupancy (because this induces enough of one type of signal), whereas other effects may require full receptor occupancy (a larger or different signal is needed). For example, IL-5 or GM-CSF at ng/ml levels can enhance eosinophil survival, but higher cytokine levels are needed to enhance cell adhesion or degranulation.

The following sections will detail how certain cell-surface receptors can respond to ligand binding by activating enzymes such as protein and lipid kinases, inducing changes in guanine-nucleotide binding protein (G protein) activity, regulating ion channels, and/or serving as docking/scaffolding sites for other signaling proteins. Conversely, intracellular receptors often act as DNA/chromatin binding molecules that promote or inhibit specific gene transcriptional activities. These events can alter protein expression/activation and induce a change in cell behavior. These cascades are not usually initiated by a single hormone/receptor system in vivo, but are often influenced by the concerted action of numerous factors that are presented to the cell simultaneously or sequentially. However, to some degree, activation of a specific pathway leads to a well-documented series of choreographed steps that are comparable across many cell types, although some cell-specific differences do exist.

MECHANISMS MEDIATING INTRACELLULAR SIGNALING

Signals emanating from an activated receptor are often mediated/amplified through 'effector' molecules and intermediates (known as intracellular or second messengers). These intermediates sometimes promote gene expression/protein synthesis, but often they regulate proteins/factors already present in the cytoplasm, thus allowing for a rapid response. Common processes and post-translational modifications associated with cell signaling include protein phosphorylation/dephosphorylation, the assembly of signaling complexes through protein–protein and protein–lipid interactions, and protein modification via processes known as ubiquitinylation, sumoylation, acetylation, and methylation. Other signaling processes encompass the modification of membrane lipids and the initiation of cytoplasmic ion fluxes (often Ca^{++}). Besides protein and lipid modification, effector molecules are often 'assembled' into modules and compartmentalized in cells, and these systems are frequently similar between cell types and across species. Interestingly, the activation/deactivation of these common signaling modules does not necessarily result in the same response between cell types (because of the differential expression of intracellular effector molecules) or even within a cell type (because a cell often integrates multiple stimuli simultaneously). The discussion below will introduce several signaling pathways that operate in many cells, but, given the scope of the topic, it is not an exhaustive listing.

PHOSPHORYLATION/DEPHOSPHORYLATION

Protein activation/inhibition can involve phosphotransfer from ATP to specific amino acids (generally serine, threonine, and/or tyrosine) by enzymes known as protein kinases. These enzymes exhibit unique substrate specificities and selectively regulate different pathways. Kinase specificity arises from the recognition of certain sequences surrounding the residue(s) to be phosphorylated, and these recognition sequences are one of the parameters used to classify kinases into different families. In general, the regulation of protein kinases leads to the control of their protein substrates, thereby transmitting the signal to downstream signaling targets. In certain cases, phosphorylation can elicit a conformational change that removes an allosteric inhibitor, allowing for protein activation (Fig. 8.2). An example of this process is the phosphorylation of protein kinase C isoforms, wherein phosphorylation alters the enzyme conformation such that a pseudosubstrate domain dissociates from the catalytic site. This process leads to kinase activation and allows substrate access to the catalytic site. Phosphorylation can also inhibit the function of certain enzymes, such as myosin light chain kinase (MLCK), wherein phosphorylation desensitizes the enzyme to activation by Ca^{++} and Ca^{++}-dependent kinases, thereby preventing it from phosphorylating myosin, which is necessary for force generation in muscle contraction.

Protein phosphorylation is a transient modification, and phosphoprotein phosphatases catalyze the removal of protein-associated phosphates.[2] Generally, dephosphorylation halts protein activation and signal amplification, e.g., mitogen-activated protein (MAP) kinase phosphatase-1 dephosphorylates and inactivates extracellular signal-regulated kinases (ERKs) and p38 MAP kinases that are linked to the control of gene transcription, cell cycle progression, and stress responses. In other cases, protein dephosphorylation leads to activation, as with the tyrosine kinase Src (Fig. 8.2).

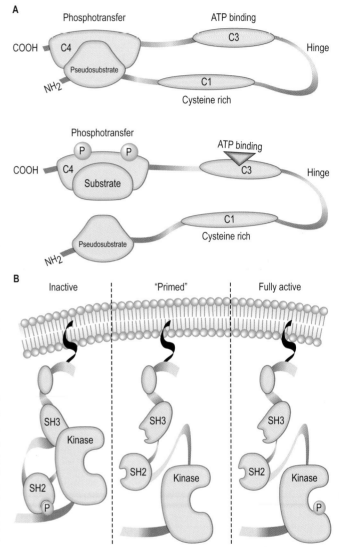

Fig. 8.2. Examples of intramolecular interactions that regulate protein function. (A) Intramolecular association of a pseudosubstrate domain in the amino terminal domain of protein kinase C zeta (PKCζ) sterically occludes the enzyme active site and blocks catalytic activity. Phosphorylation of this protein activates the enzyme by inducing a conformational change that promotes pseudosubstrate dissociation and increased substrate access to the catalytic site. ATP, adenosine triphosphate. (B) Association of two domains within Src family kinases (e.g., Src, Lyn) in the resting, 'primed', and active states. In the resting state (left) the SH2 domain of these kinases associates with a phosphorylated tyrosine on the kinase domain C-terminal region. Upon dephosphorylation of this tyrosine by specific phosphotyrosine phosphatases, the protein 'unfolds' and is in a state suitable for activation, which occurs when another tyrosine located in the kinase domain becomes phosphorylated. P, phosphorylated tyrosine.

ASSEMBLY OF SIGNALING COMPLEXES

The orchestrated assembly of various proteins and lipids is central to signal transduction. Many mechanisms are used to achieve this goal, including the promotion of protein–protein and/or protein-lipid interaction via molecular co-localization and/or phosphorylation, protein modification or effector binding to alter turnover, and the regulated trafficking of signaling molecules to discrete cellular compartments to restrict their movement and increase their potential interaction. With protein–protein/lipid interactions, many signaling molecules contain specific motifs that mediate these interactions. Examples are shown in Table 8.1, and include phosphotyrosine interaction motifs known as Src homology type 2 (SH2), phosphotyrosine binding (PTB), and immunoreceptor tyrosine-based activation motifs (ITAMs), as well as phospholipid binding domains known as Pleckstrin homology (PH) domains, and proline-rich binding domains such as Src homology type 3 (SH3) domains. Besides playing a positive role in signaling, protein modification and complex formation can exert a negative role, as in the cases where modifications (e.g., ubiquitylation) or effector molecule binding (e.g., Cbl) targets a protein for degradation by cellular proteases/proteasome, or where a recruited effector molecule is an inactivating enzyme (e.g., phosphotyrosine phosphatase SHP-1) or recruits an inactivating enzyme, such as the capacity of Dok adapter molecules to recruit protein phosphatases or G-protein inactivating molecules.

Another mechanism for controlling signaling molecules includes their modification or trafficking such that they are uniquely localized even prior to an initiating signal. Examples include lipid modifications (e.g., palmitoylation, myristoylation or isoprenylation) of proteins such as Src and certain G proteins, which allows for their membrane localization, or the recruitment of receptors, kinases/phosphatases, G proteins and adapter molecules (that link together various signaling molecules) into membrane microdomains containing high levels of cholesterol, glycolipids, and specific proteins.

COMMON SIGNALING MECHANISMS ASSOCIATED WITH PROTEIN PHOSPHORYLATION

Signaling from an activated cell-surface receptor often involves its transduction and amplification through intermediates (second messengers). Second messenger production includes the regulated synthesis/turnover of cyclic adenosine 3′,5′-monophosphate (cAMP), the initiation of Ca^{++} fluxes, and the generation of phospholipid metabolites (Fig. 8.3).

Table 8.1 Common protein motifs associated with signal transduction molecules

Motifs	Name and function	Examples
ITAM	Immunoreceptor tyrosine-based activation motif – Interacts with tyrosine kinases to propagate signals for receptors lacking a cytoplasmic tail	CD3, FcεR, Ig-α/Ig-β
ITIM	Immunoreceptor tyrosine-based inhibition motif – Region necessary for negative regulation of some immune receptor signaling	FcγRIIB, PE-CAM-1 (CD31), Siglecs
SH2	Src homology 2 domain – Binds specific phosphotyrosine-containing peptide motifs	Shc, Grb2, STATs
SH3	Src homology 3 domain – Binds to proline-rich sequences with a minimal consensus site of Pro-X-X-Pro (with proline being preceded by an aliphatic residue)	Src, Crk
PH	Pleckstrin homology domain – Binds phosphoinositides to allow a protein to be responsive to lipid messengers	Sos, PLC, Akt, Btk
SOCS box	Suppressors of cytokine signaling domain – Involved in targeting proteins for ubiquitylation	SOCS-1, SOCS-3
PTB	Phosphotyrosine binding domain – Binds Asn-Pro-X-Tyr motifs	Shc and IRS-1
SLAM	Signaling lymphocyte activation molecules – Influence the outcome of T cell-antigen presenting cell and natural killer cell-target cell interactions	CD84, CD48, CD229
DH	Dbl homology domain – Confers exchange activity to GTP exchange proteins like Ras, Rac, and Rho	Vav, Sos
DD	Death domain – 80–100 residue motifs that allow for heterodimerization of molecules containing death domains	TRAF6, IRAK
UBA	Ubiquitin-associated domain – 40 residue motif that interacts with ubiquitinated residues	C-cbl, E2 ubiquitin conjugating enzyme
RING finger	Characteristic of ubiquitin ligases that transfer ubiquitin to a substrate protein	TRAF6
PX	Phox homology domain – Binds PIP_3, targeting the proteins to the membrane	$p40^{phox}$, $p47^{phox}$ – both necessary for reactive oxygen species production
PDZ	Binds to the C-terminal 4–5 residues, frequently part of transmembrane receptors, at a Ser/Thr-X-Val sequence, or ion channels	Na^+/H^+ pumps bind to β-adrenergic receptors through these domains

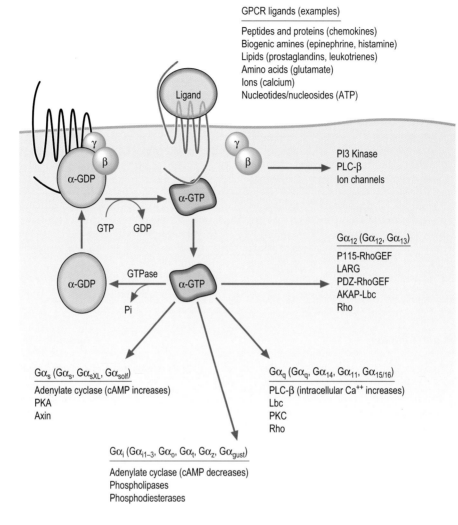

GPCR ligands (examples)

Peptides and proteins (chemokines)
Biogenic amines (epinephrine, histamine)
Lipids (prostaglandins, leukotrienes)
Amino acids (glutamate)
Ions (calcium)
Nucleotides/nucleosides (ATP)

Fig. 8.3. Heterotrimeric G proteins: receptor association, G-protein cycling and target effectors. Many signaling systems important for immune cell function entail the activation of G-protein-coupled receptors (GPCRs). Each GPCR can regulate one or more heterotrimeric G-protein complexes that are composed of α, β, and γ subunits. In the resting state, GDP is bound to Gα in the receptor-associated complex, but upon ligand-induced changes in GPCR conformation, the GDP is replaced with GTP. The Gα-GTP dissociates from Gβ/Gγ, and the subunits modulate specific effectors depending on the G-protein isoform. Gα contains intrinsic GTPase activity that hydrolyzes the bound GTP to GDP, and the Gα-GDP reassembles with Gβ/Gγ to return to the resting state.

cAMP and G proteins

cAMP is critical for the actions of many factors (such as epinephrine) and the ultimate response to cAMP depends upon the enzyme profile of the target cell. Intracellular cAMP levels represent a balance between cAMP formation from ATP via adenylate cyclases and its hydrolysis to 5'-AMP by cAMP-phosphodiesterases (PDEs). Human adenylate cyclases are located at the plasma membrane, they are differentially expressed between cell types, and they are tightly regulated. These systems are composed of a receptor, a guanine nucleotide-binding protein complex (G protein) and an adenylate cyclase isoform. The complex spans the membrane, with the G-protein-coupled receptor (GPCR)

ligand binding site on the outside and the G protein/adenylate cyclase on the inside (Figs 8.3, 8.4).[3] The GPCR, depending on its sequence, interacts with a specific heterotrimeric G-protein complex, which is composed of α, β, and γ subunits. At rest, the G-protein complex contains a GDP bound to the Gα subunit. Upon ligand binding, a receptor-mediated conformational change promotes the exchange of GTP for GDP on the Gα subunit. The resulting Gα-GTP complex dissociates from the Gβ/Gγ subunits. The Gα-GTP complex, depending on the Gα isoform, may either stimulate (Gαs) or inhibit (Gαi) adenylate cyclase. The free Gβ/Gγ subunits can also interact with certain adenylate cyclases (as well as with other effectors, see below). G-protein effects are only transiently manifested because the Gα subunits possess intrinsic GTPase activity that slowly hydrolyzes GTP to GDP. Thus, GTP hydrolysis turns off the action of the Gα subunits and promotes the re-association of the Gα-GDP, Gβ, and Gγ subunits.

Many receptors are coupled to G proteins, and there are other classes of heterotrimeric G-protein isoforms besides Gs and Gi that exhibit specific receptor coupling profiles and regulate downstream effectors other than adenylate cyclases. These other heterotrimeric G-protein-coupled systems modulate signaling molecules such as phospholipases, nucleotide exchange factors, or phosphodiesterases (Fig. 8.4). Moreover, there are other G-protein classes, including the low MW (~21 kDa) G proteins (Ras, Rac, Rho, Cdc42) that exist as monomers and are

regulated by other receptors/proteins that facilitate GDP-GTP exchange and GTPase activity. These small MW G proteins (discussed below) regulate protein kinase cascades, such as the MAP kinases, and are linked to cell growth control, differentiation, secretion, gene expression, motility, and cytoarchitecture.

cAMP and protein phosphorylation

The effects of cAMP are mediated by protein phosphorylation events catalyzed by the cAMP-dependent protein kinase (PKA). PKA is composed of two catalytic (kinase) subunits (C), and two regulatory subunits

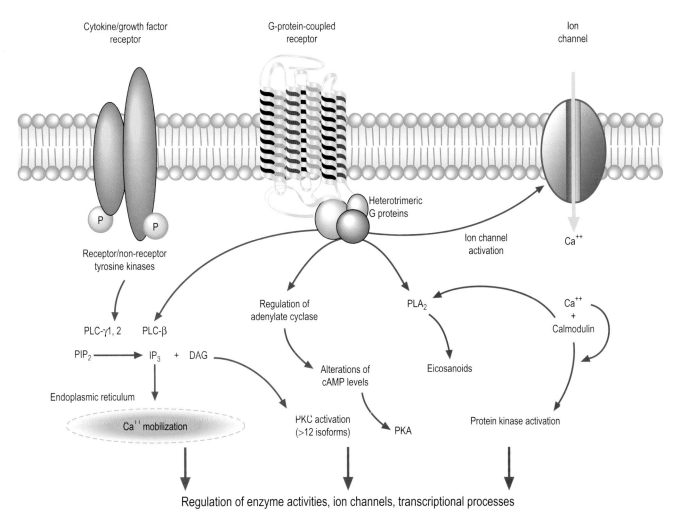

Fig. 8.4. Common signaling pathways. Several widespread systems involved in outside-in signaling are linked to the generation of second messengers, such as cAMP, cytoplasmic free Ca^{++}, and phospholipid metabolites. (Left) The activation of single transmembrane spanning receptors that possess intrinsic tyrosine kinase activity and/or activate/recruit non-receptor kinases that regulate downstream kinases and phospholipases such as PLC-γ isoforms. These PLCs catalyze the breakdown of PIP_2 to IP_3 and DAG, which promote Ca^{++} release from intracellular stores (ER) and PKC activation, respectively. (Middle) GPCRs are seven transmembrane receptors whose intracellular domains interact with specific heterotrimeric G proteins. Multiple G-protein subfamilies exist (Fig. 8.3) that regulate adenylate cyclase (with changes in cAMP levels and PKA activation) and/or phospholipases (PLCs or PLA_2) that modulate Ca^{++} fluxes or the production of pro-inflammatory eicosanoids. (Right) Ligand-gated ion channels can permit ions (such as Ca^{++}) to traverse the plasma membrane down their concentration gradient, which activates signaling networks that can involve Ca^{++} binding proteins (calmodulin) and various phospholipases (e.g., PLA_2) and protein kinases (PKCs).

(R) that bind cAMP. Inactive PKA is a complex of R_2C_2, but upon binding two cAMPs to each R, the complex dissociates and generates free C subunits that are catalytically active.

Active PKA phosphorylates many enzymes, transcription factors, and other proteins, and this amplification allows for a small amount of hormone to stimulate the production of many end products/effects. The signal can be reversed by protein dephosphorylation of the target proteins via phosphoprotein phosphatases, which are also regulated. Conversely, cAMP action can be prolonged by certain therapeutics that inhibit specific PDEs. For example, the PDE_4 inhibitor cilomilast is in therapeutic trials for asthma.

Increases in cAMP can modulate gene transcription via PKA-mediated phosphorylation of transcription factors, including the cAMP-regulatory element binding (CREB) protein. Phosphorylation of CREB regulates its interaction with DNA and other transcriptional control proteins, e.g., the CREB protein interacts with specific cAMP-regulated enhancer (CRE) regions in the IL-6 and inducible nitric oxide synthase genes and induces their expression.

Ions in cell signaling

Fluxes in intracellular ion concentrations can affect many cell processes,[4] including membrane depolarization, protease activation, and the activity of numerous phospholipases and protein and lipid kinases. As such, ion fluxes are integral to the dissemination of signals from the plasma membrane and can control events such as secretion/degranulation, gene transcription, and cytoskeletal reorganization. These events can affect processes associated with immune function, including cell chemotaxis, survival, and the degranulation of cytotoxic proteins that contribute to inflammatory responses.

Cytoplasmic free [Ca++] is normally about 10–100 nmol/l, but can be increased rapidly in response to stimuli such as epinephrine and various chemoattractants (Fig. 8.4). This change in cytoplasmic free [Ca++] can be achieved via two major mechanisms, the release of ER-sequestered Ca++ and the influx of extracellular Ca++ (which is generally around 1 mmol/l). These events can elevate intracellular free [Ca++] to 1–10 μmol/l, which is enough to activate proteins such as the Ca++-dependent protein kinases and certain phospholipases. In some cases, these Ca++ effects are mediated by the Ca++-binding protein calmodulin.

Phospholipases

Phospholipid metabolites can act as intra- and intercellular signaling molecules. Many factors activate enzymes (phospholipases) involved in the hydrolysis of either the head group or the fatty acids from the glycerol backbone of specific phospholipids. Different phospholipases hydrolyze different portions of the phospholipid: phospholipases A_1 (PLA_1) and A_2 (PLA_2) hydrolyze the ester bonds of the intact phospholipid at the C-1 and C-2 positions of the glycerol backbone, respectively. Phospholipase C (PLC) hydrolyzes the phosphodiester bond between the phosphate of the head group and the glycerol backbone, whereas phospholipase D (PLD) hydrolyzes the phosphodiester bond between the phosphate and the head group (Fig. 8.5). There are multiple isoforms of each phospholipase, and certain isoforms will act on only one type of phospholipid (e.g., phosphatidylcholine or phosphatidyl-inositol) whereas others are less specific. Some isoforms are not tightly regulated, whereas other isoforms are under strict control. For example,

several PLA_2 isoforms are activated by phosphorylation or by Ca++ or Ca++-calmodulin binding.

PLA_2 activation

Many systems that induce Ca++ mobilization result in enhanced PLA_2 activity and the release of arachidonic acid (a 20-carbon fatty acid commonly found at the C-2 position of membrane phospholipids). Arachidonic acid is a precursor for a group of poorly water-soluble factors known as the eicosanoids. These factors include the prostaglandins, lipoxins, thromboxanes, and leukotrienes such as LTA_4 and LTC_4, which can induce many effects, including bronchospasm, mucus secretion, and eosinophil recruitment.[5] These lipid derivatives are locally acting intercellular mediators that can affect inflammation, smooth muscle contraction, and platelet aggregation. In turn, the therapeutic effects of decreased PLA_2 expression and/or the attenuated action/production of various eicosanoids is important in treating certain inflammatory responses associated with allergy.

Phosphoinositide hydrolysis

Phosphatidylinositol (PI) metabolites are often important for cell responses to stimuli that mobilize intracellular Ca++. In this regard, a small pool of PI in the plasma membrane is sequentially phosphorylated to phosphatidylinositol-4-phosphate (PIP) and phosphatidyl-inositol-4, 5-bisphosphate (PIP_2) by several PI kinases (Fig. 8.5). PIP_2 can be hydrolyzed to diacylglycerol (DAG) and 1,4,5-trisphosphoinositol (IP_3) via phosphoinositide-specific PLC isoforms (PI-PLCs). With certain stimuli, ligand–receptor complex formation can activate PI-PLCs by either tyrosine phosphorylation (PLC-γ1, PLC-γ2) or via heterotrimeric G proteins (Gq) that stimulate a PIP_2-specific PLC (PLC-β). Both DAG and IP_3 serve as intracellular messengers: IP_3 interacts with Ca++ channels in the ER and rapidly promotes Ca++ release, whereas DAG activates members of a Ca++/phospholipid-dependent protein kinase family (protein kinase C, PKC) that can bind tightly to plasma and nuclear membranes. PKC phosphorylates serine/threonine residues on specific proteins (receptors, transcription factors, etc.) and modulates their activity.

Phosphoinositide 3-kinase

Besides serving as a precursor for DAG and IP_3, PIP_2 can also be phosphorylated by phosphoinositide 3-kinase (PI3 kinase) at the 3 position of the inositol ring to form PIP_3. PI3 kinase possesses phosphotyrosine binding sites (SH2 domains) and is recruited to certain plasma membrane receptors following their ligand-induced phosphorylation. At the membrane, PIP_2 is converted to PIP_3 by PI3 kinase, and PIP_3 activates 3-phosphoinositide-dependent kinases (PDKs). In turn, the PDKs phosphorylate/activate a protein kinase known as Akt (Table 8.2, Fig. 8.5). Activated PI3 kinase and Akt appear essential for mediating many hormone and cytokine effects, including nutrient uptake, gene expression, and cell survival.

Low MW G proteins

The Ras and Rho families of low MW G-proteins function as molecular switches, cycling between an inactive GDP-bound state and an active GTP-bound state, and serve to regulate the activation of various protein

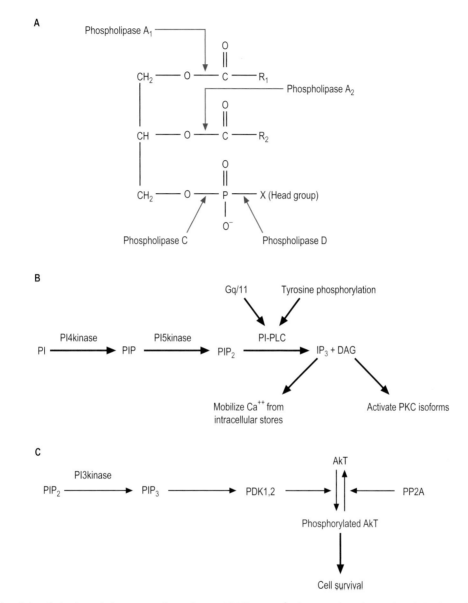

Fig. 8.5. Examples of phospholipid metabolism in signal transduction. (A) Site-specific cleavage of membrane phospholipids by phospholipases modulates the production of metabolites that serve either as second messengers (DAG, IP$_3$) or as lipid mediators in inflammation (such as arachidonic acid metabolites released via PLA$_2$). (B) Modification of phospholipids by lipid kinases (e.g., phosphoinositide (PI) kinases) and phospholipases (PI-PLCs) can also generate second messengers (IP$_3$, DAG). (C) Phosphorylation of PIP$_2$ to PIP$_3$ by PI3 kinase results in a lipid product (PIP$_3$) that activates phosphoinositide-dependent kinases (PDKs). In turn, the PDKs phosphorylate/activate Akt, which is a protein kinase that induces many effects, including cell survival.

kinase cascades (such as the MAP kinase cascades; Fig. 8.6). The cycling between the active and inactive forms of these G proteins is controlled by: (1) a group of accessory/nucleotide exchange factors (e.g., SOS or Vav) that are often recruited to tyrosine phosphorylated receptors by adapter molecules such as Shc and Grb2, whereupon they promote the accumulation of the active GTP-loaded form of the G protein and (2) by proteins that induce G-protein inactivation via stimulation of intrinsic GTPase activity (the GTPase activating proteins or GAPs are examples of this class of modulators). Many of these accessory proteins are regulated by tyrosine kinase-dependent pathways and are localized in proximity to these G proteins via association with adapter proteins. In turn, there are many downstream effectors of the low MW G proteins, and this allows them to be critically linked to the control of various biological endpoints such gene transcription and cytoskeletal reorganization.

Table 8.2 Examples of shared pathways with functions in signal transduction

Modules/ components	Selected functions
Ras-Raf-1-MEK-ERK	Receptor regulation, cytoskeletal changers, cPLA2 activation; transcription factor activation
p38 (MAP kinase)	Transcription factor activation
JNK (MAP kinase)	Transcription factor activation
Ca^{++}	Secretion, contraction, motility changes, regulation of a wide variety of enzymes (e.g., protein kinases, phospholipases, proteases)
cAMP/PKA	Response to many receptors for modulation of signaling
Shc/Grb2/SOS	Dynamically associated Ras-activating module
Calcineurin/NF-AT	Ca^{++}-dependent phosphatase in NF-AT activation
mTOR/S6 kinase	Mammalian target of rapamycin in cell proliferation and growth
Akt/PDK	Activation of transcription factors for cell survival
Pyk2/FAK	Cytoskeletal regulation; adhesion molecule–immunoreceptor cross-talk
Jak/STAT	Jak-2/STAT-5 (example of shared cytokine-signaling pathway)
NF-κB/RelA/IκBα	DNA-binding factors/transcriptional regulators
ITIM/SHIP/SHP-1	Immunoreceptor inhibitory pathway
ITAM/Src family kinases/SYK/ZAP70	Immunoreceptor stimulatory pathways

For example, active Ras can interact with multiple effector molecules such as the protein kinase Raf-1 and PI3 kinase. The recruitment of Raf-1 to the plasma membrane by active Ras and the initiation of MAP kinase cascades (Fig. 8.6) comprise a well-characterized signaling cascade crucial for transcription factor regulation.

MAP kinase cascades

The MAP kinase family is composed of serine/threonine protein kinases that are highly conserved throughout evolution and activated in response to cell stimulation by agents such as growth factors, cytokines, chemotactic factors, and phorbol esters.[6] The MAP kinase family includes the ERKs, the c-Jun NH2-terminal kinases (JNKs), and the p38 stress-activated protein kinases. These kinases are regulated by members of the low MW G-protein family, such as Ras and Rac (Fig. 8.6). For example, active Ras can interact with effector molecules including the serine/threonine kinase Raf-1. Active Ras recruits Raf-1 to the membrane, whereupon it phosphorylates and activates certain dual specificity kinases (MAPK/ERK kinases or MEKs), which phosphorylate and activate specific members of the MAP kinase family, e.g., ERK1 and ERK2. Substrates for ERKs include cytoplasmic PLA$_2$, the p90 ribosomal S6 kinase (p90 Rsk), cytoskeletal proteins, membrane-localized receptors, and certain transcription factors. As such, the accumulation of active Ras and the consequent stimulation of ERK1 and ERK2 lead to the control of many cellular processes, including the production of lipid mediators, cytoskeletal changes, and transcriptional events. In fact, the ERKs, together with the other MAP kinase family members, can trigger the activation of numerous transcription factors, such as Elk-1, CREB, ATF2, C/EBP-β, NF-AT, and c-Jun/c-Fos, which can modulate cytokine and inflammatory mediator expression.

Cytoplasmic tyrosine kinases

Cytokine and chemoattractant signaling in immune cells has been shown to be critically dependent on receptor interaction and activation of multiple cytoplasmic tyrosine kinases including Syk, ZAP-70, Lyn, and other members of the Src family of tyrosine kinases.[7,8] These enzymes are noncovalently associated with various receptors and their activity is thought to be critical for mediating many immune responses. The regulation of these enzymes generally involves their phosphorylation and recruitment into signaling complexes as generally discussed above.

GENE TRANSCRIPTION AND PROTEIN PHOSPHORYLATION

Many signaling events can promote changes in gene transcription and mRNA turnover, including the activation of PKA, PKC, and the MAP kinases, changes in Ca^{++} fluxes, and the regulation of intracellular tyrosine kinases (e.g., Src, Syk, Lyn). These events are mediated largely by the phosphorylation of transcription factors and/or proteins involved in controlling mRNA stability. There are many additional modes of regulating gene expression, but we will focus our discussion on two other common gene transcription pathways that involve protein kinase cascades and are key to immune cell regulation. These two signaling modules are the Janus kinase–Signal Transducers and Activators of Transcription (Jak–STAT) cassette and the NF-κB family of transcription factors.

Jaks/STATs

The Jak–STAT module is important for cell responses to various cytokines, chemoattractants, and growth factors (Fig. 8.6).[9] Many cytokine/hematopoietic receptors can activate specific members of the Janus cytoplasmic tyrosine kinases (Jaks1–3, Tyk2). Depending on the receptor,

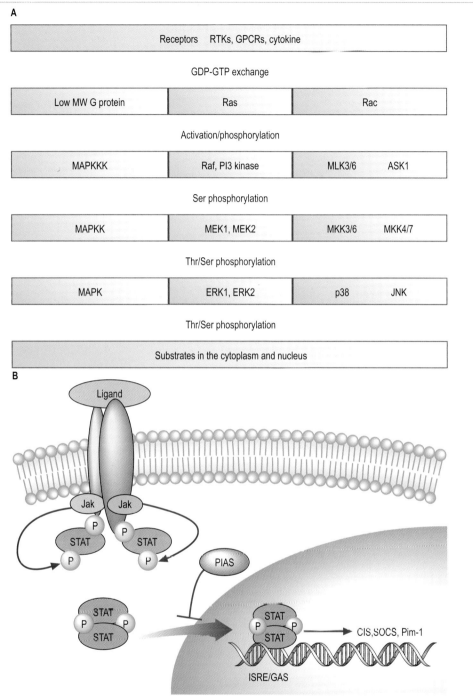

A

Receptors   RTKs, GPCRs, cytokine

GDP-GTP exchange

Low MW G protein	Ras	Rac

Activation/phosphorylation

MAPKKK	Raf, PI3 kinase	MLK3/6 ASK1

Ser phosphorylation

MAPKK	MEK1, MEK2	MKK3/6 MKK4/7

Thr/Ser phosphorylation

MAPK	ERK1, ERK2	p38 JNK

Thr/Ser phosphorylation

Substrates in the cytoplasm and nucleus

B

Ligand

Jak Jak

STAT STAT

PIAS

STAT / STAT

STAT / STAT → CIS,SOCS, Pim-1

ISRE/GAS

Fig. 8.6. Signaling modules frequently utilized by immune stimuli. (A) Examples of low MW G protein-MAP kinase signaling cascades. Many signaling cascades progress via a series of kinase (phosphorylation) reactions. Activation of MAP kinases (ERKs, JNKs, and p38) is a widely distributed cellular response. Signal initiation often occurs via cell-surface receptors that activate low MW G proteins (Ras, Rho) via receptor recruitment of adapter molecules (Grb2, Shc) and nucleotide exchange factors (SOS, Vav) resulting in the cascade of MAPKKKs, MAPKKs, and MAPKs. In the case of ERK activation, Ras activation leads to several steps of protein phosphorylation/activation resulting in specific substrate activation such as transcription factors. Similar cascades of low MW G proteins are involved in regulating the JNK and p38 MAP kinases, which control the expression of many inflammatory gene products. (B) General signaling by the Jak-STAT module. Upon ligand activation of a Jak kinase-associated receptor, the Jaks undergo reciprocal phosphorylation and tyrosine phosphorylate the receptor to create STAT binding sites. The bound STATs are tyrosine phosphorylated by the Jaks, undergo homo- or heterodimerization, and translocate into the nucleus where they bind to consensus STAT recognition sequences (ISRE/GAS, interferon-stimulated response elements/interferon-γ activation sites) and modulate gene transcription. Jak/STAT activity is opposed by phosphatases (SHP-1), the protein inhibitor of activated STATs (PIAS), and induced gene products such as CIS-1.

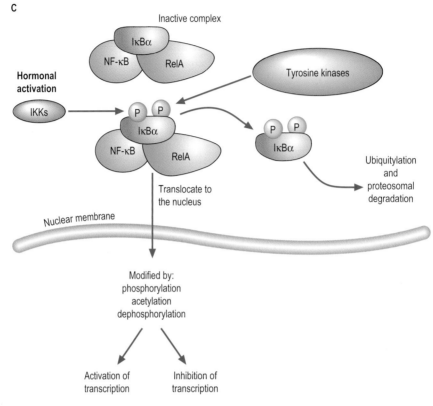

Fig. 8.6. cont'd – (C) General signaling associated with the NF-κB module. In the inactive state, cytoplasmic NF-κB/RelA dimers are associated with an IκB isoform that maintains NF-κB. Upon cell stimulation, IκB is phosphorylated by the IKKs, ubiquitylated, and undergoes proteosomal degradation, allowing the NF-κB/RelA complex to translocate into the nucleus. NF-κB is further processed in the nucleus (e.g., phosphorylation, acetylation) and associates with co-activators to initiate transcription or co-repressors to inhibit transcription.

specific members of the Jak family are constitutively, but non-covalently, associated with a specific hematopoietic receptor subunit. Ligand-induced receptor activation and dimerization of the Jaks results in their reciprocal phosphorylation/activation, and among the substrates of the active Jaks are the receptor subunits and members of the STAT family of transcription factors (STATs 1–4, 5a/b, and 6). The tyrosine phosphorylation of the receptor by the Jaks creates binding sites for the Src homology 2 (SH2) region of STATs. Once bound, the STATs are subject to Jak-dependent tyrosine phosphorylation, which promotes STAT homo- or heterodimerization. The activated STAT dimer then translocates into the nucleus, where it binds to consensus STAT binding sequences and modulates transcription. The ability of STATs to activate transcription is enhanced by their phosphorylation on serines located near the C-terminus in the transactivational domain by serine/threonine kinases.[10] Conversely, Jak/STAT activity is opposed by phosphatases such as SHP-1,[11] and the cytokine-inducible SH2-containing proteins including CIS-1. CIS-1 induction is regulated by Jak2/STAT5 pathways and appears to operate in a negative feedback mechanism.[12] Several tyrosine-phosphorylated STATs have also been suggested to act as cytoplasmic adapter proteins, thereby widening their possible role in cell signaling.

NF-κB

One signaling event initiated by many immune stimuli (e.g., TNF-α) is the activation of the NF-κB family of transcriptional regulators (Fig. 8.6).[13] In fact, the expression of many survival factors, cytokines, chemokines, and enzymes involved in inflammatory mediator production is associated with NF-κB activation. Briefly, the NF-κB or Rel family of transcription factors exist in the cytoplasm in the unstimulated state and consist of various homo- or heterodimeric pairings between family members. The activity of these dimers in the cytoplasm is suppressed by the binding of members of an inhibitory protein family, IκB, such that one IκB molecule binds per dimer. Upon the initiation of signaling events that activate cytoplasmic kinases known as the IκB kinases (IKKs), the serine phosphorylation of IκB isoforms by the IKKs targets IκB for proteasome-mediated degradation. IκB removal allows the NF-κB complex to translocate into the nucleus, where it binds to regulatory elements present in various gene promoter regions. NF-κB activation and nuclear import is also associated with the subsequent induction of IκB isoforms such that the system exhibits a self-regulatory behavior.

Acetylation/methylation and gene transcription

DNA–histone interaction is important for chromatin structure and gene regulation. Histones are subject to modifications that influence their activities, e.g., histone acetylation is thought to loosen the tightly wound DNA structure and allow for increased DNA access to transcription factors, thus allowing gene transcription to occur.[14] Histone acetyl transferases catalyze this process and act as transcriptional coactivators. Histone acetylation is reversible, and histone deacetylases are associated with the repression of transcription. Similarly, histone methylation by histone methyltransferases is another modification that can either repress or activate gene expression and is regulated by signaling pathways that impinge on transcription.

MEMBRANE MICRODOMAINS

The maintenance of specialized plasma membrane microdomains (detergent-resistant membranes, 'lipid rafts', glycolipid-enriched microdomains, caveolae) that are composed of high local concentrations of cholesterol and sphingolipids allows many eukaryotic cells to organize a subset of their receptor-signaling systems into these compartments (Fig. 8.7).[15] This arrangement facilitates the temporal and spatial regulation of cellular functions.[16] For example, studies using neutrophils have revealed that IL-8 priming promotes the recruitment of NADPH oxidase components to lipid rafts where, upon stimulation with chemoattractants, superoxide production is markedly enhanced.[17]

Many signaling molecules are localized to membrane microdomains,[18] including Ras, Src family kinases, β-arrestins, GPCRs, and glycosylphosphatidylinositol-anchored proteins such as uPAR and CD16.[19] The movement of molecules in and out of these microdomains, together with interactions between microdomains, appears important in the control of cell signaling. In many cases, disrupting these domains by altering plasma membrane cholesterol levels or by treating membranes with sphingomyelinases can result in the attenuation or potentiation of certain signaling events, such as ERK activation and phospholipase D activity, respectively.[20]

SELECTED SCAFFOLDING MOLECULES

β-Arrestins

The GPCRs are a large family of signaling molecules that are known to activate heterotrimeric G proteins to regulate downstream effectors. The GPCRs are typically desensitized by receptor phosphorylation (via the GPCR-associated kinases (GRKs) as well as other kinases) followed by the binding of a class of molecules known as the β-arrestins.[21–23] The arrestins desensitize GPCRs and attenuate G-protein binding, but can also redirect GPCR signaling to pathways involving Src family kinases and the ERKs. Arrestin interaction with a GPCR is mediated by its selectivity for the phosphorylated and activated (ligand-bound) form of the receptor.[22,23] The 'phosphate-sensing' core of arrestin interacts with phosphorylated GPCRs and facilitates their trafficking into clathrin-coated pits for internalization/degradation.[21–24] Arrestin–GPCR interaction also involves a conformational change of the arrestin molecule that allows for the binding of Src, MAP kinases (ERKs, JNKs, p38) and associated molecules such as Raf-1, Ask1, MEKs, and MKKs,[22,23] leading to MAP kinase activation.

Caveolins

In some cells, there exists Triton X-resistant plasma membrane microdomains termed caveolae that are rich in cholesterol and proteins (caveolins) that are critical for transport processes, such as cholesterol and receptor trafficking.[25] Caveolae are enriched for various receptors, effector proteins, and lipids important for cell signaling. The caveolins are 21–24-kDa integral membrane proteins that act as the coat protein of caveolae. Interestingly, a cytosolic N-terminal juxtamembrane region, known as the caveolin-1 scaffolding domain can interact with certain lipid-modified signaling molecules such as heterotrimeric G proteins, Ras, and Src family tyrosine kinases. These interactions appear to sequester the proteins within caveolae and to modulate/suppress their activities until proper ligand stimulation leads to signaling complex formation.

OTHER SIGNALING/DOWNREGULATION MECHANISMS

Ubiquitylation

Ubiquitin is a 76 amino acid peptide that can be conjugated to selected proteins to modulate their turnover/signaling.[26] Ubiquitylation involves ubiquitin conjugation to a lysine residue of a target protein or another ubiquitin molecule, thereby forming a branching structure. This modification can serve to target the protein for degradation by the 26S proteosome if the multiple ubiquitin molecules are conjugated via lysine-48. Conversely, protein conjugation to ubiquitin lysine-63 can promote protein–protein interaction between the mono-ubiquitinated substrate and proteins with ubiquitin binding domains. This modification can also be transient, as there are enzymes that can remove the ubiquitin modification, such as ubiquitin specific proteases.

Sumoylation

Another post-translational event relevant to cell signaling is sumoylation, which is a protein modification involving the addition of a member of the Small Ubiquitin-related MOdifier family (SUMO1–4).[27] These proteins are around 100 amino acids in length, but unlike ubiquitin, which can form branching structures, SUMO cannot be conjugated to itself. Sumoylation has been associated with different cellular events, including signal transduction, nuclear transport, cell cycle progression, and stress responses. As opposed to ubiquitylation, sumoylation does not promote protein degradation, but may augment protein stability and/or control protein localization. Although SUMO1–3 exhibit a wide tissue distribution, SUMO4 expression appears restricted to the kidney and immune cells. Interestingly, sumoylation of IκBα with SUMO1 and SUMO4 makes it more resistant to proteasome-mediated ubiquitylation/degradation leading to attenuated NF-κB activity.

Internalization

Ligand-induced receptor internalization via clathrin-coated pits is one mechanism by which cells downregulate signaling pathways. Other mechanisms include protease-mediated shedding of cell-surface receptors and the desensitization of receptors via complexation with certain effector molecules. As discussed above under β-Arrestins, an example

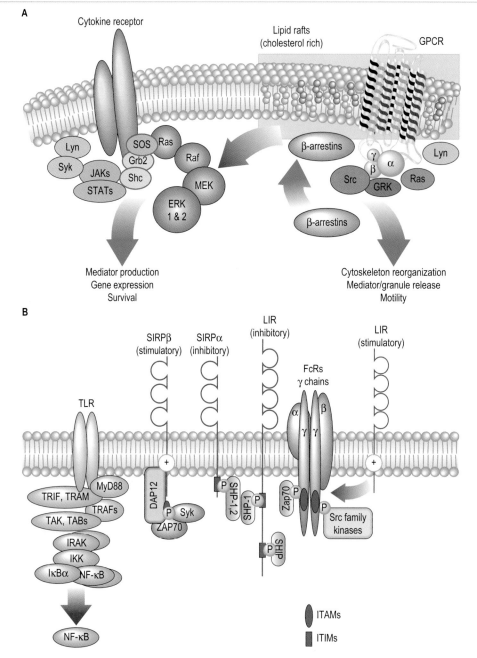

Fig. 8.7. Scaffolding of intracellular signaling cascades. (A) Effector molecule complexes are frequently assembled prior to or in response to cell stimuli and are mediated through protein–protein and/or protein–lipid interactions. Depicted here are several common groupings for cytokine receptors (Left) and the GPCRs (Right). These complexes can form around the seed of a specific receptor type or inherently be associated with membrane microdomains (lipid rafts) which often contain a diverse array of receptor types. This spatial association promotes not only rapid responses but also the capacity for cross-talk between receptor systems, such as the recruitment and activation of scaffolding molecules (such as the β-arrestins) to GPCRs that can serve to link separate systems together to co-regulate specific pathways (e.g., ERKs and Src family kinases) and thus allow for one system to 'prime' the other. (B) Examples of multi-member families of cell-surface molecules that are involved in pattern recognition behavior, cell–cell interaction responses, and the modulation of inhibitory and stimulatory cell signals. The toll-like receptors (TLRs) are a superfamily of transmembrane IL-1 receptor-like molecules that function in the innate immune system by distinguishing different pathogens based on their molecular signatures. Many other immune cell-surface receptors/signaling molecules are critical in mediating a balance between inhibitory and stimulatory cell activities, including the Fc receptors (FcRs) and their homologs, the leukocyte immunoglobulin-like receptors (LIRs), and signal-regulatory proteins (SIRPs). These proteins belong to a large class of receptors (including molecules such as the T-cell receptors, the SIGLECs, and the paired Ig-like receptors) and are characterized by their possession of common cytoplasmic tyrosine-based signaling motifs, i.e., the ITAMs (for stimulatory systems) and ITIMs (for inhibitory systems). Ligand binding to activating receptor complexes promotes ITAM tyrosine phosphorylation and the recruitment of Src family kinases that induce positive cell responses, whereas ligand binding to inhibitory receptor complexes promotes ITIM tyrosine phosphorylation and the recruitment of SH2 domain-containing phosphatases that attenuate cellular activation.

of the latter mechanism can be seen with the β-adrenergic receptors, which are GPCRs that exhibit ligand-stimulated phosphorylation (via the GRKs), followed by interaction with the β-arrestins and recruitment into endosomal vesicles where they are either recycled to the cell surface or degraded (resulting in decreased surface expression).[28]

Attenuation of Jak–STAT signaling

Signaling through the Jak–STATs by hematopoietic receptors, such as various interferon and interleukin receptors, is also subject to feedback control (Fig. 8.6). For example, certain STAT-induced genes serve as Jak–STAT inhibitors, including a family of proteins known as the suppressors of cytokine signaling (SOCS), which interact with the receptor to inhibit Jak[29] or STAT binding, or with Jak family members to inhibit their catalytic activity.[30] Also, SOCS-mediated inhibition can involve the recruitment of the ubiquitin-transferase system that targets proteins for degradation.[31] Eight members of the SOCS family have been identified, including SOCS1–7 and CIS. Interestingly, the SOCS1 knockout mouse exhibits a phenotype consistent with augmented signaling by interferon-γ, and administration of interferon-γ neutralizing antibodies corrected the phenotype, suggesting that SOCS1 serves as a critical modulator of cytokine signaling.[32] Besides the SOCS proteins, members of the Protein Inhibitor of Activated STAT (PIAS) family also appear to regulate the STATs as well as NF-κB and the tumor-suppressor protein p53. The PIAS proteins can modulate transcription via multiple mechanisms, including antagonizing the DNA-binding activity of transcription factors, promoting protein sumoylation, and recruiting transcriptional corepressors or coactivators.[33]

■ SELECTED SIGNALING SYSTEMS RELEVANT TO ALLERGY ■

The integration of multiple signaling events is needed for the proper organization and effective mediation of a specific immune response. To this end, the examples discussed below will address selected receptor types and downstream signaling pathways that are important in cellular and physiological responses to allergens and will also discuss several current therapies used to modulate these responses.

GPCRs

The GPCRs are plasma membrane-localized and composed of seven transmembrane segments. The specific G proteins that associate with these receptors can either activate or inhibit various signaling pathways (Fig. 8.3). Besides their linkage to heterotrimeric G proteins, the GPCRs may also associate with other effector molecules such as Jak2[34] and the β-arrestins.[35] These effectors can facilitate signaling or allow for receptor desensitization/downregulation. Many therapeutics target the GPCRs, as discussed below.

Chemokine receptors

Chemokines are a superfamily of polypeptides that act via GPCRs to control immune cell behavior, e.g., they promote cell adhesion, chemotaxis, and mediator release. Many chemokine-induced events are inhibited by

cell treatment with *Bordetella pertussis* toxin, which ADP ribosylates and inactivates the α-subunit of Gi/Go, suggesting that certain chemokine receptors are coupled to these G proteins. However, some chemokine-induced events are *pertussis* toxin insensitive, e.g., chemotaxis induced by IL-8 does not require Gαi but is mediated by Gβ/Gγ following receptor activation.[36] Chemokine receptors can also activate PLC isoforms, leading to IP_3 production and increased cytoplasmic Ca^{++}, which can regulate various kinases and promote cytoarchitectural changes. In certain cases, chemokine receptor signaling also activates low MW G proteins (Ras/Rho), which mediate many actin-dependent processes, such as degranulation and chemotaxis. Examples of the importance of these receptors in allergic inflammation are that the chemokines RANTES, eotaxin, and MCP-1[37] have been linked to eosinophil and macrophage activation and recruitment to the lungs of allergic asthmatics.

Leukotriene receptors

Leukotrienes are lipid-based mediators derived from the arachidonic acid liberated from membrane phospholipids following PLA_2 activation. There are two groups of leukotrienes: LTB_4 and the cysteinyl leukotrienes, including LTC_4, LTD_4, and LTE_4. These agents are implicated in asthma and other inflammatory diseases because of their potent action as immune cell chemoattractants and their ability to stimulate bronchospasm. Two receptors for LTB_4 have been identified, BLT1 and BLT2, and two receptors have been found for the cysteinyl leukotrienes, CysLT1 and CysLT2. Signaling induced by LTB_4 entails activation of Gi and Gq, thus leading to decreased cellular cAMP and increased cytoplasmic IP_3/Ca^{++} levels, respectively. Similarly, CysLT1 promotes bronchial smooth muscle contraction via increased Ca^{++} fluxes and kinase activation (PKC, MAP kinases). Antagonists of CysLT1 include montelukast, pranlukast, and zafirlukast[38] and these agents can reduce IL-4 and IL-13 production, attenuate eosinophil numbers, and decrease airway remodeling.[39]

Histamine receptors

Histamine can induce symptoms associated with acute rhinitis, bronchospasm, or cutaneous wheal and flare responses.[40] Histamine released from mast cells and basophils acts on vascular endothelium, bronchial, and smooth muscle cells. The known histamine receptors, HR1–4, are GPCRs and enjoy a wide tissue distribution. The role of HR2–4 in inflammatory/allergic processes is less clear than for HR1, which is coupled to Gαq/11 and stimulates IP_3 production and Ca^{++} fluxes/PKC activation. These events increase nitric oxide generation and leukotriene production. HR1 also promotes NF-κB activation and inflammatory cytokine/chemokine production.[40] Many antihistamines used in the treatment of allergies and asthma block HR1, including loratadine, fexofenadine, and cetirizine. Allergen-induced eosinophil accumulation in the skin, nose, and airways is also potently inhibited by antihistamines that target HR1.[41]

β-Adrenergic receptors

The β-adrenergic receptors (BAR1–3) are linked to Gs and are widely distributed; BAR2 is found in the respiratory tract, including airway smooth muscle, epithelial and endothelial cells, and mast cells. Interestingly, there exists an inverse relationship between FEV_1 and BAR2 density in the lungs.[42] When stimulated, these receptors allow for the relaxation of the bronchioles, and commonly used BAR2 agonists include the short-acting agonists albuterol and procaterol, and the long-acting agonists formoterol and salmeterol.

Proposed mechanisms for BAR2-induced smooth muscle relaxation and alleviation of bronchospasms include PKA-dependent phosphorylation of proteins that control muscle tone and/or that they inhibit Ca^{++} release from intracellular stores and/or reduce Ca^{++} entry into the cell.[43] Other studies suggest that BAR2 agonists produce airway smooth muscle relaxation via modulation of potassium channels by Gαs to counteract the excitatory response of Ca^{++} currents,[44] and can alter MLCK phosphorylation profiles to reduce smooth muscle contractile force.[45–47]

The use of BAR2 agonists is beneficial, although adverse effects include increased asthma exacerbations and decreased agonist ability to produce bronchodilation with repeated use. Possible reasons include BAR desensitization and internalization, thereby causing the patient to become refractory to prolonged or repeated agonist exposure. Also, BAR2 polymorphisms may alter receptor behavior, resulting in greater downregulation[48] and airway hyperreactivity.[42] In addition, adverse effects may be linked to agonist action on cells other than airway smooth muscle. BAR2 agonists can suppress eosinophil apoptosis[49] and upregulate HR1 expression[50], thereby aggravating the condition. However, BAR2 agonists can also promote positive effects, such as the inhibition of histamine and leukotrienes release from mast cells.[51]

Nucleoside/nucleotide receptors

Adenine nucleotides can be released from cells in a regulated manner (platelet degranulation) or as a consequence of cell damage/death. EctoATPases and nucleotidases modulate the bioavailability of extracellular nucleotides and can generate metabolites that are ligands for receptors present on many cells. Nucleotide receptors are divided into P1 and P2 classes. P1 receptors bind adenosine/AMP, whereas P2 receptors bind ATP, ADP, and pyrimidine nucleotides (UTP and UDP). The P2 family is divided into P2Y and P2X subclasses based on their predicted structures. The P1 and P2Y receptors are GPCRs, whereas the P2X receptors are ligand-gated ion channels.[52]

Mast cells, eosinophils, lymphocytes, neutrophils, and macrophages express P1 (adenosine) receptors and exhibit inflammatory mediator elaboration upon stimulation.[53] Adenosine administration by inhalation elicits bronchoconstriction in asthmatic patients, and induces mast cell release of histamine, leukotrienes, and inflammatory cytokines and chemokines. Adenosine receptor subtypes include A1, A2A/A2B, and A3. A1 receptors are ubiquitously expressed, whereas A2 receptors are expressed in mast cells, neutrophils, platelets, pancreas, smooth muscle, and the vasculature. Activation of A2 receptors promotes Gs-induced elevations in cAMP and the release of IL-8.[53] The A3 receptor is expressed in many tissues, especially the lung and liver. Its activation results in decreased cAMP and increased Ca^{++} fluxes and histamine release.[54] High levels of adenosine activate A3 and promote eosinophil apoptosis and inhibition of eosinophil and neutrophil degranulation, reactive oxygen species release, and chemotaxis.[53]

P2Y receptors are widely expressed in immune cells, they are coupled to Gq/11, Gs or Gi, and they regulate IP_3 generation, Ca^{++} fluxes, and/or cAMP formation. Of note, the leukotriene receptor antagonists montelukast and pranlukast can attenuate P2Y-mediated activation of PLC and intracellular Ca^{++} mobilization,[55] thus providing a means to modulate

P2Y-mediated inflammatory processes in allergy. The P2X receptors are ATP-gated ion channels that elevate intracellular Ca^{++} and mediate fast permeability to cations including Na^+ and K^+.[56] Of note, $P2X_7$ activation can enhance LPS-induced responses in macrophages, promote cytoskeletal reorganization and membrane blebbing (via Rho and p38),[57] activate NF-κB, and lead to the elaboration of mediators such as IL-1β and reactive oxygen species.[56] Thus, modulation of P2X and P2Y receptors may be effective at reducing inflammatory responses associated with allergy.

HEMATOPOIETIC RECEPTORS

Hematopoietic cytokine receptors control the differentiation, maturation, priming, and activation of many immune cells. These receptors are grouped into families that share common subunits. For example, the IL-5/IL-3/GM-CSF receptor family, share a common β chain necessary for signaling and forming a high-affinity receptor when associated with a ligand-specific α chain. Signaling from these receptors includes the activation of cytoplasmic tyrosine kinases (Lyn, Syk), Ras-ERK, and Jak2-STAT5. IL-5 is a cytokine that primarily targets eosinophils and contributes to eosinophilic influx and inflammation in allergic disease, whereas GM-CSF and IL-3 regulate the development, activation, and survival of many immune cells.

The IL-2 receptor family, which includes the IL-4, 7, 9, and 15 receptors, are composed of a ligand-specific α-chain and a common γ-subunit important for cell signaling.[58] The IL-2 and 15 receptors also contain a β-subunit that contributes to signaling.[59] Stimulation of receptors sharing the common γ-subunit promotes Jak1 and Jak3 phosphorylation,[60] whereas the Src family kinases Lck,[61] Lyn, and Fyn[62] are associated with the β-subunit. The IL-2 receptor also activates other signaling molecules, including PI3 kinase, PLC-γ, Ras, Raf-1, and MAP kinases.[58] The IL-4 α-subunit is shared with the IL-13 receptor, and these receptors signal through Jak1 and Tyk2 to activate STAT3 and 6.[63] Neutralizing antibodies against IL-13 have been used in mice to suppress the airway hyperresponsiveness, eosinophil infiltration, inflammatory cytokine production, serum IgE, and airway remodeling induced by ovalbumin challenge. Similarly, neutralization of IL-9 in mice reduces airway inflammation, hyperresponsiveness, and bone marrow eosinophilia, suggesting that IL-9 may be a therapeutic target in asthma.

The IL-6 receptor family includes receptors for IL-6, IL-11, leukemia inhibitory factor, oncostatin M, and ciliary neurotrophic factor, and all are known to require a common gp130 signaling subunit that is linked to the activation of Jak1, Jak2, and Tyk2.[64] Stimulation with IL-6 promotes STAT1 and STAT3 activation and heterodimerization, as well as activation of the protein tyrosine phosphatase 2 (SHP2), which links this system to Ras-ERK signaling and signal attenuation.

IL-12 is important in inflammation, and there exists two IL-12 receptors (IL-12Rβ1, IL-12Rβ2) that regulate the activation of Lck as well as Tyk2, Jak2, and STAT4. IL-12 has been administered to patients to alleviate asthma symptoms, but the occurrence of several toxic effects, including malaise and cardiac arrhythmia, have suggested that this treatment may not be beneficial.[65]

TOLL-LIKE RECEPTORS

The toll-like receptors (TLRs)[66–80] are a superfamily of transmembrane IL-1 receptor-like molecules that function in the innate immune system by distinguishing different pathogens based on their molecular signatures, i.e., the TLRs are pattern recognition receptors (Fig. 8.7). The TLRs contain leucine-rich motifs and a cytoplasmic region known as the Toll/IL-1R (TIR) domain that is necessary for cell signaling.[66] These receptors are largely expressed on the cell surface, although TLRs 7, 8, and 9 have been found at intracellular sites. Signaling via these receptors is associated with the formation of TLR homo- and heterodimers and results in the production of pro-inflammatory cytokines, chemokines, and other mediators (Chapter 2).[67] These receptors are expressed in monocytes/macrophages, dendritic cells, B cells, and mast cells, but some are found in certain non-immune cells, including cells that line mucosal surfaces (e.g., intestinal epithelial cells). Also, receptor expression is modulated by microbial invasion, microbial components, and cytokines.[68]

INHIBITORY AND STIMULATORY RECEPTORS

The balance between stimulatory and inhibitory networks is important in providing appropriate activation thresholds and sensitive tuning mechanisms for cell responses. Many cell-surface receptors/signaling molecules are critical for this balance, including the Fc receptors (FcRs) and their homologs, the leukocyte immunoglobulin-like receptors (LIRs), and the paired Ig-like receptors and signal-regulatory proteins (SIRPs). These proteins belong to a large receptor class characterized by their possession of common cytoplasmic tyrosine-based signaling motifs, namely the ITAMs (Table 8.1) that contain two repeats of the consensus sequence Y-X-X-L/I spaced by 6–8 amino acids or the immunoreceptor tyrosine-based inhibitory motifs (ITIMs) with a 6 amino acid consensus sequence (I/V/L/S)-X-Y-X-X-(L/V). Ligand binding to activating receptors leads to rapid phosphorylation of ITAM tyrosines by Src family kinases, which then initiate signaling cascades that lead to cellular activation. In contrast, tyrosine phosphorylation of the ITIMs in the inhibitory receptors generates docking sites for SH2 domain-containing phosphatases that can attenuate cellular activation. The balance between these activating and inhibitory receptors can modulate cell responses to numerous stimuli and will be discussed below.

FcRs

The FcRs are a family of multi-subunit cell-surface molecules involved in recognizing the Fc portion of immunoglobulin molecules/antibodies. Accordingly, receptors exist for each antibody class, e.g., $Fc\gamma R$ binds IgG, $Fc\alpha R$ binds IgA, $Fc\varepsilon R$ binds IgE, $Fc\alpha/\mu R$ binds IgM, and $Fc\delta R$ binds IgD. Subsets of these receptors are expressed by various leukocytes and other immune cells. Of relevance to allergy, $Fc\varepsilon R$ is expressed by mast cells and basophils, and its activation leads to the release of histamine, leukotrienes, and proteases that result in airway obstruction, smooth muscle contraction, vascular leakage, and mucus secretion. In general, therapeutic targeting of FcRs is an important issue in the treatment of allergic inflammation and is discussed elsewhere in this volume.

There are two major FcR types: one that triggers cell activation and one that leads to inhibitory signals. The FcR subtypes that trigger cell activation possess cytoplasmic ITAMs (Table 8.1, Fig. 8.7) and can be divided into two subclasses: one composed of a ligand-binding α-subunit associated with one or two intracellular signaling molecules with ITAMs, and one consisting of two related single-chain IgG receptors that have a single cytoplasmic ITAM. FcRs that are inhibitory contain cytoplasmic ITIMs and, upon their phosphorylation, they recruit phosphatases that inhibit cell activation via protein dephosphorylation.[81] Thus, negative regulation of FcRs results from co-aggregation with receptors containing ITIMs. All of these receptors are clustered at the cell surface to trigger signaling within the cell.

With the activating $Fc\varepsilon R$, ligand-induced receptor aggregation promotes rapid ITAM phosphorylation and activation of Syk and Src family kinases (Lyn, Hck, Lck).[81] The transmembrane phosphatase CD45 positively regulates the activity of Src kinases by dephosphorylating the tyrosine residues in the regulatory domain of the kinase (Fig. 8.2).[82] The $Fc\varepsilon RI$ has also been shown to stimulate the Ras-ERK pathway, via a Shc-Grb2-SOS-dependent mechanism,[83] and can activate the transcription factors NF-AT,[84] c-Fos, and c-Jun.[85]

LIRs

The LIRs, also known as immunoglobulin-like transcripts (ILTs), are a family of receptors expressed in myeloid and lymphoid cells and, although their ligands are not completely defined, some appear to recognize MHC class I molecules.[86] The LIRs contain two or four immunoglobulin-like domains in their extracellular regions and are either cell-surface transmembrane receptors with larger intracellular domains (LIRs 1, 2, 3, 5, 8), cell-surface-associated receptors with short cytoplasmic sequences (LIRs 6a, 6b, 7), or soluble molecules (LIR-4). Although the first two LIR classes have been linked to inhibitory or stimulatory signaling events, respectively, the function of LIR-4 is unclear but it may act as a soluble ligand to trigger other cell-surface receptors or as an antagonist of membrane-bound LIRs by competing for ligands.

With the inhibitory ITIM-containing LIRs, it is thought that when these receptors are brought into close proximity to activating receptors, the ITIMs become tyrosine phosphorylated by kinases recruited to the activating receptors. ITIM phosphorylation creates docking sites for SH2 domain-containing phosphatases such as SHP-1 and the inositol phosphatase SHIP, which then deliver an inhibitory signal to receptor systems such as the FcRs or cytokine receptors that utilize tyrosine kinases (Src family kinases, Syk, Jaks, etc.) and/or inositol phosphates (IP_3, PIP_3) as stimulatory signals. The utility of LIRs containing multiple cytoplasmic ITIMs is undefined, but may allow for signal amplification or the recruitment of differing signaling molecules.

The stimulatory LIRs possess short cytoplasmic domains devoid of ITIMs and a positively-charged arginine within their transmembrane domains. This arginine may direct LIR association with another surface receptor, such as the FcR common γ chain, which interacts with the FcRs for IgA, IgE, and IgG, and has a negatively-charged aspartate within its transmembrane region. The interaction of these stimulatory LIRs with FcR-γ may be required for cell-surface expression and assembly of a multimeric receptor capable of signaling. FcR-γ possesses a small extracellular domain but contains an ITAM (Table 8.1, Fig. 8.7) in its cytoplasmic region. Receptor activation may lead to the recruitment of protein kinases that phosphorylate the tyrosine residues within the ITAM region, thereby creating binding sites for the SH2 domain-containing kinases Syk and ZAP-70 and thus promote the initiation of stimulatory signals.

SIRPs

The regulation of immune responses also involves members of the SIRP family, which are expressed by myeloid cells and can interact with cell-surface-tethered proteins to either amplify or attenuate cell signaling.[87]

There exist three SIRP family members that contain three highly homologous immunoglobulin-like domains in their extracellular regions but differ in their cytoplasmic regions by the presence or absence of ITIMs.

The SIRP family comprises: (1) SIRPα, which utilizes CD47 and surfactant proteins associated with lung inflammation (such as SP-A) as ligands and is found in myeloid cells and neurons; (2) SIRPβ (also known as CD172b), which is found in macrophages and neutrophils but has no known ligand; and (3) SIRPγ (a.k.a. CD172g, SIRPβ2), which binds CD47 and is expressed in lymphocytes and natural killer cells. SIRPα initiates inhibitory signals such as reduced macrophage phagocytosis and TNF production via the presence of cytoplasmic ITIMs that, when phosphorylated, recruit phosphatases such as SHP2 to the signaling complex. Conversely, SIRPβ has a basic amino acid side chain in its transmembrane region that is essential for binding the activating adapter protein DAP12. DAP12 has a single ITAM that, when phosphorylated, binds Syk and ZAP70, and provides stimulatory signals. SIRPγ has a short cytoplasmic domain with no known motifs for recruiting signaling molecules and no charged residue to mediate association with DAP12 or other adapter proteins; thus, its signaling potential is unclear.

Because of their interaction with cell-surface-tethered proteins, the SIRPs are sometimes termed 'paired receptors'. Additional examples of inhibitory/stimulatory receptor systems include CD40/CD40L, the CD200 receptor, cytotoxic T-lymphocyte antigen-4, the intercellular adhesion molecules (ICAMs), the sialic-acid-binding immunoglobulin-like lectins (Siglecs), and the T-cell receptors (TCRs).

ADDITIONAL THERAPEUTIC CONSIDERATIONS

Therapeutics affecting protein kinases and transcription factors are used to treat asthma, airway inflammation, and other inflammatory diseases. Many kinase inhibitors, including those targeting Src kinases, Jaks, and PI3 kinase isoforms, have been examined in models of inflammation and are in development for possible human use. In terms of kinases, the p38 inhibitors VX-702 and HEP 689 have been evaluated in clinical trials for stroke and psoriasis, and other chronic inflammatory disorders. Another p38 inhibitor, BIRB796, is being evaluated in Crohn's disease, and CNI-1493, a dual inhibitor of JNK and p38, has been effective in a small study of patients with Crohn's disease.[88] A Syk inhibitor, R-112 (Rigel), is in phase II trials to treat allergic rhinitis, where it has shown effectiveness against symptoms with rapid onset. Another Syk antagonist, R-406, has entered a phase II study for rheumatoid arthritis.[88] Because Syk is involved in many processes and cell types, the selectivity, safety, and mode of delivery of these drugs are areas of intense analysis.

In terms of transcription factors, an oral small molecule inhibitor (BMS345541) that blocks IKK2-dependent phosphorylation of IκB and attenuates NF-κB-dependent transcription, reduces the incidence and severity of arthritis in mouse models. However, NF-κB is a ubiquitous transcription factor, giving rise to concerns that its inhibition may cause increased susceptibility to infections. Similarly, among the most common therapies prescribed to asthmatics to control their symptoms are inhaled or systemic glucocorticoids, which signal via intracellular receptors to regulate gene transcription.[89] Steroids used in asthma therapy include beclomethasone, budesonide, flunisolide, fluticasone, triamcinolone, and mometasone,

which inhibit inflammatory cell recruitment, lymphocyte activation, and the generation of proinflammatory mediators. For example, corticosteroid-induced upregulation of IκB attenuates NF-κB action and inhibits mediator production.[90] With decreased cytokine and chemokine production, the immune response is suppressed via attenuated lymphocyte and macrophages proliferation and migration to sites of inflammation. Also, corticosteroid therapy lowers immune cell numbers by stimulating apoptosis, perhaps via the decreased production of cytokines necessary for cell survival. However, systemic administration of these compounds results in many side effects, making their long-term use difficult.

In sum, targeting various components of signaling pathways should allow for potent treatments of allergic disease, but because of the ubiquitous nature of these molecules, these therapies face greater challenges in terms of safety and selectivity than therapies targeted towards individual receptors that are more restricted in their expression.

References

Introduction

1. Handbook of cell signaling. London: Elsevier, 2003.

Mechanisms mediating intracellular signaling

2. Mustelin T, Vang T, Bottini N. Protein tyrosine phosphatases and the immune response. Nat Rev Immunol 2005; 5:43–57.
3. Pierce KL, Premont RT, Lefkowitz RJ. Seven-transmembrane receptors. Nat Rev Mol Cell Biol 2002; 3:639–650.
4. Berridge MJ, Bootman MD, Roderick HL. Calcium signalling: dynamics, homeostasis and remodelling. Nat Rev Mol Cell Biol 2003; 4:517–529.
5. Nagai H, Teramachi H, Tuchiya T. Recent advances in the development of anti-allergic drugs. Allergol Int 2006; 55:35–42.
6. Kolch W. Coordinating ERK/MAPK signalling through scaffolds and inhibitors. Nat Rev Mol Cell Biol 2005; 6:827–837.
7. Pazdrak K, Justement L, Alam R. Mechanism of inhibition of eosinophil activation by transforming growth factor-β. Inhibition of Lyn, MAP, Jak2 kinases and STAT1 nuclear factor. J Immunol 1995; 155:4454–4458.
8. Yousefi S, Hoessli DC, Blaser K, et al. Requirement of Lyn and Syk tyrosine kinases for the prevention of apoptosis by cytokines in human eosinophils. J Exp Med 1996; 183:1407–1414.
9. Shuai K, Liu B. Regulation of JAK-STAT signalling in the immune system. Nat Rev Immunol 2003; 3:900–911.
10. Ihle JN. The Janus protein tyrosine kinase family and its role in cytokine signaling. Adv Immunol 1995; 60:1–35.
11. Jiao H, Berrada K, Yang W, et al. Direct association with and dephosphorylation of Jak2 kinase by the SH2-domain-containing protein tyrosine phosphatase SHP-1. Mol Cell Biol 1996; 16:6985–6992.
12. Yasukawa H, Sasaki A, Yoshimura A. Negative regulation of cytokine signaling pathways. Annu Rev Immunol 2000; 18:143–164.
13. Perkins ND. Integrating cell-signalling pathways with NF-κB and IKK function. Nat Rev Mol Cell Biol 2007; 8:49–62.
14. Grant PA. A tale of histone modifications. Genome Biol 2001; 2:Reviews 0003.
15. Kovarova M, Wassif CA, Odom S, et al. Cholesterol deficiency in a mouse model of Smith-Lemli-Opitz syndrome reveals increased mast cell responsiveness. J Exp Med 2006; 203: 1161–1171.
16. London E. How principles of domain formation in model membranes may explain ambiguities concerning lipid raft formation in cells. Biochim Biophys Acta 2005; 1746:203–220.
17. Guichard C, Pedruzzi E, Dewas C, et al. Interleukin-8-induced priming of neutrophil oxidative burst requires sequential recruitment of NADPH oxidase components into lipid rafts. J Biol Chem 2005; 280:37021–37032.
18. Urs NM, Jones KT, Salo PD, et al. A requirement for membrane cholesterol in the β-arrestin- and clathrin-dependent endocytosis of LPA₁ lysophosphatidic acid receptors. J Cell Sci 2005; 118:5291–5304.
19. Cunningham O, Andolfo A, Santovito ML, et al. Dimerization controls the lipid raft partitioning of uPAR/CD87 and regulates its biological functions. EMBO J 2003; 22:5994–6003.
20. Diaz O, Mebarek-Azzam S, Benzaria A, et al. Disruption of lipid rafts stimulates phospholipase D activity in human lymphocytes: implication in the regulation of immune function. J Immunol 2005; 175(12):8077–8086.
21. Olson TS, Ley K. Chemokines and chemokine receptors in leukocyte trafficking. Am J Physiol Regulat Integr Comp Physiol 2002; 283:R7–R28.
22. Gurevich VV, Gurevich EV. The molecular acrobatics of arrestin activation. Trends Pharmacol Sci 2004; 25:105–111.
23. Shenoy SK, Lefkowitz RJ. Multifaceted roles of beta-arrestins in the regulation of seven-membrane-spanning receptor trafficking and signalling. Biochem J 2003; 375:503–515.

24. Key TA, Vines CM, Wagener BM, et al. Inhibition of chemoattractant N-formyl peptide receptor trafficking by active arrestins. Traffic: 2005:87–99.
25. Parton RG, Simons K. The multiple faces of caveolae. Nat Rev Mol Cell Biol 2007; 8:185–194.
26. Weissman AM. Themes and variations on ubiquitylation. Nat Rev Mol Cell Biol 2001; 2:169–178.
27. Muller S, Hoege C, Pyrowolakis G, et al. SUMO, ubiquitin's mysterious cousin. Nat Rev Mol Cell Biol 2001; 2:202–210.
28. Luttrell LM, Lefkowitz RJ. The role of β-arrestins in the termination and transduction of G-protein-coupled receptor signals. J Cell Sci 2002; 115:455–465.
29. Seki Y, Hayashi K, Matsumoto A, et al. Expression of the suppressor of cytokine signaling-5 (SOCS5) negatively regulates IL-4-dependent STAT6 activation and Th2 differentiation. Proc Natl Acad Sci U S A 2002; 99:13003–13008.
30. Krebs DL, Hilton DJ. SOCS: physiological suppressors of cytokine signaling. J Cell Sci 2000; 113:2813–2819.
31. Yoshimura A. Negative regulation of cytokine signaling. Clin Rev Allergy Immunol 2005; 28:205–220.
32. Alexander WS, Starr R, Fenner JE, et al. SOCS1 is a critical inhibitor of interferon γ signaling and prevents the potentially fatal neonatal actions of this cytokine. Cell 1999; 98:597–608.
33. Shuai K, Liu B. Regulation of gene-activation pathways by PIAS proteins in the immune system. Nat Rev Immunol 2005; 5:593–605.

Selected signaling systems relevant to allergy

34. Ali MS, Sayeski PP, Dirksen LB, et al. Dependence on the motif YIPP for the physical association of Jak2 kinase with the intracellular carboxyl tail of the angiotensin II AT1 receptor. J Biol Chem 1997; 272:23382–23388.
35. Lefkowitz RJ. G protein-coupled receptors. III. New roles for receptor kinases and beta-arrestins in receptor signaling and desensitization. J Biol Chem 1998; 273:18677–18680.
36. Neptune ER, Iiri T, Bourne HR. Gαi is not required for chemotaxis mediated by Gi-coupled receptors. J Biol Chem 1999; 274:2824–2828.
37. Holgate ST, Bodey KS, Janezic A, et al. Release of RANTES, MIP-1 α, and MCP-1 into asthmatic airways following endobronchial allergen challenge. Am J Respir Crit Care Med 1997; 156:1377–1383.
38. Izumi T. Leukotriene receptors: classification, gene expression, and signal transduction. J Biochem 2002; 132:1–6.
39. Coffey M, Peters-Golden M. Extending the understanding of leukotrienes in asthma. Curr Opin Allergy Clin Immunol 2003; 3:57–63.
40. Jutel M, Blaser K, Akdis CA. Histamine in allergic inflammation and immune modulation. Int Arch Allergy Immunol 2005; 137:82–92.
41. Fadel R, Herpin-Richard N, Rihoux JP, et al. Inhibitory effect of cetirizine 2HCl on eosinophil migration in vivo. Clin Allergy 1987; 17:373–379.
42. Johnson M. The β-adrenoceptor. Am J Respir Crit Care Med 1998; 158:S146–S153.
43. Giembycz MA, Newton R. Beyond the dogma: novel β-adrenoceptor signalling in the airways. Eur Respir J 2006; 27:1286–1306.
44. Holgate ST. Asthma and rhinitis. London: Blackwell; 1995.
45. Miller JR, Silver PJ, Stull JT. The role of myosin light chain kinase phosphorylation in β-adrenergic relaxation of tracheal smooth muscle. Mol Pharmacol 1983; 24:235–242.
46. Price DM, Chik CL, Ho AK. Norepinephrine induction of mitogen-activated protein kinase phosphatase-1 expression in rat pinealocytes: distinct roles of α- and β-adrenergic receptors. Endocrinology 2004; 145:5723–5733.
47. Koch A, Nasuhara Y, Barnes PJ, et al. Extracellular signal-regulated kinase 1/2 control Ca(2+)-independent force development in histamine-stimulated bovine tracheal smooth muscle. Br J Pharmacol 2000; 131:981–989.
48. Reihsaus E, Innis M, MacIntyre N, et al. Mutations in the gene encoding the beta 2-adrenergic receptor in normal and asthmatic subjects. Am J Respir Cell Mol Biol 1993; 8:334–339.
49. Kankaanranta H, Lindsay MA, Giembycz MA, et al. Delayed eosinophil apoptosis in asthma. J Allergy Clin Immunol 2000; 106(1 Pt 1):77–83.
50. Mak JC, Roffel AF, Katsunuma T, et al. Up-regulation of airway smooth muscle histamine H(1) receptor mRNA, protein, and function by β(2)-adrenoceptor activation. Mol Pharmacol 2000; 57:857–864.
51. Barnes PJ. Effect of β-agonists on inflammatory cells. J Allergy Clin Immunol 1999; 104(2 Pt 2):S10–S17.
52. Burnstock G. Purinergic signalling – an overview. Novartis Found Symp 2006; 276:26–48; discussion 48–57, 275–281.
53. Polosa R. Adenosine-receptor subtypes: their relevance to adenosine-mediated responses in asthma and chronic obstructive pulmonary disease. Eur Respir J 2002; 20:488–496.
54. Baraldi PG, Cacciari B, Romagnoli R, et al. A(3) adenosine receptor ligands: history and perspectives. Med Res Rev 2000; 20:103–128.
55. Mamedova L, Capra V, Accomazzo MR, et al. CysLT1 leukotriene receptor antagonists inhibit the effects of nucleotides acting at P2Y receptors. Biochem Pharmacol 2005; 71:115–125.
56. Di Virgilio F, Chiozzi P, Ferrari D, et al. Nucleotide receptors: an emerging family of regulatory molecules in blood cells. Blood 2001; 97:587–600.
57. Guerra AN, Fisette PL, Pfeiffer ZA, et al. Purinergic receptor regulation of LPS-induced signaling and pathophysiology. J Endotoxin Res 2003; 9:256–263.
58. Sugamura K, Asao H, Kondo M, et al. The interleukin-2 receptor γ chain: its role in the multiple cytokine receptor complexes and T cell development in XSCID. Annu Rev Immunol 1996; 14:179–205.
59. Giri JG, Ahdieh M, Eisenman J, et al. Utilization of the beta and γ chains of the IL-2 receptor by the novel cytokine IL-15. EMBO J 1994; 13:2822–2830.
60. Taga T, Kishimoto T. Signaling mechanisms through cytokine receptors that share signal transducing receptor components. Curr Opin Immunol 1995; 7:17–23.
61. Hatakeyama M, Kono T, Kobayashi N, et al. Interaction of the IL-2 receptor with the src-family kinase p56lck: identification of novel intermolecular association. Science 1991; 252:1523–1528.
62. Kobayashi N, Kono T, Hatakeyama M, et al. Functional coupling of the src-family protein tyrosine kinases p59fyn and p53/56lyn with the interleukin 2 receptor: implications for redundancy and pleiotropism in cytokine signal transduction. Proc Natl Acad Sci U S A 1993; 90:4201–4205.
63. Izuhara K, Arima K. Signal transduction of IL-13 and its role in the pathogenesis of bronchial asthma. Drug News Perspect 2004; 17:91–98.
64. Ihle JN, Witthuhn BA, Quelle FW, et al. Signaling through the hematopoietic cytokine receptors. Annu Rev Immunol 1995; 13:369–398.
65. Yamagata T, Ichinose M. Agents against cytokine synthesis or receptors. Eur J Pharmacol 2006; 533:289–301.
66. Akira S. Toll-like receptor Signaling. J Biol Chem 2003; 278:38105–38108.
67. Armant MA, Fenton MJ. Toll-like receptors: a family of pattern-recognition receptors in mammals. Genome Biol 2002; 3:3011.
68. Takeda K, Kaisho T, Akira S. Toll-like receptors. Annu Rev Immunol 2003; 21:335–376.
69. Zhang G, Ghosh S. Negative regulation of toll-like receptor-mediated signaling by Tollip. J Biol Chem 2002; 277:7059–7065.
70. Gupta D, Wang Q, Vinson C, et al. Bacterial peptidoglycan induces CD14-dependent activation of transcription factors CREB/ATF and AP-1. J Biol Chem 1999; 274:14012–14020.
71. Qureshi ST, Lariviere L, Leveque G, et al. Endotoxin-tolerant mice have mutations in Toll-like receptor 4 (TLR4). J Exp Med 1999; 189:615–625.
72. Shimazu R, Akashi S, Ogata H, et al. MD-2, a molecule that confers lipopolysaccharide responsiveness on Toll-like receptor 4. J Exp Med 1999; 189:1777–1782.
73. Ogata H, Su I, Miyake K, et al. The toll-like receptor protein RP105 regulates lipopolysaccharide signaling in B cells. J Exp Med 2000; 192:23–29.
74. Gallucci S, Matzinger P. Danger signals: SOS to the immune system. Curr Opin Immunol 2001; 13:114–119.
75. Okamura Y, Watari M, Jerud ES, et al. The extra domain A of fibronectin activates Toll-like receptor 4. J Biol Chem 2001; 276:10229–10233.
76. Kurt-Jones EA, Popova L, Kwinn L, et al. Pattern recognition receptors TLR4 and CD14 mediate response to respiratory syncytial virus. Nat Immunol 2000; 1:398–401.
77. Hayashi F, Smith KD, Ozinsky A, et al. The innate immune response to bacterial flagellin is mediated by Toll-like receptor 5. Nature 2001; 410:1099–1103.
78. Hemmi H, Takeuchi O, Kawai T, et al. A Toll-like receptor recognizes bacterial DNA. Nature 2000; 408:740–745.
79. Krieg AM. Therapeutic potential of toll-like receptor 9 activation. Nat Rev Drug Discov 2006; 5:471–484.
80. Racila DM, Kline JN. Perspectives in asthma: molecular use of microbial products in asthma prevention and treatment. J Allergy Clin Immunol 2005; 116:1202–1205.
81. Daeron M. Fc receptor biology. Annu Rev Immunol 1997; 15:203–234.
82. Adamczewski M, Numerof RP, Koretzky GA, et al. Regulation by CD45 of the tyrosine phosphorylation of high affinity IgE receptor β- and γ-chains. J Immunol 1995; 154: 3047–3055.
83. Turner H, Reif K, Rivera J, et al. Regulation of the adapter molecule Grb2 by the FcεR1 in the mast cell line RBL2H3. J Biol Chem 1995; 270:9500–9506.
84. Hutchinson LE, McCloskey MA. FcεRI-mediated induction of nuclear factor of activated T-cells. J Biol Chem 1995; 270:16333–16338.
85. Razin E, Szallasi Z, Kazanietz MG, et al. Protein kinases C-β and C-ε link the mast cell high-affinity receptor for IgE to the expression of c-fos and c-jun. Proc Natl Acad Sci U S A 1994; 91:7722–7726.
86. Borges L, Cosman D. LIRs/ILTs/MIRs, inhibitory and stimulatory Ig superfamily receptors expressed in myeloid and lymphoid cells. Cytokine Growth Factor Rev 2000; 11:209–217.
87. Barclay AN, Brown MH. The SIRP family of receptors and immune regulation. Nat Rev Immunol 2006; 6:457–464.

Additional therapeutic considerations

88. Adcock IM, Chung KF, Caramori G, et al. Kinase inhibitors and airway inflammation. Eur J Pharmacol 2006; 533:118–132.
89. Goodman L SaG A. Goodman & Gilman's The pharmacological basis of therapeutics. 11th edn. New York: McGraw-Hill; 2006.
90. McKay LI, Cidlowski JA. Molecular control of immune/inflammatory responses interactions between nuclear factor-κB and steroid receptor-signaling pathways. Endocr Rev 1999; 20:435–459.

Cellular Adhesion in Inflammation

David H Broide and P Sriramarao

9

CONTENTS

- Introduction 149
- Selectins and selectin ligands 150
- Integrins 152
- Immunoglobulin gene superfamily 154
- Galectins, cadherins, and CD44 156
- Leukocyte adhesion to and across the endothelium 157
- Leukocyte adhesion in the extracellular matrix in tissues 159
- Regulation of adhesion molecule expression 160
- Human disease associated with adhesion molecule deficiency 161
- Adhesion molecules in human allergic inflammation 161
- Potential side effects of adhesion-based therapy 162
- Summary 162

SUMMARY OF IMPORTANT CONCEPTS

>> Interaction of circulating leukocytes with the endothelial cell surface is mediated by adhesion molecules expressed on circulating leukocytes and vascular endothelium

>> Cytokines (e.g. TNF, IL-1, IL-4) and mediators (e.g. histamine) released at tissue sites of allergic inflammation upregulate adhesion molecule expression by endothelium

>> Leukocyte adhesion to endothelium is a multi-step process with selectins mediating initial rolling of leukocytes on endothelium and integrins mediating subsequent firm adhesion of leukocytes to endothelium

>> The importance of leukocyte adhesion to endothelium to host defense is suggested from diseases associated with defective neutrophil adhesion to endothelium and immunodeficiency (i.e. LAD)

>> Clinical studies have demonstrated the potential benefit of anti-adhesion based therapies in multiple sclerosis, Crohn's disease, and psoriasis, but have not yet demonstrated their utility in asthma and allergic diseases

INTRODUCTION

Tissue inflammation is a characteristic feature of a wide variety of human diseases including allergy, asthma, autoimmunity, and infection. Both tissue-resident cells (i.e. mast cells, macrophages, dendritic cells), as well as peripheral blood leukocytes (eosinophils, basophils neutrophils, T cells, mononuclear cells), play a key role in the inflammatory response in tissues. This chapter describes the coordinated cellular adhesion events between circulating leukocytes and vascular endothelium which leads to the cellular recruitment of circulating leukocytes to tissue sites of inflammation where they may orchestrate a wide range of tissue inflammatory responses associated with allergy, asthma, autoimmunity, and infection.

Depending on the nature of the inciting stimulus that elicits the inflammatory response (i.e. allergen, bacteria, virus, etc.), one or more, or all of these circulating leukocyte subsets (eosinophils, basophils

neutrophils, T cells, mononuclear cells) is preferentially recruited to the inflamed tissue. For example, during episodes of acute bacterial inflammation associated with pneumonia, neutrophils are the primary cells recruited, whereas during allergic responses eosinophils and Th2 cells are recruited. Cell adhesion molecules (CAMs) are important molecules that contribute to the selective recruitment of circulating leukocytes to sites of inflammation by promoting cell–cell and cell–matrix interactions. Based on shared structural features and functions, CAMs have been subdivided into three main families; selectins, integrins, and immunoglobulin gene super family (IgSF) members. Adhesion molecules belonging to one of these families, with some exceptions, promote a series of leukocyte interactions with endothelial cells within blood vessels that mediate subsequent leukocyte migration across the endothelium followed by directed leukocyte migration into tissues. This chapter summarizes the structural and functional characteristics of the CAM families, focusing in particular on those CAMs associated with allergic inflammation or immunodeficiencies.

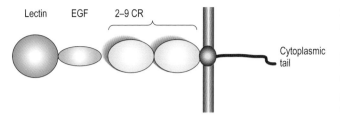

Fig. 9.1. Selectin. Selectins (E-, L-, or P-selectin) have a structure composed of an extracellular lectin domain that mediates cell adhesion, an epidermal growth factor-like region (EGF), two to nine consensus repeats (2–9 CR) similar to those found in complement regulatory proteins, and a cytoplasmic tail.

■ SELECTINS AND SELECTIN LIGANDS ■

SELECTIN STRUCTURE AND FUNCTION

Selectins are a family of CAMs which bind to specific sugar determinants on the surface of adjacent cells which act as adhesion counterreceptors.[1] The selectin family includes leukocyte-expressed L-selectin (CD62L), endothelial-expressed E-selectin (CD62E), and P-selectin (CD62P) which is expressed by both platelets and endothelial cells.[1] While selectins are primarily involved in leukocyte trafficking to tissues, they can also function in transmitting signals that lead to leukocyte activation. All three selectins contain a critical 120-amino acid N-terminal Ca^{2+}-dependent (C-type) lectin homologue domain that mediates cell adhesion, an epidermal growth factor-like region, two to nine consensus repeats similar to those found in complement regulatory proteins, a transmembrane region, and a 17–35 amino acid cytoplasmic tail (Fig. 9.1). The extracellular domains (lectin and EGF domains) of the three selectins share significant homology. In contrast, there is little homology among the transmembrane and intracytoplasmic domains between the various selectins. Whereas all three selectins utilize the lectin domain to mediate adhesion, the endogenous intracytoplasmic portion of the molecule is required for the adhesive function of L-selectin but is not needed for adhesion mediated by E-selectin or P-selectin.[2,3] In addition to the cell surface expression of selectins, soluble forms of all three selectins have been detected in blood and other body fluids. As yet, the biologic activities of soluble selectins and/or the diagnostic value of measuring levels of soluble selectins in disease states are not well understood.

L-selectin

The expression of L-selectin is restricted to leukocytes. L-selectin was originally identified as a peripheral lymph node homing receptor responsible for lymphocyte adhesion to high endothelial venules in lymph nodes.[4] L-selectin is constitutively expressed on the tips of the microvilli of most leukocytes, including neutrophils, eosinophils, monocytes, naïve T and B cells as well as on the surface of some activated T cells and memory T cells upon activation by appropriate stimuli including chemotactic factors.[4] L-selectin mediates leukocyte margination and tethering to endothelium under conditions of shear stress associated with blood flow. L-selectin is irreversibly and rapidly shed from the leukocyte cell surface by endogenous membrane-bound proteases.

E-selectin

The expression of E-selectin is restricted to endothelial cells. E-selectin is not expressed on the surface of unstimulated endothelium but is induced within several hours following exposure to either interleukin-1 (IL-1), tumor necrosis factor-α (TNF-α), or bacterial endotoxin.[5] Endothelial-expressed E-selectin functions as a ligand for various myeloid cells as well as subsets of T lymphocytes bearing the cutaneous lymphocyte antigen.[3,5,6] Under conditions of physiologic blood flow, E-selectin preferentially supports adhesion of neutrophils and subsets of T cells but not eosinophils in vivo.[7] Surface expression of E-selectin in vitro is relatively transient, with endothelial expression levels peaking at 4–6 h and approaching baseline levels by 24 h.[5] While most expressed E-selectin is re-internalized and degraded, a small amount is shed.[8] Molecular studies of the E-selectin promoter have revealed that transcription is under the control of several transcription factors, including nuclear factor kappa B (NF-κB)[9] and its expression at sites of inflammation in vivo appears to be more prolonged than noted in vitro. Furthermore, expression of E-selectin can be potentiated by interferon gamma (IFN-γ) and inhibited by transforming growth factor beta (TGF-β).[3]

P-selectin

P-selectin functions as a vascular ligand for most myeloid and lymphoid cells.[1,3,10] While P-selectin, like E-selectin, is expressed by activated endothelium, it is also expressed by activated platelets. P-selectin is stored preformed in intracellular granules and can be rapidly translocated to the cell surface when endothelial cells are stimulated with agents such as C5a, histamine, thrombin, phorbol esters or leukotriene C4.[10] In contrast to this rapid translocation of preformed P-selectin, exposure of endothelial cells to cytokines such as IL-13 results in P-selectin mRNA transcription and a more gradual and continued increase in P-selectin expression.[11] Leukocyte interaction with endothelial P-selectin has been shown to alter leukocyte cellular functions, including superoxide production, integrin-mediated phagocytosis, and production of cytokines and chemokines.[12,13] In contrast, leukocyte activation can reduce leukocyte adhesion to P-selectin expressed by endothelium by altering the topographic location of P-selectin ligands on the leukocyte cell surface, as well as by stimulus-induced shedding.[14]

SELECTIN LIGANDS

All known selectin ligands are transmembrane glycoproteins, which present oligosaccharide structures to selectins.[15,16] Selectins and their ligands form transient interactions and bonds which mediate the initial steps of the leukocyte endothelial adhesion cascade. All three selectins can recognize glycoproteins and/or glycolipids containing the tetrasaccharide sialyl-Lewis^X (sialyl-CD15, sLe^X) and in some cases its isomer sialyl-Lewis^a.[16] The sialyl-Lewis^X tetrasaccharide is found on all circulating myeloid cells and is composed of fucosylated and sialylated carbohydrate moieties such as sialic acid, galactose, fucose, and N-acetylgalactosamine. Biosynthesis of selectin ligands such as sLe^X is dependent upon the sequential activity of specific sialyl- and fucosyl-transferases.[16,17] Despite some common ligands, a number of important differences exist among ligands for different selectins. For example, ligands for P-selectin on human leukocytes are protease sensitive and endo-β-galactosidase resistant. In contrast, E-selectin ligands are protease resistant and endo-β-galactosidase sensitive,[18] suggesting that the former is an sLe^X-containing glycoprotein, whereas the latter may be an extended chain, sLe^X-containing glycolipid.

Many selectin ligands have been described which are able to mediate adhesion to L-, E-, and P- selectins in vitro. Which of these selectin ligands is important in selectin-mediated adhesion in vivo in specific disease states still requires further study. One of the best described selectin ligands is P-selectin glycoprotein ligand-1 (PSGL-1), the key ligand for P-selectin. PSGL-1 (CD162) is a dimeric sialomucin widely expressed by leukocytes including eosinophils.[18] Eosinophils in nasal polyps utilize PSGL-1 to adhere to endothelial cells in polyp tissue.[19]

Various carbohydrate ligands have been described for L-selectin on lymph node endothelia including CD34, the mucosal addressin cell adhesion molecule-1 (MAdCAM-1), the glycosylation-dependent cell adhesion molecule-1 (GlyCAM-1), and the sulfated glycoprotein 200 (Sgp200).[20] Most L-selectin ligands contain mucins rich in O-linked sugars that contain sLe^X. L-selectin has also been shown to interact with PSGL-1 under conditions of flow in vitro as well as with cutaneous lymphocyte antigen (CLA) and a sLe^X-like or sialyl-6-sulfo-Lewis^X-like structure on high endothelial venules.[20]

Several sialylated ligand structures have been identified as possible E-selectin ligands. These sialylated ligands for E-selectin may be carried on CD65, CD66, L-selectin, or additional surface molecules on neutrophils and B lymphocytes.[21] For subsets of memory (CD45RO+) skin-homing T lymphocytes, CLA, a modified form of PSGL-1, functions as a ligand for E-selectin but not for P-selectin.[21] E-selectin ligand-1 (ESL-1), a variant of the fibroblast growth factor receptor,[22] has been identified as an E-selectin ligand on mouse leukocytes. There is also evidence of glycolipid E-selectin ligands (such as polylactosaminolipids, which have been termed *myeloglycans*) on leukocytes.[21]

ENZYMES INVOLVED IN SELECTIN LIGAND SYNTHESIS

Selectin ligands are either synthesized by leukocytes (e.g., eosinophils, neutrophils, basophils, T cells, mononuclear cells) to bind to selectins expressed by endothelial cells (e.g., P-selectin, E-selectin), or alternatively selectin ligands may be synthesized by endothelial cells to bind to selectins expressed by circulating leukocytes (e.g., L-selectin). The ability of leukocytes or endothelial cells to express selectin ligands is dependent upon their expression of several enzymes termed glycosyltransferases which are needed to synthesize selectin ligands. Several Golgi resident enzymes termed glycosyltransferases, including sialyl-transferases and fucosyl-transferases (FucT), have been identified which play an important role in the biosynthesis of the selectin ligand sLe^X, a carbohydrate structure composed of four sugar molecules. sLe^X is expressed by selectin ligands and is able to bind to all three selectins (E-, P-, L-selectin). Several isoforms of FucTs have been cloned, and both FucT-IV and FucT-VII are especially important for leukocyte synthesis of sLe^X.[23]

SELECTIN DEFICIENT MICE: INSIGHTS INTO ROLE OF SELECTINS IN ALLERGIC INFLAMMATION

Mice deficient in either P-selectin (expressed by endothelial cells), or L-selectin (expressed by leukocytes), have been generated and studied in mouse models of allergic inflammation and asthma. P-selectin deficient

mice challenged with inhaled allergen have decreased airway hyperreactivity and attenuated influx of eosinophils and lymphocytes in bronchoalveolar lavage.[24] Studies using intravital microscopy to visualize adhesion of eosinophils to endothelium in the microcirculation in vivo have demonstrated that eosinophils have significant reductions in the first step of adhesion to inflamed endothelium (i.e. deficient leukocyte 'rolling' on P-selectin deficient endothelium).[25] Similarly, L-selectin deficient mice show a marked decrease of airway hyperreactivity and a mild attenuation of T cell recruitment in bronchoalveolar lavage (BAL) in a mouse model of asthma.[26] E-selectin appears to be more important to the adhesion of neutrophils to endothelium as compared to the adhesion of eosinophils to endothelium.[7] In primate models of asthma anti-E-selectin Abs do not inhibit eosinophilic inflammation or airway hyperreactivity.

SELECTIN LIGAND DEFICIENT MICE: INSIGHTS INTO ROLE OF SELECTIN LIGANDS IN INFLAMMATION

Support for a critical role of glycosyltransferases (which synthesize selectin ligands such as sLe^X) to leukocyte trafficking in vivo has been provided in animal models of inflammation. Studies have demonstrated that mice deficient in FucT-VII have a significantly increased peripheral blood leukocyte count due to an almost complete absence of leukocyte rolling in inflamed venules.[23,27] The FucT-VII deficient leukocytes have a significant reduction in levels of expression of selectin ligands that bind to P-selectin and E-selectin expressed by endothelial cells. These studies underscore the importance of the leukocyte enzyme FucT-VII in selectin ligand synthesis. FucT-VII appears to be more important than FucT-IV in leukocyte adhesion to endothelium as FucT-IV deficient mice have normal numbers of peripheral blood leukocytes and exhibit normal rolling on inflamed endothelium.

HUMAN GENETIC DISEASE ASSOCIATED WITH SELECTIN LIGAND DEFICIENCY: INSIGHTS INTO ROLE OF SELECTINS IN INFLAMMATION

Genetic defects in fucose metabolism caused by a defect in the Golgi associated guanosine diphosphate fucose transporter (GFTP) in patients with leukocyte adhesion deficiency (LAD)-II result in impaired leukocyte sLe^X synthesis (fucose is an essential sugar component of the selectin ligand sLe^X), with resultant impaired leukocyte adhesion to endothelium, and consequent impaired leukocyte tissue recruitment predisposing to infection.[28] Patients with leukocyte adhesion deficiency (LAD)-II have both an immunodeficiency characterized by elevated leukocyte counts and recurrent bacterial infections as well as mental retardation suggesting a role for fucose in both sLe^X synthesis and brain development. A patient with an immunodeficiency similar in clinical expression to LAD who had an E-selectin deficiency has also been described.[29]

TARGETING SELECTINS IN HUMAN ALLERGIC INFLAMMATION

At present, there are limited published studies of selectin inhibitors in human subjects with allergic inflammation or asthma. Human studies have examined whether a single intravenous dose of a pan-selectin antagonist TBC1269 administered 15 minutes before allergen challenge could inhibit the early and late asthmatic responses in mild asymptomatic asthmatics.[30] TBC1269 had only minor inhibitory effects on allergen-induced sputum eosinophilia and did not attenuate the early or late asthmatic response to allergen challenge in asthmatic subjects. Further studies are needed to determine whether selectin antagonists as a class are not of benefit in asthma or whether studies of selectin antagonists in subjects with persistent asthma, as opposed to studies in allergen challenge models of asthma, would demonstrate different results.

■ INTEGRINS ■

INTEGRIN STRUCTURE AND FUNCTION

Integrins belong to a large family of structurally related non-covalently linked α and β heterodimeric cell adhesion receptors.[31,32] The α and β subunits are type I transmembrane proteins containing large extracellular domains (700–1100 amino acids) and relatively small cytoplasmic domains (30–50 amino acids).[31,32] The extracellular portion of integrin α subunits is composed of three or four domains that resemble calcium binding sites, with each domain being approximately 60 amino acids in length. At a functional level, integrins regulate cell behavior by both creating transmembrane linkages between the extracellular matrix and the cell cytoskeleton, as well as by transmitting extracellular signals to the intracellular compartment promoting cellular activation.[31,32] As single-chain transmembrane structures, integrins possess intracytoplasmic domains with distinct sites for attachment to cytoskeletal elements such as actin, talin, α-actinin, filamin, and paxillin.[31,32] During adhesion, integrins and associated cytoskeletal proteins localize on the cell surface within contact sites called focal adhesions.[31,32] Conserved sequences in the cytoplasmic carboxyl terminus of several β subunits influence the avidity of binding as well. Integrins are expressed by all multicellular organisms, and the mammalian genome is composed of 18 α and 8 β ($\beta1$ to $\beta8$) subunit genes. To date, 24 different $\alpha\beta$ receptors have been reported.

Figure 9.2 shows the structure of a typical $\alpha\beta$ integrin heterodimer. The binding affinity of the $\alpha\beta$ heterodimers appears to rest within the

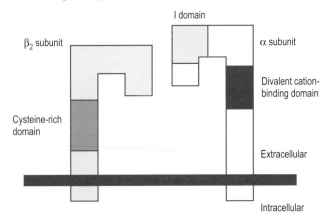

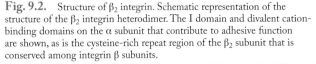

Fig. 9.2. Structure of β_2 integrin. Schematic representation of the structure of the β_2 integrin heterodimer. The I domain and divalent cation-binding domains on the α subunit that contribute to adhesive function are shown, as is the cysteine-rich repeat region of the β_2 subunit that is conserved among integrin β subunits.

specific divalent cation-binding sites of the β hairpin loop.[31,32] In addition to these domains, many β_1 and all β_2 integrins contain an 'inserted' or I domain, that is a conserved structural feature and key recognition site for integrin-binding activity.[31,32] In addition to the extracellular portion of integrins, β subunits contain 56 cysteine residues that are localized into four tandem domains which appear to maintain the heterodimer in an extended and rigid conformation. Intracytoplasmic integrin assembly and subsequent surface expression of integrins require an intact β subunit. This is known to be true in humans because genetic mutations in the β_2 subunit (especially near the N-terminal portion) have been identified in LAD-I, in which leukocyte surface expression of β_2 integrins is greatly impaired or absent.[28]

INTEGRIN EXPRESSION AND LIGANDS

Most integrins are characterized by their ability to interact with multiple ligands, and conversely a single integrin ligand (extracellular matrix proteins and other CAMs) can interact with multiple integrins. The profile of integrins expressed either by leukocytes or structural cells (i.e. endothelial cells, epithelial cells, etc.) varies from one cell type to the other. The expression of integrins on various leukocytes and mast cells is represented in Table 9.1. Cells relevant to allergic disease such as eosinophils and basophils express common α_4 ($\alpha_4\beta_1$ and $\alpha_4\beta_7$) and β_2 ($\alpha_L\beta_2$, $\alpha_M\beta_2$, $\alpha_X\beta_2$, $\alpha_d\beta_2$) integrins, but differ with respect to expression of some integrins. Eosinophils express $\alpha_6\beta_1$ while basophils express $\alpha_5\beta_1$.[3] Endothelial and epithelial cells express multiple integrin receptors which mediate their adhesion to specific integrin ligands expressed by basement membrane matrix and other proteins. For example, endothelial cells express several β_1 integrins ($\alpha_2\beta_1$, $\alpha_3\beta_1$, $\alpha_5\beta_1$, $\alpha_6\beta_1$) as well as $\alpha_v\beta_3$,[33] while respiratory epithelial cells express these as well as $\alpha_9\beta_1$, $\alpha_v\beta_1$, $\alpha_6\beta_4$, $\alpha_v\beta_5$, and $\alpha_v\beta_6$.[34]

The levels of surface expression of integrins can also be altered during hematopoiesis or due to cellular activation.[31,32] For example, the maturation of mast cells from stem cell precursors over 14 weeks is associated with declines in $\alpha_4\beta_1$ and $\alpha_5\beta_1$ integrin expression and the de novo appearance of $\alpha_v\beta_3$, $\alpha_2\beta_1$, and $\alpha_3\beta_1$ integrins at various times during the culture.[35] Other integrins, such as $\alpha_M\beta_2$ and $\alpha_d\beta_2$, exist both on the cell surface and within intracytoplasmic granules which can rapidly translocate to the cell surface after cell activation. Thus individual leukocyte subsets (i.e. eosinophils, basophils, mast cells, neutrophils) may exhibit either shared or selective expression of individual integrin family members. In addition, leukocyte subsets may exhibit differences in their relative levels of integrin expression, as well as demonstrate variations in the cell type-specific stimuli that alter their adhesion and migration responses. However, for all leukocytes, several of the leukocyte endothelial adhesion cascade steps (i.e. firm adhesion, locomotion) are largely dependent on the engagement of β_2 integrins. In fact, defects in β_2 integrin expression or function lead to impaired leukocyte recruitment responses, especially in neutrophils.[28]

INTEGRIN SIGNALING

In addition to playing an important role in mediating cellular adhesion, integrins also have important functions as signal-transducing molecules.[31,32] Integrins function as bi-directional signaling molecules. For example, cell surface receptors such as integrins bind specific extracellular ligands and subsequently transduce the extracellular signal

Table 9.1 Integrin adhesion molecule expression on human leukocytes[a] and mast cells

Subunit (CD, name)	Ligands	Lympho[b]	Mono	Neutro	Eosino	Baso	Mast[b]
$\alpha_1\beta_1$ (49a/29, VLA-1)	Laminin, collagen	+	−	−	−	−	−
$\alpha_2\beta_1$ (49b/29, VLA-2)	Collagen, laminin	+	+	−	−	−	−
$\alpha_3\beta_1$ (49c/29, VLA-3)	Collagen, laminin, fibronectin	+	−	−	−	−	+
$\alpha_4\beta_1$ (49d/29, VLA-4)	VCAM-1, fibronectin CS-1 domain	+	+	−	+	+	+
$\alpha_5\beta_1$ (49e/29, VLA-5)	Fibronectin	+	+	+	−	+	+
$\alpha_6\beta_1$ (49f/29, VLA-6)	Laminin	+	+	+	+		
$\alpha_L\beta_2$ (11a/18, LFA-1)	ICAM-1,-2,-3,-4, and -5	+	+	+	+	+	
$\alpha_M\beta_2$ (11b/18, Mac-1)	ICAM-1 and -2, C3bi, fibrinogen, heparin	−	+	+	+	+	
$\alpha_X\beta_2$ (11c/18, p150,95)	C3bi, fibrinogen	+	+	+	+	+	+
$\alpha_d\beta_2$ (α_d/18)	ICAM-3, VCAM-1	+	+	+	+	+	−
$\alpha_V\beta_3$ (51/61)	Vitronectin, PECAM-1, other RGD peptides	−	−	−	−	−	+
$\alpha_4\beta_7$ (49d/β_7, ACT-1)	MAdCAM-1, VCAM-1, fibronectin CS-1 domain	+	+	−	+	+	−
$\alpha_E\beta_7$ (103/β_7, HML-1)	E-cadherin	+	−	−	−	−	−

[a]Lymphocytes, monocytes, neutrophils, eosinophils, basophils.
[b]Expression may be restricted to subsets of these cells.
+, Present; −, absent; CD, cluster of differentiation nomenclature; VLA, very late (activation) antigen; LFA, leukocyte function-associated antigen; VCAM, vascular cell adhesion molecule; CS-1, connecting segment-1; ICAM, intercellular adhesion molecule; RGD, arginine-glycine-aspartic acid; PECAM, platelet-endothelial cell adhesion molecule; MadCAM, mucosal-addressin cell adhesion molecule.

from the cell surface to the interior of the cell (classic 'outside-in signaling' from the cell surface to the cell interior). However, in addition to classic 'outside-in signaling,' integrins can also mediate 'inside-out signaling' in which activation of the cytoplasmic tail of the integrin sends a signal to the extracellular domain of the integrin to change its conformation. 'Outside-in' integrin signal transduction does not occur through kinase or phosphatase activity of the integrins themselves because intracytoplasmic domains of integrins lack kinase or phosphatase activity of their own, and also lack sequence homology with known signaling proteins.[31,32] Therefore, subsequent to integrin ligation by extracellular ligands, transmembrane 'outside-in' integrin signal transduction is initiated via adapter or linker proteins that activate cytoplasmic kinases resulting in transcription factor activation. 'Outside-in' signaling through integrins can influence cell proliferation, differentiation, migration, gene transcription, and apoptosis.[31,32]

In addition to 'outside-in' signaling by integrins, integrins also mediate 'inside-out' signaling which is important in a key step of the adhesion of leukocytes to endothelium. These intracellular signals are generated in the leukocyte from activation of a non-integrin receptor (e.g. cytokine or chemokine) by external stimuli such as cytokines or chemokines. This leukocyte integrin activation process, referred to as 'inside-out signaling', ultimately changes the integrin conformation to increases leukocyte integrin affinity for ligands expressed by inflamed endothelium. Chemokines, such as eotaxin and IL-8, are potential in situ regulators of

integrin activity on leukocytes (i.e. eosinophils and neutrophils, respectively) interacting with vessel walls or migrating across the extracellular matrix.[36] Thus, when a rolling leukocyte adheres and rolls over the endothelium-expressing chemokines, the leukocyte can recognize the endothelial-presented chemokines via its seven transmembrane spanning chemokine receptor, which elicit a leukocyte integrin activation signal by activating heterotrimeric G proteins, mainly of the Gi family. This process is extremely rapid and can occur in subseconds, the time frame of individual adhesive contacts engaged by a continuously rolling leukocyte.[36] In addition to the important role of integrin signaling in mediating leukocyte endothelial adhesion, 'inside-out' integrin signaling also plays a role in host defense as the immune deficiency syndrome LAD-III is due to a genetic defect in 'inside out' integrin signaling in leukocytes.[28]

INTEGRIN DEFICIENT MICE: INSIGHTS INTO ROLE OF INTEGRINS IN INFLAMMATION

As targeting individual integrin genes (i.e. integrins $\alpha_4, \alpha_5, \beta_1$; or integrin ligand such as fibronectin) has generated lethal mutations in mice, the study of the role of these individual integrin genes in mice using these integrin deficient mice has not been possible. However, studies with several different neutralizing antibodies (Abs) to individual integrins in animal models of asthma has provided insight into the potential utility of targeting integrins to inhibit allergic inflammation and airway responsiveness. In animal models of asthma, the trafficking of inflammatory cells from the circulation into the airway and airway responsiveness can be inhibited by antibodies to either β_1 or α_4 integrins.[37–39] Interestingly, some studies using animal models of asthma suggest that the beneficial response from targeting $\alpha_4\beta_1$ is due to inhibiting leukocyte activation of integrin-expressing inflammatory cells already resident in the airway, rather than due to the minor inhibitory effect of anti-$\alpha_4\beta_1$ inhibiting leukocyte trafficking from the bloodstream into the airway.[38]

TARGETING INTEGRINS IN HUMAN ALLERGIC INFLAMMATION

Initial studies in humans with asthma have focused on inhibiting VLA-4 ($\alpha_4\beta_1$) based on promising results of studies with VLA-4 antagonists in inhibiting airway responsiveness in animal models of asthma.[37–39] In a pilot study, 16 adult subjects with mild-to-moderate atopic asthma were treated with either the VLA-4 antagonist (IVL745) or placebo twice daily by inhalation for 7 days prior to inhalation allergen challenge.[40] The VLA-4 antagonist did not inhibit the early or the late asthmatic response (measured by changes in FEV_1), methacholine hyperresponsiveness, or exhaled NO. The VLA-4 antagonist did modestly suppress the 7-day sputum eosinophil count by approximately 50% and was well tolerated in this short-term study.

In a second study, a single inhaled dose of the VLA-4 antagonist GW559090X was used to determine whether it could protect against allergen-induced changes in airway responses in 15 patients with mild intermittent asthma.[41] The VLA-4 antagonist was administered 30 min prior to allergen challenge. The VLA-4 antagonist did not inhibit the early or late phase response to inhalation allergen challenge (measured as FEV_1). No sputum eosinophils were measured in this study.

Although VLA-4 antagonists have not yet been shown to be effective in the treatment of asthma, VLA-4 antagonists such as natalizumab have shown clinical efficacy in multiple sclerosis,[42] and Crohn's disease.[43] Natalizumab binds to α_4 and thereby inhibits the interaction both between $\alpha_4\beta_1$ and VCAM-1, as well as between $\alpha_4\beta_7$ and MadCAM-1 (Fig. 9.3). In multiple sclerosis by inhibiting the interaction of leukocyte $\alpha_4\beta_1$ and blood vessel VCAM, natalizumab blocks leukocyte trafficking across the blood-brain barrier and thereby reduces inflammation within multiple sclerosis lesions. In Crohn's disease, the major cells associated with the inflammatory process are neutrophils which do not express α_4 integrin. Thus in Crohn's disease natalizumab may function by inhibiting T lymphocytes that induce cytokines and chemokines needed to sustain neutrophil recruitment.

In addition to targeting β_1 integrins with VLA-4 antagonists, human studies in asthma have also evaluated targeting β_2 integrins expressed by leukocytes with antibodies such as efalizumab.[44] Efalizumab is a humanized anti-α_L mAb, which targets leukocyte CD11a (also known as LFA-1). By targeting CD11a, efalizumab inhibits the α chain of the leukocyte β_2 integrin (CD11a/CD18, or $\alpha_L\beta_2$, or LFA-1) binding to ICAM-1 expressed by blood vessels (Fig. 9.3). In studies of mild asthmatics treated with weekly subcutaneous injections of efalizumab or placebo for approximately 4 months, efalizumab significantly reduced the post-allergen challenge increase in sputum EG2-positive eosinophils as well as metachromatic cells, but did not inhibit the early and late phase fall in FEV_1 after allergen challenge.[44] Although efalizumab therapy has not

proven to be effective in pilot studies in asthma, efalizumab therapy has resulted in significant improvements in plaque psoriasis in subjects with moderate-to-severe disease.[45]

■ IMMUNOGLOBULIN GENE SUPERFAMILY ■

The immunoglobulin gene superfamily (IgSF) of CAMs consists of more than 25 molecules.[46] The structure of this family of CAMs includes a series of globular domains, formed by disulfide bonds, resembling those found in immunoglobulins.[46] Firm adhesion of leukocytes to endothelial cells, as well as leukocyte activation is mediated by receptors of the immunoglobulin gene superfamily. These CAMs are involved in leukocyte adhesion at relatively low shear forces but cause a stronger attachment of leukocytes to the endothelium than the selectins. Figure 9.3 shows the structures of several important IgSF family members involved in leukocyte endothelial cell adhesion, as well as in endothelial cell-endothelial cell, and leukocyte-leukocyte adhesion. Other members of the IgSF include CD2, CD3, CD4, CD8, CD58, MHC class I and II, and the T cell receptor.[46] We will discuss the role of five molecules that belong to this IgSF family that are expressed by endothelial cells: intercellular adhesion molecule-1, -2 and -3 (ICAM-1, ICAM-2, and ICAM-3), vascular cell adhesion molecule-1 (VCAM-1), and platelet-endothelial cell adhesion molecule-1 (PECAM-1) (Fig. 9.3).

Intercellular adhesion molecule-1

The extracellular portion of ICAM-1 (CD54) is organized into five Ig-like domains. ICAM-1 is expressed constitutively in low amounts along the luminal, intercellular, and subluminal surface of endothelial cells, as well as by leukocytes, epithelial cells, and fibroblasts.[3,46] Levels of endothelial ICAM-1 expression greatly increase following stimulation by cytokines (IL-1, TNF-α, IFN-γ), or bacterial endotoxin. IFN-γ selectively induces ICAM-1 expression without affecting expression of other adhesion molecules.[3,46] ICAM-1 expression can be induced on eosinophils as well as other cells, including respiratory epithelial cells.[3,46] Ligands for the most N-terminal domain of ICAM-1 include LFA-1, fibrinogen, and most serotypes of rhinovirus, whereas the third domain is recognized by Mac-1.[3,46]

Intercellular adhesion molecule-2

ICAM-2 (CD102) has only two Ig-like extracellular domains that possess 34% homology to the first two domains of ICAM-1.[3,46] The ligand binding site for LFA-1 is located in the first N-terminal domain in ICAM-1. In addition to endothelial cells, ICAM-2 is constitutively expressed on mononuclear cells, basophils, mast cells, and platelets, and expression appears to be unaffected by cytokines.[3,46]

Intercellular adhesion molecule-3

ICAM-3 (CD50) also functions as an LFA-1 ligand[3,46] but it can also be recognized by $\alpha_d\beta_2$ integrin. ICAM-3 has approximately 50% homology to ICAM-1 and approximately 35% homology to ICAM-2.

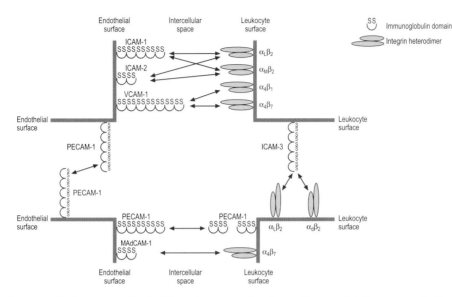

Fig. 9.3. Structure of immunoglobulin gene superfamily. Schematic representation of several immunoglobulin gene superfamily molecules expressed on endothelial cells and leukocytes. The counterligands, most of which are integrins, are also shown. Arrows denote ligand-counterligand interactions but do not indicate domains used for binding (see text). Note that mucosal-addressin cell adhesion molecule (MAdCAM-1) expression appears to be limited to endothelium in the lamina propria of the gut and to Peyer's patches, whereas others, such as vascular cell adhesion molecule-1 (VCAM-1), require specific stimuli to induce expression. ICAM, intercellular adhesion molecule; PECAM, platelet-endothelial cell adhesion molecule.

ICAM-3, like ICAM-1, has five Ig-like extracellular domains, and is constitutively expressed on all leukocytes and on mast cells. ICAM-3 cross-linking results in calcium mobilization, tyrosine phosphorylation, enhanced adhesion, chemokine secretion, and modulation of basophil mediator release.[3,46]

Vascular cell adhesion molecule-1

VCAM-1 (CD106) is a cytokine-inducible endothelial cell adhesion molecule that can be expressed in two alternatively spliced versions, existing primarily in a seven-domain form rather than the rarer six-domain form.[46] Extensive homology exists among the three N-terminal VCAM-1 domains and VCAM-1 domains 4 to 6, probably a result of gene duplication.[46] Within the extracellular portions of VCAM-1, domains 1 and 4 are most homologous to each other; these are the domains that carry the IDSPL amino acid sequence recognized by VLA-4 and $\alpha_d\beta_2$ integrin.[46]

VCAM-1 expression has been detected on cell types other than endothelium, including macrophages, dendritic cells, astrocytes, bone marrow stromal cells, and respiratory epithelial cell lines.[46] VCAM-1 can be induced de novo within several hours after exposure to IL-1, TNF-α, or bacterial endotoxin with expression reaching maximal levels by 24–48 h.[46] IL-1, TNF-α, or bacterial endotoxin induce increased expression of not only VCAM-1 but also other endothelial CAMs, including ICAM-1 and E-selectin. In contrast, IL-4 or IL-13 induce selective induction of VCAM-1 expression.[3,46] The combination of IL-4 with TNF-α is synergistic due to transcriptional activation and stabilization of VCAM-1 mRNA.[3] Patterns of VCAM-1 induction may differ among endothelial cell types.

For example, human dermal microvascular endothelial cells express VCAM-1 only after stimulation with TNF-α and not with IL-1 or IL-4.[3]

In addition to supporting α_4 integrin-mediated leukocyte rolling and adhesion,[47] VCAM-1 clustering also leads to signal transduction events that are associated with increased vascular permeability, as well as Rac1 and Rho signaling-dependent leukocyte transendothelial migration.[3,46]

Platelet-endothelial cell adhesion molecule-1

PECAM-1 (CD31) is a cell adhesion molecule expressed on endothelial cells and circulating leukocytes that plays an important role in mediating neutrophil and monocyte transendothelial migration in vivo.[48] PECAM-1 is not only constitutively expressed on endothelial cells and platelets but also on most leukocytes. PECAM is part of the immunoglobulin gene superfamily as its structure contains six immunoglobulin domains.[48] PECAM-1 is found at particularly high concentrations at inter-endothelial cell interfaces suggesting a role in transendothelial migration which has been confirmed in in vivo studies of neutrophil and mononuclear cell endothelial transmigration in mice. PECAM expressed by leukocytes can either bind to PECAM expressed by endothelial cells (homotypic binding), or PECAM can bind to an alternate ligand the integrin $\alpha_v\beta_3$ (heterotypic binding).[48] Studies with blocking antibodies suggest a critical role for PECAM-1 during neutrophil transendothelial migration in vitro and in vivo.[48] In contrast, although eosinophils express PECAM and bind to PECAM, eosinophil transmigration into the lung or cornea following allergen challenge is PECAM independent.[49] Anti-PECAM Abs do not inhibit airway responsiveness in a mouse model of asthma.[49]

INSIGHTS INTO THE ROLE OF IMMUNOGLOBULIN GENE SUPERFAMILY IN INFLAMMATION

Studies in mice deficient in ICAM-1[50] as well as in primates treated with anti-ICAM-1 Abs[51] have demonstrated an important role for ICAM-1 in eosinophilic airway inflammation in animal models of allergen-induced asthma. Intravital microscopy studies in mice deficient in ICAM-1 have demonstrated reduced firm adhesion of eosinophils to inflamed blood vessels in vivo.[25]

TARGETING IMMUNOGLOBULIN GENE SUPERFAMILY MEMBERS IN HUMAN ALLERGIC INFLAMMATION

At present, there are no published results of agents targeting immunoglobulin gene superfamily members in human subjects with asthma. However, agents targeting one of the immunoglobulin gene superfamily members (i.e. ICAM-1) have been used in clinical trials in rheumatoid arthritis, transplant rejection, and stroke which provides some insight into the safety and effectiveness of such an approach in human disease.[52,53] For example, in rheumatoid arthritis initial clinical trials with R6.5 (BIRR-1, Enlimomab), a murine IgG2a mAb to human ICAM-1 proved to be beneficial in reducing disease activity in a subset of patients with rheumatoid arthritis.[53] However, adverse effects such as fever (50%), and cutaneous reactions (22% pruritus; 9% urticaria) were frequent, and leukopenia was also noted.[52]

■ GALECTINS, CADHERINS, AND CD44 ■

GALECTINS

Galectins are a family of β-galactose-recognizing proteins that exhibit a conserved $\approx$130 amino acid carbohydrate-recognition domain (CRD).[54] Among the various galectins, galectin-3 has been shown to be involved in allergic inflammation and airway hyperreactivity in a mouse model of asthma.[55] Based on their conserved structural features, galectins can be subdivided into those containing one CRD that exist as dimers (galectin-1, -2, -5, -7, -10, -11, -13, -14, and -15); those containing two CRDs separated by a single-chain polypeptide linker of up to 70 amino acids (galectin-4, -6, -8, -9, and -12); and finally galectin-3, which is distinct and contains a long 120 amino acid N-terminal domain joined to the CRD (Fig. 9.4). Galectin-3 can form pentamers after binding to multivalent carbohydrates.[54]

Although galectins appear to exhibit a wide array of functions in different physiological and pathological conditions, in the context of inflammation, their ability to regulate cell adhesion is noteworthy. Endothelial cell-expressed galectin-3 mediates rolling and adhesion of human carcinoma cells under flow conditions in vitro.[54] Furthermore, galectin-3 can directly bind to polylactosamine residues on integrins via its CRD.[54]

Galectin	Type	Structure
1, 2, 5, 7, 10, 11, 13, 14, and 15	One-CRD	
4, 6, 8, 9, and 12	Two-CRD	
3	Chimeric	

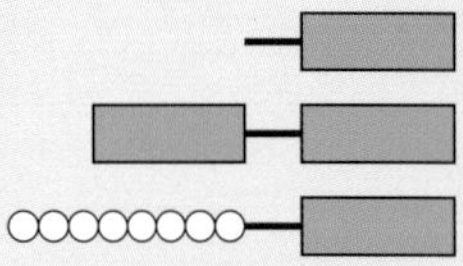

Fig. 9.4. Structure of galectin. Galectins are a family of lectins that contain conserved carbohydrate-recognition domains (CRDs), which play a vital role in the ability of galectins to recognize and interact with specific galactose-containing oligosaccharide structures. Galectins are subdivided into three major groups: one-CRD; two distinct CRDs in sequence with a linker; and galectin-3, which is unusual in that it is composed of repeating tandem units fused onto the CRD to form a chimeric galectin.

CADHERINS

Cadherins are transmembrane proteins that mediate intercellular adhesion in epithelial and endothelial cells. To date, over 80 proteins within the cadherin family, having different structures, functions, and localizations, have been identified.[56] The cadherin family of adhesion molecules include E-, N-, P-, T-, and VE-cadherins, protocadherins, seven-transmembrane cadherin, and FAT-family cadherin. Cadherins are found on structural cells, including endothelium and epithelium and are potentially involved in maintaining tissue integrity, cell–cell recognition, signaling, communication, growth, and angiogenesis.[56] Cadherins are composed of five extracellular domains (N-terminus), a transmembrane domain, and a cytoplasmic domain (C-terminus) and are involved in homotypic or heterotypic adhesion between adjacent cells and provide linkage through α and β catenins and vinculin to the actin cytoskeleton through their cytoplasmic domains.[56] The adherens junction functional unit in endothelial or epithelial cells is composed of the cadherin/catenin complex where the β or α catenin can physically interact with the catenin-binding domain near the C-terminus of cadherin. This complex in turn links to the actin cytoskeleton network via α catenin as the linker protein to mediate cellular function.[56] At endothelial cell adherence junctions, for example, structures within desmosomes contain VE-cadherin, with linkage to intermediate filaments via plakoglobin, plakophilins, desmocollin, and desmoglein. In the skin, diseases such as pemphigus are associated with autoimmune responses targeted against certain cadherins.[56]

CD44

CD44 is found in high levels on most leukocytes, endothelial cells, epithelial cells, and other cells and has been implicated in a variety of biological processes including lymphopoiesis, angiogenesis, wound healing, leukocyte extravasation at inflammatory sites, and tumor metastasis.[57] The adhesive function of CD44, like other molecules involved in inducible adhesion, is tightly regulated. The ligand binding properties of CD44 can be modulated by multiple factors such as post-translational modifications, isoform expression, aggregation state, and protein associations that are regulated by cell type and the activation state of the cell. Many splice-variant forms of CD44 of differing molecular weights have been identified. The most extensively characterized ligand for CD44 is hyaluronan, which is a component of the extracellular matrix.[57] Interactions between CD44 and hyaluronan can mediate both cell–cell and cell–extracellular matrix adhesion. CD44 has also been shown to mediate interactions between lymphocytes and airway smooth muscle cells, inducing growth of the latter cell type.[57] Cytokines including IL-3, IL-5, and granulocyte-macrophage colony stimulating factor (GM-CSF) appear to increase CD44 expression on eosinophils. However, the functional significance of CD44 expression on eosinophils has not been identified as these cells do not appear to interact with hyaluronate, its natural ligand.[58] In mouse models of asthma, administration of an anti-CD44 mAb prevented both lymphocyte and eosinophil accumulation in the lung, and reduced airway hyperresponsiveness.[59]

TARGETING ADHESION MOLECULES IN HUMAN ALLERGIC INFLAMMATION

At present there are no studies evaluating the therapeutic benefit of targeting galectins, CD44, or cadherins in human asthma and allergy.

■ LEUKOCYTE ADHESION TO AND ACROSS THE ENDOTHELIUM ■

The recruitment of circulating leukocytes from the bloodstream to the extravascular sites of inflammation involves a series of overlapping and sequential steps and is mediated by selectins and integrins (Fig. 9.5).[60,61]

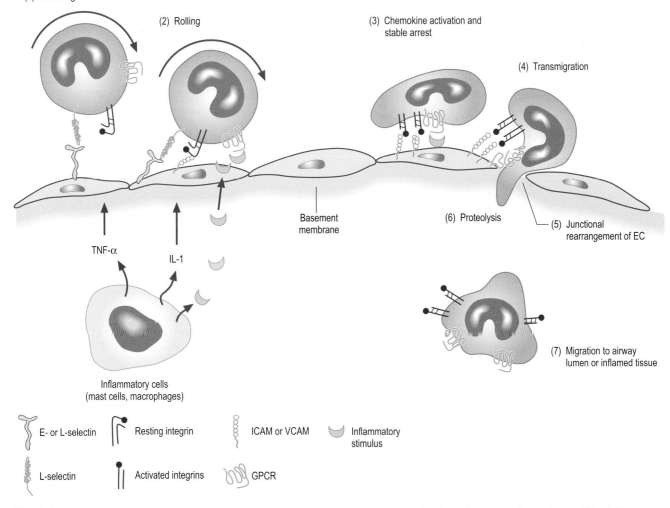

Fig. 9.5. Leukocyte endothelial cell adhesion. The sequential steps of leukocyte adhesion to endothelium that occur under conditions of blood flow in vivo are depicted. Leukocytes initially tether to endothelium (step 1), roll along endothelium (step 2), become firmly adherent following chemokine activation (step 3), transmigrate between endothelial cells (step 4) which is associated with junctional rearrangement of endothelium (step 5), proteolysis (step 6), and migration of leukocyte in the extracellular matrix of tissues (step 7).

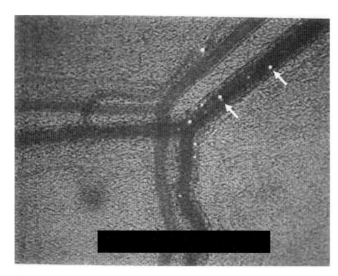

Fig. 9.6. Intravital videomicroscopy of eosinophil endothelial cell adhesion in vivo. This figure demonstrates the use of intravital videomicroscopy to visualize fluorescently labeled eosinophils rolling on inflamed endothelium (arrows). The interior of the blood vessel is black, whereas the wall of the blood vessel and surrounding tissue is gray in color.

Under condition of physiologic shear stress, leukocytes, including eosinophils, neutrophils, monocytes, and lymphocytes, engage in multiple activation and adhesive interactions with endothelial cells before emigrating into the peripheral tissues. The first step of this adhesion cascade involves the ability of freely flowing leukocytes to undergo a rapid and reversible capture by endothelium that is facilitated by weak adhesive interactions between selectins and carbohydrates leading to leukocyte rolling on the endothelial cell surface. Depending on the type of leukocyte and target endothelial bed, most of these transient rolling adhesions last from a few seconds to minutes.[62] Leukocyte rolling on endothelium can be visualized microscopically in vivo using intravital videomicroscopy in several vascular beds including the mesentery, lymph nodes, cremaster, liver, brain, and lungs (Fig. 9.6). While both P-selectin and E-selectin support neutrophil rolling under conditions of flow, eosinophil rolling in post-capillary venules appears to be mediated predominantly by P-selectin[25] but not E-selectin.[7] It has been suggested that rolling may actually be two separable events, tethering and rolling, in which L-selectin on the leukocyte presents oligosaccharide ligands to either E-selectin or P-selectin expressed by endothelial cells to initiate tethering before stable rolling can occur through interaction of vascular selectins with other leukocyte ligands. In addition to selectins, α_4 integrins ($\alpha_4\beta_1$ and $\alpha_4\beta_7$) can also mediate rolling of circulating eosinophils and T-lymphocytes through interactions with ligands including VCAM-1 and potentially MAdCAM.[47,63,64] While integrin-mediated rolling most likely stabilizes the L-selectin-initiated capture and rolling, α_4 integrins may independently support leukocyte rolling.[47,63]

The next step in the adhesion cascade is stable arrest or 'firm adhesion' and requires activation of one or more of the four main integrins: $\alpha_4\beta_1$, $\alpha_4\beta_7$, $\alpha_M\beta_2$, and $\alpha_L\beta_2$.[60–62] While the molecular basis of integrin activation and cell sticking (arrest) is not completely understood, it is believed that leukocyte integrin activation occurs due to their exposure to leukocyte-activating factors (such as chemoattractants and chemokines) produced by or displayed on the surface of endothelial cells.[60–62] Studies have shown that a combination of chemokines and G protein-coupled receptors (GPCRs) are involved in promoting integrin-dependent arrest under shear flow.[60–62] In addition to chemokines, several effector molecules such as CD44, CD47, CD98, and tetraspanins, regulate the conformational switch of integrins, leading to their ability to microcluster and anchor to actin cytoskeleton, leading to increases in the avidity of integrins on the leukocyte surface and their increased binding to counterligands such as ICAM-1 and VCAM-1.[3] Cytokines, chemokines, and other chemotactic factors can potentiate the processes of adhesion and transendothelial migration by directly activating leukocyte migration responses. In addition, endothelial-expressed oxidases such as vascular adhesion protein-1 (VAP-1) may also contribute to stabilization of rolling and subsequent integrin-mediated arrest of leukocytes through modification of endothelial and leukocyte ligands.

The vascular endothelium is normally impermeable to leukocytes and macromolecules, forming a non-adhesive barrier between blood and tissue. However, during episodes of inflammation the endothelium undergoes changes in vascular permeability and facilitates programmed transmigration of leukocytes through the basement membrane.[60] The paracellular (junctional) route of leukocyte transmigration is the dominant pathway for leukocyte diapedesis. However, in some studies neutrophils have been reported to utilize a transcellular process of migration across endothelium in vivo. The active participation of apical and junctional ICAM-1 and VCAM-1 has been demonstrated in leukocyte transmigration across endothelium.[60] Depending on the site of inflammation, transmigration can be facilitated by the engagement of junctional endothelial ligands such as CD99, junctional adhesion molecules (JAMs), and PECAM-1.[48] In addition, a critical role for GTPase, Rap1, and RhoA has been implicated during leukocyte transmigration. The Rac family of GTPases, specific protein kinases, phophotidylinositol-3-OH kinase (PI$_3$K) isoforms and focal adhesion kinases promote motility and directed migration of leukocytes across endothelial barriers.[65] Among these, the PI$_3$K isoforms including PI$_3$Kγ and PI$_3$Kδ appear to be involved in the directed migration of distinct immune cells including granulocytes, macrophages, dendritic cells, eosinophils, and mast cells during varied inflammatory conditions.[66] Transendothelial leukocyte migration appears to be additionally dependent on the engagement of VE-cadherins and β catenins (cytoskeletal linkers) that result in localized and temporal loss of junctional endothelial cell assemblies and adherens junctions.[56]

Subsequent to endothelial adhesion, leukocytes emigrate between endothelial cells and penetrate the basement membrane to enter the extravascular space. This process is potentially mediated through the engagement of Rap1 GTPases on transmigrating leukocytes leading to increased avidity of leukocyte β_1 and β_2 integrins for ECM proteins promoting their motility through the basement lamina.[60] For example, $\alpha_1\beta_1$, $\alpha_2\beta_1$, and $\alpha_6\beta_1$ have been shown to be important in the location and retention of various leukocyte subsets in different inflamed tissues.[60] Furthermore, specific proteases such as matrix metalloproteinase-9 (MMP-9) that are upregulated in leukocytes in response to stimulation with chemoattractants may contribute to motility through the basement membrane lamina. Additionally, cytokines, chemokines, and other chemotactic factors, through activation of β_2 integrins ($\alpha_m\beta_2$, $\alpha_L\beta_2$, $\alpha_x\beta_2$), potentiate the processes of adhesion and transendothelial migration.[67]

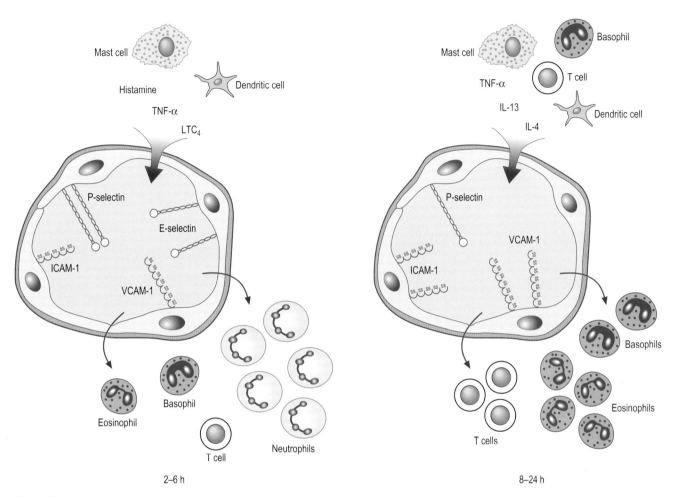

Fig. 9.7. Regulation of adhesion molecule expression. Hypothetic model by which IgE-dependent cellular activation could result in profiles of cytokines and other mediators that selectively stimulate endothelial expression of intercellular adhesion molecule-1 (ICAM-1), vascular cell adhesion molecule-1 (VCAM-1), and other adhesion molecules during allergic inflammatory reactions. TNF, tumor necrosis factor; LTC, leukotriene C; IL, interleukin.

■ LEUKOCYTE ADHESION IN THE EXTRACELLULAR MATRIX IN TISSUES ■

Following the adhesion of leukocytes to adhesion molecules expressed by endothelial cells at sites of allergic inflammation, leukocytes diapedese between endothelial cells and migrate along a chemokine gradient into tissues where they come in contact with extracellular matrix proteins.[68] Leukocytes express adhesion receptors which allow them to bind to extracellular matrix proteins (e.g., fibronectin, laminin, vitronectin, tenascin, collagen). The adhesion of leukocytes to extracellular matrix proteins is frequently associated with modulation of leukocyte functional responses (e.g., changes in leukocyte activation status, mediator release, survival, etc.).[68]

Most leukocyte adhesion receptors for extracellular matrix proteins belong to the β_1 integrin family (Table 9.1). For example, eosinophils can bind to the extracellular matrix protein fibronectin through $\alpha_4\beta_1$ integrins (VLA-4) expressed by eosinophils. The counter-receptor to VLA-4 expressed in the extracellular matrix is the CS 1 region of fibronectin.[68,69] Eosinophil adhesion to fibronectin through VLA-4 activates a variety of eosinophil functions, including production of superoxide anion, leukotriene release, degranulation, as well as release of GM-CSF (augments eosinophil survival in an autocrine fashion).[68,69] Basophils and mast cells also express VLA-4 and can thus bind to fibronectin in the extracellular matrix.[70] Basophils from asthmatic (but not normal) donors release histamine on antibody cross-linking of β_1 integrins, whereas IgE-dependent basophil and mast cell mediator release is inhibited by β_1 integrin cross-linking.[70] Studies of rat, mouse, or culture-derived human mast cells, demonstrate that mast cell interactions with fibronectin enhances IgE-dependent histamine and cytokine release.[70] In vivo studies demonstrate that administration of α_4 integrin antibodies to sensitized rats inhibits mast cell activation and prevents acute allergic airway responses.[70] Thus, integrin engagement can affect a wide range of biologic activities on eosinophils, basophils, and mast cells.

Table 9.2 Human disease associated with adhesion molecule deficiency

Human syndrome	Adhesion molecule defect	Clinical phenotype
LAD-I	β_1 integrin structure	Absent or near-absent expression of all β_1 integrins; blood neutrophilia with tissue neutropenia, delayed umbilical cord separation, recurrent soft tissue infections (e.g., skin, periodontal), impaired pus formation and wound healing; reduced or absent neutrophil adhesion, transendothelial migration, and chemotactic responses; normal rolling adhesion
LAD-I variants	β_1 integrin function	β_1 integrins expressed but dysfunctional; biologic consequences identical to those of LAD-I
LAD-II	GFTP gene and sLe^X	Defect in fucosylation of many structures, including sialyl-Lewis-X (sLe^X); developmental abnormalities (e.g., severe mental retardation, short stature, distinctive facial appearance). Bombay (hh) blood phenotype, impaired pus formation, pneumonia, periodontitis, and otitis; neutrophil studies, reduced or absent sLe^X expression, reduced rolling adhesion, normal firm adhesion
LAD-III	Integrin signaling	LAD-III is a very rare disorder characterized by severe recurrent infections, a bleeding tendency and marked leukocytosis. Leukocytes and platelets have normal expression of CD18 (defective in LAD-I), normal expression of CD15a (defective in LAD-II), but defective integrin signaling
E-selectin	E-selectin	Case report of child with clinical presentation similar to LAD disease but whose neutrophils expressed normal levels of β_1 integrins, L-selectin, and sLe^X; staining of inflamed tissue revealed no E-selectin

LAD-I, leukocyte adhesion deficiency type I; LAD-II, leukocyte adhesion deficiency type II; LAD-III, leukocyte adhesion deficiency type III.

Human skin mast cells express α_3 integrins that are used for adhesion to and migration on laminin.[71] Laminins are extracellular matrix proteins that may be important in attachment of inflammatory cells in the extracellular matrix. Laminin-1 binds to several cell surface receptors including integrin receptors expressed on leukocytes (e.g. $\alpha_6\beta_1$, $\alpha_6\beta_4$ and $\alpha_7\beta_1$). Mast cell interactions with laminin may be important in their tissue localization in vivo.[71] Eosinophils can also bind to laminin through α_6 integrins.

■ REGULATION OF ADHESION MOLECULE EXPRESSION ■

A variety of pro-inflammatory mediators (histamine, cytokines) are released at sites of allergic inflammation that may regulate the expression of adhesion molecules expressed by inflamed endothelium (Fig. 9.7). In the absence of an inflammatory stimulus, endothelial cells do not express adhesion molecules and thus circulating leukocytes do not adhere to such non-inflamed blood vessels. However, following an allergic stimulus, resident tissue mast cells rapidly release histamine and TNF from preformed cytoplasmic granule stores, as well as LTC$_4$ from membrane lipids which induce adhesion molecule expression by

endothelium. Subsequently several cell types including macrophages (TNF), mast cells (TNF, IL-4, IL-13), and T cells (IL-4, IL-13) transcribe and release cytokines which also upregulate expression of adhesion molecules by endothelium. The kinetics of expression of endothelial adhesion molecules varies with preformed P-selectin being rapidly expressed within 30 min after stimulation with histamine (or other activating stimuli such as TNF-α, lipopolysaccharide, thrombin, complement C5a), whereas E-selectin (4–6 h), and ICAM-1 and VCAM-1 (8–24 h) have peaks of expression at later timepoints. In addition some cytokines (e.g., TNF and IL-1) induce several adhesion molecules (E-selectin, ICAM-1, VCAM-1), whereas other cytokines (IL-4, IL-13) are selective for VCAM-1 expression and do not induce E-selectin or ICAM-1.

Cytokines not only regulate adhesion molecule expression on endothelium but also influence adhesion molecules which are constitutively expressed on circulating leukocytes by inducing their upregulation, shedding, or change in affinity. For example, exposure of eosinophils to IL-3, IL-5, or GM-CSF augments adhesion molecule function, induces L-selectin shedding and CD11b upregulation, and enhances chemoattractant-induced adhesion responses and transendothelial migration, with little or no effect on neutrophils.[72] Cytokines and chemokines may also be important in regulating the functional state of integrins expressed by leukocytes.

■ HUMAN DISEASE ASSOCIATED WITH ADHESION MOLECULE DEFICIENCY ■

LAD-I

Of the LAD syndromes, LAD-I is the most common (described in over 300 patients) (Table 9.2).[28] LAD-I is due to a genetic defect in the β subunit (CD18) of the integrin.[28] The absence of β_2 integrin expression on neutrophils results in blood neutrophilia with tissue neutropenia. Hallmarks of LAD-I are delayed separation of the umbilical cord, recurrent severe bacterial infection without pus formation, marked leukocytosis, and the absence or marked decrease in CD18 expression on the leukocyte surface. Patients with severe LAD-I do not survive childhood and the only curative therapy is bone marrow transplantation.[28] Patients with a milder form of LAD-I have been described who have point mutations which disrupted integrin function rather than integrin expression as is noted in the majority of LAD-I patients.

LAD-II

LAD-II is a rare condition[28] (Table 9.2), which is characterized by recurrent infection, growth and mental retardation, and lack of expression of the fucose-containing structures (CD15a) and the red blood cell H antigen. Subsequent studies have demonstrated that LAD-II is associated with a generalized defect in fucose metabolism due to a defect in a Golgi-associated guanosine diphosphate-fucose transporter (GFTP) protein.[28] As fucose-containing sLe^X is an adhesion molecule ligand for selectins expressed on leukocytes as well as on endothelial cells, neutrophils from LAD-II subjects are unable to adhere to P-selectin and E-selectin expressed by endothelial cells. LAD-II patients suffer from infection to a lesser degree than those with LAD-I. They have a defect in the first phase of the adhesion cascade, the selectin-mediated rolling phase. The primary defect is a genetic mutation in the GFTP transporter of fucose from the cytoplasm into the Golgi apparatus. Thus, glycans like CD15a or the H antigen (Bombay) which incorporate fucose, are not expressed on myeloid cells. This is a general genetic defect in fucose metabolism in all cells in the body (defect not confined to hematopoietic or endothelial cells) and thus there is associated severe growth and mental retardation. In a case report, fucose administration significantly improved both the clinical state as well as the leukocyte adhesion abnormality.[28]

LAD-III

The recently described LAD-III syndrome (Table 9.2) is also very rare[28] with clinical symptoms characterized by severe recurrent infections, bleeding tendency and marked leukocytosis with normal expression of CD18 (defective in LAD-I) and normal expression of CD15a (defective in LAD-II). In LAD III several integrins (β_1, β_2, and β_3) expressed by either leukocytes or platelets are defective in signaling, resulting in their inability to adhere.[73] Hence LAD-III patients have a tendency for bleeding in addition to the severe recurrent infections.

Although integrin expression and structure are normal in LAD-III, patients with LAD-III have marked defects in integrin activation signaling by physiological inside-out stimuli such as chemokines.[28] This defect in inside-out integrin signaling is evident in leukocytes (neutrophils, lymphocytes) as well as in platelets. In LAD-III patients integrin signals do not enhance platelet aggregation, or neutrophil adhesion to ICAM-1 or fibronectin. Agonists that directly stimulate integrin activity bypassing inside-out signaling are able to reconstitute integrin-dependent adhesion, suggesting that leukocytes from LAD-III patients express structurally intact integrins.

■ ADHESION MOLECULES IN HUMAN ALLERGIC INFLAMMATION ■

ALLERGEN CHALLENGE STUDIES IN THE SKIN

The skin provides an accessible organ to biopsy in research studies examining the expression of adhesion molecules in blood vessels following allergen challenge. These allergen challenge studies in the skin confirm that adhesion molecules are expressed in skin blood vessels following challenge. Intradermal injection with allergen induces endothelial cells in the skin to express E-selectin and VCAM-1, and also increases endothelial expression of ICAM-1.[74,75] Studies have attempted to use correlations to gain insight into which cytokines upregulate adhesion molecules in the skin following allergen challenge. In a skin allergen challenge study the number of IL-13-positive cells, but not IL-4-positive cells, correlated with both VCAM-1 staining and eosinophils at both 6 and 24h after challenge[76] suggesting that IL-13 rather than IL-4 was important for VCAM-1 expression and eosinophil recruitment in the skin. Unfortunately, correlative studies cannot establish a cause and effect relationship between levels of expression of adhesion molecules, cytokines, and recruited inflammatory cells. Studies using neutralizing Abs to individual cytokines or adhesion molecules are therefore needed to extend our insight into these initial correlative clinical studies. An important role for IL-1 and TNF in inducing E selectin expression in skin endothelial cells was suggested from studies in which E-selectin expression induced in skin sites was inhibited when the skin biopsy was immediately placed into culture with a mixture of Abs that neutralize IL-1 and TNF-α.[75]

ALLERGIC RHINITIS

Increases in levels of nasal mucosa VCAM-1 have been observed 24h after local intranasal allergen challenge, with the number of infiltrating eosinophils correlating with the extent and intensity of VCAM-1 staining.[77] However, when allergic rhinitis subjects were pretreated with intranasal beclomethasone, allergen-induced symptoms and superficial mucosal eosinophils were reduced without affecting the number of infiltrating submucosal eosinophils or endothelial VCAM-1 expression.[78] Interestingly, local nasal provocation of subjects with allergic rhinitis resulted in both nasal and bronchial eosinophilia, in association with increased expression of ICAM-1, VCAM-1, and E-selectin on both nasal and bronchial blood vessels.[79] This finding suggests that nasal challenge can result in endothelial activation and eosinophil recruitment at multiple levels throughout the airway.

In perennial rhinitis, studies of nasal tissue detected increased expression of ICAM-1 and VCAM-1, but not E-selectin, compared to non-allergic control subjects.[3] Seasonal exposure to pollen is associated with increases in nasal epithelial cell expression of ICAM-1 along with increased numbers of eosinophils, neutrophils, and metachromatic cells.[3] In nasal polyps, evidence suggests roles for P-selectin and VCAM-1 in eosinophil recruitment.[3,19] Studies have also implicated TNF-α as a possible inducer of VCAM-1 in the nasal mucosa.[80]

ASTHMA

In asthma endobronchial allergen challenge increases endothelial VCAM-1 staining and epithelial ICAM-1 staining, which correlates significantly with eosinophil influx.[81] Increased levels of soluble forms of E-selectin, ICAM-1, and VCAM-1 have been noted in BAL fluids in asthmatics following allergen challenge.[82] Allergen challenge in asthma is also associated with changes in levels of adhesion molecules expressed by circulating leukocytes. For example analysis of levels of adhesion molecules expressed on granulocytes recovered from blood and from BAL after antigen challenge revealed increased expression of CD11b, diminished levels of L-selectin, and little or no change in expression of LFA-1, CD32, or VLA-4.[81,82]

In asthmatic subjects, baseline E-selectin expression is increased on endothelial cells of bronchial mucosal biopsies compared with healthy subjects, and is further increased 5–6 h after allergen challenge, coinciding with the recruitment of eosinophils, neutrophils, and lymphocytes into the airway mucosa.[82] In addition, sLe^X glycans, the ligand for selectins, are increased in lung endothelial cells in asthmatic subjects.[82]

While studies of allergen challenge in asthma demonstrate induced expression of adhesion molecules, studies of levels of adhesion molecule expression in asthma unrelated to allergen challenge are somewhat contradictory, perhaps because of differences in patient severity and treatments. Several studies have examined adhesion molecule expression in the airways of mild asthmatics which are less confounded with therapy than studies of patients with moderate to severe asthma. One study examining mild asthmatics used bronchial mucosal biopsies from subjects with mild allergic asthma and normal subjects and found similar levels of endothelial ICAM-1 and E-selectin, despite an increased number of eosinophils in the mucosa of the mild asthmatic patients.[82] Treatment of mild asthmatics with inhaled corticosteroids reduced the tissue eosinophilia without changing ICAM-1 or E-selectin expression. Another study of mild asthmatics compared endothelial adhesion molecule expression in airway biopsies from subjects with mild allergic and non-allergic asthma as well as normal controls.[81] Endothelial staining for ICAM-1 and E-selectin, but not VCAM-1, was significantly increased in the mild asthmatic who were not allergic, but was not increased in the mild asthmatics who were allergic.[81] Epithelial staining for ICAM-1 was increased in both groups of mild asthmatic subjects.

In contrast to studies of mild asthmatics, studies of moderately symptomatic asthmatic patients have noted strong endothelial staining for VCAM-1 as well as for ICAM-1, which correlated with levels of IL-4 in the airway.[82] Increased serum levels of soluble ICAM-1 and E-selectin, but not VCAM-1, have been measured in asthmatic patients admitted for exacerbations.[82] However, in other studies increased levels of soluble VCAM-1 have been reported in asthmatic patients.[82]

Studies have also examined the effect of asthma medications on levels of adhesion molecule expression. VCAM-1 staining of airways from asthmatic patients before and after 8 weeks treatment with inhaled budesonide or formoterol revealed that only the budesonide-treated subjects had a reduction in VCAM-1 expression,[83] while both treatments reduced eosinophil numbers. In another study, prednisone reduced levels of soluble E-selectin in BAL fluid.[84]

ESINOPHILIC ESOPHAGITIS

Pediatric patients with eosinophilic esophagitis have increased levels of VCAM 1 staining of blood vessels,[85] further supporting the role of VCAM-1 in eosinophilic inflammation.

◼ POTENTIAL SIDE EFFECTS OF ADHESION-BASED THERAPY ◼

The potential side effects of adhesion-based therapy has been best studied in autoimmune diseases rather than asthma. For example, blocking the adhesive functions of α_4 integrins has been shown to be an effective therapeutic approach in the treatment of autoimmune diseases, but also carries the risk of defects in development, hematopoiesis, and immune surveillance. Until 2006, approximately 8000 patients had received the α_4-integrin antagonist natalizumab for the treatment of multiple sclerosis or Crohn's disease.[86] Although major side effects have been infrequent, the occurrence of three cases of progressive multifocal leukoencephalopathy (PML) and their association with anti-α_4 therapy[87,88] led to suspension of natalizumab from sales and clinical trials in the USA in February 2005.[89] In June 2006 the FDA approved an application for resumed marketing of natalizumab with a special restricted distribution program.[86] Long-term α_4-integrin blockade in some patients can lead to impaired immune surveillance of the central nervous system (CNS) by inhibiting α_4 integrin-mediated immune cell trafficking to the CNS, and thus allowing JC virus replication.[90]

◼ SUMMARY ◼

Advances in our understanding of the cellular and molecular pathways involved in leukocyte adhesion have provided insight into molecular causes of immunodeficiencies (i.e. LAD-I, LAD-II, LAD-III), as well as provide insight into potential adhesion-based therapeutic targets in asthma and allergy. At present clinical studies have demonstrated the potential benefit of adhesion-based therapies in multiple sclerosis, Crohn's disease, and psoriasis, but have not yet, in the initial small-scale studies, demonstrated their utility in asthma and allergic diseases. This will require further study.

References

Selectins and selectin ligands

1. Sperandio M. Selectins and glycosyltransferases in leukocyte rolling in vivo. FEBS J 2006; 273:4377.
2. Kansas GS, Ley K, Munro JM, et al. Regulation of leukocyte rolling and adhesion to high endothelial venules through the cytoplasmic domain of L-selectin. J Exp Med 1993; 177:833.
3. Bochner BS, ed. Adhesion molecules in allergic disease. New York: Marcel Dekker; 1997.
4. Butcher EC, Picker LJ. Lymphocyte homing and homeostasis. Science 1996; 272:60.

5. Bevilacqua MP, Pober JS, Mendrick DL, et al. Identification of an inducible endothelial-leukocyte adhesion molecule. Proc Natl Acad Sci USA 1987; 84:9238.
6. Bochner BS, Sterbinsky SA, Bickel CA, et al. Differences between human eosinophils and neutrophils in the function and expression of sialic acid-containing counterligands for E-selectin. J Immunol 1994; 152:774.
7. Sriramarao P, Norton CR, Borgstrom P, et al. E-selectin preferentially supports neutrophil but not eosinophil rolling under conditions of flow in vitro and in vivo. J Immunol 1996; 157:4672.
8. Newman W, Beall LD, Carson CW, et al. Soluble E-selectin is found in supernatants of activated endothelial cells and is elevated in the serum of patients with septic shock. J Immunol 1993; 150:644.
9. Montgomery DF, Osborn L, Hession C, et al. Activation of endothelial-leukocyte adhesion molecule 1 (ELAM-1) gene transcription. Proc Natl Acad Sci U S A 1991; 88:6523.
10. Lorant DE, Topham MK, Whatley RE, et al. Inflammatory roles of P-selectin. J Clin Invest 1993; 92:559.
11. Khew-Goodall Y, Butcher CM, Litwin MS, et al. Chronic expression of P-selectin on endothelial cells stimulated by the T-cell cytokine, interleukin-3. Blood 1996; 84:1432.
12. Cooper D, Butcher CM, Berndt MC, et al. P-selectin interacts with a $\beta2$-integrin to enhance phagocytosis. J Immunol 1994; 153:3199.
13. Weyrich AS, McIntyre TM, McEver RP, et al. Monocyte tethering by P-selectin regulates monocyte chemotactic protein-1 and tumor necrosis factor-alpha secretion. J Clin Invest 1995; 95:2297.
14. Lorant DE, McEver RP, Mcintyre TM, et al. Activation of polymorphonuclear leukocytes reduces their adhesion to P-selectin and causes redistribution of ligands for P-selectin on their surfaces. J Clin Invest 1995; 96:171.
15. Lowe JB, Ward PA. Therapeutic inhibition of carbohydrate-protein interactions in vivo. J Clin Invest 1997; 99:822.
16. Varki A. Selectin ligands: will the real ones please stand up? J Clin Invest 1997; 99:158.
17. Phillips ML, Nudelman E, Gaeta FC, et al. ELAM-1 mediates cell adhesion by recognition of a carbohydrate ligand, sialyl-Lex. Science 1990; 250:1130.
18. Wein M, Sterbinsky SA, Bickel CA, et al. Comparison of eosinophil and neutrophil ligands for P-selectin: ligands for P-selectin differ from those for E-selectin. Am J Respir Cell Mol Biol 1995; 12:315.
19. Symon FA, Walsh GM, Watson SR, et al. Eosinophil adhesion to nasal polyp endothelium is P-selectin-dependent. J Exp Med 1994; 180:371.
20. Rosen SD. Ligands for L-selectin: homing, inflammation, and beyond. Ann Rev Immunol 2004; 22:129.
21. Leung DYM, Picker LJ. Adhesion pathways controlling recruitment responses of lymphocytes during allergic inflammatory reactions in vivo. In: Bochner BS, ed. Adhesion molecules in allergic diseases. New York: Marcel Dekker; 1997:297.
22. Steegmaier M, Levinovitz A, Isenmann S, et al. The E-selectin ligand ESL-1 is a variant of a receptor for fibroblast growth factor. Nature 1995; 373:615.
23. Homeister JW, Thall AD, Petryniak B, et al. The $\alpha(1,3)$fucosyltransferases FucT-IV and Fuc T-VII exert collaborative control over selectin-dependent leukocyte recruitment and lymphocyte homing. Immunity 2001; 15:115.
24. De Sanctis GT, Wolyniec WW, Green FH, et al. Reduction of allergic airway responses in P-selectin-deficient mice. J Appl Physiol 1997; 83:681.
25. Broide DH, Humber D, Sullivan S, et al. Inhibition of eosinophil rolling and recruitment in P-selectin- and intracellular adhesion molecule-1-deficient mice. Blood 1998; 91:2847.
26. Fiscus LC, Van Herpen J, Steeber DA, et al. L-Selectin is required for the development of airway hyperresponsiveness but not airway inflammation in a murine model of asthma. J Allergy Clin Immunol 2001; 107:1019.
27. Maly P, Thall AD, Petryniak B, et al. The $\alpha(1,3)$ fucosyltransferase Fuc-TVII controls leukocyte trafficking through an essential role in L-, E-, and P-selectin ligand biosynthesis, Cell 1996; 86:643.
28. Etzioni A, Alon R. Leukocyte adhesion deficiency III: a group of integrin activation defects in hematopoietic lineage cells. Curr Opin Allergy Clin Immunol 2004; 4:485.
29. DeLisser HM, Christofidou-Solomidou M, Sun J, et al. Loss of endothelial surface expression of E-selectin in a patient with recurrent infections. Blood 1999; 94:884.
30. Avila PC, Boushey HA, Wong H, et al. Effect of a single dose of the selectin inhibitor TBC1269 on early and late asthmatic responses. Clin Exp Allergy 2004; 34:77.

Integrins

31. Hynes RO. The emergence of integrins: a personal and historical perspective. Matrix Biol 2004; 23:333.
32. Humphries JD, Byron A, Humphries MJ. Integrin ligands at a glance. J Cell Sci 2006; 119:3901.
33. Bochner BS, Schleimer RP. Endothelial cells and cell adhesion. In: Kaplan AP, ed. Allergy. 2nd edn. Philadelphia: WB Saunders; 1997:251.
34. Polito AJ, Proud D. Epithelial cells: phenotype, substratum and mediator production. In: Bochner BS, ed. Cell adhesion molecules in allergic disease. New York: Marcel Dekker; 1997:43.
35. Tachimoto H, Hudson SA, Bochner BS. Acquisition and alteration of adhesion molecules during cultured human mast cell differentiation. J Allergy Clin Immunol 2000; 107:302.
36. Kitayama J, Mackay CR, Ponath PD, et al. The C-C chemokine receptor CCR3 participates in stimulation of eosinophil arrest on inflammatory endothelium in shear flow. J Clin Invest 1998; 101:2017.
37. Abraham WM, Sielczak MW, Ahmed A, et al. Alpha 4-integrins mediate antigen-induced late bronchial responses and prolonged airway hyperresponsiveness in sheep. J Clin Invest 1994; 93:776.
38. Henderson WR, Chi EY, Albert RK, et al. Blockade of CD49d (alpha4 integrin) on intrapulmonary but not circulating leukocytes inhibits airway inflammation and hyperresponsiveness in a mouse model of asthma. J Clin Invest 1997; 100:3083.

39. Rabb HA, Olivenstein R, Issekutz TB, et al. The role of the leukocyte adhesion molecules VLA-4, LFA-1, and Mac-1 in allergic airway responses in the rat. Am J Respir Crit Care Med 1994; 149:1186.
40. Norris V, Choong L, Tran D, et al. Effect of IVL745, a VLA-4 antagonist, on allergen-induced bronchoconstriction in patients with asthma. J Allergy Clin Immunol 2005; 116:761.
41. Ravensberg AJ, Luijk B, Westers P, et al. The effect of a single inhaled dose of a VLA-4 antagonist on allergen-induced airway responses and airway inflammation in patients with asthma. Allergy 2006; 61:1097.
42. Miller DH, Khan OA, Sheremata WA, et al. A controlled trial of natalizumab for relapsing multiple sclerosis. N Engl J Med 2003; 348:15.
43. Ghosh S, Goldin E, Gordon FH, et al. Natalizumab for active Crohn's disease. N Engl J Med 2003; 348:24.
44. Gauvreau GM, Becker AB, Boulet LP, et al. The effects of an anti-CD11a mAb, efalizumab, on allergen-induced airway responses and airway inflammation in subjects with atopic asthma. J Allergy Clin Immunol 2003; 112:331.
45. Lebwohl M, Tyring SK, Hamilton TK, et al. Efalizumab Study Group. A novel targeted T-cell modulator, efalizumab, for plaque psoriasis. N Engl J Med 2003; 349:2004.

Immunoglobulin gene superfamily

46. Springer TA. Adhesion receptors of the immune system. Nature 1990; 346:425.
47. Sriramarao P, von Andrian UH, Butcher EC, et al. L-selectin and very late antigen-4 integrin promote eosinophil rolling at physiological shear rates in vivo. J Immunol 1994; 153:4238.
48. Newman PJ. The biology of PECAM-1. J Clin Invest 1997; 99:3.
49. Miller M, Sung KL, Muller WA, et al. Eosinophil tissue recruitment to sites of allergic inflammation in the lung is platelet endothelial cell adhesion molecule independent. J Immunol 2001; 167:2292.
50. Broide DH, Sullivan S, Gifford T, et al. Inhibition of pulmonary eosinophilia in P-selectin- and ICAM-1-deficient mice. Am J Respir Cell Mol Biol 1998; 18:218.
51. Wegner CD, Gundel RH, Reilly P, et al. Intercellular adhesion molecule-1 in the pathogenesis of asthma. Science 1990; 247:456.
52. Kavanaugh AF, Davis LS, Nichols LA, et al. Treatment of refractory rheumatoid arthritis with a monoclonal antibody to intercellular adhesion molecule 1. Arthritis Rheum 1994; 37:992.
53. Sherman DG. The Enlimomab acute stroke trial: final results. Neurology 1997; 48:A270.

Galectins, cadherins, and CD44

54. Liu FT. Regulatory roles of galectins in the immune response. Int Arch Allergy Immunol 2005; 136:385.
55. Zuberi RI, Hsu DK, Kalayci O, et al. Critical role for galectin-3 in airway inflammation and bronchial hyperresponsiveness in a murine model of asthma. Am J Pathol 2004; 165:2045.
56. Gumbiner BM. Regulation of cadherin adhesive activity. J Cell Biol 2000; 148:399.
57. Pure E, Cuff CA. A crucial role for CD44 in inflammation. Trends Mol Med 2001; 7:213.
58. Matsumoto K, Appiah-Pippim J, Schleimer RP, et al. CD44 and CD69 represent different types of cell surface activation markers for human eosinophils. Am J Respir Cell Mol Biol 1998; 18:860.
59. Katoh S, Matsumoto N, Kawakita K, et al. A role for CD44 in an antigen-induced murine model of pulmonary eosinophilia. J Clin Invest 2003; 111:1563.

Leukocyte adhesion to and across the endothelium

60. Luster AD, Alon R, von Andrian UH. Immune cell migration in inflammation: present and future therapeutic targets. Nat Immunol 2005; 6:1182.
61. Broide DH, Sriramarao P. Eosinophil trafficking to sites of allergic inflammation. Immunol Rev 2001; 179:163.
62. Ley K. Integration of inflammatory signals by rolling neutrophils. Immunol Rev 2002; 186:8.
63. Berlin C, Bargatze RF, Campbell JJ, et al. $\alpha4$ integrins mediate lymphocyte attachment and rolling under physiologic flow. Cell 1995; 80:413.
64. Sriramarao P, DiScipio RG, Cobb RR, et al. VCAM-1 is more effective than MAdCAM-1 in supporting eosinophil rolling under conditions of shear flow. Blood 2000; 95:592.
65. Vicente-Manzanares M, Sanchez-Madrid F. Role of the cytoskeleton during leukocyte responses. Nat Rev Immunol 2004; 4:110.
66. Wymann MP, Marone R. Phosphoinositide 3-kinase in disease timing, location, and scaffolding. Curr Opin Cell Biol 2005; 17:141.
67. DiScipio RG, Schraufstatter IU, Sikora L, et al. Comparison of C3a and C5a-mediated stable adhesion of rolling eosinophils in postcapillary venules and transendothelial migration in vitro and in vivo. J Immunol 1999; 162:1127.

Leukocyte adhesion in the extracellular matrix in tissues

68. Hunt SW III, Kellermann S-A, Shimizu Y. Integrins, integrin regulators and the extracellular matrix: the role of signal transduction and leukocyte migration. In: Bochner BS, ed. Cell adhesion molecules in allergic disease. New York: Marcel Dekker; 1997:73.
69. Neeley SP, Hamann KJ, Dowling TL, et al. Augmentation of stimulated eosinophil degranulation by VLA-4 (CD49d)-mediated adhesion to fibronectin. Am J Respir Cell Mol Biol 1994; 11:206.

70. Warner JA, Rich K, Goldring K. Integrin-dependent responses in human basophils. In: Bochner BS, ed. Adhesion molecules in allergic diseases. New York: Marcel Dekker; 1997:139.
71. Vliagoftis H, Metcalfe DD. Cell adhesion molecules in mast cell adhesion and migration. In: Bochner BS, ed. Adhesion molecules in allergic diseases. New York: Marcel Dekker; 1997:151.

Regulation of adhesion molecule expression

72. Neeley SP, Hamann KJ, White SR, et al. Selective regulation of expression of surface adhesion molecules Mac-1, L-selectin, and VLA-4 on human eosinophils and neutrophils. Am J Respir Cell Mol Biol 1993; 8:633.

Human disease associated with adhesion molecule deficiency

73. McDowall A, Inwald D, Leitinger B, et al. A novel form of integrin dysfunction involving [beta]1, [beta]2 and [beta]3 integrins. J Clin Invest 2003; 111:51.

Adhesion molecules in human allergic inflammation

74. Kyan-Aung U, Haskard DO, Poston RN, et al. Endothelial leukocyte adhesion molecule-1 and intercellular adhesion molecule-1 mediate the adhesion of eosinophils to endothelial cells in vitro and are expressed by endothelium in allergic cutaneous inflammation in vivo. J Immunol 1991; 146:521.
75. Leung DYM, Pober JS, Cotran RS. Expression of endothelial-leukocyte adhesion molecule-1 in elicited late phase allergic reactions. J Clin Invest 1991; 87:1805.
76. Ying S, Meng Q, Barata LT, et al. Associations between IL-13 and IL-4 (mRNA and protein), vascular cell adhesion molecule-1 expression, and the infiltration of eosinophils, macrophages, and T cells in allergen-induced late-phase cutaneous reactions in atopic subjects. J Immunol 1997; 158:5050.
77. Lee B-J, Naclerio RM, Bochner BS, et al. Nasal challenge with allergen upregulates the local expression of vascular endothelial adhesion molecules. J Allergy Clin Immunol 1994; 94:1006.
78. Baroody FM, Rouadi P, Driscoll PV, et al. Intranasal beclomethasone reduces allergen-induced symptoms and superficial mucosal eosinophilia without affecting submucosal inflammation. Am J Respir Crit Care Med 1998; 157:899.

79. Braunstahl GJ, Overbeek SE, Kleinjan A, et al. Nasal allergen provocation induces adhesion molecule expression and tissue eosinophilia in upper and lower airways. J Allergy Clin Immunol 2001; 107:469.
80. Weinberger MS, Davidson TM, Broide DH. Differential expression of vascular cell adhesion molecule mRNA and protein in nasal mucosa in response to IL-1 or tumor necrosis factor. J Allergy Clin Immunol 1996; 97:662.
81. Bentley AM, Durham SR, Robinson DS, et al. Expression of endothelial and leukocyte adhesion molecules intercellular adhesion molecule-1, E-selectin, and vascular cell adhesion molecule-1 in the bronchial mucosa in steady-state and allergen-induced asthma. J Allergy Clin Immunol 1993; 92:857.
82. Montefort S, Holgate ST. Expression of cell adhesion molecules in asthma. In: Bochner BS, ed. Adhesion molecules in allergic diseases. New York: Marcel Dekker; 1997:315.
83. Wilson SJ, Wallin A, Della-Cioppa G, et al. Effects of budesonide and formoterol on NFκB, adhesion molecules, and cytokines in asthma. Am J Respir Crit Care Med 2001; 164:1047.
84. Liu MC, Proud D, Lichtenstein LM, et al. Effects of prednisone on the cellular responses and release of cytokines and mediators after segmental allergen challenge of asthmatic subjects. J Allergy Clin Immunol 2001; 108:29.
85. Aceves SS, Newbury RO, Dohil R, et al. Esophageal remodeling in pediatric eosinophilic esophagitis. J Allergy Clin Immunol 2007; 119:206.

Potential side effects of adhesion-based therapy

86. Kummer C, Ginsberg MH. New approaches to blockade of alpha4-integrins, proven therapeutic targets in chronic inflammation. Biochem Pharmacol 2006; 72:1460.
87. Langer-Gould A, Atlas SW, Green AJ, et al. Progressive multifocal leukoencephalopathy in a patient treated with natalizumab. N Engl J Med 2005; 353:375.
88. Van Assche G, Van Ranst M, Sciot R, et al. Progressive multifocal leukoencephalopathy after natalizumab therapy for Crohn's disease. N Engl J Med 2005; 353:362.
89. Steinman L. Blocking adhesion molecules as therapy for multiple sclerosis: natalizumab. Nat Rev Drug Discov 2005; 4:510.
90. Berger JR, Koralnik IJ. Progressive multifocal leukoencephalopathy and natalizumab – unforeseen consequences. N Engl J Med 2005; 353:414.

Cytokines in Allergic Inflammation

Larry Borish and Lanny J Rosenwasser

10

CONTENTS

- Introduction: definition, evolution of cytokine biology, and nomenclature 165
- Cytokine production by antigen-presenting cells 166
- Cytotoxic immunity 168
- Humoral immunity 168
- Cellular immunity 168
- Allergic immunity 169
- Antiinflammatory cytokines 171
- T helper lymphocyte families 173
- Cytokines involved in Th1 differentiation 173
- Cytokines involved in Th2 differentiation 173
- Cytokines and immune responses to allergens 176
- Summary 176

SUMMARY OF IMPORTANT CONCEPTS

>> Cytokines are families of secreted proteins that mediate immune and inflammatory reactions in local or distant tissues

>> Each cytokine within a cytokine family has a unique set of receptors on cells that respond to the cytokine. Genetic factors may control some aspects of cytokine biology

>> Tissue expression of cytokines may indicate targets for treatment of disease and disease modification

>> A new set of biotherapeutic agents has begun to be developed utilizing monoclonal antibodies and antagonists to cytokines and cytokine receptors

◼ INTRODUCTION: DEFINITION, EVOLUTION OF CYTOKINE BIOLOGY, AND NOMENCLATURE ◼

Cytokines are secreted proteins with growth, differentiation, and activation functions that regulate and determine the nature of immune responses. Cytokines are involved in virtually every facet of immunity and inflammation, including innate immunity, antigen presentation, bone marrow differentiation, cellular recruitment and activation, and adhesion molecule expression. Which cytokines are produced in response to an immune insult determines initially whether an immune response develops and subsequently whether that response is cytotoxic, humoral, cell mediated, allergic, or tolerogenic.

The identification and classification of new cytokines has undergone three phases of development. Initially, cytokines were identified purely by their biological activities and termed 'factors' reflecting that activity, for example 'T cell growth factor'. The development of cloning strategies and the ability to generate purified recombinant proteins, for example interleukin (IL)-2, rapidly resulted in the recognition of how confused the 'factor' phase was, with the recognition of the tremendously pleiotropic and redundant activities of cytokines. Subsequently cytokines were identified based on their unique expression patterns, for example, in activated T helper lymphocytes. This 'recombinant' phase led to much of our understanding of cytokines. Currently, however, cytokine biology has evolved into a third phase, driven primarily by genomics and, in particular, the human genome project. With the identification of the complete repertoire of human genes, a major effort is now being applied to assigning a function for the huge library of previously unrecognized proteins. One of the more effective approaches to achieve this objective is through sequence comparison with previously known genes and predicting that homologous proteins should have related functions. In the current, 'genomic' phase of cytokine development, numerous candidate cytokines have been identified based on their homologies to previously described cytokines. In the exact reverse of the 'factor' phase of cytokine development, the predicted protein is expressed and its activities assessed in a series of biological assays, including, most importantly, assessment of the phenotype of mice genetically engineered as either knockout or overexpressing mice. At present, at least 70 candidate cytokines have been proposed. After identification and consensus regarding each candidate's biological activity, a cytokine nomenclature is assigned. For this chapter, cytokines are grouped according to those that are predominantly mononuclear phagocytic derived or T lymphocytic derived; that predominantly mediate cytotoxic (antiviral and anticancer), humoral, cell-mediated, or allergic immunity; and that are immunosuppressive. A discussion of the complementary family of secreted immune proteins, the chemokines, can be found in Chapter 11.

CYTOKINE PRODUCTION BY ANTIGEN-PRESENTING CELLS

Cytokines primarily derived from dendritic cells, mononuclear phagocytic cells, and other antigen-presenting cells (APCs) are particularly effective in promoting the cellular infiltrate and damage to resident tissue characteristic of inflammation (Fig. 10.1). The processing of antigens as they are taken up by APCs, metabolized and presented to T helper (Th) lymphocytes provides one pathway for this class of cytokine production. Alternatively, APCs are potently triggered to produce cytokines through the innate immune system using pattern recognition receptors (see Chapter 1) that recognize stereotypic components of pathogens that do not occur on mammalian cells. These receptors, such as the lipopolysaccharide

(LPS) and other toll-like receptors (TLRs), contribute to the ability of the immune system to distinguish pathogens from non-pathogenic proteins to which the immune system may become exposed. The cytokines predominantly produced by APCs include tumor necrosis factor (TNF), IL-1, IL-6, CCL8 (IL-8) and other members of the chemokine family, IL-12, IL-15, IL-18, IL-23, and IL-27.

TUMOR NECROSIS FACTOR

TNF represents two homologous proteins primarily derived from mononuclear phagocytes (TNF-α) and lymphocytes (TNF-β).[1] The active form of both cytokines is a homotrimer. In addition to mononuclear phagocytes, TNF-α may be produced by neutrophils, activated lymphocytes, natural killer (NK) cells, endothelial cells, and mast cells. The most potent inducer of TNF by monocytes is LPS acting through TLR4 and CD14γ. TNF-α is processed as a membrane-bound protein from which the soluble active factor is derived via cleavage using the enzyme TNF-α converting enzyme (TACE).[2] TNF-β (lymphotoxin-α) can be synthesized and processed as a typical secretory protein but is usually linked to the cell surface by forming heterotrimers with a third, membrane-associated, member of this family, lymphotoxin-β. TNF-α and TNF-β bind to the same two distinct cell surface receptors – TNFR I (p75) and TNFR II (p55) – with similar affinities and produce similar, although not identical, effects.[3] TNFs induce antitumor immunity through direct cytotoxic effects on cancerous cells and by stimulating antitumor immune responses. TNF interacts with endothelial cells to

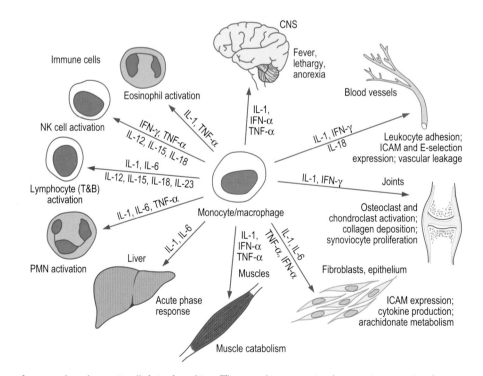

Fig. 10.1. Actions of mononuclear phagocytic cell-derived cytokines. These cytokines are uniquely potent in generating the symptoms and initiating the immune responses associated with infection and inflammatory disorders. CNS, central nervous system; IL, interleukin; TNF, tumor necrosis factor; NK, natural killer; IFN, interferon; ICAM, intracellular adhesion molecule.

induce intercellular adhesion molecule-1 (ICAM-1), vascular cell adhesion molecule-1 (VCAM-1), and E-selectin, permitting the egress of granulocytes into inflammatory loci. TNF is a potent activator of neutrophils, mediating adherence, chemotaxis, degranulation, and the respiratory burst. Enthusiasm for the potential therapeutic value of TNF has been tempered by its severe side effects. TNF is responsible for the severe cachexia that occurs in chronic infections and cancer.[1] Furthermore, TNF induces vascular leakage, has negative inotropic effects, and is the primary endogenous mediator of toxic shock and sepsis.[4] Anti-TNF has recently been shown to have some potential role in the treatment of asthma, although large-scale clinical trials are thus far in progress to truly assess the role of TNF blockade in the treatment of asthma and bronchial hyperactivity.

INTERLEUKIN-1

The IL-1 family represents five peptides (IL-1α, IL-1β, the IL-1 receptor antagonist [IL-1ra], IL-18, and IL-33).[5] IL-1α and IL-1β have similar biologic activities, and both of these proteins along with IL-1ra interact with similar affinities to the two IL-1 receptors (IL-1Rs). Type I receptors transduce the biologic effects attributed to IL-1.[6] These are in contrast to type II receptors, which are expressed on B cells, neutrophils, and bone marrow cells and which have a minimal intracellular domain. The capture and sequestration of IL-1 by these inactive type II receptors serves an antiinflammatory function and hence are referred to as decoy receptors. The capacity of IL-1ra to bind to the type I (pro-inflammatory) IL-1R without transducing biologic activities is the basis for its capacity to function as a cytokine antagonist.[7] IL-1 is primarily produced by cells of the mononuclear phagocytic lineage but is also produced by endothelial cells, keratinocytes, synovial cells, osteoblasts, neutrophils, glial cells, and numerous other cells. IL-1 production may be stimulated by a variety of agents, including endotoxin, other cytokines, microorganisms, and antigens. Both IL-1α and IL-1β, as well as the related proteins IL-18 and IL-33, are synthesized as a minimally active precursor that is without a secretory leader sequence. The mechanism for their secretion depends on their cleavage by a specific converting enzyme, termed interleukin-1 converting enzyme (ICE) or caspase 1, which cleaves the pro-cytokines into their active secreted forms.[8] The identification of the IL-1 receptor antagonist (anakinra) suggest that this too may play a role in the treatment of a variety of allergic and asthmatic conditions, including adult-onset Still's disease, familial cold urticaria syndromes, periodic fevers, and even severe asthma.

One of the most important biologic activities of IL-1 is its ability to activate T lymphocytes by enhancing the production of IL-2 and expression of IL-2 receptors. In the absence of IL-1, a diminished immune response or a state of tolerance develops. IL-1 augments B cell proliferation and increases immunoglobulin synthesis. The production of IL-1 during the immune response produces a spectrum of changes associated with being ill. IL-1 interacts with the central nervous system to produce fever, lethargy, sleep, and anorexia. An IL-1-hepatocyte interaction inhibits production of 'housekeeping' proteins (e.g., albumin) and stimulates the synthesis of acute phase response peptides (e.g., amyloid peptide, C-reactive peptide, complement). IL-1 stimulates endothelial cell adherence of leukocytes through the upregulation of ICAM-1, VCAM-1, and E-selectin. IL-1 contributes to the hypotension of septic shock. TNF and IL-1 share numerous biologic activities, the major distinction being that TNF has no direct effect on lymphocyte proliferation.

The IL-1ra is secreted naturally in inflammatory processes. Its production is upregulated by many cytokines, including IL-4, IL-6, IL-13, and transforming growth factor (TGF)-β. Production of IL-1ra modulates the potentially deleterious effects of IL-1 in the natural course of inflammation.

INTERLEUKIN-6

Mononuclear phagocytic cells are the most important source of IL-6;[9] however, IL-6 is also produced by T and B lymphocytes, fibroblasts, endothelial cells, keratinocytes, hepatocytes, and bone marrow cells. Under the influence of IL-6, B lymphocytes differentiate into mature plasma cells and secrete immunoglobulins. IL-6 mediates T cell activation, growth, and differentiation. As discussed below, IL-6 is the major determinant of differentiation of IL-17-producing Th17 lymphocytes. In addition to lymphocyte activation, IL-6 shares several activities with IL-1, including the induction of pyrexia and the production of acute phase proteins. IL-6 is the most important inducer of hepatocyte synthesis of acute-phase proteins. In contrast to these pro-inflammatory effects, IL-6 mediates several antiinflammatory effects. Whereas both IL-1 and TNF induce synthesis of each other, as well as IL-6, IL-6 terminates this up-regulatory inflammatory cascade and inhibits IL-1 and TNF synthesis, while stimulating synthesis of IL-1ra.

INTERLEUKINS-12, 18, AND 23

IL-12 is derived most importantly from dendritic cells but also from Langerhans' cells, mononuclear phagocytic cells, B cells, PMNs, and mast cells.[10] The biologically active form is a heterodimer. The larger subunit (p40) is homologous to the soluble receptor for IL-6, whereas the smaller subunit (p35) is homologous to IL-6. Homodimers and monomers of the p40 peptide act as competitive antagonists by binding to IL-12Rs without transducing activating signals. IL-12 stimulates IFN-γ production and activates and induces proliferation, cytotoxicity, and cytokine production of NK cells. Other activities attributed to IL-12 include proliferation of T helper and cytotoxic lymphocytes. Its roles in T helper immune deviation and counter-regulatory role in allergic inflammation are discussed later.

IL-18 was originally derived from the liver and is also produced by lung tissue, pancreas, kidney, and skeletal muscle but not lymphocytes or NK cells.[11] Similar to IL-1, IL-18 requires a specific converting enzyme (ICE or caspase 1) to permit secretion and activation. In contrast to most cytokines, IL-18 is constitutively expressed and release of its active form is regulated through activation of this converting enzyme. However, its major biologic activity is more similar to that of IL-12 than IL-1. IL-18 has an important role in cellular adhesion, being the final common pathway utilized by IL-1 and TNF that leads to ICAM-1 expression. IL-18 binds to a unique heterodimer receptor. IL-18R expression is upregulated by IL-12 and thereby these two cytokines synergize to stimulate IFN-γ release. Soluble IL-18 receptors are derived from a unique gene that has lost its signaling domain and thereby functions as a natural decoy antiinflammatory receptor.[12]

IL-23 is a heterodimer consisting of a unique IL-23α chain and the p40 chain of IL-12.[13] IL-23 is primarily secreted by activated dendritic cells. As with IL-12 and IL-18 it is an inducer of IFN-γ. However, in contrast to IL-12 and IL-18 and their influence on Th1 immune deviation, more recent studies suggest that IL-23 might have more important influences on Th17 differentiation (discussed below). Its receptor consists of a heterodimer comprising a unique IL-23Rα chain and the IL-12Rβ1 chain.

INTERLEUKIN-15

IL-15 has activity similar to that of IL-2 and is primarily distinguished from IL-2 through its use of a unique α chain as part of its receptor signaling complex.[14] Both receptors share the use of the IL-2Rβ and common γ chain. Mononuclear phagocytic cells, epithelium, fibroblasts, and placenta are other sources of IL-15, whereas activated T lymphocytes, the most important source of IL-2, do not express IL-15. As discussed later, IL-15 similar to IL-2 is a T cell growth factor, is chemotactic for T lymphocytes, differentiates NK cells, and stimulates B cell growth and differentiation. IL-15 provides a mechanism by which mononuclear phagocytic cells can regulate T and NK cell proliferation and function in a fashion similar to T cell-derived IL-2.

INTERLEUKIN-27

The cells responsible for most of the production of IL-27 are macrophages and dendritic cells. Pro-inflammatory functions of IL-27 include its ability to synergize with IL-12 to induce IFN-γ production from human NK and T helper cells. As will be discussed later, these activities lead to a role for IL-27 in contributing to IL-12-mediated Th1 immune deviation.

CYTOTOXIC IMMUNITY

Immune responses directed against virus-infected and neoplastic cells are primarily mediated by CD8+ cytotoxic lymphocytes and NK cells. Cytokines that activate cytotoxic immunity include IL-2, IL-4, IL-5, IL-6, IL-7, IL-10, IL-12, IL-15, and IL-27 – which are discussed elsewhere – as well as IL-11, IL-32, and, most importantly, TNF and the IFNs.

INTERLEUKIN-11

In addition to its functions in promoting cytotoxic immune response, IL-11 was originally described as a stimulatory factor for hematopoietic cells. It contributes to lymphoid production in the bone marrow and synergizes with other growth factors to produce erythrocytes and platelets. IL-11 increases the production of acute phase proteins and induces lymphoid cell differentiation. IL-11 is also an important stimulatory factor for connective tissue cells such as fibroblasts. A role for IL-11 in asthma remodeling is suggested by studies demonstrating expression of IL-11 in severe asthma[15] and the capacity of this cytokine to stimulate fibroblast proliferation and collagen deposition.

INTERLEUKIN-32

IL-32 was recently discovered in a search for IL-18-inducible genes.[16,17] The highest levels of expression are observed in natural killer and T cells; however, expression could also be observed in epithelial cells in response to IFN-γ and IL-1β. It is not homologous to any other known cytokine. In addition to a putative role in cytotoxicity, its biological activities

include induction of several proinflammatory cytokines (such as TNF-α) and chemokines (including CXCL8 (IL-8) and macrophage inflammatory protein 2, MIP-2) from differentiated macrophages.

INTERFERONS

There are three members of the IFN family (α, β, and γ), and their nomenclature is based on their ability to 'interfere' with viral growth. Type I interferons (IFN-α/β) are primarily derived from monocytes, macrophages, B lymphocytes, and NK cells. The most important source of IFN-α is plasmacytoid DC (pDC), reflecting their activation by viral RNA acting through TLR7 or immunostimulatory bacterial DNA acting through TLR9. Type I IFNs have significant antiviral activity mediated through their ability to inhibit viral replication within virus-infected cells, protect uninfected cells from infection, and stimulate antiviral immunity by cytotoxic (CD8+) lymphocytes NK cells. IFN-α has other important biologic actions, including upregulation of class I MHC antigens and mediation of antitumor activity. Other IFN-like factors with antiviral immunity include IL-28 and IL-29. These 'type III' interferons are members of the IL-10 family and will be discussed below.

IFN-γ is primarily made by T cells and NK cells and to a lesser degree by macrophages. The biologic activities of IFN-γ include only modest antiviral activity and its derivation primarily from T lymphocytes suggests that it is more of an interleukin than an IFN. IFN-γ and its roles in cellular and allergic immunity are discussed later.

HUMORAL IMMUNITY

At least two cytokines contribute to B lymphocyte maturation in the bone marrow, the lymphoid stem cell growth factors IL-7 and IL-11. IL-7 is critically important to the development of B and T lymphocytes through its production by stromal tissue of the bone marrow and thymus, from which it interacts with lymphoid precursors. In addition, IL-7 stimulates the proliferation and differentiation of cytotoxic T and NK cells and stimulates the tumoricidal activity of monocytes and macrophages.

After B cells egress from the bone marrow, isotype switching, the activation of mature B cells into immunoglobulin-secreting B cells, and their final differentiation into plasma cells are processes that are under T cell control.[18] Cytokines that trigger isotype switching include IL-4 and IL-13, which induces the IgE isotype, TGF-β, which triggers IgA, and IL-10, which contributes to the generation of IgG4. Other cytokines that influence B cell maturation include IFN-γ, IL-1, IL-2, IL-5, IL-6, IL-12, IL-15, and IL-21.

CELLULAR IMMUNITY

INTERLEUKIN-2

Stimulation of T cells by antigen in the presence of accessory signals provided by the cytokines IL-1 and IL-6 and the cognate interaction of the B7 molecules (CD80 or CD88) with CD28 induces the simultaneous secretion of IL-2 and the expression of high-affinity IL-2R.

Subsequently, the binding of secreted IL-2 to these IL-2R-positive T cells induces clonal T cell proliferation. The requirement for both IL-2 production and IL-2R expression for T cell proliferation ensures that only T cells specific for the antigen inciting the immune response become activated. While newly activated effector T lymphocytes are induced to express the CD25 chain of the IL-2R, CD25 is constitutively expressed on regulatory T lymphocytes. IL-2 thereby also has antiinflammatory activities through its ability to activate and induce proliferation of regulatory T cells. In addition to its role as a T cell growth factor, IL-2 is also involved in activation of NK cells, B cells, cytotoxic T cells, and macrophages.

INTERLEUKIN-21

IL-21 shares homology to both IL-2 and IL-15 and, similar to IL-2, is predominantly produced by activated T lymphocytes.[19] IL-21 receptors are expressed on activated B, T, and NK cells. It shares numerous biological activities with IL-2 and IL-15, including the capacity to activate natural killer cells and promote the proliferation of B and T lymphocytes.

INTERFERON-γ

The most important cytokine responsible for cell-mediated immunity is IFN-γ.[20] It is primarily produced by T helper lymphocytes but is also derived from cytotoxic T cells and NK cells. IFN-γ mediates increased MHC class I and II expression. IFN-γ stimulates antigen presentation and cytokine production by monocytes and also stimulates monocyte effector functions, including adherence, phagocytosis, secretion, the respiratory burst, and nitric oxide production. The net result is the accumulation of macrophages at the site of cellular immune responses, with their activation into mononuclear phagocytes capable of killing intracellular pathogens. In addition to its effects on mononuclear phagocytes, IFN-γ stimulates killing by NK cells and neutrophils. It stimulates adherence of granulocytes to endothelial cells through the induction of ICAM-1, an activity shared with IL-1 and TNF. As with other IFNs, IFN-γ inhibits viral replication. As discussed later, IFN-γ is an inhibitor of allergic responses through its capacity to suppress IL-4-mediated effects.

INTERLEUKIN-16

Additional cytokines that are secreted by T helper lymphocytes and contribute to cell-mediated immunity are TNF-β, IL-16, and IL-17. IL-16 is a T cell-derived product that is chemotactic for CD4+ lymphocytes, eosinophils, and monocytes and utilizes the CD4 molecule as its receptor.[21] Its production is upregulated by TNF-α, TGF-β, IL-4, IL-9, and IL-13 as well as by histamine.

INTERLEUKIN-17

IL-17 comprises a structurally related family of 6 proteins (IL17A through F) having no known sequence similarity to any other cytokine.[22] (Because of its unique spectrum of activities, IL-17E is now termed IL-25 and is discussed later.) IL-17 family members have overlapping but not identical biologic activities. Similarly cell sources for these different family members are distinct. IL-17A (generally referred to as IL-17) is mainly expressed in CD4+ T cells and to a lesser extent from neutrophils,

eosinophils, and CD8+ T cells. The selective production of IL-17 by clonal T helper lymphocytes has led to the recognition of the Th17 cell as a distinct lymphocyte subset, as will be discussed below. The cellular sources for IL-17B and IL-17C have not been determined. Similar to IL-17A, its most closely structurally related family member, IL-17F is also expressed in activated CD4+ T cells, but can also be produced by activated basophils and cord blood-derived mast cells, suggesting a wider tissue distribution.[22] In contrast to IL-17A and IL-17F, IL-17D is expressed in resting CD4+ T and B cells.

Both IL-17 (IL-17A) and IL-17F can induce expression of a variety of cytokines and chemokines from epithelial and vascular endothelial cells, including IL-6, granulocyte colony-stimulating factor (G-CSF), granulocyte macrophage-colony stimulating factor (GM-CSF), and CXCL10 (interferon-inducible protein-10, IP-10). IL-17 has a particularly important role in activation of fibroblasts that may contribute to a central role for this cytokine in fibrotic autoimmune diseases. IL-11 and the neutrophil-activating factors IL-6 and CXCL8 (IL-8) are secreted by fibroblasts in response to IL-17 (and IL-17F). In addition to direct activation of fibroblasts, IL-17 induces expression of the profibrotic cytokines IL-6 and IL-11, whereas IL-17F induces TGF-β expression. IL-17 activates macrophages, fibroblasts, and stromal cells, inducing their expression of ICAM-1 and secretion of prostaglandin E_2, and nitric oxide. As a result of these activities, IL-17 is increasingly recognized to have important roles in murine models of autoimmune diseases such as experimental allergic encephalitis.[23] In immunity, the ability of IL-17 to induce neutrophil differentiation, recruitment, and activation make it uniquely important in the T cell activation of protective immunity to extracellular bacterial pathogens, such as *Klebsiella*. The IL-17 family members are expressed in asthma.[24] Their ability to induce neutrophil but not eosinophil migration makes it plausible that these cytokines play roles in severe persistent asthma, in which accumulation of neutrophils is a hallmark of disease. Both IL-17 and IL-17F induce goblet cell hyperplasia and mucus hypersecretion. Through these effects and the ability to promote fibrosis and remodeling, IL-17 is likely to contribute to the development of airway hyperreactivity, remodeling, and subepithelial fibrosis.

ALLERGIC IMMUNITY

A final possible outcome of proinflammatory T cell activation is the development of allergic (and presumably antiparasite) immunity. Several features specifically associated with the asthmatic state are regulated by cytokines. These include the regulation of IgE, eosinophilia, and mast cell proliferation.

REGULATION OF IgE

The inappropriate production of IgE in response to allergen defines atopy. The regulation of IgE is primarily a function of the relative activities of IL-4, IL-13, and IFN-γ.

Interleukin-4

In addition to T helper lymphocytes, IL-4[25] is derived from basophils, natural T cells (NKT), and possibly eosinophils and mast cells. In both eosinophils and basophils, IL-4 exists as a preformed, granule-associated peptide that can be rapidly released in allergic inflammatory responses. IL-4 stimulates MHC class II, B7 (CD80/CD86), CD40, surface IgM, and low-affinity IgE receptor (CD23) expression by B cells, thereby enhancing the antigen-presenting capacity of B cells. IL-4 induces the immunoglobulin isotype switch from IgM to IgE.[26,27] Other B cell-activating cytokines, such as IL-2, IL-5, IL-6, and IL-9 synergize with IL-4 to increase the secretion of IgE. IL-4 has been identified in the serum, bronchoalveolar lavage fluid, and lung tissue of asthmatic subjects, in nasal polyp tissue, and in the nasal mucosa of subjects with allergic rhinitis.

In addition to these effects on B cells, IL-4 has important influences on T lymphocyte growth, differentiation, and survival, producing important influences on allergic inflammation. As will be discussed later, IL-4 drives the initial differentiation of naive Th0 lymphocytes toward a Th2 phenotype. IL-4 is also important in maintaining allergic immune responses by preventing apoptosis of T lymphocytes.[28,29] The production of IL-4 by Th2 lymphocytes renders these cells refractory to the anti-inflammatory influences of corticosteroids.

Other activities of IL-4 include enhancing the expression of MHC molecules and low-affinity IgE receptors (CD23) on macrophages. In contrast to these proinflammatory effects on monocytes, IL-4 down-regulates antibody-dependent cellular cytotoxicity (ADCC), inhibits expression of $Fc\gamma$ receptors, inhibits their differentiation into macrophages, and downregulates production of nitric oxide, IL-1, IL-6, and TNF-α while stimulating production of IL-1ra and IL-10.[30] Another important activity of IL-4 in allergic inflammation is its ability to induce expression of vascular cell adhesion molecule 1 (VCAM-1) on endothelial cells. This produces enhanced adhesiveness of endothelium for T cells, eosinophils, basophils, and monocytes, but not neutrophils, as is characteristic of allergic reactions.[31] IL-4, but not IL-13 receptors, are present on mast cells where they function to stimulate IgE receptor expression. An additional important influence of IL-4 on allergic inflammation is its ability to induce mast cell expression of the enzyme LTC_4 synthase, thereby determining the capacity of mast cells to produce cysteinyl leukotrienes.[32] IL-4 stimulates mucin production and contributes to the excessive mucus production in the asthmatic airway. Functional IL-4 receptors are heterodimers consisting of the IL-4Rα chain interacting with either the shared γ chain or the IL-13Rα1 chain.[33] This shared use of the IL-4Rα chain by IL-13 and IL-4 and the activation by this chain of the signaling protein Stat6 explains many of the common biological activities of these two cytokines.

Interleukin-13

IL-13 is homologous to IL-4 and shares much of its biologic activities on mononuclear phagocytic cells, endothelial cells, epithelial cells, and B cells. Thus IL-13 induces the IgE isotype switch and VCAM-1 expression.[34] Functional IL-13 receptors are a heterodimer containing the IL-4Rα chain and a unique IL-13Rα chain. The two IL-13Rα chains that have been described include the active form of the receptor IL-13Rα1 and a decoy receptor, IL-13Rα2, which lacks the motif required for initiating intracellular signaling cascades.[35] IL-13Rα1 expression is more limited than IL-4 receptors and includes endothelial cells, B cells, mononuclear phagocytes, and basophils but not mast cells or T cells. This more limited distribution of IL-13Rα1 explains the unique ability of IL-4 to induce Th2 lymphocyte differentiation and mast cell activation. However, IL-13 is more widely produced than IL-4 and is more readily identified in allergic inflammatory tissue.[36] IL-13 has a singularly important role in causing mucus hypersecretion and non-specific airway hyperreactivity (AHR) in mouse models and its expression results in the characteristic airway metaplasia of asthma with the replacement of epithelial cells with goblet cells.[36]

Interleukin-9

IL-9 was originally described as a mast cell growth factor[37] and contributes to mast cell-mediated allergic responses through its ability to stimulate the production of mast cell proteases. IL-9 supports the growth and survival of antigen-specific T lymphocytes and increases their expression of the IgE high-affinity receptor. IL-9 is derived from eosinophils and Th2-like lymphocytes. Its selective production by Th2 cells suggests a role in allergic inflammation and, in human T lymphocytes, this is a feature shared only with IL-4, IL-5, IL-13, and IL-25. IL-9 has other important activities in allergic inflammation, including inducing expression of CCL11 (eotaxin-1), IL-5 receptors, and chemokine receptor 4. It synergizes with IL-4 to enhance the production of IgE and with IL-5 to enhance the production of eosinophils.

Interferon-γ

The third cytokine central to the regulation of IgE synthesis is IFN-γ. IFN-γ functions as an inhibitor of allergic responses through its capacity to inhibit the isotype switch to IgE and IL-4-mediated expression of low-affinity IgE receptors. The downregulation of IL-4- and IL-13-dependent IgE production is a direct effect of IFN-γ, but physiologically, this results as a consequence of the biologic activity of the IFN-γ inducers, IL-12 and IL-18.

EOSINOPHILIA

Another characteristic feature of allergic diseases is the presence of increased numbers of activated eosinophils.

Interleukin-5

IL-5 is the most important eosinophilopoietin.[38] In addition to stimulating eosinophil production, IL-5 is chemotactic for eosinophils and activates mature eosinophils, inducing eosinophil secretion and enhanced cytotoxicity. Another mechanism by which IL-5 promotes accumulation of eosinophils is through its ability to upregulate responses to chemokines and $\alpha_d\beta_2$ integrins on eosinophils, thereby promoting their adherence to VCAM-1-expressing endothelial cells. IL-5 prolongs eosinophil survival by blocking apoptosis.[39] Administration of IL-5 to humans causes mucosal eosinophilia and an increase in bronchial hyperreactivity. IL-5-dependent activation of eosinophils is now thought to be less central to the pathophysiology of asthma as a result of the disappointing results in trials using IL-5 antagonists, perhaps due to redundant cytokine profiles with GM-CSF. These results reflect IL-5-independent pathways towards persistent eosinophil-mediated inflammation but also non-eosinophil-mediated contributions to asthma. Other activities of IL-5 include maturation of cytotoxic T lymphocytes and basophil differentiation. In addition to Th2-like lymphocytes, other sources for IL-5 include mast cells, NKT cells, and perhaps eosinophils themselves. IL-5 interacts with specific

IL-5Rs that consist of a heterodimer containing IL-5Rα and a β chain (CD131) shared with GM-CSFR and IL-3R.[40]

Interleukin-3 and GM-CSF

In addition to IL-5, two colony-stimulating factors (CSFs), IL-3[41] and GM-CSF,[42] contribute to the activity of eosinophils in allergic inflammation through their capacities to prolong eosinophil survival and to generate activated eosinophils. IL-3 is an important factor that supports the growth of precursors for a variety of hematopoietic cells, including dendritic cells, erythrocytes, granulocytes (especially basophils), macrophages, mast cells, and lymphoid cells. The major source of IL-3 is T lymphocytes, but in allergic inflammation it is also derived from eosinophils and mast cells.

Like IL-3, GM-CSF is an important CSF that supports the maturation of dendritic cells, neutrophils, and macrophages. GM-CSF also synergizes with other CSFs to support the production of platelets and erythrocytes. GM-CSF is an activating factor for mature granulocytes and mononuclear phagocytic cells. The role of GM-CSF in allergic immunity is derived from its shared ability with IL-3 and IL-5 to inhibit apoptosis of eosinophils and thereby prolong the survival of eosinophils at sites of allergic inflammation. GM-CSF is particularly important in the allergic airway as mature, activated eosinophils lose their expression of IL-5Rs and responsiveness to IL-5 but instead upregulate GM-CSF receptors. Thus GM-CSF, and not IL-5, may be responsible for the persistent survival and function of eosinophils in the asthmatic airway. These observations provide one explanation for the failure of IL-5 antagonism in asthma trials. GM-CSF activates mature eosinophils, increasing their degranulation, cytotoxicity, and response to chemoattractants. As noted, all three of these eosinophil-activating cytokines – IL-5, IL-3, and GM-CSF – bind to $\alpha\beta$ heterodimer receptors, which have unique α chains but share the common β chain.

MAST CELL PROLIFERATION AND ACTIVATION

Increased numbers of mast cells characterize allergic diseases, and, as with elevated IgE concentrations and eosinophilia, this is a T cell dependent process. The most important cytokine responsible for mast cell growth and proliferation is stem cell factor (SCF or c-kit ligand).[43] It is by far the most important factor needed when growing mast cells from CD34+ precursors in culture. SCF is derived from bone marrow stromal cells, endothelial cells, and fibroblasts. SCF induces histamine release from human mast cells but inconsistently from basophils and remains the only cytokine with this property. The importance of this factor in humans is supported by clinical observations that the local administration of SCF is associated with mast cell histamine release[44] and when administered systemically is associated with cutaneous mast cell proliferation and urticaria. In addition to being essential for mast cell differentiation, SCF interacts with other hematopoietic growth factors to stimulate myeloid, lymphoid, and erythroid progenitor cells. Several cytokines, including, and especially, IL-3 IL-5, IL-6, IL-9, IL-10, IL-11, and nerve growth factor, may also contribute to mast cell proliferation.[45] In addition to the factors that stimulate mast cell proliferation, several cytokines have been demonstrated to induce histamine release from basophils, including several members of the chemokine family (discussed in Chapter 11).

NEWER Th2 CELL-DERIVED CYTOKINES INVOLVED IN THE DEVELOPMENT OF ALLERGIC INFLAMMATION: IL-25 AND IL-31

Interleukin-25

IL-25 was originally described as a member of the IL-17 family (IL-17E) but because of its unique spectrum of activities has now been given its distinct nomenclature. IL-25 contributes to IgE secretion through its ability to stimulate IL-4 and IL-13 production.[46] Similar to IL-4, IL-5, and IL-9, it is derived from Th2-like lymphocytes. It stimulates release of IL-4, IL-5, and IL-13 from non-lymphoid cells and from Th2 lymphocytes themselves. Intraperitoneal injection of mice with IL-25 leads to enhanced IL-4 and IL-13 production, which is associated with increased IgE production. IL-25 stimulation of IL-5 production promotes eosinophilopoiesis, and mice treated with IL-25 demonstrate eosinophilic inflammation. IL-25 increases expression of CCL5 (RANTES) and CCL11 (eotaxin 1), which might further contribute to the homing of eosinophils to the lungs.[22]

Interleukin-31

IL-31 is another cytokine that was identified on the basis of sequence homology. It is a member of the hematopoietin family of cytokines that includes IL-3, IL-5, and GM-CSF. It is primarily expressed by T helper lymphocytes under Th2-skewing conditions. Its biological activities include induction of expression of chemokines that are involved in recruitment of neutrophils, monocytes, and T cells. Overexpression of IL-31 in mice produces an inflammatory infiltrate suggestive of atopic dermatitis.[47–49,50] Similarly, the murine model of airway hyperreactivity demonstrates increased expression of the IL-31 receptor.

ANTIINFLAMMATORY CYTOKINES

In addition to cytokines that stimulate cytotoxic, cellular, humoral, and allergic inflammation, several cytokines have predominantly antiinflammatory effects, including, as previously discussed, IL-1ra, but also TGF-β and members of the IL-10 family.

TRANSFORMING GROWTH FACTOR-β

TGF-β represents a family of peptides that regulate cell growth, having both stimulatory and inhibitory effects on different cell types.[51] It is produced primarily by chondrocytes, osteocytes, fibroblasts, platelets, monocytes, and T cells. The TGF-β-producing T helper lymphocyte has been proposed to represent a distinct phenotype termed the T repressor (Tr1) or type 3 T helper (Th3) cell (Table 10.1 and see Table 10.3 below). TGF-β is synthesized as an inactive precursor that requires proteolytic cleavage for activation and is an important stimulant of fibrosis, inducing formation of the extracellular matrix, and it promotes wound healing and scar formation. In immunity, it is inhibitory for B lymphocytes and T helper and cytotoxic lymphocytes. It inhibits immunoglobulin secretion by B lymphocytes and cytotoxicity of mononuclear phagocytes and NK cells. In general, it inhibits

Table 10.1 Cytokine production patterns of T cell subtypes

Th1	Th17
IFN-γ	IL-17
TNF-β	IL-21
	IL-22
Th2	
IL-4	**Th3 cells**
IL-5	TGF-β
IL-9	IL-10
IL-13	
IL-25	**Treg/Tr1**
IL-31	IL-10
Both	
TNF-α	
GM-CSF	
IL-2	
IL-3	
IL-10	

the proliferation of many different cell types. Production of TGF-β by apoptotic cells creates an immunosuppressive milieu and is one explanation for the absence of inflammation and autoimmunity as a consequence of apoptotic cell death.[52] In contrast to these antiinflammatory effects, TGF-β is a chemoattractant for macrophages and supports the α isotype switch to IgA by B cells.[53] Production of TGF-β in gut lymphoid tissue by Th3 cells is responsible for secretory IgA production and is also critical for the maintenance of immune non-responsiveness to otherwise benign gut pathogens and food allergens. TGF-β is also constitutively produced in the healthy lung and can help promote B and T cell non-responsiveness. TGF-β production by regulatory cells may lessen allergic inflammation through a capacity to inhibit IgE synthesis and mast cell proliferation. In contrast, in allergic inflammation, eosinophils comprise the most important source of TGF-β,[54] and their expression of TGF-β has been ascribed as a cause of the fibrosis observed in asthma. These conflicting pro- and antiinflammatory influences reflect the distinctive actions of TGF-β as a function of which cells are producing it, the stage of the immune response during which it is acting, different signaling pathways it engages, and other divergent influences.

INTERLEUKIN-10 FAMILY: IL-10, 19, 20, 22, 24, 26, 28, AND 29

IL-10 is a product of numerous cells, including Th1 and Th2 lymphocytes,[55] cytotoxic T cells, B lymphocytes, mast cells, dendritic cells, and mononuclear phagocytic cells. The primary T cell source for IL-10 is regulatory T lymphocytes, described below. IL-10 inhibits production of IFN-γ and IL-2 by Th1 lymphocytes; IL-4 and IL-5 by Th2 lymphocytes;[55] IL-1β, IL-6, IL-8, IL-12, and TNF-α by mononuclear phagocytes; and IFN-γ and TNF-α by NK cells. In addition, IL-10 inhibits MHC class II, CD23, ICAM-1, and CD80/CD86 expression by dendritic cells and other antigen presenting cells. Reduction of CD80/CD86 expression inhibits the ability of the APC to provide the accessory signal necessary for T helper

activation,[56] and this is primarily responsible for the inhibition of Th1 and Th2 cytokine production. Constitutive expression of IL-10 by immature dendritic cells and mononuclear phagocytic cells in the respiratory tract of normal subjects has a central role in the induction and maintenance of tolerance to allergens and otherwise benign bioaerosols. In contrast, asthma and allergic rhinitis are associated with diminished IL-10 expression in the allergic airway, which will contribute to the development of an inflammatory milieu[57] and create a permissive influence on expression of mature dendritic cells. Support for a modulating role for IL-10 in human allergic disease is further derived from observations that IL-10 inhibits eosinophil survival and IL-4-induced IgE synthesis. These inhibitory effects of IL-10 are in contrast to its effect on B lymphocytes, in which it functions as an activating factor that stimulates cell proliferation and immunoglobulin secretion. IL-10 enhances isotype switching to IgG4 and functions as a growth cofactor for cytotoxic T cells. Thus, IL-10 inhibits cytokines associated with cellular immunity and allergic inflammation while stimulating humoral and cytotoxic immune responses. TNF-α and other cytokines stimulate IL-10 secretion, suggesting a homeostatic mechanism whereby an inflammatory stimulus induces TNF-α secretion, which in turn stimulates IL-10 secretion, which feeds back to terminate TNF-α synthesis.

Newer members of the IL-10 family include IL-19, IL-20, IL-22, IL-24, IL-26, IL-28, and IL-29.[58] These cytokines and their receptors share structural homology and intron–exon structure with IL-10/IL-10 receptors but also loosely share homologies with interferons/interferon receptors and many display antiviral activity. In contrast to IL-10, none of these cytokines significantly inhibit cytokine synthesis, an activity that remains unique for IL-10.

IL-19 is expressed by monocytes in response to LPS.[58] It acts upon monocytes to stimulate their secretion of IL-6 and TNF-α and to produce reactive oxygen species. IL-19 contributes to Th2 immune deviation as well as the development of airway inflammation in murine models of asthma and its increased expression has been observed in asthmatics.[59]

IL-20, another recently described member of the IL-10 family, is predominantly expressed by monocytes and skin keratinocytes, and it is overexpressed in psoriasis. It induces keratinocyte proliferation and overexpression in mice is lethal secondary to defective skin formation.

IL-22 is derived from T lymphocytes, in particular Th17 and Th1 cells, as well as NK cells, and mast cells, and its expression is induced by IL-9 and LPS. The predominant biological activity described for IL-22 is induction of acute phase responses in hepatocytes, including serum amyloid A (SAA) protein. It also activates innate immune defenses on skin, airway, and gastrointestinal cells. Consistent with the interferon-like activities of these cytokines, it induces MHC class I antigen expression. IL-22 receptors are widely expressed on barrier sights but not on immune cells. It therefore has been proposed as a means of enhancing innate immune defenses without producing the toxicity associated with widespread immune cell activation.

IL-24 is the fourth new member of the IL-10 family and is produced by monocytes as well as by Th2 lymphocytes in an IL-4-inducible fashion. It was originally discovered as a factor expressed on melanoma cells that had been fully differentiated into a non-proliferating states. It has numerous antineoplastic activities, including the ability to inhibit proliferation, induce tumor apoptosis, and engage an antitumor immune response. In preliminary phase I/II studies, IL-24 has been shown to induce anticancer responses. Its lack of activity against non-cancerous cells suggests that it will be well tolerated.

IL-26, which is primarily generated by monocytes and T memory cells, is considered important in the transformation of human T cells after their infection by herpes virus.[60] Engagement of the IL-26 receptor is associated with induction of IL-8 and IL-10, as well as cell surface expression of ICAM-1. It is located in the chromosome 12q15 gene cluster, along with IFN-γ and IL-22, in an area thought to contribute to allergic and autoimmune diseases. In contrast, IL-19, IL-20, and IL-24 cluster in the IL-10 region on chromosome 1.

Finally, **IL-28** and **IL-29** are also closely related to the type I IFNs, but their genomic organization is more similar to that of members of the IL-10 family. Both cytokines have antiviral properties, and pretreating hepatocellular cells prevents viral infection.[61]

These cytokines have unique heterodimer receptor complexes, which are widely shared. IL-19, IL-20, and IL-24 share IL-20Rα/IL-20Rβ (type I IL-20R). IL-22 has a unique receptor and IL-20 and IL-24 (but not IL-19) can also use this IL-22Rα/IL-20Rβ receptor (type II IL-20R). A soluble form of the IL-22 receptor functions as a natural antagonist for IL-22. IL-26 has a unique receptor consisting of a heterodimer of the IL-22Rα chain and the IL-10Rβ chain.[62] Finally, IL-28 binds to a heterodimer consisting of a unique IL-28Rα chain combined with the IL-10Rα. All of these receptors have unique patterns of expression, which determines in part their unique activities. In contrast to IL-10 receptors, IL-20Rα, IL-20Rβ, and IL-22R are absent or expressed at extremely low levels on cells of the hematopoietic lineage. These receptors are mainly found on epithelial, stromal cells and fibroblasts.

■ T HELPER LYMPHOCYTE FAMILIES ■

Th1, Th2, AND Th17-LIKE LYMPHOCYTES

Subclasses of T helper lymphocytes can be identified on the basis of their repertoire of cytokines (Table 10.1).[63] Naive Th0 cells produce primarily IL-2 but may also synthesize cytokines characteristic of both Th1 and Th2 lymphocytes. In humans, type 1 helper cells produce interferon-γ and TNF-β but not IL-4 and IL-5. Type 2 helper cells produce IL-4, IL-5, IL-9, IL-13, and IL-25 but not IFN-γ or TNF-β. Both classes can produce GM-CSF, TNF-α, IL-2, IL-3, and, to a lesser extent, IL-10. Although distinct Th1/Th2 cytokine profiles are seldom apparent in human cells, there remains an inverse relationship between the tendency of T lymphocytes to produce IFN-γ as opposed to IL-4 or IL-5. Type 1 T helper lymphocytes activate T cells and monocytes, promote cell-mediated immune responses, and are important in antibody-dependent immunity. Type 2 T helper lymphocytes produce IL-4, IL-5, and IL-13 that function in the relative absence of IFN-γ to induce anti-parasite and allergic immune responses. More recently, a third class of T helper lymphocyte, the Th17 cell, has been described based on its unique cytokine repertoire (IL-17 expression but also IL-21 and IL-22), distinct differentiation pathway, and counter-regulatory influences on Th1 and Th2 differentiation.

■ CYTOKINES INVOLVED IN Th1 DIFFERENTIATION ■

One of the more important questions in understanding the cause of allergic disorders is to determine the basis for Th1/Th2 differentiation in response to allergen. The most critical element in determining T helper differentiation is the cytokine milieu in which the T lymphocyte is activated (Table 10.2). Th1 differentiation is induced and maintained through the influences of IL-12, IL-18, and IL-27, with IL-12 providing the most important role.[64] IL-12 interacts with naive T helper lymphocytes to activate STAT4, leading to expression of T-bet. T-bet is a nuclear transcription factor that is the master regulator responsible for the differentiation of Th1 cells. Actions of T-bet include production of IFN-γ and the IL-12 receptor. Simultaneously it blocks alternative T helper differentiation pathways by suppressing expression of Th2 cytokines, such as IL-4, and acting as a negative regulator of Th17 differentiation. Similar to IL-12, IL-27 also activates STAT4, leading to increased expression of T-bet and IFN-γ. Addition of recombinant IL-27 to naive T cells in culture under Th2-polarizing conditions results in decreased expression of GATA-3, the transcription factor that is the master regulator for Th2 development, along with a decrease in production of IL-4 and other Th2 cytokines.[65] Once Th1 cells become differentiated, newly synthesized IFN-γ, acting through STAT-1, also increases expression of T-bet and functions as a negative regulator of Th17 and Th2 differentiation. IL-18 upregulates IL-12R expression and is a growth factor for Th1 cells. IL-12-producing dendritic cells are the most important mediator of Th1-like immune deviation. In addition, insofar as mononuclear phagocytes are an additional source of IL-12, this suggests a mechanism whereby antigens more likely to be processed by macrophages, including bacterial antigens and intracellular parasites, produce Th1 responses.

■ CYTOKINES INVOLVED IN Th2 DIFFERENTIATION ■

The major determinant of Th2 differentiation are the cytokines IL-4, IL-19, IL-25, IL-33, and thymic stromal lymphopoietin (Table 10.2).[66] IL-4 interacts with naive Th0 cells to activate STAT6. Activated STAT6 promotes expression of GATA3, the master regulator of Th2 cells and suppresses expression of T-bet. GATA3 potentiates IL-4 expression and suppresses expression of Th1 differentiation and cytokine (IFN-γ) production. IL-4 and GATA3 similarly inhibit differentiation of Th17 lymphocytes. Other transcription factors, including especially MAF and NFAT, contribute to IL-4 and other Th2 cytokine production once Th2 differentiation is established.

The original source of the IL-4 responsible for Th2 differentiation is unclear but is likely to be provided by the naive Th0 lymphocytes themselves. However, recently NKT cells have also been shown to be capable of robust IL-4 secretion.[67,68] NKT cells are CD4+ lymphocytes that express an invariant rearrangement of the T cell receptor (Vα24-Jα18 in humans) and are specialized to recognize glycolipid antigens presented in the context of CD1d, a molecule closely related structurally to MHC class I. Whatever the source is for the IL-4, the end result is that in a milieu in which allergic

Table 10.2 Cytokines and transcription factors involved in T cell subtype differentiation

	Cytokines involved in differentiation	Transcription factors involved in differentiation
Th1	**IL-12:** activates stat4 leading to expression of T-bet **IL-27:** activates stat4 leading to increased expression of T-bet and IFN-γ **IFN-γ:** increases expression of T-bet by increasing expression of stat1; negative regulator of Th17 and Th2 differentiation	**T-bet:** master regulator of Th1 cells; potentiates production of IFN-γ and IL-12Rβ2; suppresses expression of Th2 cytokines (IL-4); negative regulator of Th17 differentiation **Stat4:** produced in response to IL-12 and potentiates production of IFN-γ **Stat1:** increases expression of T-bet; negative regulator of IL-17-producing cells
Th2	**IL-4:** activates stat6 leading to expression of GATA3; negative regulator of Th17 differentiation **IL-19, IL-25, IL-33, TSLP:** promote differentiation and survival of Th2-like cells	**GATA3:** master regulator of Th2 cells; potentiates IL-4 expression; suppresses expression of Th1 differentiation and cytokines expression (IFN-γ) **MAF:** contributes to IL-4 production once Th2 program is established; inhibition of Th17 differentiation **Stat6:** promotes Th2-cell differentiation; negative regulator of T-bet expression and Th1 differentiation **NFAT:** increased transcription of IL-4
Treg	**TGF-β:** differentiation factor for the generation of Treg cells **IL-10:** important for differentiation of peripheral Tr1 cells, role in Treg development uncertain **IL-2:** promotes survival, proliferation, and survival of Treg cells via their constitutive expression of CD25	**Foxp3:** master regulator of thymus-derived Treg cells
Th17	**IL-6:** differentiation factor for the generation of Th17 cells **TGF-β** and **IL-23** support the differentiation and function of Th17 cells in the additional presence of IL-6	**RORγt** (retinoic acid-related orphan nuclear receptor) is the master regulator of Th17 cell differentiation

inflammation is present (e.g., bronchial lymphatic tissue), more and more extensive allergenic responses against bystander antigens are expected to develop.

IL-19, IL-33 AND THYMIC STROMAL LYMPHOPOIETIN (TSLP) INVOLVEMENT IN Th2 IMMUNE DEVIATION

IL-19, a member of the IL-10 family, is primarily produced by mononuclear phagocytic cells and its expression is upregulated by IL-4 and downregulated by IFN-γ. Reflecting these contrasting influences of IL-4 and IFN-γ, IL-19 promotes Th2 immune deviation and in the presence of IL-19, increased IL-4 and fewer IFN-γ producing cells are observed.[69] IL-19 expression is important to the development of airway inflammation in murine models of asthma and its increased expression has been observed in humans.[59] As previously discussed, IL-25 may also contribute to Th2 immune deviation.[70]

Similar to IL-18, IL-33[71] is an IL-1-like cytokine that signals through an IL-1 receptor-related protein (originally termed ST2[72]). As with IL-1 and IL-18, IL-33 is produced as an inactive precursor and its secretion and activation are dependent upon cleavage by caspase-1.[73] IL-33 is constitutively expressed by bronchial epithelial cells, fibroblasts, and smooth muscle cells and is inducible in lung and dermal fibroblasts, keratinocytes, activated dendritic cells, and macrophages. IL-33 receptors are expressed on T cells[74] (specifically Th2-like cells), macrophages, hematopoietic stem cells, mast cells, and fibroblasts. Administration of IL-33 enhances Th2 cytokine production, including IL-5 and IL-13, causes elevated IgE, and generates profound mucosal eosinophilic inflammation in the lung and gastrointestinal tract.[71,75] Administration of an IL-33 receptor antagonist reduces production of Th2 cytokines and airway inflammation in murine asthma models.[72,76]

Recently, the cytokine thymic stromal lymphopoietin (TSLP) has also been demonstrated to be an important contributor to Th2 immune deviation.[77] TSLP activates DC in such a way as to promote Th2 cytokine production in induced effector T cells. The TSLP receptor is primarily expressed by DCs. TSLP induces expression of foxp3, the transcription factor that serves as the master regulator of Treg cells in thymocytes.[78] TSLP is therefore thought to also have a role in inducing natural Treg cells. However, in the periphery, TSLP induces Th2 cells with the unique profile of being high in TNF-α but not IL-10, a profile suggestive of allergic inflammation.[79] TSLP is highly expressed in the keratinocytes of patients with atopic dermatitis and in tonsils.[80] The ectopic expression of TSLP in the lungs of mice produces severe airway hyperreactivity[81,82] and, similarly, ectopic expression in the skin produces severe skin inflammation suggestive of atopic dermatitis.[83]

Th17 LYMPHOCYTES

The selective production of IL-17 by clonal T helper lymphocytes has led to the recognition of the Th17 cell as a distinct lymphocyte subset.[84] The presence of distinct pathways involved in differentiation of IL-17-producing T lymphocytes (Table 10.2) and that counter-regulate development of the alternative Th1 and Th2-like pathways, further supports the concept that these Th17-producing CD4+ T helper lymphocytes comprise a distinct lineage. Differentiation of Th17 cells is not dependent upon the cytokines or transcription factors that mediate Th1/Th2 cell development. IL-6 is considered the most important cytokine responsible for differentiation of Th17 cells. The transcription factor retinoic acid receptor-related orphan nuclear receptor γt (RORγt) is the master regulatory of Th17 cells.[85] TGF-β and IL-23 act in synergy with IL-6 to promote Th17 differentiation and function of these cells.[86] In the absence of IL-6, TGF-β promotes differentiation into regulatory T cell pathways. IL-6 thereby acts as a 'switch' which converts TGF-β from Treg- to Th17-inducing pathways.[87] The Th17-inducing action of IL-6 on naive T cells is antagonized by IFN-γ and IL-4, consistent with the model that Th17 cells comprise a separate lineage of T helper lymphocytes. IL-17 production is important to the development of remodeling and fibrosis in several models of autoimmune diseases. Although involved in protective adaptive immunity against specific classes of pathogens, such as extracellular bacteria, Th17 cells have also been implicated in a growing list of autoimmune disorders, including inflammatory bowel disease and multiple sclerosis. The increased expression of IL-17 in asthma suggests a role for Th17 CD4+ T cells in asthma, in particular in asthma associated with irreversible obstruction.

IL-10 AND REGULATORY T LYMPHOCYTE FAMILIES, INCLUDING Tr1, Treg, AND Th3 CELLS

In addition to traditional Th1 and Th2 subclasses of helper lymphocytes, much progress has been made in the past several years in identifying and clarifying the characteristics and functions of several families of regulatory T lymphocytes (Table 10.3).[88] These include IL-10-producing lymphocytes, termed Tr1 cells, thymic-derived CD25+ regulatory T cells (Treg) cells, and TGF-β-producing Th3 cells. Thymus-derived Treg cells are characterized by their constitutive expression of the IL-2 receptor (CD25) and the transcription factor foxp3. Similar to the role assumed by T-bet in Th1 differentiation, GATA3 in Th2 differentiation, and RORγt in Th17 differentiation, foxp3 serves as a master regulator of Treg cells (Table 10.2). Treg cells are produced in response to expression in the thymus of self-antigens and are thereby important for prevention of autoimmunity. Th3 cells are primarily gut-derived and ascribed to generating mucosal tolerance. Reflecting their prominent production of TGF-β, in addition to tolerance, they are relevant to antigen-specific IgA production. Although critically important for self tolerance and mucosal immunity, respectively, these cell types are less likely to be involved in either tolerance to allergens in healthy subjects or the immune benefits associated with allergen immunotherapy. In contrast, a class of regulatory T cells has been described which can develop in the periphery and be differentiated from pre-existing T effector lymphocytes or possibly circulating naive

Th0 cells. These regulatory cells are characterized by their prominent production of IL-10 and are termed Tr1 cells. In contrast to Treg cells, Tr1 expression of foxp3 and CD25 is controversial. The induction of IL-10-producing Tr1 cells may play a key role in reducing allergen-specific T cell responsiveness in normal subjects and after immunotherapy. A prominent role of IL-10-producing CD4+ cells was first described in studies involving bee venom immunotherapy.[89] Subsequent investigations have extended the importance of IL-10 (and TGF-β) production by CD4+ T cells to inhalant allergy immunotherapy[90] and confirmed that this occurred in parallel to suppression of Th2 proliferation and cytokine production.[91] In this latter study, IL-10 responses in healthy non-atopic individuals exposed to allergen were similar to those in the immunotherapy-treated group, implying restoration of tolerant T cell responses in the atopic individual. As noted, this area of research remains controversial and, for example, although a role for CD25 expression has been ascribed to these IL-10-producing cells, it is unclear whether this reflects the constitutive expression of this component of the IL-2 receptor, the signature characteristic of Treg cells, or their derivation from activated effector T cells. However, what is consistent is that each of these studies has identified cells capable of making high levels of IL-10 (±TGF-β) consistent with the Tr1 cell type, and current concepts focus on the integral role of these IL-10-producing cells in immune tolerance to allergens in healthy subjects and allergic subjects after successful immunotherapy.

Table 10.3 CD4+ T cells with regulatory activity

Regulatory T cell subtype	Characteristics
Treg	CD25+ foxp3+ thymus-derived
	Not dependent upon IL-10 for their biological activity
	Mediate self-tolerance/prevent autoimmune disease
	Not likely to be relevant to acquired tolerance to allergens
Th3	Characterized by TGF-β (±IL-10) production
	Mediate mucosal tolerance/antigen-specific IgA production
	Not relevant to inhalant allergy or immunotherapy
Tr1	Peripheral-derived regulatory T cells
	IL-10 responsible for their biological activity (±TGF-β)
	Thought to be derived from Th1-/Th2-like effector lymphocytes
	±CD25 expression (reflecting their effector function/activation)
	±Foxp3 expression
	Proposed mechanism of immunotherapy

CYTOKINES AND IMMUNE RESPONSES TO ALLERGENS

Bronchial biopsies of patients with allergic asthma, skin test challenge sites from atopic patients, and the nasal mucosa in allergic rhinitis are all characterized by T helper lymphocytes displaying a Th2-like cytokine profile. However, although there may be a reduced presence of the Th1 cytokines, allergic inflammatory tissue is also characterized by the presence of IFN-γ, and it is likely that IFN-γ exacerbates allergic inflammation through its ability to activate accessory cell function, stimulate cytokine secretion, induce adhesion molecule expression, and activate both eosinophils and neutrophils. The concept that IFN-γ promotes allergic inflammation is supported by data that IFN-γ-producing Th1 lymphocytes exacerbate murine asthma.[92] Th1-like processes are most prevalent in patients with severe persistent asthma especially in the concomitant presence of irreversible obstruction and neutrophilic inflammation.

The pattern of cytokine response to allergens observed in non-allergic individuals is even more complex. Normal individuals are exposed to the same concentrations of allergens as their allergic counterparts living in the same environment. Remaining healthy requires active systems that prevent the development of inflammation. It is frequently stated that the immune response to allergens in non-allergic subjects is characterized by Th1-like lymphocyte responses. However, functional Th1 responses stimulate the recruitment and activation of mononuclear phagocytes and are associated with cellular immunity and granuloma formation, features not present in healthy subjects. If present in vivo,

these Th1-like cells must therefore be present in a milieu that prevents cellular inflammation from developing. The absence of inflammation in normal subjects is maintained by influences that promote the development of tolerance. Immune responses to allergens do develop in non-atopic subjects but these responses are generally of a lower order of magnitude than those observed in allergic subjects. Thus, non-allergic subjects demonstrate decreased allergen-induced T cell proliferation and lower allergen-specific IgG antibody responses compared with their allergic counterparts.[93] One influence contributing to immune non-responsiveness is diminished accessory cell function. In contrast to asthmatic lungs, in the healthy lung, dendritic cells are immature and characterized by reduced or absent expression of CD80/CD86, are unable to present allergen to T helper lymphocytes, and cannot stimulate cellular activation and proliferation.[94] These immature dendritic cells, when presented with antigen, promote the development of IL-10-producing tolerogenic T cell responses (Tr1 cells). The cytokine milieu of the non-asthmatic respiratory tract is characterized by elevated concentrations of IL-10 and TGF-β, which may also help mitigate inflammatory responses.

SUMMARY

Cytokines important in the pathophysiology of allergic disorders are summarized in Table 10.4. The IgE isotype switch results from the activities of IL-4 and IL-13 and is inhibited by IFN-γ and TGF-β. IL-2, IL-5, IL-6, and IL-9 synergize with IL-4 and IL-13 to enhance IgE secretion. IL-4 is responsible for the differentiation of IL-4-producing

Table 10.4 Cytokines in allergy and asthma

Function	Cytokine	Activity
IgE synthesis regulation	IL-4, IL-13	Induces ϵ isotype switch
	IFN γ, TGF-β	Inhibition of Il -4 and IL-13 production
	IL-25	Enhanced production of IL-4 and IL-13
	IL-4, IL-19, IL-33, TSLP	Generation of IL-4-producing (Th2-like) lymphocytes
Eosinophilia	IL-5	Eosinophilopoiesis
	IL-5, IL-3, GM-CSF, IL-4, TNF-α, IFN-γ	Inhibition of apoptosis
	IL-5, IL-3, GM-CSF, IL-1, TNF-α, IFN-γ	Eosinophil chemotaxis, degranulation, and activation
Mast cell development	Stem cell factor	Mast cell growth and differentiation; histamine release
	IL-3, IL-4, IL-9, IL-10, IL-11, nerve growth factor	Cofactors for mast cell growth
Adhesion molecule expression	IL-1, IL-4, IL-13, TNF-α	Induction of VCAM-1
	IL-1, TNF-α, IFN-γ	Induction of ICAM-1
Airway fibrosis and remodeling	IL-4, IL-6, IL-9, IL-11, IL-13, IL-17, TGF-β	Promote fibroblast proliferation and collagen deposition; subepithelial fibrosis

Table 10.5 Cytokines contributing to inflammation in allergic diseases

Cytokine	Primary sources	Secondary sources	Stimuli for production	Primary targets	Effects	Secondary targets	Effects	Comments
Interleukin-28 (IL-28) (IFN λ1)	Keratinocytes, epithelial cells			Virally-infected cells	Interference with viral replication			Type 3 IFN
Interleukin-29 (IL-29) (IFN λ2)	Keratinocytes, epithelial cells			Virally-infected cells	Interference with viral replication			Type 3 IFN
Interleukin-31 (IL-31) is associated with cutaneous lymphocyte antigen-positive skin homing T cells in patients with atopic dermatitis	T cells CLA(+) T cells		Allergenic antigens	Epithelial cells Nerve cells	Itching			Target for atopic dermatitis therapy
Interleukin-32 (IL-32) is a novel cytokine with a possible role in disease	Macrophages Synovial cells		IL-1 TNF	T cells Synovial cells Cartilage	Arthritis			Target for therapy
Interleukin-33 (IL-33) is a chemoattractant for human Th2 cells. An IL-I family member requires caspase-processing and signals through the ST2 receptor	Macrophages Dendritic cells		IL-1 TNF	Th2 cells	Allergy Asthma			Target for therapy

lymphocytes and other cytokines including IL-19, IL-25, IL-33, and TSLP contribute to this process. IL-12, IL-18, and IFN-γ inhibit the differentiation of IL-4-producing Th2-like cells, promoting instead Th1 differentiation; whereas IL-6, with TGF-β and IL-23, serves an analogous role of driving T helper differentiation into the Th17 phenotype. IL-5 is the most important eosinophilopoietin and, with GM-CSF and IL-3, prolongs the survival of mature eosinophils. These three cytokines are primarily responsible for generating the activated eosinophils that characterize the asthmatic state. Mast cell differentiation and proliferation results from the activity of stem cell factor and other cytokines, including IL-3, IL-6, IL-9, IL-10, IL-11, and nerve growth factor promote mast cell expansion. Many cytokines contribute to the inflammatory state of allergic inflammatory disorders (Table 10.5). IL-1, TNF, and IFN-γ increase the expression of endothelial cell adhesion molecules such as ICAM-1 and support the egress of mononuclear cells, neutrophils, and eosinophils into the lungs. Induction of VCAM-1 by TNF-α, IL-4, and IL-13 promotes the selective recruitment of eosinophils, basophils, and lymphocytes. Many cytokines and chemokines then contribute to the activation of these leukocytes once they reach the airways. Cytokines important in promoting fibrosis and airway remodeling are IL-6, IL-11, IL-17, and TGF-β.

References

Cytokine production by antigen-presenting cells

1. Beutler B, Cerami A. The biology of cachectin/TNF – a primary mediator of the host response. Annu Rev Immunol 1989; 7:625–655.
2. Perez C, Albert I, DeFay K, et al. A nonsecretable cell surface mutant of tumor necrosis factor (TNF) kills by cell-to-cell contact. Cell 1990; 63:251–258.
3. Tartaglia LA, Goeddel DV. Two TNF receptors. Immunol Today 1992; 13:151–153.
4. Tracey KJ, Fong Y, Hesse DG, et al. Anti-cachectin/TNF monoclonal antibodies prevent septic shock during lethal bacteraemia. Nature 1987; 330:662–664.
5. Dinarello CA, Wolff SM. The role of interleukin-1 in disease. N Engl J Med 1993; 328:106–113.
6. Sims JE, Gayle MA, Slack JL, et al. Interleukin 1 signaling occurs exclusively via the type I receptor. Proc Natl Acad Sci U S A 1993; 90:6155–6159.
7. Arend WP. Interleukin-1 receptor antagonist. Adv Immunol 1993; 54:167–227.
8. Cerretti DP, Kozlosky CJ, Mosley B, et al. Molecular cloning of the interleukin-1 beta converting enzyme. Science 1992; 256:97–100.
9. Akira S, Taga T, Kishimoto T. Interleukin-6 in biology and medicine. Adv Immunol 1993; 54:1–78.
10. Brunda MJ. Interleukin-12. J Leukoc Biol 1994; 55:280–288.
11. Dinarello CA. Interleukin-18, a proinflammatory cytokine. Eur Cytokine Netw 2000; 11:483–486.
12. Novick D, Schwartsburd B, Pinkus R, et al. A novel IL-18BP ELISA shows elevated serum IL-18BP in sepsis and extensive decrease of free IL-18. Cytokine 2001; 14:334–342.
13. Oppmann B, Lesley R, Blom B, et al. Novel p19 protein engages IL-12p40 to form a cytokine, IL-23, with biological activities similar as well as distinct from IL-12. Immunity 2000; 13:715–725.
14. Grabstein KH, Eisenman J, Shanebeck K, et al. Cloning of a T cell growth factor that interacts with the beta chain of the interleukin-2 receptor. Science 1994; 264:965–968.

REFERENCES

Cytotoxic immunity

15. Minshall E, Chakir J, Laviolette M, et al. IL-11 expression is increased in severe asthma: association with epithelial cells and eosinophils. J Allergy Clin Immunol 2000; 105: 232–238.
16. Kim SH, Han SY, Azam T, et al. Interleukin-32: a cytokine and inducer of TNFalpha. Immunity 2005; 22:131–142.
17. Dinarello CA. IL-32, a novel cytokine with a possible role in disease. Ann Rheum Dis 2006; 65.

Humoral immunity

18. Finkelman FD, Holmes J, Katona IM, et al. Lymphokine control of in vivo immunoglobulin isotype selection. Annu Rev Immunol 1990; 8:303–333.

Cellular immunity

19. Parrish-Novak J, Dillon SR, Nelson A, et al. Interleukin 21 and its receptor are involved in NK cell expansion and regulation of lymphocyte function. Nature 2000; 408:57–63.
20. Farrar MA, Schreiber RD. The molecular cell biology of interferon-gamma and its receptor. Annu Rev Immunol 1993; 11:571–611.
21. Cruikshank WW, Center DM, Nisar N, et al. Molecular and functional analysis of a lymphocyte chemoattractant factor: association of biologic function with CD4 expression. Proc Natl Acad Sci U S A 1994; 91:5109–5113.
22. Kawaguchi M, Adachi M, Oda N, et al. IL-17 cytokine family. J Allergy Clin Immunol 2004; 114:1265–1274.
23. Chen Y, Langrish CL, McKenzie B, et al. Anti-IL-23 therapy inhibits multiple inflammatory pathways and ameliorates autoimmune encephalomyelitis. J Clin Invest 2006; 116:1317–1326.
24. Molet S, Hamid Q, Davoine F, et al. IL-17 is increased in asthmatic airways and induces human bronchial fibroblasts to produce cytokines. J Allergy Clin Immunol 2001; 108:430–438.

Allergic immunity

25. Paul WE, Ohara J. B-cell stimulatory factor-1/interleukin 4. Annu Rev Immunol 1987; 5:429–459.
26. Coffman RL, Ohara J, Bond MW, et al. B cell stimulatory factor-1 enhances the IgE response of lipopolysaccharide-activated B cells. J Immunol 1986; 136:4538–4541.
27. Romagnani S. Regulation and deregulation of human IgE synthesis. Immunol Today 1990; 11:316–321.
28. Vella A, Teague TK, Ihle J, et al. Interleukin 4 (IL-4) or IL-7 prevents death of resting T cells: Stat-6 is probably not required for the effect of IL-4. J Exp Med 1997; 186:325–330.
29. Enelow R, Baramki DF, Borish LC. Inhibition of effector T lymphocytes mediated through antagonism of IL-4. J Allergy Clin Immunol 2004; 113:560–562.
30. Steinke JW, Negri J, Enelow R, et al. Proinflammatory effects of IL-4 antagonism. J Allergy Clin Immunol 2006; 118:756–758.
31. Schleimer RP, Sterbinsky SA, Kaiser J, et al. IL-4 induces adherence of human eosinophils and basophils but not neutrophils to endothelium. Association with expression of VCAM-1. J Immunol 1992; 148:1086–1092.
32. Hsieh FH, Lam BK, Penrose JF, et al. T helper cell type 2 cytokines coordinately regulate immunoglobulin E-dependent cysteinyl leukotriene production by human cord blood-derived mast cells: profound induction of leukotriene C(4) synthase expression by interleukin 4. J Exp Med 2001; 193:123–133.
33. Izuhara K, Shirakawa T. Signal transduction via the interleukin-4 receptor and its correlation with atopy. Int J Mol Med 1999; 3:3–10.
34. Zurawski G, de Vries JE. Interleukin 13, an interleukin 4-like cytokine that acts on monocytes and B cells, but not on T cells. Immunol Today 1994; 15:19–26.
35. Donaldson DD, Whitters MJ, Fitz LJ, et al. The murine IL-13 receptor alpha 2: molecular cloning, characterization, and comparison with murine IL-13 receptor alpha 1. J Immunol 1998; 161:2317–2324.
36. Zhu Z, Homer RJ, Wang Z, et al. Pulmonary expression of interleukin-13 causes inflammation, mucus hypersecretion, subepithelial fibrosis, physiologic abnormalities, and eotaxin production. J Clin Invest 1999; 103:779–788.
37. Hultner L, Druez C, Moeller J, et al. Mast cell growth-enhancing activity (MEA) is structurally related and functionally identical to the novel mouse T cell growth factor P40/TCGFIII (interleukin 9). Eur J Immunol 1990; 20:1413–1416.
38. Clutterbuck EJ, Hirst EM, Sanderson CJ. Human interleukin-5 (IL-5) regulates the production of eosinophils in human bone marrow cultures: comparison and interaction with IL-1, IL-3, IL-6, and GMCSF. Blood 1989; 73:1504–1512.
39. Rothenberg ME, Petersen J, Stevens RL, et al. IL-5-dependent conversion of normodense human eosinophils to the hypodense phenotype uses 3T3 fibroblasts for enhanced viability, accelerated hypodensity, and sustained antibody-dependent cytotoxicity. J Immunol 1989; 143:2311–2316.
40. Kitamura T, Sato N, Arai K, et al. Expression cloning of the human IL-3 receptor cDNA reveals a shared beta subunit for the human IL-3 and GM-CSF receptors. Cell 1991; 66:1165–1174.
41. Rothenberg ME, Owen WF Jr, Silberstein DS, et al. Human eosinophils have prolonged survival, enhanced functional properties, and become hypodense when exposed to human interleukin 3. J Clin Invest 1988; 81:1986–1992.
42. Owen WF Jr, Rothenberg ME, Silberstein DS, et al. Regulation of human eosinophil viability, density, and function by granulocyte/macrophage colony-stimulating factor in the presence of 3T3 fibroblasts. J Exp Med 1987; 166:129–141.

43. Anderson DM, Lyman SD, Baird A, et al. Molecular cloning of mast cell growth factor, a hematopoietin that is active in both membrane bound and soluble forms. Cell 1990; 63: 235–243.
44. Lukacs NW, Strieter RM, Lincoln PM, et al. Stem cell factor (c-kit ligand) influences eosinophil recruitment and histamine levels in allergic airway inflammation. J Immunol 1996; 156:3945–3951.
45. Matsuda H, Kannan Y, Ushio H, et al. Nerve growth factor induces development of connective tissue-type mast cells in vitro from murine bone marrow cells. J Exp Med 1991; 174:7–14.
46. Fort MM, Cheung J, Yen D, et al. IL-25 induces IL-4, IL-5, and IL-13 and Th2-associated pathologies in vivo. Immunity 2001; 15:985–995.
47. Dillon SR, Sprecher C, Hammond A, et al. Interleukin 31, a cytokine produced by activated T cells, induces dermatitis in mice. Nat Immunol 2004; 5:752–760.
48. Neis MM, Peters B, Dreuw A, et al. Enhanced expression levels of IL-31 correlate with IL-4 and IL-13 in atopic and allergic contact dermatitis. J Allergy Clin Immunol 2006; 118: 930–937.
49. Sonkoly E, Muller A, Lauerma AI, et al. IL-31: a new link between T cells and pruritus in atopic skin inflammation. J Allergy Clin Immunol 2006; 117:411–417.
50. Bilsborough J, Leung DY, Maurer M, et al. IL-31 is associated with cutaneous lymphocyte antigen-positive skin homing T cells in patients with atopic dermatitis. J Allergy Clin Immunol 2006; 117:418–423.

Antiinflammatory cytokines

51. Sporn MB, Roberts AB. Transforming growth factor-beta: recent progress and new challenges. J Cell Biol 1992; 119:1017–1021.
52. Chen W, Frank ME, Jin W, et al. TGF-beta released by apoptotic T cells contributes to an immunosuppressive milieu. Immunity 2001; 14:715–725.
53. Sonoda E, Matsumoto R, Hitoshi Y, et al. Transforming growth factor beta induces IgA production and acts additively with interleukin 5 for IgA production. J Exp Med 1989; 170:1415–1420.
54. Kay AB, Phipps S, Robinson DS. A role for eosinophils in airway remodelling in asthma. Trends Immunol 2004; 25:477–482.
55. Del Prete G, De Carli M, Almerigogna F, et al. Human IL-10 is produced by both type 1 helper (Th1) and type 2 helper (Th2) T cell clones and inhibits their antigen-specific proliferation and cytokine production. J Immunol 1993; 150:353–360.
56. Ding L, Linsley PS, Huang LY, et al. IL-10 inhibits macrophage costimulatory activity by selectively inhibiting the up-regulation of B7 expression. J Immunol 1993; 151:1224–1234.
57. Borish L, Aarons A, Rumbyrt J, et al. Interleukin-10 regulation in normal subjects and patients with asthma. J Allergy Clin Immunol 1996; 97:1288–1296.
58. Conti P, Kempuraj D, Frydas S, et al. IL-10 subfamily members: IL-19, IL-20, IL-22, IL-24 and IL-26. Immunol Lett 2003; 88:171–174.
59. Liao SC, Cheng YC, Wang YC, et al. IL-19 induced Th2 cytokines and was up-regulated in asthma patients. J Immunol 2004; 173:6712–6718.
60. Fickenscher H, Pirzer H. Interleukin-26. Int Immunopharmacol 2004; 4:609–613.
61. Sheppard P, Kindsvogel W, Xu W, et al. IL-28, IL-29 and their class II cytokine receptor IL-28R. Nat Immunol 2003; 4:63–68.
62. Sheikh F, Baurin VV, Lewis-Antes A, et al. Cutting edge: IL-26 signals through a novel receptor complex composed of IL-20 receptor 1 and IL-10 receptor 2. J Immunol 2004; 172:2006–2010.

T helper lymphocyte families

63. Mosmann TR, Coffman RL. TH1 and TH2 cells: different patterns of lymphokine secretion lead to different functional properties. Annu Rev Immunol 1989; 7:145–173.

Cytokines involved in Th1 differentiation

64. Manetti R, Parronchi P, Giudizi MG, et al. Natural killer cell stimulatory factor (interleukin 12 [IL-12]) induces T helper type 1 (Th1)-specific immune responses and inhibits the development of IL-4-producing Th cells. J Exp Med 1993; 177:1199–1204.
65. Villarino AV, Huang E, Hunter CA. Understanding the pro- and anti-inflammatory properties of IL-27. J Immunol 2004; 173:715–720.

Cytokines involved in Th2 differentiation

66. Seder RA, Paul WE, Davis MM, et al. The presence of interleukin 4 during in vitro priming determines the lymphokine-producing potential of CD4+ T cells from T cell receptor transgenic mice. J Exp Med 1992; 176:1091–1098.
67. Bilenki L, Yang J, Fan Y, et al. Natural killer T cells contribute to airway eosinophilic inflammation induced by ragweed through enhanced IL-4 and eotaxin production. Eur J Immunol 2004; 34:345–354.
68. Akbari O, Faul JL, Hoyte EG, et al. CD4+ invariant T-cell-receptor+ natural killer T cells in bronchial asthma. N Engl J Med 2006; 354:1117–1129.
69. Gallagher G, Eskdale J, Jordan W, et al. Human interleukin-19 and its receptor: a potential role in the induction of Th2 responses. Int Immunopharmacol 2004; 4:615–626.
70. Tamachi T, Maezawa Y, Ikeda K, et al. IL-25 enhances allergic airway inflammation by amplifying a TH2 cell-dependent pathway in mice. J Allergy Clin Immunol 2006; 118: 606–614.

71. Schmitz J, Owyang A, Oldham E, et al. IL-33, an interleukin-1-like cytokine that signals via the IL-1 receptor-related protein ST2 and induces T helper type 2-associated cytokines. Immunity 2005; 23:479–490.
72. Coyle AJ, Lloyd C, Tian J, et al. Crucial role of the interleukin 1 receptor family member T1/ST2 in T helper cell type 2-mediated lung mucosal immune responses. J Exp Med 1999; 190:895–902.
73. Dinarello CA. An IL-1 family member requires caspase-1 processing and signals through the ST2 receptor. Immunity 2005; 23:461–462.
74. Komai-Koma M, Xu D, Li Y, et al. IL-33 is a chemoattractant for human Th cells: Eur J Immunol 2007; 37(10):2779–2786.
75. Xu D, Chan WL, Leung BP, et al. Selective expression of a stable cell surface molecule on type 2 but not type 1 helper T cells. J Exp Med 1998; 187:787–794.
76. Lohning M, Stroehmann A, Coyle AJ, et al. T1/ST2 is preferentially expressed on murine Th2 cells, independent of interleukin 4, interleukin 5, and interleukin 10, and important for Th2 effector function. Proc Natl Acad Sci U S A 1998; 95:6930–6935.
77. Wang YH, Ito T, Homey B, et al. Maintenance and polarization of human TH2 central memory T cells by thymic stromal lymphopoietin-activated dendritic cells. Immunity 2006; 24:827–838.
78. Watanabe N, Wang YH, Lee HK, et al. Hassall's corpuscles instruct dendritic cells to induce CD4+CD25+ regulatory T cells in human thymus. Nature 2005; 436:1181–1185.
79. Ito T, Wang YH, Duramad O, et al. TSLP-activated dendritic cells induce an inflammatory T helper type 2 cell response through OX40 ligand. J Exp Med 2005; 202:1213–1223.
80. Soumelis V, Reche PA, Kanzler H, et al. Human epithelial cells trigger dendritic cell mediated allergic inflammation by producing TSLP. Nat Immunol 2002; 3:673–680.
81. Al-Shami A, Spolski R, Kelly J, et al. A role for TSLP in the development of inflammation in an asthma model. J Exp Med 2005; 202:829–839.
82. Zhou B, Comeau MR, De Smedt T, et al. Thymic stromal lymphopoietin as a key initiator of allergic airway inflammation in mice. Nat Immunol 2005; 6:1047–1053.
83. Yoo J, Omori M, Gyarmati D, et al. Spontaneous atopic dermatitis in mice expressing an inducible thymic stromal lymphopoietin transgene specifically in the skin. J Exp Med 2005; 202:541–549.

84. Dong C. Diversification of T-helper-cell lineages: finding the family root of IL-17-producing cells. Nat Rev Immunol 2006; 6:329–333.
85. Iwakura Y, Ishigame H. The IL-23/IL-17 axis in inflammation. J Clin Invest 2006; 116:1218–1222.
86. Mangan PR, Harrington LE, O'Quinn DB, et al. Transforming growth factor-beta induces development of the T(H)17 lineage. Nature 2006; 441:231–234.
87. Bettelli E, Carrier Y, Gao W, et al. Reciprocal developmental pathways for the generation of pathogenic effector TH17 and regulatory T cells. Nature 2006; 441:235–238.
88. Sakaguchi S. Regulatory T cells: key controllers of immunologic self-tolerance. Cell 2000; 101:455–458.
89. Akdis CA, Blesken T, Akdis M, et al. Role of interleukin 10 in specific immunotherapy. J Clin Invest 1998; 102:98–106.
90. Francis JN, Till SJ, Durham SR. Induction of IL-10+CD4+CD25+ T cells by grass pollen immunotherapy. J Allergy Clin Immunol 2003; 111:1255–1261.
91. Jutel M, Pichler WJ, Skrbic D, et al. Bee venom immunotherapy results in decrease of IL-4 and IL-5 and increase of IFN-gamma secretion in specific allergen-stimulated T cell cultures. J Immunol 1995; 154:4187–4194.

Cytokines and immune responses to allergens

92. Randolph DA, Carruthers CJ, Szabo SJ, et al. Modulation of airway inflammation by passive transfer of allergen-specific Th1 and Th2 cells in a mouse model of asthma. J Immunol 1999; 162:2375–2383.
93. Platts-Mills T, Vaughan J, Squillace S, et al. Sensitisation, asthma, and a modified Th2 response in children exposed to cat allergen: a population-based cross-sectional study. Lancet 2001; 357:752–756.
94. von Bubnoff D, Geiger E, Bieber T. Antigen-presenting cells in allergy. J Allergy Clin Immunol 2001; 108:329–339.

Chemokines in Cell Movement and Allergic Inflammation

11

Zamaneh Mikhak and Andrew D Luster

SUMMARY OF IMPORTANT CONCEPTS

>> The movement of cells within the body is a highly regulated process and is critical for many vital biological functions ranging from embryogenesis to inflammation

>> Chemokines are *chemoattractant cytokines* that direct cell movement by binding and activating seven transmembrane-spanning, pertussis toxin-sensitive, G-protein-coupled receptors

>> Approximately 50 chemokines interact with approximately 20 chemokine receptors to provide the navigational cues that fine tune leukocyte migration in the body during homeostasis and inflammation

>> Each inflammatory disease is characterized by a specific set of infiltrating leukocytes, responding to a specific subset of chemokines produced in the tissue

>> Chemokines important in allergic inflammation include the IL-4-STAT6-inducible chemokines, CCL17 and CCL22, which activate CCR4 on Th2 cells, and CCL11 and CCL26, which activate CCR3 on eosinophils and basophils

INTRODUCTION

The movement of cells within the body is a highly regulated process. Complex rules that dictate cell trafficking apply to every vital biological function from embryogenesis to inflammation. Chemokines provide the navigational cues that direct leukocytes to the right place at the right time for immunosurveillance and effective inflammatory responses. This chapter focuses on the chemokine system and its role in allergic inflammation.

CHEMOKINES

Chemokines are 8–10 kDa chemoattractant cytokines that signal through seven-transmembrane-domain, pertussis toxin-sensitive, G-protein-coupled receptors.[1–3] All chemokines share the same overall structure. They all have a minimum of three β-pleated sheets, an α-helix in their C-terminal domain, and disulfide bonds connecting their conserved cysteine residues (Fig. 11.1). Chemokines are classified into four families based on the arrangement of the first two N-terminal cysteine residues within their amino acid sequence: the CXC (or α) family, the CC (or β) family, the CX3C (or δ) family, and the C (or γ) family. The CXC family of chemokines has one amino acid in between the two N-terminal cysteine residues. Some members of this family, such as IL-8 (CXCL8), play important roles in neutrophil recruitment, while others, such as IP-10 (CXCL10), are important for lymphocytes recruitment. The CC chemokines, in which the first two cysteine residues are adjacent to each other, are the largest group. Many members of this family, such as MCP-1 (CCL2), are potent monocyte chemoattractants. TARC (CCL17) and MDC (CCL22) in this family attract Th2 cells, while the eotaxins (CCL11, CCL24, and CCL26) attract eosinophils and participate in allergic inflammation. There is only one member in the CX3C family, fractalkine (CX3CL1), and this chemokine has three amino acids between its first two cysteine residues. The fourth family is the C family of chemokines, with only a single cysteine residue in the N-terminus and one member, lymphotactin (XCL1) and its splice variant SCM-1β (XCL2). While all chemokines are soluble chemoattractants, CXCL16 and CX3CL1 are initially produced as cell membrane proteins and thus function as both cell adhesion receptors and, when cleaved from

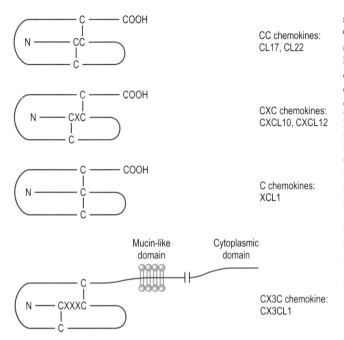

CC chemokines: CL17, CL22

CXC chemokines: CXCL10, CXCL12

C chemokines: XCL1

CX3C chemokine: CX3CL1

Fig. 11.1. Chemokines are 8–10 kDa chemoattractant cytokines. Chemokines share the same overall structure with intramolecular disulfide bonds connecting their conserved cysteine residues. Chemokines are classified into four families based on the amino acid sequence arrangement of the first two N-terminal cysteine residues: CC family, CXC family, C family, and CX3C family.

the cell surface, as soluble chemoattractants. Chemokines can be stored in granules and secreted quickly on stimulation. After release, chemokines, which are positively charged, bind sulfated proteoglycans present on cell surfaces or in the extracellular matrix. This binding ensures that chemokines remain locally concentrated after release. Endothelial cells, which are exposed to a variety of leukocytes under-flow, are a source of chemokines themselves but also can bind chemokines found in the extracellular matrix, or transport chemokines from their non-luminal side to their luminal side.

To date, a total of 47 chemokines and 19 chemokine receptors have been identified (Tables 11.1, 11.2). There are two systems of nomenclature for chemokines in the literature. One system is based on acronyms and originated when each chemokine was discovered, when the biological role of chemokines was not clear, although their association with inflammation was appreciated. The second system of nomenclature is based on chemokine structure with respect to their conserved cysteine residues. In the later nomenclature, chemokines are named $CCLn$, $CXCLn$, $XCLn$ or $CX3CLn$, where L stands for ligand and n for an arbitrary number. Chemokine receptors are named based on the family of chemokines they bind as $CCRn$, $CXCRn$, $CX3CRn$ or $XCRn$, where R stands for receptor and n indicates the rank in order of discovery.[4,5]

In addition to the structural classification, conceptually, chemokines can be divided into functional categories as inflammatory chemokines and homeostatic chemokines. Inflammatory chemokines are produced during an inflammatory response by activated or injured tissue resident cells or activated leukocytes. These chemokines attract effector innate or

adaptive leukocytes into sites of active inflammation. Examples include CXCL1 and CXCL8 that attract neutrophils or CXCL9, CXCL10, and CXCL11 that attract Th1 cells. In contrast, homeostatic chemokines are produced by healthy tissue constitutively. These chemokines direct leukocytes to correct anatomic locations for effective embryogenesis, hematopoiesis, and immune surveillance. Examples of homeostatic chemokines include CCL19 and CCL21, which draw lymphocytes into lymph nodes,[6] CCL25, which brings lymphocytes into gut associated lymphoid tissues (GALT),[7] and CCL27, which is involved in the homing of lymphocytes to the skin.[8] Although conceptually helpful, the distinction between inflammatory and homeostatic chemokines is not absolute as many homeostatic chemokines can be upregulated during inflammation. For example, CCL27 expression is increased in the skin lesions of patients with psoriasis and atopic dermatitis.[9,10]

Leukocytes, platelets, tissue resident cells, such as keratinocytes and fibroblasts as well as structural cells, such as endothelial cells and epithelial cells, all produce a variety of chemokines. Macrophages can produce a plethora of chemokines, while B cells are the source of only a few (Tables 11.3, 11.4). The type of chemokine produced depends on the combination of the type of the cell, the anatomic location of the cell, and the stimulus. For example, high endothelial venules in the lymph node produce CCL19 and CCL21, while the endothelial cells in the skin produce CCL1, CCL17, CCL26, and CX3CL1.[11] While human monocytes produce CCL3 and CCL5 in response to a variety of stimuli, ranging from exposure to bacterial cell wall endotoxins to infection with dsRNA viruses, monocyte production of CCL1 is more selective and occurs after engagement of Fcγ receptor II[12] along with exposure to LPS or IL-1β.

■ CHEMOKINE RECEPTORS AND SIGNALING ■

One of the first chemokines to be identified, IFNγ inducible protein-10 or IP-10 (CXCL10), was discovered in 1985 when it was detected in response to recombinant IFNγ in human mononuclear cells, fibroblasts, and endothelial cells.[13] The significant amino acid homology between CXCL10 and PF4 as well as beta-thromboglobulin, two platelet-derived chemotactic proteins, pointed to the possibility that CXCL10 may be involved in chemotaxis and similarities in their genomic organization suggested that they may belong to a larger family of proteins involved in inflammation.[13,14] RANTES (CCL5), IL-8 (CXCL8), and MCP-1 (CCL2) were the next chemokines discovered.[15–17] CXCL8 was first identified as a neutrophil activating factor. Experiments to understand the mechanism of neutrophil activation by CXCL8 revealed that treatment of neutrophils with *Bordetella pertussis* toxin abrogated signaling through CXCL8, much the same way fMLP signaling was abrogated by this toxin, implying that the receptor for CXCL8 was a G-protein-coupled receptor, specifically coupled to the Gαi subunit.[16] The cloning of the IL-8 receptor in 1991 confirmed that this receptor belongs to the superfamily of G-protein-coupled receptors.[18,19] With approximately 1000 members, G-protein-coupled receptors are widely used to sense small changes in concentrations of biologically active substances in the body and participate in many pathways of signal transduction and numerous biological responses. The chemoattractant receptors, which mediate chemotaxis, constitute a distinct subfamily of the G-protein-coupled receptor superfamily.

Table 11.1 CC chemokines and their receptors in humans and mice

Chemokine	Other names	Chemokine receptor
CCL1	I-309, (mouse TCA3)	CCR8
CCL2	MCP-1, (mouse JE)	CCR2
CCL3	MIP-1α	CCR1, CCR5
CCL4	MIP-1β, HC21	CCR5
CCL5	RANTES	CCR1, CCR3, CCR5
CCL6	C-10, MRP-1	CCR1
CCL7	MCP-3, Fic, MARC	CCR2, CCR3
CCL8	MCP-2	CCR1, CCR2, CCR3, CCR5
CCL9/10	MIP-1γ, MRP-2, CCF18	CCR1
CCL11	Eotaxin-1	CCR3
CCL12	(mouse MCP-5)	CCR2
CCL13	MCP-4, Ckβ10	CCR2, CCR3, CCR5
CCL14	HCC-1	CCR1
CCL15	Leukotactin-1, HCC-2, MIP-5, MIP-1d	CCR1, CCR3
CCL16	HCC-4, NCC-4, LEC	CCR1
CCL17	TARC	CCR4
CCL18	DC-CK1, PARC, AMAC-1, MIP-4	?
CCL19	ELC, MIP-3β, exodus-3	CCR7
CCL20	MIP-3α, LARC, exodus-1	CCR6
CCL21	SLC, exodus-2, 6Ckine, TCA4, CKβ9	CCR7
CCL22	MDC, STCP-1, ABCD-1	CCR4
CCL23	MPIF1, MIP-3, CKβ8	CCR1
CCL24	Eotaxin-2, MPIF2, CKβ6	CCR3
CCL25	TECK	CCR9
CCL26	Eotaxin-3, MPIF-2	CCR3
CCL27	CTAK, ILC, Eskine	CCR10
CCL28	MEC	CCR10

G-protein-coupled receptors have an extracellular NH_2 terminus, seven transmembrane domains, and a cytoplasmic COOH terminus. The intracytoplasmic loops of the transmembrane domains are stretched along the inner aspect of the plasma membrane and the COOH terminus is laterally positioned, giving these receptors more surface area than expected from their 40 kDa size for interaction with GTP-binding proteins as well as other downstream effector and scaffolding molecules.[20] G-protein-coupled receptors signal through heterotrimeric GTP-binding proteins consisting of α, β, and γ subunits. After binding to its ligand, the G-protein-coupled receptor changes the conformation of its transmembrane α helices and exposes its GTP-binding sites. Following GTP binding, the GTP-bound Gα subunit and the G$\beta\gamma$ subunits dissociate from the receptor and signal through distinct pathways downstream. There are four subclasses of mammalian Gα subunits, α_s, α_i, α_q or $\alpha_{12/13}$, and the type of downstream signal generated by the Gα subunit depends on the subclass involved.

In the case of chemokine receptors, the dissociated GTP-coupled Gαi subunit inactivates adenylate cyclase and activates phospholipases as well as phosphodiesterases but Gαi is thought not to be necessary for induction of chemotaxis.[21] Instead, it is the G$\beta\gamma$ subunit that mediates chemotaxis. However, only the G$\beta\gamma$ subunit that was once associated with a Gα_i subunit is capable of inducing chemotaxis.[20,22] The G$\beta\gamma$ subunit activates phospholipase C (PLC-β2 and β3), which results in increased levels of inositol-1,4,5-triphosphate and a transient rise in intracellular free Ca^{++}. The increase in intracellular free Ca^{++} is a widely used test to assess chemokine receptor responsiveness but is not necessary for chemotaxis. Another effector molecule generated through the signaling of G$\beta\gamma$ subunit is phosphatidylinositol 3-kinase (PI3K), which triggers PKB activation and its subsequent translocation to the membrane of the leading edge of the cells.[23] In neutrophils, PI3K activates the small GTPase Rac, which together with PKB induce actin polymerization in the leading edge.[24,25] In lymphocytes,

Table 11.2 CXC, C, and CX3C chemokines and their receptors in humans and mice

Chemokine	Other names	Chemokine receptor
CXCL1	GROα, MGSA-α (mouse KC)	CXCR1, CXCR2
CXCL2	GROβ, MGSA-β, MIP-2α ((mouse MIP-2)	CXCR2
CXCL3	GROγ, MGSA-γ, MIP-2β (mouse MIP-2)	CXCR2
CXCL4	PF4	?
CXCL5	ENA-78 (mouse LIX)	CXCR2
CXCL6	GCP-2	CXCR1, CXCR2
CXCL7	NAP-2, CTAPIII	CXCR2
CXCL8	IL-8, NAP-1, MDNCF	CXCR1, CXCR2
CXCL9	MIG	CXCR3
CXCL10	IP-10, (mouse CRG-2), (rat mob-1)	CXCR3
CXCL11	ITAC, βR1, IP-9, H174	CXCR3, CXCR7
CXCL12	SDF-1, PBSF	CXCR4, CXCR7
CXCL13	BLC, BCA-1	CXCR5
CXCL14	BRAK	?
CXCL15	Lungkine	?
CXCL16		CXCR6
XCL1	Lymphotactin a, SCM-1α	XCR1
XCL2	Lymphotactin b, SCM-1β	XCR1
CXC3L1	Fractalkine neurotactin	CX3CR1

PI3K-independent pathways result in Rac activation with the involvement of the scaffold protein DOCK-2.[26] Along with PIK3K, PKB and Rac, Rap1 is generated downstream of chemokine receptor binding and is important for integrin activation in the leading edge.[27] While the leading edge organizes to propel the cell forward, Rho family of GTPases translocates to the trailing edge of the cell and regulates the formation of actin-myosin complexes that are needed for the retraction of the trailing edge.[24,28] There are numerous other signaling pathways downstream of chemokine receptor engagement including mitogen-activated protein kinase (MAPK), receptor tyrosine kinases, Ras, Raf, extracellular signal-regulated kinase (ERK), and MAPK-ERK kinase (MEK)[20,29] (Fig. 11.2). Complexity of chemokine receptor signaling is further increased with receptor homodimerization and heterodimerization, which may change the signaling properties of the receptors. For example, CCR2 and CCR5 have been shown to heterodimerize, a process which increases the sensitivity of the heterodimeric chemokine receptor to its ligands, recruits new signaling pathways, renders the chemokine receptor pertussis toxin resistant, and induces cell adhesion not chemotaxis.[30] The diversity of signaling pathways downstream of chemokine receptor binding makes it possible for different chemokine receptors, expressed on the same cell, to signal through distinct pathways and for the same chemokine receptor to induce a variety of inflammatory responses.

Signaling through chemokine receptors is rapid and transient. The cessation of signaling is through receptor phosphorylation, desensitization and internalization. As mentioned above, the dissociated G subunit activates phospholipase C. One of the downstream events from phospholipase C is activation of protein kinase C, which together with G-protein-coupled receptor kinases, phosphorylates chemokine receptors.[20,31] The phosphorylated chemokine receptor binds arrestins, an event that leads to receptor desensitization. The receptor-arrestin complex is then internalized through the clathrin-mediated internalization pathway.[20] This desensitization process is more complex than implied above as the arrestin-bound chemokine receptor can activate new signaling pathways.[32]

There are seven CXCRs, 10 CCRs, one XCR, and one CX3CR. Most chemokine receptors bind to more than one chemokine, resulting in a level of redundancy that ensures adequate leukocyte recruitment. While many chemokine receptors are redundant, CXCR4 is vital for successful embryogenesis.[33,34] Expression of chemokine receptors depends on the cell type as well as the state of activation and differentiation of the cell. For example, CCR3 is the chemokine receptor most highly expressed in eosinophils and basophils. While naive T cells express CXCR4 and CCR7, Th1 differentiated and activated T cells express CXCR3, CXCR6, and CCR5 but Th2 differentiated and activated T cells express CCR4, CCR8, and CCR3.[35–39] This selective expression of chemokine receptors by different cells allows for differential recruitment of leukocytes into tissue sites based on the types of chemokines generated. The coordinated expression of Stat1-dependent chemokines, CXCL9, CXCL10, and CXCL11, and Stat6-dependent chemokines, CCL1, CCL17, and

Table 11.3 Chemokine expression by inflammatory cells

Chemokine	Eosinophils	Basophils	Mast cells	T cells	B cells	Neutrophils	Monocyte/ macrophages	Dendritic cells
CCL1			X	X			X	X
CCL2	X		X			X	X	X
CCL3	X	X	X			X	X	
CCL4	X	X	X	X		X	X	
CCL5	X		X	X			X	
CCL6	X						X	
CCL7			X				X	
CCL8			X				X	
CCL9/10							X	X
CCL11	X		X	X				
CCL12			X				X	X
CCL13				X				X
CCL14								
CCL15				X	X		X	X
CCL16							X	
CCL17	X		X				X	X
CCL18							X	X
CCL19						X		X
CCL20			X	X		X	X	
CCL21								
CCL22	X		X	X	X		X	X
CCL23							X	X
CCL24				X			X	
CCL25								X
CCL26								
CCL27								
CCL28								
CXCL1	X					X	X	
CXCL2			X			X	X	
CXCL3						X	X	
CXCL4			X					
CXCL5	X		X					
CXCL6							X	
CXCL7							X	
CXCL8		X	X	X		X	X	
CXCL9						X	X	
CXCL10			X			X	X	
CXCL11						X	X	
CXCL12								X
CXCL13							X	X

(Continued)

Table 11.3 Chemokine expression by inflammatory cells—cont'd

Chemokine	Eosinophils	Basophils	Mast cells	T cells	B cells	Neutrophils	Monocyte/ macrophages	Dendritic cells
CXCL14					X		X	
CXCL15								
CXCL16					X		X	X
XCL1	X		X	X				
XCL2				X				
CXC3L1				X				X

CCL22, differentially recruit Th1 and Th2 cells into sites of Th1 and Th2 inflammation, respectively.[40,41]

REGULATORY MECHANISMS FOR THE CHEMOKINE RESPONSE

Chemokines control leukocyte positioning throughout the body in time and space. At the initial level, the chemokine network is regulated by the stimuli that initiate chemokine production. Some chemokines are produced and released upon activation of transcriptional signals, while others are stored in granules and are available for rapid release after degranulation signals.[42] However, since most chemokines are soluble molecules and function at a distance from their site of generation, there must exist local and post-transcriptional regulatory pathways to closely titrate chemokine bioavailability and fine tune chemokine responses.

After secretion, chemokines bind the negatively charged cell surface or extracellular glycosaminoglycans.[43] In addition, chemokines can be secreted bound to glycosaminoglycans as large molecular weight complexes.[42] The binding of chemokines to glycosaminoglycans concentrates chemokines at the location of secretion, prevents their diffusion, and establishes the gradient for leukocyte chemotaxis.[44] Chemokine binding to glycosaminoglycans on endothelial cell surfaces maintains a high concentration of chemokines on the capillary bed even under shear forces generated by blood flow. Moreover, chemokines have been shown to oligomerize on glycosaminoglycans.[45] Mutations that prevent glycosaminoglycan binding and oligomerization render CCL2, CCL4, and CCL5 ineffective in vivo while maintaining in vitro chemotactic activity.[46] The role of oligomerization was revealed by studies that showed mutant CXCL10 is not retained on endothelial cells and does not induce transendothelial migration.[47] Therefore, factors that influence glycosaminoglycans affect the chemokine response.

A number of specific proteases have been identified that regulate the chemokine response by either altering the glycosaminoglycan composition of the extracellular matrix or by working directly on chemokines. Three groups of proteases have been most intensely studied (Fig. 11.3). The first group is the matrix metalloproteases, which are zinc-dependent endopeptidases that degrade the extracellular matrix during inflammation, release glycosaminoglycans, and modulate

chemokine binding to glycosaminoglycans. For instance, following bleomycin injury, CXCL1 binds to the proteoglycan, syndecan-1, and recruits neutrophils from the bloodstream into the lung parenchyma. MMP-7 then sheds CXCL1-syndecan-1 complexes from damaged lung epithelial cells into the alveoli, a process that is required for neutrophil movement from the injured lung into the alveolar space. Consequently, MMP-7-deficient mice are more tolerant of bleomycin-induced lung injury since their neutrophils are trapped in the lung interstitium and fail to enter the lung air space.[48] Similarly, MMP-2-deficient mice show decreased leukocyte mobilization from the lung into the BAL in an asthma model.[49] In addition, MMPs can degrade or inactivate chemokines.[50,51] For example, MMP-9-deficient mice display more severe allergic airway inflammation with increases in CCL11, CCL22, eosinophil, and T-cell recruitment to the lung and the BAL.[52] MMPs can also degrade chemokines and transform them into receptor antagonist. For example, MMP-truncated CCL7, CCL8, and CCL13 have been shown to act as antagonists for their receptors in transwell cell migration assays.[53]

The second group of proteases is the ADAM (a disintegrin and metalloprotease) – family of proteases. ADAM10 cleaves the cell membrane bound forms of CXCL16 and CX3CL1 and releases these chemokines as soluble chemoattractants.[54,55] The third group is CD26, a membrane bound serine protease and a T lymphocyte surface marker, which cleaves two amino acids from the NH2 terminus of chemokines that have a proline or alanine at the second position, such as CXCL12 and CCL22.[56] CD26 processing of chemokines has varying effects on the chemokine response depending on the chemokine and the chemokine receptor involved. For example, CD26 reduces the chemotactic potency of CXCR3 ligands without affecting their role in angiogenesis.[57] CD26-truncated CCL4 maintains its ability to down regulate CCR5 and to prevent HIV entry into cells and becomes a CCR1 and CCR2 agonist.[58] CD26 is upregulated in both activated and anergic T cells.[59] Non-anergic T cells fail to transmigrate across the endothelial cell monolayer, which was pre-incubated with CD26-expressing anergic T cells.[59] It has been postulated that the expression of CD26 on T cells allows T cells to modify their chemokine environment and influence the movement of their neighboring leukocytes.

In addition to chemokine receptors, a number of other serpentine receptors, which are not G-protein-coupled, have been shown to function as decoy receptors (Fig. 11.4). Decoy receptors are proteins that bind

Table 11.4 Chemokine expression by tissue resident cells

Chemokines	Endothelial cells	Epithelial cells	Fibroblasts	Keratinocytes
CCL1	X			X
CCL2	X	X	X	X
CCL3			X	
CCL4			X	
CCL5			X	X
CCL6				
CCL7	X	X	X	
CCL8			X	
CCL9/10				
CCL11	X	X	X	X
CCL12				
CCL13				X
CCL14				
CCL15				
CCL16				X
CCL17	X	X	X	X
CCL18				X
CCL19	X			
CCL20	X			X
CCL21	X			
CCL22		X		
CCL23				
CCL24				
CCL25	X	X		
CCL26	X			X
CCL27	X			X
CCL28	X	X		
CXCL1	X		X	
CXCL2	X		X	
CXCL3	X		X	
CXCL4				
CXCL5	X			
CXCL6	X		X	
CXCL7	X			
CXCL8	X	X	X	
CXCL9				
CXCL10	X		X	
CXCL11				
CXCL12	X	X		
CXCL13	X			
CXCL14			X	

(Continued)

Table 11.4 Chemokine expression by tissue resident cells—cont'd

Chemokines	Endothelial cells	Epithelial cells	Fibroblasts	Keratinocytes
CXCL15	X			
CXCL16				
XCL1				
XCL2				
CX3CL1	X	X		

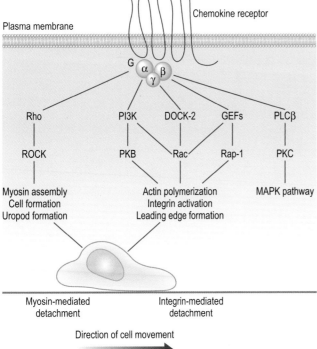

Fig. 11.2. Signaling pathways downstream of G-protein-coupled chemokine receptors. These pathways are thought to lead to myosin-mediated detachment and integrin-mediated attachment, resulting in directional cell movement.

cell membrane and endosomes. When in the endosome, at a lower pH, the affinity of D6 decreases for its ligand, which results in ligand shedding and degradation.[63,64] D6 knockout mice have increased levels of CCL3 and CCL5 and enhanced cutaneous inflammatory responses to phorbol esters.[65] In addition, D6 is expressed in the placenta at the interface of maternal and fetal blood. D6 knockout mice produce higher levels of CC chemokines in response to LPS and antiphospholipid antibodies, have more leukocyte infiltration in placenta, and experience more fetal loss.[66]

Duffy antigen receptor for chemokines (DARC) was first recognized as a blood group antigen and an entry receptor for some malaria strains.[67] Later, it was recognized that many CC and CXC chemokines bind to DARC without signaling.[68,69] DARC, which is expressed not only on erythrocytes but also endothelial cells,[70] influences the chemokine response in three ways. First, it binds chemokines on the abluminal side of the endothelium, internalizes the chemokines, and transports them to the luminal side of the endothelium, where chemokines can interact with the chemokine receptors of leukocytes. For example, CXCL1 transport across the endothelium was increased in DARC transfected human endothelial cells and this was associated with an increase in neutrophil chemotaxis across the endothelium. Consistent with this finding, DARC-deficient mice had decreased neutrophil influx into the lung in response to CXCL8.[71] Second, DARC on erythrocytes can function as a chemokine buffer system in the blood. It can bind free chemokines when chemokines are present in excess, thus preventing the interaction of blood chemokines with chemokine receptors on circulating leukocytes and subsequent chemokine receptor desensitization.[72] Third, DARC can function as a decoy receptor, thus dampening the chemokine response. This is supported by the observation that DARC-deficient mice experience an exaggerated inflammatory response to LPS.[73] CCX-CKR is a non-signaling high-affinity receptor for CCL21, CCL19, and CCL25 and a low-affinity receptor for CXCL13. CCX-CKR is expressed on dendritic cells and T cells, implying a role for this receptor in the regulation of the adaptive immune response.[74]

Understanding the net effect of the chemokine network is further complicated by the observation that chemokines that are ligands for one chemokine receptor could function as antagonists for another chemokine receptor. Similarly, chemokine receptors can bind chemokines that are not their ligands, and therefore, act as decoy receptors. For example, CXCL11, a CXCR3 ligand, functions as a CCR3 antagonist and CXCR3 functions as a decoy receptor for CCL11.[75] Furthermore, CCL7

ligands with high affinity and specificity but cannot transmit downstream signals. They thus prevent ligand binding to its actual functioning receptor. Three types of decoy receptors have been identified and extensively studied: D6, DARC, and CCX-CKR. D6, which is a seven transmembrane domain receptor, expressed on lymphatic vessels, binds to majority of inflammatory CC chemokines without signaling.[60–62] For example, D6 binds to CCR4 ligands, CCCL17 and CCL22, with high affinity but does not bind the homeostatic ligands of CCR6 and CCR7.[62] Bound or unbound, D6 is constantly recycled between the

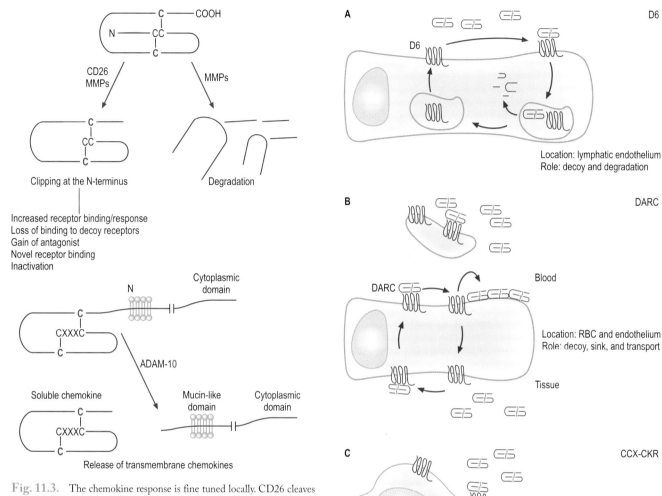

Fig. 11.3. The chemokine response is fine tuned locally. CD26 cleaves two amino acids from the N-terminus of chemokines with varying effects on the chemokine response depending on the chemokine involved. Matrix metalloproteases degrade and inactivate chemokines. ADAM-10 cleaves membrane-bound chemokines and releases these chemokines as soluble chemoattractants.

Location: lymphatic endothelium
Role: decoy and degradation

Location: RBC and endothelium
Role: decoy, sink, and transport

Location: dendritic cells and T cells
Role: decoy

Fig. 11.4. D6, DARC, and CCX-CKR are decoy-type receptors. Decoy receptors bind ligands with high affinity and specificity but do not transmit downstream signals. (A) D6 binds a majority of inflammatory CC chemokines and is continuously recycled between the cell membrane and endosomes. When in the endosome, at a lower pH, the affinity of D6 decreases for its ligands, resulting in ligand release and subsequent degradation. (B) DARC binds chemokines on the abluminal side of the endothelium, internalizes the chemokines, and transports them to the luminal side of the endothelium, where chemokines, can interact with leukocyte chemokine receptors. In addition, DARC on erythrocytes can function as a chemokine buffer system in the blood. (C) CCX-CKR is a non-signaling high-affinity receptor for many chemokines.

is a CCR5 antagonist[76] and CCL26 is a CCR1, CCR2, and CCR5 antagonist.[77] It should be noted that these observations have been made in vitro, and therefore, in vivo significance of these observations is uncertain at this point.

Finally, the chemokine response can be regulated at the level of signaling. For example, dendritic cells that are exposed to inflammatory stimuli mature, downregulate CCR1, CCR2, and CCR5, upregulate CCR7, and traffic to draining lymph nodes. However, when dendritic cells are exposed to an inflammatory signal, such as LPS, along with IL-10, they retain high levels of CCR1, CCR2, and CCR5 and fail to upregulate CCR7. Although these receptors can bind their ligands, they are uncoupled from signaling pathways and do not induce chemotaxis, thus functioning as decoy receptors.[78] Regulators of G protein signaling (RGS) proteins provide another regulatory pathway for chemokine

signaling. RGS proteins regulate the decay of the GTP-bound $G\alpha$ subunit and are able to terminate the signaling cascade downstream of G-protein-coupled receptors.[20] As a result, for example, mice transgenic for RGS 16 have a defect in migration of CXCR4, CCR3, and CCR5 bearing cells.[79]

BIOLOGICAL ROLE OF CHEMOKINE–CHEMOKINE RECEPTOR INTERACTIONS ■

LEUKOCYTE RECRUITMENT

Unstimulated leukocytes circulating in the blood in un-inflamed tissues are not adherent to other cells, the endothelium or the extracellular matrix. After injury or pathogen entry, resident cells at tissue sites make chemokines, which interact with their corresponding chemokine receptors on leukocytes and attract these leukocytes in order to repair the damage and/or fight pathogens. Different leukocytes express different chemokine receptors. Therefore, the type of inflammation that develops depends on the types of chemokines that are produced and the types of responding leukocytes. This recruitment process is integral to both the innate and adaptive immune response and host survival. The interaction of chemokines with chemokine receptors is critical for two distinctly regulated stages of recruitment: leukocyte extravasation out of the bloodstream and into the tissue and leukocyte navigation within tissue to the right anatomic location. While leukocyte extravasation occurs under conditions of blood flow, leukocyte navigation within tissue takes place under static conditions.

In order to traffic into inflamed tissues, leukocytes must cross the endothelium through sequential steps of rolling, tethering, firm adhesion, and diapedesis (Fig. 11.5). While rolling primarily relies on selectins and their carbohydrate ligands, firm adhesion is mediated through integrins. Lymphocytes express β integrins, such as LFA-1 (lymphocyte function associated 1), and α_4 integrins, such as VLA4 (very late antigen 4) and $\alpha_4\beta_7$ integrin. The binding of LFA1 to ICAM mediates lymphocyte trafficking to peripheral lymph nodes and attachment of lymphocytes to antigen presenting cells. The interaction of $\alpha_4\beta_7$ with MADCAM1 mediates lymphocyte trafficking to mucosal surfaces while VLA4-VCAM1 interaction results in lymphocyte trafficking to other inflamed tissues.[80]

Pertussis toxin treatment of lymphocytes does not interfere with rolling but prevents the sticking of activated lymphocytes to high endothelial venules, a rapid process that occurs 1–3 s into rolling.[81] This indicates that there must be in situ agonists that work on activated lymphocytes through G-protein-coupled receptors to mediate firm adhesion by rapid synthesis of high-energy bonds under-flow. The finding that chemokines bind proteoglycans and other proteins on endothelial cells and epithelial cells supported the hypothesis that chemokines could act as the intermediate step between rolling and integrin-dependent firm adhesion.[82–84] Interaction of selectins with their ligands results in rolling of leukocytes on the endothelial surface. This exposes the chemokine receptors on leukocytes to chemokines on endothelial cells. The intracellular events that follow chemokine–chemokine receptor binding ultimately alter integrin clustering and distribution on the cell surface of leukocytes and change integrin affinity through inside-out signaling. The clustered integrins bind with high affinity to their ligands, providing the rapid high-energy bonds that result in firm adhesion and inducing directional cell movement through outside-in signaling. Therefore, chemokines trigger leukocyte extravasation into lymph nodes or sites of inflammation through their influence on integrins.

The immune system can generate different types of inflammatory responses, such as allergic and granulomatous, because specific classes of leukocytes can be differentially recruited into inflamed tissues depending on the insult, injury or pathogen. This specificity of leukocyte recruitment is made possible by the exact combination of selectins, chemokine–chemokine receptors, and integrins present. Specific combinations of chemokines and integrin-mediated adhesion mechanisms have been

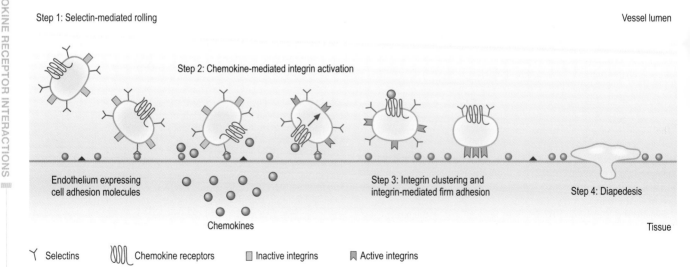

Fig. 11.5. Multi-step model of leukocyte entry into tissue. In order to traffic into tissues, leukocytes must cross the endothelium, a process that involves the sequential steps of rolling, tethering, firm adhesion, and diapedesis. Interaction of selectins with their ligands results in rolling of leukocytes on the endothelial surface. This exposes the chemokine receptors on leukocytes to chemokines on endothelial cells. The intracellular events that follow chemokine–chemokine receptor binding ultimately alter integrin clustering and distribution on the cell surface of leukocytes and change integrin affinity. The clustered integrins bind with high affinity to their ligands, result in firm adhesion and induce diapedesis.

shown for different subsets of leukocytes. For example, CCL5, CCL7, and CCL11 cause VLA-4 and Mac-1 mediated adhesion in eosinophils. CXCL8 mediates Mac-1 mediated adhesion in neutrophils, while CCL2, CCL3, CCL5, CXCL8, and CXCL12 induce β_1 and β_2 integrin mediated adhesion in monocytes.[85]

In addition to leukocyte extravasation, chemokines are also critical in navigating leukocytes within tissue to their right anatomic location. For example, the development of the adaptive immune response requires that naive lymphocytes not only enter the lymph node, where antigen encounter is most efficient, but also find their correct position within the lymph node. CCL21, CXCL12, and CXCL13 are expressed on the apical surface of endothelial cells. Interaction of these chemokines with their respective chemokine receptors on lymphocytes results in clustering of LFA1 on lymphocytes, increased affinity of this integrin for its ligand, ICAM, and arrest of lymphocytes. Once in the lymph node, lymphocytes face a non-uniform distribution of chemokines. CXCL13 is expressed in B follicular regions while CCL21 is expressed in T follicular areas. As a result, B cells that bear CXCR5, the receptor for CXCL13, home to B follicular areas and T cells that bear CCR7, the receptor for CCL21, traffic to T follicular regions.[10]

Chemokines navigate leukocytes in tissue by inducing and controlling cell polarity. Actin polymerizes in the front, in the direction of maximum concentration of chemokine, and forms the leading edge, which makes new attachments to the extracellular matrix. This is accompanied by the formation of the uropod in the rear and detachment from the extracellular matrix mediated through actin-myosin contractions.[80] Navigation to the right anatomic location requires that leukocytes move in the direction of maximum chemokine concentration or respond to different chemokines at different stages of navigation. The exact mechanism of this directional sensing in mammalian cells is not completely clear. Although there are conflicting reports, one possibility is that chemokine receptors are concentrated in the leading edge.[86] The other possibility is that chemokine receptors remain uniformly distributed throughout the cell but non-uniform distribution of intracellular signaling proteins is responsible for directional movement of the cells.[87] In this model, PI3K accumulates at the leading edge and raises the levels of lipid second messenger, phosphatidylinositol triphosphate, while PTEN accumulates on the sides and the rear of the cell and degrades phosphatidylinositol triphosphate.

HOMEOSTASIS AND T-CELL DIFFERENTIATION

The lymph node is the hub of the adaptive immune system. This is where mature activated dendritic cells bring antigens from peripheral tissue for presentation. It is also where T and B lymphocytes search for their cognate antigen. To maintain homeostasis, dendritic cells must scrutinize and present every antigen while T lymphocytes must evaluate every presented antigen to find a match for their T-cell receptor. This requires constant and orchestrated trafficking of dendritic cells, and T and B lymphocytes in and out of the lymph node and in and out of specific anatomic locations within the lymph node. Naive T and B cells enter the lymph node from the blood via the high endothelial venules while dendritic cells and memory T cells enter the lymph node via afferent lymphatics (Fig. 11.6).[10] Dendritic cells, naive T cells, central memory cells, and B cells rely on CCR7 for entry into the lymph node.[6,88] CCR7 on T cells interacts with CCL19 and CCL21 expressed on high endothelial venules, which leads to upregulation of LFA-1 on lymphocytes and extravasation of lymphocytes into the lymph node.

B-cell entry into the lymph node is mediated by both CXCR4 and CCR7 while B cell entry into Peyer's patches depends on CXCR4, CCR7, and CXCR5.[89] Interestingly, central memory T cells, but not naive T cells, can home to the lymph node via a CCR7-independent pathway by expression of CXCR4.[90] Moreover, effector T cells and memory T cells can exit inflamed tissue and enter draining lymph nodes via the afferent lymphatics through a CCR7-dependent process.[91,92] B cells express CXCR5 and travel into B-cell follicles.[93] Dendritic cells and T cells traffic to the T-cell zones via the influence of CCR7 and CCL19 and CCL21. Lymphocytes spend several hours in the lymph node searching for their antigen. If there is no antigen encounter, lymphocytes leave the lymph node using the receptor for sphingosine-1-phosphate, $S1P_1$, a G-protein-coupled receptor required for T-cell exit from the lymph node and re-entry into the blood via efferent lymphatics.[94]

In the setting of inflammation, the chemokine dynamics that orchestrate leukocyte trafficking in and out of lymph nodes and direct lymph node compartmentalization change (Fig. 11.7). CCL21 expression increases in lymphatic vessels leading to increased dendritic cell recruitment into lymph nodes. This upregulation of CCL19 and CCL21 may also attract NK cells, NKT cells, and $\gamma\delta$ T cells, which have been shown to express CCR7 and L-selectin.[95,96] In addition, NK cells can be recruited to stimulated lymph nodes via a CCR7-independent and CXCR3-dependent process.[97] T-cell receptor engagement leads to downregulation of $S1P_1$, and as a result, T cells are retained in the lymph node for a few cycles of division.[94] At this point, the cytokine milieu of the lymph node will dictate the direction of T-cell polarization. For example, NK cell production of IFNγ can polarize T cells to a Th1 phenotype.[97] TCR engagement also upregulates CXCR5 and downregulates CCR7 responsiveness on antigen-activated T cells.[98] Simultaneously, recognition of antigen by the B-cell receptor leads to increased CCR7 expression and increased responsiveness to CCL19 and CCL21.[99] Antigen-activated T- and B-cell subgroups move to the edge of the lymphoid follicle where T-cell help for B-cell activation can occur.[10]

Finally, B cells downregulate CCR7 and CXCR5 and upregulate CCR6, for homing to mucosal surfaces, or CXCR3 for trafficking to other inflamed peripheral tissues, and CXCR4 for homing to the bone marrow.[100] Activation and differentiation of T cells modify the chemokine expression patterns on effector T cells. Th1 cells acquire CXCR3, CCR5, and CXCR6 while Th2 cells acquire CCR4, CCR8.[35–39] Dendritic cells appear to dictate the expression of tissue-specific homing receptors. For example, dendritic cells from Peyer's patches direct CD8+ T cells to express CCR9, the receptor for CCL25 expressed in the GALT[101] while skin Langerhans cells induce the expression of cutaneous-associated antigen (CLA) and CCR4 on CD8+ cells.[102] In addition, cutaneous dendritic cell metabolize locally produced vitamin D_3 to its active form, which in turn signals T cells to express CCR10 and migrate towards CCL27 secreted by skin keratinocytes.[103]

CHEMOKINE CONTROL OF CELL MOVEMENT IN DEVELOPMENT

Studies of CXCL12 and CXCR4 deficient mice expanded the biological importance of chemokines beyond their role in the control of leukocyte movement, demonstrating that chemokines also plays a role in embryogenesis, hematopoiesis, and angiogenesis. CXCL12 is constitutively expressed in several tissues and CXCR4 is found both on leukocytes and tissue cells. Mice with CXCL12 deficiency die perinatally and

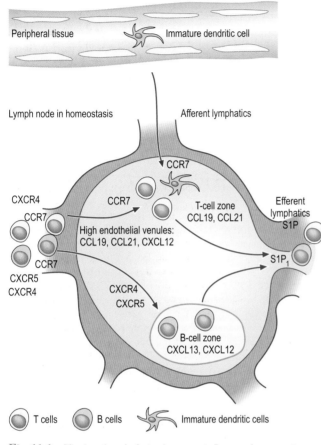

Fig. 11.6. The lymph node during homeostasis. Immune homeostasis requires constant and orchestrated trafficking of dendritic cells, and T and B lymphocytes in and out of the lymph node and in and out of specific anatomic locations within the lymph node. Naïve T and B cells enter the lymph node from the blood via the high endothelial venules while dendritic cells and memory T cells enter the lymph node via afferent lymphatics. Dendritic cells, naïve T cells, central memory cells, and B cells rely on CCR7 for entry into the lymph node. CCR7 on T cells interacts with CCL19 and CCL21 expressed on high endothelial venules, which leads to upregulation of LFA-1 on lymphocytes and extravasation of lymphocytes into the lymph node. CXCR4 and CXCR5 are additional chemokine receptors that mediate lymphocyte homing to the lymph node. B cells express CXCR5 and travel into B-cell follicles. Dendritic cells and T cells traffic to the T-cell zones via the influence of CCR7 and CCL19 and CCL21. Lymphocytes spend several hours in the lymph node searching for their antigen. If there is no antigen encounter, lymphocytes leave the lymph node using the receptor for sphingosine-1-phosphate, $S1P_1$, a G-protein-coupled receptor required for T-cell exit from the lymph node and re-entry into the blood via efferent lymphatics.

have reduced numbers of B cell and myeloid progenitors.[104] CXCL12 is chemotactic for pre-B cells, pro-B cells[105] as well as CD34+ cells.[106] It is required for the colonization of the bone marrow with hematopoietic precursors during embryogenesis, attracting B-cell progenitors to the bone marrow and directing them to their correct bone marrow compartment, where the stromal microenvironment can support the development of B cells.[105,106] The fact that CXCL12-deficient mice have ventricular septal defect suggests that CXCL12 may also play a role in morphogenesis.

In addition, CXCR4 knockout mice show abnormal CNS development due to aberrant neuronal migration[33] and intestinal obstruction and hemorrhage due to incorrect branching of intestinal vasculature during embryonic development.[34] More recent studies have linked CXCR4 to the homing of early progenitor cells to the outer cortex of the thymus[107] and CCR7 to the medullary localization of double positive thymocytes within the thymus.[108] CXCR7 has been recently shown to form a heterodimer with CXCR4, a process that enhances CXCL12 signaling. Similar to the phenotype observed in CXCL12-deficient mice, mice with CXCR7 deficiency die soon after birth due to cardiac defects such as ventricular septal defect and heart valve malformation.[109]

■ ROLE IN HUMAN DISEASE ■

Newly formed naive T cells from the thymus and freshly generated innate immune cells and B cells from the bone marrow enter the bloodstream. While innate immune cells are equipped with chemoattractant receptors that enable them to traffic to sites of injury and infection quickly, naive T and B cells are relatively unresponsive to the chemoattractant cues from peripheral tissue and continue to recirculate between secondary lymphoid organs. Arrival of mature activated antigen-bearing dendritic cells in the draining lymph node leads to T-cell activation and differentiation, B-cell proliferation, and plasma cell formation. Differentiated effector lymphocytes are now decorated with new chemokine receptors and are able to home to peripheral tissue, the chemokine profile of which has been altered by interaction with the innate immune cells that arrived there first. Each disease has a characteristic inflammatory infiltrate, a specific subset of leukocytes that have been attracted to the site of tissue injury based on the chemokines secreted in the tissue. The sequential arrival of each of these leukocyte subsets alters the chemokine milieu of the tissue and attracts the next set of leukocytes responsible for disease pathogenesis. The following section will focus on the role of chemokines and chemokine receptors in the pathogenesis of a spectrum of allergic inflammatory disorders.

ASTHMA

It is the coordinated infiltration of lung tissue with IL-4, IL-5, and IL-13 producing Th2 cells, eosinophils, and mast cells that characterizes allergic airway inflammation seen in asthma (Fig. 11.8). The structural and tissue resident cells of the lung, such as epithelial cells, endothelial cells, smooth muscle cells, fibroblasts, macrophages, histiocytes, and mast cells, produce the first wave of chemokines responsible for allergic inflammation.

In response to pathogens or pathogen-associated products such as LPS, toll-like receptors are activated and result in production of TNF and IL-1 within an hour of exposure. TNF and IL-1 have been shown to upregulate the epithelial cell expression of CCL13, a potent eosinophil and monocyte chemoattractant protein in vitro. In addition, exposure of epithelial cells to respiratory viruses increases the production of numerous eosinophil, neutrophil, and monocyte attracting chemokines, including CCL3, CCL5, CCL11, CXCL1, CXCL5, and CXCL8.[110] Airway epithelial cell exposure to IL-4 results in secretion of CCL26, which binds to surface proteins on epithelial cells and is responsible for transepithelial migration of eosinophils.[84] Bronchial mucosal biopsies of asthmatic individuals localize CCL11 production to epithelial and endothelial cells while CCR3 is expressed

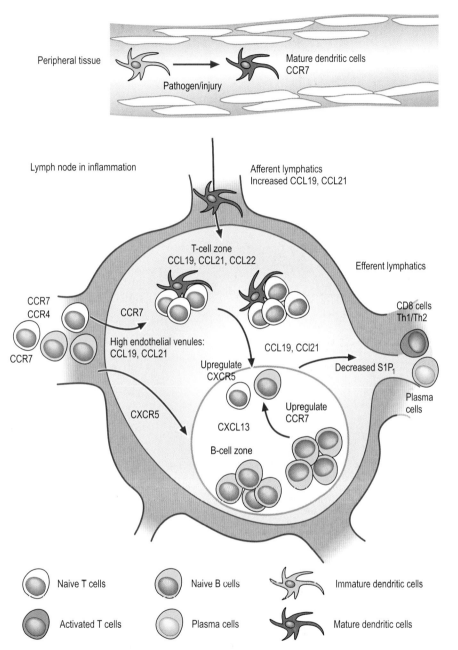

Fig. 11.7. The lymph node during inflammation. In the setting of inflammation, the chemokine dynamics that orchestrate leukocyte trafficking in and out of lymph nodes and direct lymph node compartmentalization change. CCL21 expression increases in lymphatic vessels, leading to increased dendritic cell recruitment into lymph nodes. T-cell receptor engagement leads to downregulation of $S1P_1$, and as a result, T cells are retained in the lymph node for a few cycles of division. At this point, the cytokine milieu of the lymph node will dictate the direction of T-cell polarization. TCR engagement also upregulates CXCR5 and downregulates CCR7 responsiveness on antigen-activated T cells. Simultaneously, recognition of antigen by the B-cell receptor leads to increased CCR7 expression and increased responsiveness to CCL19 and CCL21. Antigen-activated T- and B-cell subgroups meet inside the lymphoid follicle where T-cell help for B-cell activation can occur.

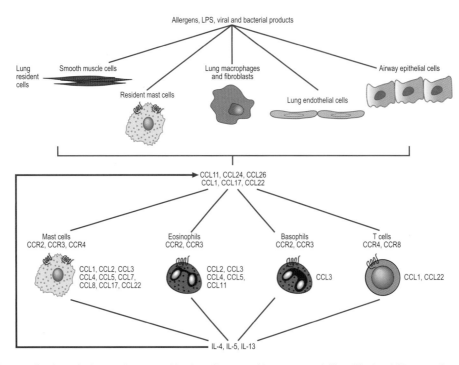

Fig. 11.8. Chemokines and asthma. Asthma is characterized by the infiltration of lung tissue with IL-4, IL-5, and IL-13 producing Th2 cells, eosinophils, basophils, and mast cells. Allergens and pathogens activate lung resident cells to produce the first wave of CC chemokines, which attracts eosinophils, basophils, mast cells, and T lymphocytes to the lung. These cells produce IL-4, IL-5, and IL-13, which in turn upregulate the production of CC chemokines and attract more inflammatory cells.

predominantly by infiltrating eosinophils.[111] Furthermore, smooth muscle cells express CCL11, CCL2, CCL8, CCL7, and CCL5 after exposure to IL-1 and TNF.[112]

In fibroblasts, synergism between TNF and IL-4 leads to production of eotaxins while TNF synergy with IFNγ results in production of CCL5.[113] TGF-β is another inducer of CCL11 production in human airway fibroblasts.[114] Finally, resident mast cells bear toll-like receptors that become activated by LPS, viral particles, and peptidoglycan. For example, TLR2 activation of bone marrow-derived mast cells leads to secretion of IL-4, IL-5, and IL-13 while TLR4 activation of these cells results in IL-13, CCL1, CCL5, and CCL8 secretion.[115,116] These reports support the observation that low levels of LPS signaling through TLR4, in a TNF-dependent fashion, is required for Th2 responses to inhaled antigens.[117] Basophils also bear TLR2 and secrete IL-4 and IL-13 after exposure to peptidoglycan.[118]

Overall, CCL5, CCL11, and monocyte chemoattractant proteins, CCL2, CCL7, and CCL13, have been detected in the bronchial epithelium, the bronchoalveolar lavage fluid, and/or bronchial biopsies of asthmatics. Following segmental allergen challenge, eosinophils, basophils, and mast cells bear CCR2 and CCR3 and respond to the highly expressed levels of their ligands generated during the initial phase of allergic airway inflammation (Fig. 11.8).[1,111,119–122]

CCR3 ligands, CCL5, CCL7, CCL11, and CCL13 all leads to eosinophil degranulation and IL-5 augments the degranulation seen in response to CCR3 ligands.[123] The degranulation of mast cells, eosinophils, and basophils results in a flood of cytokines, chemokines, lipid

mediators, reactive oxygen radicals, and proteases that augment the allergic response. The released cysteinyl leukotrienes recruit more eosinophils, prolong eosinophil survival, and promote eosinophil adhesion.[124] Activated eosinophils generate CCL2, CCL3, CCL4, CCL5, and CCL11, which further amplify the allergic response.[125] Activated basophils release CCL3,[126] leukotrienes, and prostaglandins, which lead to vasodilatation and increased vascular permeability. In addition to releasing histamine, tryptase, chymase, proteases, and arachidonic acid metabolites, activated mast cells release a large number of chemokines, such as CCL1, CCL2, CCL3, CCL4, CCL5, CCL8, CCL17, and CCL22.[116,127,128] More importantly, the degranulation of eosinophils and basophils results in release of IL-4,[129] which augments the production of CCL11, CCL24, CCL26, CCL1, CCL17, and CCL22.

The release of TNF and IL-1 also activates dendritic cells, which subsequently express CCR7 and traffic to the draining lymph nodes for antigen presentation.[6,130] Activation and differentiation of naive T cells into Th2 cells is marked by downregulation of L-selectin and CCR7 along with appearance of CCR4 and CCR8 on Th2 cells, which enables Th2 cells to move down the concentration gradient in response to CCL1, CCL17, and CCL22. It should be noted that concurrent with chemokine receptor expression, Th2 cells express BLT1 and DP2, which are receptors for leukotriene B4 and prostaglandin D_2, respectively, lipid mediators that are generated early during the allergic inflammatory process.[131]

Once the allergic response is established, allergen-specific IgE occupies the Fc epsilon receptor I on mast cells. Re-exposure to allergen and the subsequent cross linking of IgE upregulates the production of CCL1, CCL2, CCL3, CCL4, CCL7, CCL17, CCL22, and XCL1[116,132] as well as CCR1, CCR2, CCR3, and CCR5 expression.[127] The release of CCL1, CCL17, and CCL22 upon mast cell degranulation sets the stage for Th2 cell recruitment and provides a link between the innate immune response to allergen and the adaptive immune response through antigen-specific Th2 cells. It also explains why the atopic asthmatic response is often biphasic. The early phase occurs within the first hour and is due to mast-cell degranulation and the late phase begins between 4 and 24h of allergen exposure and is due to lymphocyte recruitment.

Once in the peripheral tissue, Th2 cells are an efficient source of IL-4, IL-5, and IL-13, all of which propagate the allergic responses. IL-5 leads to release of eosinophils from the bone marrow. IL-4 and IL-13 induce lung residing macrophages, epithelial cells, and endothelial cells to produce CCL11, CCL24, CCL26, CCL1, CCL17, and CCL22 in a Stat6-dependent fashion. Additionally, Th2 cells are themselves a source of CC chemokines as anti-CD3 activated Th2 cells have been shown to produce CCL1 and upregulate CCL22 mRNA in a Stat6-dependent fashion.[133] The Th2 cell release of IL-4 and IL-13 and the subsequent Stat6 induction of Th2-attracting chemokines magnify the allergic response significantly. As a result, mice deficient in Stat6 have dramatically impaired Th2 cell trafficking and show decreased allergic airway inflammation.[41]

It is becoming increasingly clear that Th1 inflammatory processes and Th1-associated chemokines and chemokine receptors also participate in the pathogenesis of asthma. For example, mice that overexpress CXCL10, a CXCR3 ligand, have exaggerated allergic airway inflammation while mice that lack CXCL10 have reduced airway inflammation.[134] Moreover, following segmental allergen challenge, the ligands for CXCR1, CXCR2, CXCR3, CCR5 are elevated in the bronchoalveolar lavage fluid of asthmatics[135,136] in addition to the ligands for CCR4.[135,137] At the same time, lung and alveolar T cells are enriched for CCR5 and CXCR3.[138–140]

ALLERGIC RHINITIS

Like asthma, allergic rhinitis is characterized by the coordinated production of cytokines, adhesion molecules, and chemoattractants that result in the recruitment, and eventual activation, of predominantly CD4+ T cells and eosinophils. The chemokines implicated in allergic rhinitis include: CCL2, CCL3, CCL5, CCL11, CCL26, and CXCL8.[141–143] In patients with allergic rhinitis, allergen challenge leads to a rise in CCL11 levels in nasal lavage fluid and a corresponding increase in nasal eosinophils. Using nasal endothelial cells in a chemotaxis assay, CCL11 proved to be more potent than CCL5 and CCL13 in eosinophil chemotaxis. Pretreatment of eosinophils with anti-CCR3 monoclonal antibody blocked eosinophil endothelial transmigration in response to nasal mucosa homogenate.[144] CCL26 protein levels are increased in the nasal mucosal epithelium from allergic patients compared to non-allergic patients and cell-surface bound CCL26 is critical for eosinophil transepithelial migration.[84] When adenoid CD4+ cells from atopic children were stimulated with allergen, approximately 45% produced IL-4, 54% expressed CCR4, 10% expressed CCR3, and <1% expressed CCR8.[145] Consistent with this observation, relief of nasal obstruction after allergen immunotherapy in patients with allergic rhinitis correlated with a decrease in serum levels of CCL17, the ligand for CCR4.[146] In addition, patients with active allergic rhinitis have increased mRNA expression of CXCR1 and CXCR2 and ex-vivo bradykinin stimulation of nasal epithelial cells from

these patients increases the surface expression of CXCR1.[147] Moreover, CD4+ cells from the nasal mucosa of atopic donors express CXCR1 and migrate towards CXCL8.[148] Finally, immunohistochemical studies of the inferior turbinate biopsy samples from allergic rhinitis patients and non-atopic controls shows staining for TGF-β and TGF-β receptor in the epithelium of atopic patients and a correlation between TFG-β staining and infiltrating mast cell numbers.[149]

ATOPIC DERMATITIS

Atopic dermatitis is a pruritic chronic inflammatory disease of the skin. Its pathophysiology begins with an itch-scratch cycle that causes mechanical trauma to the skin and leads to generation of a number of pro-inflammatory cytokines, including IL-1, TNF, and GM-CSF.[150,151] Recruitment of dendritic cells and their activation by antigens, allergen triggering of mast cells, recruitment of memory T cells and their recognition of allergen, bacterial colonization, and inflammatory responses to bacterial superantigens all propagate and establish skin inflammation in atopic dermatitis (Fig. 11.9).

Histologically, atopic dermatitis is marked by an inflammatory infiltrate composed of predominantly CD4+ memory T lymphocytes but also dendritic cells, mast cells and eosinophils, located in the perivascular, subepidermal, and intraepidermal areas.[152] The chemokines found in the skin of atopic dermatitis patients include: CCL1, CCL2, CCL3, CCL4, CCL5, CCL11, CCL13, CCL18, CCL20, CCL22, CCL26, and CCL27. In addition, disease activity has been correlated with serum levels of CCL11, CCL17, CCL22, CCL26, CCL27, and CX3CL1.[11]

Mice sensitized epicutaneously with staphylococcal enterotoxin B develop eosinophilic skin infiltration with upregulation of Th2-type cytokines.[153] Exposure to staphylococcal enterotoxin B induces CCL18 and CCL1, two chemokines abundantly expressed in the skin of patients with atopic dermatitis.[11,154] Skin dendritic cells of patients with atopic dermatitis, and not patients with other inflammatory skin conditions, produce high levels of CCL18 upon exposure to relevant allergen or staphylococcal enterotoxin B.[155] Although the receptor for CCL18 is not identified, CLA+ T cells from the peripheral blood of patients with atopic dermatitis have been shown to migrate towards CCL18.[154]

Epithelial cells and keratinocytes in the lesions of atopic dermatitis produce high levels of thymic stromal lymphopoietin (TSLP). This cytokine activates CD11c+ dendritic cells and triggers CCL17 and CCL22 production and primes CD4+ cells to produce IL-4, IL-5, IL-13, and TNF.[156] Transgenic mice that overexpress TSLP develop atopic dermatitis-like lesions, thus underscoring the importance of this cytokine in atopic dermatitis.[157,158] TSLP-activated and CD40L-engaged CD11c+ dendritic cells induce CD8+ cells to produce not only IL-5 and IL-13 but also IFNγ.[159] This is in agreement with the observation that chronic lesions of atopic dermatitis have both Th1 and Th2 inflammatory processes.

The number of dendritic cells is increased in the lesions of atopic dermatitis. Dendritic cell precursors must migrate from the blood into peripheral tissue, where they function as sentinels for the immune system. There are several chemokine receptors that can participate in this migration step since dendritic cell precursors express CCR1, CCR2, CCR5, CXCR4, CX3CR1.[11] Unlike their precursors, Langerhans cells have a restricted repertoire of chemokine receptors and express only CCR6 abundantly. Meanwhile, keratinocytes stimulated with IL-1 or TNF express high levels of CCL20, the ligand for CCR6, and CCL20 production is induced in the lesions of atopic dermatitis but not in normal skin.[160]

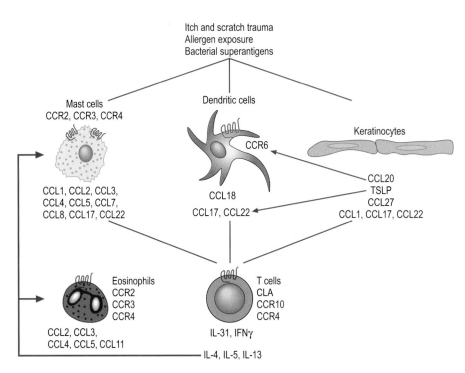

Fig. 11.9. Chemokines and atopic dermatitis. Atopic dermatitis begins with an itch–scratch cycle that causes mechanical trauma to the skin and leads to generation of pro-inflammatory cytokines. Recruitment of dendritic cells and their activation by antigens, allergen activation of mast cells and memory T cells, bacterial colonization, and inflammatory responses to bacterial superantigens lead to production of CC chemokines that attract eosinophils and T lymphocytes. Eosinophils and T lymphocytes release Th2 and Th1 cytokines, which further augment the inflammatory cascade.

T cells are required for the development of atopic dermatitis.[161] Skin homing memory T cells express CLA, which interacts with E-selectin on inflamed endothelium, and initiates rolling. The specific homing of CLA^+ T cells to the skin is controlled by the interaction of CCR10 on memory skin-homing T cells with CCL27, the ligand for CCR10, which is displayed on the skin vascular endothelium.[162] CCL27 is constitutively expressed only by epidermal keratinocytes, and CCL27 neutralization diminishes lymphocyte recruitment to the skin.[9] Skin homing memory $CD4^+$ cells also express CCR4 and the skin endothelium expresses CCL17. While CCR4 deficiency alone and anti-CCL27 neutralizing antibody alone do not decrease the trafficking of $CD4^+$ T cells that are isolated from the draining lymph node of inflamed skin, CCL27 neutralization abrogates the homing of CCR4-deficient $CD4^+$ cells.[163] This implies that the trafficking of skin homing $CD4^+$ T cells depends on both CCR10 and CCR4.

Eosinophil numbers are also increased in lesions of atopic dermatitis. Eosinophils express CCR3 and migrate towards CCR3 ligands, CCL5, CCL11, CCL13, and CCL26, which are expressed in lesional skin and CCR3-deficient mice fail to recruit eosinophils into the skin in an atopic dermatitis model.[164] Mast cell activation following trauma or after allergen cross-linking of IgE results in release of histamine, neuropeptides, proteases, kinins, and cytokines, all of which contribute to pruritus. IL-31, a newly identified cytokine produced predominantly by Th2 cells,[165] is found in higher levels in lesions of atopic dermatitis in response to staphylococcal superantigens,[166] is produced by CLA^+ T

cells,[167] and induces the production of CCL1, CCL17, and CCL22 in keratinocytes. Mice that over express IL-31 in lymphocytes have been shown to develop pruritus and dermatitis.[165] The generation of pruritus sets in motion a positive feedback loop that amplifies the pathophysiologic processes that lead to atopic dermatitis.

EOSINOPHILIC GASTROINTESTINAL DISORDERS

Numerous gastrointestinal disorders are associated with eosinophilic infiltration (Fig. 11.10). These include IgE-mediated food allergy, eosinophilic esophagitis, eosinophilic gastroenteritis, eosinophilic colitis, allergic colitis, gastroesophageal reflux, and to a much lesser extent inflammatory bowel disease.[168] Eosinophilic gastrointestinal disorders are not associated with peripheral blood eosinophilia, implying specific recruitment of eosinophils to the gastrointestinal system. This is in contrast to hypereosinophilic syndrome, in which there is both peripheral blood and tissue (including gastrointestinal) eosinophilia.

CCL11 is one of the primary chemoattractants for eosinophil homing to the gastrointestinal track both during homeostasis[169] and inflammation. CCL11-deficient mice are protected from eosinophilic infiltration after ingestion of enteric-coated antigen.[170] Consistently, CCR3-deficient mice have diminished eosinophil recruitment to the jejunum both at baseline and after infection with *T spiralis*.[171] In a mouse model of ovalbumin-induced food allergy, CCL5 mRNA expression

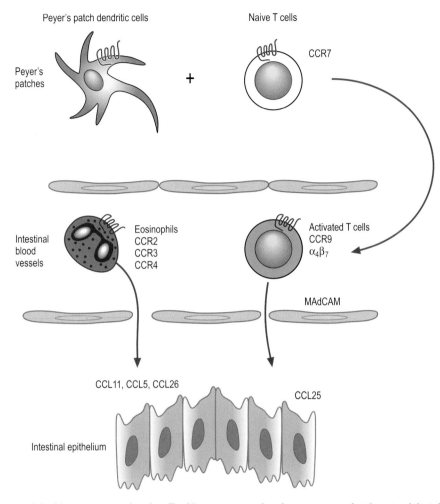

Peyer's patch dendritic cells

Naive T cells

Peyer's patches

CCR7

Intestinal blood vessels

Eosinophils
CCR2
CCR3
CCR4

Activated T cells
CCR9
$\alpha_4\beta_7$

MAdCAM

CCL11, CCL5, CCL26

CCL25

Intestinal epithelium

Fig. 11.10. Chemokines and food hypersensitivity disorders. Food hypersensitivity disorders are associated with eosinophilic infiltration of the gastrointestinal tract and depend on food-specific T cells for cytokine and IgE production. Eosinophil homing to the gastrointestinal tract is mediated through the interaction of CCR3 with CCL11, CCL5, and CCL26 produced in the gut. The homing of naive T cells to Peyer's patches is mediated by the interaction of CCR7 with CCL21 expressed on Peyer's patch high endothelial venules. After activation by Peyer's patch dendritic cells, gut homing T cells express CCR9, which responds to CCL25 secreted in the gut, and $\alpha_4\beta_7$ integrin, which interacts with MAdCAM, the addressin on gut mucosal endothelial cells.

in the gut correlated with the level of eosinophilic infiltration and degranulation.[172] In a recent study, CCL26 was shown to be highly upregulated in patients with eosinophilic esophagitis, compared with controls, and the level of CCL26 mRNA and protein correlated with the number of infiltrating eosinophils and mast cells.[173] In addition to CCL11, CCL5, and CCL26, eosinophilic homing to the gastrointestinal track depends on the interaction of $\alpha_4\beta_7$ integrin on eosinophils with MAdCAM on the intestinal mucosal endothelium.[174]

Food hypersensitivity disorders also depend on T cells for the production of food-specific IgE and cytokine release. The homing of naive T cells to Peyer's patches is mediated by the interaction of CCR7 with CCL21 expressed on Peyer's patch high endothelial venules.[175] After activation by Peyer's patch dendritic cells, gut homing T cells express CCR9, which responds to CCL25 secreted in the gut, and $\alpha_4\beta_7$ integrin, which interacts with MAdCAM, the addressin on gut mucosal

endothelial cells.[101] T cells sensitized in the gut also can differentiate for homing to other organs, thus explaining how food allergy may manifest in extraintestinal organ systems. For example, in patients with atopic dermatitis or urticaria due to milk protein allergy, incubation of peripheral blood mononuclear cells with casein results in the expansion of CLA+ T cells. This CLA+ T-cell expansion is not observed in patients whose food allergy does not involve skin manifestations.[176,177] Food allergen-specific T-cells have been shown to be a source of IL-5. For example, T-cell lines specific for ovomucoid, generated from peripheral blood mononuclear cells of egg allergic patients, consistently express IL-5.[178] IL-5 results in eosinophil expansion in the bone marrow, promotes the release of eosinophils from the bone marrow into the circulation and prolongs eosinophil survival and subsequently contributes to the eosinophilic infiltration seen in eosinophilic gastrointestinal disorders.

Table 11.5 Chemokines and chemokine receptors in non-allergic inflammatory diseases

Disease	Chemokines	Predominant chemokine receptors on infiltrating cells
Hypersensitivity pneumonitis	CXCL10 CXCL8 CCL18	CXCR3
Sarcoidosis	CXCL10 CCL5	CXCR3, CXCR6, CCR5
Inflammatory bowel disease	CCL2, CCL3, CCL4, CCL5, CCL7, CXCL5, CXCL8, CXCL10, CXCL12, and CX3CL1, CCL25	CCR9, CCR5, CXCR3
Rheumatoid arthritis	CXCL8, CCL2, CCL3, and CCL5 CCL19, CCL21, CXCL12 and CXCL13	CCR2, CCR4, CCR5, CXCR3, CXCR6, CXCR4, CCR7
Atherosclerosis	CCL2 CXCL9, CXCL10, CXCL11 CX3CL1 CCL5 CCL11	CCR2 CXCR3 CX3CR1 CCR5 CCR3

NON-ALLERGIC INFLAMMATORY DISEASES

Chemokines and chemokine receptors also participate in the pathogenesis of a very broad spectrum of non-allergic inflammatory diseases, including hypersensitivity pneumonitis, sarcoidosis, inflammatory bowel disease, rheumatoid arthritis, and atherosclerosis. Refer to Table 11.5 for a brief summary of chemokines and chemokine receptors that are associated with these non-allergic inflammatory disorders.[1,2,179]

◼ CLINICAL MANIFESTATIONS OF GENE MUTATIONS AFFECTING THE CHEMOKINE SYSTEM ◼

Although the chemokine system is crucial for regulated leukocyte movement and generation of inflammatory responses, mutations in a single chemokine or chemokine receptor have proven to lead to subtle effects in many animal models of disease. This is most likely secondary to the redundancy that is prominent in the chemokine response. There are a few examples of clinically relevant specific mutations involving chemokine receptor genes. Surprisingly, some of these mutations have proven to be beneficial not harmful.

HIV

During HIV infection, the viral gp120 glycoprotein binds the host CD4 molecule as well as CCR5 and/or CXCR4 co-receptors. Following this binding, the viral gp41 glycoprotein is activated, which leads to virus and host cell membrane fusion. Acute infection is almost always associated with viral interaction with CCR5. However, the virus uses CXCR4 with disease progression and early usage of CXCR4 is associated with a poorer prognosis.[180] Individuals who lack a functional CCR5 due to a mutation in the coding region, the null CCR5δ32 allele, are protected from HIV infection despite having functional CXCR4.[181,182] This allele

is enriched in long-term survivors of HIV infection testifying to the survival advantage of this chemokine receptor mutation.[182]

WEST NILE VIRUS

West Nile virus (WNV) can cause fatal encephalitis in mice and humans. Following subcutaneous infection with WNV, the levels of CCR5 and CCL5 expression increase in the mouse brain along with an influx of inflammatory cells. WNV infection is fatal in mice deficient in CCR5 and is associated with increased viral load. Adoptive transfer of splenocytes from WNV infected wild-type mice into CCR5-deficient mice improves survival, demonstrating that CCR5 plays a critical role in the eradication of WNV infection.[183] Consistent with these findings, epidemiologic studies have revealed that patients who are homozygous for the CCR5delta32 mutation are more likely to have symptomatic WNV infection and a fatal outcome.[184]

DARC

DARC deficiency is another chemokine receptor deficiency that has proven to be beneficial. The agent for malaria, *Plasmodium vivax* and *Plasmodium knowlesi*, enter erythrocytes by binding to Duffy blood group antigen or DARC. A mutation in the promoter region of the gene for DARC prevents the transcription of this chemokine receptor in erythrocytes but not other tissues. As a result, in West Africa, where this mutation is present in 95% of the population, the prevalence of malaria is very low.[185]

WHIM SYNDROME

WHIM syndrome is characterized by warts, hypogammaglobulinemia, immune deficiency and myelokathexis or retention of mature neutrophils in the bone marrow.[186] Patients with WHIM syndrome present with neutropenia and recurrent bacterial infections in early infancy. Despite baseline neutropenia, neutrophil function is normal and patients are able to generate reactive leukocytosis during acute infections. T- and B-cell lymphopenia, T-cell dysfunction, and hypogammaglobulinemia occur in a large number of patients, who nonetheless tolerate viral infections well except for HPV. Lymphoproliferative disorders and lymphoma can be a complication. The bone marrow is hypercellular with increased cellular apoptosis.[187] The disease causing mutations in WHIM syndrome are in the carboxy terminus cytoplasmic tail of CXCR4 and are thought to lead to decreased receptor phosphorylation, decreased binding to β-arrestins, and diminished internalization, resulting in prolonged responsiveness to CXCL12.[187] As a result, neutrophils of patients with WHIM syndrome respond vigorously to stromal CXCL12 in the bone marrow and, therefore, are retained in the bone marrow.[188] Another model of mutation pathogenesis for WHIM syndrome is that prolonged signaling through CXCR4 leads to heterologous desensitization of CXCR2. CXCL12 has been shown to attenuate the response of neutrophils to CXCL1, a CXCR2 ligand and an inflammatory chemokine, which drives neutrophils out of the bone marrow.[189]

■ CONCLUSION ■

There has been a wealth of new information on the role of chemokines and chemokine receptors in health and disease in the past two decades. The chemokine response has proven to participate in both homeostasis and inflammation. Unique chemokine signatures are required for the sequential and specific recruitment of leukocyte subsets in the pathogenesis of every disease. Understanding these disease-specific chemokine navigational cues may lead to new therapeutic targets.

References

Chemokines

1. Luster AD. Chemokines – chemotactic cytokines that mediate inflammation. N Engl J Med 1998; 338:436–445.
2. Rot A, von Andrian UH. Chemokines in innate and adaptive host defense: basic chemokinase grammar for immune cells. Annu Rev Immunol 2004; 22:891–928.
3. Charo IF, Ransohoff RM. The many roles of chemokines and chemokine receptors in inflammation. N Engl J Med 2006; 354:610–621.
4. Murphy PM, Baggiolini M, Charo IF, et al. International Union of Pharmacology. XXII. Nomenclature for chemokine receptors. Pharmacol Rev 2000; 52:145–176.
5. Zlotnik A, Yoshie O. Chemokines: a new classification system and their role in immunity. Immunity 2000; 12:121–127.
6. Forster R, Schubel A, Breitfeld D, et al. CCR7 coordinates the primary immune response by establishing functional microenvironments in secondary lymphoid organs. Cell 1999; 99:23–33.
7. Svensson M, Marsal J, Ericsson A, et al. CCL25 mediates the localization of recently activated CD8alphabeta(+) lymphocytes to the small-intestinal mucosa. J Clin Invest 2002; 110:1113–1121.
8. Homey B, Wang W, Soto H, et al. Cutting edge: the orphan chemokine receptor G protein-coupled receptor-2 (GPR-2, CCR10) binds the skin-associated chemokine CCL27 (CTACK/ALP/ILC). J Immunol 2000; 164:3465–3470.
9. Homey B, Alenius H, Muller A, et al. CCL27-CCR10 interactions regulate T cell-mediated skin inflammation. Nat Med 2002; 8:157–165.
10. Sallusto F, Mackay CR. Chemoattractants and their receptors in homeostasis and inflammation. Curr Opin Immunol 2004; 16:724–731.
11. Homey B, Steinhoff M, Ruzicka T, et al. Cytokines and chemokines orchestrate atopic skin inflammation. J Allergy Clin Immunol 2006; 118:178–189.
12. Sironi M, Martinez FO, D'Ambrosio D, et al. Differential regulation of chemokine production by Fcgamma receptor engagement in human monocytes: association of CCL1 with a distinct form of M2 monocyte activation (M2b, Type 2). J Leukoc Biol 2006; 80:342–349.

Chemokine receptors and signaling

13. Luster AD, Unkeless JC, Ravetch JV. Gamma-interferon transcriptionally regulates an early-response gene containing homology to platelet proteins. Nature 1985; 315:672–676.
14. Luster AD, Ravetch JV. Genomic characterization of a gamma-interferon-inducible gene (IP-10) and identification of an interferon-inducible hypersensitive site. Mol Cell Biol 1987; 7:3723–3731.
15. Schall TJ, Jongstra J, Dyer BJ, et al. A human T cell-specific molecule is a member of a new gene family. J Immunol 1988; 141:1018–1025.
16. Thelen M, Peveri P, Kernen P, et al. Mechanism of neutrophil activation by NAF, a novel monocyte-derived peptide agonist. FASEB J 1988; 2:2702–2706.
17. Rollins BJ, Morrison ED, Stiles CD. Cloning and expression of JE, a gene inducible by platelet-derived growth factor and whose product has cytokine-like properties. Proc Natl Acad Sci U S A 1988; 85:3738–3742.
18. Holmes WE, Lee J, Kuang WJ, et al. Structure and functional expression of a human interleukin-8 receptor. Science 1991; 253:1278–1280.
19. Murphy PM, Tiffany HL. Cloning of complementary DNA encoding a functional human interleukin-8 receptor. Science 1991; 253:1280–1283.
20. Thelen M. Dancing to the tune of chemokines. Nat Immunol 2001; 2:129–134.
21. Neptune ER, Iiri T, Bourne HR. Galphai is not required for chemotaxis mediated by Gi-coupled receptors. J Biol Chem 1999; 274:2824–2828.
22. Neptune ER, Bourne HR. Receptors induce chemotaxis by releasing the betagamma subunit of Gi, not by activating Gq or Gs. Proc Natl Acad Sci U S A 1997; 94:14489–14494.
23. Meili R, Ellsworth C, Lee S, et al. Chemoattractant-mediated transient activation and membrane localization of Akt/PKB is required for efficient chemotaxis to cAMP in Dictyostelium. EMBO J 1999; 18:2092–2105.
24. Meili R, Firtel RA. Two poles and a compass. Cell 2003; 114:153–156.
25. Tanaka T, Bai Z, Srinoulprasert Y, et al. Chemokines in tumor progression and metastasis. Cancer Sci 2005; 96:317–322.
26. Fukui Y, Hashimoto O, Sanui T, et al. Haematopoietic cell-specific CDM family protein DOCK2 is essential for lymphocyte migration. Nature 2001; 412:826–831.
27. Katagiri K, Maeda A, Shimonaka M, et al. RAPL, a Rap1-binding molecule that mediates Rap1-induced adhesion through spatial regulation of LFA-1. Nat Immunol 2003; 4:741–748.
28. Vicente-Manzanares M, Cruz-Adalia A, Martin-Cofreces NB, et al. Control of lymphocyte shape and the chemotactic response by the GTP exchange factor Vav. Blood 2005; 105:3026–3034.
29. Sodhi A, Montaner S, Gutkind JS. Viral hijacking of G-protein-coupled-receptor signalling networks. Nat Rev Mol Cell Biol 2004; 5:998–1012.
30. Mellado M, Rodriguez-Frade JM, Vila-Coro AJ, et al. Chemokine receptor homo- or heterodimerization activates distinct signaling pathways. EMBO J 2001; 20:2497–2507.
31. Richardson RM, DuBose RA, Ali H, et al. Regulation of human interleukin-8 receptor A: identification of a phosphorylation site involved in modulating receptor functions. Biochemistry 1995; 34:14193–14201.
32. Luttrell LM, Daaka Y, Lefkowitz RJ. Regulation of tyrosine kinase cascades by G-protein-coupled receptors. Curr Opin Cell Biol 1999; 11:177–183.
33. Zou YR, Kottmann AH, Kuroda M, et al. Function of the chemokine receptor CXCR4 in haematopoiesis and in cerebellar development. Nature 1998; 393:595–599.
34. Tachibana K, Hirota S, Iizasa H, et al. The chemokine receptor CXCR4 is essential for vascularization of the gastrointestinal tract. Nature 1998; 393:591–594.
35. Campbell DJ, Kim CH, Butcher EC. Chemokines in the systemic organization of immunity. Immunol Rev 2003; 195:58–71.
36. Qin S, Rottman JB, Myers P, et al. The chemokine receptors CXCR3 and CCR5 mark subsets of T cells associated with certain inflammatory reactions. J Clin Invest 1998; 101:746–754.
37. Bonecchi R, Bianchi G, Bordignon PP, et al. Differential expression of chemokine receptors and chemotactic responsiveness of type 1 T helper cells (Th1s) and Th2s. J Exp Med 1998; 187:129–134.
38. Sallusto F, Lenig D, Mackay CR, et al. Flexible programs of chemokine receptor expression on human polarized T helper 1 and 2 lymphocytes. J Exp Med 1998; 187:875–883.
39. D'Ambrosio D, Iellem A, Bonecchi R, et al. Selective up-regulation of chemokine receptors CCR4 and CCR8 upon activation of polarized human type 2 Th cells. J Immunol 1998; 161:5111–5115.
40. Mikhak Z, Fleming CM, Medoff BD, et al. STAT1 in peripheral tissue differentially regulates homing of antigen-specific Th1 and Th2 cells. J Immunol 2006; 176:4959–4967.
41. Mathew A, MacLean JA, DeHaan E, et al. Signal transducer and activator of transcription 6 controls chemokine production and T helper cell type 2 cell trafficking in allergic pulmonary inflammation. J Exp Med 2001; 193:1087–1096.

Regulatory mechanisms for the chemokine response

42. Wagner L, Yang OO, Garcia-Zepeda EA, et al. Beta-chemokines are released from HIV-1-specific cytolytic T-cell granules complexed to proteoglycans. Nature 1998; 391:908–911.
43. Luster AD, Greenberg SM, Leder P. The IP-10 chemokine binds to a specific cell surface heparan sulfate site shared with platelet factor 4 and inhibits endothelial cell proliferation. J Exp Med 1995; 182:219–231.
44. Handel TM, Johnson Z, Crown SE, et al. Regulation of protein function by glycosaminoglycans – as exemplified by chemokines. Annu Rev Biochem 2005; 74:385–410.
45. Hoogewerf AJ, Kuschert GS, Proudfoot AE, et al. Glycosaminoglycans mediate cell surface oligomerization of chemokines. Biochemistry 1997; 36:13570–13578.
46. Proudfoot AE, Handel TM, Johnson Z, et al. Glycosaminoglycan binding and oligomerization are essential for the in vivo activity of certain chemokines. Proc Natl Acad Sci U S A 2003; 100:1885–1890.
47. Campanella GS, Grimm J, Manice LA, et al. Oligomerization of CXCL10 is necessary for endothelial cell presentation and in vivo activity. J Immunol 2006; 177:6991–6998.
48. Li Q, Park PW, Wilson CL, et al. Matrilysin shedding of syndecan-1 regulates chemokine mobilization and transepithelial efflux of neutrophils in acute lung injury. Cell 2002; 111:635–646.
49. Corry DB, Rishi K, Kanellis J, et al. Decreased allergic lung inflammatory cell egression and increased susceptibility to asphyxiation in MMP2-deficiency. Nat Immunol 2002; 3:347–353.
50. McQuibban GA, Gong JH, Tam EM, et al. Inflammation dampened by gelatinase A cleavage of monocyte chemoattractant protein-3. Science 2000; 289:1202–1206.
51. McQuibban GA, Butler GS, Gong JH, et al. Matrix metalloproteinase activity inactivates the CXC chemokine stromal cell-derived factor-1. J Biol Chem 2001; 276:43503–43508.

52. McMillan SJ, Kearley J, Campbell JD, et al. Matrix metalloproteinase-9 deficiency results in enhanced allergen-induced airway inflammation. J Immunol 2004; 172:2586–2594.
53. McQuibban GA, Gong JH, Wong JP, et al. Matrix metalloproteinase processing of monocyte chemoattractant proteins generates CC chemokine receptor antagonists with anti-inflammatory properties in vivo. Blood 2002; 100:1160–1167.
54. Gough PJ, Garton KJ, Wille PT, et al. A disintegrin and metalloproteinase 10-mediated cleavage and shedding regulates the cell surface expression of CXC chemokine ligand 16. J Immunol 2004; 172:3678–3685.
55. Hundhausen C, Misztela D, Berkhout TA, et al. The disintegrin-like metalloproteinase ADAM10 is involved in constitutive cleavage of CX3CL1 (fractalkine) and regulates CX3CL1-mediated cell-cell adhesion. Blood 2003; 102:1186–1195.
56. Lambeir AM, Proost P, Durinx C, et al. Kinetic investigation of chemokine truncation by CD26/dipeptidyl peptidase IV reveals a striking selectivity within the chemokine family. J Biol Chem 2001; 276:29839–29845.
57. Proost P, Schutyser E, Menten P, et al. Amino-terminal truncation of CXCR3 agonists impairs receptor signaling and lymphocyte chemotaxis, while preserving antiangiogenic properties. Blood 2001; 98:3554–3561.
58. Guan E, Wang J, Roderiquez G, et al. Natural truncation of the chemokine MIP-1 beta /CCL4 affects receptor specificity but not anti-HIV-1 activity. J Biol Chem 2002; 277:32348–32352.
59. James MJ, Belaramani L, Prodromidou K, et al. Anergic T cells exert antigen-independent inhibition of cell-cell interactions via chemokine metabolism. Blood 2003; 102:2173–2179.
60. Nibbs RJ, Wylie SM, Yang J, et al. Cloning and characterization of a novel promiscuous human beta-chemokine receptor D6. J Biol Chem 1997; 272:32078–32083.
61. Nibbs RJ, Kriehuber E, Ponath PD, et al. The beta-chemokine receptor D6 is expressed by lymphatic endothelium and a subset of vascular tumors. Am J Pathol 2001; 158:867–877.
62. Bonecchi R, Locati M, Galliera E, et al. Differential recognition and scavenging of native and truncated macrophage-derived chemokine (macrophage-derived chemokine/CC chemokine ligand 22) by the D6 decoy receptor. J Immunol 2004; 172:4972–4976.
63. Weber M, Blair E, Simpson CV, et al. The chemokine receptor D6 constitutively traffics to and from the cell surface to internalize and degrade chemokines. Mol Biol Cell 2004; 15:2492–2508.
64. Comerford I, Nibbs RJ. Post-translational control of chemokines: a role for decoy receptors?. Immunol Lett 2005; 96:163–174.
65. Jamieson T, Cook DN, Nibbs RJ, et al. The chemokine receptor D6 limits the inflammatory response in vivo. Nat Immunol 2005; 6:403–411.
66. Martinez de la Torre Y, Buracchi C, Borroni EM, et al. Protection against inflammation- and autoantibody-caused fetal loss by the chemokine decoy receptor D6. Proc Natl Acad Sci U S A 2007; 104:2319–2324.
67. Miller LH, Mason SJ, Dvorak JA, et al. Erythrocyte receptors for (Plasmodium knowlesi) malaria: Duffy blood group determinants. Science 1975; 189:561–563.
68. Neote K, Darbonne W, Ogez J, et al. Identification of a promiscuous inflammatory peptide receptor on the surface of red blood cells. J Biol Chem 1993; 268:12247–12249.
69. Neote K, Mak JY, Kolakowski LF, Jr, et al. Functional and biochemical analysis of the cloned Duffy antigen: identity with the red blood cell chemokine receptor. Blood 1994; 84:44–52.
70. Patterson AM, Siddall H, Chamberlain G, et al. Expression of the duffy antigen/receptor for chemokines (DARC) by the inflamed synovial endothelium. J Pathol 2002; 197:108–116.
71. Lee JS, Frevert CW, Wurfel MM, et al. Duffy antigen facilitates movement of chemokine across the endothelium in vitro and promotes neutrophil transmigration in vitro and in vivo. J Immunol 2003; 170:5244–5251.
72. Darbonne WC, Rice GC, Mohler MA, et al. Red blood cells are a sink for interleukin 8, a leukocyte chemotaxin. J Clin Invest 1991; 88:1362–1369.
73. Dawson TC, Lentsch AB, Wang Z, et al. Exaggerated response to endotoxin in mice lacking the Duffy antigen/receptor for chemokines (DARC). Blood 2000; 96:1681–1684.
74. Gosling J, Dairaghi DJ, Wang Y, et al. Cutting edge: identification of a novel chemokine receptor that binds dendritic cell- and T cell-active chemokines including ELC, SLC, and TECK. J Immunol 2000; 164:2851–2856.
75. Xanthou G, Duchesnes CE, Williams TJ, et al. CCR3 functional responses are regulated by both CXCR3 and its ligands CXCL9, CXCL10 and CXCL11. Eur J Immunol 2003; 33:2241–2250.
76. Blanpain C, Migeotte I, Lee B, et al. CCR5 binds multiple CC-chemokines: MCP-3 acts as a natural antagonist. Blood 1999; 94:1899–1905.
77. Petkovic V, Moghini C, Paoletti S, et al. Eotaxin-3/CCL26 is a natural antagonist for CC chemokine receptors 1 and 5. A human chemokine with a regulatory role. J Biol Chem 2004; 279:23357–23363.
78. D'Amico G, Frascaroli G, Bianchi G, et al. Uncoupling of inflammatory chemokine receptors by IL-10: generation of functional decoys. Nat Immunol 2000; 1:387–391.
79. Lippert E, Yowe DL, Gonzalo JA, et al. Role of regulator of G protein signaling 16 in inflammation-induced T lymphocyte migration and activation. J Immunol 2003; 171:1542–1555.

Biological role of chemokine–chemokine receptor interactions

80. Kinashi T. Intracellular signalling controlling integrin activation in lymphocytes. Nat Rev Immunol 2005; 5:546–559.
81. Bargatze RF, Butcher EC. Rapid G protein-regulated activation event involved in lymphocyte binding to high endothelial venules. J Exp Med 1993; 178:367–372.
82. Rot A. Endothelial cell binding of NAP-1/IL-8: role in neutrophil emigration. Immunol Today 1992; 13:291–294.
83. Tanaka Y, Adams DH, Hubscher S, et al. T-cell adhesion induced by proteoglycan-immobilized cytokine MIP-1 beta. Nature 1993; 361:79–82.
84. Yuan Q, Campanella GS, Colvin RA, et al. Membrane-bound eotaxin-3 mediates eosinophil transepithelial migration in IL-4-stimulated epithelial cells. Eur J Immunol 2006; 36:2700–2714.
85. Laudanna C, Kim JY, Constantin G, et al. Rapid leukocyte integrin activation by chemokines. Immunol Rev 2002; 186:37–46.
86. Manes S, Gomez-Mouton C, Lacalle RA, et al. Mastering time and space: immune cell polarization and chemotaxis. Semin Immunol 2005; 17:77–86.
87. Franca-Koh J, Kamimura Y, Devreotes PN. Leading-edge research: PtdIns(3,4,5)P(3) and directed migration. Nat Cell Biol 2007; 9:15–17.
88. Sallusto F, Lenig D, Forster R, et al. Two subsets of memory T lymphocytes with distinct homing potentials and effector functions. Nature 1999; 401:708–712.
89. Okada T, Ngo VN, Ekland EH, et al. Chemokine requirements for B cell entry to lymph nodes and Peyer's patches. J Exp Med 2002; 196:65–75.
90. Scimone ML, Felbinger TW, Mazo IB, et al. CXCL12 mediates CCR7-independent homing of central memory cells, but not naive T cells, in peripheral lymph nodes. J Exp Med 2004; 199:1113–1120.
91. Bromley SK, Thomas SY, Luster AD. Chemokine receptor CCR7 guides T cell exit from peripheral tissues and entry into afferent lymphatics. Nat Immunol 2005; 6:895–901.
92. Debes GF, Arnold CN, Young AJ, et al. Chemokine receptor CCR7 required for T lymphocyte exit from peripheral tissues. Nat Immunol 2005; 6:889–894.
93. Ohl L, Henning G, Krautwald S, et al. Cooperating mechanisms of CXCR5 and CCR7 in development and organization of secondary lymphoid organs. J Exp Med 2003; 197:1199–1204.
94. Matloubian M, Lo CG, Cinamon G, et al. Lymphocyte egress from thymus and peripheral lymphoid organs is dependent on S1P receptor 1. Nature 2004; 427:355–360.
95. Johnston B, Kim CH, Soler D, et al. Differential chemokine responses and homing patterns of murine TCR alpha beta NKT cell subsets. J Immunol 2003; 171:2960–2969.
96. Brandes M, Willimann K, Lang AB, et al. Flexible migration program regulates gamma delta T-cell involvement in humoral immunity. Blood 2003; 102:3693–3701.
97. Martin-Fontecha A, Thomsen LL, Brett S, et al. Induced recruitment of NK cells to lymph nodes provides IFN-gamma for T(H)1 priming. Nat Immunol 2004; 5:1260–1265.
98. Breitfeld D, Ohl L, Kremmer E, et al. Follicular B helper T cells express CXC chemokine receptor 5, localize to B cell follicles, and support immunoglobulin production. J Exp Med 2000; 192:1545–1552.
99. Reif K, Ekland EH, Ohl L, et al. Balanced responsiveness to chemoattractants from adjacent zones determines B-cell position. Nature 2002; 416:94–99.
100. Kunkel EJ, Butcher EC. Plasma-cell homing. Nat Rev Immunol 2003; 3:822–829.
101. Mora JR, Bono MR, Manjunath N, et al. Selective imprinting of gut-homing T cells by Peyer's patch dendritic cells. Nature 2003; 424:88–93.
102. Dudda JC, Simon JC, Martin S. Dendritic cell immunization route determines CD8+ T cell trafficking to inflamed skin: role for tissue microenvironment and dendritic cells in establishment of T cell-homing subsets. J Immunol 2004; 172:857–863.
103. Sigmundsdottir H, Pan J, Debes GF, et al. DCs metabolize sunlight-induced vitamin D_3 to 'program' T cell attraction to the epidermal chemokine CCL27. Nat Immunol 2007; 8:285–293.
104. Nagasawa T, Hirota S, Tachibana K, et al. Defects of B-cell lymphopoiesis and bone-marrow myelopoiesis in mice lacking the CXC chemokine PBSF/SDF-1. Nature 1996; 382:635–638.
105. D'Apuzzo M, Rolink A, Loetscher M, et al. The chemokine SDF-1, stromal cell-derived factor 1, attracts early stage B cell precursors via the chemokine receptor CXCR4. Eur J Immunol 1997; 27:1788–1793.
106. Aiuti A, Webb IJ, Bleul C, et al. The chemokine SDF-1 is a chemoattractant for human CD34+ hematopoietic progenitor cells and provides a new mechanism to explain the mobilization of CD34+ progenitors to peripheral blood. J Exp Med 1997; 185:111–120.
107. Plotkin J, Prockop SE, Lepique A, et al. Critical role for CXCR4 signaling in progenitor localization and T cell differentiation in the postnatal thymus. J Immunol 2003; 171:4521–4527.
108. Kwan J, Killeen N. CCR7 directs the migration of thymocytes into the thymic medulla. J Immunol 2004; 172:3999–4007.
109. Sierro F, Biben C, Martinez-Munoz L, et al. Disrupted cardiac development but normal hematopoiesis in mice deficient in the second CXCL12/SDF-1 receptor, CXCR7. Proc Natl Acad Sci U S A 2007; 104:14759–14764.

Role in human disease

110. Message SD, Johnston SL. Host defense function of the airway epithelium in health and disease: clinical background. J Leukoc Biol 2004; 75:5–17.
111. Ying S, Robinson DS, Meng Q, et al. Enhanced expression of eotaxin and CCR3 mRNA and protein in atopic asthma. Association with airway hyperresponsiveness and predominant co-localization of eotaxin mRNA to bronchial epithelial and endothelial cells. Eur J Immunol 1997; 27:3507–3516.
112. Ghaffar O, Hamid Q, Renzi PM, et al. Constitutive and cytokine-stimulated expression of eotaxin by human airway smooth muscle cells. Am J Respir Crit Care Med 1999; 159:1933–1942.
113. Teran LM, Mochizuki M, Bartels J, et al. Th1- and Th2-type cytokines regulate the expression and production of eotaxin and RANTES by human lung fibroblasts. Am J Respir Cell Mol Biol 1999; 20:777–786.
114. Wenzel SE, Trudeau JB, Barnes S, et al. TGF-beta and IL-13 synergistically increase eotaxin-1 production in human airway fibroblasts. J Immunol 2002; 169:4613–4619.
115. Supajatura V, Ushio H, Nakao A, et al. Differential responses of mast cell Toll-like receptors 2 and 4 in allergy and innate immunity. J Clin Invest 2002; 109:1351–1359.
116. Okumura S, Kashiwakura J, Tomita H, et al. Identification of specific gene expression profiles in human mast cells mediated by Toll-like receptor 4 and FcepsilonRI. Blood 2003; 102:2547–2554.
117. Eisenbarth SC, Piggott DA, Huleatt JW, et al. Lipopolysaccharide-enhanced, toll-like receptor 4-dependent T helper cell type 2 responses to inhaled antigen. J Exp Med 2002; 196:1645–1651.
118. Bieneman AP, Chichester KL, Chen YH, et al. Toll-like receptor 2 ligands activate human basophils for both IgE-dependent and IgE-independent secretion. J Allergy Clin Immunol 2005; 115:295–301.
119. Liu LY, Jarjour NN, Busse WW, et al. Chemokine receptor expression on human eosinophils from peripheral blood and bronchoalveolar lavage fluid after segmental antigen challenge. J Allergy Clin Immunol 2003; 112:556–562.
120. Sousa AR, Lane SJ, Nakhosteen JA, et al. Increased expression of the monocyte chemoattractant protein-1 in bronchial tissue from asthmatic subjects. Am J Respir Cell Mol Biol 1994; 10:142–147.

121. Rojas-Ramos E, Avalos AF, Perez-Fernandez L, et al. Role of the chemokines RANTES, monocyte chemotactic proteins-3 and -4, and eotaxins-1 and -2 in childhood asthma. Eur Respir J 2003; 22:310–316.
122. Lilly CM, Nakamura H, Belostotsky OI, et al. Eotaxin expression after segmental allergen challenge in subjects with atopic asthma. Am J Respir Crit Care Med 2001; 163:1669–1675.
123. Fujisawa T, Kato Y, Nagase H, et al. Chemokines induce eosinophil degranulation through CCR-3. J Allergy Clin Immunol 2000; 106:507–513.
124. Busse W, Kraft M. Cysteinyl leukotrienes in allergic inflammation: strategic target for therapy. Chest 2005; 127:1312–1326.
125. Oliveira SH, Taub DD, Nagel J, et al. Stem cell factor induces eosinophil activation and degranulation: mediator release and gene array analysis. Blood 2002; 100:4291–4297.
126. Li H, Sim TC, Grant JA, et al. The production of macrophage inflammatory protein-1 alpha by human basophils. J Immunol 1996; 157:1207–1212.
127. Oliveira SH, Lukacs NW. Stem cell factor and IgE-stimulated murine mast cells produce chemokines (CCL2, CCL17, CCL22) and express chemokine receptors. Inflamm Res 2001; 50:168–174.
128. Selvan RS, Butterfield JH, Krangel MS. Expression of multiple chemokine genes by a human mast cell leukemia. J Biol Chem 1994; 269:13893–13898.
129. Voehringer D, Shinkai K, Locksley RM. Type 2 immunity reflects orchestrated recruitment of cells committed to IL-4 production. Immunity 2004; 20:267–277.
130. Sallusto F, Schaerli P, Loetscher P, et al. Rapid and coordinated switch in chemokine receptor expression during dendritic cell maturation. Eur J Immunol 1998; 28:2760–2769.
131. Luster AD, Tager AM. T-cell trafficking in asthma: lipid mediators grease the way. Nat Rev Immunol 2004; 4:711–724.
132. Rumsaeng V, Vliagoftis H, Oh CK, et al. Lymphotactin gene expression in mast cells following Fc(epsilon) receptor I aggregation: modulation by TGF-beta, IL-4, dexamethasone, and cyclosporin A. J Immunol 1997; 158:1353–1360.
133. Zhang S, Lukacs NW, Lawless VA, et al. Cutting edge: differential expression of chemokines in Th1 and Th2 cells is dependent on Stat6 but not Stat4. J Immunol 2000; 165:10–14.
134. Medoff BD, Sauty A, Tager AM, et al. IFN-gamma-inducible protein 10 (CXCL10) contributes to airway hyperreactivity and airway inflammation in a mouse model of asthma. J Immunol 2002; 168:5278–5286.
135. Bochner BS, Hudson SA, Xiao HQ, et al. Release of both CCR4-active and CXCR3-active chemokines during human allergic pulmonary late-phase reactions. J Allergy Clin Immunol 2003; 112:930–934.
136. Virchow JC Jr., Walker C, Hafner D, et al. T cells and cytokines in bronchoalveolar lavage fluid after segmental allergen provocation in atopic asthma. Am J Respir Crit Care Med 1995; 151:960–968.
137. Pilette C, Francis JN, Till SJ, et al. CCR4 ligands are up-regulated in the airways of atopic asthmatics after segmental allergen challenge. Eur Respir J 2004; 23:876–884.
138. Campbell JJ, Brightling CE, Symon FA, et al. Expression of chemokine receptors by lung T cells from normal and asthmatic subjects. J Immunol 2001; 166:2842–2848.
139. Kallinich T, Schmidt S, Hamelmann E, et al. Chemokine-receptor expression on T cells in lung compartments of challenged asthmatic patients. Clin Exp Allergy 2005; 35:26–33.
140. Thomas SY, Banerji A, Medoff BD, et al. Multiple chemokine receptors, including CCR6 and CXCR3, regulate antigen-induced T cell homing to the human asthmatic airway. J Immunol 2007; 179:1901–1912.
141. Alam R. Chemokines in allergic inflammation. J Allergy Clin Immunol 1997; 99:273–277.
142. Elsner J, Escher SE, Forssmann U. Chemokine receptor antagonists: a novel therapeutic approach in allergic diseases. Allergy 2004; 59:1243–1258.
143. Minshall EM, Cameron L, Lavigne F, et al. Eotaxin mRNA and protein expression in chronic sinusitis and allergen induced nasal responses in seasonal allergic rhinitis. Am J Respir Cell Mol Biol 1997; 17:683–690.
144. Terada N, Hamano N, Kim WJ, et al. The kinetics of allergen-induced eotaxin level in nasal lavage fluid: its key role in eosinophil recruitment in nasal mucosa. Am J Respir Crit Care Med 2001; 164:575–579.
145. Banwell ME, Robinson DS, Lloyd CM. Adenoid-derived TH2 cells reactive to allergen and recall antigen express CC chemokine receptor 4. J Allergy Clin Immunol 2003; 112:1155–1161.
146. Takeuchi H, Yamamoto Y, Kitano H, et al. Changes in thymus- and activation-regulated chemokine (TARC) associated with allergen immunotherapy in patients with perennial allergic rhinitis. J Investig Allergol Clin Immunol 2005; 15:172–176.
147. Eddleston J, Christiansen SC, Jenkins GR, et al. Bradykinin increases the in vivo expression of the CXC chemokine receptors CXCR1 and CXCR2 in patients with allergic rhinitis. J Allergy Clin Immunol 2003; 111:106–112.
148. Francis JN, Jacobson MR, Lloyd CM, et al. CXCR1+CD4+ T cells in human allergic disease. J Immunol 2004; 172:268–273.
149. Salib RJ, Kumar S, Wilson SJ, et al. Nasal mucosal immunoexpression of the mast cell chemoattractants TGF-beta, eotaxin, and stem cell factor and their receptors in allergic rhinitis. J Allergy Clin Immunol 2004; 114:799–806.
150. Mihara K, Kuratani K, Matsui T, et al. Vital role of the itch-scratch response in development of spontaneous dermatitis in NC/Nga mice. Br J Dermatol 2004; 151:335–345.
151. Wood LC, Jackson SM, Elias PM, et al. Cutaneous barrier perturbation stimulates cytokine production in the epidermis of mice. J Clin Invest 1992; 90:482–487.
152. Leung DY, Bieber T. Atopic dermatitis. Lancet 2003; 361:151–160.
153. Laouini D, Kawamoto S, Yalcindag A, et al. Epicutaneous sensitization with superantigen induces allergic skin inflammation. J Allergy Clin Immunol 2003; 112:981–987.
154. Gunther C, Bello-Fernandez C, Kopp T, et al. CCL18 is expressed in atopic dermatitis and mediates skin homing of human memory T cells. J Immunol 2005; 174:1723–1728.
155. Pivarcsi A, Gombert M, Dieu-Nosjean MC, et al. CC chemokine ligand 18, an atopic dermatitis-associated and dendritic cell-derived chemokine, is regulated by staphylococcal products and allergen exposure. J Immunol 2004; 173:5810–5817.
156. Soumelis V, Reche PA, Kanzler H, et al. Human epithelial cells trigger dendritic cell mediated allergic inflammation by producing TSLP. Nat Immunol 2002; 3:673–680.
157. Li M, Messaddeq N, Teletin M, et al. Retinoid X receptor ablation in adult mouse keratinocytes generates an atopic dermatitis triggered by thymic stromal lymphopoietin. Proc Natl Acad Sci U S A 2005; 102:14795–14800.
158. Yoo J, Omori M, Gyarmati D, et al. Spontaneous atopic dermatitis in mice expressing an inducible thymic stromal lymphopoietin transgene specifically in the skin. J Exp Med 2005; 202:541–549.
159. Gilliet M, Soumelis V, Watanabe N, et al. Human dendritic cells activated by TSLP and CD40L induce proallergic cytotoxic T cells. J Exp Med 2003; 197:1059–1063.
160. Nakayama T, Fujisawa R, Yamada H, et al. Inducible expression of a CC chemokine liver- and activation-regulated chemokine (LARC)/macrophage inflammatory protein (MIP)-3 alpha/CCL20 by epidermal keratinocytes and its role in atopic dermatitis. Int Immunol 2001; 13:95–103.
161. Woodward AL, Spergel JM, Alenius H, et al. An obligate role for T-cell receptor alphabeta+ T cells but not T-cell receptor gammadelta+ T cells, B cells, or CD40/CD40L interactions in a mouse model of atopic dermatitis. J Allergy Clin Immunol 2001; 107:359–366.
162. Campbell JJ, Butcher EC. Chemokines in tissue-specific and microenvironment-specific lymphocyte homing. Curr Opin Immunol 2000; 12:336–341.
163. Reiss Y, Proudfoot AE, Power CA, et al. CC chemokine receptor (CCR)4 and the CCR10 ligand cutaneous T cell-attracting chemokine (CTACK) in lymphocyte trafficking to inflamed skin. J Exp Med 2001; 194:1541–1547.
164. Ma W, Bryce PJ, Humbles AA, et al. CCR3 is essential for skin eosinophilia and airway hyperresponsiveness in a murine model of allergic skin inflammation. J Clin Invest 2002; 109:621–628.
165. Dillon SR, Sprecher C, Hammond A, et al. Interleukin 31, a cytokine produced by activated T cells, induces dermatitis in mice. Nat Immunol 2004; 5:752–760.
166. Sonkoly E, Muller A, Lauerma AI, et al. IL-31: a new link between T cells and pruritus in atopic skin inflammation. J Allergy Clin Immunol 2006; 117:411–417.
167. Bilsborough J, Leung DY, Maurer M, et al. IL-31 is associated with cutaneous lymphocyte antigen-positive skin homing T cells in patients with atopic dermatitis. J Allergy Clin Immunol 2006; 117:418–425.
168. Rothenberg ME. Eosinophilic gastrointestinal disorders (EGID). J Allergy Clin Immunol 2004; 113:11–28; quiz 9.
169. Matthews AN, Friend DS, Zimmermann N, et al. Eotaxin is required for the baseline level of tissue eosinophils. Proc Natl Acad Sci U S A 1998; 95:6273–6278.
170. Hogan SP, Mishra A, Brandt EB, et al. A pathological function for eotaxin and eosinophils in eosinophilic gastrointestinal inflammation. Nat Immunol 2001; 2:353–360.
171. Gurish MF, Humbles A, Tao H, et al. CCR3 is required for tissue eosinophilia and larval cytotoxicity after infection with Trichinella spiralis. J Immunol 2002; 168:5730–5736.
172. Lee JB, Matsumoto T, Shin YO, et al. The role of RANTES in a murine model of food allergy. Immunol Invest 2004; 33:27–38.
173. Blanchard C, Wang N, Stringer KF, et al. Eotaxin-3 and a uniquely conserved gene-expression profile in eosinophilic esophagitis. J Clin Invest 2006; 116:536–547.
174. Mishra A, Hogan SP, Brandt EB, et al. Enterocyte expression of the eotaxin and interleukin-5 transgenes induces compartmentalized dysregulation of eosinophil trafficking. J Biol Chem 2002; 277:4406–4412.
175. Warnock RA, Campbell JJ, Dorf ME, et al. The role of chemokines in the microenvironmental control of T versus B cell arrest in Peyer's patch high endothelial venules. J Exp Med 2000; 191:77–88.
176. Abernathy-Carver KJ, Sampson HA, Picker LJ, et al. Milk-induced eczema is associated with the expansion of T cells expressing cutaneous lymphocyte antigen. J Clin Invest 1995; 95:913–918.
177. Beyer K, Castro R, Feidel C, et al. Milk-induced urticaria is associated with the expansion of T cells expressing cutaneous lymphocyte antigen. J Allergy Clin Immunol 2002; 109:688–693.
178. Eigenmann PA, Huang SK, Sampson HA. Characterization of ovomucoid-specific T-cell lines and clones from egg-allergic subjects. Pediatr Allergy Immunol 1996; 7:12–21.
179. Viola A, Luster AD. Chemokines and their receptors: drug targets in immunity and inflammation. Annu Rev Pharmacol Toxicol 2007.

Clinical manifestations of gene mutations affecting the chemokine system

180. Margolis L, Shattock R. Selective transmission of CCR5-utilizing HIV-1: the 'gatekeeper' problem resolved? Nat Rev Microbiol 2006; 4:312–317.
181. Liu R, Paxton WA, Choe S, et al. Homozygous defect in HIV-1 coreceptor accounts for resistance of some multiply-exposed individuals to HIV-1 infection. Cell 1996; 86:367–377.
182. Dean M, Carrington M, Winkler C, et al. Genetic restriction of HIV-1 infection and progression to AIDS by a deletion allele of the CKR5 structural gene. Hemophilia Growth and Development Study, Multicenter AIDS Cohort Study, Multicenter Hemophilia Cohort Study, San Francisco City Cohort, ALIVE Study. Science 1996; 273:1856–1862.
183. Glass WG, Lim JK, Cholera R, et al. Chemokine receptor CCR5 promotes leukocyte trafficking to the brain and survival in West Nile virus infection. J Exp Med 2005; 202:1087–1098.
184. Glass WG, McDermott DH, Lim JK, et al. CCR5 deficiency increases risk of symptomatic West Nile virus infection. J Exp Med 2006; 203:35–40.
185. Hadley TJ, Peiper SC. From malaria to chemokine receptor: the emerging physiologic role of the Duffy blood group antigen. Blood 1997; 89:3077–3091.
186. Zuelzer WW. 'Myelokathexis' – a new form of chronic granulocytopenia. Report of a case. N Engl J Med 1964; 270:699–704.
187. Diaz GA. CXCR4 mutations in WHIM syndrome: a misguided immune system? Immunol Rev 2005; 203:235–243.
188. Gulino AV, Moratto D, Sozzani S, et al. Altered leukocyte response to CXCL12 in patients with warts hypogammaglobulinemia, infections, myelokathexis (WHIM) syndrome. Blood 2004; 104:444–452.
189. Martin C, Burdon PC, Bridger G, et al. Chemokines acting via CXCR2 and CXCR4 control the release of neutrophils from the bone marrow and their return following senescence. Immunity 2003; 19:583–593.

REFERENCES

Lipid Mediators of Hypersensitivity and Inflammation

R Stokes Peebles Jr and Joshua A Boyce

12

CONTENTS

SUMMARY OF IMPORTANT CONCEPTS

>> Lipid mediators can act to either propagate or suppress allergic inflammation depending upon the specific mediator and the receptor through which it signals

>> Signaling through prostanoid receptors that increase cAMP generally restrain allergic inflammation

>> LTB₄ and the cysteinyl leukotrienes are important pro-inflammatory mediators

>> Isoprostanes (IsoPs) are formed by the free radical-catalyzed peroxidation of arachidonic acid formation and are not only a dependable marker of oxidant injury both in vivo and in vitro but also are mediators that are biologically active and may regulate oxidant injury

>> Sphingosine-1-phosphate is produced by mast cells and other cell types and is a major regulator of T lymphocyte function in preventing apoptosis, promoting CD4⁺CD25⁺ T regulatory cell activity, and enhancing chemotaxis

INTRODUCTION

Lipid mediators were first recognized as important products of allergic reactions in the 1940 report by Kellaway and Trethewie, describing contraction of airway smooth muscle in the lungs of egg protein-sensitized guinea pigs with re-exposure to the egg protein.[1] These investigators did not know at the time that the 'slow reacting substance' responsible for the smooth muscle contraction they witnessed were leukotrienes generated by various cell types in response to both IgE-dependent and -independent stimuli, and have profound immunologic and physiologic roles in allergic responses. Moreover, recent evidence suggests that lipid mediators are profoundly important as regulators of the initial dendritic cell response to antigens during primary sensitization. Therefore, our understanding of the scope of the mechanisms by which lipid mediators modulate allergic inflammation is more far reaching than was previously appreciated. In this chapter, we will review the pathways of lipid mediator generation, examine studies that confirm the presence of these products in allergic inflammatory states, and discuss in vivo intervention studies in humans and recent murine reports which elucidate the activity of these mediators in the pathogenesis of allergic disease.

GENERATION OF LIPID MEDIATOR PRECURSORS BY PHOSPHOLIPASE A₂

The phospholipases A_2 (PLA_2) are enzymes which hydrolyze fatty acids at the sn-2 position of membrane phospholipids, forming free fatty acids including arachidonic acid and lysoglycero-phospholipids.[2] Arachidonic acid serves as the precursor for the synthesis of all prostaglandins and leukotrienes, collectively known as eicosanoids because the Greek word for 20 is *eikosi*, the number of carbon atoms in arachidonic acid.[3] The lysoglycero-phospholipids are precursors for lysophosphatidic acid

A | IMMUNOLOGY

EICOSANOID FORMATION

Table 12.1 Phospholipase A_2 family

Group	Subgroups	Enzyme type
I	A–B	$sPLA_2$
II	A–F	$sPLA_2$
III		$sPLA_2$
IV	A–F	$cPLA_2$
V		$sPLA_2$
VI	A–F	$iPLA_2$
VII	A–B	PAF–AH
VIII	A–B	PAF–AH
IX		$sPLA_2$
X		$sPLA_2$
XI	A–B	$sPLA_2$
XII		$sPLA_2$
XIII		$sPLA_2$
XIV		$sPLA_2$
XV		$LPLA_2$

$sPLA_2$, secreted; $cPLA_2$, cytosolic; $iPLA_2$, Ca^{2+} independent; PAF-AH, platelet-activating factor acetylhydrolase activity; $LPLA_2$, lysosomal PLA_2.

(LPA) and sphingosine-1-phosphate (S_1P).[2] Both the generation and biologic function of the eicosanoids and the lysoglycero-phospholipids metabolites will be discussed in detail later in this chapter. The PLA_2s are categorized into five major classes, secretory PLA_2s ($sPLA_2$), cytosolic PLA_2s ($cPLA_2$), Ca^{2+} independent PLA_2 ($iPLA_2$), platelet-activating factor acetylhydrolases (PAF-AH), and lysosomal PLA_2s.[2] The current classification scheme of the PLA_2s is based upon the catalytic mechanism of the individual PLA_2, as well as their functional and structural properties, and consists of 15 groups (Table 12.1). Although these 15 groups of PLA_2 have now been identified, the groups that lead to lipid mediator generation are, at least to this point, limited to group IIA, group IVA, group VI, and, very recently, group X.[4]

The $sPLA_2$ are secreted from their cellular source, are small enzymes (14–18 kDa) that utilize an active site histidine and a His/Asp dyad, and require μM levels of Ca^{2+} for their catalytic activity.[2] After cellular release, the $sPLA_2$s can participate in either paracrine or autocrine generation of arachidonic acid from the outer leaflet of plasma membranes. Group IIA $sPLA_2$ is important in the generation of lysophosphatidyl choline for synthesis of LPA.[5] Recently, mice lacking group X $sPLA_2$ showed strikingly diminished bronchial inflammation, airway remodeling, pulmonary Th2 cytokine levels, and levels of multiple lipid mediators in a model of chicken ovalbumin (OVA)-induced airway disease.[4]

The $cPLA_2$ are present in the cytosol and are larger than the $sPLA_2$ (61–114 kDa).[2] There are six subgroups (denoted A–F) of $cPLA_2$ enzymes in group IV and these use a catalytic serine in a Ser/Asp dyad. The group IVA $cPLA_2$ does not require Ca^{2+} for its catalytic activity, but Ca^{2+} is important for this enzyme's translocation to intracellular membranes after binding to a C2-domain. Group IVA $cPLA_2$ not

only hydrolyzes glycerophospholipids at the sn-2 position to liberate arachidonic acid, but also has lysophospholipase and transacylase activities.[2] The generation of group IVA knock-out mice has revealed that this enzyme also regulates nociception,[6] inflammation, intestinal ulceration, acute lung injury, polyposis, ischemia reperfusion brain injury, anaphylaxis, and parturition.[7]

The Ca^{2+} independent PLA_2 are termed $iPLA_2$ and are in group VI.[2] Similar to the $cPLA_2$, the $iPLA_2$ use a catalytic serine and there are also six subgroups (denoted A–F) of $iPLA_2$ enzymes in group VI. Group VIA and group VIB $iPLA_2$ act to generate arachidonic acid release for eicosanoid production, while group VIA has roles in glycerophospholipid remodeling, protein expression, acetylcholine-modulated endothelium-dependent relaxation of vessels, apoptosis, and lymphocyte proliferation. The platelet-activating factor acetylhydrolases (PAF-AH) hydrolyze the acetyl group from the sn-2 position of PAF.[2] There are two groups of PAF-AH, classified as groups VII and VIII. As these PLA_2 are not involved in eicosanoid formation, these groups will not be discussed in this chapter.

Thus, the PLA_2 enzymes, while critical for the generation of arachidonic acid, LPA, and S_1P from membrane phospholipids, also have many other important far-reaching biologic functions.

■ EICOSANOID FORMATION ■

CYCLOOXYGENASE PATHWAY

Arachidonic acid is oxidatively metabolized by the cyclooxygenase and lipoxygenase pathways.[8] Cyclooxygenase catalyzes two reactions, first a cyclooxygenase reaction that inserts two molecules of oxygen into arachidonic acid to produce prostaglandin (PG)G_2, followed by an endoperoxidase reaction that reduces PGG_2 to PGH_2 (Fig. 12.1). PHG_2 is the precursor for the prostanoids PGD_2, PGE_2, $PGF_{2\alpha}$, and PGI_2, and thromboxane A_2 (TXA_2). Each prostanoid is produced by tissue-specific enzymes and isomerases, which will be discussed below. There are two cyclooxygenase enzymes, COX-1 and COX-2, which are products of separate genes and have different biologic functions based on their different temporal and tissue-specific expression.[8] The human COX-1 gene is located on chromosome 9, is constitutively expressed in most tissues, and although inducible in some contexts is presumed to be involved in homeostatic prostanoid synthesis.[8] On the other hand, COX-2 expression is inducible and usually transient. The human COX-2 gene is present on chromosome 1. COX-2 expression can be induced by lipopolysaccharide (LPS) produced by Gram-negative bacteria, in addition to interleukin (IL)-1, IL-2, and TNF.[9] COX-2 expression can be induced in macrophages, endothelial cells, airway epithelial cells,[10,11] airway smooth muscle cells,[12,13] and airway fibroblasts.[14] The multitude and diversity of stimuli that induce COX-2 expression, and the myriad of cells capable of expressing it, ensures that its function is a frequent concomitant of inflammatory diseases. COX-2 is also constitutively expressed in some contexts, such as in cultured human lung epithelial cells,[15] cortical thick ascending limb of the kidney,[16] pancreatic islet cells,[17] human brain cortical cells in Rett syndrome,[18] and in human gastric carcinoma.[19] The capacity of non-steroidal antiinflammatory drugs to inhibit COX-2 activity may constitute their major therapeutic effect, while inhibition of COX-1 may result in some of their undesired side effects.[20,21]

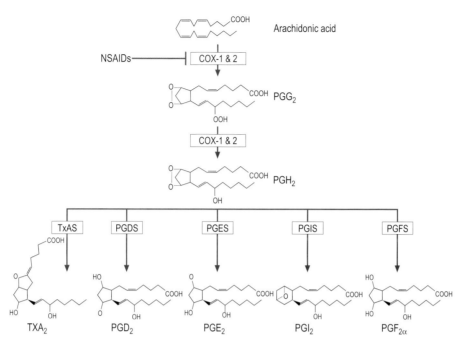

Fig. 12.1. Prostanoid generation. Biosynthesis of prostaglandins. Arachidonic acid is metabolized by cyclooxygenase-1 or -2 to the unstable endoperoxide PGH_2, the common precursor for the five principal prostaglandins. Thromboxane A_2, PGD_2, PGE_2, PGI_2, and $PGF_{2\alpha}$ are generated by individual prostaglandin synthase enzymes (TxAS, PGDS, PGES, PGIS, and PGFS) and elicit their biological effects by activating cell surface G protein-coupled receptors. NSAIDs, non-steroidal antiinflammatory drugs. (Reproduced from Hata AN and Breyer RD. Pharmacology and signalling of prostaglandin receptors: Multiple roles in inflammation and immune modulation. Pharmacology and Therapeutics 2004; 103:147–166, with permission. Copyright, Elsevier.)

There have been contradictory reports about the expression of COX-2 in the asthmatic lung. One study reported a fourfold amplification in bronchial epithelial COX-2 immunostaining in asthmatic subjects compared with healthy controls;[22] however, another study discerned no difference in the level of immunostaining in asthmatics, chronic bronchitics, or controls who had no lung disease.[23] COX-2 mRNA expression and immunoreactive protein was increased in the airway epithelium of asthmatics that have not been treated with corticosteroids compared with non-asthmatic controls, while corticosteroid-treated asthmatics had decreased COX-2 expression compared with their non-treated counterparts.[24] The relationship between the cytokines implicated in the allergic response and COX-2 expression is complex. For instance, IL-4 downregulated COX-2 expression and prostanoid synthesis in human monocytes and macrophages, and monocytes were more susceptible to this effect than alveolar macrophages.[25] IL-4 also suppresses COX-2 expression by mouse bone marrow-derived mast cells. IL-13 treatment of human bronchial epithelial cells suppressed the expression of both COX-2 and microsomal PGE synthase.[26] Thus, in asthmatic subjects, increased levels of TNF might result in COX-2 induction, while IL-4 and IL-13 might inhibit this enzyme's expression. Prednisone treatment for 1 week increased COX-2 expression in monocytes and alveolar macrophages from allergic subjects; however, this same treatment in normal subjects resulted in inhibition of COX-2 expression in these same cell types.[27] It is possible that while corticosteroids inhibit COX-2, they might act indirectly by reducing IL-4 (and perhaps IL-13), in so doing permitting TNF induction of COX-2.

In vitro, COX-2 immunoreactivity in airway epithelial cells is reduced by corticosteroid treatment, while corticosteroids have little effect on COX-1 immunoreactivity.[28] Corticosteroids decrease basal and bradykinin-induced levels of PGE_2 in airway epithelial cells, implying that COX-2 is the primary producer of PGE_2 in airway epithelium.[28] COX-1 and COX-2 mRNA is present in resting human T lymphocytes.[29] T cell activation does not affect COX-1 expression in T cells, while T cell stimulation upregulates COX-2 mRNA levels with increased COX-2 protein and cyclooxygenase activity.[29] COX-1 and COX-2 are important in T cell development.[30] Therefore, COX expression exists in both resident airway cells and cells of the adaptive immune response.

Human studies of the COX pathway in allergic inflammation

There is abundant data that COX products are increased as a result of allergic inflammation. For instance, COX products in the bronchoalveolar (BAL) fluid of allergic asthmatics are significantly increased compared with healthy non-asthmatic controls, and allergic antigen challenge of the airways further augments prostanoid production. BAL fluid levels of PGD_2 and $PGF_{2\alpha}$ were 12- to 22-fold greater in asthmatics than in non-allergic subjects, and 10-times greater in allergic asthmatics than in non-asthmatic subjects who had allergic rhinitis.[31] Segmental allergen challenge led to a 17- to 208-fold increase in the levels of PGD_2, thromboxane B_2, and 6-keto-$PGF_{1\alpha}$, a PGI_2 metabolite in allergic asthmatics.[32] When these subjects were treated with prednisone for 3 days prior to segmental allergen challenge, there was no alteration in the BAL fluid prostanoid concentrations, revealing that corticosteroids do not inhibit activation of the COX pathway that occurs with an allergic inflammatory stimulus.[33]

Intervention studies examining the importance of the COX enzymes in allergic airway disease have been performed by treating subjects with indomethacin, which blocks both COX-1 and COX-2, before allergen challenge. Indomethacin did not effect lung function prior to allergen challenge in either allergic asthmatics or subjects with allergic rhinitis who did not have asthma.[34] However, indomethacin treatment reduced the forced expiratory volume in 1 s (FEV_1) and specific airway conductance in non-asthmatic subjects with allergic rhinitis in response to inhaled allergen challenge.[34] Indomethacin administration prior to allergen challenge caused a small but significant decrease in specific airway conductance in the allergic asthmatic subjects compared with placebo treatment, yet indomethacin had no effect on allergen-induced alterations in FEV_1.[34] Indomethacin treatment had no significant effect on airway responsiveness to histamine, nor did it change the immediate or late phase pulmonary response to allergen challenge in allergic asthmatics.[35,36] In subjects with exercise-induced asthma, indomethacin did not alter bronchoconstriction after exercise, but did prevent refractoriness after exercise.[37] The apparent complex effect of COX inhibition on lung function reflects the diversity of the individual prostanoids (see below), some of which counteract one another's actions.

Mouse studies of the COX pathway in allergic inflammation

Mice with targeted deletions of COX-1 and COX-2 genes have been subjected to models of sensitization and challenge with OVA. COX-1 deficient mice showed heightened lung eosinophilia, serum IgE levels, augmented airway responsiveness, increased numbers of CD4+ and CD8+ T cells, and exaggerated levels of Th2 cytokines, and amplified concentrations of eotaxin and thymus- and activation-regulated chemokine (TARC) compared with both mice deficient in COX-2 and wild-type control mice.[38,39] Thus, COX-1-derived prostanoids may be homeostatic during allergen-induced pulmonary inflammation. One study reported that COX-2 deficient mice on a C57BL/6 genetic background had increased serum IgE levels, vascular cell adhesion molecule-1 (VCAM-1), and intercellular adhesion molecule-1 (ICAM-1) levels compared with control mice, but no difference in pulmonary eosinophilia or airway responsiveness.[38,39] Another group reported that COX-2 deficient mice, also on a C57BL/6 background, had greater allergen-induced lung eosinophilia compared with wild-type mice.[40] Based on these findings that COX-1 inhibition augments allergic airway inflammation and airway responsiveness, one would suspect that overexpression of COX-1 would have the opposite effect. However, COX-1 overexpression targeted to the airway epithelium decreased basal airway responsiveness yet had no effect on the degree of allergic inflammation.[41]

Pharmacologic inhibition of COX enzymes produces profound effects on the development of allergic inflammation. Mice treated with oral indomethacin during the induction of allergic airway disease had increased Th2 cytokines in the lungs, increased pulmonary eosinophilia, and greater airway responsiveness to methacholine compared with vehicle-treated mice.[42] Although BAL leukotriene levels were increased as a result of indomethacin treatment, 5-LO deficient mice also had increased allergen-induced inflammation with indomethacin treatment, effectively ruling out a causative role for enhanced leukotriene production in the exaggerated inflammatory response.[43] The

heightened allergic inflammation with indomethacin administration was dependent on CD4+ cells, but independent of IL-4, IL-4 receptor alpha signaling, and STAT6, elements deemed critical in the canonical Th2 signaling pathway.[44] This augmented allergic phenotype is not specific to indomethacin as both COX-1 and COX-2 inhibitors independently augmented lung levels of IL-13 and airway responsiveness compared with vehicle-treated mice.[45] COX-2 inhibition during epicutaneous sensitization with OVA in a mouse model of atopic dermatitis increased eosinophil skin infiltration, elevated total and antigen-specific IgE, and resulted in a systemic Th2 response to antigen.[46] As several studies reveal that COX inhibition during the development of allergic disease resulted in increased allergen-induced inflammation and airway responsiveness, these results imply that a COX product may restrain allergic inflammation and might be a therapeutic target for the treatment of allergic diseases such as asthma and atopic dermatitis.

It is critical to recognize that in these mouse studies COX inhibition was present throughout the entire development of allergic disease, from the initial stage of antigen presentation and throughout all allergen challenges. In the human studies using indomethacin, COX inhibition occurred only at the time of an antigen challenge, long after the regulatory elements of allergic inflammation in the lung had been set in place. It is also important to note that prostanoids such as PGD_2 that are bronchoconstrictive in humans fail to constrict mouse airways.[47] Thus, animal models of allergic pulmonary disease, whether COX functions are ablated pharmacologically or by gene deletion, are better suited to identify immunologic functions of prostanoids, rather than the direct effects on end-organ physiology seen in human studies.[47]

■ INDIVIDUAL PROSTANOIDS ■

PGD_2

PGD_2 is the major mast cell-derived prostanoid, being released in nanogram quantities by this cell type in response to IgE-mediated activation.[48,49] There are two distinct forms of PGD_2-synthesizing enzymes, hematopoietic- and lipocalin-PGD_2 synthases (H-PGDS and L-PGDS, respectively); only the former is involved in PGD_2 production by mast cells and other hematopoietic cell types.[50] L-PGDS is present in the choroid plexus, leptomeninges, oligodendrocytes, organs of the male genital tract, and in the hearts of humans and monkeys.[50] L-PGDS gene expression in the central nervous system can be modulated by glucocorticoid, thyroid, and estrogen hormones, while L-PGDS expression in the heart is modulated by estrogen.[50] H-PGDS is expressed to the greatest degree in humans in placenta, lung, adipose tissue, and fetal liver, while it is expressed in lower levels in the heart, lymph nodes, bone marrow, and appendix.[50] H-PGDS is also expressed in mast cells, CD4+ Th2 (but not Th1) T lymphocytes, CD8+ Tc2 cells, histiocytes, megakaryocytes, dendritic cells, and Kupffer cells.[50] PGD_2 can be metabolized to $PGF_{2\alpha}$, $9\alpha,11\beta-PGF_{2\alpha}$ (the stereoisomer of $PGF_{2\alpha}$), and the J series of prostanoids which includes PGJ_2, $\Delta^{12}-PGJ_2$, and 15d-PGJ_2.[51]

As is the case for all eicosanoids, PGD_2 signals through distinct seven transmembrane, G-protein coupled receptors (GPCRs), termed DP_1 and DP_2 (Table 12.2).[50] DP_1 is expressed on mucus-secreting goblet cells in the nasal and colonic mucosa, nasal serous glands, vascular endothelium, Th2 cells, dendritic cells, and eosinophils.[50] DP_1 stimulation activates

Table 12.2 PGD_2 receptor expression, signaling, and function

	DP₁	DP₂
Expression	Mucus-secreting goblet cells in nasal and colonic mucosa, nasal serous glands, vascular endothelium, Th2 cells, dendritic cells, eosinophils	Immune cells such as CD4⁺ Th2 and CD8⁺ Tc2 cells, basophils, and eosinophils
Receptor signaling	Stimulation activates adenyl cyclase, resulting in intracellular increase in cAMP levels and PKA activity	Decreases intracellular cAMP
Function	Promotes sleep, survival of eosinophils, secretion of mucus, vasodilation, and vascular permeability; decreases cytokine secretion and chemotaxis	Chemotaxis of CD4⁺ Th2 and CD8⁺ Tc2 cells, basophils, and eosinophils; induces release of eosinophils from bone marrow, initiates their respiratory burst, and primes them for degranulation; increases microvascular permeability; depletion of goblet cells; constricts coronary arteries

adenyl cyclase, resulting in an intracellular increase in cAMP levels and PKA activity.[52] Signaling through DP_1 has been reported to promote sleep, survival of eosinophils, secretion of mucus, vasodilation, and vascular permeability, while decreasing cytokine secretion and chemotaxis.[50] DP_2 is also known as chemoattractant receptor-like molecule expressed on Th2 cells (CRTH2). In addition to PGD_2, other DP_2 agonists include Δ^{12}-PGJ_2; 15-deoxy-$\Delta^{12,14}PGJ_2$ (15d-PGJ_2); 13,15-dihydro-15-keto-PGD_2; 11-dehydro-TXB_2; and the COX inhibitor indomethacin.[50] DP_2 is expressed on immune cells such as CD4⁺ Th2 and CD8⁺ Tc2 cells, eosinophils, and basophils. These cells each respond chemotactically to PGD_2 in a DP_2-dependent manner.[50] DP_2 signaling in eosinophils also induces the release of eosinophils from bone marrow, initiates their respiratory burst, increases the chemotactic response to other chemokines such as eotaxin, and primes them for degranulation.[50,53,54] In addition, DP_2 signaling is reported to increase microvascular permeability, depletion of goblet cells, and constrict coronary arteries.[50] In contrast to DP_1 signaling, activation of DP_2 results in decreased intracellular cAMP.[55] Thus, PGD_2 signaling through DP_2, through suppression of cAMP, would be predicted to facilitate allergic inflammation through its effect on chemotaxis, and mediator release by effector cells.

Human studies of PGD₂ in allergic inflammation

Inhalation challenge of allergic human asthmatic subjects with specific allergen increases the levels of PGD_2 in the BAL fluid.[56] PGD_2 is increased in the nasal lavage from subjects with allergic rhinitis,[57] in tears from persons suffering from allergic conjunctivitis,[58] and in the fluid from experimentally produced skin blisters in patients with late phase reactions of the skin.[59] PGD_2 is a potent bronchoconstrictor and vasodilator, and potentiates airway responsiveness.[60] Intranasal administration of PGD_2 increased nasal resistance 10-times more potently than histamine and 100-times greater than bradykinin.[61] PGD_2 induced vascular leakage in the conjunctiva and skin,[62] and led to eosinophil influx in the conjunctiva[63] and trachea,[64] suggesting that it may have a direct pathogenic role in allergic disease. The vascular effects of PGD_2 are thought to largely reflect dilation mediated by DP_1, whereas recruitment of effector cells is more likely to reflect chemotaxis via DP_2.[65,66] Although both receptors may function in

the effector phase of inflammatory responses, DP_1 receptor signaling potently inhibited TNF-α-induced migration of Langerhans cells from human skin explants and strongly blunted the chemotactic responses of human Langerhans cell precursors and the maturation of maturing Langerhans cells to the chemokines CCL19 and CCL20.[67] Thus DP_1 may negatively regulate allergen sensitization if it is present during the initial inductive stages of the response. This is supported by studies in mice (see below).

Mouse studies of PGD₂ in allergic inflammation

Mouse studies reveal a complex role of PGD_2 in experimental allergic disease.[68] Transgenic mice that overexpress L-PGDS had greater BAL fluid levels of Th2 cytokines, eotaxin, eosinophils, and lymphocytes following allergen sensitization and challenge compared with nontransgenic littermates.[69] Aerosolized PGD_2 administered 1 day prior to inhalational challenge with low-dose antigen amplified the numbers of eosinophils, lymphocytes, and macrophages, as well as IL-4 and IL-5, in BAL fluid of sensitized mice.[70] These results suggest that PGD_2 augments pulmonary Th2 responses.

Rodent studies of DP_1 function in allergic inflammation have been somewhat contradictory. Allergen sensitized and challenged DP_1-deficient mice had significantly reduced BAL concentrations of IL-4, IL-5, and IL-13 compared with control mice, and diminished AHR, without a difference in the levels of IFN-γ in BAL fluid.[68] These DP_1-deficient mice had decreased BAL cellular influx with less eosinophils and lymphocytes compared with control mice, suggesting that DP_1 signaling was important in the full expression of allergic inflammation.[68] However, in a recent study of allergic lung inflammation in mice, the DP_1 agonist BW245C suppressed the function of lung dendritic cells, including lung migration and the ability of dendritic cells to stimulate T cell proliferation.[71,72] Mice treated with BW245C or mice receiving adoptively transferred DP_1-treated dendritic cells had increased numbers of Foxp3⁺ CD4⁺ regulatory T cells that suppressed inflammation in an interleukin 10-dependent mechanism.[72] The reduction in allergic inflammation caused by the DP_1 agonist on dendritic cell function was mediated by cyclic AMP-dependent protein kinase A.[72] In addition, chimeric mice that lacked DP_1 expression on hematopoietic cells had strongly enhanced airway inflammation

Table 12.3 PGE_2 receptor expression, signaling, and function

	EP_1	EP_2	EP_3	EP_4
Receptor expression	T cells, B cells, dendritic cells, smooth muscle	T cells, B cells, dendritic cells, mast cells, basophils, uterus, lung, spleen, smooth muscle	T cells, B cells, dendritic cells, smooth muscle	T cells, B cells, dendritic cells, kidney, lung, smooth muscle
Effect of receptor signaling	↑ intracellular Ca^{2+}	↑ cAMP concentration	↓ cAMP synthesis	↑ cAMP concentration
Function	Smooth muscle contraction	Inhibition of dendritic cell differentiation and T cell stimulatory capacity; smooth muscle relaxation	Smooth muscle contraction	Enhances migration of antigen-stimulated dendritic cells to lymph nodes; inhibition of IL-12 production by monocytes and macrophages; promotes initiation of contact hypersensitivity reactions; smooth muscle relaxation

when challenged with allergen, indicating an important homeostatic role of DP_1 and endogenous PGD_2.[72] Collectively, this data suggests that DP_1 signaling facilitates effector responses through structural cells, but may dampen responses of dendritic cells so as to restrain the allergic inflammatory process at the sensitization phase.

Studies examining DP_2 support the notion that signaling through this receptor amplifies allergic inflammation, PGD_2 exerts in vitro chemotactic activity on mouse eosinophils through DP_2 activation.[73] In addition, 13,14-dihydro-15-keto-PGD_2, a specific DP_2 agonist augmented eosinophil recruitment at inflammatory sites in vivo in two models of allergic inflammation, atopic dermatitis and allergic asthma, while DP_1 activation tended to ameliorate the pathology.[73] A pair of DP_2 antagonists, TM30089 and ramatroban, downregulated allergen-induced pulmonary inflammation in vivo by reducing peribronchial eosinophilia and mucus cell hyperplasia.[74] Thus, PGD_2 signaling through DP_2 increases allergic inflammation, and interference with this receptor attenuates such inflammatory responses.

PGE_2

There are three distinct enzymes that can metabolize PGH_2 to PGE_2. These are microsomal PGE synthase-1 (mPGES-1), mPGES-2, and cytosolic PGE synthase (cPGES). mPGES-1 is membrane-associated, localized to the perinuclear area, glutathione-dependent, and has a trimeric structure.[75] PGE_2 production was substantially greater in cells co-transfected with both mPGES-1 and COX-2 than cells co-transfected with mPGES-1 and COX-1, suggesting that mPGE-1 preferentially couples with COX-2 to immediately generate PGE_2 when COX-2 is active in cells, as well as the delayed PGE_2 production that occurs when COX-2 is induced.[75] mPGES-1 can metabolize PGH_2 produced from COX-1, but this seemingly occurred when arachidonic acid levels were higher or when this substrate was provided exogenously.[75] mPGES-1 activity was upregulated by IL-1β, requiring the early growth response-1 (Egr-1) transcription factor, while it was decreased by 15d-PGJ_2.[76] The expression of cPGES is mostly constitutive and not induced by inflammatory

stimuli.[76] Compared with mPGES-1, cPGES coupled more efficiently with COX-1 than with COX-2 for PGE_2 generation.[77] Although this suggests that $cPGE_2$ may provide PGE_2 necessary for cellular homeostasis,[76] mice lacking mPGES-1 show strikingly diminished levels of basal PGE_2 production in most organs.[78] Although cPGES is localized to the cytosol, there was evidence that it translocates from the cytosol to the nuclear membrane to assemble with COX-1 in PGE_2 production, although it has a slight preference to interact with COX-2.[76] Heat shock protein 90, casein kinase II, and bradykinin upregulated $cPGE_2$ activity, while dexamethasone decreased cPGES activation.[76] In contrast to mPGES-1, mPGES-2 is not dependent on glutathione.[76] mPGES-2 is expressed constitutively in many cells and tissues, but can be induced in colorectal adenocarcinoma cells to high levels.[76] In transfected cells, mPGES-2 uses PGH_2 derived from COX-1 and COX-2 with equal efficiency.

The effects of PGE_2 both in vivo and in vitro are complex, relating to the fact that this prostanoid signals through four distinct GPCRs, termed EP receptors 1 through 4 (Table 12.3). Each EP receptor has a distinct G protein coupling preference and downstream signal activation, and some of these signals counteract with one another. All four receptor subtypes are present in the lung and other organs associated with allergic responses.[79,80] Signaling through the EP_1 receptor increased inositol triphosphate and diacylglycerol, resulting in increased cell Ca^{2+} and smooth muscle contraction.[81] Activation of the EP_2 and EP_4 receptors increased intracellular cAMP concentrations and relaxed smooth muscle.[82] Stimulation of the EP_2 receptor inhibited mast cell and basophil mediator release. EP_2 is expressed most abundantly in the uterus, lung, and spleen.[79] EP_4 receptor expression is greatest in the kidney and peripheral blood leukocytes, but there is high level of expression in the thymus, lung, and a number of other tissues.[83] EP_3 receptors caused smooth muscle contraction by decreasing the rate of cAMP synthesis.[84] EP_3 receptors are unique because of the diversity created by multiple splice variants that produce alternate sequences in the C-terminal tail of this receptor subtype; however, the functional importance of these alternative splice variants is not well understood.[79] Usually these splice variants of EP_3 decrease cAMP generation, in contrast to signaling through EP_2

and EP_4 which increase cAMP.[79] Thus, PGE_2 activity can be diverse and possibly competing, dependent upon the relative contributions of the receptors that are stimulated in a given context.

Human studies of PGE_2 in allergic inflammation

PGE_2 is a predominant COX product of the airway epithelium and smooth muscle.[85,86] There is abundant evidence to support the proposition that endogenous PGE_2 may be bronchoprotective in human asthma.[87] PGE_2 produced by epithelial cells inhibited vagal cholinergic contraction of airway smooth muscle.[88] There was a negative correlation between the sputum levels of PGE_2 from asthmatics and their sputum eosinophil count, suggesting that PGE_2 may have anti-inflammatory properties.[89] PGE_2 inhalation also inhibited the pulmonary immediate and late phase responses to inhaled allergen.[90,91] Inhaled PGE_2 decreased the change in methacholine airway reactivity and reduced the number of eosinophils after inhaled allergen challenge.[90] In addition, PGE_2 inhibited both exercise-induced and aspirin-induced bronchoconstriction in patients sensitive to these challenges.[92,93] Interestingly, although PGE_2 significantly protects against decrements in pulmonary function in challenge models, it does not alter baseline FEV_1 or methacholine reactivity.[91] The results from these studies suggest that PGE_2 has greater immunomodulatory properties than directly affecting airway caliber. This is supported by the observation that PGE_2 inhalation prior to segmental allergen challenge significantly reduced the BAL levels of PGD_2, an important product of mast cell activation, and the concentrations of cys-LTs.[94]

PGE_2 is rapidly metabolized and this has prompted investigators to utilize the more stable orally active PGE_1 analogue, misoprostol, in studies of allergen-induced airway inflammation and lung function in humans, but the results have largely been negative. Misoprostol did not have an impact on pulmonary function, β_2 agonist use, or asthma severity score in aspirin-sensitive asthmatics.[95] In mild asthmatics, misoprostol had no effect on either baseline lung function or histamine reactivity, but did elicit significant gastrointestinal side effects in one-third of the subjects enrolled in the study.[96]

In vitro studies have not supported human in vivo studies that propose PGE_2 decreases allergic inflammation. PGE_2 in vitro inhibited lymphocyte production of the Th1 cytokines IL-2 and interferon-γ (IFN-γ), thus promoting T cell differentiation toward a Th2 cytokine profile.[97–100] These in vitro results suggesting PGE_2 promoted Th2 cytokine production may be regulated at antigen presentation. Myeloid dendritic cells matured in the presence of IFN-γ produced Th1 $CD4^+$ T lymphocyte responses, while dendritic cells matured in PGE_2 elicited Th2 T cell responses.[101] PGE_2 induction of Th2 cytokine production mostly through its activity at the time of antigen presentation would not necessarily contradict in vivo human studies that have suggested PGE_2 is anti-inflammatory. Acute antigen challenge models probably more precisely reflect effector cell function, since allergic sensitization to an antigen occurs much earlier in life.

Besides PGE_2's activity in the development of $CD4^+$ Th1 and Th2 cell development, this prostanoid has important immunomodulatory effects on other inflammatory cells presumed to be pathogenic in asthma. In a cell culture system, both PGE_2 and cAMP inhibited spontaneous eosinophil apoptosis, as did an EP_2 agonist.[102] Thus, by prolonging eosinophil survival, PGE_2 could potentially increase the inflammatory potential of these cells in asthma. However, PGE_2 was also reported to decrease eosinophil chemotaxis, aggregation, degranulation, and IL-5-mediated survival.[103,104] Therefore, the relevance of these in vitro findings to in vivo disease states is still to be determined.

PGE_2 also modulated the expression of a very important growth factor, granulocyte-macrophage-colony stimulating factor (GM-CSF), from human airway smooth muscle cells.[105] The COX inhibitor-indomethacin upregulated GM-CSF production by cultured human airway smooth muscle cells; however, exogenous PGE_2 decreased this indomethacin-induced GM-CSF production, suggesting that PGE_2 restrained GM-CSF expression and the inflammation that is associated with this cytokine.[105] In contrast, PGE_2 increased IL-6 and GM-CSF production as a result of IgE-mediated mast cell degranulation by signaling through EP_1 and EP_3 receptors.[106] PGE_2 has also been reported to have contrasting activities on the mast cell production of differing mediators. PGE_2 has been reported to either reduce[107–109] or enhance[110,111] the release of histamine and other inflammatory mediators. These differences may relate to the relative dominance of EP_3 (activating) versus EP_2 (inhibitory) signaling in a given mast cell population. For instance, PGE_2 can activate human mast cells through EP_3, but inhibit activation through the EP_2-PKA signaling pathway.[112]

Mouse studies of PGE_2 in allergic inflammation

In the OVA-sensitized and challenged model, mice that are deficient in the EP_3 receptor had enhanced allergic inflammation compared with WT mice, while there were no differences in the pulmonary allergic inflammation between WT, EP_1-deficient, EP_2-deficient, and EP_4-deficient mice.[113] Compared with WT mice, EP_3-deficient mice had greater airway numbers of eosinophils, neutrophils, and lymphocytes in BAL fluid, as well as augmented BAL concentrations of IL-4, IL-5, and IL-13.[113] Administration of the EP_3 agonist AE-248 to OVA-sensitized and challenged WT mice significantly suppressed allergic airway cellularity and tended to decrease airway mucus expression and airways responsiveness to methacholine.[113] In ex vivo experiments, lungs from OVA-sensitized and challenged EP_3-deficient or WT mice were harvested and then challenged with OVA.[113] In these studies, lungs from WT mice treated with an EP_3 agonist produced significantly decreased histamine and cys-LT, suggesting that PGE_2 may signal through EP_3 on mast cells in vivo to inhibit mediator release.[113] It is important to note that the results of these studies could not have been predicted from in vivo analyses, since EP_3 receptor signaling causes mast cell activation in vitro, whereas EP_2 receptor signaling is inhibitory.[112] PGE_2 also regulates airway tone in mice. Immunologically naïve mice that lack 15-hydroxyprostaglandin dehydrogenase, the major catabolic enzyme of PGE_2, and that therefore have elevated levels of PGE_2, had a decreased bronchoconstrictor response to methacholine.[114] Similarly, mice that had elevated PGE_2 levels as a result of overexpression of PGE_2 synthase in the lung had decreased methacholine-induced airway constriction.[114] Thus PGE_2 protects against lower airway bronchoconstriction, and other studies suggest that this effect is mediated through EP_2. Pre-treatment with aerosolized PGE_2 blunted methacholine-induced bronchoconstriction in WT mice, but not in EP_2-deficient animals.[115] In addition, methacholine-induced bronchoconstriction was reversed by aerosolized PGE_2 in WT, but not EP_2-deficient, mice.[115] These findings were confirmed by another group that reported that PGE_2-induced bronchodilation was a consequence of direct activation of EP_2 receptors on airway smooth muscle, while

PGE_2 signaling through EP_1 and EP_3 led to bronchoconstriction.[116] Collectively, these studies suggest that PGE_2 regulates homeostasis of bronchomotor tone and pulmonary immune responses through different respective receptors.

$PGF_{2\alpha}$

$PGF_{2\alpha}$ is produced by PGF synthase (PGFS).[117] PGFS has two activities: (1) catalyzing the formation of $PGF_{2\alpha}$ from PGH_2 by PGH_2 9,11-endoperoxide reductase in the presence of NADPH, and (2) forming $PGF_{2\alpha}$ from PGD_2 by PGD_2 11-ketoreductase.[117] The PGFS binding sites for PGH_2 and PGD_2 are proposed to be distinct.[117] PGFS is expressed in lung and peripheral blood lymphocytes, suggesting a possible role in allergic diseases such as asthma.[118] PGFS may also have a role in the nervous system, since it has been identified in neurons and vascular endothelial cells in the rat spinal cord.[119] PGFS in inhibited by non-steroidal antiinflammatory drugs (NSAIDs) such as indomethacin and this may partially explain the protective effect of this class of drugs in some gastrointestinal tumors in which PGFS activity is high.[117] $PGF_{2\alpha}$ binds a sole receptor, termed FP (Table 12.4), which is the most promiscuous of the prostanoid GPCRs in binding the principal prostaglandins, with PGD_2 and PGE_2 both binding FP at nanomolar concentrations.[120] Selective FP agonists such as fluprostenol and latanoprost have been produced that are used in clinical settings because of these agents' ocular hypotensive properties.[120] $PGF_{2\alpha}$ plays a critical function in reproduction, renal physiology, and modulation of intraocular pressure. Tissue distribution of FP receptor mRNA expression is highest in the ovarian corpus luteum, followed by the kidney, with lower-level expression in the lung, stomach, and heart.[121] FP expression has not been reported in the spleen, thymus, or on immune cells. As a result, in contrast to the other prostaglandins, there is very little evidence to suggest an important contribution of $PGF_{2\alpha}$-FP receptor signaling in inflammatory and immunological processes.[120]

Human studies of $PGF_{2\alpha}$

$PGF_{2\alpha}$ has not been studied to nearly the same extent as PGD_2 or PGE_2 in allergic disease and asthma. $PGF_{2\alpha}$ inhalation leads to a dose-related decrease in specific airway conductance in both control and asthmatic subjects.[122–124] There has been a wide variation in the pulmonary function response to $PGF_{2\alpha}$ reported in asthmatics, in contrast to the relatively small inter-individual variation in healthy control subjects.[124] Subjects who inhaled $PGF_{2\alpha}$, experienced wheezing, coughing, and chest irritation within 3 to 4 min, while watery sputum also occurred shortly thereafter.[124] Maximal decrease in specific airway conductance after $PGF_{2\alpha}$ occurred 6 min after inhalation and recovery took place within 30 min.[124] Asthmatic subjects experienced an approximate 150 times greater sensitivity to $PGF_{2\alpha}$ than did healthy controls, yet asthmatics were only 8.5 times more sensitive to histamine than non-asthmatic subjects.[124] There was decreased variation in individual responses to histamine compared with inhaled $PGF_{2\alpha}$ challenge, but sensitivity to both drugs correlated with each other.[124] In general, women had a diminished bronchoconstrictor response to $PGF_{2\alpha}$ compared with men.[124] Both PGE_2 and isoprenaline shortened recovery from the decrease in pulmonary function caused by inhalation of $PGF_{2\alpha}$; however, neither atropine, cromolyn sodium, nor flufenamic acid prevented $PGF_{2\alpha}$-induced bronchoconstriction.[124]

$PGF_{2\alpha}$ (and PGE_2 as well) decreased exhaled nitric oxide (NO) concentrations in both healthy controls and asthmatic subjects; however, the meaning of this outcome is unknown.[125] Although FP is not expressed on immune cells, there is some evidence that $PGF_{2\alpha}$ may have a role on airway inflammation. In subjects with asthma, the magnitude of sputum eosinophilia correlated with the log sputum $PGF_{2\alpha}$ concentrations, while there was a negative correlation between sputum eosinophilia and PGE_2 levels and no correlation between the number of sputum eosinophils and sputum levels of cys-LTs, thromboxane, and PGD_2.[89]

Mouse studies of $PGF_{2\alpha}$ in allergic inflammation

To our knowledge, there are no published studies examining the effect of $PGF_{2\alpha}$ administration or signaling through the FP receptor in the mouse allergen challenge model.

PGI_2

PGI_2 is converted from PGH_2 by PGI synthase (PGIS). The gene encoding PGIS is located on chromosome 20q13.11–13.[126] PGIS is strongly expressed in the heart, lung, smooth muscle, kidney, and ovary and expressed at moderate levels in the brain, pancreas, and prostate.[126] There is low-level PGIS expression in the placenta, spleen, and leukocytes.[126] PGI_2 signals through its receptor, IP, a GPCR (Table 12.4).[79] Binding of PGI_2 to its receptor activates adenylate cyclase via G_s in a dose-dependent manner, increasing the production of cAMP.[127] This increase in intracellular cAMP mediates PGI_2's effect of inhibiting platelet aggregation, and dispersing existing platelet aggregates both in vitro and in human circulation.[127] Northern blot analysis reveals that IP mRNA is expressed to the greatest degree in the thymus, while a high level of IP mRNA expression is also found in spleen, heart, lung, and neurons in the dorsal root ganglia. IP is also expressed on mouse bone marrow-derived dendritic cells (BMDC).[128] The PGI_2 analogs iloprost and cicaprost decreased BMDC production of proinflammatory cytokines (IL-12, TNF-α, IL-1α, IL-6) and chemokines (MIP-1α, MCP-1), while these analogs increased the production of the antiinflammatory cytokine IL-10 by BMDCs.[128] The modulatory effect was associated with IP-dependent upregulation of intracellular cAMP and downregulation of NF-kB activity.[128] Iloprost and cicaprost also suppressed LPS-induced expression of CD86, CD40, and MHC class II molecules by BMDCs and inhibited the ability of BMDCs to stimulate antigen-specific CD4 T cell proliferation and production of IL-5 and IL-13.[128] IP is also expressed in T cells of mice, along with the PGE_2 receptor (EP) subtypes and the thromboxane receptor (TP).[129] IP has also been found in kidney smooth muscle and epithelial cells.[130] Messenger RNA for IP is expressed in both CD4+ Th1 and Th2 cells.[131] Thus, IP has been located on several different cell types, including those critical to the adaptive immune response.

Human studies of PGI_2 in allergic inflammation

PGI_2 and PGD_2 were the predominant COX products produced in antigen-induced anaphylactic reactions of human lung parenchyma, on the order of 3- to 7-times greater concentrations than of the other prostanoids.[132] The PGI_2 metabolite 6-keto-$PGF_{1\alpha}$ was produced in concentrations two-to-three-fold higher than all the other prostanoids in both

Table 12.4 $PGF_{2\alpha}$, PGI_2, thromboxane A_2 receptor expression, signaling, and function

	FP	IP	TP
Receptor expression	Ovarian corpus luteum, kidney eye, lung, stomach, heart	Th1 and Th2, dendritic cells, endothelium, platelets	Vascular tissues such as lung, heart, kidney, smooth muscle,
Effect of receptor signaling	↑ intracellular Ca^{2+}	↑ cAMP concentration	Phospholipase C activation, calcium release, activation of protein kinase C TPα – activates adenylate cyclase TPβ – inhibits adenylate cyclase
Function	Smooth muscle contraction, cardiac hypertrophy	Inhibition of dendritic cell differentiation and T cell stimulatory capacity	Potentiates smooth muscle contraction, inhibits T dendritic cell-T cell interaction

airway and subpleural lung fragments in an in vitro anaphylaxis assay of passively sensitized human lung.[133] Plasma 6-keto-$PGF_{1\alpha}$ was also increased following antigen challenge in which asthmatic subjects were pretreated with indomethacin.[134] Thus, PGI_2 is produced in abundance in allergic inflammatory responses in the lung, presumably a reflection of activated endothelial cells.

Most of the published intervention studies examining the modulatory effect of PGI_2 in human asthma were performed over 15 years ago and the limitations of these older reports is that PGI_2 (half-life 3–5 min) was used, rather than the more recently developed stable analogs. Therefore, these studies may not accurately reflect the therapeutic capability of the currently available class of PGI_2 agents. Pre-treatment with PGI_2 had no effect on allergen-induced immediate phase bronchoconstriction.[135] In another study, PGI_2 protected against both exercise and ultrasonic water-induced bronchospasm, yet again had no effect on allergen-induced airway reactivity.[136] Inhaled PGI_2 also had no effect on specific airway conductance, but did result in consistent bronchodilation in two of the asthmatic subjects. In this study, there was a significant effect of PGI_2 on the cardiovascular system. Inhaled PGI_2 resulted in a fall in both diastolic (20 + 3 mmHg) and systolic (8 ± 2 mmHg) blood pressure, as well as an increased pulse rate (29 ± 3 beats/min).[137] Intravenous PGI_2 administration had no effect on the fall in airflow induced by aspirin in subjects with aspirin-induced asthma.[138] Somewhat contradictory results of the effect of inhaled PGI_2 in subjects with mild asthma have been reported.[139] In these studies PGI_2 did not alter specific airway conductance, but resulted in a concentration-dependent decrease in FEV_1. In contrast, these same investigators found that PGI_2 protected against bronchoconstriction induced by either PGD_2 or methacholine. The authors proposed that these disparate findings might be explained by PGI_2's marked vasodilator effect, resulting in airway narrowing through mucosal blood engorgement, while this same phenomenon possibly reduced the spasmogenic properties of other inhaled mediators by increasing their clearance from the airways. An oral PGI_2 analog (OP-41483) had no affect on FEV_1 or airways responsiveness to methacholine in stable asthmatics.[140] Since this last report, which was published in 1991, to our knowledge, there have been no other published manuscripts examining PGI_2 in human allergic inflammation in the lung or asthma. The therapeutic potential of newer, more stable PGI_2 analogs in asthma remains unexplored.

Mouse studies of PGI_2 in allergic inflammation

Three studies using mouse models suggest that PGI_2 and signaling through IP are involved in homeostatic control of allergic inflammation. In a model of short-term OVA challenge, IP-deficient mice showed increased lung production of IL-4 and IL-5, serum antigen-specific and total IgE levels, and airway leukocyte accumulation compared with wild type mice.[141] In another study, the period of allergen challenge was extended to generate signatures of 'chronic' allergen exposure. In this study, IP-deficient mice had greater airway eosinophils and lymphocytes, Th2 cytokine levels, and hydroxyproline concentrations compared with wild-type mice.[142] In vitro, treatment of polarized murine Th2 CD4+ T lymphocytes with a stable PGI_2 analog augmented the production of IL-10, a cytokine that restrains allergic responses.[143] Mice that lacked the ability to signal through IP had augmented inflammatory and physiologic changes compared with WT mice in the model of bleomycin-induced fibrosis.[144] Thus, published work indicates that signaling through IP downregulates allergic inflammation in the lung and may attenuate pathways required for fibrosis and remodeling as well.

THROMBOXANE A_2

Thromboxane A_2 (TXA_2) is the principal product of arachidonic acid metabolism formed by platelets and is a potent platelet aggregating agent.[145] Thromboxane synthase ($TXAS$) is an endoplasmic reticulum membrane protein that catalyzes the conversion of prostaglandin H_2 to thromboxane A_2.[146] TXAS is a member of the cytochrome P450 superfamily and is localized to band q33-q34 of the long arm of chromosome 7 in humans.[146] TXAS is expressed abundantly in lung, liver, kidney, and blood cells, including megakaryocytes and monocytes.[146] Lower, but significant, levels of TXAS mRNA are observed in kidney, placenta, and thymus.[146] TXA_2 is principally produced by platelets, monocytes, macrophages, neutrophils, and lung parenchyma.[147] After it is formed, TXA_2 is non-enzymatically hydrolyzed to thromboxane B_2, which is further metabolized to the principle urinary metabolites 2,3-dinor-thromboxane B_2 and 11-dehydro-thromboxane B_2.[148] The TXA_2 receptor is termed TP (Table 12.4) and there are two isoforms, TPα and TPβ, which are produced by alternative splicing occurring in the carboxy-terminal region after the seventh transmembrane domain.[149] Both of these isoforms functionally couple to a Gq protein, resulting in phospholipase C activation, calcium release, and activation of protein kinase C.[150] However, these receptor isoforms couple oppositely to adenylate cyclase as $TP\alpha$ activates adenylate cyclase while $TP\beta$ inhibits this enzyme.[151] The TP receptors are localized to both plasma membrane and cytosolic compartments and are mainly distributed in tissues rich in vasculature such as lung, heart, and kidney.[120] These GPCRs are involved in a multitude of physiological and pathological processes such as vasoconstriction implicated in vascular diseases such as hypertension, stroke, atherosclerosis, and myocardial infarction.[152]

Human studies of TXA_2 in allergic inflammation

TXA_2 has a half-life of approximately $30\,s$,[49] and because of this lability there is a paucity of in vivo studies examining the effect of TXA_2 in the human airway. TXA_2 was a potent stimulant of in vitro smooth muscle constriction,[145] there are data that suggests that TXA_2 might have a role in the physiology associated with acute asthma exacerbations. Levels of TXA_2 metabolites were increased 4–6-fold in the urine of patients admitted to the hospital with asthma compared with non-smoking controls admitted for other diagnoses.[153] Allergic asthmatics subjected to inhaled allergen challenge had a significant increase in urinary excretion of TXA_2 products,[36,154] yet others have not found similar results.[153] Allergic asthmatics pre-treated with indomethacin before inhaled allergen challenge had resulted in a significant decline in urinary TXA_2 metabolites; however, no change in pulmonary function was noted.[36] Subjects that experience ozone-induced airway hyperresponsiveness had significant increases in BAL concentrations of TXA_2 and airway neutrophilia.[155] Similarly, LTB_4 inhalation also resulted in increased levels of TXA_2 and neutrophils in BAL fluid.[156]

TXA_2 antagonists have been used in challenge models to determine thromboxane's effect on allergen-induced pulmonary function. In a non-randomized, uncontrolled study the TP antagonist seratrodast (AA-2414) significantly reduced bronchial reactivity in asthmatic subjects after 4 weeks of once-daily therapy compared with a pre-treatment baseline.[157] In this study, seratrodast had no effect on either exhaled nitric oxide or on the percentage of eosinophils in sputum.[157] In a follow-up double-blind, placebo-controlled study of asthmatics treated for 4 weeks, seratrodast treatment resulted in significant improvements in symptom score, peak expiratory flow (PEF) rates, diurnal variation of PEF, and bronchial responsiveness compared with the placebo group.[158] These improvements were associated with a significant reduction in the number of submucosal eosinophils on bronchial biopsy.[158] Seratrodast treatment resulted in a significant decrease in the number of cells in the epithelium expressing RANTES and macrophage inflammatory protein (MIP)-1α, as well as a diminished number of cells in the submucosa expressing monocyte chemotactic protein-3, RANTES, MIP-1α, and eotaxin.[158] These findings suggest that thromboxane antagonism may reduce allergic inflammation in the lung, although the mechanisms are not well defined.

Mouse studies of TXA_2 in allergic inflammation

Both the TXA_2 synthase inhibitor OKY-046 and the TP receptor antagonist S-1452 significantly decreased the number of total cells and eosinophils in BAL fluid in a dose-responsive relationship in OVA-sensitized and challenged mice.[159] Treatment with either the TXA_2 synthase inhibitor or the TP receptor antagonist significantly inhibited antigen-specific activation of splenic mononuclear cells from sensitized mice in ex vivo experiments as defined by pro-inflammatory cytokine production.[159]

■ LIPOXYGENASE PATHWAY ■

As is the case for prostanoids, arachidonic acid liberated by group IV $cPLA_2$ is the precursor for lipoxygenase (LO) pathway products.[160] Two major enzymes, 5-LO and 15-LO, metabolize arachidonate in the initial steps that form distinctive respective mediator classes (Fig. 12.2). The latter enzyme catalyzes the hydroperoxidation of arachidonic acid by the insertion of one molecule of oxygen at position 15 to form 15-HPETE, as well as the insertion of molecular oxygen into other polyunsaturated fatty acids and phospholipids. The 15-LO pathway is responsible for forming 15-hydroxyeicosatetraenoic acid (15-HETE) and the dihydroxy acids 8, 15-diHETE and 14,15-diHETE. 15-HETE is a precursor of the lipoxins, a group of mediators with putative antiinflammatory functions.[161–163] 5-LO translocates in a Ca^{2+}-dependent manner from either the cytoplasm or the nucleus to the perinuclear membrane and catalyzes the insertion of molecular oxygen into arachidonic acid to produce 5-hydroperoxyeicosatetraenoic acid (5-HPETE). 5-HPETE can then either be dehydrated to leukotriene (LTA_4) by 5-LO, or reduced to 5-hydroxyeicosatetraenoic acid (5-HETE) and further converted to the 5-oxo-ETEs.[160,164] Both of these catalytic functions require 5-LO activating protein (FLAP), an integral perinuclear membrane protein that transfers free arachidonic acid to 5-LO and is essential for the 5-LO function of generating LTA_4.[160] FLAP is a member of the structurally homologous microsome-associated proteins involved in eicosanoid and glutathione metabolism (MAPEG) family, which includes mPGES-1 and LTC_4 synthase (LTC_4S).

LEUKOTRIENES

Leukotrienes, named for their cells of origin (leukocytes) and three positionally conserved double bonds (trienes), are potent inflammatory mediators generated from the unstable precursor LTA_4.[165] There are two distinct classes of leukotrienes; LTB_4 is a dihydroxyl compound formed by a cytosolic LTA_4 hydrolase (LTA_4H). LTA_4H is expressed by mast cells, macrophages, and neutrophils, the major cellular sources of LTB_4 in vivo. The human gene encoding LTA_4H maps to chromosome 12q22.[166] LTA_4 can also be conjugated to reduced glutathione to form LTC_4, the parent molecule of the cys-LTs by leukotriene C_4 synthase (LTC_4S), an integral perinuclear protein and member of the MAPEG family.[112,167] The major cellular sources of cys-LTs are eosinophils, basophils, mast cells, and macrophages, each of which express LTC_4S. LTC_4S expression is sharply up-regulated in human mast cells by IL-4/STAT6-dependent transcription, potentially reflecting a mechanism for upregulating cys-LT production in allergic inflammation.[168] The gene encoding LTC_4S in humans maps to chromosome 5q35, distal to the Th2 cytokine gene cluster.[169] Both LTB_4 and LTC_4 are exported by specific respective transporter proteins. LTC_4 is converted to LTD_4 extracellularly by cleavage of glutamic acid and is cleaved from the glutathione moiety by γ-glutamyl-transpeptidase, or by a more specific γ-glutamyl-leukotrienease.[170] A dipeptidase then cleaves glycine from LTD_4 to form LTE_4.[170]

Leukotrienes in human studies of allergic inflammation and asthma

LTB_4 and the cys-LTs were increased in exhaled breath condensate from asthmatic subjects compared with healthy controls.[171] After allergen challenge, there was a significant increase in leukotriene levels in the BAL fluid of allergic subjects and this was associated with increased

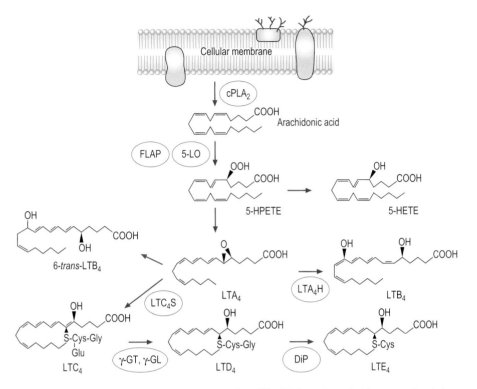

Fig. 12.2. Leukotriene generation. Biosynthesis and molecular structures of cys-LTs. cPLA$_2$ catalyzes the liberation of arachidonic acid from cell membranes. 5-LO translocates to the nuclear envelope, requiring the integral membrane protein FLAP to convert arachidonic acid to the precursor LTA$_4$. LTA$_4$ can spontaneously convert to the inactive metabolite 6-*trans* LTB$_4$, specifically hydrolyzed by LTA$_4$ hydrolase (LTA$_4$H) to LTB$_4$, or conjugated to reduce glutathione by LTC$_4$S, forming LTC$_4$, the first committed molecule of the cys-LTs (red). Following specific export, LTC$_4$ is converted by the extracellular enzymes γ-GT and γ-GL to LTD$_4$ by dipeptidase (Dip). Enzymes essential for cys-LT synthesis are in bold. (Reproduced from Kanaoka Y and Boyce JA. Cysteinyl leukotrienes and their receptors: cellular distribution and function in immune and inflammatory responses. Journal of Immunology 2004; 173:1503–1510, with permission. Copyright, American Association of Immunologists)

eosinophilic inflammation and bronchial responsiveness.[172] Leukotrienes can be measured in induced sputum and the levels of these mediators were not only increased in asthmatic subjects compared with non-asthmatic control subjects but also correlated with severity of disease.[89] Urinary LTE$_4$ is also increased in asthmatic subjects compared with controls.[173] Therefore, leukotrienes can be measured in a wide range of biologic fluids and reflect ongoing inflammation in the lung and the physiologic changes associated with asthma. Corticosteroid treatment had no impact on leukotriene levels in asthmatics, suggesting that leukotriene generation is relatively impervious to this class of anti-inflammatory medications.[27,171]

5-LO inhibitors block the formation of both LTB$_4$ and the cys-LTs, and as such provide insight into the role of both of these groups of mediators in the pathogenesis of both allergic disease and asthma. As mentioned above, both 5-LO and FLAP are critical to the generation of leukotrienes. While there is abundant clinical experience with 5-LO inhibitors, no FLAP inhibitors have been approved for human use. Zileuton is a 5-LO inhibitor and its activity is presumed to be related to its ability to chelate iron at the active site of 5-LO, thus preventing its redox potential.[174] In a study of asthmatics with mild-to-moderate disease, zileuton administration produced a 350 ml (15% from pre-treatment baseline) increase in FEV$_1$ within 1 h and was statistically increased compared with placebo. After a 4-week study period, there was also a significant improvement in peak expiratory flow rate in the

zileuton-treated subjects (600 mg four times daily) compared with placebo. Of note, after the 4 weeks of treatment, zileuton reduced urinary LTE$_4$ levels by only approximately 40% compared with the placebo group, indicating that even the highest clinically recommended dose of the 5-LO inhibitor did not fully block leukotriene generation.[175] In another 13-week study of asthmatic subjects who had FEV$_1$ between 40% and 80% predicted, zileuton significantly decreased the need for rescue β-agonists, reduced daytime and night-time symptoms, and increased symptom-free days and nights compared with placebo.[176] In this trial, zileuton also significantly reduced the number of subjects requiring corticosteroid therapy for an asthma exacerbation.[176] In a trial to investigate the role of 5-LO inhibition on inflammation following segmental allergen challenge, zileuton inhibited urinary LTE$_4$ production by 86% and prevented the increase in BAL eosinophils that was noted in the placebo-treated subjects.[177] The fact that 5-LO inhibition blunts allergen-induced inflammation while improving lung function and symptoms in asthmatic subjects validates the role of leukotrienes in asthma pathogenesis.

Murine studies of leukotriene inhibition

Unlike human airways, mouse airways are resistant to the bronchoconstrictive effects of the cys-LTs.[47] Nonetheless, mouse models of allergen-induced pulmonary inflammation have uncovered key roles for these mediators in the induction and amplification of this process. Mice that lack 5-LO as a result of targeted gene disruption have decreased allergen-induced BAL eosinophilia, serum IgE, and airway responsiveness compared with wild-type mice.[178] A similar phenotype was described for mice lacking group IVA PLA_2, which generates neither leukotrienes nor prostaglandins.[179] Similarly, zileuton reduced allergen-induced leukotriene release in the BAL and eosinophil recruitment to the lungs, while dose dependently reducing AHR, mucus accumulation, and remodeling.[180] Specific inhibitors of 5-LO and FLAP independently blocked airway mucus release and airway infiltration by eosinophils, indicating a key role for leukotrienes in these features of allergic pulmonary inflammation; however, they had no effect on allergen-induced airway responsiveness.[181] Zileuton treatment blocked airway responsiveness and inflammation that occurred as a result of intratracheal instillation of IL-13, monocyte chemoattractant protein (MCP)-1, MCP-5, and KC, the mouse homolog of IL-8.[182] Thus, the effects of pharmacologic and genetic deletion of 5-LO pathway products in mice are profound and reflect the composite loss of both cys-LT and LTB_4-mediated actions (see below).

LTB_4

LTB_4 exerts its biologic effects by signaling through two distinct GPCRs, BLT_1 and BLT_2.[183] LTB_4 binds with much greater affinity to BLT_1 compared with BLT_2.[183] Other eicosanoids, specifically 12(s)-HETE, 12(S)-HPETE, and 15(S)-HETE can bind BLT_2, but do not bind BLT_1.[183] BLT_1 is predominantly expressed on activated leukocytes, with decreased expression in spleen, thymus, bone marrow, lymph nodes, heart, skeletal muscle, brain, and liver.[183] BLT_2 is expressed in most human tissues with the greatest degree in spleen, liver, ovary, and peripheral blood white cells.[183] Among the leukocytes, there are some significant differences in LTB_4 receptor expression.[183] For instance, neutrophils and eosinophils both express high levels of both BLT_1 and BLT_2, while mononuclear cells express high levels of BLT_2, but very low levels of BLT_1.[183] BLT_1 expression is upregulated on activated cells and expression is increased by both IFN-γ and glucocorticoids.[183] The primary known function of LTB_4 receptor signaling is leukocyte recruitment.[183] LTB_4 is a leukocyte chemoattractant and also changes leukocyte rolling to firm attachment through its upregulation of the integrin CD11b/CD18 on neutrophils.[183] With these properties, exogenous LTB_4 administration in both the skin and airways caused neutrophils migration to those sites.

Human studies of LTB_4 in allergic inflammation

To date, there are no intervention studies using specific BLT_1 or BLT_2 antagonists or agonists to examine the role of signaling through these receptors in modulating allergic inflammation in humans. However, there are recent studies which suggest that signaling through these receptors may regulate the allergic phenotype. For instance, in healthy subjects, T cells that express BLT_1 are rare in peripheral blood, but do express the activation markers CD38 and HLA-DR.[184] When compared with T cells that do not express BLT_1, a larger proportion of peripheral blood expressing T cells also express the effector cytokines IFN-γ and IL-4, as well as inflammatory chemokine receptors, CCR1, CCR2, CCR6, and CXCR1.[184] T cell BLT_1 expression is tightly regulated by inflammation and only expressed transiently after naive T lymphocytes are activated by dendritic cells. The number of peripheral blood T cells expressing BLT_1 was increased in frequency in the airways of asymptomatic allergic asthmatics.[184] LTB_4, via

BLT_1, is strongly chemotactic for mast cell progenitors in vitro.[185] Activated mature mast cells produced LTB_4 which was highly chemotactic for 2-week-old mast cells that expressed high levels of mRNA for BLT_1 while expression of this receptor was not present on mature mast cells.[185] There was also accumulation of immature cells in vivo in response to intradermally injected LTB_4, and LTB_4 was extremely potent in recruiting mast cell progenitors from freshly isolated bone marrow cell suspensions.[185] Additionally, LTB_4 was a potent chemoattractant for human cord blood-derived immature, but not mature, mast cells.[185] To date, there are no published studies in humans or human cells examining the effect of signaling through BLT_2 on the regulation of allergic inflammation.

Mouse studies of LTB_4 in allergic inflammation

BLT_1 expression was low in naïve murine CD4+ T cells, but strong in activated Th0, Th1, and Th2 cells, while BLT_2 was not expressed in these cell populations.[186] LTB_4 induced CD4+ T cell chemotaxis in wild-type mice, but not in BLT_1-deficient mice, signifying the receptor specificity for this chemotaxis.[186] BLT_1-deficent mice had decreased number of both CD4+ and CD8+ T cells in BAL fluid after 1 and 2 days, but not after 3 days of allergen challenge in which mice had been sensitized first with an intraperitoneal injection of OVA and the adjuvant aluminum hydroxide, while there was no difference in the numbers of CD4+ and CD8+ cells in the lung parenchyma. BLT_1-deficient and wild-type mice did not differ in the expression of chemokines responsible for T cell recruitment, suggesting that reduced effector T cell trafficking into the airway in BLT_1-deficient mice was a direct consequence of the absence of LTB_4-BLT_1 signaling.[186] In this model, there were no differences in serum IgE levels between the BLT_1-deficient and wild-type mice, and neither airway eosinophilia nor mucus expression was reported. However, adoptively transferred antigen-specific transgenic T cells did not require BLT_1 for antigen-induced recruitment to the lungs of naïve mice.[186] Thus, the role of BLT_1 signaling in the setting of allergen challenge is dependent on the model used. Another group using OVA/aluminum hydroxide sensitization model found that BLT_1-deficient mice were protected from AHR, eosinophilic inflammation, and hyperplasia of goblet cells.[187] These BLT_1-deficient mice also had reduced IgE production and levels of IL-5 and IL-13 in bronchoalveolar lavage fluid, suggesting BLT_1 signaling was critical for the generation of a Th2-type immune response.[187] Another group found similar results in allergen-sensitized and challenged BLT_1-deficient mice and was able to increase allergic inflammation by transfer of allergen-primed wild-type T cells into the BLT_1-deficient mice that were subsequently allergen challenged.[188] Signaling through BLT_1 has also been proposed to mediate CD8-dependent allergic airway inflammation and AHR. CD8-deficient mice that were adoptively transferred CD8+ cells from allergen-sensitized wild-type, but not BLT_1-deficient mice developed allergen inflammation and AHR.[189,190] There have been no reports of murine studies examining the BLT_2 receptor in regulating allergic inflammation, although dendritic cells from mice deficient in both BLT_1 and BLT_2 had a marked defect in the ability to migrate to draining lymph nodes compared with dendritic cells from wild-type mice.[191]

CYSTEINYL LEUKOTRIENES

Cys-LTs signal through at least two GPCRs, $CysLT_1$ and $CysLT_2$ (Table 12.5).[165] Recently, a third receptor, formerly known as GPR17 was found to bind cys-LTs.[192] In humans, $CysLT_1$ maps to the X chromosome,

Table 12.5 Cysteinyl leukotriene receptor expression, signaling, and function

	CysLT$_1$	CysLT$_2$
Ligands	LTD$_4$ >LTC$_4$=LTE$_4$	LTC$_4$=LTD$_4$ >LTE$_4$
Chromosome	Human: Xq13.2–21.1	Human: 13q14.12–q21.1
	Mouse: X–D	Mouse: 14-D1
Expression		
Human	Tissues: spleen, lung, placenta, small intestine Cell types: bronchial smooth muscle, monocyte/macrophages, mast cells, eosinophils, CD34$^+$ hematopoietic progenitor cells, neutrophils, HUVEC	Tissues: spleen, lung, heart, lymph node, brain Cell types: monocyte/macrophages, mast cells, eosinophils, cardiac, Purkinje cells, pheochromocytes and ganglion cells in adrenal medulla, bronchial smooth muscle, HUVEC, coronary smooth muscle
Mouse	Tissues: lung, skin, small intestine Cell types: monocyte/macrophages, fibroblasts	Tissues: spleen, lung, small intestine, kidney, brain, skin Cell types: monocyte/macrophages, fibroblasts, endothelial cells, cardiac, Purkinje cells
Function	Dilates blood vessels with increased vascular permeability; amplifies mucus expression, bronchial smooth muscle constriction, augments transendothelial migration of CD34$^+$ hematopoietic cells and eosinophils, increases IgE-mediated mast cell production of IL-5 and TNF	Activation of endothelial cells

while CysLT$_2$ maps to chromosome 13q14.[165] CysLT$_1$ binds LTD$_4$ with high affinity and LTC$_4$ and LTE$_4$ equally with lower affinity.[165] In contrast, CysLT$_2$ binds LTC$_4$ and LTD$_4$ equally and with greater affinity than LTE$_4$.[165] In humans, CysLT$_1$ is expressed in the spleen, lung, placenta, and small intestine.[165] Specific cell types on which CysLT$_1$ is expressed include bronchial smooth muscle, glandular epithelium, monocyte/macrophages, mast cells, basophils, eosinophils, dendritic cells, B and T lymphocytes, CD34$^+$ hematopoietic progenitors, neutrophils, and human umbilical vein endothelial cells.[165,193,194] CysLT$_1$ expression can be upregulated on peripheral blood mononuclear cells by IL-4 and IL-13, or on an eosinophilic leukemic cell line by IL-5, with a resulting increase in expression of CysLT$_1$ leading to enhanced chemotaxis to LTD$_4$.[165] CysLT$_2$ is expressed in the lung, spleen, heart, lymph nodes, and brain. Cells expressing CysLT$_2$ include monocyte/macrophages, mast cells, eosinophils, cardiac, Purkinje cells, bronchial smooth muscle, coronary smooth muscle, and human umbilical vein endothelial cells. The specific CysLT$_1$ receptor antagonists such as montelukast, zafirlukast, and pranlukast have been critical in determining the effects of signaling through this receptor in biological systems and in humans in vivo. Signaling through CysLT$_1$ dilates blood vessels with a resultant increase in vascular permeability, amplified mucus expression, bronchial smooth muscle constriction, and inflammatory cell recruitment. Specifically, CysLT$_1$ signaling augments transendothelial migration of CD34$^+$ hematopoietic cells and eosinophil chemotaxis in vitro. In addition, cys-LTs increase IgE-mediated mast cell production of IL-5 and TNF via the CysLT$_1$ receptor and regulate mast cell proliferation by inducing transactivation of the c-Kit receptor tyrosine kinase.[195] The consequences of CysLT$_2$-mediated signaling are far less well understood than that of CysLT$_1$ signaling because there are no specific CysLT$_2$ receptor antagonists. Therefore, CysLT$_2$ receptor-mediated properties in humans are inferred from studies in which the

effects of the cys-LTs are not abrogated by CysLT$_1$ receptor antagonists. A primary role of CysLT$_2$ signaling may be activation of endothelial cells in vascular responses, as indicated by the CysLT$_2$-dominant signaling reported in human umbilical vein endothelial cells.[165]

Human studies of cysteinyl leukotrienes in allergic inflammation

Site-directed allergen challenge increases the concentrations of cys-LTs in the skin, eye, nose, and lung, and these levels are strongly correlated with allergic symptoms.[171,196,197] Direct administration of cys-LTs into the human airways confirmed that these lipids are the most potent known bronchoconstrictors, are pro inflammatory, and that their effects are receptor mediated. In asthmatic subjects, inhaled LTE$_4$ increased airway eosinophils and this was blocked by treatment with the CysLT$_1$ receptor antagonist zafirlukast.[198] CysLT$_1$ antagonists have been used in clinical trials of allergic conditions such as asthma, rhinitis, and urticaria, and these studies revealed that signaling through this receptor is involved in the pathogenesis of these diseases. In a 12-week study of asthmatics with FEV$_1$ 50–85% predicted, montelukast significantly improved pulmonary function and symptoms compared with placebo, but was not as effective as inhaled corticosteroids for the same endpoints.[199] CysLT$_1$ receptor antagonists have also been shown to inhibit both early and late phase pulmonary reactions to allergen challenge as well as the airway obstruction medicated by exercise, SO$_2$, hyperpnea, adenosine, and mannitol.[200–205] In clinical studies of rhinitis, CysLT$_1$ receptor antagonists have reduced rhinorrhea, nasal congestion, and sneezing, while improving daytime and night-time symptoms, although there is variability between studies in the effectiveness of this medication class on these individual endpoints.[194] CysLT$_1$ antagonists have also been shown to reduce the symptoms of chronic urticaria compared with placebo.[206–208] Several of these clinical trials identified significant suppression of blood and/or tissue eosinophil counts by the administration of $CysLT_1$ antagonists, implying a role for cys-LTs in regulating eosinophil homeostasis.[194]

Mouse studies of cys-LTs in allergic inflammation

In a 'mast cell-dependent' model of OVA-induced pulmonary inflammation, BALB/c mice lacking LTC_4S showed strikingly diminished AHR, goblet cell metaplasia, OVA-specific IgE, and cytokine production by restimulated lymph node cells when compared with wild-type, allergen-treated control mice.[209] These mice also showed strikingly decreased mast cell numbers in the bronchial epithelium compared with wild-type controls.[209] In another model of OVA-induced allergic pulmonary inflammation, wild-type BALB/c mice were treated with a long (76 day) period of allergen challenge to induce changes of airway remodeling.[210] In this study, the administration of the $CysLT_1$ receptor-selective antagonist montelukast during the challenge phase decreased lung expression of IL-4 and IL-5, and decreased bronchial eosinophil numbers, while inhibiting smooth muscle hypertrophy and collagen deposition.[210] In this model, inflammation subsided after cessation of the allergen challenge, but the smooth muscle hypertrophy and collagen deposition persisted out to 3 months.[210] Interestingly, montelukast reversed the remodeling signatures when administered from days 73–163 (after the challenge phase of the experiment), whereas dexamethasone did not.[210] Thus cys-LTs orchestrate both sensitization and remodeling events in models of allergic pulmonary inflammation in mice, consistent with their abundant generation by mast cells and eosinophils, as well as the broad distribution of their receptors on both hematopoietic and structural cells in the lung.

When pulsed ex vivo with dust mite antigen, mouse myeloid dendritic cells exposed to exogenous LTD_4 had augmented production of IL-10 and attenuated IL-12 generation compared with antigen pulsing alone.[211] Treatment of these DCs with $CysLT_1$ receptor-selective antagonists during antigen pulsing attenuated IL-10 generation and augmented IL-12 production.[211] Myeloid dendritic cells treated with $CysLT_1$ antagonists during stimulation with dust mite allergen in vitro were substantially less able to support an eosinophil-dominated inflammatory response to inhaled allergen following when adoptively transferred into the tracheas of naïve recipient mice.[211] Thus, as is the case for PGD_2, cys-LTs participate in the regulation of dendritic cell maturation responses. Whether cys-LTs, like LTB_4, also act on T cells remains to be determined.

■ ISOPROSTANES ■

Isoprostanes (IsoPs) are prostaglandin-like molecules that are not formed by the action of the COX enzymes, but instead are formed by the free radical-catalyzed peroxidation of arachidonic acid.[212] IsoP formation is not only a dependable marker of oxidant injury both in vivo and in vitro but also these mediators are biologically active and may regulate oxidant injury.[212] There are several classes of IsoPs that differ based on the functional groups present on the prostane ring.[212] The classes include the F_2-IsoPs, the D_2/E_2-IsoPs, the A_2/J_2-IsoPs, the isothromboxanes, and the isoketals (IsoKs).[212] These classes are distinguished by the type of isoprostane ring that each contains.[212] A_2/J_2-IsoPs are formed from the dehydration of E_2/D_2-IsoPs. F_2-IsoP can be detected in all normal

biologic fluids in both humans and animals, while the D_2/E_2-IsoPs, the A_2/J_2-IsoPs, and the isothromboxanes cannot.[212] However, levels of all of these classes are substantially increased in vivo following oxidant injury such as carbon tetrachloride administration, with the exception of the A_2/J_2-IsoPs and the IsoKs which still cannot be detected.[212] The neuroprostanes are similar to the IsoPs in that they contain various prostane ring functional groups. However, the neuroprostanes are formed from docosahexaenoic acid that is present in high levels of neural tissue.[212]

IsoPs have been shown to have potent biologic activity and perhaps regulate adverse effects of oxidant injury. The biologic activities of $15\text{-}F_{2t}$-IsoP (also known as 8-isoprostane or 8-iso-$PGF_{2\alpha}$) and $15\text{-}E_{2t}$-IsoP have been particularly well studied and these were potent vasoconstrictors in the kidney, lung, heart, retina, portal vein, and lymphatics.[213–219] At least part of the vasoconstrictive properties of $15\text{-}F_{2t}$-IsoP resulted from its interaction with the thromboxane receptor TP.[220] $15\text{-}F_{2t}$-IsoP also promoted the release of endothelin and vascular smooth muscle cell proliferation.[221,222] Other activities ascribed to $15\text{-}F_{2t}$-IsoP include osteoclastic differentiation resulting in bone resorption and augmented resistance to aspirin-induced blockade of platelet aggregation.[223–225]

As the F_2-IsoPs can be easily detected in human biologic fluid at baseline, changes in the levels of these compounds have been used as an in vivo index of endogenous lipid peroxidation or oxidant stress. The fact that the F_2-IsoPs can be measured in urine further increases the usefulness of these products as a non-invasive marker of oxidant stress activity and the activity of antioxidant compounds in vivo. Similar to the prostaglandins, measurement of F_2-IsoPs in the urine is the most dependable method to assess total endogenous levels of these products as blood levels may reflect only recent trends because the biologic half-life of these mediators is very short, on the order of 16 min. The preferred method of measurement of the IsoPs is gas chromatography/negative ion chemical ionization mass spectroscopy. Immunoassays are commercially available; however, the presence of substances in biologic fluids that interfere with these assays may confound results obtained with this technique. It is important to note that biologic material in which IsoPs are to be measured should be stored at −70°C or with the addition of antioxidants to avoid production of IsoPs ex vivo.

Human studies of isoprostanes in allergic inflammation

Levels of IsoPs have been studied in asthma and other allergic diseases such as asthma. Compared with healthy non-asthmatic controls, exhaled breath condensates of the F_2-IsoP series member $15\text{-}F_{2t}$-IsoP were greater in children with asthma, whether they had either mild persistent asthma, stable mild-to-moderate persistent asthma that was treated with inhaled corticosteroids, or unstable asthma.[226] Similarly, steroid-naive asthmatic children and children in stable condition with mild-to-moderate persistent asthma who were being treated with inhaled corticosteroids had greater levels of $15\text{-}F_{2t}$-IsoP compared with healthy non-asthmatic children.[227,228] In children experiencing an asthma exacerbation, oral corticosteroids significantly reduced exhaled breath condensate levels of $15\text{-}F_{2t}$-IsoP, although not to the same concentrations as measured in non-asthmatics, suggesting that corticosteroids may not be fully effective in reducing oxidative stress in children with an exacerbation of asthma.[229] IsoPs have also been measured in exhaled breath condensates in adults. In women with mild allergic asthma, the levels of $15\text{-}F_{2t}$-IsoP were inversely correlated with the percent predicted FEV_1.[230] Exhaled breath condensate levels of $15\text{-}F_{2t}\text{-}IsoP$ were also elevated in steroid-naïve subjects with aspirin-induced asthma compared with both subjects with aspirin-induced asthma treated with steroids and healthy control subjects.[231] Induced sputum has also been used as a biologic fluid in which IsoPs may be measured. Adults who either had asthmatic or bronchiectasis had greater levels of sputum $15\text{-}F_{2t}\text{-}IsoP$ than in healthy control subjects.[232] In addition, $15\text{-}F_{2t}\text{-}IsoP$ levels decreased in the induced sputum in asthmatics as they recovered from an exacerbation.[232] Urinary levels of IsoPs were also elevated in asthmatic subjects experiencing allergen challenge. $15\text{-}F_{2t}\text{-}IsoP$ was elevated from as early as 2 h, and as long as 8 hours, following inhaled allergen challenge in subjects with mild allergic asthma.[233] In contrast, no increase in the urinary excretion of 8-isoprostane occurred after methacholine challenge.[233] Therefore, IsoP levels are increased during ongoing allergic inflammatory responses and decrease with treatment.

Mouse studies of isoprostanes in allergic inflammation

IsoP measurements have also been performed in mouse models of allergic lung inflammation. In the OVA model, F_2-isoprostanes in whole lung were increased on the ninth day of daily aerosol allergen challenge.[234] Increased immunoreactivity to $15\text{-}F_{2t}\text{-}IsoP$ or to isoketal protein adducts was found in epithelial cells 24 h after the first aerosol challenge and after 5 days of allergen exposure in macrophages.[234] Collagen surrounding airways and blood vessels, and airway and vascular smooth muscle, also exhibited increased $15\text{-}F_{2t}\text{-}IsoP$ immunoreactivity after OVA challenge.[234] Dietary vitamin E restriction in conjunction with allergic inflammation led to increased whole lung F_2-isoprostanes while supplemental vitamin E suppressed their formation.[234] Similar changes in immunoreactivity to F_2-isoprostanes were seen.[234] Airway responsiveness to methacholine was also increased by vitamin E depletion and decreased slightly by supplementation with the antioxidant.[234] Therefore, IsoPs are also increased in the mouse model of allergic inflammation and these are reduced with antioxidant treatment.

■ SPHINGOSINE-1-PHOSPHATE ■

There are two primary members of lysosphingolipids (LPLs) that have immunomodulatory functions. These are the lysoglycero-phospholipids, such as lysophosphatidic acid (LPA), and the lysosphingolipids, of which sphingosine-1-phosphate (S_1P) is a key member.[5] S_1P is synthesized intracellularly with the primary sources among immune cells being mast cells, platelets, and macrophages; however, a variety of non-immune cells can also produce this mediator.[235] The first step in S_1P production is the sphingomyelinase conversion of endogenous membrane-derived sphingomyelin to ceramide; then ceramidase converts ceramide to sphingosine.[5] Sphingosine is then converted to S_1P through phosphorylation by either of two Sph kinases, SphK1 or SphK2.[5] In mouse bone marrow-derived mast cells SphK2 was the principal regulator of intracellular signaling events such as calcium flux and downstream calcium-dependent activation of protein kinase C, NF-kB, eicosanoid production, and cytokine secretion.[236] SphK1 had no apparent role in these intracellular activities, but instead regulated the concentration of extracellular S_1P and the sensitivity of mast cells to antigen-driven degranulation.[236] S_1P can be transformed back into sphingosine by S_1P phosphatase or removed

from the production pathway by a S_1P lyase.[235] S_1P functions within cells as a modulator of calcium homeostasis and as a regulator of cellular survival and proliferation.[235] The receptors responsible for these intracellular functions are not clearly defined. S_1P can be transported extracellularly and functions to activate cell motility.[235] This function is mediated by S_1P signaling through five GPCRs S_1P_{1-5}.[235] The principal functional receptor for leukocyte chemotaxis to S_1P is S_1P_1, which is expressed on T and B lymphocytes, mononuclear phagocytes, dendritic cells, mast cells, and NK cells.[237] S_1P signaling through S_1P_1 is a major regulator of T lymphocyte function in preventing apoptosis, promoting $CD4^+CD25^+$ T regulatory cell activity, and enhancing chemotaxis.[237] S_1P_1 signaling promotes thymocyte emigration and movement of lymphocytes from lymph nodes, but not from the spleen, into efferent lymph and subsequently to blood.[237] S_1P_1 receptors also regulate the chemotaxis of mast cells toward antigen, while S_1P_2 receptors facilitate IgE-dependent mast cell degranulation. It is thus likely that S_1P generated by mast cells plays an important autocrine role in their function.[238]

Human studies of S_1P in allergic inflammation

Segmental allergen challenge in allergic asthmatics induced a two-fold increased in S_1P levels in BAL fluid 24 h after the challenge; however, there was no change in BAL S_1P levels in non-allergic non-asthmatic controls after challenge.[239] In in vitro experiments using human airway smooth muscle cells, S_1P administration resulted in a dose-dependent increase in both DNA synthesis and cell proliferation.[239] S_1P also induced IL-6 production by human smooth muscle airway cells that was further increased by treatment of the cells with both S_1P and TNF. However, S_1P inhibited TNF-induced RANTES expression. Therefore, further work will need to be performed to conclusively define the role of S_1P in the human allergic inflammatory response.

Mouse studies of S_1P in allergic inflammation

The pharmacologic agent FTY720 downregulates the activity of S_1P_1 in addition to S_1P_2 and S_1P_5, but not S_1P_3 or S_1P_4, and has been used in animal models to test the activity of signaling through the receptors in which it exerts inhibitory activity.[237] In a model in which OVA-specific polarized Th2 cells were adoptively transferred into naïve mice, orally administered FTY720 inhibited the influx of T lymphocytes and eosinophils into the lungs when these mice were subsequently challenged with aerosolized OVA.[240] In mice that were sensitized with an intraperitoneal injection of OVA formulated with aluminum hydroxide, oral FTY720 at the time of OVA challenge inhibited the airway accumulation of lymphocytes and eosinophils, prevented the induction of bronchial hyperresponsiveness, and reduced goblet cell hyperplasia.[240] Intratracheal administration of FTY720 significantly reduced the number of BAL macrophages, neutrophils, lymphocytes, and eosinophils when it was given 30 min prior to OVA aerosolization in mice that had been previously sensitized to OVA.[241] In addition, intratracheal FTY720 inhibited allergen-induced AHR and parenchymal lung inflammation.[241] Although FTY720 had no effect on the number of blood circulating lymphocytes or lymphocytes in peripheral lymph nodes, the number of T cells in lung-draining lymph nodes was significantly reduced.[241] The effect of FTY720 seemed to be predominantly mediated by its inhibition of the migration of lung dendritic cells to the mediastinal lymph nodes, which in turn blunted the formation of allergen-specific Th2 cells in lymph nodes.[241] In addition, FTY720-treated dendritic cells were intrinsically less effective in activating naive and effector Th2 cells due to a inhibited capacity to form stable interactions with T cells and thus to produce an immunological synapse.[241] Thus, inhibition of signaling through several S_1P receptors downregulates allergic inflammation in the mouse. Very recently, FTY720 was reported to potently and selectively inhibit group IVA PLA_2.[242] It is thus possible that some of its immunosuppressive effects may be mediated by interference with eicosanoid generation.

■ SUMMARY ■

The lipid mediators are a diverse array of potent molecules that can be rapidly generated by structural cells as well as leukocytes in response to environmental perturbations. The spectrum of homeostatic, immunologic, and inflammatory functions served by these mediators can now be better understood due to the identification of the GPCRs and enzyme systems responsible for the actions and synthesis of each, and the development of receptor-deficient mice and receptor-selective agonists. While the development of specific enzyme inhibitors and receptor antagonists for therapeutic use is still in its infancy, the success of the COX and 5-LO inhibitors and the $CysLT_1$ antagonists strongly support the role of eicosanoids in human disease. It is likely that additional reagents under development, such as FTY720, will both provide efficacious treatment for human disease and new insights into the biologic importance of lipid mediators in both health and disease.

References

1. Kellaway CH, Trethewie ER. The liberation of a slow-reacting smooth muscle-stimulating substance in anaphylaxis. Q J Exp Physiol Cog Med Sci 1940; 30:121–145.

Generation of lipid mediator precursors by phospholipase A_2

2. Schaloske RH, Dennis EA. The phospholipase A2 superfamily and its group numbering system. Biochim Biophys Acta 2006; 1761:1246–1259.
3. Diaz BL, Arm JP. Phospholipase A(2). Prostaglandins Leukot Essent Fatty Acids 2003; 69: 87–97.
4. Henderson WR Jr, Chi EY, Bollinger JG, et al. Importance of group X-secreted phospholipase A2 in allergen-induced airway inflammation and remodeling in a mouse asthma model. J Exp Med 2007; 204:865–877.
5. Lin DA, Boyce JA. Lysophospholipids as mediators of immunity. Adv Immunol 2006; 89: 141–167.
6. Lucas KK, Svensson CI, Hua XY, et al. Spinal phospholipase A2 in inflammatory hyperalgesia: role of group IVA cPLA2. Br J Pharmacol 2005; 144:940–952.
7. Uozumi N, Shimizu T. Roles for cytosolic phospholipase A2alpha as revealed by gene-targeted mice. Prostaglandins Other Lipid Mediat 2002; 68–69:59–69.

Cyclooxygenase pathway

8. Kang YJ, Mbonye UR, Delong CJ, et al. Regulation of intracellular cyclooxygenase levels by gene transcription and protein degradation. Prog Lipid Res 2007; 46:108–125.
9. Broide DH, Lotz M, Cuomo AJ, et al. Cytokines in symptomatic asthma airways. J Allergy Clin Immunol 1992; 89:958–967.
10. Mitchell JA, Belvisi MG, Akarasereenont P, et al. Induction of cyclo-oxygenase-2 by cytokines in human pulmonary epithelial cells: regulation by dexamethasone. Br J Pharmacol 1994; 113:1008–1014.
11. Newton R, Kuitert LM, Slater DM, et al. Cytokine induction of cytosolic phospholipase A2 and cyclooxygenase-2 mRNA is suppressed by glucocorticoids in human epithelial cells. Life Sci 1997; 60:67–78.
12. Belvisi MG, Saunders MA, Haddad E, et al. Induction of cyclo-oxygenase-2 by cytokines in human cultured airway smooth muscle cells: novel inflammatory role of this cell type. Br J Pharmacol 1997; 120:910–916.
13. Pang L, Knox AJ. Effect of interleukin-1 beta, tumour necrosis factor-alpha and interferon-gamma on the induction of cyclo-oxygenase-2 in cultured human airway smooth muscle cells. Br J Pharmacol 1997; 121:579–587.

14. Endo T, Ogushi F, Sone S, et al. Induction of cyclooxygenase-2 is responsible for interleukin-1 beta-dependent prostaglandin E2 synthesis by human lung fibroblasts. Am J Respir Cell Mol Biol 1995; 12:358–365.
15. Asano K, Lilly CM, Drazen JM. Prostaglandin G/H synthase-2 is the constitutive and dominant isoform in cultured human lung epithelial cells. Am J Physiol 1996; 271:L126–L131.
16. Harris RC, Breyer MD. Physiological regulation of cyclooxygenase-2 in the kidney. Am J Physiol Renal Physiol 2001; 281:F1–11.
17. Robertson RP. Dominance of cyclooxygenase-2 in the regulation of pancreatic islet prostaglandin synthesis. Diabetes 1998; 47:1379–1383.
18. Kaufmann WE, Worley PF, Taylor CV, et al. Cyclooxygenase-2 expression during rat neocortical development and in Rett syndrome. Brain Dev 1997; 19:25–34.
19. Ristimaki A, Honkanen N, Jankala H, et al. Expression of cyclooxygenase-2 in human gastric carcinoma. Cancer Res 1997; 57:1276–1280.
20. Griswold DE, Adams JL. Constitutive cyclooxygenase (COX-1) and inducible cyclooxygenase (COX-2): rationale for selective inhibition and progress to date. Med Res Rev 1996; 16: 181–206.
21. Jouzeau JY, Terlain B, Abid A, et al. Cyclo-oxygenase isoenzymes. How recent findings affect thinking about nonsteroidal anti-inflammatory drugs. Drugs 1997; 53:563–582.
22. Sousa A, Pfister R, Christie PE, et al. Enhanced expression of cyclo-oxygenase isoenzyme 2 (COX-2) in asthmatic airways and its cellular distribution in aspirin-sensitive asthma. Thorax 1997; 52:940–945.
23. Demoly P, Jaffuel D, Lequeux N, et al. Prostaglandin H synthase 1 and 2 immunoreactivities in the bronchial mucosa of asthmatics. Am J Respir Crit Care Med 1997; 155:670–675.
24. Redington AE, Meng QH, Springall DR, et al. Increased expression of inducible nitric oxide synthase and cyclo-oxygenase-2 in the airway epithelium of asthmatic subjects and regulation by corticosteroid treatment. Thorax 2001; 56:351–357.
25. Dworski R, Sheller JR. Differential sensitivities of human blood monocytes and alveolar macrophages to the inhibition of prostaglandin endoperoxide synthase-2 by interleukin-4. Prostaglandins 1997; 53:237–251.
26. Trudeau J, Hu H, Chibana K, et al. Selective downregulation of prostaglandin E2-related pathways by the Th2 cytokine IL-13. J Allergy Clin Immunol 2006; 117:1446–1454.
27. Dworski R, Fitzgerald GA, Oates JA, et al. Effect of oral prednisone on airway inflammatory mediators in atopic asthma. Am J Respir Crit Care Med 1994; 149:953–959.
28. Aksoy MO, Li X, Borenstein M, et al. Effects of topical corticosteroids on inflammatory mediator-induced eicosanoid release by human airway epithelial cells. J Allergy Clin Immunol 1999; 103:1081–1091.
29. Iniguez MA, Punzon C, Fresno M. Induction of cyclooxygenase-2 on activated T lymphocytes: regulation of T cell activation by cyclooxygenase-2 inhibitors. J Immunol 1999; 163:111–119.
30. Rocca B, Spain LM, Pure E, et al. Distinct roles of prostaglandin H synthases 1 and 2 in T-cell development. J Clin Invest 1999; 103:1469–1477.
31. Liu MC, Bleecker ER, Lichtenstein LM, et al. Evidence for elevated levels of histamine, prostaglandin D2, and other bronchoconstricting prostaglandins in the airways of subjects with mild asthma. Am Rev Respir Dis 1990; 142:126–132.
32. Liu MC, Hubbard WC, Proud D, et al. Immediate and late inflammatory responses to ragweed antigen challenge of the peripheral airways in allergic asthmatics. Cellular, mediator, and permeability changes. Am Rev Respir Dis 1991; 144:51–58.
33. Liu MC, Proud D, Lichtenstein LM, et al. Effects of prednisone on the cellular responses and release of cytokines and mediators after segmental allergen challenge of asthmatic subjects. J Allergy Clin Immunol 2001; 108:29–38.
34. Fish JE, Ankin MG, Adkinson NF Jr, et al. Indomethacin modification of immediate-type immunologic airway responses in allergic asthmatic and non-asthmatic subjects: evidence for altered arachidonic acid metabolism in asthma. Am Rev Respir Dis 1981; 123:609–614.
35. Kirby JG, Hargreave FE, Cockcroft DW, et al. 1989. Effect of indomethacin on allergen-induced asthmatic responses. J Appl Physiol 66:578–583.
36. Sladek K, Dworski R, Fitzgerald GA, et al. Allergen-stimulated release of thromboxane A2 and leukotriene E4 in humans. Effect of indomethacin. Am Rev Respir Dis 1990; 141: 1441–1445.
37. O'Byrne PM, Jones GL. The effect of indomethacin on exercise-induced bronchoconstriction and refractoriness after exercise. Am Rev Respir Dis 1986; 134:69–72.
38. Carey MA, Germolec DR, Bradbury JA, et al. Accentuated T helper type 2 airway response after allergen challenge in cyclooxygenase-1-/- but not cyclooxygenase-2-/- mice. Am J Respir Crit Care Med 2003; 167:1509–1515.
39. Zeldin DC, Wohlford-Lenane C, Chulada P, et al. Airway inflammation and responsiveness in prostaglandin H synthase-deficient mice exposed to bacterial lipopolysaccharide. Am J Respir Cell Mol Biol 2001; 25:457–465.
40. Nakata J, Kondo M, Tamaoki J, et al. Augmentation of allergic inflammation in the airways of cyclooxygenase-2-deficient mice. Respirology 2005; 10:149–156.
41. Card JW, Carey MA, Bradbury JA, et al. Cyclooxygenase-1 overexpression decreases basal airway responsiveness but not allergic inflammation. J Immunol 2006; 177:4785–4793.
42. Peebles RS Jr, Dworski R, Collins RD, et al. Cyclooxygenase inhibition increases interleukin 5 and interleukin 13 production and airway hyperresponsiveness in allergic mice. Am J Respir Crit Care Med 2000; 162:676–681.
43. Peebles RS Jr, Hashimoto K, Sheller JR, et al. Allergen-induced airway hyperresponsiveness mediated by cyclooxygenase inhibition is not dependent on 5-lipoxygenase or IL-5, but is IL-13 dependent. J Immunol 2005; 175:8253–8259.
44. Hashimoto K, Sheller JR, Morrow JD, et al. Cyclooxygenase inhibition augments allergic inflammation through CD4-dependent, STAT6-independent mechanisms. J Immunol 2005; 174:525–532.
45. Peebles RS Jr, Hashimoto K, Morrow JD, et al. Selective cyclooxygenase-1 and -2 inhibitors each increase allergic inflammation and airway hyperresponsiveness in mice. Am J Respir Crit Care Med 2002; 165:1154–1160.
46. Laouini D, Elkhal A, Yalcindag A, et al. COX-2 inhibition enhances the TH2 immune response to epicutaneous sensitization. J Allergy Clin Immunol 2005; 116:390–396.
47. Martin TR, Gerard NP, Galli SJ, et al. Pulmonary responses to bronchoconstrictor agonists in the mouse. J Appl Physiol 1988; 64:2318–2323.

PGD_2

48. Lewis RA, Austen KF. Mediation of local homeostasis and inflammation by leukotrienes and other mast cell-dependent compounds. Nature 1981; 293:103–108.
49. Roberts LJ, Sweetman BJ, Lewis RA, et al. Increased production of prostaglandin D2 in patients with systemic mastocytosis. N Engl J Med 1980; 303:1400–1404.
50. Herlong JL, Scott TR. Positioning prostanoids of the D and J series in the immunopathogenic scheme. Immunol Lett 2006; 102:121–131.
51. Fitzpatrick FA, Wynalda MA. Albumin-catalyzed metabolism of prostaglandin D2. Identification of products formed in vitro. J Biol Chem 1983; 258:11713–11718.
52. Boie Y, Sawyer N, Slipetz DM, et al. Molecular cloning and characterization of the human prostanoid DP receptor. J Biol Chem 1995; 270:18910–18916.
53. Gervais FG, Cruz RP, Chateauneuf A, et al. Selective modulation of chemokinesis, degranulation, and apoptosis in eosinophils through the PGD2 receptors CRTH2 and DP. J Allergy Clin Immunol 2001; 108:982–988.
54. Heinemann A, Schuligoi R, Sabroe I, et al. Delta 12-prostaglandin J2, a plasma metabolite of prostaglandin D2, causes eosinophil mobilization from the bone marrow and primes eosinophils for chemotaxis. J Immunol 2003; 170:4752–4758.
55. Sawyer N, Cauchon E, Chateauneuf A, et al. Molecular pharmacology of the human prostaglandin D2 receptor, CRTH2. Br J Pharmacol 2002; 137:1163–1172.
56. Murray M, Webb MS, O'Callaghan C, et al. Respiratory status and allergy after bronchiolitis. Arch Dis Child 1992; 67:482–487.
57. Naclerio RM, Meier HL, Kagey-Sobotka A, et al. Mediator release after nasal airway challenge with allergen. Am Rev Respir Dis 1983; 128:597–602.
58. Proud D, Sweet J, Stein P, et al. Inflammatory mediator release on conjunctival provocation of allergic subjects with allergen. J Allergy Clin Immunol 1990; 85:896–905.
59. Charlesworth EN, Kagey-Sobotka A, Schleimer RP, et al. Prednisone inhibits the appearance of inflammatory mediators and the influx of eosinophils and basophils associated with the cutaneous late-phase response to allergen. J Immunol 1991; 146:671–676.
60. Johnston SL, Freezer NJ, Ritter WS, et al. Prostaglandin D2-induced bronchoconstriction is mediated only in part by the thromboxane prostanoid receptor. Eur Respir J 1995; 8: 411–415.
61. Doyle WJ, Boehm S, Skoner DP. Physiologic responses to intranasal dose-response challenges with histamine, methacholine, bradykinin, and prostaglandin in adult volunteers with and without nasal allergy. J Allergy Clin Immunol 1990; 86:924–935.
62. Flower RJ, Harvey EA, Kingston WP. Inflammatory effects of prostaglandin D2 in rat and human skin. Br J Pharmacol 1976; 56:229–233.
63. Woodward DF, Hawley SB, Williams LS, et al. Studies on the ocular pharmacology of prostaglandin D2. Invest Ophthalmol Vis Sci 1990; 31:138–146.
64. Emery DL, Djokic TD, Graf PD, et al. Prostaglandin D2 causes accumulation of eosinophils in the lumen of the dog trachea. J Appl Physiol 1989; 67:959–962.
65. Hirai H, Tanaka K, Yoshie O, et al. Prostaglandin D2 selectively induces chemotaxis in T helper type 2 cells, eosinophils, and basophils via seven-transmembrane receptor CRTH2. J Exp Med 2001; 193:255–262.
66. Monneret G, Gravel S, Diamond M, et al. Prostaglandin D2 is a potent chemoattractant for human eosinophils that acts via a novel DP receptor. Blood 2001; 98:1942–1948.
67. Angeli V, Staumont D, Charbonnier AS, et al. Activation of the D prostanoid receptor 1 regulates immune and skin allergic responses. J Immunol 2004; 172:3822–3829.
68. Matsuoka T, Hirata M, Tanaka H, et al. Prostaglandin D2 as a mediator of allergic asthma. Science 2000; 287:2013–2017.
69. Fujitani Y, Kanaoka Y, Aritake K, et al. Pronounced eosinophilic lung inflammation and Th2 cytokine release in human lipocalin-type prostaglandin D synthase transgenic mice. J Immunol 2002; 168:443–449.
70. Honda K, Arima M, Cheng G, et al. Prostaglandin D2 reinforces Th2 type inflammatory responses of airways to low-dose antigen through bronchial expression of macrophage-derived chemokine. J Exp Med 2003; 198:533–543.
71. Hammad HH, de Heer J, Soullie T, et al. Prostaglandin D2 inhibits airway dendritic cell migration and function in steady state conditions by selective activation of the D prostanoid receptor 1. J Immunol 2003; 171:3936–3940.
72. Hammad H, Kool M, Soullie T, et al. Activation of the D prostanoid 1 receptor suppresses asthma by modulation of lung dendritic cell function and induction of regulatory T cells. J Exp Med 2007; 204:357–367.
73. Spik I, Brenuchon C, Angeli V, et al. Activation of the prostaglandin D2 receptor DP2/CRTH2 increases allergic inflammation in mouse. J Immunol 2005; 174:3703–3708.
74. Uller L, Mathiesen JM, Alenmyr L, et al. Antagonism of the prostaglandin D2 receptor CRTH2 attenuates asthma pathology in mouse eosinophilic airway inflammation. Respir Res 2007; 8:16.

PGE_2

75. Murakami M, Naraba H, Tanioka T, et al. Regulation of prostaglandin E2 biosynthesis by inducible membrane-associated prostaglandin E2 synthase that acts in concert with cyclooxygenase-2. J Biol Chem 2000; 275:32783–32792.
76. Park JY, Pillinger MH, Abramson SB. Prostaglandin E2 synthesis and secretion: the role of PGE2 synthases. Clin Immunol 2006; 119:229–240.
77. Tanioka T, Nakatani Y, Semmyo N, et al. Molecular identification of cytosolic prostaglandin E2 synthase that is functionally coupled with cyclooxygenase-1 in immediate prostaglandin E2 biosynthesis. J Biol Chem 2000; 275:32775–32782.
78. Boulet L, Ouellet M, Bateman KP, et al. Deletion of microsomal prostaglandin E2 (PGE2) synthase-1 reduces inducible and basal PGE2 production and alters the gastric prostanoid profile. J Biol Chem 2004; 279:23229–23237.
79. Breyer RM, Bagdassarian CK, Myers SA, et al. Prostanoid receptors: subtypes and signaling. Annu Rev Pharmacol Toxicol 2001; 41:661–690.
80. Reinheimer T, Harnack E, Racke K, et al. Prostanoid receptors of the EP3 subtype mediate inhibition of evoked [3H]acetylcholine release from isolated human bronchi. Br J Pharmacol 1998; 125:271–276.
81. Funk CD, Furci L, Fitzgerald GA, et al. Cloning and expression of a cDNA for the human prostaglandin E receptor EP1 subtype. J Biol Chem 1993; 268:26767–26772.
82. Coleman RA, Smith WL, Narumiya S. International Union of Pharmacology classification of prostanoid receptors: properties, distribution, and structure of the receptors and their subtypes. Pharmacol Rev 1994; 46:205–229.
83. An S, Yang J, Xia M, et al. Cloning and expression of the EP2 subtype of human receptors for prostaglandin E2. Biochem Biophys Res Comm 1993; 197:263–270.
84. Adam M, Boie Y, Rushmore TH, et al. Cloning and expression of three isoforms of the human EP3 prostanoid receptor. FEBS Lett 1994; 338:170–174.
85. Churchill L, Chilton FH, Resau JH, et al. Cyclooxygenase metabolism of endogenous arachidonic acid by cultured human tracheal epithelial cells. Am Rev Respir Dis 1989; 140:449–459.
86. Delamere F, Holland E, Patel S, et al. Production of PGE2 by bovine cultured airway smooth muscle cells and its inhibition by cyclo-oxygenase inhibitors. Br J Pharmacol 1994; 111:983–988.
87. Pavord ID, Tattersfield AE. Bronchoprotective role for endogenous prostaglandin E2. Lancet 1995; 345:436–438.
88. Barnett K, Jacoby DB, Nadel JA, et al. The effects of epithelial cell supernatant on contractions of isolated canine tracheal smooth muscle. Am Rev Respir Dis 1988; 138:780–783.
89. Pavord ID, Ward R, Woltmann G, et al. Induced sputum eicosanoid concentrations in asthma. Am J Respir Crit Care Med 1999; 160:1905–1909.
90. Gauvreau GM, Watson RM, O'Byrne PM. Protective effects of inhaled PGE2 on allergen-induced airway responses and airway inflammation. Am J Respir Crit Care Med 1999; 159:31–36.
91. Pavord ID, Wong CS, Williams J, et al. Effect of inhaled prostaglandin E2 on allergen-induced asthma. Am Rev Respir Dis 1993; 148:87–90.
92. Melillo E, Woolley KL, Manning PJ, et al. Effect of inhaled PGE2 on exercise-induced bronchoconstriction in asthmatic subjects. Am J Respir Crit Care Med 1994; 149:1138–1141.
93. Sestini P, Armetti L, Gambaro G, et al. Inhaled PGE2 prevents aspirin-induced bronchoconstriction and urinary LTE4 excretion in aspirin-sensitive asthma. Am J Respir Crit Care Med 1996; 153:572–575.
94. Hartert TV, Dworski RT, Mellen BG, et al. Prostaglandin E(2) decreases allergen-stimulated release of prostaglandin D(2) in airways of subjects with asthma. Am J Respir Crit Care Med 2000; 162:637–640.
95. Wasiak W, Szmidt M. A six week double blind, placebo controlled, crossover study of the effect of misoprostol in the treatment of aspirin sensitive asthma. Thorax 1999; 54:900–904.
96. Harmanci E, Ozakyol A, Ozdemir N, et al. Misoprostol has no favorable effect on bronchial hyperresponsiveness in mild asthmatics. Allerg Immunol (Paris) 1998; 30:298–300.
97. Betz M, Fox BS. Prostaglandin E2 inhibits production of Th1 lymphokines but not of Th2 lymphokines. J Immunol 1991; 146:108–113.
98. Snijdewint FG, Kalinski P, Wierenga EA, et al. Prostaglandin E2 differentially modulates cytokine secretion profiles of human T helper lymphocytes. J Immunol 1993; 150:5321–5329.
99. Katamura K, Shintaku N, Yamauchi Y, et al. Prostaglandin E2 at priming of naive $CD4^+$ T cells inhibits acquisition of ability to produce IFN-gamma and IL-2, but not IL- 4 and IL-5. J Immunol 1995; 155:4604–4612.
100. Hilkens CM, Vermeulen HR, van Neerven J, et al. Differential modulation of T helper type 1 (Th1) and T helper type 2 (Th2) cytokine secretion by prostaglandin E2 critically depends on interleukin-2. Eur J Immunol 1995; 25:59–63.
101. Vieira PL, de Jong EC, Wierenga EA, et al. Development of Th1-inducing capacity in myeloid dendritic cells requires environmental instruction. J Immunol 2000; 164:4507–4512.
102. Peacock CD, Misso NL, Watkins DN, et al. PGE 2 and dibutyryl cyclic adenosine monophosphate prolong eosinophil survival in vitro. J Allergy Clin Immunol 1999; 104:153–162.
103. Kita H, Abu-Ghazaleh RI, Gleich GJ, et al. Regulation of Ig-induced eosinophil degranulation by adenosine 3',5'-cyclic monophosphate. J Immunol 1991; 146:2712–2718.
104. Teixeira MM, al-Rashed S, Rossi AG, et al. Characterization of the prostanoid receptors mediating inhibition of PAF-induced aggregation of guinea-pig eosinophils. Br J Pharmacol 1997; 121:77–82.
105. Lazzeri N, Belvisi MG, Patel HJ, et al. Effects of prostaglandin E2 and cAMP elevating drugs on GM-CSF release by cultured human airway smooth muscle cells. Relevance to asthma therapy. Am J Respir Cell Mol Biol 2001; 24:44–48.
106. Gomi K, Zhu FG, Marshall JS. Prostaglandin E2 selectively enhances the IgE-mediated production of IL-6 and granulocyte-macrophage colony-stimulating factor by mast cells through an EP1/EP3-dependent mechanism. J Immunol 2000; 165:6545–6552.
107. Hogaboam CM, Bissonnette EY, Chin BC, et al. Prostaglandins inhibit inflammatory mediator release from rat mast cells. Gastroenterology 1993; 104:122–129.
108. Kaliner M, Austen KF. Cyclic AMP, ATP, and reversed anaphylactic histamine release from rat mast cells. J Immunol 1974; 112:664–674.
109. Peachell PT, MacGlashan DW Jr, Lichtenstein LM, et al. Regulation of human basophil and lung mast cell function by cyclic adenosine monophosphate. J Immunol 1988; 140:571–579.
110. Leal-Berumen I, O'Byrne P, Gupta A, et al. Prostanoid enhancement of interleukin-6 production by rat peritoneal mast cells. J Immunol 1995; 154:4759–4767.
111. Nishigaki N, Negishi M, Honda A, et al. Identification of prostaglandin E receptor 'EP2' cloned from mastocytoma cells EP4 subtype. FEBS Lett 1995; 364:339–341.
112. Feng C, Beller EM, Bagga S, et al. Human mast cells express multiple EP receptors for prostaglandin E2 that differentially modulate activation responses. Blood 2006; 107:3243–3250.
113. Kunikata T, Yamane H, Segi E, et al. Suppression of allergic inflammation by the prostaglandin E receptor subtype EP3. Nat Immunol 2005; 6:524–531.
114. Hartney JM, Coggins KG, Tilley SL, et al. Prostaglandin E2 protects lower airways against bronchoconstriction. Am J Physiol Lung Cell Mol Physiol 2006; 290:L105–L113.
115. Sheller JR, Mitchell D, Meyrick B, et al. EP(2) receptor mediates bronchodilation by PGE(2) in mice. J Appl Physiol 2000; 88:2214–2218.
116. Tilley SL, Hartney JM, Erikson CJ, et al. Receptors and pathways mediating the effects of prostaglandin E2 on airway tone. Am J Physiol Lung Cell Mol Physiol 2003; 284:L599–L606.

$PGF_{2\alpha}$

117. Komoto J, Yamada T, Watanabe K, et al. Prostaglandin F2alpha formation from prostaglandin H2 by prostaglandin F synthase (PGFS) crystal structure of PGFS containing bimatoprost. Biochemistry 2006; 45:1987–1996.

118. Suzuki-Yamamoto T, Nishizawa M, Fukui M, et al. cDNA cloning, expression and characterization of human prostaglandin F synthase. FEBS Lett 1999; 462:335–340.

119. Suzuki-Yamamoto T, Toida K, et al. Immunocytochemical localization of lung-type prostaglandin F synthase in the rat spinal cord. Brain Res 2000; 877:391–395.

120. Hata AN, Breyer RM. Pharmacology and signaling of prostaglandin receptors: multiple roles in inflammation and immune modulation. Pharmacol Ther 2004; 103:147–166.

121. Breyer MD, Breyer RM. G protein-coupled prostanoid receptors and the kidney. Annu Rev Physiol 2001; 63:579–605.

122. Mathe AA, Hedqvist P, Holmgren A, et al. Bronchial hyperreactivity to prostaglandin F2 and histamine in patients with asthma. Br Med J 1973; 1:193–196.

123. Smith AP, Cuthbert MF. Prostaglandins and resistance to beta adrenoceptor stimulants. Br Med J 1972; 2:166.

124. Smith AP, Cuthbert MF, Dunlop LS. Effects of inhaled prostaglandins E1, E2, and F2alpha on the airway resistance of healthy and asthmatic man. Clin Sci Mol Med 1975; 48:421–430.

125. Kharitonov SA, Sapienza MA, Barnes PJ, et al. Prostaglandins E2 and F2alpha reduce exhaled nitric oxide in normal and asthmatic subjects irrespective of airway caliber changes. Am J Respir Crit Care Med 1998; 158:1374–1378.

PGI_2

126. Nakayama, T. Prostacyclin analogues: prevention of cardiovascular diseases. Cardiovasc Hematol Agents Med Chem 2006; 4:351–359.

127. Breyer RM, Kennedy CR, Zhang Y, et al. Structure-function analyses of eicosanoid receptors. Physiologic and therapeutic implications. Ann N Y Acad Sci 2000; 905:221–231.

128. Zhou W, Hashimoto K, Goleniewska K, et al. Prostaglandin I2 analogs inhibit proinflammatory cytokine production and T cell stimulatory function of dendritic cells. J Immunol 2007; 178:702–710.

129. Narumiya S, Sugimoto Y, Ushikubi F. Prostanoid receptors: structures, properties, and functions. Physiol Rev 1999; 79:1193–1226.

130. Komhoff M, Lesener B, Nakao K, et al. Localization of the prostacyclin receptor in human kidney. Kidney Int 1998; 54:1899–1908.

131. Zhou W, Blackwell TS, Goleniewska KJ, et al. Prostaglandin I2 analogs inhibit Th1 and Th2 effector cytokine production by CD4 T cells. J Leukoc Biol 2007; 81:809–817.

132. Schulman ES, Newball HH, Demers LM, et al. Anaphylactic release of thromboxane A2, prostaglandin D2, and prostacyclin from human lung parenchyma. Am Rev Respir Dis 1981; 124:402–406.

133. Schulman ES, Adkinson NF Jr, Newball HH. Cyclooxygenase metabolites in human lung anaphylaxis: airway vs. parenchyma. J Appl Physiol 1982; 53:589–595.

134. Shephard EG, Malan L, Macfarlane CM, et al. Lung function and plasma levels of thromboxane B2, 6-ketoprostaglandin F1 alpha and beta-thromboglobulin in antigen-induced asthma before and after indomethacin pretreatment. Br J Clin Pharmacol 1985; 19:459–470.

135. Bianco S, Robuschi M, Grugni A, et al. Effect of prostacyclin on antigen induced immediate bronchoconstriction in asthmatic patients. Prostaglandins Med 1979; 3:39–45.

136. Bianco S, Robuschi M, Ceserani R, et al. Effects of prostacyclin on aspecifically and specifically induced bronchoconstriction in asthmatic patients. Eur J Respir Dis Suppl 1980, 106.81–87.

137. Hardy C, Robinson C, Lewis RA, et al. Airway and cardiovascular responses to inhaled prostacyclin in normal and asthmatic subjects. Am Rev Respir Dis 1985; 131:18–21.

138. Nizankowska E, Czerniawska-Mysik G, Szczeklik A. Lack of effect of i. v. prostacyclin on aspirin-induced asthma. Eur J Respir Dis 1986; 69:363–368.

139. Hardy CC, Bradding P, Robinson C, et al. Bronchoconstrictor and antibronchoconstrictor properties of inhaled prostacyclin in asthma. J Appl Physiol 1988; 64:1567–1574.

140. Fujimura M, Ozawa S, Matsuda T. Effect of oral administration of a prostacyclin analog (OP-41483) on pulmonary function and bronchial responsiveness in stable asthmatic subjects. J Asthma 1991; 28:419–424.

141. Takahashi Y, Tokuoka S, Masuda T, et al. Augmentation of allergic inflammation in prostanoid IP receptor deficient mice. Br J Pharmacol 2002; 137:315–322.

142. Nagao K, Tanaka H, Komai M, et al. Role of prostaglandin I2 in airway remodeling induced by repeated allergen challenge in mice. Am J Respir Cell Mol Biol 2003; 29:314–320.

143. Jaffar Z, Wan KS, Roberts K. A key role for prostaglandin I2 in limiting lung mucosal Th2, but not Th1, responses to inhaled allergen. J Immunol 2002; 169:5997–6004.

144. Lovgren AK, Jania LA, Hartney JM, et al. COX-2-derived prostacyclin protects against bleomycin-induced pulmonary fibrosis. Am J Physiol Lung Cell Mol Physiol 2006; 291:L144–L156.

Thromboxane A_2

145. Whittle BJ, Moncada S. Pharmacological interactions between prostacyclin and thromboxanes. Br Med Bull 1983; 39:232–238.

146. Miyata A, Yokoyama C, Ihara H, et al. Characterization of the human gene (TBXAS1) encoding thromboxane synthase. Eur J Biochem 1994; 224:273–279.

147. Ruan KH. Advance in understanding the biosynthesis of prostacyclin and thromboxane A2 in the endoplasmic reticulum membrane via the cyclooxygenase pathway. Mini Rev Med Chem 2004; 4:639–647.

148. Roberts LJ, Sweetman BJ, Oates JA. Metabolism of thromboxane B2 in man. Identification of twenty urinary metabolites. J Biol Chem 1981; 256:8384–8393.

149. Raychowdhury MK, Yukawa M, Collins LJ, et al. Alternative splicing produces a divergent cytoplasmic tail in the human endothelial thromboxane A2 receptor. J Biol Chem 1994; 269:19256–19261.

150. Huang JS, Ramamurthy SK, Lin X, et al. Cell signalling through thromboxane A2 receptors. Cell Signal 2004; 16:521–533.

151. Hirata T, Ushikubi F, Kakizuka A, et al. Two thromboxane A2 receptor isoforms in human platelets. Opposite coupling to adenylyl cyclase with different sensitivity to Arg60 to Leu mutation. J Clin Invest 1996; 97:949–956.

152. Grosser T, Fries S, Fitzgerald GA. Biological basis for the cardiovascular consequences of COX-2 inhibition: therapeutic challenges and opportunities. J Clin Invest 2006; 116:4–15.

153. Taylor IK, Ward PS, O'Shaughnessy KM, et al. Thromboxane A2 biosynthesis in acute asthma and after antigen challenge. Am Rev Respir Dis 1991; 143:119–125.

154. Lupinetti MD, Sheller JR, Catella F, et al. Thromboxane biosynthesis in allergen-induced bronchospasm. Evidence for platelet activation. Am Rev Respir Dis 1989; 140:932–935.

155. Seltzer J, Bigby BG, Stulbarg M, et al. O3-induced change in bronchial reactivity to methacholine and airway inflammation in humans. J Appl Physiol 1986; 60:1321–1326.

156. O'Byrne PM, Leikauf GD, Aizawa H, et al. Leukotriene B4 induces airway hyperresponsiveness in dogs. J Appl Physiol 1985; 59:1941–1946.

157. Aizawa H, Inoue H, Nakano H, et al. Effects of thromboxane A2 antagonist on airway hyperresponsiveness, exhaled nitric oxide, and induced sputum eosinophils in asthmatics. Prostaglandins Leukot Essent Fatty Acids 1998; 59:185–190.

158. Hoshino M, Sim J, Shimizu K, et al. Effect of AA-2414, a thromboxane A2 receptor antagonist, on airway inflammation in subjects with asthma. J Allergy Clin Immunol 1999; 103:1054–1061.

159. Shi H, Yokoyama A, Kohno N, et al. Effect of thromboxane A2 inhibitors on allergic pulmonary inflammation in mice. Eur Respir J 1998; 11:624–629.

Lipoxygenase pathway

160. Brock TG. Regulating leukotriene synthesis: the role of nuclear 5-lipoxygenase. J Cell Biochem 2005; 96:1203–1211.

161. Levy BD, De Sanctis GT, Devchand PR, et al. Multi-pronged inhibition of airway hyper-responsiveness and inflammation by lipoxin A(4). Nat Med 2002; 8:1018–1023.

162. Levy BD. Lipoxins and lipoxin analogs in asthma. Prostaglandins Leukot Essent Fatty Acids 2005; 73:231–237.

163. Levy BD, Bonnans C, Silverman ES, et al. Diminished lipoxin biosynthesis in severe asthma. Am J Respir Crit Care Med 2005; 172:824–830.

164. Powell WS, Rokach J.. Biochemistry, biology and chemistry of the 5-lipoxygenase product 5-oxo-ETE. Prog Lipid Res 2005; 44:154–183.

Leukotrienes

165. Kanaoka Y, Boyce JA. Cysteinyl leukotrienes and their receptors: cellular distribution and function in immune and inflammatory responses. J Immunol 2004; 173:1503–1510.

166. Mancini JA, Evans JF. Cloning and characterization of the human leukotriene A4 hydrolase gene. Eur J Biochem 1995; 231:65–71.

167. Lam BK, Penrose JF, Freeman GJ, et al. Expression cloning of a cDNA for human leukotriene C4 synthase, an integral membrane protein conjugating reduced glutathione to leukotriene A4. Proc Natl Acad Sci U S A 1994; 91:7663–7667.

168. Hsieh FH, Lam BK, Penrose JF, et al. T helper cell type 2 cytokines coordinately regulate immunoglobulin E-dependent cysteinyl leukotriene production by human cord blood-derived mast cells: profound induction of leukotriene C(4) synthase expression by interleukin 4. J Exp Med 2001; 193:123–133.

169. Penrose JF, Spector J, Baldasaro M, et al. Molecular cloning of the gene for human leukotriene C4 synthase. Organization, nucleotide sequence, and chromosomal localization to 5q35. J Biol Chem 1996; 271:11356–11361.

170. Lam BK, Austen KF. Leukotriene C4 synthase: a pivotal enzyme in cellular biosynthesis of the cysteinyl leukotrienes. Prostaglandins Other Lipid Mediat 2002; 68–69:511–520.

171. Mondino C, Ciabattoni G, Koch P, et al. Effects of inhaled corticosteroids on exhaled leukotrienes and prostanoids in asthmatic children. J Allergy Clin Immunol 2004; 114: 761–767.

172. Sedgwick JB, Calhoun WJ, Gleich GJ, et al. Immediate and late airway response of allergic rhinitis patients to segmental antigen challenge. Characterization of eosinophil and mast cell mediators. Am Rev Respir Dis 1991; 144:1274–1281.

173. Sampson AP, Castling DP, Green CP, et al. Persistent increase in plasma and urinary leukotrienes after acute asthma. Arch Dis Child 1995; 73:221–225.

174. McGill KA, Busse WW. Zileuton. Lancet 1996; 348:519–524.

175. Israel E, Rubin P, Kemp JP, et al. The effect of inhibition of 5-lipoxygenase by zileuton in mild-to-moderate asthma. Ann Intern Med 1993; 119:1059–1066.

176. Israel E, Cohn J, Dube L, et al. Effect of treatment with zileuton, a 5-lipoxygenase inhibitor, in patients with asthma. A randomized controlled trial. Zileuton Clinical Trial Group. JAMA 1996; 275:931–936.

177. Kane GC, Pollice M, Kim CJ, et al. A controlled trial of the effect of the 5-lipoxygenase inhibitor, zileuton, on lung inflammation produced by segmental antigen challenge in human beings. J Allergy Clin Immunol 1996; 97:646–654.

178. Irvin CG, Tu YP, Sheller JR, et al. 5-Lipoxygenase products are necessary for ovalbumin-induced airway responsiveness in mice. Am J Physiol 1997; 272:L1053–1058.

179. Nagase T, Uozumi N, Ishii S, et al. A pivotal role of cytosolic phospholipase A(2) in bleomycin-induced pulmonary fibrosis. Nat Med 2002; 8:480–484.

180. Vargaftig BB, Singer M. Leukotrienes mediate part of Ova-induced lung effects in mice via EGFR. Am J Physiol Lung Cell Mol Physiol 2003; 285:L808–L818.

181. Henderson WR Jr, Lewis DB, Albert RK, et al. The importance of leukotrienes in airway inflammation in a mouse model of asthma. J Exp Med 1996; 184:1483–1494.

182. Vargaftig BB, Singer M. Leukotrienes, IL-13, and chemokines cooperate to induce BHR and mucus in allergic mouse lungs. Am J Physiol Lung Cell Mol Physiol 2003; 284:L260–L269.

LTB_4

183. Tager AM, Luster AD. BLT1 and BLT2: the leukotriene B(4) receptors. Prostaglandins Leukot Essent Fatty Acids 2003; 69:123–134.
184. Islam SA, Thomas SY, Hess C, et al. The leukotriene B4 lipid chemoattractant receptor BLT1 defines antigen-primed T cells in humans. Blood 2006; 107:444–453.
185. Weller CL, Collington SJ, Brown JK, et al. Leukotriene B4, an activation product of mast cells, is a chemoattractant for their progenitors. J Exp Med 2005; 201:1961–1971.
186. Tager AM, Bromley SK, Medoff BD, et al. Leukotriene B4 receptor BLT1 mediates early effector T cell recruitment. Nat Immunol 2003; 4:982–990.
187. Terawaki K, Yokomizo T, Nagase T, et al. Absence of leukotriene B4 receptor 1 confers resistance to airway hyperresponsiveness and Th2-type immune responses. J Immunol 2005; 175:4217–4225.
188. Miyahara N, Takeda K, Miyahara S, et al. Requirement for leukotriene B4 receptor 1 in allergen-induced airway hyperresponsiveness. Am J Respir Crit Care Med 2005; 172: 161–167.
189. Miyahara N, Takeda K, Miyahara S, et al. Leukotriene B4 receptor-1 is essential for allergen-mediated recruitment of CD8+ T cells and airway hyperresponsiveness. J Immunol 2005; 174:4979–4984.
190. Taube C, Miyahara N, Ott V, et al. The leukotriene B4 receptor (BLT1) is required for effector CD8+ T cell-mediated, mast cell-dependent airway hyperresponsiveness. J Immunol 2006; 176:3157–3164.
191. Del Prete A, Shao WH, Mitola S, et al. Regulation of dendritic cell migration and adaptive immune response by leukotriene B4 receptors: a role for LTB4 in up-regulation of CCR7 expression and function. Blood 2007; 109:626–631.

Cysteinyl leukotrienes

192. Ciana P, Fumagalli M, Trincavelli ML, et al. The orphan receptor GPR17 identified as a new dual uracil nucleotides/cysteinyl-leukotrienes receptor. EMBO J 2006; 25:4615–4627.
193. Gauvreau GM, Plitt JR, Baatjes A, et al. Expression of functional cysteinyl leukotriene receptors by human basophils. J Allergy Clin Immunol 2005; 116:80–87.
194. Peters-Golden M, Gleason MM, Togias A. Cysteinyl leukotrienes: multi-functional mediators in allergic rhinitis. Clin Exp Allergy 2006; 36:689–703.
195. Jiang Y, Kanaoka Y, Feng C, et al. Cutting edge: interleukin 4-dependent mast cell proliferation requires autocrine/intracrine cysteinyl leukotriene-induced signaling. J Immunol 2006; 177:2755–2759.
196. Bisgaard H, Ford-Hutchinson AW, Charleson S, et al. Production of leukotrienes in human skin and conjunctival mucosa after specific allergen challenge. Allergy 1985; 40:417–423.
197. Creticos PS, Peters SP, Adkinson NF Jr, et al. Peptide leukotriene release after antigen challenge in patients sensitive to ragweed. N Engl J Med 1984; 310:1626–1630.
198. Laitinen A, Lindqvist A, Halme M, et al. Leukotriene E(4)-induced persistent eosinophilia and airway obstruction are reversed by zafirlukast in patients with asthma. J Allergy Clin Immunol 2005; 115:259–265.
199. Malmstrom K, Rodriguez-Gomez G, Guerra J, et al. Oral montelukast, inhaled beclomethasone, and placebo for chronic asthma. A randomized, controlled trial. Montelukast/Beclomethasone Study Group. Ann Intern Med 1999; 130:487–495.
200. Brannan JD, Anderson SD, Gomes K, et al. Fexofenadine decreases sensitivity to and montelukast improves recovery from inhaled mannitol. Am J Respir Crit Care Med 2001; 163:1420–1425.
201. Lazarus SC, Wong HH, Watts MJ, et al. The leukotriene receptor antagonist zafirlukast inhibits sulfur dioxide-induced bronchoconstriction in patients with asthma. Am J Respir Crit Care Med 1997; 156:1725–1730.
202. Leigh R, Vethanayagam D, Yoshida M, et al. Effects of montelukast and budesonide on airway responses and airway inflammation in asthma. Am J Respir Crit Care Med 2002; 166:1212–1217.
203. Pearlman DS, van Adelsberg J, Philip G, et al. Onset and duration of protection against exercise-induced bronchoconstriction by a single oral dose of montelukast. Ann Allergy Asthma Immunol 2006; 97:98–104.
204. Rorke S, Jennison S, Jeffs JA, et al. Role of cysteinyl leukotrienes in adenosine 5'-monophosphate induced bronchoconstriction in asthma. Thorax 2002; 57:323–327.
205. Rundell KW, Spiering BA, Baumann JM, et al. Effects of montelukast on airway narrowing from eucapnic voluntary hyperventilation and cold air exercise. Br J Sports Med 2005; 39:232–236.
206. Di Lorenzo G, Pacor ML, Mansueto P, et al. Randomized placebo-controlled trial comparing desloratadine and montelukast in monotherapy and desloratadine plus montelukast in combined therapy for chronic idiopathic urticaria. J Allergy Clin Immunol 2004; 114:619–625.
207. Erbagci Z. The leukotriene receptor antagonist montelukast in the treatment of chronic idiopathic urticaria: a single-blind, placebo-controlled, crossover clinical study. J Allergy Clin Immunol 2002; 110:484–488.
208. Pacor ML, Di Lorenzo G, Corrocher R. Efficacy of leukotriene receptor antagonist in chronic urticaria. A double-blind, placebo-controlled comparison of treatment with montelukast and cetirizine in patients with chronic urticaria with intolerance to food additive and/or acetylsalicylic acid. Clin Exp Allergy 2001; 31:1607–1614.
209. Kim DC, Hsu FI, Barrett NA, et al. Cysteinyl leukotrienes regulate Th2 cell-dependent pulmonary inflammation. J Immunol 2006; 176:4440–4448.
210. Henderson WR Jr, Tang LO, Chu SJ, et al. A role for cysteinyl leukotrienes in airway remodeling in a mouse asthma model. Am J Respir Crit Care Med 2002; 165:108–116.
211. Machida I, Matsuse H, Kondo Y, et al. Cysteinyl leukotrienes regulate dendritic cell functions in a murine model of asthma. J Immunol 2004; 172:1833–1838.

Isoprostanes

212. Fam SS, Morrow JD. The isoprostanes: unique products of arachidonic acid oxidation – a review. Curr Med Chem 2003; 10:1723–1740.
213. Fukunaga M, Takahashi K, Badr KF. Vascular smooth muscle actions and receptor interactions of 8-iso-prostaglandin E2, an E2-isoprostane. Biochem Biophys Res Commun 1993; 195: 507–515.
214. Hoffman SW, Moore S, Ellis EF. Isoprostanes: free radical-generated prostaglandins with constrictor effects on cerebral arterioles. Stroke 1997; 28:844–849.
215. Kang KH, Morrow JD, Roberts LJ, et al. Airway and vascular effects of 8-epi-prostaglandin F2 alpha in isolated perfused rat lung. J Appl Physiol 1993; 74:460–465.
216. Lahaie I, Hardy P, Hou X, et al. A novel mechanism for vasoconstrictor action of 8-isoprostaglandin F2 alpha on retinal vessels. Am J Physiol 1998; 274:R1406–R1416.
217. Marley R, Harry D, Anand R, et al. 8-Isoprostaglandin F2 alpha, a product of lipid peroxidation, increases portal pressure in normal and cirrhotic rats. Gastroenterology 1997; 112:208–213.
218. Mobert J, Becker BF, Zahler S, et al. Hemodynamic effects of isoprostanes (8-iso-prostaglandin F2alpha and E2) in isolated guinea pig hearts. J Cardiovasc Pharmacol 1997; 29:789–794.
219. Sinzinger H, Oguogho A, Kaliman J. Isoprostane 8-epi-prostaglandin F2 alpha is a potent contractor of human peripheral lymphatics. Lymphology 1997; 30:155–159.
220. Takahashi K, Nammour TM, Fukunaga M, et al. Glomerular actions of a free radical-generated novel prostaglandin, 8-epi-prostaglandin F2 alpha, in the rat. Evidence for interaction with thromboxane A2 receptors. J Clin Invest 1992; 90:136–141.
221. Fukunaga M, Makita N, Roberts LJ, et al. Evidence for the existence of F2-isoprostane receptors on rat vascular smooth muscle cells. Am J Physiol 1993; 264:C1619–C1624.
222. Fukunaga M, Yura T, Badr KF. Stimulatory effect of 8-Epi-PGF2 alpha, an F2-isoprostane, on endothelin-1 release. J Cardiovasc Pharmacol 1995; 26(Suppl 3):S51–S52.
223. Cranshaw JH, Evans TW, Mitchell JA. Characterization of the effects of isoprostanes on platelet aggregation in human whole blood. Br J Pharmacol 2001; 132:1699–1706.
224. Csiszar A, Stef G, Pacher P, et al. Oxidative stress-induced isoprostane formation may contribute to aspirin resistance in platelets. Prostaglandins Leukot Essent Fatty Acids 2002; 66:557–558.
225. Tintut Y, Parhami F, Tsingotjidou A, et al. 8-Isoprostaglandin E2 enhances receptor-activated NFkappa B ligand (RANKL)-dependent osteoclastic potential of marrow hematopoietic precursors via the cAMP pathway. J Biol Chem 2002; 277:14221–14226.
226. Zanconato S, Carraro S, Corradi M, et al. Leukotrienes and 8-isoprostane in exhaled breath condensate of children with stable and unstable asthma. J Allergy Clin Immunol 2004; 113:257–263.
227. Shahid SK, Kharitonov SA, Wilson NM, et al. Exhaled 8-isoprostane in childhood asthma. Respir Res 2005; 6:79.
228. Baraldi E, Ghiro L, Piovan V, et al. Increased exhaled 8-isoprostane in childhood asthma. Chest 2003; 124:25–31.
229. Baraldi E, Carraro S, Alinovi R, et al. Cysteinyl leukotrienes and 8-isoprostane in exhaled breath condensate of children with asthma exacerbations. Thorax 2003; 58:505–509.
230. Battaglia S, den Hertog H, Timmers MC, et al. Small airways function and molecular markers in exhaled air in mild asthma. Thorax 2005; 60:639–644.
231. Antczak A, Montuschi P, Kharitonov S, et al. Increased exhaled cysteinyl-leukotrienes and 8-isoprostane in aspirin-induced asthma. Am J Respir Crit Care Med 2002; 166:301–306.
232. Wood LG, Garg ML, Simpson JL, et al. Induced sputum 8-isoprostane concentrations in inflammatory airway diseases. Am J Respir Crit Care Med 2005; 171:426–430.
233. Dworski R, Roberts LJ, Murray JJ, et al. Assessment of oxidant stress in allergic asthma by measurement of the major urinary metabolite of F2-isoprostane, 15-F2t-IsoP (8-iso-PGF2alpha). Clin Exp Allergy 2001; 31:387–390.
234. Talati M, Meyrick B, Peebles RS Jr, et al. Oxidant stress modulates murine allergic airway responses. Free Radic Biol Med 2006; 40:1210–1219.

Sphingosine-1-phosphate

235. Beaven MA. Division of labor: specialization of sphingosine kinases in mast cells. Immunity 2007; 26:271–273.
236. Olivera A, Mizugishi K, Tikhonova A, et al. The sphingosine kinase-sphingosine-1-phosphate axis is a determinant of mast cell function and anaphylaxis. Immunity 2007; 26:287–297.
237. Goetzl EJ, Rosen H. Regulation of immunity by lysosphingolipids and their G protein-coupled receptors. J Clin Invest 2004; 114:1531–1537.
238. Jolly PS, Bektas M, Olivera A, et al. Transactivation of sphingosine-1-phosphate receptors by FcepsilonRI triggering is required for normal mast cell degranulation and chemotaxis. J Exp Med 2004; 199:959–970.
239. Ammit AJ, Hastie AT, Edsall LC, et al. Sphingosine 1-phosphate modulates human airway smooth muscle cell functions that promote inflammation and airway remodeling in asthma. FASEB J 2001; 15:1212–1214.
240. Sawicka E, Zuany-Amorim C, Manlius C, et al. Inhibition of Th1- and Th2-mediated airway inflammation by the sphingosine 1-phosphate receptor agonist FTY720. J Immunol 2003; 171:6206–6214.
241. Idzko M, Laut M, Panther E, et al. Lysophosphatidic acid induces chemotaxis, oxygen radical production, CD11b up-regulation, Ca2+ mobilization, and actin reorganization in human eosinophils via pertussis toxin-sensitive G proteins. J Immunol 2004; 172:4480–4485.
242. Payne SG, Oskeritzian CA, Griffiths R, et al. The immunosuppressant drug FTY720 inhibits cytosolic phospholipase A2 independently of sphingosine-1-phosphate receptors. Blood 2007; 109:1077–1085.

Neuronal Control of Airway Function in Allergy

13

Bradley J Undem and Brendan J Canning

CONTENTS

SUMMARY OF IMPORTANT CONCEPTS

>> Symptoms of allergic airway disease such as sneezing, rhinorrhea, unproductive coughing, episodic bronchospasm, and sensations of breathlessness are in part or entirely neuronally mediated

>> The vagus nerves supply the lower respiratory tract with the vast majority of its afferent (sensory) innervation, and all of its preganglionic parasympathetic innervation. The innervation from spinal afferent nerves or from sympathetic nerves is relatively sparse by comparison

>> The afferent nerves provide the communication pathway between the lungs and central nervous system. Their activity initiates protective and autonomic reflexes, provides some control over the rate and depth of breathing, and can cause or contribute to urge-to-cough sensations and to sensations of dyspnea

>> The parasympathetic branch of the autonomic nervous system controls airway smooth muscle tone via cholinergic contractile innervation and via noncholinergic relaxant innervation. The autonomic nervous system also regulates glandular secretion and blood flow through the bronchial and pulmonary vasculature

>> Allergic inflammation can modulate airway innervation by stimulating or influencing the excitability of primary afferent terminals, by altering gene expression in sensory ganglion neurons, by increasing synaptic transmission within the CNS and within autonomic ganglia, and by increasing transmitter secretion at the level of the nerve-effector junction

■ INTRODUCTION ■

Both the immune system and nervous system are critical to host defense. With respect to the airways, the immune system uses cellular and humoral mechanisms to protect the peripheral air spaces from invasion and colonization by microorganisms. The nervous system protects the airways by orchestrating reflexes such as sneezing, coughing, mucus secretion, and bronchospasm. The difference in mechanisms of defense means that these two systems act in a complementary, non-redundant manner. The two systems (in addition to the endocrine system), however, can also be viewed as integrated systems. Immune tissues are directly innervated by the autonomic nervous system, providing the pathways by which the brain can influence immune function. Stimulation of nerves can also indirectly augment immune function by stimulating inflammation in so-called neurogenic inflammatory reactions. On the other hand, mediators released during immune reactions can act on the nervous system to modulate its activity. These nerve-immune interactions can be beneficial to the host. For example, in experimental animals, chemical denervation of airway C-fiber sensory nerves has been found to decrease substantially the host's ability to clear *Mycoplasma* infection of the airways.[1] Deleterious nerve-immune interactions can also occur in allergy when the immune response is inappropriate. In this case, the immune response triggered by allergen exposure can recruit the nervous system in a way that is not beneficial to the host but rather causes or exacerbates the symptoms of allergic disease: irritation, pruritus, sneezing, coughing, hypersecretion, reversible bronchospasm, and dyspnea.

This chapter provides an overview of the neurophysiology of the lower airway wall, followed by a review of the literature on the mechanisms by which this neurophysiology is altered during allergic reactions. Although this discussion focuses on the airways, the fundamental principles are likely to extend to any organ in which allergic reactions take place.

LOWER AIRWAY INNERVATION

EXTRINSIC INNERVATION

Vagus nerves

The airways and lungs are innervated bilaterally by the vagus nerves (cranial nerve X). The vagi are mixed nerves, with the majority of vagal fibers being afferent (or sensory) in nature.[2] Vagal afferent nerve fibers have their cell bodies in one of two ganglia: the jugular (superior vagal) or nodose (inferior vagal) ganglia.[3,4] These ganglia are of distinct embryonic origin, which has important influence over the physiologic properties of the nerves they project to the viscera.[5,6] The remaining vagal nerves are preganglionic parasympathetic nerves innervating parasympathetic ganglia and motor nerve fibers innervating the striated muscle of the larynx, upper airways, and esophagus. Vagal afferent nerve fibers terminate in integrative centers in the brainstem, primarily the nucleus tractus solitarius (nTS). The parasympathetic nerves and the vagal motor nerve fibers arise from discrete brainstem nuclei, including the dorsal motor nucleus of the vagus nerve (dmnX) and the nucleus ambiguus (nA). Although these brainstem structures have viscerotopic organization, considerable overlap among the sites of afferent nerve subtype termination and of efferent projection is apparent. This overlap contributes in part to the nonselective clustering of autonomic reflexes (e.g., effects on heart rate, respiratory pattern, and airway caliber) initiated by selective activation of specific afferent nerve subtypes.[7,8]

Spinal nerves

The majority of postganglionic sympathetic nerves projecting to the airways arise bilaterally from the superior cervical ganglia and the stellate ganglia.[3] Spinal afferent nerves also project to the airways. Studies in animals suggest that spinal afferent nerves regulate airway sympathetic reflexes and perhaps respiratory pattern.[9,10]

The superior laryngeal nerves, recurrent laryngeal nerves, and the bronchial branches of the vagus nerves carry the vagal and spinal nerve fibers projecting to the airways. Both afferent and efferent vagal nerves project bilaterally, although ipsilateral innervation is much more extensive. No evidence shows contralateral projections of postganglionic sympathetic nerves.

INTRINSIC INNERVATION

Afferent and efferent nerve fibers occupy multiple nerve plexuses in the airway wall from the larynx to the terminal bronchioles.[11–13] Afferent nerve fibers are found just beneath and between epithelial cells in an epithelial nerve plexus. The epithelial plexus is composed primarily of afferent nerve endings, but efferent innervation of the epithelium has been described.[14] Both afferent and efferent nerves are found in the plexus of the lamina propria, where most effectors of the airways (airway smooth muscle, mucus glands, arterioles) are located (Fig. 13.1).[15] Airway parasympathetic ganglia occupy a serosal nerve plexus of the extrapulmonary airways, a plexus that merges with the lamina propria plexus in the intrapulmonary airways.[12,13,16–18] Occasionally, ganglia may also be found elsewhere in the airway wall. Parasympathetic ganglia containing as few as one neuron to more than 100 neurons are randomly and sparsely dispersed in the serosal nerve plexus and are associated primarily with the

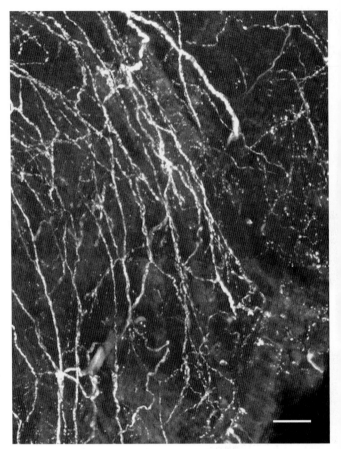

Fig. 13.1. Fluorescence photomicrograph of confocal microscope image stacks showing dense neural network in biopsy specimen from asthmatic airway. (Nerves stained with protein gene product 9.5; ×calibration bar: 50 μm.) Reproduced from Goldie RG, Fernandes L, Rigby P. Airway nerves–detection and visualisation. Current Opinion in Pharmacology 2002; 2:273. Copyright, Elsevier.

extrapulmonary airways. Ganglia associated with the intrapulmonary airways are typically localized to branch points in the bronchial tree. No ganglia are found in or adjacent to the bronchioles.

Except for afferent nerve endings terminating in neuroepithelial bodies of the epithelium,[19] most airway afferent nerves do not assume structures characteristic of muscle spindle sensory nerves, or touch-sensitive sensory nerves of the somatic system or of special sensory nerve terminals (visual, aural, gustatory, smell). Rather, airway afferent nerves form apparently nonspecialized (based on appearance) receptive fields in the epithelium and in and around various structures of the airway wall. Swellings associated with airway afferent nerve terminals in the epithelium contain synaptic vesicles with neurotransmitters that may be released during axonal reflexes. Afferent nerve fibers may also innervate other effector tissues in the airway wall, including glands,[20,21] airway smooth muscle,[3] blood vessels,[22] and airway parasympathetic ganglia.[23,24]

Postganglionic autonomic nerves innervate structures throughout the airway wall, including glands,[25] blood vessels,[22] airway smooth muscle,[26] and perhaps adjacent airway parasympathetic ganglia.[17,27] Morphologic analyses reveal little change in nerve fiber densities in the smooth muscle from the large bronchi to the bronchioles.[16,26,28] The neurochemistry of these nerve fibers, however, may differ considerably in the large and small airways.

Airway parasympathetic ganglia

Postganglionic parasympathetic nerve terminals are found throughout the airways. Parasympathetic ganglia, however, are few in number and contain only a handful of neurons. Airway parasympathetic tone is thus determined by the actions of relatively few ganglia neurons in fewer still ganglia.[17]

Airway ganglia neurons are not simply relays between the central nervous system (CNS) and the effector tissues of the airway wall. Rather, airway ganglia neurons subserve an important integrative role (Fig. 13.2). This function is facilitated by the complex morphology of the ganglia neurons and by the many biophysical properties of the neurons that facilitates integration of synaptic input.[17,18,29,30]

Synaptic transmission between preganglionic and postganglionic parasympathetic nerves in the bronchi is mediated primarily, if not exclusively, by acetylcholine acting on nicotinic receptors.[18,31] When activated, nicotinic receptors on the airway ganglia neuronal dendrite initiate depolarizations known as fast excitatory postsynaptic potentials (fEPSPs). In the airway ganglia, most fEPSPs are subthreshold for action potential formation. Summation of several fEPSPs may be necessary to reach threshold for action potential generation (Fig. 13.2). The filtering capacity of airway ganglia neurons can be modulated by a number of mechanisms, either through modulatory effects of noncholinergic neurotransmitters or through alterations in the excitability of the ganglia neurons.

Airway ganglia neurons are innervated by preganglionic nerve fibers carried by the vagus nerves. Neurons are often innervated by several convergent preganglionic fibers, which in turn may diverge extensively in the airways and innervate multiple airway ganglia. This divergence may facilitate coordination of airway reflexes.[17] Airway ganglia neurons may also innervate adjacent ganglia neurons.[27] Collaterals of afferent nerves containing neuropeptides are also found in airway ganglia and can regulate synaptic transmission in the ganglia through peripheral reflexes.[32–35]

REFLEX REGULATION OF AIRWAYS

Afferent nerve subtypes

Multiple afferent nerve subtypes innervate the airways. These nerve subtypes can be subclassified based on their neurochemistry, responsiveness to physical and chemical stimuli, myelination, conduction velocity, sites of termination in the CNS, and ganglionic origin.[2,36,37] Airway low-threshold mechanoreceptors have at least two subtypes: rapidly adapting receptors (RARs) respond to the dynamic physical effects of lung inflation and slowly adapting receptors (SARs) respond to the sustained physical effects of lung inflation. Some airway mechanoreceptors can also be activated indirectly by bronchoconstrictors, such as histamine, acetylcholine, and leukotrienes.[38,39] When activated, airway mechanoreceptors may initiate alterations in autonomic nerve activity and cough and may play an integral role in controlling respiratory rate and tidal volume.[2,36,37] Not surprisingly, therefore, many airway mechanoreceptors are active during the respiratory cycle (Fig. 13.3).[40] This continuous activity of airway mechanoreceptors may be of fundamental importance

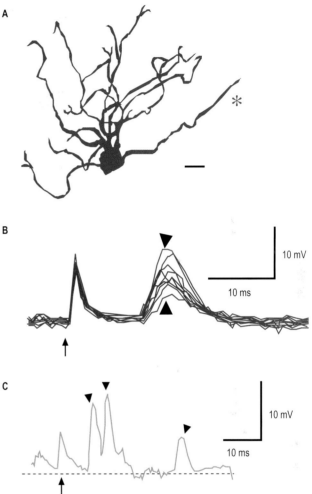

Fig. 13.2. (A) Drawing of single neuron injected with Neurobiotin and processed for peroxidase histochemistry; asterisk (*) indicates axon (calibration bar: 20 μm). (B) Fast excitatory postsynaptic potentials (fEPSPs) in human bronchial ganglia. Overlay of traces shows responses by human bronchial ganglia neuron to 10 consecutive peribronchial nerve stimulations (shock artifact at vertical arrow; stimulus = 1.0 ms, 20 V, 0.5 Hz). fEPSPs are subthreshold for action potential generation and graded in amplitude (arrowheads). (C) Single stimulus (shock artifact at vertical arrow) to preganglionic nerve trunk elicits three temporally distinct fEPSPs (arrowheads), indicating convergence of preganglionic axons. Reproduced from Kajekar R, Rohde HK, Myers AC. American Journal of Respiratory and Critical Care Medicine. 2001; 164:1927. Official Journal of the American Thoracic Society. Copyright, American Thoracic Society.

to the maintenance of baseline autonomic tone, respiratory pattern, and possibly, how subsequently evoked reflexes proceed.[41]

Afferent nerves that are similar to the nociceptors of the somatic nervous system also innervate the airways. These nociceptors, most of which are unmyelinated C fibers, are generally unresponsive to mechanical stimuli and are thus essentially quiescent during tidal breathing[42] (Fig. 13.3). These nociceptors, however, are activated by inflammatory mediators such as bradykinin, adenosine, and 5-hydroxytryptamine

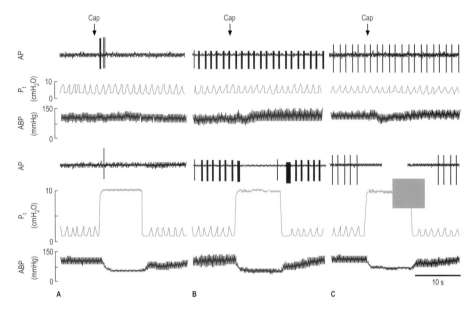

Fig. 13.3. Representative experimental records illustrating three basic phenotypes of afferent nerves in the lungs through the action potential (AP) discharge in response to capsaicin (Cap) injection, tidal breathing, and hyperinflation of rat lungs. (A) Pulmonary C fiber arising from an ending in right upper lobe of anesthetized, open-chest rat (conduction velocity of fiber = 1.05 m/s). Note that C fiber responds to capsaicin, but not to mechanical effects of tidal breathing (top) or even hyperinflation (bottom). (B) Fiber with rapidly adapting receptor (RAR) located in right upper lobe (conduction velocity = 21.4 m/s). Note that RAR does not respond to capsaicin, but does respond with AP discharge during tidal breathing. The fiber adapts to the mechanical stimulus of prolonged hyperinflation. (C) Slowly adapting receptor (SAR) located in right lower lobe (conduction velocity = 23.5 m/s). Note that SAR does not respond to capsaicin, but does respond during tidal breathing and in a non-adapting manner to prolonged hyperinflation. Upper panels, Capsaicin (1 g/kg in 0.2 ml solution) was first slowly injected into the catheter (dead space 0.3 ml) and then flushed into the right atrium (arrow) as a bolus with saline (0.4 ml). Lower panels, Hyperinflation was generated by maintaining a constant tracheal pressure (P_t) at 30 cmH$_2$O for 10 s while the respirator was turned off. ABP, arterial blood pressure. Reproduced from Ho CY, GU Q, Lin YS et al. Respir Physiol 2001; 127:113, with permission. Copyright, Elsevier.

(5-HT, serotonin) and may also be activated by low pH, hypertonic saline, or the vanilloid capsaicin.[2,5,6,43–45] Capsaicin activates airway nociceptors by opening the ion channel and receptor TRPV1 (transient receptor potential vanilloid 1).[46] TRPV1 may play an important role in regulating signaling by nociceptors. Endogenous ligands for TRPV1 include 12-lipoxygenase (12-LO) and 15-LO products and the endogenous cannabinoid anandamide.[47,48] When activated, airway nociceptors initiate alterations in autonomic nerve activity and cough and have unique effects on respiratory pattern.

Autonomic nerve subtypes

Both sympathetic and parasympathetic nerves innervate the airways. Sympathetic nerves primarily innervate the bronchial vasculature, whereas airway parasympathetic nerves innervate the vasculature but also the glands and airway smooth muscle.[49,50]

For almost a century, autonomic control of the airways was viewed as a balance between the opposing actions of the sympathetic and parasympathetic nerves. It was further assumed that the actions of the parasympathetic nervous system were mediated by acetylcholine, whereas the sympathetic nerves used norepinephrine to regulate airway function. Despite the accuracy of some aspects of this model and its great predictive value, it has become apparent that autonomic control is much more complex than being described simply as the opposing actions of acetylcholine and norepinephrine. Multiple neurotransmitters have been localized to

the autonomic nerves innervating the airways. These neurotransmitters have multiple effects on the end organs in the airways, and their role as true neurotransmitters and neuromodulators has been confirmed.[49,50]

Autonomic regulation of airway smooth muscle tone

Postganglionic parasympathetic nerves innervate airway smooth muscle from the trachea to the terminal bronchioles. When activated, airway parasympathetic cholinergic nerves initiate marked contractions of airway smooth muscle throughout the airway tree. Sympathetic innervation of human airway smooth muscle is either sparse or nonexistent. A comparable paucity of sympathetic innervation of the intrapulmonary airways in other species has been noted. Indeed, even though human airway smooth muscle expresses abundant beta adrenoceptors (primarily β_2-adrenoceptors), direct functional evidence of sympathetic (adrenergic) innervation of human airway smooth muscle is lacking. It seems likely, therefore, that hormonal catecholamines are the primary ligand for the β-adrenoceptors expressed on human airway smooth muscle.[9,50]

The only functional relaxant innervation of airway smooth muscle in many species, including humans, is provided by the parasympathetic nervous system. Parasympathetic nerve-mediated relaxation of airway smooth muscle may be mediated by vasoactive intestinal peptide (VIP), pituitary adenylate cyclase-activating peptide (PACAP), and polypeptide with histidine at N-terminal and methionine at C-terminal

(PHM, human form of PHI, with isoleucine at C-terminal), as well as the gaseous transmitter nitric oxide (NO, synthesized from arginine by neuronal NO synthase). These nonadrenergic, noncholinergic (NANC) relaxant responses can be evoked in airways from the trachea to the small bronchi.[50,51]

It was long assumed that the neurotransmitters mediating NANC relaxation of airway smooth muscle were co-released with acetylcholine from a single population of postganglionic parasympathetic nerves. It was further hypothesized that the function of these neurotransmitters was to serve as a break on the parasympathetic nerves, preventing excessive constriction during periods of elevated parasympathetic nerve activity. Studies in guinea pigs, however, reveal that at least in this species, noncholinergic parasympathetic neurotransmitters are not necessarily co-released with acetylcholine from postganglionic parasympathetic nerves. Rather, data support the hypothesis that an entirely distinct parasympathetic pathway regulates noncholinergic nerve activity in the airways.[52,53] Preganglionic nerve subtypes and reflexes also differentially regulate these distinct parasympathetic pathways.[52,54-56] Morphologic and physiologic studies in ferrets and guinea pigs indicate that the parasympathetic ganglia mediating cholinergic and noncholinergic responses in the airways are also distinct.[13,52,57,58] Distinct parasympathetic pathways also likely regulate cholinergic and noncholinergic responses in cats.[54,55] Separate cholinergic and noncholinergic parasympathetic ganglion neurons have also been identified in human airways.[16,50]

Many stimuli initiate reflex alterations in airway parasympathetic nerve activity.[50] The homeostatic role of these alterations is not readily apparent, but these may serve to optimize the efficiency of gas exchange and may facilitate clearance mechanisms during cough by regulating airflow velocity. Bronchoconstrictors such as histamine, prostaglandin D_2 (PGD_2), leukotrienes, and even methacholine, for example, initiate both cough and reflex bronchospasm.[56,59,60] Nociceptor stimulants such as capsaicin, bradykinin, hypertonic saline, and acidic solutions also initiate reflex bronchospasm.[48,56,59-61] Other stimuli initiating reflex bronchospasm include chemoreceptor stimulation, esophageal afferent nerve stimulation, and upper airway afferent nerve stimulation.[48,52,56]

Stimuli initiating reflex bronchodilation include stimulants that activate airway mechanoreceptors and airway nociceptors.[50,54,56,60-62] By contrast, chemoreceptor stimulation is without apparent effect on noncholinergic parasympathetic nerve activity.[54,56] Activation of skeletal muscle afferent nerves, as might occur during exercise, also initiates reflex bronchodilation, primarily through withdrawal of baseline cholinergic tone.[63,64]

Direct evidence for airway sympathetic reflexes following spinal or vagal afferent nerve activation has been reported in studies using guinea pigs.[9] Adrenoceptors and thus the endogenous catecholamines play an important role in regulating human airway caliber and responsiveness. Circulating catecholamines are likely more important in regulating human airway function than the sparse sympathetic adrenergic innervation of the human airways.[50]

Autonomic regulation of glands

Airway glands are regulated primarily by the parasympathetic nervous system. Acetylcholine (ACh) is the primary neurotransmitter regulating airway glandular secretion, but other peptide neurotransmitters may also play a role in mucus secretion. Sympathetic nerves play little or no role in mucus secretion. Neurotransmitters associated with sympathetic nerves have subtle if any effect on secretion but may play a role in regulating parasympathetic nerve activity.[25,65]

Reflexes initiating parasympathetic nerve-dependent mucus secretion are induced by many of the same stimuli that initiate reflex bronchospasm. Therefore, the postganglionic parasympathetic nerve-regulating mucus secretion and smooth muscle tone in the airways may be derived from the same subpopulations of airway parasympathetic nerves. Evidence suggests, however, that the neurochemistry of the postganglionic parasympathetic nerves innervating glands may differ from those innervating airway smooth muscle. The trophic influence of these end organs on the phenotype of the autonomic nerves has not been studied.

Autonomic regulation of bronchial vasculature

Sympathetic and parasympathetic nerves regulate bronchial vascular tone.[22,66-68] Sympathetic nerves mediate vasoconstriction through the actions of norepinephrine and neuropeptide Y, whereas parasympathetic nerves mediate vasodilatation through the actions of ACh, NO, and perhaps peptides (e.g., VIP). Reflex regulation of bronchial vascular tone is poorly described, in large part due to the difficulty in studying the bronchial vasculature. Airway nociceptor stimulation, however, is known to initiate parasympathetic reflex dilation of the bronchial vasculature.[69]

Axon reflexes

Activation of some sensory nerves, primarily nociceptors, causes the release of proinflammatory transmitters, such as substance P and perhaps adenosine triphosphate (ATP), from their peripheral endings that act on the tissue of innervation, thereby initiating neurogenic inflammation.[70] This peripheral release of neurotransmitters from sensory nerve collaterals and the resulting end-organ effects comprise the axon reflex. Afferent nerves innervating the airway mucosa of most species, including humans, express the anatomic attributes of the sensory nerves mediating axon reflexes in somatic tissues. Many of these afferent nerve endings contain potent proinflammatory peptides such as substance P, neurokinin A, and calcitonin gene-related peptide (CGRP). When administered exogenously, these putative neurotransmitters have profound effects in the airways, initiating bronchospasm, mucus secretion, vasodilation, plasma exudation, and inflammatory cell recruitment.[71] These observations naturally led to the hypothesis that axonal reflexes contribute to the pathogenesis of inflammatory airway disease.

Axon reflexes have been well defined in the airways of rats and guinea pigs, and evidence indicates that axon reflexes may regulate human upper airway responses to bradykinin and capsaicin. The role of axon reflexes in the lower airways is less clear. Morphologic studies of the afferent innervation of the human airway mucosa reveal a dense plexus of afferent nerves innervating the epithelium but a general sparseness of neurokinin-containing nerve fibers.[50,59] Capsaicin evokes contractions of isolated human airway smooth muscle preparations and mucus secretion from airway mucosal explants, but these effects are unlikely to be mediated by neurokinins.[72-74] Bronchospasm initiated by putative C-fiber stimulants in human subjects and in species other than rats or guinea pigs are caused primarily by CNS-dependent parasympathetic reflexes.[75,76]

Cough and dyspnea

Cough plays an essential role in the clearance of inhaled pathogens, aeroallergens, irritants, particulate matter, secretions, and aspirate, and thus protects the airway mucosa from damage. However, cough may also be 'dry' or non-productive.[77] This irritating type of cough is a common symptom of patients with allergic inflammation of the airways. Vagal afferent nerves regulate the cough reflex. In general, stimuli that initiate reflex bronchospasm also initiate cough. The afferent nerves mediating cough are likely both the airway mechanoreceptors, which are activated by inhaled particulate, accumulated mucus, and bronchospasm, and the airway nociceptors, which are activated by irritants such as acid (including aspirate), bradykinin, and capsaicin.[59]

Dyspnea is associated with airways obstruction and other respiratory reflexes and sensations but the relationships are complex. The exact mechanisms underlying the sensation of dyspnea are unclear but likely involve the afferent innervation of the airways and lungs. Much of our understanding of this respiratory sensation comes from clinical studies. In general, more severe asthma (based on basal percentage predicted FEV_1) is associated with a blunted sensation of dyspnea and/or airways obstruction.[78] Allergic inflammation and mediators associated with allergic inflammation may, however, acutely alter the sensations of dyspnea. Doses of histamine and methacholine that are equally effective at inducing airways obstruction produce differing levels of dyspnea, with histamine producing more symptoms than methacholine.[79] Lidocaine inhalation prevents the histamine-induced enhancement of dyspnea produced by resistive loading.[80] These results imply that histamine but not methacholine has a direct effect on airway sensory nerve activity and/or excitability. Consistent with the notion that mediators associated with allergic inflammation can enhance the excitability of the vagal afferent nerves triggering the sensation of dyspnea, prostaglandin E_2 inhalation does not induce dyspnea or airways obstruction in healthy adults, but worsens the sensations of dyspnea associated with exercise.[81] Intravenous adenosine also causes dyspnea but does not induce airways obstruction in nonasthmatics.[82] Inhalation of ATP (and to a lesser extent AMP) induces coughing, dyspnea, and airways obstruction in asthmatics, but neither dyspnea nor airways obstruction in nonasthmatics.[83]

■ AIRWAY NEUROPHYSIOLOGY AND THE ALLERGIC REACTION ■

The symptoms of allergic disease are largely the result of altered neuronal activity. Whether the symptom is pruritus or 'itchy airways' resulting in excessive coughing, eye irritation, gastrointestinal irritation, runny nose, or the rapid and reversible bronchospasm that leads to dyspneic sensations, the nervous system serves as the principal transducer between immunologic aspects of allergic inflammation and the symptomatology of immediate hypersensitivity. This may occur as the result of allergen-induced mediator production and release from resident cells interacting with receptors on sensory and autonomic nerves. Relatively little is known about the specific pharmacology of allergen-immune-nerve interactions, but the mediators likely include histamine, arachidonic acid metabolites, and neurotrophins, as well as chemokines and cytokines.[2,84–86]

As outlined earlier, the peripheral nervous system functions in terms of reflex arcs. Although an increase in airway reflex activity is self-evident to those coughing and sneezing during their allergy season, it is difficult to measure hyperreflexia experimentally in humans. Studies in the human nose have provided a clear-cut example of upregulation in reflex physiology by allergy. In these studies, a sensory nerve irritant (bradykinin) was applied to one nostril of a subject before and during their allergy season. When subjects were not experiencing allergies, bradykinin had very little effect on airway physiology. Applying bradykinin to the nose of the same subjects during their allergy season, however, led to excessive sneezing and reflex secretions (Fig. 13.4).[87] This observation has been repeated in other laboratories and may be observed with other types of sensory nerve stimulants.[88–90] This same type of hyperreflexia can be seen in the lower airways when cough is used as the outcome variable.[91]

Reflexes can be conceptually subdivided into four components (Fig. 13.5). First, a reflex begins with stimulation of afferent or sensory nerves that innervate all tissues in the body. Second, action potentials (APs) travel along the afferent axon until they reach the central terminals, where APs evoke the release of neurotransmitters at the synapse with secondary neurons in the CNS. Synaptic activation of secondary neurons is then transmitted to other centers in the CNS, leading to sensations, respiratory reflexes, or increases or decreases in the activity of

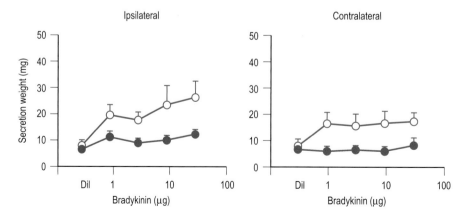

Fig. 13.4. Effect of nasal provocation with bradykinin in nine patients with seasonal allergy challenged in season (open circles) and out of season (closed circles). Left, ipsilateral responses; Right, contralateral responses; Dil, diluent. Significant increase in contralateral secretion weights was seen in subjects challenged in season (p <0.01) but not out of season. Reproduced from Riccio MM, Proud D. Evidence that enhanced nasal reactivity to bradykinin in patients with symptomatic allergy is mediated by neural reflexes. Journal of Allergy and Clinical Immunology. 1996; 97:1252, with permission. Copyright, Elsevier.

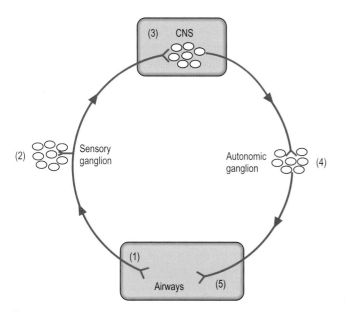

Fig. 13.5. Airway central reflex pathway, showing points along the pathway that may be modulated by allergic inflammation. (1) Mediators released during an allergic reaction may activate primary afferent nerves, leading to action potential (AP) discharge. Alternatively, mediators may increase excitability of afferent nerve endings such that the threshold for other stimuli (e.g., mechanical stimulation) is decreased. (2) Mediators released during the allergic reaction may interact with nerve terminals whereby signals are sent to the cell bodies in the sensory ganglia, leading to changes in gene expression, as when allergen inhalation increases expression of the preprotachykinin gene in vagal sensory ganglia. (3) Allergic inflammation of airways can lead to increases in excitability of secondary neurons in the brainstem, where changes in accommodation have been observed. Changes in amount and type of transmitter released from the central terminals of afferent nerves may also lead to augmented synaptic transmission (central sensitization). (4) Allergic inflammation has been shown to increase synaptic transmission in the bronchial ganglia, thereby decreasing the capacity of the ganglia to act as filters of preganglionic input. This, in theory, would lead to a generalized increase in parasympathetic tone in the airways. (5) Allergic inflammation has been associated with increases in the amount of acetylcholine released per AP, and with decreases in the amount or efficacy of the nonadrenergic, noncholinergic (NANC) parasympathetic transmitters vasoactive intestinal peptide (VIP) and nitric oxide (NO).

preganglionic autonomic fibers. Third, APs in preganglionic fibers reach the terminals of these fibers, where they evoke the release of ACh at the synapse of autonomic ganglion neurons. Fourth, synaptic activation of postganglionic autonomic neurons leads to autonomic transmitter release at effector cells (e.g., smooth muscle, vasculature). The allergic reaction appears particularly adept at influencing reflex physiology in the airways by modifying each of the four steps in the pathway of reflex action.

PRIMARY AFFERENT NERVES IN AIRWAYS

Most, if not all, airway afferent nerves are sensitive to mechanical perturbation. Allergic reactions can lead indirectly to mechanosensitive afferent nerve activation by releasing mediators that cause bronchial smooth muscle contraction. For example, histamine leads to activation of afferent RARs and SARs by a mechanism that can be inhibited by bronchodilators.[37,50] This finding may explain the AP discharge in RARs observed after allergen challenge in rabbit airways.[92] In various experimental models of allergy, allergen provocation can also directly influence the activity of afferent nerve fibers. With respect to nociceptive-like fibers, chemical mediators such as bradykinin are effective in evoking AP discharge and initiating airway reflexes.[75,84,93,94] Mediators released during allergic reactions can also affect the electrical excitability of afferent fibers. In this context, 'excitability' refers to processes that do not overtly lead to AP discharge but rather increase the sensitivity of the nerve fiber to other stimulants. In isolated guinea pig nerve-airway preparations, allergen challenge did not evoke AP discharge in sensory nerves but did cause a fourfold decrease in the amount of mechanical force required to activate the nerve fibers (Fig. 13.6).[95] The specific mediator(s) responsible for this increase in mechanosensitivity has not yet been defined. Mediators associated with allergic reactions can also increase airway afferent nerve responses to mechanical stimulation in vivo.[42,96] The mechanism by which the allergic reaction leads to increases in afferent nerve excitability is unknown but likely involves the interaction of inflammatory mediators with specific ion channels in the nerve membrane.[97–99]

In addition to causing an increase in AP discharge, allergic reactions can also modify neuropeptide release from the peripheral nerve terminals of nociceptive-type afferent nerves. As discussed earlier, neuropeptides may also be released from peripheral terminals as a consequence of axon reflexes resulting in neurogenic inflammation.[11,100] Allergen provocation can augment this process by increasing neuropeptide secretion. In airways isolated from sensitized guinea pigs, antigen challenge leads to a pronounced enhancement of AP-induced neuropeptide release.[101] This effect occurs at very low concentrations of antigen and persists for more than 2 h. Histamine and cysteinyl leukotrienes (cysLTs) are the mediators responsible for these effects.[101–103] In fact, cysLTs are more potent at affecting sensory neuropeptide secretion than contracting airway smooth muscle.[102] Both histamine and cysLTs have been shown to interact directly with sensory nerves by decreasing resting potassium currents leading to membrane depolarizations.[103,104]

Substance P and related sensory neuropeptides are metabolized in the airways by neutral endopeptidase.[105] Allergic inflammation may also increase neurogenic inflammatory reactions by decreasing airway neutral endopeptidase activity.[106]

CENTRAL NERVOUS SYSTEM INTEGRATION

An increase in the activity of primary afferent nerves will result in an increase in the activity of the secondary neurons to which the primary nerves project. Because most vagal afferent nerves project to neurons in the nucleus tractus solitarius (nTS), allergen provocation in visceral tissues will likely lead to an increase in the activity of neurons within the nTS. For example, intestinal anaphylaxis in rats leads to stimulation of numerous neurons in the rat nTS.[107] Investigators studying the mechanism underlying various pain syndromes observe that peripheral inflammation not only leads to synaptic activation of secondary neurons but also can lead to increases in efficacy of synaptic transmission such that neurotransmission is magnified within the spinal cord. This process is referred to as central sensitization.[108] Given the similarities between visceral hyperreflexia and somatosensory hyperalgesia, allergic inflammation may also lead to central sensitization. Evidence shows

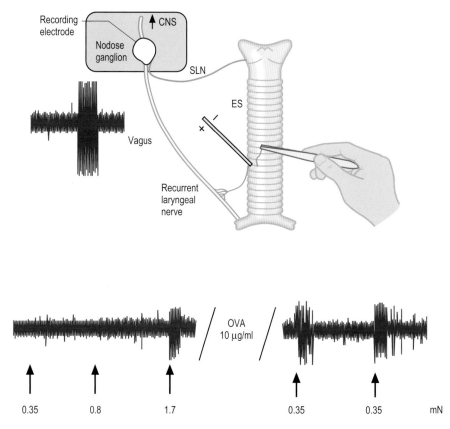

Fig. 13.6. Mechanical sensitivity of an afferent rapidly adapting receptor (RAR)-like fiber in isolated guinea pig trachea before and after allergen challenge. Mechanical sensitivity was determined using von Frey filaments and expressed in millinewtons (mN) before and 15 min after allergen challenge in trachea isolated from actively sensitized guinea pigs. Allergen (OVA, ovalbumin) exposure did not evoke action potential discharge in RAR-like fibers (not shown) but did cause on average a significant fourfold decrease in amount of force required to activate the mechanical receptive field. Reproduced from Riccio MM, Myers AC, Undem BJ. J Physiol 1996; 491:499. Copyright, Blackwell.

synergistic interactions between airway afferent nerves mediating reflex bronchospasm and cough.[48,109] Likewise, in an allergic monkey model, sensitization to and repeated inhalation exposure with house-dust mite allergen led to profound changes in the electrophysiologic properties of secondary neurons in brainstem (nTS neurons).[110] The nTS neurons from control monkeys responded to prolonged suprathreshold current pulses with about 20 APs, whereas nTS neurons isolated from allergen-exposed monkeys responded to the depolarizing current pulse with more than 100 APs (Fig. 13.7). These data support the hypothesis that airway inflammation can alter afferent input into the CNS such that plastic changes occur in the basic electrophysiologic properties of neurons within the nTS.

Because nociceptors and RARs mediate similar reflex effects in the airways, these afferent nerve subtypes might act synergistically to initiate these reflexes. Such synergistic interactions are facilitated by the likely convergence of the central nerve terminals of these afferent nerves in key integrative sites in the brainstem.[6,7] These interactions would be analogous to the processes initiating hyperalgesia and pain sensations in somatic tissues.[108,111] The parallels between hyperalgesia and airway hyperresponsiveness (AHR) seem obvious. Such interactions between afferent nerve subtypes may explain in part how extrapulmonary disorders such as gastroesophageal reflux disease,[112] allergic rhinitis,[113] and upper respiratory tract infections[114] initiate pulmonary symptoms such as cough and reflex bronchospasm and perhaps AHR.

AUTONOMIC GANGLIONIC NEUROTRANSMISSION

By increasing primary afferent nerve activity and increasing synaptic transmission in the CNS, allergic inflammation will likely lead to an increase in activity of autonomic preganglionic nerves. In addition, however, experimental evidence supports the hypothesis that allergic inflammation may also increase autonomic tone, by increasing the efficacy of synaptic transmission within autonomic ganglia. This process of ganglionic sensitization is analogous to the previously discussed central sensitization.[17]

As described above, airway parasympathetic ganglia filter or integrate input from the CNS.[17,18,115] Any process that increases the efficacy of synaptic transmission, resulting in increases in EPSP amplitude, will result in a decrease in filtering and a generalized increase in airway parasympathetic tone.[116] Allergen challenge to bronchi isolated from actively

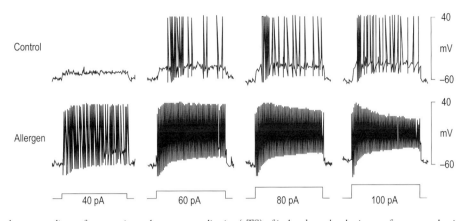

Fig. 13.7. Current-clamp recordings of neurons in nucleus tractus solitarius (nTS) of isolated monkey brainstem from control animals and animals chronically exposed to inhalation of house-dust mite allergen. Membrane potential is recorded in response to 500-ms injections of increasing amounts of current (40–100 pA). Note that neurons in nTS of the allergen-exposed animal responded to the current injection with many more action potentials than observed in control monkeys. In other words, chronic inhalation of allergen led to increased excitability of neurons in the central nervous system. Reproduced from Chen CY, Bonham AC, Schelegle ES, et al. Extended allergen exposure in asthmatic monkeys induces neuroplasticity in nucleus tractus solitarius. J All Clin Immunol 2001; 108:557 with permission. Copyright, Elsevier.

sensitized guinea pigs increases the excitability of bronchial ganglion neurons.[117] This response occurs through several mechanisms and may involve many different mediators. Histamine released from mast cells in or near the ganglia results in decreases in potassium conductance and a membrane depolarization, whereas PGD_2 challenge inhibits accommodation of airway ganglia neurons such that the same stimulus results in many more APs.[117,118] In unpublished experiments, we have also noted that when mast cell-activating anti-immunoglobulin E (IgE) is added to human bronchial preparations, the membrane potentials of bronchial parasympathetic ganglion neurons depolarize in a manner similar to that observed in guinea pigs.

No studies have systematically compared the effect of allergen challenge on synaptic efficacy in the cholinergic versus noncholinergic parasympathetic ganglia. However, work in the sympathetic system suggests that regardless of the nature of the autonomic ganglia, mediators associated with allergen challenge will lead to an increase in synaptic efficacy and a generalized increase in autonomic tone. For example, exposing the superior cervical, mesenteric, or myenteric ganglia to a sensitizing antigen results in ganglionic mast cell activation and a pronounced increase in synaptic neurotransmission.[119–121] Autonomic synaptic efficacy is affected by very low concentrations of antigen. The antigen-induced effect is persistent; a brief (5-min) antigen challenge of an isolated superior cervical ganglion potentiates synaptic transmission for longer than 3 h (as long as the experiment lasted). This process has been termed antigen-induced long-term potentiation.[122]

POSTGANGLIONIC NEUROEFFECTOR TRANSMISSION

The final place in an autonomic reflex loop that can be modulated is at the postganglionic neuroeffector junction. This junction is the site where APs arising from the ganglionic synapse invade the postganglionic varicosities, causing neurotransmitter release, which then affects the effector cells. In the airways, allergen challenge is associated with an elevation in the amount of ACh released from the airway postganglionic nerve

varicosities.[123,124] Several mediators have been found to interact with postganglionic nerve fibers to enhance transmitter release.[49] In addition to conventional autacoid effects, allergen-induced eosinophilic inflammation may augment ACh release by inhibiting the function of cholinergic muscarinic M_2 receptors.[123–125] The prejunctional M_2 receptors serve as negative-feedback 'autoreceptors', such that when the released ACh acts on these receptors, signals are produced that lead to an inhibition of further ACh release.[126] Allergen challenge inhibits this process, apparently through an inhibitory effect of eosinophil-derived major basic protein (MBP) on M_2 receptor function.[127]

Few studies have examined the effect of allergen challenge on the release of noncholinergic transmitters from postganglionic parasympathetic nerve endings. Allergen challenge has been shown to attenuate subsequently evoked noncholinergic relaxant responses in animals.[128,129] The mechanism for this effect of allergen challenge is unclear.[50] Elevated levels of superoxide, perhaps derived from infiltrating eosinophils, may attenuate relaxant responses mediated by neuronal NO.[129,130] Alternatively, mast cell tryptase or other peptidases may attenuate relaxant responses mediated by VIP and other relaxant neuropeptides.[106] The bronchoprotective effects of deep inspiration have been associated with NO formation, although the NO source is unknown.[131,132] Interestingly, the bronchoprotective effect of endogenous NO may be inhibited in asthmatic patients.[133,134] Some studies indicate that the inflammation associated with asthma may decrease VIP levels in the airways or perhaps NO synthase in the lung.[135,136] More recently, a role for arginase and S-nitrosothiol dehydrogenase in NO metabolism and asthma pathogenesis has been suggested.[137–141] These enzymes may regulate the actions of neuronally derived nitric oxide.

Neurotrophins including nerve growth factor (NGF) brain-derived neurotrophic factor (BDNF) are associated with allergic inflammation and have been implicated in the pathogenesis of allergic asthma.[85] NGF has a variety of effects on airway nerves and non-neural cells, including induction of neuropeptide expression in sensory nerves, facilitation of synaptic transmission in airway parasympathetic ganglia and effects on inflammatory cells and airways responsiveness.[142–145] NGF may also increase nerve-mediated contractions of airway smooth muscle through postganglionic effects on parasympathetic nerves.[146,147] BDNF may mediate the allergen-induced enhancement of field stimulation evoked cholinergic contractions in mice.[148]

Airway nerves may also precipitate altered neuroeffector transmission by directly or indirectly regulating the allergic response. Vagus nerve stimulation and the resulting bronchospasm induces eosinophil recruitment to the airways.[149] This effect is prevented by atropine, suggesting that the effects of nerve stimulation may be indirect and due to the resulting airways obstruction. More recently, however, the chemoattractant eotaxin has been localized to airway nerves.[150,151]

■ CONCLUSIONS ■

Many of the signs and symptoms of patients with allergic disease are the result of inappropriate neural function. Depending on the site of allergen exposure, these manifestations may include cutaneous reactions and excessive itching, gastrointestinal disturbances, sneezing, rhinorrhea, coughing, bronchospasm, and sensations of breathlessness. The molecular mechanisms by which allergen exposure affects the nervous system have not been elucidated in detail. The experimental evidence from human studies and animal models, however, indicates that allergic inflammation may affect reflex physiology at multiple sites (Fig. 13.5). The effects include changes in excitability of primary afferent terminals, changes in gene expression in sensory ganglion neurons, increases in synaptic transmission within the CNS and within autonomic ganglia, and changes in transmitter secretion at the level of the nerve-effector junction. Future research into the mediators and mechanisms of allergen-induced neuromodulation will not only increase our basic understanding of the pathophysiology of allergic disease but also may suggest novel therapeutic strategies.

References

1. Bowden JJ, Baluk P, Lefevre PM, et al. Sensory denervation by neonatal capsaicin treatment exacerbates Mycoplasma pulmonis infection in rat airways. Am J Physiol 1996; 270:L393.

Lower airway innervation

2. Coleridge HM, Coleridge, JC, Schultz HD. Afferent pathways involved in reflex regulation of airway smooth muscle. Pharmcol Ther 1989; 42:1.
3. Kummer W, Fischer A, Kurkowski R, et al. The sensory and sympathetic innervation of guinea-pig lung and trachea as studied by retrograde neuronal tracing and double-labelling immunohistochemistry. Neuroscience 1992; 49:715.
4. Springall DR, Cadieux A, Oliveira H, et al. Retrograde tracing shows that CGRP-immunoreactive nerves of rat trachea and lung originate from vagal and dorsal root ganglia. J Auton Nerv Syst 1987; 20:155.
5. Riccio MM, Kummer W, Biglari B, et al. Interganglionic segregation of distinct vagal afferent fibre phenotypes in guinea-pig airways. J Physiol 1996; 496:521.
6. Undem BJ, Chuaychoo B, Lee MG, et al. Subtypes of vagal afferent C-fibres in guinea-pig lungs. J Physiol 2004; 556:905.
7. Kubin L, Alheid GF, Zuperku EJ, et al. Central pathways of pulmonary and lower airway vagal afferents. J Appl Physiol 2006; 101:618.
8. Haxhiu MA, Kc P, Moore CT, et al. Brain stem excitatory and inhibitory signaling pathways regulating bronchoconstrictive responses. J Appl Physiol 2005; 98:196.
9. Oh EJ, Mazzone SB, Canning BJ, et al. Reflex regulation of airway sympathetic nerves in guinea-pigs. J Physiol 2006; 573:549.
10. Soukhova G, Wang Y, Ahmed M, et al. Bradykinin stimulates respiratory drive by activating pulmonary sympathetic afferents in the rabbit. J Appl Physiol 2003; 95:241.
11. McDonald DM, Mitchell RA, Gabella G, et al. Neurogenic inflammation in the rat trachea. II. Identity and distribution of nerves mediating the increase in vascular permeability. J Neurocytol 1988; 17:605.
12. Yamamoto Y, Ootsuka T, Atoji Y, et al. Morphological and quantitative study of the intrinsic nerve plexuses of the canine trachea as revealed by immunohistochemical staining of protein gene product 9.5. Anat Rec 1998; 250:438.

13. Dey RD, Altemus JB, Rodd A, et al. Neurochemical characterization of intrinsic neurons in ferret tracheal plexus. Am J Respir Cell Mol Biol 1996; 14:207.
14. Dey RD, Satterfield B, Altemus JB. Innervation of tracheal epithelium and smooth muscle by neurons in airway ganglia. Anat Rec 1999; 254:166.
15. Goldie RG, Fernandes L, Rigby P. Airway nerves: detection and visualisation. Curr Opin Pharmacol 2002; 2:273.
16. Fischer A, Hoffmann B. Nitric oxide synthase in neurons and nerve fibers of lower airways and in vagal sensory ganglia of man: correlation with neuropeptides. Am J Respir Crit Care Med 1996; 154:209.
17. Myers AC. Transmission in autonomic ganglia. Respir Physiol 2001; 125:99.
18. Kajekar R, Rohde HK, Myers AC. The integrative membrane properties of human bronchial parasympathetic ganglia neurons. Am J Respir Crit Care Med 2001; 164:1927.
19. Adriaensen D, Brouns I, Pintelon I, et al. Evidence for a role of neuroepithelial bodies as complex airway sensors: comparison with smooth muscle-associated airway receptors. J Appl Physiol 2006; 101:960.
20. Kuo HP, Rohde JA, Tokuyama K, et al. Capsaicin and sensory neuropeptide stimulation of goblet cell secretion in guinea-pig trachea. J Physiol 1990; 431:629.
21. Ramnarine SI, Haddad EB, Khawaja AM, et al. On muscarinic control of neurogenic mucus secretion in ferret trachea. J Physiol 1996; 494:577.
22. Haberberger R, Schemann M, Sann H, et al. Innervation pattern of guinea pig pulmonary vasculature depends on vascular diameter. J Appl Physiol 1997; 82:426.
23. Myers A, Undem B, Kummer W. Anatomical and electrophysiological comparison of the sensory innervation of bronchial and tracheal parasympathetic ganglion neurons. J Auton Nerv Syst 1996; 61:162.
24. Kummer W. Ultrastructure of calcitonin gene-related peptide-immunoreactive nerve fibres in guinea-pig peribronchial ganglia. Regul Pept 1992; 37:135.
25. Rogers DF. Motor control of airway goblet cells and glands. Respir Physiol 2001; 125: 129.
26. Canning BJ, Fischer A. Localization of cholinergic nerves in lower airways of guinea pigs using antisera to choline acetyltransferase. Am J Physiol 272:L731,1997.
27. Zhu W, Dey RD. Projections and pathways of VIP- and nNOS-containing airway neurons in ferret trachea. Am J Respir Cell Mol Biol 2001; 24:38.
28. Ward JK, Barnes PJ, Springall DR, et al. Distribution of human i-NANC bronchodilator and nitric oxide-immunoreactive nerves. Am J Respir Cell Mol Biol 1995; 13:175.
29. Coburn RF, Kalia MP. Morphological features of spiking and nonspiking cells in the paratracheal ganglion of the ferret. J Comp Neurol 1986; 254:341.
30. Myers AC, Undem BJ, Weinreich D. Electrophysiological properties of neurons in guinea pig bronchial parasympathetic ganglia. Am J Physiol 259:L403, 1990.
31. Mitchell RA, Herbert DA, Baker DG, et al. In vivo activity of tracheal parasympathetic ganglion cells innervating tracheal smooth muscle. Brain Res 1987; 437:157.
32. Myers AC, Undem BJ. Electrophysiological effects of tachykinins and capsaicin on guinea-pig bronchial parasympathetic ganglion neurons. J Physiol 1993; 470:665.
33. Canning BJ, Undem BJ. Evidence that antidromically stimulated vagal afferents activate inhibitory neurons innervating guinea pig trachealis. J Physiol 1994; 480:613.
34. Canning BJ, Reynolds SM, Anukwu LU, et al. Endogenous neurokinins facilitate synaptic neurotransmission in guinea pig airway parasympathetic ganglia. Am J Physiol (Regul Integr Comp Physiol) 283:R320, 2002.
35. Myers AC, Goldie RG, Hay DW. A novel role for tachykinin neurokinin-3 receptors in regulation of human bronchial ganglia neurons. Am J Respir Crit Care Med 2005; 171:212.
36. Canning BJ. Anatomy and neurophysiology of the cough reflex: ACCP evidence-based clinical practice guidelines. Chest 129:33S, 2006.
37. Taylor-Clark T, Undem BJ. Transduction mechanisms in airway sensory nerves. J Appl Physiol 2006; 101:950.
38. Bergren DR, Myers DL, Mohrman M. Activity of rapidly-adapting receptors to histamine and antigen challenge before and after sodium cromoglycate. Arch Int Pharmacodyn Ther 1985; 273:88.
39. Dixon M, Jackson DM, Richards IM. The effects of 5-hydroxytryptamine, histamine and acetylcholine on the reactivity of the lung of the anaesthetized dog. J Physiol 1980; 307:85.
40. Ho CY, Gu Q, Lin YS, et al. Sensitivity of vagal afferent endings to chemical irritants in the rat lung. Respir Physiol 2001; 127:113.
41. Kesler BS, Canning BJ. Regulation of baseline cholinergic tone in guinea-pig airway smooth muscle. J Physiol 1999; 518:843.
42. Lee LY, Shuei Lin Y, Gu Q, et al. Functional morphology and physiological properties of bronchopulmonary C-fiber afferents. Anat Rec A Discov Mol Cell Evol Biol 2003; 270:17.
43. Fox AJ, Urban L, Barnes PJ, et al. Effects of capsazepine against capsaicin- and proton-evoked excitation of single airway C-fibres and vagus nerve from the guinea-pig. Neuroscience 1995; 67:741.
44. Kajekar R, Myers AC. Effect of bradykinin on membrane properties of guinea pig bronchial parasympathetic ganglion neurons. Am J Physiol Lung Cell Mol Physiol 278:L485, 2000.
45. Pedersen KE, Meeker SN, Riccio MM, et al. Selective stimulation of jugular ganglion afferent neurons in guinea pig airways by hypertonic saline. J Appl Physiol 1998; 84:499.
46. Caterina MJ, Schumacher MA, Tominaga M, et al. The capsaicin receptor: a heat-activated ion channel in the pain pathway. Nature 1997; 389:816.
47. Hwang SW, Cho H, Kwak J, et al. Direct activation of capsaicin receptors by products of lipoxygenases: endogenous capsaicin-like substances. Proc Natl Acad Sci U S A 2000; 97:6155.
48. Mazzone SB, Canning BJ. Synergistic interactions between airway afferent nerve subtypes mediating reflex bronchospasm in guinea pigs. Am J Physiol (Regul Integr Comp Physiol) 2002; 283: R86.
49. Barnes PJ. Modulation of neurotransmission in airways. Physiol Rev 1992; 72:699.
50. Canning BJ. Reflex regulation of airway smooth muscle tone. J Appl Physiol 2006; 101:971.
51. Ellis JL, Undem BJ. Pharmacology of non-adrenergic, non-cholinergic nerves in airway smooth muscle. Pulm Pharmacol 1994; 7:205.
52. Canning BJ, Undem BJ. Evidence that distinct neural pathways mediate parasympathetic contractions and relaxations of guinea-pig trachealis. J Physiol 1993; 471:25.

53. Canning BJ, Undem BJ, Karakousis PC, et al. Effects of organotypic culture on parasympathetic innervation of guinea pig trachealis. Am J Physiol 271:L698, 1996.
54. Ichinose M, Inoue H, Miura M, et al. Possible sensory receptor of nonadrenergic inhibitory nervous system. J Appl Physiol 1987; 63:923.
55. Lama A, Delpierre S, Jammes Y. The effects of electrical stimulation of myelinated and non-myelinated vagal motor fibres on airway tone in the rabbit and the cat. Respir Physiol 1988; 74:265.
56. Mazzone SB, Canning BJ. Evidence of differential reflex regulation of cholinergic and noncholinergic nerves innervating the airways. Am J Respir Crit Care Med 2002; 165:1076.
57. Moffatt JD, Dumsday B, McLean JR. Non-adrenergic, non-cholinergic neurons innervating the guinea-pig trachea are located in the oesophagus: evidence from retrograde neuronal tracing. Neurosci Lett 1998; 248:37.
58. Fischer A, Canning BJ, Undem BJ, et al. Evidence for an esophageal origin of VIP-IR and NO synthase-IR nerves innervating the guinea pig trachealis: a retrograde neuronal tracing and immunohistochemical analysis. J Comp Neurol 1998; 394:326.
59. Canning BJ, Mori N, Mazzone SB. Vagal afferent nerves regulating the cough reflex. Respir Physiol Neurobiol 2006; 152:223.
60. Canning BJ, Reynolds SM, Mazzone SB. Multiple mechanisms of reflex bronchospasm in guinea pigs. J Appl Physiol 2001; 91:2642.
61. Kesler BS, Mazzone SB, Canning BJ. Nitric oxide dependent modulation of smooth muscle tone by airway parasympathetic nerves. Am J Respir Crit Care Med 2002; 165:481.
62. Inoue H, Ichinose M, Miura M, et al. Sensory receptors and reflex pathways of nonadrenergic inhibitory nervous system in feline airways. Am Rev Respir Dis 1989; 139:1175.
63. McCallister LW, McCoy KW, Connelly JC, et al. Stimulation of groups III and IV phrenic afferents reflexly decreases total lung resistance in dogs. J Appl Physiol 1986; 61:1346.
64. Solomon IC, Motekaitis AM, Wong MK, et al. NMDA receptors in caudal ventrolateral medulla mediate reflex airway dilation arising from the hindlimb. J Appl Physiol 1994; 77:1697.
65. Davis B, Roberts AM, Coleridge HM, et al. Reflex tracheal gland secretion evoked by stimulation of bronchial C-fibers in dogs. J Appl Physiol 1982; 53:985.
66. Zimmerman MP, Pisarri TE. Bronchial vasodilation evoked by increased lower airway osmolarity in dogs. J Appl Physiol 2000; 88:425.
67. Pisarri TE, Giesbrecht GG. Reflex tracheal smooth muscle contraction and bronchial vasodilation evoked by airway cooling in dogs. J Appl Physiol 1997; 82:1566.
68. Widdicombe J. The tracheobronchial vasculature: a possible role in asthma. Microcirculation 1996; 3:129.
69. Pisarri TE, Coleridge JC, Coleridge HM. Capsaicin-induced bronchial vasodilation in dogs: central and peripheral neural mechanisms. J Appl Physiol 1993; 74:259.
70. McDonald DM, Bowden JJ, Baluk P, et al. Neurogenic inflammation: a model for studying efferent actions of sensory nerves. Adv Exp Med Biol 1996; 410:453.
71. Baluk P. Neurogenic inflammation in skin and airways. J Invest Dermatol Symp Proc 1997; 2:76.
72. Baker B, Peatfield AC, Richardson PS. Nervous control of mucin secretion into human bronchi. J Physiol 1985; 365:297.
73. Rogers DF, Barnes PJ. Opioid inhibition of neurally mediated mucus secretion in human bronchi. Lancet 1989; 1:930.
74. Ellis JL, Sham JS, Undem BJ. Tachykinin-independent effects of capsaicin on smooth muscle in human isolated bronchi. Am J Respir Crit Care Med 1997; 155:751.
75. Roberts AM, Kaufman MP, Baker DG, et al. Reflex tracheal contraction induced by stimulation of bronchial C-fibers in dogs. J Appl Physiol 1981; 51:485.
76. Fuller RW, Dixon CM, Barnes PJ. Bronchoconstrictor response to inhaled capsaicin in humans. J Appl Physiol 1985; 58:1080.
77. Irwin RS, Baumann MH, Bolser DC, et al. American College of Chest Physicians (ACCP). Diagnosis and management of cough executive summary: ACCP evidence-based clinical practice guidelines. Chest 129:1S, 2006.
78. Manning HL, Schwartzstein RM. Respiratory sensations in asthma: physiological and clinical implications. J Asthma 2001; 38:447.
79. Tetzlaff K, Leplow B, ten Thoren C, et al. Perception of dyspnea during histamine- and methacholine-induced bronchoconstriction. Respiration 1999; 66:427.
80. Taguchi O, Kikuchi Y, Hida W, et al. Effects of bronchoconstriction and external resistive loading on the sensation of dyspnea. J Appl Physiol 1991; 71:2183.
81. Taguchi O, Kikuchi Y, Hida W, et al. Prostaglandin E2 inhalation increases the sensation of dyspnea during exercise. Am Rev Respir Dis 1992; 145:1346.
82. Burki NK, Dale WJ, Lee LY. Intravenous adenosine and dyspnea in humans. J Appl Physiol 2005; 98:180.
83. Basoglu OK, Pelleg A, Essilfie-Quaye S, et al. Effects of aerosolized adenosine 5'-triphosphate vs adenosine 5'-monophosphate on dyspnea and airway caliber in healthy nonsmokers and patients with asthma. Chest 2005; 128:1905.

Airway neurophysiology and the allergic reaction

84. Undem BJ, Carr MJ. Pharmacology of airway afferent nerve activity. Respir Res 2001; 2:234.
85. Nockher WA, Renz H. Neurotrophins in allergic diseases: from neuronal growth factors to intercellular signaling molecules. J Allergy Clin Immunol 2006; 117:583.
86. Oh SB, Tran PB, Gillard SE, et al. Chemokines and glycoprotein120 produce pain hypersensitivity by directly exciting primary nociceptive neurons. J Neurosci 2001; 21:5027.
87. Riccio MM, Proud D. Evidence that enhanced nasal reactivity to bradykinin in patients with symptomatic allergy is mediated by neural reflexes. J Allergy Clin Immunol 1996; 97:1252.
88. Baraniuk JN, Silver PB, Kaliner MA, et al. Perennial rhinitis subjects have altered vascular, glandular, and neural responses to bradykinin nasal provocation. Int Arch Allergy Immunol 1994; 103:202.
89. Riccio MM, Reynolds CJ, Hay DW, et al. Effects of intranasal administration of endothelin-1 to allergic and nonallergic individuals. Am J Respir Crit Care Med 1995; 152:1757.
90. Sanico AM, Atsuta S, Proud D, et al. Plasma extravasation through neuronal stimulation in human nasal mucosa in the setting of allergic rhinitis. J Appl Physiol 1998; 84:537.
91. Chang AB. Cough, cough receptors, and asthma in children. Pediatr Pulmonol 1999; 28:59.
92. Mills JE, Widdicombe JG. Role of the vagus nerves in anaphylaxis and histamine-induced bronchoconstrictions in guinea-pigs. Br J Pharmacol 1970; 39:724.
93. Fox AJ, Barnes PJ, Urban L, et al. An in vitro study of the properties of single vagal afferents innervating guinea-pig airways. J Physiol 1993; 469:21.
94. Kajekar R, Proud D, Myers AC, et al. Characterization of vagal afferent subtypes stimulated by bradykinin in guinea pig trachea. J Pharmacol Exp Ther 1999; 289:682.
95. Riccio MM, Myers AC, Undem BJ. Immunomodulation of afferent neurons in guinea-pig isolated airway. J Physiol 1996; 491:499.
96. Lee LY, Morton RF. Histamine enhances vagal pulmonary C-fiber responses to capsaicin and lung inflation. Respir Physiol 1993; 93:83.
97. Undem BJ, Hubbard W, Weinreich D. Immunologically induced neuromodulation of guinea pig nodose ganglion neurons. J Auton Nerv Syst 1993; 44:35.
98. Lee LY, Gu Q, Gleich GJ. Effects of human eosinophil granule-derived cationic proteins on C-fiber afferents in the rat lung. J Appl Physiol 2001; 91:1318.
99. Carr MJ, Undem BJ. Ion channels in airway afferent neurons. Respir Physiol 2001; 125:83.
100. McDonald DM. Neurogenic inflammation in the rat trachea. I. Changes in venules, leucocytes and epithelial cells. J Neurocytol 1988; 17:583.
101. Ellis JL, Undem BJ. Antigen-induced enhancement of noncholinergic contractile responses to vagus nerve and electrical field stimulation in guinea pig isolated trachea. J Pharmacol Exp Ther 1992; 262:646.
102. Ellis JL, Undem BJ. Role of peptidoleukotrienes in capsaicin-sensitive sensory fibre-mediated responses in guinea-pig airways. J Physiol 1991; 436:469.
103. McAlexander MA, Myers AC, Undem BJ. Inhibition of 5-lipoxygenase diminishes neurally evoked tachykinergic contraction of guinea pig isolated airway. J Pharmacol Exp Ther 1998; 285:602.
104. Undem BJ, Weinreich D. Electrophysiological properties and chemosensitivity of guinea pig nodose ganglion neurons in vitro. J Auton Nerv Syst 1993; 44:17.
105. Borson DB. Roles of neutral endopeptidase in airways. Am J Physiol 260:L212, 1991.
106. Lilly CM, Kobzik L, Hall AE, et al. Effects of chronic airway inflammation on the activity and enzymatic inactivation of neuropeptides in guinea pig lungs. J Clin Invest 1994; 93:2667.
107. Castex N, Fioramonti J, Fargeas MJ, et al. c-fos Expression in specific rat brain nuclei after intestinal anaphylaxis: involvement of 5-HT3 receptors and vagal afferent fibers. Brain Res 1995; 688:149.
108. Woolf CJ, Salter MN. Neuronal plasticity: increasing the gain in pain. Science 2000; 288:1765.
109. Mazzone SB, Mori N, Canning BJ. Synergistic interactions between airway afferent nerve subtypes regulating the cough reflex in guinea-pigs. J Physiol 2005; 569:559.
110. Chen CY, Bonham AC, Schelegle ES, et al. Extended allergen exposure in asthmatic monkeys induces neuroplasticity in nucleus tractus solitarius. J Allergy Clin Immunol 2001; 108:557.
111. Ma QP, Woolf CJ. Involvement of neurokinin receptors in the induction but not the maintenance of mechanical allodynia in rat flexor motoneurons. J Physiol 1995; 486:769.
112. Theodoropoulos DS, Pecoraro DL, Efstratiadis SE. The association of gastroesophageal reflux disease with asthma and chronic cough in the adult. Am J Respir Med 2002; 1:133.
113. Togias A. Rhinitis and asthma: evidence for respiratory system integration. J Allergy Clin Immunol 2003; 111:1171.
114. Empey DW, Laitinen LA, Jacobs L, et al. Mechanisms of bronchial hyperreactivity in normal subjects after upper respiratory tract infection. Am Rev Respir Dis 1976; 113:131.
115. Myers AC, Undem BJ. Analysis of preganglionic nerve evoked cholinergic contractions of the guinea pig bronchus. J Auton Nerv Syst 1991; 35:175.
116. Undem BJ, Weinreich D. Neuroimmune interactions in the lung. In: Bienenstock J, Goetzl EJ, Blennerhassett MG, eds. Autonomic neuroimmunology. London: Taylor and Francis: 2003; 279.
117. Myers AC, Undem BJ, Weinreich D. Influence of antigen on membrane properties of guinea pig bronchial ganglion neurons. J Appl Physiol 1991; 71:970.
118. Myers AC, Undem BJ. Antigen depolarizes guinea pig bronchial parasympathetic ganglion neurons by activation of histamine H1 receptors. Am J Physiol 1995; 268:L879.
119. Weinreich D, Undem BJ, Taylor G, et al. Antigen-induced long-term potentiation of nicotinic synaptic transmission in the superior cervical ganglion of the guinea pig. J Neurophysiol 1995; 73:2004.
120. Cavalcante de Albuquerque AA, Leal-Cardoso JH, Weinreich D. Antigen-induced synaptic plasticity in sympathetic ganglia from actively and passively sensitized guinea-pigs. J Auton Nerv Syst 1996; 61:139.
121. Frieling T, Palmer JM, Cooke HJ, et al. Neuroimmune communication in the submucous plexus of guinea pig colon after infection with Trichinella spiralis. Gastroenterology 1994; 107:1602.
122. Weinreich D, Undem BJ, Leal-Cardoso JH. Functional effects of mast cell activation in sympathetic ganglia. Ann NY Acad Sci 1992; 664:293.
123. Fryer AD, Wills-Karp M. Dysfunction of M2-muscarinic receptors in pulmonary parasympathetic nerves after antigen challenge. J Appl Physiol 1991; 71:2255.
124. Costello RW, Evans CM, Yost BL, et al. Antigen-induced hyperreactivity to histamine: role of the vagus nerves and eosinophils. Am J Physiol 1999; 276:L709.
125. Ten Berge RE, Krikke M, Teisman AC, et al. Dysfunctional muscarinic M2 auto-receptors in vagally induced bronchoconstriction of conscious guinea pigs after the early allergic reaction. Eur J Pharmacol 1996; 318:131.
126. Blaber LC, Fryer AD, Maclagan J. Neuronal muscarinic receptors attenuate vagally-induced contraction of feline bronchial smooth muscle. Br J Pharmacol 1985; 86:723.
127. Evans CM, Fryer AD, Jacoby DB, et al. Pretreatment with antibody to eosinophil major basic protein prevents hyperresponsiveness by protecting neuronal M2 muscarinic receptors in antigen-challenged guinea pigs. J Clin Invest 1997; 100:2254.
128. Miura M, Ichinose M, Kimura K, et al. Dysfunction of nonadrenergic non-cholinergic inhibitory system after antigen inhalation in actively sensitized cat airways. Am Rev Respir Dis 1992; 145:70.

129. Miura M, Yamauchi H, Ichinose M, et al. Impairment of neural nitric oxide-mediated relaxation after antigen exposure in guinea pig airways in vitro. Am J Respir Crit Care Med 1997; 156:217.
130. Ricciardolo FL, Timmers MC, Geppetti P, et al. Allergen-induced impairment of broncho-protective nitric oxide synthesis in asthma. J Allergy Clin Immunol 2001; 108:198.
131. Skloot G, Permutt S, Togias A. Airway hyperresponsiveness in asthma: a problem of limited smooth muscle relaxation with inspiration. J Clin Invest 1995; 96:2393.
132. Silkoff PE, Sylvester JT, Zamel N, et al. Airway nitric oxide diffusion in asthma: role in pulmonary function and bronchial responsiveness. Am J Respir Crit Care Med 2000; 161:1218.
133. Ricciardolo FL, Geppetti P, Mistretta A, et al. Randomised double-blind placebo-controlled study of the effect of inhibition of nitric oxide synthesis in bradykinin-induced asthma. Lancet 1996; 348:374.
134. Ricciardolo FL, Di Maria GU, Mistretta A, et al. Impairment of broncho protection by nitric oxide in severe asthma. Lancet 1997; 350:1297.
135. Ollerenshaw S, Jarvis D, Woolcock A, et al. Absence of immunoreactive vasoactive intestinal polypeptide in tissue from the lungs of patients with asthma. N Engl J Med 1989; 320:1244.
136. Samb A, Pretolani M, Dinh-Xuan AT, et al. Decreased pulmonary and tracheal smooth muscle expression and activity of type 1 nitric oxide synthase (nNOS) after ovalbumin immunization and multiple aerosol challenge in guinea pigs. Am J Respir Crit Care Med 2001; 164:149.
137. Gaston B, Sears S, Woods J, et al. Bronchodilator S-nitrosothiol deficiency in asthmatic respiratory failure. Lancet 1998; 351:1317.
138. Zimmermann N, King NE, Laporte J, et al. Dissection of experimental asthma with DNA microarray analysis identifies arginase in asthma pathogenesis. J Clin Invest 2003; 111:1863.
139. Morris CR, Poljakovic M, Lavrisha L, et al. Decreased arginine bioavailability and increased serum arginase activity in asthma. Am J Respir Crit Care Med 2004; 170:148.
140. Que LG, Liu L, Yan Y, et al. Protection from experimental asthma by an endogenous bronchodilator. Science 2005; 308:1618.
141. Maarsingh H, Leusink J, Bos IS, et al. Arginase strongly impairs neuronal nitric oxide-mediated airway smooth muscle relaxation in allergic asthma. Respir Res 2006; 7:6.
142. Hunter DD, Myers AC, Undem BJ. Nerve growth factor-induced phenotypic switch in guinea pig airway sensory neurons. Am J Respir Crit Care Med 2000; 161:1985.
143. de Vries A, Engels F, Henricks PA, et al. Airway hyper-responsiveness in allergic asthma in guinea-pigs is mediated by nerve growth factor via the induction of substance P: a potential role for trkA. Clin Exp Allergy 2006; 36:1192.
144. Nassenstein C, Dawbarn D, Pollock K, et al. Pulmonary distribution, regulation, and functional role of Trk receptors in a murine model of asthma. J Allergy Clin Immunol 2006; 118:597.
145. Hazari MS, Pan JH, Myers AC. Nerve growth factor acutely potentiates synaptic transmission in vitro and induces dendritic growth in vivo on adult neurons in airway parasympathetic ganglia. Am J Physiol Lung Cell Mol Physiol 2007; 292:L992.
146. Bachar O, Adner M, Uddman R, et al. Nerve growth factor enhances cholinergic innervation and contractile response to electric field stimulation in a murine in vitro model of chronic asthma. Clin Exp Allergy 2004; 34:1137.
147. Wu ZX, Dey RD. Nerve growth factor-enhanced airway responsiveness involves substance P in ferret intrinsic airway neurons. Am J Physiol Lung Cell Mol Physiol 2004; 291:431.
148. Braun A, Lommatzsch M, Neuhaus-Steinmetz U, et al. Brain-derived neutrotrophic factor (BDNF) contributes to neuronal dysfunction in a model of allergic airway inflammation. Br J Pharmacol 2004; 141:431.
149. Saito Y, Okazawa M. Eosinophilic leukocyte accumulation during vagally induced bronchoconstriction. Am J Respir Crit Care Med 1997; 156:1614.
150. Chou DL, Daugherty BL, McKenna EK, et al. Chronic aeroallergen during infancy enhances eotaxin-3 expression in airway epithelium and nerves. Am J Respir Cell Mol Biol 2005; 141:431.
151. Fryer AD, Stein LH, Nie Z, et al. Neuronal eotaxin and the effects of CCR3 antagonist on airway hyperreactivity and M2 receptor dysfunction. J Clin Invest 2006; 116:228.

Biochemical Events in Basophil/ Mast Cell Activation and Mediator Release

Donald W MacGlashan Jr

CONTENTS

SUMMARY OF IMPORTANT CONCEPTS

>> The IgE-mediated response in mast cells and basophils is tuned so that these cells can release significant mediators (e.g., histamine, LTC4) with fewer than 500–1000 molecules of antigen-specific IgE antibodies bound per cell

>> IgE receptor expression can be regulated by the presence of IgE antibody. This relationship represents an important feedback loop in the cell's responsiveness to antigenic stimulation

>> The IgE receptor has no intrinsic enzymatic activity but relies on the presence of Src-family kinases and Syk (spleen tyrosine kinase) to initiate signaling. Therefore, the receptor plus these kinases represent the core IgE-dependent signaling complex

>> Termination of the ongoing IgE-mediated reaction involves several different mechanisms, including other receptors and negative feedback signaling such as that found embodied in SHIP (SH2-containing 5′ inositol phosphatase). The IgG receptor, CD32, provides another Ig-dependent mechanism of downregulating the IgE response that works by recruiting to the signaling complex termination-enzymes like SHIP

>> There are therapies in development that exploit the dependence of early signaling on Syk or negative regulation like that offered by CD32

INTRODUCTION

The mast cell and basophil are considered critical components of an allergic response because they express the high-affinity IgE receptor (FcεRI) and, in response to aggregation of this receptor by antigens acting through bound IgE, secrete mediators known to be responsible for the symptoms and pathology of allergic diseases. It is now known that in humans there are other cells that also express a variant form of FcεRI, introducing a broader range of reactions – that are initiated by antigens binding to cell surface IgE – into the pathological processes that lead to atopy. Nevertheless, the response of the mast cell and basophil are considered critical and as such, the reaction that drives the secretion of mediators from these cells is considered to be a therapeutic target for controlling allergies and asthma (for which IgE-mediated secretion is considered an important trigger).

While stimulating mast cells and basophils through the IgE receptor is an important component of an allergic reaction, both cell types express a variety of receptors that also induce secretion of mediators that cause allergic symptoms. Some of these receptors are now considered part of the innate immune response and mast cells have been implicated in mediating several non-allergic diseases by virtue of their responsiveness to these other types of stimulation. For example, mast cell and basophils respond to anaphylatoxin products such as C5a and C3a. These are generally thought to operate as classical 7-transmembrane spanning receptors and therefore operate through GTP-binding proteins to initiate secretion. There are more recently recognized mechanisms of activation, such as the LIR receptors. The mechanisms underlying early signal transduction of these receptors are less clear. Nevertheless, secretion from mast cells and basophils and their participation in other disease entities is not restricted to IgE-mediated reactions.

When discussing activation of these two cell types, it is also important to consider the functional outcome of stimulation. Classically, mediator secretion is the measured outcome of activation but increasingly other endpoints warrant exploration. Even within the realm of mediator secretion, it is apparent that not all forms of stimulation result in the same profile of mediators released. It is possible to classify three types of secretion: (1) rapid from pre-formed pools, (2) rapid but newly synthesized, and (3) slow but newly synthesized. Granule contents such as histamine represent the first group while arachidonic acid metabolites such as leukotriene C4 or prostaglandin D2 represent the second group. Cytokines, chemokines, and growth factors represent the third group although there is some evidence that a small fraction of these mediators may be pre-formed and released during degranulation (from an unidentified pool). Except under special circumstances, it is not uncommon find that GTP-binding protein-linked receptors are poor at inducing the third class of mediators while the immunoreceptors are good at inducing all three classes of mediators. Therefore identifying the stimulus in a given situation may determine the expected types of mediators. There are other functions, such as adhesion and migration, that are also part of the mast cell or basophil repertoire and are critical to the behavior of these cell types but will be only briefly considered in this chapter.

It is also worth noting at this point that mast cells and basophils only share some attributes. Although there remains some controversy about the bone marrow lineage of the two cell types, it is generally felt that the immediate progenitors are not the same and that there is no phenotypic plasticity that can cause a mast cell to become a basophil and vice-versa. Consequently, a general statement about the signal transduction reactions that follow FcεRI aggregation or other forms of stimulation is not strictly possible. There are several known differences whose biological and clinical significance are not understood. Nevertheless, this chapter will discuss the signaling as if the mechanisms are shared between the two cell types and note where differences are thought to exist.

IgE-MEDIATED SIGNALING: THE AGGREGATION REACTION

For the last few decades, it was thought that the IgE receptor, like all immunoreceptors, must be aggregated to induce secretion. In recent years, there have been studies that call into question this paradigm of secretion and these experiments will be discussed in some detail because they speak to a fundamental behavior of this receptor system and the issues raised may impinge on a variety of clinical conditions.

Early studies noted that simply sensitizing a mast cell or basophil did not seem to result in secretion. For the early studies, only secretion of class I mediators was known. Even today, most IgE molecules, in monomeric form, do not induce measurable secretion. The earliest studies found that covalently crosslinked IgE, as small as dimers, could readily induce secretion.[1] During the last couple of decades, a variety of studies have revealed an ever-increasing subtlety to this aggregation reaction. Four examples highlight some of the issues. First, not all aggregate sizes result in similar activation. Depending on the cell type studied (animal source and basophil vs mast cell), dimeric aggregates induce a qualitatively and quantitatively different secretion compared to trimeric and larger aggregates.[2,3] On the other side of aggregate size distribution, very large aggregates appear to be poor inducers of secretion.[4] Second, studies in rat basophilic leukemia cells (RBL cells, a longstanding model of IgE-mediated secretion) demonstrated that the antigen ligand for IgE could be a freely mobile univalent molecule incapable of inducing secretion in solution form but quite capable when located in a lipid membrane.[5-7] These studies suggested that at points of contact between the RBL cell and the ligand-containing lipid membrane, receptor would cluster at high enough concentrations to initiate signal transduction and therefore secretion. Third, if the ligand that binds to IgE is made very long

and rigid but of reasonably high affinity, the aggregated receptors do not need to be in close proximity to each other to induce signal transduction. In this instance, there is a stabilized aggregate with receptor separated by 400 Å nearly three times the radius of gyration of the receptor-bound IgE.[8] Finally, not all crosslinking reagents induce secretion. There are some receptor antibodies that appear to induce aggregation of the receptor but do not induce secretion.[9,10] It is possible that certain adjacent receptor orientations do not effectively stimulate signal transduction. Some of these studies suggest an even more subtle result, that some but not all early signaling reactions occur.[10] These various results suggest some interesting characteristics and may even highlight some possible conditions whereby different antigens induce qualitatively different mast cell or basophil responses, despite all inducing some form of aggregation. Notably, aggregate size and the dynamics of aggregate formation are determinants of the ensuing reaction. Antigens presented on cell surfaces or other solid surfaces may induce reactions that would not be readily anticipated on the basis of solution phase experiments. Also, stable aggregation per se may not be necessary, simply concentrating the receptor in a restricted region of the membrane may be sufficient to induce secretion. While the average concentration of receptor in these types of situations would be required to be high, specific receptors could wander in and out of a locally high concentration region.

It is in this context that recent studies on secretion induced by monomeric IgE binding might be viewed.[11,12] A fraction of the available monoclonal IgE antibodies have been found to induce signaling that leads to survival and/or secretion of some mediators. Although there are limited reports of this occurring in human mast cells, the observation is most commonly made with monoclonal IgE antibodies binding to murine mast cells. These observations are important for a variety of reasons. First, if monomeric IgE can induce secretion, the underlying paradigm that explains why aggregates are needed must be modified. Second, if this is a characteristic of only some IgE antibodies, it raises the possibility that some severe disease might be explained by the presence of IgE and no antigen. A telling observation of at least one of these activating IgE antibodies (the term cytokinergic IgE has been proposed), whose antigen-specificity is known to be dinitrophenol hapten (DNP), is that monovalent DNP inhibits the reaction. This is normally considered a characteristic of an aggregation reaction induced by multivalent antigen and it suggests that although the IgE is bound monomerically, its ligand binding site may be interacting with an unknown cell surface structure to effectively induce a form of aggregation or receptor clustering (see above). This explanation is aided by the observation that experiments in which cytokinergic IgE antibodies are tested use cells in which FcεRI is highly expressed. Biophysical considerations raise the possibility that there are a reasonable number of spontaneous clusters of receptors that may be partially stabilized by a monomeric IgE interacting weakly with a cell surface structure.

The observations regarding monomeric IgE signaling are not exclusively related to the induction of secretion. In some cases, monomeric IgE antibodies that only poorly induce secretion, nevertheless induce mast cell survival.[13,14] In addition, it has been demonstrated in all systems studied that monomeric IgE stabilizes the presence of FcεRI on the cell surface.[15-19] These two mechanisms appear distinct. In the case of survival, this has only been observed in murine mast cells and studies with selected knockout mice suggest that the early elements of signal transduction required for standard secretion are still required for the survival effects.[14] In contrast, these early elements are not needed for IgE to protect FcεRI from removal from the cell surface. The mechanism underlying this protective effect of IgE may be passive in that no explicit signaling is required, i.e., IgE induces a conformational change in receptor or acts sterically to inhibit receptor recognition by another cell surface element responsible for removing receptor from the cell surface.[18,19] This mechanism of expression regulation remains unknown although it is now known that receptor endocytosis occurs when receptor is removed from the surface.

◼ IgE RECEPTOR STRUCTURE ◼

Before discussing the consequences of receptor aggregation, it is worth noting several features of receptor composition. Rodents and humans express three subunits that have no known enzymatic activities. An interesting distinguishing characteristic of the human and rodent receptors is that rodent cells require all three subunits for expression while in humans, only two subunits are required.[20,21] The three subunits are labeled α, β, and γ, and the γ subunit is expressed as a disulfide-linked dimer. The α subunit has a large two-domain chain that binds IgE antibody monomerically, a transmembrane segment, and short cytoplasmic tail. Although IgE is composed of two heavy chains, two IgE antibodies cannot bind to the α subunit due to unique use of both IgE heavy chains in the binding pocket of FcεRIα.[22,23] The β chain is the optional subunit in humans. It is generally not expressed in non-mast cells/basophils such as dendritic cells, Langerhans cells, monocytes, macrophages (and more controversially, eosinophils, neutrophils, platelets, and smooth muscle cells). The β subunit is a member of the family of four membrane crossing membrane proteins, the MS4A family. The role for the β subunit is complex; it may serve as a chaperone for the α subunit[24] and therefore influence expression levels and it may act to enhance the very earliest steps of signal transduction.[25] Indeed, the classical model of aggregation-induced signaling begins with phosphorylation of the β subunit on its sole ITAM (immunotyrosine activation motif). There is a also splice variant of the β chain that cannot function as a chaperone and it is rapidly degraded, but in the process of being transiently expressed may act as 'spoiler' for the normal splice variant that is present.[26] The consequence is that too much expressed β chain variant (β_T) and receptor expression is diminished. The γ subunits express tandem ITAMs, which are required to initiate a robust signaling reaction. However, the γ subunit, in the absence of the β subunit, also acts as a required chaperone for cell surface expression of the α subunit. The topological disposition of all four subunits ($\alpha\beta\gamma2$) in the cell membrane is not known, so the precise interactions among the components remains abstract.

◼ BRIEF OVERVIEW OF THE EARLY STAGES OF FcεRI-MEDIATED SIGNALING ◼

Because the IgE receptor subunits have no known enzymatic activity, one might consider that an extended view of the receptor would include the tyrosine kinases that are required for the initiation of signaling. However, the precise disposition of the kinases remains unclear. At least three are early participants, the Src-family kinase, Lyn, and the ZAP-70 family kinase, Syk (spleen tyrosine kinase), are considered key components,

and recent studies suggest that the Src-family kinase, fyn, is required as well (at least in mast cells[27]). There may be other Src-family kinases involved. The confusion about the extended view of the receptor comes from a variety of studies that suggest that Lyn kinase, which is modified with two myristic acid chains so that it localizes in the plasma membrane, may be located in lipid rafts (more on this below) prior to association with FcεRI.[28] An alternative view is that Lyn interacts with FcεRI through its so-called unique domain.[29,30] Syk is presumably cytosolic until recruited to the receptor after γ subunit phosphorylation and the precise disposition of fyn is not known. Therefore, while these components are required elements, their locations are not clearly known in the resting state. Until recently, there was a canonical model of aggregation-induced signaling that did not implicate a role for fyn but this model no longer appears adequate in describing the early reaction. Relative to the previous model, which was best visualized when Lyn kinase is thought to already have an association with the β subunit through its unique domain, the current model of the earliest steps in signaling is actually less clear. However, it seems likely that some aspects of the previous model remain a partial description of the earliest steps in signaling. In this model, Lyn kinase is in its inactive conformation (see below). Aggregation brings into proximity the ITAM of an adjacent FcεRIβ. Note that in this model, Lyn kinase apparently does not readily 'see' the β subunit to which it is associated. Presumably, there are steric reasons why Lyn can only transphosphorylate an adjacent β subunit. Once transphosphorylation of a participating β subunit occurs, Lyn kinase may use its SH2 domain to associate strongly with FcεRIβ and thereby induce its full enzymatic activity. In this bound configuration, Lyn kinase can phosphorylate the γ subunits and these phosphorylated ITAMs recruit Syk kinase into the developing reaction complex.[31,32]

There are many studies that demonstrate the critical role of Syk kinase.[33,34] Its absence eliminates many of the subsequent signaling steps, although not all. All secretion is inhibited without Syk due to multiple branching pathways being eliminated. Notably, there is no increase in cytosolic calcium, which is considered another critical element for secretion, if not other functional endpoints. Syk phosphorylates a variety of components that participate in the next level of the reaction complex assembly that occurs around the aggregated FcεRI. At this point the model becomes remarkably complex and its details are not fully understood. There are adaptor molecules, e.g., Shc, LAT, NLAT, SLP-76, VAV, GAB2, whose roles are to provide a scaffold for the developing signaling reaction complex. Phosphorylation of these adaptor proteins by Syk, Lyn or fyn is the switch for the recruitment of other critical signaling elements. Another early critical enzyme is PI3 kinase. This kinase phosphorylates plasma membrane inositol lipids. Notably, PI3 kinase creates a local concentration of phosphatidylinositol 3,4,5-trisphosphate (PIP3). This highly phosphorylated lipid leads to recruitment of other enzymes to the surrounding membrane through PH (pleckstrin homology) domains. For example, the Bruton's tyrosine kinase, Btk, has a PH domain that directs it to PIP3-rich regions of the membrane, those presumably surrounding the FcεRI reaction complex. Figure 14.1 shows the current scheme and some of the sections that follow will develop the details further.

The steps described above constitute activation of signaling. However, there must be counter-regulation or the reaction would never end. Signal termination is less well-explored but some of the outlines are in place and these will be discussed below. As crude as the description is thus far, it is possible to already see places for modulation. Like any signaling

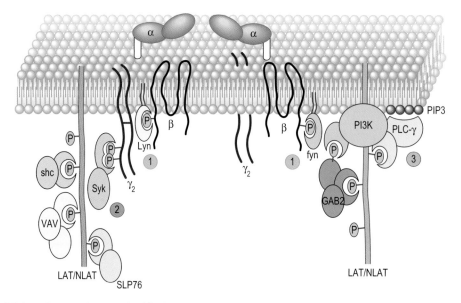

Fig. 14.1. Early FcεRI-dependent signaling complex. The IgE molecules bound to the α subunit are left out of the picture. The approximate order of assembly of the complex is shown with the numbers 1–3. In the earliest step of the reaction (1), a Src-family kinase, probably Lyn kinase, initiates phosphorylation of either the β or γ subunit of the IgE receptor. This allows recruitment of Syk kinase (step 2) which becomes more active after binding to the γ subunit. Syk begins phosphorylating other substrates, including itself, such as LAT and NLAT which act as scaffolds for recruitment of other adaptors and enzymes. Notably, PI3 kinase (PI3K) is recruited leading to conversion of PIP2 to PIP3 (step 3), which leads to further assembly of proteins near the cell membrane.

reaction, there is likely considerable amplification of the reaction by the various enzymatic activities. Therefore, modulation is possible by simply limiting the extent of amplification. However, it was considered possible that amplification of the reaction would be so intense that the cell would effectively fully degranulate, a so-called all-or-nothing response. There is compelling evidence that this does not happen. Essentially every step that can be studied at the single cell level has been found to be graded according to the magnitude of the stimulation. Each cell is capable of a less than a full response,[35–37] at least for physiological stimuli.

In the context of disease presentation, there is an important consideration: how many aggregated receptors are required to induce half-maximal secretion? The mast cell and basophil are exposed to a large number of antigen-specific IgE antibodies. In order for any given antigen to induce secretion, there must be enough cell-bound antigen-specific IgE to induce secretion and each clone of IgE is in competition with other clones for the limited number of receptors on the mast cell. Each new antigen to which the animal becomes sensitized must compete with the existing pool of cell-bound IgE or the cell is unable to respond. This situation is mitigated by the cell through two mechanisms. One has been noted above; monomeric IgE antibody stabilizes any surface FcεRI. The current model suggests that these cells constitutively synthesize receptor; the rate of production appears to be on the order of 45 000 per day. IgE does not modulate this synthetic rate although cytokines may. But even in the absence of changes in the rate of synthesis, this situation results in the accumulation of receptor on the cell surface. FcεRI can be expressed at remarkably high densities; it is not uncommon to observe 500 000 receptors per cell and 1 000 000 receptors have also been observed, although rarely. When considering the radius of gyration of bound IgE, 1 000 000 receptors looks like the 'overhead' view shown in Figure 14.2.

The second mechanism that deals with the clonal binding problem above is the adjustment of the cellular sensitivity. It is not possible to know precisely how many aggregates are required because the tools do not exist for making such measurements. Even if this measurement could be made, it would be harder still to quantify the lifetime of the aggregates or their size, characteristics which are clearly important in the strength of subsequent signaling. However, it is possible to simply measure the density of antigen-specific IgE and ask about the density required to generate a half-maximal response following stimulation with an optimal concentration of an antigen. (*Note* that an optimal concentration for a simple antigen – one for which the affinity is reasonably restricted – is defined by the single-site affinity or avidity of the antigen for its IgE.[38,39]) Studies have shown that the typical human basophil requires approximately 2000 antigen-specific IgE antibodies per cell for the half-maximal response.[40,41] However, there is considerable variation among subject's basophils, ranging from 300 to 30 000. Early studies of RBL cells noted that in some cases, as few as 50 covalently crosslinked trimers of IgE could induce modest secretion (more dimeric IgE was required) and studies of human basophils have also noted that as few as 25 molecules of antigen-specific IgE were sufficient to mediate an observable response from the basophils of some subjects. Like the dimer/trimer difference in RBL cells, bivalent haptens require higher densities of IgE than multivalent haptenated proteins. This cellular sensitivity can be modulated. Notably, cytokines change sensitivity. In addition, the maximal response and the sensitivity are weakly interdependent parameters of the cell response, i.e., how much mediator release one observes shows a weak correlation to cellular sensitivity. Therefore, the cell can regulate whether it can sense an environmental antigen by several mechanisms. Combining these various parameters of the reaction, one can see that

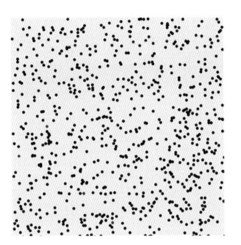

Fig. 14.2. Receptor distribution in a 0.2 μm square of the cell surface at resting conditions, i.e., prior to aggregation. The black circles represent the radius of gyration of surface bound IgE (~130 Å). The dynamics of the motion can't be observed but at the high density of receptors shown here, ~1 million receptors per basophil, there is considerable spontaneous, although transient, clustering (view obtained from a stochastic computer model of receptor aggregation).

if a cell expressed 500000 receptors and could respond with some mediator release using only 100 molecules of antigen-specific IgE, that 1/5000 of total IgE could be specific for a given antigen and the mast cell or basophil could still respond.

It should be noted that the control of IgE expression by IgE is only a log-linear relationship.[42,43] As more IgE is generated by an immune response, the cell doesn't respond by loading a compensatory number of receptors; a 10-fold increase in IgE results in only a two-fold increase in receptor in the range of 10–30000 ng/ml of IgE. So it is possible to swamp the cell with non-specific IgE and this may be a mechanism for parasites, for example, to counter the compensatory mechanisms of the mast cell.

FOCUS ON SPECIFIC STEPS

Protein domain structure and signaling

A useful way to view the activation cascade in any cell is as an assembly of protein domains. Each of the signaling proteins to be discussed is a mixture of functional domains. Enzymes are composed of the catalytic domain and several smaller domains that mediate the interaction with other proteins. Adaptor proteins have no enzymatic function but usually consist of 4–5 of the smaller domains that bind or are bound to by other proteins. For immunoreceptors, there are several well-described domains based on the Src-family kinases. SH2 (Src-homology 2) domains are generally around 100 amino acids in length and bind to specific phosphorylated tyrosine peptide sequences in other proteins. SH2 domains are distinguished by the particular phosphorylated tyrosine sequence to which they can bind. SH3 (Src-homolog 3) domains are somewhat smaller and have selected interactions with proline-rich regions of other proteins. Related to the SH2 domain is the PTB domain, which also

binds to selected phosphorylated tyrosine peptide sequences in other proteins. PH (pleckstrin-homology) domains are found in various signaling proteins and mediate recruitment of some proteins to phosphorylated lipids in the plasma membrane. Many of these interactions are mediated by phosphorylation events; each phosphorylation, often of tyrosines, provides a site for SH2 and PTB domains – with their associated protein/catalytic domains – to bind.

Src-family kinases

The Src family is composed of nine known kinases that are present throughout all metazoan cells. The study of enzymes modulated by specific intradomain interactions and domain-target interactions can be largely traced to the detailed study of Src-family kinases. The domain structure of these kinases is characterized by a unique, SH4, SH3, SH2, catalytic and phosphorylated tyrosine latch sequence. The SH4 domain is generally acylated with two myristic acid chains and/or a mixture of myristic and palmitic acid. For most of the Src kinases, these two fatty acid chains allow the kinase to intimately associate with cell membranes. This feature may help define one of the critical aspects of immunoreceptor signaling, the role of lipid rafts in organizing the signaling complex (see below). The unique domain of Src-family kinases may allow the kinase to weakly associate with other proteins in a manner that is selective for the particular Src-family member. For example, the unique domain of Lyn kinase appears to allow weak association with FcεRIβ and this association may be important in the very first step of phosphorylation of the FcεRβ ITAM on an adjacent FcεRI, the so-called transphosphorylation step.[44] Under these circumstances, Lyn enzymatic activity might be very low because one of the hallmarks of the Src-family kinases is that in their folded state there is limited enzymatic activity. In this configuration, the SH3 and SH2 domains interact with the backside of the catalytic domain and allosteric effects induce a conformation that is catalytically inactive (or weakly active). Study of the SH2 domain of the Src-family kinases resulted in classification of this 100 amino acid sequence as a model of a protein domain that could bind to selected phosphotyrosine sequences. In Lyn, the binding of the SH2 domain to an adjacent FcεRβ phosphorylated ITAM would induce an unfolding that would allow full activity of the enzyme but there are data to suggest that Lyn might already be in an active state, associated with the β subunit, in resting cells. Another characteristic of this family is the placement of a tyrosine on the C-terminal peptide that, when phosphorylated, binds to the intramolecular SH2, latching the conformation in an inactive state. In rodent mast cells, the phosphorylation state of this tyrosine can be regulated by a specific tyrosine kinase, Csk. An unresolved issue is how this latch sequence becomes unphosphorylated although, the phosphatase CD45 has been implicated in this step (see below).

Recent studies of the IgE-mediated aggregation reaction in murine mast cells derived from bone marrow cultures (BMMC) have led to a model of the signaling complex that is dependent on both Lyn and fyn kinases. The current information suggests that the Lyn remains integral to receptor (β and γ), Syk and LAT phosphorylation; in fyn knockout mice, phosphorylation of these elements is similar to that found in wild-type mice.[45] However, in fyn -/- mast cells (BMMC), phosphorylation of phospholipase D (see below), PDK-1 and Akt (see below), and a decreased activation of PKC isozymes (see below) because of the decreased PDK-1 activation, have been observed,[27,45] Functionally, mast cells derived from fyn knockout mice show decreased IgE-mediated degranulation and a decrease in the generation of some, but not all cytokines. Perhaps more surprisingly, although removing Lyn dramatically results in early reductions in the phosphorylation of early signaling elements, functional responses are sometimes much greater.[46,47] The reasons for this counterintuitive result are multifaceted. There may be compensatory events in these knockout mice that result in exaggerated responses when Lyn is absent,[46] but there are also indications that Lyn may have mixed roles in signaling, both activating and deactivating the signaling complex. For example, Lyn may be required for phosphorylation of SHIP (see below) that may act to downregulate events downstream of the early signaling complex.[47] The complementary nature of Lyn and fyn activity is highlighted by studies that indicate that cytoskeletal changes needed for degranulation involve two necessary pathways, one that is fyn dependent and one that is Lyn dependent.[48] Recent studies have suggested that the precise role of Lyn depends on how strongly the mast cell is activated through FcεRI.[49] The emerging picture is that the canonical model that requires Lyn kinase for starting the reaction is probably correct but fyn is involved in starting some additional pathways (e.g., GAB2-dependent pathways) that become necessary for proper degranulation and the generation of some cytokines (e.g., NF-κB-dependent cytokines, see below). In addition, because Lyn kinase is also involved in establishing the activity of some negative regulators of the reaction, the precise timing and strength of activation will determine the duration of response due to the differential roles of Lyn in establishing activating and deactivating events. However, it is also apparent from a variety of studies that the precise disposition of the Src-family kinases may differ between different strains of mice and certainly between mice and man. There are also indications in murine mast cells that the β subunit may have both positive and negative roles. This occurs because the ITAM on the β chain is not quite a canonical ITAM; it has a third tyrosine that if phosphorylated, opposes the ability of the ITAM to bind the Lyn SH2 domain. Lyn can phosphorylate this third tyrosine and therefore, once again, act in a positive or negative role. The current picture developed for BMMC has not been established for mast cells and basophils from man.

A side trip on a lipid raft

A hallmark of signal transduction is the assembly of large signaling complexes composed of many different proteins. Included in the signaling complex is the plasma membrane and immunoreceptors are now thought to signal in a membrane environment that is different in composition from the rest of the bulk membrane.[50] Stimulation of immunoreceptors leads to a change in the migration of the receptor in detergent-solubilized membranes analyzed on sucrose density gradients, inducing association with a detergent-resistant component of the membrane. These membrane structures have been termed lipid rafts (or GEMs, DIGs, DRMs). Their composition is dependent on cholesterol and agents that remove cholesterol from the plasma membrane markedly interfere with immunoreceptor function.[51] These regions also are rich in sphingomyelin and glycolipids, as well as glycosylphosphatidyl inositol (GPI)-anchored proteins. In addition to an enrichment of certain lipids, some inner membrane-associated proteins such as Src-family kinases and LAT (see below) also associate strongly with lipid raft regions. There remains considerable debate about the pre-existence of the rafts; some models hold that raft formation accompanies aggregation of immunoreceptor while in other models, the rafts exist before stimulation and sorting of receptor and other protein components occurs during stimulation. There are also indications that up to 40% of the plasma membrane

may consist of these domains. Initiation of signaling requires the domains and maintenance of signaling requires continued association of receptors with the domains.[52] However, normally, receptors are only transiently associated and therefore only transiently active. Agents that disrupt actin polymerization disallow the segregation of receptors from the rafts and therefore markedly enhance the duration and magnitude of signaling.[51]

Syk kinase

Src-family kinases like Lyn and fyn are the initiators of receptor phosphorylation, but it is Syk kinase that serves the role of receptor kinase (it is not clear whether the other member of this enzyme family, ZAP-70, plays a role in mast cell/basophil activation). Many, but not all, downstream measures of the cell response are dependent on the activity of Syk kinase. Association of Syk kinase to the FcεRIγ ITAMs through its tandem SH2 domains is a critical step in regulating the full activity of this enzyme. Once bound, the enzyme is capable of self-phosphorylation of two activation site tyrosines and this further increases its enzymatic activity. Elimination of Syk (by various means, such as knock-outs or siRNA treatment) abrogates most cell functions and transfection with just the tandem-SH2-domains acts as in inhibitor of the Syk interaction with FcεRIγ ITAMs and also abrogates downstream activities.[34,53] In addition to the activation site tyrosines, there are six other tyrosines that can be phosphorylated. Some of these act as recruitment motifs for other adaptor proteins and some act to recruit negative regulatory proteins such as the cbl family (see below). Phosphorylated tyrosines in the linker region between the tandem SH2 domains and the catalytic domain mediate recruitment of cbl, PLC-γ1, and VAV. Because Syk is a critical early kinase in FcεRI-dependent signaling, there are a growing number of efforts to develop a selective inhibitor of this enzyme as a means of regulating mast cell and basophil secretion in allergic patients. There has been one clinical trial of a second-generation Syk inhibitor.[54] Because Syk is also a critical kinase in other immune cells, this approach to suppress allergic reactions has potential drawbacks. Current trials have taken the appropriately cautious approach of using inhibitors topically in the hope that their use will have only local impact on general immune function. It is notable that unlike many pharmacological agents, Syk inhibitors completely abrogate all forms of secretion.

Phosphatidylinositol 3-kinase

In mammalian cells, a large family of enzymes act as kinases to phosphorylate membrane lipids. A well-recognized lipid kinase is the PI3K family composed of three classes that are segregated on the basis of substrates and sequence homology. Class 1A members of this large family are the PI3 kinases composed of an 85 kDa regulatory subunit and a 110 kDa catalytic subunit. The class 1A enzymes typically interact and mediate signaling from receptor tyrosine kinases or immunoreceptors while class 1B PI3Ks interact with G-protein-linked receptors. The catalytic subunit (p110) has three forms, α, β, δ (the γ form is the one class 1B) and the p85 regulatory subunit has an α and β form and some splice variants of these two forms (p55γ). The distribution of the various forms of class 1A enzymes among different tissues is complex. RBL cells express all three forms of p110,[55] but there is some controversy about the isoforms that are needed during IgE-mediated secretion.[55,56] Human basophils have been found to express only p110δ,[57] and a specific inhibitor of p110δ completely inhibits secretion (unpublished data). Whether the limited expression of p110δ in basophils is related to the end-stage nature of these cells is not known. The p85 subunit has a couple of SH2 domains, a p110 binding domain, and a tyrosine phosphorylation site that allows interactions with other adaptors. The p110 subunit not only has the catalytic domain and p85 binding domain but also a p21ras binding domain whose exact functionality is not clear. For example, a change in the interaction of p110δ and p21ras in stimulated human basophils was not observed.[57]

While there are genetic tools for demonstrating a role of these enzymes in secretion, it is notable that there are two relatively selective inhibitors of the class 1A enzymes, LY292004 and wortmannin. Use of these drugs has demonstrated that secretion of all classes of mediators from mast cells and basophils is dependent on this enzyme. Inhibition is complete with these agents, much as second- and third-generation Syk inhibitors result in complete inhibition. The precise interactions that drive the recruitment of PI3K to the signaling complex probably varies somewhat from mast cell to basophil but from the many cell types in which this enzyme is studied, SH2 domains in the p85 subunit bind directly to phosphorylated receptor subunits or to closely linked adaptor proteins that are associated with the phosphorylated receptor. This recruitment and binding of the p85 subunit alters the enzymatic activity of the p110 subunit and brings it into close proximity with the plasma membrane where it can phosphorylate membrane lipid head groups.

There are several interesting dynamics in these reactions. First, it is now apparent from studies of type 2 diabetes that cells express the p85α subunit independently from the p110 subunit.[58,59] Too much p85α expression and the free subunit competes with the p85-p110 combination for binding to the receptor or receptor–adaptor complex. This competition results in less PI3K activity. It is not clear whether a similar dynamic balance exists in mast cells or basophils but in a recent survey of signal element expression in the general population's basophils, expression of the p85 subunit was found to be very consistent even when the ability of the basophils to release histamine was very broad. In addition, the ratio of p85a/p110d was not correlated with function. Whether a similar result would occur in human mast cells studies is not known but studies of p85 overexpression in rat basophilic leukemia cells (a rat mast cell tumor line) do show suppression of downstream responses.

The reaction that this enzyme catalyzes in shown in Figure 14.3. It is interesting that PI3K competes for the same phospholipid substrate that generates the small soluble mediator, inositol trisphosphate (IP3), that is critical for releasing intracellular calcium from its internal stores (see below). PI3K phosphorylates phosphatidylinositol 4,5 phosphate (PtdIns(4,5)P2 or PIP2) to generate phosphatidylinositol 3,4,5-trisphosphate (PtdIns(3,4,5)P3 or PIP3). This removes some PIP2 from the membrane, PIP2 that could be used to generate IP3 through the action of PLCγ1/2 (see below). It also removes PIP2 which is a potential regulator of actin strand ends. On the other hand, PIP3 recruits PH-domain-containing proteins such as btk (Bruton's tyrosine kinase), PLCγ, VAV (an GTPase-activating adaptor protein), PDK-1, and Akt (regulating cell survival) to the cell membrane. Figure 14.3 also shows that there are two major ways in which PIP3 is metabolized and these will be discussed in further detail below.

Phospholipase C

If PI3K starts the process of lipid conversion, its activity is quickly paralleled by the activity of phospholipase C. This enzyme family currently consists of 13 members divided into six groups, PLC-β (4 members),

PLC-γ (2 members), PLC-δ (4 members), PLC-ε, PLC-ζ, PLC-ν (1 member each). All members share the catalytic core domains (so-called X&Y), and a PH domain, but only the X&Y domains share significant homology among the isozymes. Differences in the family members include the addition or subtraction of various other domains like the tandem SH2 domains of the PLC-γ subgroup leading to molecular weights ranging from 85 kDa (PLC-δs) to 260 kDa (PLC-ε). Among the most recently recognized domain structures are the Ras binding domains (see below) which have introduced a new level of regulation to the PLC family. Classically, the PLC-γ and PLC-β groups have been regulated by tyrosine kinases or heterotrimeric GTP-binding proteins, respectively. The addition of yet another way of regulating the catalytic activity of these enzymes may lead to a re-evaluation of early signal transduction regulation.

During IgE-mediated stimulation of mast cells and basophils, it is PLC-γ1 and PLC-γ2 activity that appears to be critical. These two isozymes include a tandem SH2 and SH3 domains located between the core X&Y domains and these domains mediate association of PLC-γ with phosphorylated adaptor proteins such as LAT and SLP-76. PLC-γ appears to undergo a two stage activation, with the N-SH2 domain initiating association with adaptor proteins and localizing the PLC so that it is tyrosine phosphorylated (Y783), followed by an intramolecular association of the C-SH2 domain with Y783 that leads to activation of the enzyme.

Activation of mast cells or basophils through 7-transmembrane receptors like the C5a or FMLP receptors results in changes to heterotrimeric GTP-binding proteins. PLC-β1 is activated by associating with $G_q\alpha$ through its long C-terminal tail while Gβγ interacts with PLC-β through its PH domain.

Several interesting relationships exist between PI3K and PLC. First, the presence of a PH domain in PLC suggests that PLC localizes to the plasma membrane after the action of PI3K on local lipids to generate PIP3. However, the catalytic action of PLC is to remove the head group from phosphatidylinositol lipids, notably generating inositol 3,4,5 trisphosphate (IP3) and diacylglycerols (DAG) from PIP2. As noted above, this action, in effect, competes with PI3K for a common substrate. It is not known whether this competition has any functional consequence because PIP2 is in approximately a 100-fold molar excess to PIP3, suggesting that no serious substrate depletion is occurring in normal cells. A third relationship is perhaps more subtle: both PI3K and PLC can be regulated by ras proteins. In human basophils, PI3K activity influences p21ras activity,[60] which may, therefore, influence PLC activity. However, in human mast cells derived from long-term cultures, inhibitors of PI3K don't inhibit phosphorylation of PLC-γ1 or the early calcium response, and surprisingly, only inhibit degranulation by 50%.[61] There are indications that in murine mast cells, the activation of PLCγ is dependent on the presence of VAV1.[62] Since these dependencies are not universal in all cell types, it is clear that there remains more to learn about regulation of PLCγ in mast cells and basophils.

One of the most well-studied early signaling reactions in any cell type, and for any receptor that ultimately generates an elevation in cytosolic calcium, is the catalytic activity of PLC to generate IP3 and DAG. IP3 is one of several small molecule second messengers that mediate the release of free Ca^{++} from internal cellular stores by mediating the permeability of the IP3 receptor on the cell's endoplasmic reticulum. While IP3 is a major regulator of the IP3 receptor, there exists a network of inositol phosphates, regulated by a partially

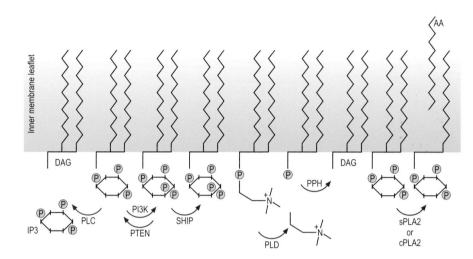

Fig. 14.3. Some example membrane lipid transformations that are part of the early signaling steps in mast cells and basophils. Note that only two head groups are shown, inositol and choline, and no detail concerning the fatty acid chains is indicated. On the left side of the picture is shown the critical reaction mediated by the lipid kinase, PI3 kinase, and the counter-reaction phosphatases, PTEN and SHIP (see text). From membrane resident PIP2, PI3K creates PIP3 which acts to recruit a variety of proteins that contain PH domains that recognize PIP3. A second set of reactions is shown in the middle of the picture where phospholipase D clips off the head group of membrane lipids. In the example shown, a choline head group, which is a preferred substrate of PLD, is removed. The phosphatidic acid that results can be used a number of ways, one of which is to generate DAG (by PPH), a headless phospholipid that may mediate membrane fusion events and act as a cofactor in the activation of PKC. On the far right is shown the generation of fatty acids from membrane phospholipids by either secretory or cytosolic phospholipase A2. In the example that is shown, arachidonic acid is removed from the second position of the phospholipids and, depending of the region of the cell in which it is produced and the other enzymes that are available, it may lead to the generation of prostaglandins or leukotrienes.

understood group of enzymes, that have varying effects on calcium signaling. The simplistic view is confined to the action of IP3 on calcium release and on its metabolism. The other by-product of the action of PLC is the generation of a variety of molecular species of diacylglycerol. There are several molecular species of phosphatidylinositol 4,5-bisphosphate due to the various fatty acids that contribute to formation of this lipid. However, there are dominant molecular species containing C16 and C18 saturated and unsaturated fatty acids. These diacylglycerol species are known to act as co-regulators of several protein kinase C isozymes (see below). Therefore, the action of PLC is to generate two critical second messengers. The substrate specificity of isolated PLC for different inositol lipids is only partially understood and an in situ specificity is essentially unknown. DAG generation has been studied in mast cells or basophils but it is often the observation that overall changes can be quite subtle when exploring IgE-mediated secretion. Rat peritoneal mast cells, RBL cells, and human basophils have been examined but only in rat peritoneal mast cells are IgE-mediated changes marked. In RBL cells, it has been suggested that the rapid life cycle of the cell establishes a general background of DAG generation that masks the IgE-mediated signal. In human basophils, stimulation with G-protein-linked receptors like fMLP induces marked stimulation indices for DAG generation but for IgE-mediated stimulation a molecular species analysis is required to tease out the response. These various studies demonstrate that a general measurement of DAG is not a sufficient way to analyze these events; both head group and fatty acid molecular species analysis is required. This suggests that these reactions are relatively localized such that whole membrane analysis masks critical changes.

Tec-family kinases

The Tec-family kinase, Bruton's tyrosine kinase (Btk), appears to be another early tyrosine kinase that influences early signaling reactions, at least in murine mast cells where it has been extensively explored.[63] Btk deficiency results in immunodeficiency disorders because Btk plays a wide variety of roles in hematopoietic cells. Unlike the dependency of most mast cell signaling reactions on the presence of Syk, absence of Btk has more subtle effects on mast cell function. Btk activity itself is dependent on Syk and PI3K. There are SH2, SH3, and PH domains in Btk but the PH domain is critical for proper recruitment to the plasma membrane via interaction with PIP3. Once activated, Btk influences the activity of PLC-γ and therefore the sustained cytosolic calcium response (see below). However, the primary outcome of a Btk knockout is a reduced expression of cytokines following IgE-mediated activation, with only a modest effect on histamine release. There are reciprocal effects of Btk on PKCβ enzymes and phosphorylation of Btk by PKCβ.[64] Btk appears to influence activation of the stress-activated kinases like JNK/SAPK1/2 which may explain its influence on specific cytokine production.[63] More recently, Btk has been observed to influence the ability of stem cell factor (SCF) to augment an IgE-mediated response in murine mast cells.[65]

The [Ca++]i response

One of the earliest aspects of secretion to attract study was its dependence on extracellular calcium. Besides noting the requirement for extracellular calcium, early studies noted an increased transport of ⁴⁵Ca++ into cells during stimulation. It is now clear that elevations in free cytosolic calcium are required for many of the enzymes that participate in secretion. For example, in response to several types of secretagogues, mast cells and basophils secrete leukotriene C4. Generation of this mediator from any cell type requires the production of free arachidonic acid from phospholipid pools and metabolism of arachidonic acid by several membrane associated enzymes. Cytosolic PLA2 (type IV phospholipase A2), FLAP (5-lipoxygenase activating protein), 5-lipoxygenase, and LTC4 synthase all require Ca^{++} for activity. Resting levels of $[Ca^{++}]_i$ are 50–100 nM while these enzymes function well with >200–300 nM $[Ca^{++}]_i$. Many secretory reactions require an elevation of $[Ca^{++}]_i$ and therefore all physiological secretagogues induce its elevation. This is, therefore, a commonly shared signaling element. Some of its targets, such as calmodulin are also shared elements because Ca^{++}/calmodulin is itself a regulatory signaling element for a variety of proteins (e.g., calcineurin, see below).

It is not the signaling element itself (in this case, Ca^{++}) that is unique to the different types of secretagogues but the nature of the pathways that lead to its elevation. And, even here, there are many shared steps. For example, for many secretagogues, there are two phases to the calcium elevation that follows stimulation. For the purposes of discussion, three secretagogues that operate on human basophils will be examined: anti-IgE antibody (which aggregates all surface-bound IgE and its high-affinity receptor, FcεRI), FMLP (a bacterial tripeptide with a receptor on all granulocytes), and C5a (a complement split product). The reasons for these choices will become clear. The two-phase type of response typifies $[Ca^{++}]_i$ signaling for a vast number of cell types. There is a very rapid initial response which in some cases is noticeably distinct from a second phase of the response (as is the case for both FMLP and anti-IgE Ab). The first phase is dependent on the release of Ca^{++} from an internal store often associated with a structure that resembles, or is, the endoplasmic reticulum. Part of the linkage between the plasma membrane receptor and this store of calcium is shared among secretagogues while part is unique to each secretagogue. The ER (endoplasmic reticulum) has a calcium channel protein that is sensitive to the presence of inositol-3,4,5-trisphosphate (IP3). This IP3 receptor has multiple control elements, with Ca^{++} itself acting in both a positive and negative feedback loop to modulate further activation of the receptor. In all leukocytes (and probably most other non-voltage dependent calcium responses in all cells), the emptying of the internal store of calcium is a trigger to initiate the influx of Ca^{++} from outside the cell. There have been many candidate processes and/or proteins that have been postulated to mediate the communication of empty ER to the plasma membrane but in 2006, a variety of groups put together a very likely mechanism to explain this process. It was first noted that a protein family called STIM (stromal interaction protein), in particular STIM1, is likely to be the sensor in the ER membrane for the depleted state of the ER calcium pool.[66] When the stores are empty, STIM1 appears to coalesce in regions of the ER that are adjacent to the plasma membrane, presumably interacting with the calcium-release-activated calcium (CRAC) channels responsible for the influx of extracellular calcium. Several labs have identified such a CRAC channel, alternatively named CRACM1 or Orai1 (Orai being the Greek *gatekeeper of heaven*).[67,68] Recent studies have shown the interdependence of STIM1 and Orai1/CRACMA and the dependence of calcium influx on their combined presence (see Fig. 14.4 for a synopsis).[69–71] These results have recently been recapitulated in mast cells or basophils. Since the electrical and chemical gradient between the extracellular medium and the cytosol have a role in mediating the extent of the cytosolic calcium

response (see below), it is not clear how this would work for a STIM1-CRACM1 process that directly links the ER rather than the cytosol to the outside environment.

There is a second possible pathway to the generation of a calcium response.[72] In addition to the IP3 receptor-mediated release of calcium from internal stores, sphingosine-1-phosphate (S1P) can act as a second messenger to release internal stores of calcium. However, there is only limited understanding of this pathway. Recent studies have demonstrated that reduced expression of the long form of sphingosine kinase, the enzyme responsible for the generation of S1P from sphingosine, results in markedly reduced elevations in cytosolic calcium following stimulation through FcεRI but not through stimulation of a GTP-binding protein-linked receptor (adenosine was the non-IgE-dependent stimulus in these studies). It should be noted that there is a family of three cell surface receptors specific for extracellular S1P, two of which are coupled through a GTP-binding protein, G_q, that also result in a calcium response but that this mode of inducing a calcium response is distinct from the internal second messenger status of S1P (knocking-out these receptors does not alter the internal behavior of S1P). The internal proteins responsible for mediating the actions of S1P are not yet described.

The dual nature of the $[Ca^{++}]_i$ elevation is not always present. Stimulation of human basophils with C5a leads to an initial $[Ca^{++}]_i$ elevation that easily matches, if not exceeds, the response following stimulation with FMLP and yet C5a most often only results in this initial transient elevation in $[Ca^{++}]_i$. These results suggest that the second phase of the $[Ca^{++}]_i$ response reflects not only the signals being sent from the ER to the plasma membrane but a sustained signal to continue the emptying from the ER. Only then will the second phase of the response be apparent. Depending on what cell type is being studied, the influx of Ca^{++} from the extracellular medium may have a route directly into the ER or first enter the cytoplasm and then the ER. A transient activation of the C5a receptor will therefore, result in a measurable initial phase but an influx that is difficult to detect because the only calcium necessary is that needed to restore the internal pool and this never makes it back into the cytoplasm. These conclusions are supported by a series of studies where the filling state of the internal pool can be manipulated by thapsigargin, an inhibitor of the calcium pump that promotes the transfer of cytoplasmic Ca^{++} back into the ER (a process which is distinct from the influx mechanism discussed above). This attribute of the C5a-induced response has the functional consequence that C5a does not induce LTC4 generation. This occurs because the phosphorylation of cPLA2 (see below) is a somewhat later event and since an elevation in Ca^{++} and cPLA2 phosphorylation must occur simultaneously, the asynchrony of the two events following C5a disallows LTC4 generation. If cPLA2 phosphorylation is accelerated or the cytosolic calcium response is prolonged, then LTC4 release occurs.[73]

An IgE-mediated elevation of $[Ca^{++}]_i$ is similar in profile to the one induced by FMLP (for human basophils), i.e., a first and second phase are present. However, the overall response is much slower. While a concentration of FMLP that is optimal for inducing degranulation or LTC4 secretion results in the initial release of internal stores of calcium within 1–2 s, stimulation with anti-IgE results in an elevation only after 15–300 s. Although not universal among preparations of human basophils and somewhat distinct from human mast cells, the $[Ca^{++}]_i$ elevation that follows anti-IgE is often characterized by a series of transient spikes in $[Ca^{++}]_i$ when observed at the level of single cells. Calcium spiking can also be observed in stimulated RBL cells[74] If EGTA is present

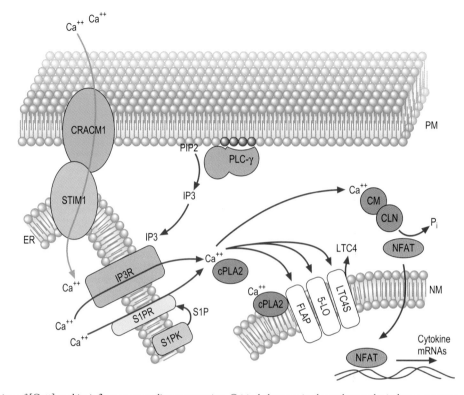

Fig. 14.4. Regulation of $[Ca^{++}]_i$ and its influence on mediator generation. Critical elements in the pathways the induce a receptor-mediated $[Ca^{++}]_i$ elevation. Picking up from Figure 14.1, PLC-γ hydrolyzes the inositol head group from membrane phospholipids to generate inositol 3,4,5-trisphosphate (IP3). PLC is attracted to PIP3 (red circles) generated on the inner leaflet of the membrane by PI3K. IP3 binds to an ER receptor, IP3R, to discharge free Ca^{++} to the cytosolic compartment. A newer possible mechanism of ER discharge involves the generation of sphingosine-1-phosphate by S1P kinase. How S1PK is activated is unknown and the ER-based S1P receptor remains unknown. Once the ER is empty, STIM1 signals a plasma membrane calcium transport process (possibly by direct interaction) mediated by CRACM1 to restore ER free Ca^{++}, which continues to be discharged to the cytosol provided the signaling continues. Free cytosolic calcium mediates many signaling steps, including those that lead to LTC4 generation (the cPLA2, FLAP, 5LO, LTC4 synthase complex) and cytokine generation by activating various transcriptional factors indirectly via the action of calmodulin-dependent calcineurin (a phosphatase). In the example shown, calcineurin dephosphorylates NFAT, thereby allowing its translocation to the nucleus. ER, endoplasmic reticulum; PM, plasma membrane; NM, nuclear membrane.

in the extracellular medium, these transient spikes occur several times and then dampen out. If extracellular Ca^{++} is present, then the transient spiking persists and often the transients merge into a sustained second phase. It is possible to observe spiking following a stimulus like FMLP, but it only occurs at concentrations of FMLP that do not induce secretion (but may induce chemotaxis). Many cell types display regular or irregular $[Ca^{++}]_i$ oscillations (or spiking) following activation and in some cases this particular behavior may have a functional relevance. But this is difficult to prove and such behavior may only represent the highly non-linear characteristics of this particular signal transduction pathway. Although these single cell characteristics distinguish stimulation with anti-IgE and FMLP, the IgE-mediated response remains one composed of the same two phases.

It is generally felt that the resting plasma membrane potential in mast cells (basophils haven't been studied) is relatively low but the relative negative potential (inside relative to outside) is important for assisting in the chemical potential gradient that brings calcium into the mast cell during stimulation. As calcium flows down this chemical gradient, the charge it brings into the cell can reverse the electrical potential, decreasing

the electrochemical gradient and suppressing further influx. To counter this possibility, human mast cells appear to express a calcium-dependent K efflux channel.[75] Activation of this channel moves potassium out of the cell, re-establishing an electrical gradient and therefore enhancing calcium influx. Specific inhibition of this channel suppresses the calcium response and enhancing $K_{Ca}I$ channel activity, enhances the calcium response and secretion in rat mast cells. Oddly, a gene-chip analysis of several sources of human mast cells did not identify this channel.[76] The expression study did make note of the presence of a large conductance potassium channel mRNA. As with all mRNA expression profiles, the absence of the mRNA does not imply an absence of the protein but more work is needed to understand these expression patterns.

Various Cl^- channels have been described in mast cells, usually rat peritoneal mast cells. If Cl^- flows into the cell, then these channels would enhance the calcium response and if flowing outward, they would down-modulate the calcium response. Studies differ in their conclusions about the role of these anion channels. Expression studies have identified several other ion channels in mast cells but only 1 or 2 Trp channels; in one study only TrpV2 and TrpM2.[76] There are hints in the published and unpublished literature that Trp channels may influence the mast cell response. It is notable that skin mast cells have a different temperature sensitivity to activation when compared to lung mast cells. In accord with their presence in skin, the temperature maximum occurs at 32°C and decreases at higher temperatures. The cytosolic calcium response follows this temperature sensitivity, suggesting a role for a temperature-sensitive Trp channel in regulating the skin mast cell calcium response.

A variety of studies have shown that LTC4 secretion from human basophils is completely dependent on the $[Ca^{++}]_i$ response. This is unlike degranulation for which there are specialized conditions where a calcium response does not appear necessary. A clear example is that stimulation with phorbol esters (which presumably strongly and directly activate some PKC isozymes present in basophils) results in strong degranulation without a $[Ca^{++}]_i$ response, LTC4 release, or free AA generation.[77] This degranulation response to phorbol esters, however, does not occur in mast cells, rodent or human. The absence of free AA generation occurs despite the fact that there is strong activation by PKC of the essential pathway leading to phosphorylation of cytosolic PLA2. This point will be returned to shortly. There are other ways to demonstrate that the $[Ca^{++}]_i$ response may not be necessary even when the stimulus is FMLP, C5a, or anti-IgE antibody. Histamine release occurs during the initial calcium response following FMLP and degranulation is almost completely insensitive to the enforced absence of second phase (by including EGTA during the reaction). However, the initial phase also appears unnecessary and is certainly not sufficient.[78] It is difficult to completely rule out a role for calcium during normal receptor-mediated activation because most of the experimental maneuvers that are used to test the requirement perturb the system in ways that make interpretation problematic. For example, extracellular Ca^{++} may be necessary for the proper maintenance of many homeostatic functions including the detailed structure of membranes themselves. These considerations apply only to human basophils as mast cells have different requirements.

Protein kinase C

This relatively large family of enzymes mediates serine and threonine phosphorylation of a wide variety of substrates. There are several subfamilies defined by their requirements for activation. The first subfamily (α, β_I, β_{II}, γ) is the classically described kinase that is sensitive to the presence of free calcium, diacylglycerol, and phospholipids. There are three other subfamilies, the novel (δ, ε, η, Φ) are regulated by diacylglycerol and phospholipids, the atypical (ζ, λ) enzymes are not sensitive to either calcium or diacylglycerol, and the fourth subfamily (μ and ν) is less well characterized. Following stimulation, some PKC members can be observed to translocate from the cytosol to the plasma membrane. PKC isozymes are expressed in all cells although the precise profile is probably unique to each cell type. As serine/threonine kinases, they mediate a wide variety of phosphorylation events. Since the 'classic' subfamily is sensitive to the presence of both free calcium and diacylglycerols and since both of these second messengers are generated during the early steps of stimulation, it follows that they have a role in secretion. But the role is not well understood and varies depending on the source of mast cells or basophils. As noted above, human basophils are unique in that direct activation of PKC isozymes with phorbol esters results in degranulation without a rise in cytosolic calcium and no AA metabolites or cytokine generation. But human mast cells and rodent mast cells do not display this characteristic.

For rodent mast cells, there are many different indications that PKC isozymes are required for secretion[64,79–82] but for human mast cells and basophils, second- and third-generation PKC inhibitors do not inhibit secretion but instead may lead to modest enhancement of the response.[83,84] Downregulation of PKC expression by overnight treatment with phorbol esters had little effect on IgE-mediated secretion from human lung mast cells but a more marked effect on secretion from human skin mast cells. The ability of PKC enzymes to contribute to downregulation is a common theme in other cell types as well, where PKC-dependent phosphorylation of some receptors results in loss of the receptor from the cell surface. It has also been found that third-generation PKC inhibitors markedly upregulate the activation of ERK in human basophils, an effect that mimics the priming effects of IL-3 in these cells.[85] Resolution of these issues is likely to take some time even with murine models[86–88] and longer for human cell models.

Phospholipase D and phospholipase A2

The metabolism of phospholipids is an integral part of the signal transduction process. However, lipid biochemistry is a difficult area of study and the details of the transformations occurring during signaling are often lacking. It is clear that the generation of PIP3, the generation of IP3 (and other soluble inositol phosphates), and the generation of diacylglycerols are important. Likewise, the generation of arachidonic acid, used in the generation of LTC4 and PGD2 (see below), and the co-generation deacylated phospholipids that can generate platelet activating factor are critical to mediator secretion. Metabolism of sphingolipids is an area just beginning to receive attention in studies of mast cells and basophils. Some of the complexity in lipid research lies in the fact that phospholipids differ in fatty acid composition and that enzymes show selectivity for the composition of head group and fatty acid. As noted above, phospholipase C can generate IP3 and diacylglycerols and the diacylglycerols may be important in the activation of protein kinase C and in the ability of the plasma membrane to fuse with granules (see below). However, it appears that in mast cells, the primary generation of diacylglycerols does not result from the action of PLC but the activity of phospholipase D in a two-stage process of PLD acting on the phospholipids to generate phosphatidic acid followed by phosphate removal by phosphatidate phosphohydrolase (PPH, see Fig. 14.3).[89] Lysophosphatidic acid can be generated from the phosphatidic acid[90] and also play a role in membrane fusion and the phosphatidic acid can interact and regulate the behavior of actin and its polymerization. There are two family members of this protein family and both have been found expressed in mast cells, at least of the rodent variety. The two PLDs contain a lipid-binding Phox domain as well as a PH domain. It is not clear which of these domains is critical to the function of the PLDs in IgE-mediated signaling. But these and other PLD domains also mediate interaction with other proteins. In RBL cells, the location of the two PLDs in resting cells appears to differ, with PLD1 initially located on granule membranes.[91,92] The enzyme is phosphorylated and activated by the action of Src-family kinases.[93] Degranulation appears dependent on PLD activity. More recently, PLD2 has been demonstrated, in RBL cells, to regulate the recruitment of Syk to the early reaction complex in a lipase-independent manner.[94] This is an unexpected behavior for PLD and suggests that it can, in effect, act as an adaptor molecule.

Another class of lipases has, at a minimum, a role in generating free arachidonic acid but may also be important in conditioning the membrane for other changes that are required for secretion. Phospholipase

A2 enzymes remove arachidonic acid from the second position of the glycerol backbone of phospholipids that contain arachidonic acid and in the process also generate lysophospholipids that may be involved in membrane fusion events. There are four groups of PLA2 enzymes expressed in cells and there has been considerable confusion about the role of these enzymes both in the generation of free arachidonic acid and in generating the signaling reaction itself: (1) a growing family of secretory PLA2 enzymes (sPLA2, with 12 members so far), (2) the calcium-sensitive cytosolic PLA2 (cPLA2) enzymes with six known isoforms, (3) the calcium-independent cytosolic PLA2 enzyme (iPLA2), and (4) PAF acetyl hydrolases (PAF-AH). The principal confusion comes from the observations that many cells involved in inflammation, including mast cells and basophils, express all forms of PLA2 enzymes, but in particular express stored sPLA2 enzymes,[95,96] the profile of expression being unique to each cell type. The sPLA2 enzymes are secreted during activation and the extracellular sPLA2, which requires relatively high calcium concentrations for activation, can act on the available cell membranes to generate free arachidonic acid.[96] Some of the sPLA2 family members also bind to extracellular receptors to generate a canonical signal transduction reaction (signaling cascades similar to G-protein linked receptors)[97,98] although a high-affinity receptor for known sPLA2 enzymes has not yet been found in man. This type of activation occurs in the absence of enzymatic activity; lipase-dead mutant sPLA2 enzymes can still activate cells. This mixture of effects and the fact that they are released by mast cells or basophils gives the appearance that the enzymes are important in general signaling. Separating these effects from the normal immunoreceptor or G-protein linked receptor activation might be problematic in some cases although it seems clear that the cells still need their normal activation cascade to result in sPLA2 release. The role of cPLA2 enzymes in the generation of free arachidonic acid is also well studied and will be covered in greater detail below.

Actin cytoskeleton and components of its polymerization

It was noted in the section on lipid rafts that polymerization of actin in the cell influences the persistence of early signals because polymerized actin appears to change the way that the signaling complex stays sorted in lipid rafts. The cytoskeleton plays many roles in the cell dynamics of growth, adhesion, and secretory activation. The signaling steps have been studied extensively in other cell types and with some degree of refinement in mast cell models. Signaling to the polymerization of actin brings up the topic of small G-protein molecular switches that are involved in a wide variety of signaling steps, some of which will be discussed in greater detail below. GTP-binding proteins use the binding of GTP as a molecular switch the way phosphorylation acts as a molecular switch for a wide variety of other proteins. GTP-binding proteins have very slow turnover numbers for the hydrolysis of GTP but this rate is controlled by various types of regulator proteins that determine the lifetime of the on-state of the G-protein. The rho family of G-proteins includes Rho, Rac, and Cdc42.[99] Each of these family members has a different role in regulating the cytoskeleton. Working backwards from signaling elements that drive actin polymerization, one finds the WASP/Arp2/3 complex which controls actin polymerization itself,[100] i.e., the extension of the actin assembly. WASP was discovered as a protein that was altered in Wiskott–Aldrich patients (an immunodeficiency disorder characterized by disordered lymphocyte motility). WASP is activated by

the small G-proteins Rac and Cdc42 which themselves are regulated by the guanine nucleotide exchange factor modulator, VAV. These exchange factors enhance or inhibit the intrinsic GTPase activity of the small G-proteins. VAV itself is known to be phosphorylated and participates in the structure of the early signaling complex and VAV is linked to this complex by interaction with SLP-76, an adaptor protein phosphorylated by Syk.[62,101,102] VAV has multiple domains, one SH2 domain, 2 SH3 domains, 1 PH domain, a Dbl domain and a calponin homology domain. This is, therefore, a complex adaptor and GTPase regulator of the early signaling complex. The adaptor protein Nck also associates with SLP-76 and is itself a regulator of WASP function. The small G-proteins, Rac and Rho also regulate the activation of kinases such as PAK2 and pyk2 which participate in actin polymerization in concert with focal adhesion kinase (FAK). Integration of the various elements into a coordinated signal to properly configure the shape and activity of the cytoskeleton remains a subject of future studies.

SELF-REGULATION OR SIGNAL TERMINATION

The rapid downregulation of the C5a $[Ca^{++}]_i$ response discussed previously and its possible relationship to the action of a PKC isozyme raises the very important topic of self-regulation. For each of the pathways presented, there appears to exist the means to turn off the response. For GTP-binding protein linked receptors such as the FMLP and C5a receptors or chemokine receptors, there are both specific and non-specific methods of downregulating the receptor's ability to respond. Specific methods include a family of specific receptor kinases. There are multiple sites of phosphorylation on the cytoplasmic tail of 7-transmembrane receptors and there are specific and non-specific kinases that mediate the phosphorylation of these sites. PKC might be considered a non-specific method of phosphorylation since a particular PKC member may be able to phosphorylate several types of receptor while β-ARK (β-adrenergic receptor kinase) would be considered a receptor-specific kinase, able only (using the word loosely) to phosphorylate the β-adrenergic receptor. Phosphorylation of this type of receptor is often a signal for another family of proteins, the β-arrestins, to bind to the receptor and mediate their removal from the cell surface, a topic of considerable depth.[103] It is probably safe to say that all receptors are removed from the cell surface following the correct conditions of stimulation. The timing varies enormously, however, and in some cases, removal is not synonymous with loss of activity. The canonical sequence is endocytosis via clathrin-dependent, caveolin-dependent, or clathrin/caveolin-independent pathways to an early endosome. Signaling may persist in the early endosome and receptors can be dissociated from their ligands and recycled back to cell surface. Alternatively, receptors become post-translationally modified (e.g., ubiquitinylation, see below) and further processed to the late endosome and ultimately degraded in lysosomes or proteasomes. Seven-transmembrane receptors are usually endocytosed very rapidly (minutes) while immunoreceptors show a broader range of time constants for loss. The fate of the IgE receptor seems very dependent on the cell model being studied. Both early and more recent studies in RBL cells demonstrate that aggregation of the receptor results in 50% loss from the cell surface in 5 minutes and this loss is temporally consistent with the loss of signaling. However, studies of human basophils showed that there was no loss in the first hours of stimulation although function was lost in tens of minutes. More recent studies do find that loss occurs but with a half-life from the surface of approximately 12h and degradation takes much longer.

Studies in human mast cells haven't been done. For FcεRI, aggregation is required to induce only one form of loss, but, as noted above, this receptor is also lost from the cell surface when its native ligand is not bound, a behavior unlike most receptors. Until recently, it has not been known if this loss mechanism resulted in endocytosis or shedding. However, at least in human basophils, endocytosis occurs and some recycling can be observed.

There are also means to downregulate responses downstream of the receptor, including modification of the GTP-binding proteins themselves, a shared resource that then affects other receptor responses.

For IgE-mediated secretion, there is downregulation that is specific to the receptors being aggregated (i.e., specific for the antigen used to stimulate the cell, which under natural conditions can aggregate only a fraction of the IgE present on the cell surface) and there is downregulation that alters the cell's response to other antigens. Downregulation of the IgE-mediated response acquired the term cellular desensitization and although this process(es) alters the IgE-mediated response, it does not alter in a significant way, the ability of the cell to respond to other non-FcεRI receptors. Recent studies have identified at least one form of this desensitization process. A feature of the human basophil response that appears to distinguish it from rodent mast cell models is that PI3 kinase regulates the activity of p21ras. There are reasonably selective inhibitors of PI3 kinase, some of which are even specific for isozymes of PI3 kinase, which can be shown to inhibit the activation of p21ras when the basophil is stimulated through FcεRI but not when it is activated by FMLP or IL-3.[60]

What makes this particular point in the pathway more interesting is that the PIP3 product of PI3 kinase activity is removed by the action of well-described phosphatases. There is a ubiquitous phosphatase called PTEN (phosphatase and tensin homolog deleted in chromosome 10) that metabolizes PIP3 by removing the 3' phosphate, i.e., the precise reversal of the action of PI3 kinase. PTEN is found in the cytosol and nucleus and there exists a very dynamic equilibrium between its association with the plasma membrane and its location in the cytosol. It has a catalytic domain and a C2 domain that mediates its binding to the plasma membrane.[104] The C2 domain is found in many proteins and basic groups in this domain are known to mediate interaction with the anionic surface of the plasma membrane. Neither the presence of PIP3 nor PTEN's enzymatic activity play a role in binding to the membrane. Instead, PTEN is constitutively active and binding to the membrane determines whether the enzyme has access to its ligand. Membrane binding is masked by multiple phosphorylations on its C-terminal tail and this may be the primary way to regulate substrate access. It is suggested that since only a small fraction of PTEN is associated with the membrane at any given time and that its association is otherwise not dependent on the presence of PIP3, that this characteristic allows PTEN to maintain the basal state of PIP3 without interfering in some types of signaling that require PIP3.[104] Therefore, control of C-terminal phosphorylation is one way that a PTEN set-point can be maintained. PTEN has been identified as an enzyme that is dysregulated in some tumor cells.

In addition to PTEN, there are 2 primary genes in the SHIP (SH2-containing inositol 5'-phosphatase) family, SHIP1 and SHIP2, and there are various molecular weight variants (or splice variants) of SHIP1 and SHIP2 whose specific functions are not well understood. Figure 14.3 outlines these events. SHIP is composed of three well-characterized domains. At the N-terminal end is an SH2 domain and a C-terminal

proline-rich domain that also contains two tyrosines that are phosphorylated when SHIP participates in a signal complex and can bind to signaling elements like Shc, dok-1, and dok-2 that recognize this peptide motif. This latter domain can also interact, as a proline-rich domain, with other SH2 domains. Finally, the central portion of the protein is the catalytic subunit which can hydrolyze, in vitro, PIP3 and the small inositol specific, IP4 (inositol-1,3,4,5 tetraphosphate). Together, these domains provide a means of recruiting SHIP to a signaling complex and may allow SHIP to act like an adaptor protein. In human basophils, translocation of SHIP1 has been observed during IgE-mediated stimulation. Figure 14.5 shows a hypothetical role for SHIP where the SH2 domain brings SHIP to the plasma membrane whereupon it is phosphorylated, possibly by a Src-family kinase like Lyn. In RBL cells, there are indications that SHIP1 is associated with FcεRIβ prior to stimulation.[105] This phosphorylation allows SHIP to recruit negative adaptor proteins like dok-1 that may mediate the downregulation of the ras-MAPK pathway. In this scenario, SHIP acts in two capacities, its catalytic site metabolizing PIP3 and its adaptor function serving to downregulate an important MAPK pathway. SHIP2 has a similar domain structure although it has only one phosphorylated tyrosine motif and its proline-rich region is considerably different from SHIP1. SHIP2 is also more widely expressed than SHIP1, whose expression is largely limited to hematopoietic cells.[106]

The PIP3 lipids recruit various proteins involved in cell survival. For example, PDK-1 and PDK-2 kinases are recruited and phosphorylate Akt. This reaction is common to signaling that initiates secretion but it also is a branch point for pathways that lead to cell survival and proliferation driven by growth hormones. Underexpression of PTEN or its dysregulation can accentuate the presence of growth factor signaling which may account for the role of PTEN in tumor cell behavior. The emerging pattern is that these lipid phosphatases determine the steady-state concentration of PIP3, although the relative role of PTEN or SHIPs appears to depend on the cell being studied. This overall dynamic is therefore of great interest and seems to be a focal point for cellular regulation. In human basophils, secretion of LTC4 ceases after 15 minutes while IL-4 secretion requires several hours. Since secretion of IL-4 requires the creation and maintenance of FcεRI aggregates, just as with histamine and LTC4 secretion, the implication is that some elements of signaling are sustained while others are transient. Indeed, Syk, shc, Grb2/SOS association with shc, and PI3 kinase activation are all sustained when the cells are stimulated with anti-IgE antibody while all elements of the p21ras pathway are transient.[57] This set of observations suggests that somewhere between PI3 kinase activity and p21ras activation is a region of regulation. Preliminary studies suggest that it may be the maintenance of PIP3 levels and that SHIP is the critical regulatory element. Studies in murine mast cells suggest that SHIP expression is an important regulator of secretion.[107] More recent studies in human basophils indicate that SHIP expression determines a hyper-releasable state.[108]

In addition to the lipid phosphatases there are several phosphotyrosine phosphatases that have been identified to participate in the early signaling reaction in mast cells and basophils. SHP-1 and SHP-2 are both well-described phosphatases containing two SH2 domains that allow their recruitment to the early signaling complex. SHP-2 is often found associated with growth factor receptor signaling complexes. In human basophils, SHP-2 is phosphorylated following stimulation with IL-3 but not with anti-IgE antibody. In contrast, SHP-1 is phosphorylated following stimulation with anti-IgE

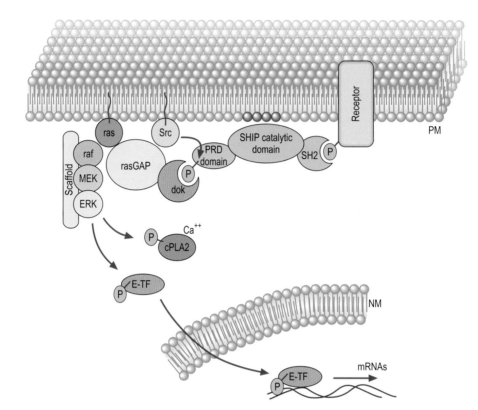

Fig. 14.5. One possible way that SHIP may regulate secretion. The SH2 domain of SHIP interacts with phosphorylated receptor or a phosphorylated adaptor protein which brings the catalytic domain of SHIP into proximity with PIP3 (generated by PI3K) to downregulate this important second messenger (see Fig. 14.3). In addition, localizing SHIP to the membrane allows a kinase, possibly a Src-family kinase, to phosphorylate the C-terminal domain of SHIP, thereby allowing association of dok and its associated rasGAP protein. Proteins like rasGAP induce the catalytic activity of p21ras GTPase, leading to its inactivity as a modulator of Raf and therefore a general shutdown of the raf-MEK-ERK enzyme cascade. Since ERK activity regulates lipid metabolism and transcriptional factors (E-TF), SHIP recruitment to receptor complex ultimately shuts off the generation of a number of mediators. The catalytic removal of PIP3 also decreases recruitment of activation enzymes (like PLC-γ) to the plasma membrane.

antibody but not with IL-3 in basophils. The precise role of SHP enzymes is not always clear although in mast cells SHP-1 appears to regulate signaling to JNK (see below) and the generation of cytokines but not degranulation.[109]

The phosphatase family is large and since so many proteins are regulated by the molecular switch of phosphorylation and since all processes are self-limiting, there exist phosphatases that each have a role in reversing the various kinase activities that are stimulated during secretory activation. In this context, there is an unidentified phosphatase in mast cells that dephosphorylates FcεRIβ and γ ITAMs during and possibly before activation. Hematopoietic cells also express CD45, a receptor-like transmembrane phospho-tyrosine phosphatase that has the potential of regulating the activation of Src-family kinases by hydrolyzing the activation-loop phospho-tyrosine of this family of kinases. For human basophils, aggregation of cell surface CD45 with monoclonal antibodies selectively suppresses IgE-mediated activation,[110] although what is happening during aggregation of CD45 is not clear. Its role in mast cell activation is less clear; there is evidence that genetically inactivating CD45 in mice influences FcεRI-mediated activation but some studies show that it is not regulator of Syk signaling in RBL cells.[111–113]

Adaptor proteins for negative regulation

Since a great deal of effort has been invested in discovering the activating pathways in most cell types, there have consequently been many adaptor proteins discovered that play a positive role in the activating pathways. However, it is now apparent that there are parallel pathways of inactivation that modulate the magnitude of the reaction to suit the particular conditions surrounding the cell. In these pathways, there have been adaptor proteins discovered as well. Table 14.1 shows some of these positive and negative adaptor proteins that have relevance to hematopoietic cells. For the negative adaptor proteins, the dok (downstream of kinase) family is slowly expanding and providing the otherwise absent linkage needed to understand downregulation. There are a family of five dok proteins (1–5) that appear to regulate the recruitment of negative signaling molecules to the reaction complex. For example, dok-1 and dok-2 can bind p120rasGAP (GTPase activating protein) which acts as negative regulator of ras activity. A recent family member, dok-3, has a PH domain that may be critical to the timing of downregulation. Dok-3 is thought to recruit SHIP to the plasma membrane but to do so, it may use its PH domain to associate with the plasma membrane.[114] Since the PH domain is not able to associate with the membrane until PI3 kinase has been active enough to generate PIP3, the downregulatory activity of dok-3, and therefore of SHIP, can't begin until the activating pathway is already well underway. Translocation of dok-3 via its PH domain brings it into proximity of Src-family kinases and following phosphorylation, SHIP is attracted by its SH2-domain, locating SHIP in the region of PIP3 generation by PI3 kinase and presumably downregulating this critical step in signaling. Alternatively, dok-3 may act to isolate Grb2 from the reaction complex.[115] How broadly these schemes apply to immunoreceptor signaling throughout hematopoietic cells, or to mast cells and basophils specifically, is not yet known although dok-1 proteins are associated with FcεRI in resting RBL cells and recruit rasGAP to the signaling complex during activation.[116] As noted below, dok-1 is also associated with the inhibitory signaling induced by co-clustering MAFA and FcεRI.[117]

Co-receptors of negative regulation

It is important to note that the downregulation discussed thus far has been focused on regulation that occurs during active secretion. It is notable that other receptors can recruit downregulatory molecules like SHIP to the membrane prior to activation. An illustrative example

of this process occurs in B cells where one type of IgG receptor (FcγRIIb1) recruits SHIP to its cytoplasmic tail (via a so-called ITIM – immunoreceptor tyrosine inhibition motif) when aggregated (phosphorylation of the ITIM may be accomplished by the action of Lyn kinase) and if the IgG receptor is co-aggregated with the B cell receptor, the SHIP that is brought into the activation complex inhibits or limits the extent of the reaction. A similar mechanism operates in murine mast cells[118,119] and has recently been demonstrated for human basophils.[120] This is an active area of investigation because many receptors are being found that express ITIM motifs or domains that may recruit negative regulatory proteins. It will surely be found that when a cell is surrounded by other cell types in the tissue that its behavior will be the sum result of both positive and negative influences. Some of the negative influences will probably come from ligands found on neighboring cells. A good example of this possibility comes from studies of gp49 deficient mice. The cell surface protein gp49B1 has two negative regulatory ITIMs on its cytoplasmic tail and can act to limit an IgE-mediated reaction on mast cells which express it. Mast cells isolated from gp49 -/- knockout mice do not appear to express a different phenotype, i.e., secretion is similar to wild-type mast cells isolated from the same strain of mouse. However, it is has recently been shown that in vivo mast

Table 14.1 Some positive and negative adaptor proteins that have relevance to hematopoietic cells

	Function
Positive adaptors	
Shc	Binds to several ITAMs, often a linking element for Grb2/SOS
LAT/NLAT	Found in T cells, mast cells and basophils – early scaffold protein for linking PLC-γ
SLP-76	Linker for early signaling complex in T cells and mast cells
Grb2	Often found constitutively associated with SOS, contains SH2 and SH3 domains
SOS	Induces the activation of GTPase, notably p21ras, linking immunoreceptor to ras
VAV	Induces the activation of rho-like GTPases, has a PH domain that mediates is translocation
Blnk	Linker involved in early BCR signaling in B cells
Negative adaptors	
dok-1	Associates with ITIM motifs to recruit rasGAP, a protein that induces GTPase activity, turning off ras
dok-2	Binds to ITIMs, also recruits rasGAP
dok-3	Has a PH domain and after phosphorylation, recruits SHIP and/or CSK
SHIP	Although not strictly an adaptor, it appears to sometimes serve this role by recruiting dok-1
Negative regulating co-receptors	
FcγRMB	Low-affinity IgG receptor with cytoplasmic ITIM
LIR	Leukocyte inhibitory receptors (five family members), now termed LILR (also CD85a-m)
KIR	Killer (cell) Ig-like/inhibitory receptor
MAFA	Mast cell function associated antigen
SIRPs	Signal regulatory proteins
gp49B	See text
siglecs	Sialic acid-binding Ig-related lectins (15 family members, some with cytoplasmic ITIMs)

cell-dependent reactions are much stronger in knockout mice.[121] One potential ligand for gp49B1 appears to be the integrin $\alpha_v\beta_3$,[122] which is expressed on many tissue cell types. The juxtaposition of the mast cell to cells expressing this ligand appears to act as a break on their secretion (the wild-type condition), so that the absence of the gp49B1 results in a stronger response to stimulation, but only in a context where the ligand for gp49B1 is appropriately presented to the mast cell, as with the in vivo studies. Mast cells and basophils express other receptors known to operate by possession of ITIM-like motifs on their cytoplasmic tails. These include the FcgRIIb receptor, various LIR (leukocyte inhibitory receptors), MAFA (mast cell function associated antigen),[117,123] CD200R,[124] LMIR1 (leukocyte mono-Ig-like receptor),[125] and Siglec-8.[126] It is not well understood when these receptors are operative in vitro or in vivo and often the ligands remain unknown as well.

Downregulation by ubiquitinylation

An important mechanism of signal regulation includes the processing of signaling proteins by 26S proteasome-mediated degradation. The 26S proteasome is a very large macromolecular complex responsible for proteolytic digestion of intracellular proteins and one of its principal methods for identifying proteins for processing is the attachment of the 8 kDa protein ubiquitin to the target protein. To accomplish ubiquitinylation of the target protein, cells express a large family of ubiquitin ligating enzymes. Monomeric ubiquitin generated by an E1 ligase is transferred to one of 25 known E2 ligases found in cells. It is the association of E2 ligases with highly selective E3 ligases that confers a selective ligation of ubiquitin to target proteins. The current model has the E3 ligase bound to its target protein and to an E2 ligase. The E2 ligase transfers ubiquitin to the E3 ligase and E3 transfers the ubiquitin to the target protein via an isopeptide bond which links the amino terminal side chain of target protein lysines to ubiquitin. Proteins that are targeted for degradation are generally polyubiquinated, often with a chain of ubiquitins. Mono-ubiquitinylation is usually not sufficient to allow recognition of the protein by the 26S proteasome. In the IgE-mediated signaling reaction, the family of Cbl ligases takes the role of the needed E3 ligase. The Cbl family is composed of 7 members of which c-Cbl and b-Cbl have been studied in some detail in RBL cells,[127–129] in murine mast cells,[130] and to a lesser extent in human basophils.[131] Cbl is composed of a N-terminal tyrosine-binding domain (TKB), a central ring-finger domain that binds an E2 ligase, a central proline-rich domain (PRO) that binds to SH3 domains and a C-terminal leucine zipper domain. The TKB and PRO domains, are involved in binding to the target proteins. In mast cells and basophils, Syk is a clear target of Cbl. The TKB domain of Cbl has been shown to bind to phosphorylated Y323 of Syk, the interlinker tyrosine originally described to be a negative regulatory site of Syk. This tyrosine appears to be phosphorylated by a Src-family kinase rather than by Syk itself. The working model is that Syk phosphorylated on this tyrosine binds to Cbl and becomes ubiquitinylated. A classical ladder of Syk-polyubiquitin species (with a molecular weight separation of multiples of 8–9 kDa) can be observed on Western blots of activated RBL cells and human basophils. There may be other pro-activating roles for Cbl in the early signaling complex. There are also indications from studies in RBL cells that Lyn kinase and FcεRIα become ubiquitinylated during activation.[132] Cbl itself is phosphorylated during activation and an interesting feature of phosphorylation in stimulated human basophils is that phosphorylation is persistent for much longer than many other early signaling elements. One could speculate that since Cbl is acting as a downregulator of Syk expression, its persistent activation reflects the long-term consequence and slow processing of Syk for elimination. In human basophils, the downregulation of Syk expression is too slow for its elimination to have a significant impact on the release of class I and II mediators. However, it seems likely that it may be responsible for some non-specific desensitization (see below) of the cell and possibly regulate late cytokine secretion (class III mediators). Whether c-Cbl or b-Cbl mediates this process probably depends on the cell being studied. Recent studies in RBL cells suggests that b-Cbl is the form most responsible for downregulating Syk expression,[127,129,130] while in basophils it is clear that c-Cbl associates with Syk during activation.[131]

PUTTING THE PIECES TOGETHER

It is apparent that there are many components in the early signaling complex and each of the components usually has multiple amino acids that can be phosphorylated. Of the many questions that arise, it is reasonable to ask how many of the potential states that can be described are important for signaling. In other words, how much do we need to know about the details of this system to adequately predict its behavior. Recent mathematical studies have begun to address this question. In a model that consisted of dimeric aggregated FcεRI with two phosphorylation sites per receptor (one for FcεRIβ and one for FcεRIγ with a single γ site acting as a lumped version of the two actual ITAM sites), one Lyn kinase with no phosphorylation states but able to bind through its unique domain or through its SH2 domain, and one Syk kinase with two possible phosphorylation states, one can describe 354 possible species of complex with 3680 possible unidirectional reactions.[133] Note that this model excludes many possible phosphorylation sites for Syk, Lyn and receptor and therefore already represents a scaled-down version of the core signaling complex. In such a complex network of possible states, the first question is whether at optimal stimulation, there is only a subset of states that are visited during the reaction. This is indeed the case, with only small portion of the possible 354 states being 'visited' during the reaction. However, as the reaction conditions change, either altering the amount of Syk or Lyn available or the amount of dimeric IgE (to induce dimeric aggregates), it becomes apparent that many of the other states are visited, although for each condition, only a small portion of possible states are involved. In other words, to make accurate predictions about the outcomes of different starting conditions, all the possible states must be included in the model. Some testing of the model against experimental evidence has been done in studies of RBL cells.[133]

The modeling technique that is discussed in these studies has been termed a domain-oriented microscopic view of signal transduction. A description of the various signaling elements in this chapter has focused on domain structure because it now appears that much of our understanding of signaling comes from understanding which domains are present. The experimentalist uses this approach extensively by swapping domains to explore the role they play in the signaling reaction. These models, while very complex, and yet still simple relative to reality, nevertheless make some interesting predictions regarding the IgE-mediated signaling reaction in mast cells and basophils. For example, one very difficult aspect of the reaction to predict without a reasonably comprehensive model is the effect of different levels of Syk or Lyn on the output of the signaling complex.[134] There are many non-linear effects in this system that are related to protecting phosphorylation of sites of the various components and these cannot be appreciated by other modeling techniques. For example, Syk is not only activated by binding to γ subunit ITAMs but also protects the ITAM phosphorylation sites of the γ subunit from dephosphorylation. In basophils, the expression of Syk appears to be an important predictor of response (see below), so these models make explicit predictions about the general behavior of the system under conditions where Syk is limiting and Lyn is not.[135] A different approach to modeling can be seen in the phenomenological model of signaling that has been called kinetic proofreading. The general idea is that if a ligand dissociates rapidly, before some of the early signaling modifications are completed, e.g., phosphorylation, then a signal does not propagate completely. In effect, this model examines the impact of different rates of ligand dissociation and state changes in the affected components on the final outcome (for example, what is the predicted outcome of comparing two ligands with equal affinity constants but one ligand has a fast forward and reverse binding constant while the other has a slow forward binding constant compensated by a slow reverse binding constant?). Ligands that dissociate more slowly result in much stronger signals even though they may actually result in lower equilibrium values of ligand-bound receptor. Some experimental systems provide support for kinetic proofreading, including FcεRI-mediated signaling.[136] However, there are also several experimental results that do not fit with this phenomenological description. The domain-oriented models not only recapitulate the kinetic proofreading phenomenon but also show how some responses escape this phenomenon.[137] For example, cytokine synthesis is largely independent of kinetic proofreading while histamine release is not. The microscopic domain-oriented models provide some predictions on what to look for that would allow this type of outcome while the phenomenological and heuristic models do not. Another example of the power of the domain-oriented approach involves the multi-point attachment sites of adaptor molecules. Because the response depends on several components being assembled in a single adaptor molecule in order to juxtaposition the required elements, one can see that too much adaptor protein might actually inhibit a reaction because excess adaptor would bind components more sparsely (same number of total bound species but not necessarily co-located on the same adaptor). This situation has been modeled for the FcεRI-mediated reaction described above but where Syk concentration is varied and the Lyn concentration is saturating and it demonstrates an inhibitory region in the ligand concentration–dependence curve that is no longer concordant with the magnitude of aggregation.[134] Such situations are found in the IgE mediated reaction, e.g., the dose response curve for polyclonal anti-IgE antibody stimulation, although the biological basis for experimental observations has not been determined.

Feedback augmentation or inhibition of signaling

The hallmark of the mast cell and basophil response is the secretion of numerous mediators. There is the plethora of granule contents, a variety of lipid species that are well-described mediators, like PGD2 or LTC4, but also lipids that are less abundant. Later in the reaction, there are cytokines and other proteins secreted. A reasonable question is whether some of these molecules feedback in an autocrine fashion to modulate the mast cell/basophil response,[138] either an ongoing response or a response that might occur in the future. For example, basophils express histamine and LTC4 receptors and like many 7-transmembrane receptors, these receptors initiate rapid

changes internally, negative in the case of H_2 receptors, or positive in the case of LTCR1. Likewise, there are several, or even many, cytokine chemokine, and growth factor receptors. The answer to the general question is mixed. Thus far, the inclusion of histamine receptor or LTC4 antagonists hasn't been found to alter the ongoing response in basophils. On the other hand, histamine can be shown to rapidly induce an increase in cAMP levels, which, if applied before stimulation, can reduce secretion.[139] Application of LTC4 to basophils causes very modest transient elevations in cytosolic calcium,[140] so the absence of clear effects on ongoing secretion is puzzling. Studies in mast cells have now shown that a variety of Edg receptors (that bind several different species of lipids) augment the ongoing response. For example, sphingosine-1-phosphate that is generated in the early IgE-mediated reaction can feed-forward, when released from the cell, to further drive a cytosolic calcium response (and other signaling pathways).[141,142]

LATTER SIGNALING EVENTS

Thus far, the discussion has primarily covered signaling elements that assemble in the earliest steps of the reaction. As one moves away in time (ms to s to min) from these initial events, the model is more spotty. Generally, further downstream events are better known when they are specifically related to well-described functional endpoints. For each of the classes of mediators, there is additional detail. Although histamine release was one of the first mediators to be studied, there is actually not a lot known about the very complex granule fusion biochemistry beyond some general principles being learned about granule fusion in other cell types. In the last few years, several groups have begun working on the protein assemblies that mediate granule fusion in RBL cells but the connections between some of these steps and earlier signaling steps are not well described. Considerably more is known about class II mediators like LTC4 and PGD2 because of its linkage to the ras-ERK pathway. Finally, class III mediators like IL-4 have been studied in great detail in other cell types and much of this knowledge has been translated to mast cells.

Degranulation

Granule release is complicated by the observation that there are, in fact, several morphological forms of degranulation. Two clear cut modalities of degranulation have been termed piece-meal and anaphylactic (AND).[143] Piece-meal degranulation appears to involve a constant transport of large granule contents in small vesicles shuttling between the granule and the plasma membrane. Anaphylactic degranulation involves the wholesale fusion of a granule with the plasma membrane so that its interior becomes congruent with the extracellular space. The type of degranulation that occurs depends on the stimulus and time point being examined. Some stimuli, such as FMLP (a 7-transmembrane receptor/GTP binding protein-dependent receptor) induce both types of degranulation with piece-meal dominating the early phase of release (first seconds) and the AND form becoming more visibly apparent at latter times (10s of seconds).[144] It is in this context that the signaling steps must be considered.

The general model of granule fusion has been worked out using a wide variety of cell models. The basic scheme involves the establishment of a macromolecular complex of proteins on both the vesicle and plasma membranes. These integral membrane proteins are the so-called SNAREs (soluble NSF attachment proteins): a t-SNARE (target-SNARE) and v-SNARE (vesicle SNARE). The SNAREs are composed of proteins of the syntaxin and SNAP families. A critical conceptual piece of this model is that t-SNAREs and v-SNAREs must co-assemble to form a single so-called trans-complex (i.e., one membrane group associating with a different membrane group). But SNAREs can form a cis-complex, i.e., SNAREs in the same membrane forming these complexes. If SNAREs were free of outside influences, the cis-conformations would disallow the formation of trans-complexes. Therefore, an integral component of the process is the catalytic activity of NSF (N-ethylmaleimide-sensitive factor) and other soluble NSF-attachment proteins, which dynamically maintain enough SNARE in a non-cis-conformation so that they can from trans-complexes when needed for granule fusion. Studies in RBL cells (and occasionally in bone-marrow-derived mast cells), have outlined the family members present in the SNARE complexes.[145] On the plasma membrane side, SNAP-23 and syntaxin-4 have been identified and on the granule side, syntaxin-3, VAMP-3 (vesicle-associated membrane protein), VAMP-7, and VAMP-8 have also been identified. Studies in RBL cells have shown that NSF is required to maintain a state of readiness for granule fusion, as predicted from the canonical model.[146] Like most signaling proteins, there are various possible phosphorylation states for SNARE proteins but there has been some controversy about changes in the state of SNAP-23 and syntaxin-4 phosphorylation[147] during stimulation of RBL cells through FcεRI. Recent studies show changes in phosphorylation of SNAP-23 on a time scale consistent with degranulation.[148] Modification of the relevant phosphorylated amino acids alters fusion events. More recent studies have found that SNAP-23 is partially associated with lipid rafts prior to stimulation and this association increases during stimulation.[149] Syntaxin-4 is not associated with rafts until stimulation and it likely becomes associated by its attachment to SNAP-23. If this process of lipid raft association is relevant to granule fusion, then the linkage between early events and histamine release might be considerably short, i.e., any process establishing lipid rafts and active kinases in the lipid rafts might be sufficient to drive phosphorylation of SNAP-23 and induction of SNARE trans-complexes. However, this viewpoint has not been formally established.

Arachidonic acid metabolites and the ERK pathway

LTC4, prostaglandin D2, and related lipid mediators require the generation of free arachidonic acid from cellular pools of lipids and phospholipids. As noted previously, generation of free arachidonic acid results from the action of phospholipase A2. Although there remain some issues regarding the type of PLA2 responsible for the bulk of free AA generation, the consensus view based on available evidence is that cytosolic PLA2 (cPLA2) is the enzyme responsible. Unlike iPLA2 or PAF-AH, cPLA2 requires elevated cytosolic calcium although its calcium requirements are in the submicromolar range (compared to the perimicromolar range for sPLA2s). The (85 kDa) enzyme consists of a calcium-binding domain and catalytic domain. For full activation, the cytosolic calcium must be elevated above resting levels of 50–80 nM (which induces translocation rather than altering enzymatic activity) and the enzyme must be phosphorylated (Ser 505, 517 or 727). The dual requirement for activation introduces some interesting biology to the generation of AA. Phosphorylation can be asynchronous with the calcium elevation and the enzyme doesn't generate free AA.[73] Translocation to cellular membranes, notably ER or nuclear membranes, occurs during activation, placing the enzyme in the vicinity of the correct phospholipids. Since LTC4 generating enzymes also must be membrane bound and appear to locate on nuclear membranes, the LTC4 generating complex is brought together by calcium elevations. Available evidence suggests that the mitogen activated kinase (MAPK), ERK 1/2, is responsible for phosphorylation of cPLA2.[150–152] Mice lacking cPLA2 develop normally but inflammatory reactions are blunted.[153]

The MAP kinases are a family of kinases that are ubiquitous and often involved in some way with many forms of signaling. The three canonical terminal MAP kinases are ERK (extracellular regulated kinase), JNK (c-Jun NH2-terminal kinase), and p38. However, these three are part of an extended family; there are 9 ERK members, 3 JNK members, and 4 p38 members. ERK 1/2 is the most intensively studied of the MAP kinases and the signaling cascade to ERK is very well described. In a limited way it also provides a model for the nature of the signaling to JNK and p38 but the inputs to the various MAPK pathways should not be considered similar. For example, in fyn knockout mice, the ERK pathway is intact while activation of p38 and JNK is suppressed.[45] The MAP kinases each are phosphorylated by a MAPKK and these kinases in turn phosphorylated by a MAPKKK. There is a canonical tyrosine-x-threonine peptide within each MAPK that is dual phosphorylated to initiate activation. For ERK 1/2, the antecedent kinase is MEK 1/2 and the antecedent kinase for MEK is Raf-1. There are at least 7 members of the MEK family and a poorly determined number of MAPKKK members. This signaling unit has been described as a ultrasensitive enzyme cascade.[154] The terminology refers the behavior of each subsequent component to a linear input signal that starts at the top of the cascade. As one moves down the chain, the activation curve becomes progressively more sigmoidal, with ERK activation appearing very step-like (Fig. 14.6). Whether this behavior is universal and a part of mast cell activation has yet to be determined. The precise nature of the activation is known to be dependent on many factors. First, the Raf-1/ERK sequence is built upon a complex scaffold of proteins that determine which ERK is activated. Second, there are many input pathways to modulate each of the steps. Working backwards, Raf-1 (MAPKKK) is activated by the ubiquitous p21ras small GTP-binding protein. As noted previously, these molecular switch proteins depend on GTP binding for allosteric activation and because they are GTPases, their relative activity is modulated by proteins that change the turnover rate of the catalytic site. For p21ras, for which there are multiple family members, there are several entry points. Ras has a fatty acid chain that allows it to be associated with the plasma membrane. For IgE-mediated secretion, one entry point to ras activation is the association between SOS (son-of-sevenless) and Grb2 (SOS is a quanine nucleotide exchange factor, inducing p21ras into the GTP bound form to increase its activity). The Grb2-SOS dimer is sometimes considered constitutively dimeric although certain forms of activation can reduce the association.[155] Grb2 is a multi-domain adaptor protein (1 SH2 domain and 2 SH3 domains) that can associate with Shc, another multi-domain adaptor (1 SH2 domain and an N-terminal PTB domain) that is phosphorylated by Syk. The phosphorylation of Shc results in recruitment of Grb2-SOS to the plasma membrane and therefore juxtaposition with p21ras, initiating the ras/ERK cascade. Therefore, in broad outline, the entire pathway from receptor aggregation to LTC4 generation has been described. Factors modulating this cascade remain less clear. Although ERK activation leads to cPLA2 phosphorylation, the dimer of ERK also translocates to the nucleus to mediate transcriptional events. The other MAP kinases also mediate various transcription reactions.

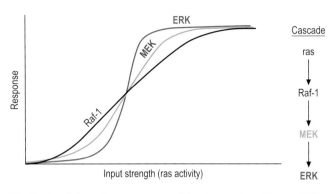

Fig. 14.6. Schematic representation of the ultrasensitive p21ras to ERK pathway. Each signaling element downstream of ras may show a progressively sigmoidal response pattern relative to the linear input signal at the top of the cascade (ras activity).

Cytokine generation

The class III mediators are perhaps the largest class because the ability of the mast cell and basophil to make new proteins long after the fast mediators have stopped being secreted is an open-ended set of possibilities. The number of proteins synthesized and used for the purpose of modifying the extracellular environment is steadily growing; there have been at least 30 cytokines, chemokines and growth factors described as being generated following IgE-mediated activation of mast cells and at least 15 generated from activated basophils, a cell with a far more limited lifespan than mast cells. This does not even consider the proteins that are synthesized that contribute to phenotypic plasticity, a well-documented behavior of mast cells and to a lesser extent, basophils. As a consequence of this complexity, there are many signaling pathways that are only partially understood or completely unknown that lead to the generation of class III mediators. However, there is some progress for several types of cytokines. Notably, cytokine generation that is under the control of the transcription factor NF-κB (nuclear factor-κB) has a somewhat complete path from FcεRI aggregation to gene transcription. While details are ultimately critical, the knowledge obtained from studies in many other cell types about how NF-κB regulates gene transcription is generally applicable to mast cells (the likely difference between mast cells and basophils and other cell types is the nature of the 'open' chromatin, i.e., the genes that are readily available for modification as the profile of chromatin availability partially defines the phenotype of the cell). What is needed for this discussion is how to connect activation of NF-κB to FcεRI aggregation.

The NF-κB transcription factor consists of 5 known family members, NF-κB1, NF-κB2, RelA, RelB, and c-Rel. These members combine into various homo- or heterodimers but a dominant form includes the p50/RelA heterodimer. In the resting state, this transcription factor is found in the cytoplasm linked to a IkB (inhibitor of kB) protein. It is the phosphorylation of IkB by the IkB kinase (IKK) complex that induces dissociation of IkB from NF-κB and the degradation of IkB by the 26S proteosome due to its targeted ubiquitinylation after phosphorylation. The dissociated NF-κB is free to migrate to the nucleus where it mediates gene transcription. Although there may be other factors involved in the transcription of specific genes, NF-κB is a necessary factor in the expression of some new genes.

Recent studies have suggested that the IKK complex is activated by a pair of molecules, Bcl10 and Malt1, initially described in Malt lymphomas and now known to be required for some signaling steps in B and T cell responses to antigen. Knocking out Bcl10 or Malt1 in mice doesn't effect mast cell development or the generation of many early signaling steps in FcεRI-dependent activation. Neither histamine nor leukotriene release or early signaling steps in mast cells were altered in these knockout mice but secretion of TNF-α and IL-6, cytokines whose generation is dependent on NF-kB, was impaired.[156,157] It was noted above that the MAP kinases also mediate gene transcription after translocating to the nucleus and it was found that eliminating Bcl10/Malt1 did not alter activation of the MAP kinases. The Bcl10/Malt1 complex is phosphorylated by PKCβ and since PKCβ is activated by elevations in cytosolic calcium and the presence of diacylglycerol (see above); there is a reasonably well understood sequence of events that leads to NF-κB-dependent cytokine generation.

A similar gene transcriptional pathway could be described for those genes whose transcription is dependent on NFAT (nuclear factor of activated T cells) gene transcriptional factors (e.g., IL-4). Activation of the various NFAT family members (five known) is dependent on calcineurin, a calcium, calmodulin-dependent phosphatase that dephosphorylates NFAT. In the resting state, NFAT is heavily phosphorylated by several kinases including casein kinase I, p38, JNK, GSK3 (glycogen synthase kinase 3), and DYRK (dual specificity tyrosine phosphorylation regulated kinase). Current evidence suggests that different domains of NFAT are phosphorylated by these various kinases, maintaining the resting state. The apparent absolute dependence of dephosphorylation of NFAT by calcineurin and its absolute dependence on the calcium-calmodulin co-factor suggests that this pathway is relatively short. Any elevation of cytosolic calcium would lead to NFAT dephosphorylation. However, not all stimuli that elevate cytosolic calcium, fMLP in particular in human basophils, lead to cytokine secretion. Therefore, either the fMLP calcium elevation is too short-lived or there are other signaling pathways following aggregation of FcεRI that allow dephosphorylated NFAT to act on its target genes.

CONTROL OF SIGNALING BY REGULATION OF EXPRESSION

Natural expression levels

An important concept in any biological process is the notion of set-points. The question is where does the particular sensitivity of a biological system come from? This question has been asked of all receptor-mediated signaling events and has also been asked about IgE-mediated secretion from mast cells and basophils. It was noted above that the typical peripheral blood human basophil and human lung mast cell require approximately 2000 antigen-specific IgE molecules (per cell) to trigger a half-maximal response to antigenic stimulation. In this description, half-maximal response refers to histamine release, i.e. release of a pre-formed mediator. This particular set-point may not apply to secretion of other classes of mediators. It also refers to the notion that maximal release is variable. The definition used the term half-maximal because not all cells have the capability of full degranulation even when optimally stimulated through the IgE receptor. As noted previously, this is not a subpopulation issue, at least not in wild-type cells. All cells respond (although there is a single cell distribution), they simply do not respond such that they fully degranulate. It is apparent that there is a process that limits secretion. There is also a mechanism that establishes the set-point for the response. In studies of human mast cells and basophils, the range of responsiveness is considerable but studies in mast cells are confounded by the difficulty in isolating the cells from a broad range of subjects. In contrast, studies of circulating basophils are relatively straightforward and a wide variety of clinical states can be examined. Here it is found that stimulating the isolated basophils (the preparations can range from whole blood to purified basophils) with an optimal concentration of anti-IgE Ab (a concentration that establishes the optimum number of aggregates) results in histamine release that ranges from 0 to 100%. Similarly, it can be shown that cellular sensitivity, i.e., the density of cell surface antigen-specific IgE needed for an optimal concentration of antigen to induce a half-maximal response, ranges from 300 to 30 000 molecules per basophil. These distributions are reasonably Gaussian but the tails of the distributions are interesting for their implications concerning system responsiveness. The origins of this kind of biological variation has been a topic of study. Some early studies identified a phenotype of basophils that were called 'non-releasers'.[158] These cells were normally responsive to non-IgE-mediated stimulation (e.g., FMLP or C5a) but unresponsive to stimulation through FcεRI. The cells expressed normal levels of FcεRI occupied with IgE but there was no apparent response to a stimulus that aggregates the IgE (mediator secretion, adherence, etc.). This phenotype was ultimately discovered to poorly express Syk,[159,160] which, as noted previously, is critical for secretion. However, this absence of Syk is simply the low tail of a population distribution of Syk kinase expression. A survey of the general population shows that the maximal response to anti-IgE Ab correlates quite well with expression of Syk kinase.[135] A total of 20 signaling elements have been studied thus far (some published and some unpublished) and the population variance of Syk expression is the greatest of the group. Indeed, for many of the other proteins, the population distribution is as narrow as one could expect given the inherent variability of the measurement technique. This narrowness in the distribution in a heterogeneous population is, in itself, an interesting observation, the significance of which is not known. The survey also established a quantity of Syk kinase per basophil, the value ranged from 6000 to 60 000 molecules per cell, a number that is interesting because the receptor density averages approximately 150 000 in this population. In contrast, Lyn kinase showed a very narrow distribution centered on approximately 100 000 molecules per cell. Given the established importance of Syk in generating the secretory reaction, it seems likely that this population distribution of Syk is a reasonable, although causally unproven, explanation for the population variation in responsiveness.

The same survey asked a related question about the expression of SHIP1 (SH2-containing inositol 5'-phosphatase, see above). Studies in mice with this gene knocked-out demonstrated that mast cells were hyper-responsive to IgE-mediated stimulation.[107] As discussed above, SHIPs role in secretion may be multifaceted, acting as an adaptor and a downregulator of the reaction being driven by PI3 kinase through its generation of PIP3. The mouse studies suggested that the dominant role was therefore one of downregulation and that regulation of SHIP expression might be a means for the cell to adjust the set-point of the response. The basophil population survey found that SHIP expression was more variable than many other signaling elements, with the exception of Syk, and a multi-regression analysis of Syk and SHIP, the expression of the two elements together, accounted for more variance in maximum

histamine release than either alone. In this analysis, SHIP had a weak inverse relationship; however, SHIP expression levels only accounted for one-sixth of the variance in the correlation as Syk expression. Therefore, regulation of SHIP expression in this study had only a very modest inverse impact on secretion. This may not always be the case. Histamine-releasing factor (HRF-p23) is a cytokine that in a selected subpopulation of individuals induces mediator release from human basophils.[161] It also appears that this same subpopulation is sensitive to other ligands that normally only 'prime' the basophil response but in this unique group of subjects, also directly induce secretion. Current evidence supports the hypothesis that this cytokine has a distinct receptor that otherwise shares many of the signaling characteristics of IgE-mediated release. For example, HRF induces Syk phosphorylation and secretion is inhibited by newer generations of Syk inhibitors. In individuals that respond to HRF with secretion, SHIP expression is 4–5-fold lower than the normal population.[108] Therefore, there appear to be at least some in vivo conditions that modulate SHIP expression which may predispose the basophil to respond to stimuli that otherwise only prime the basophil response.

One of the tasks of signal transduction biologists is to discover pathways that are unique to a particular situation because such pathways might be a target for therapeutic intervention that does not have collateral effects. In a similar context, it is also useful to discover which of the many signaling elements that are being described as necessary in the cell response are explicitly regulated by natural mechanisms. The survey information above addresses this later point. The apparently specific modulation of Syk in circulating human basophils suggests that nature has focused its attention on this element as a way to modulate secretion. Discovering how this modulation occurs is the next task. The distribution of Syk expression in peripheral blood basophils has not been explored in tissue mast cells, so this particular mechanism for controlling the mast cell response among subjects is not yet identified.

Downregulation of expression

Whether or not Syk expression is a generally important point of regulation for IgE-mediated secretion in mast cells and basophils, there is a general search for information regarding the change in expression levels of signaling elements in mast cells and basophils following a variety of methods of conditioning the cell response. For example, long-term exposure of these cells to cytokines to induce phenotypic changes is a common approach. It is likely that any overt phenotypic change is accompanied by a change in the expression level of some protein rather than simply inducing post-translational modifications of existing elements (which does occur following short exposures). Of particular interest are changes in IgE-mediated secretion due to changes in signal element expression level. Work with cytokines is complicated by the conditions of cell handling. For example, tumor cell lines are often driven by changes in growth receptors or closely associated molecules. Similarly, long-term cultures of mast cells, murine or human, are complicated by (1) the cells are undergoing differentiation rather than already being mature and (2) there is a complex pre-existing cytokine environment used to produce the cultured cells. Therefore, study of cytokine modulation that alters signal element expression is inseparable from how these molecules are altering the maturing cell. Some insights have come from study of peripheral blood basophils. These cells are arguably in their resting mature state prior to cytokine exposure and therefore, the subsequent influence of cytokines may properly reflect the nature of the changes in the signal transduction apparatus. Initial exposure of basophils to a cytokine like IL-3 results in some fast post-translational modifications that immediately influence mediator release. For example, IL-3 induces activation of the ras-ERK pathway and modifies the rate that components in this pathway are dephosphorylated.[85] The activation of ERK and therefore phosphorylation of cPLA2 primes the cell to any stimulus that induces an elevation in cytosolic calcium resulting in synergistic activity of cPLA2 and augmented arachidonic acid generation and LTC4 release. Culturing the basophils for 24 hours results in a return of the resting behavior of the ERK pathway when responding to secretagogues but an augmentation of the cytosolic calcium response occurs. The basis for augmentation at 24 h is not yet known but the enhanced cytosolic calcium response enhances all mediator release and other outcomes. On a 2–4 day timeframe, continued exposure to IL-3 begins to change the phenotype of the basophil. For example, IL-3 converts a non-releasing basophil (see above) to one that releases to IgE-mediated stimulation.[162] This change is accompanied by an increase in Syk expression.[163] However, changes in other signaling elements are even greater than the change in Syk expression.[135] For example, SHIP1 expression is increased 2–6-fold while Syk changes only 50–80%. IL-3 also induces some very late cytokine secretion without stimulation from a secretagogue (FMLP, IgE aggregation, etc.). For example, IL-13 is induced as is the generation of gramicidin B which is added to the granule contents, suggesting that even the granules show phenotypic plasticity.[164] However, no signal element has yet been identified to decrease.

To observe downregulation of signaling components, mast cells and basophils are stimulated to aggregate the IgE receptor.[131,165] As noted above, stimulation of Syk kinase ultimately leads to its ubiquitinylation and degradation. In human basophils, 20-fold reductions in Syk expression could be observed. There were also very modest changes in the expression of Lyn kinase and after 2–3 days, nearly complete removal of involved aggregated cell surface receptor. An examination of 22 other signaling elements did not reveal any changes; therefore, the ability of the cell to downregulate signaling species appears restricted to only the earliest elements involved in the core receptor signaling complex.[135] Recent studies have shown that Syk expression can be reduced by non-IgE-dependent receptor activation. This is especially true of receptors that also use Syk kinase in their early signaling complex but also occurs to a limited extent with FMLP receptors that do not activate Syk. These observations raise the possibility that signal element expression can be modulated by other receptors expressed on the basophil or mast cell surface.

THERAPEUTIC SIGNIFICANCE

This chapter has focused on signaling pathways that are often shared by several receptors. Each new pathway element, initially thought to be specific, is often found to be involved in multiple signaling events. This economy of resources by the cell makes sense from one perspective but it complicates our ability to understand the nature of specific responses. It also makes elements that are shared less appealing as therapeutic targets. The problem of finding specific therapeutic targets is compounded when more than one cell type is considered. Many of the signaling elements that are well described today are not unique to one particular cell type. So even if the signaling element appears uniquely involved in

one receptor signal transduction pathway in one cell type, it is likely to be used by other cell types in a different way. For example, for the moment, Syk kinase has a central role in IgE-mediated signaling in human basophils and mast cells. Other secretory receptor pathways in basophils are now known to use this kinase but unless Syk kinase has a role in basophil or mast cell development, or an unknown physiological role for mast cells, this might be considered a good target for a therapeutic. However, Syk is certainly a central kinase in immunoreceptor function in other cells of the immune system as well as cells outside of the immune system. Therefore, developing a therapeutic agent that targets Syk kinase has a good chance of being non-selective in its effects. This is a particular problem for non-life-threatening (or only marginally so) diseases that are chronic in nature. One approach to this general problem is to less aggressively inhibit the activity of any one target but, with a more detailed understanding of the entire signaling pathway, choose to target several elements which, taken together, specifically characterize one cell type and therefore result in only its inhibition. For example, one might speculate that specific, but partial, inhibition of both Syk kinase and PI3 kinase δ might afford some selectivity to inhibition of the human basophil response. For the IgE-mediated response in basophils, both kinase activities appear to be required but the particular pattern of expression and requirement might be somewhat unique to the basophil. Other cells use Syk and PI3 kinase but often use other PI3 kinase family members, or if they use PI3 kinase δ, may not use Syk. This is not the usual approach to drug development because for FDA approval, each agent must be efficacious for the indication desired. But, there are many instances of combined drug therapies for disease treatment, so it remains a possibility. There are also several instances where drugs that inhibit a signal element common in many cell types (e.g., PKCβ1) nevertheless appear to still have some selective therapeutic benefit.[166,167]

There is an alternative, although related, approach. The unique phenotype that characterizes a cell type results from unique patterns of gene expression. It may be possible to find unique expression controls for certain signaling elements that track with the phenotype of the cell. There are two possible examples of this kind of control in human basophils and it would expected that similar kinds of control would be found for other cell types. The first relates to the expression of Syk, as discussed above. The varied level of Syk expression is only found in the basophil; when Syk expression is low in the basophil, it is not low in other leukocytes. Since regulation of expression appears to be post-translational it may be possible to discover the mechanism that leads to highly downregulated expression of Syk and exploit this process as a therapeutic.

A second example comes from even more recent studies of SHIP expression in basophils. In this case, the basophil phenotype is its ability to respond to stimuli that do not normally induce secretion. The stimulus that brought attention to this phenotype is called HRF (histamine-releasing factor), as noted previously. The reduction in SHIP levels in the hyper-releasable basophils of certain subjects supports the notion that SHIP levels do control secretion in humans as well. As in the studies of non-releasers showing low Syk expression in basophils, low SHIP expression is restricted to the basophil. Other circulating leukocytes, from donors with either the hyper-releaser phenotype or normo-releaser phenotype, express similar levels of SHIP. Like Syk expression in basophils, there may be unique pathways in basophils that regulate SHIP1 expression and these pathways could be exploited.

These two examples demonstrate that it is possible to selectively regulate the levels of two critical signaling elements that appear, at this time, to be primarily functional in the FcεRI-dependent signaling pathways. How this level of control is exerted in the basophil is not yet known but the studies provide a natural example of selective regulation. A similar approach may apply to every cell type; one only needs to find those elements that appear sensitive to their cell context.

References

IgE-mediated signaling: the aggregation reaction

1. Segal DM, Taurog JD, Metzger H. Dimeric immunoglobulin E serves as a unit signal for mast cell degranulation. Proc Natl Acad Sci U S A 1977; 74:2993–2997.
2. Fewtrell C, Metzger H. Larger oligomers of IgE are more effective than dimers in stimulating rat basophilic leukemia cells. J Immunol 1980; 125:701–710.
3. MacGlashan DW Jr, Schleimer RP, Lichtenstein LM. Qualitative differences between dimeric and trimeric stimulation of human basophils. J Immunol 1983; 130:4–6.
4. Magro AM, Alexander A. Histamine release: studies of the inhibitory region of the dose-response curve. J Immunol 1974; 112:1762–1764.
5. Cooper AD, Balakrishnan K, McConnell HM. Mobile haptens in liposomes stimulate serotonin release by rat basophil leukemia cells in the presence of specific immunoglobulin E. J Biol Chem 1981; 256:9379–9381.
6. Weis RM, Balakrishnan K, Smith BA, et al. Stimulation of fluorescence in a small contact region between rat basophil leukemia cells and planar lipid membrane targets by coherent evanescent radiation. J Biol Chem 1982; 257:6440–6445.
7. Balakrishnan K, Hsu FJ, Cooper AD, et al. Lipid hapten containing membrane targets can trigger specific immunoglobulin E-dependent degranulation of rat basophil leukemia cells. J Biol Chem 1982; 257:6427–6433.
8. Kane P, Holowka D, Baird B. Characterization of model antigens composed of biotinylated haptens bound to avidin. Immunol Invest 1990; 19:1–25.
9. Posner RG, Subramanian K, Goldstein B, et al. Simultaneous cross-linking by two nontriggering bivalent ligands causes synergistic signaling of IgE Fc epsilon RI complexes. J Immunol 1995; 155:3601–3609.
10. Paar JM, Harris NT, Holowka D, et al. Bivalent ligands with rigid double-stranded DNA spacers reveal structural constraints on signaling by Fc epsilon RI. J Immunol 2002; 169:856–864.
11. Kalesnikoff J, Huber M, Lam V, et al. Monomeric IgE stimulates signaling pathways in mast cells that lead to cytokine production and cell survival. Immunity 2001; 14:801–811.
12. Asai K, Kitaura J, Kawakami Y, et al. Regulation of mast cell survival by IgE. Immunity 2001; 14:791–800.
13. Kitaura J, Xiao W, Maeda-Yamamoto M, et al. Early divergence of Fc epsilon receptor I signals for receptor up-regulation and internalization from degranulation, cytokine production, and survival. J Immunol 2004; 173:4317–4323.
14. Kawakami T, Kitaura J. Mast cell survival and activation by IgE in the absence of antigen: a consideration of the biologic mechanisms and relevance. J Immunol 2005; 175:4167–4173.
15. Hsu C, MacGlashan DW Jr. IgE Antibody up-regulates high affinity IgE binding on murine bone marrow derived mast cells. Immunol Lett 1996; 52:129–134.
16. MacGlashan DW Jr, White-Mckenzie J, Chichester K, et al. In vitro regulation of FcεRIα expression on human basophils by IgE antibody. Blood 1998; 91:1633–1643.
17. Lantz CS, Yamaguchi M, Oettgen HC, et al. IgE regulates mouse basophil FcεRI expression in vivo. J Immunol 1997; 158:2517–2521.
18. Borkowski TA, Jouvin MH, Lin SY, et al. Minimal requirements for IgE-mediated regulation of surface Fc epsilon RI. J Immunol 2001; 167:1290–1296.
19. MacGlashan DW Jr, Xia HZ, Schwartz LB, Gong JP. IgE-regulated expression of FcεRI in human basophils: control by regulated loss rather than regulated synthesis. J Leuk Biol 2001; 70:207–218.

IgE receptor structure

20. Miller L, Blank U, Metzger H, et al. Expression of high-affinity binding of human immunoglobulin E by transfected cells. Science 1989; 244:334–337.
21. Hiraoka S, Furumoto Y, Koseki H, et al. Fc receptor beta subunit is required for full activation of mast cells through Fc receptor engagement. Int Immunol 1999; 11:199–207.
22. Garman SC, Wurzburg BA, Tarchevskaya SS, et al. Structure of the Fc fragment of human IgE bound to its high-affinity receptor Fc epsilonRI alpha. Nature 2000; 406:259–266.
23. Henry AJ, Cook JP, McDonnell JM, et al. Participation of the N-terminal region of Cepsilon3 in the binding of human IgE to its high-affinity receptor FcepsilonRI. Biochemistry 1997; 36:15568–15578.
24. Donnadieu E, Jouvin MH, Kinet JP. A second amplifier function for the allergy-associated Fc(epsilon)RI-beta subunit. Immunity 2000; 12:515–523.
25. Dombrowicz D, Lin S, Flamand V, et al. Allergy-associated FcRbeta is a molecular amplifier of IgE- and IgG-mediated in vivo responses. Immunity 1998; 8:517–529.
26. Donnadieu E, Jouvin MH, Rana S, et al. Competing functions encoded in the allergy-associated F(c)epsilonRIbeta gene. Immunity 2003; 18:665–674.

Brief overview of the early stages of FcεRI-mediated signaling

27. Parravicini V, Gadina M, Kovarova M, et al. Fyn kinase initiates complementary signals required for IgE-dependent mast cell degranulation. Nat Immunol 2002; 3:741–748.
28. Field KA, Holowka D, Baird B. Compartmentalized activation of the high affinity immunoglobulin E receptor within membrane domains. J Biol Chem 1997; 272:4276–4280.
29. Vonakis BM, Chen H, Haleem-Smith H, et al. The unique domain as the site on Lyn kinase for its constitutive association with the high affinity receptor for IgE. J Biol Chem 1997; 272:24072–24080.
30. Vonakis BM, Haleem-Smith H, Benjamin P, et al. Interaction between the unphosphorylated receptor with high affinity for IgE and Lyn kinase. J Biol Chem 2001; 276:1041–1050.
31. Kihara H, Siraganian RP. Src homology 2 domains of Syk and Lyn bind to tyrosine-phosphorylated subunits of the high affinity IgE receptor. J Biol Chem 1994; 269:22427–22432.
32. Zhang J, Billingsley ML, Kincaid RL, et al. Phosphorylation of Syk activation loop tyrosines is essential for Syk function. An in vivo study using a specific anti-Syk activation loop phosphorylation antibody. FASEB J 2001; 15:A1020.
33. Zhang J, Berenstein EH, Evans RL, et al. Transfection of Syk protein tyrosine kinase reconstitutes high affinity IgE receptor-mediated degranulation in a Syk-negative variant of rat basophilic leukemia RBL-2H3 cells. J Exp Med 1996; 184:71–79.
34. Vilarino N, MacGlashan D Jr. Transient transfection of human peripheral blood basophils. J Immunol Methods 2005; 296:11–18.
35. MacGlashan DW Jr. Single-cell analysis of Ca++ changes in human lung mast cells: graded vs. all-or-nothing elevations after IgE-mediated stimulation. J Cell Biol 1989; 109:123–134.
36. MacGlashan DW Jr, Bochner B, Warner JA. Graded changes in the response of individual human basophils to stimulation: distributional behavior of early activation events. J Leukoc Biol 1994; 55:13–23.
37. MacGlashan DW Jr. Graded changes in the response of individual human basophils to stimulation: distributional behavior of events temporally coincident with degranulation. J Leukoc Biol 1995; 58:177–188.
38. Dembo M, Goldstein B, Sobotka AK, et al. Histamine release due to bivalent penicilloyl haptens: control by the number of cross-linked IgE antibodies on the basophil plasma membrane. J Immunol 1978; 121:354–358.
39. MacGlashan DW Jr, Dembo M, Goldstein B. Test of a theory relating to the cross-linking of IgE antibody on the surface of human basophils. J Immunol 1985; 135:4129–4134.
40. MacGlashan DW Jr. Releasability of human basophils: cellular sensitivity and maximal histamine release are independent variables. J Allergy Clin Immunol 1993; 91:605–615.
41. MacGlashan DW Jr. Syk, but not SHIP-1, expression regulates IgE mediated responsiveness of human basophils in the general population. J Allergy Clin Immunol 2006; 117:S123–S139.
42. Malveaux FJ, Conroy MC, Adkinson NFJ, et al. IgE receptors on human basophils. Relationship to serum IgE concentration. J Clin Invest 1978; 62:176–181.
43. Saini SS, Klion AD, Holland SM, et al. The relationship between serum IgE and surface levels of FcepsilonR on human leukocytes in various diseases: correlation of expression with FcepsilonRI on basophils but not on monocytes or eosinophils. J Allergy Clin Immunol 2000; 106:514–520.
44. Pribluda VS, Pribluda C, Metzger H. Transphosphorylation as the mechanism by which the high-affinity receptor for IgE is phosphorylated upon aggregation. Proc Natl Acad Sci U S A 1994; 91:11246–11250.
45. Gomez G, Gonzalez-Espinosa C, Odom S, et al. Impaired FcepsilonRI-dependent gene expression and defective eicosanoid and cytokine production as a consequence of Fyn deficiency in mast cells. J Immunol 2005; 175:7602–7610.
46. Odom S, Gomez G, Kovarova M, et al. Negative regulation of immunoglobulin E-dependent allergic responses by Lyn kinase. J Exp Med 2004; 199:1491–1502.
47. Hernandez-Hansen V, Smith AJ, Surviladze Z, et al. Dysregulated FcepsilonRI signaling and altered Fyn and SHIP activities in Lyn-deficient mast cells. J Immunol 2004; 173:100–112.
48. Nishida K, Yamasaki S, Ito Y, et al. FcεRI-mediated mast cell degranulation requires calcium-independent microtubule-dependent translocation of granules to the plasma membrane. J Cell Biol 2005; 170:115–126.
49. Xiao W, Nishimoto H, Hong H, et al. Positive and negative regulation of mast cell activation by Lyn via the FcepsilonRI. J Immunol 2005; 175:6885–6892.
50. Holowka D, Gosse JA, Hammond AT, et al. Lipid segregation and IgE receptor signaling: a decade of progress. Biochim Biophys Acta 2005; 1746:252–259.
51. Holowka D, Sheets ED, Baird B. Interactions between Fc(epsilon)RI and lipid raft components are regulated by the actin cytoskeleton. J Cell Sci 2000; 113:1009–1019.
52. Swamy MJ, Ciani L, Ge M, et al. Coexisting domains in the plasma membranes of live cells characterized by spin-label ESR spectroscopy. Biophys J 2006; 90:4452–4465.
53. Taylor JA, Karas JL, Ram MK, et al. Activation of the high-affinity immunoglobulin E receptor Fc epsilon RI in RBL-2H3 cells is inhibited by Syk SH2 domains. Mol Cell Biol 1995; 15:4149–4157.
54. Meltzer EO, Berkowitz RB, Grossbard EB. An intranasal Syk-kinase inhibitor (R112) improves the symptoms of seasonal allergic rhinitis in a park environment. J Allergy Clin Immunol 2005; 115:791–796.
55. Smith AJ, Surviladze Z, Gaudet EA, et al. p110beta and p110delta phosphatidylinositol 3-kinases up-regulate Fc(epsilon)RI-activated Ca²⁺ influx by enhancing inositol 1,4,5-trisphosphate production. J Biol Chem 2001; 276:17213–17220.
56. Windmiller DA, Backer JM. Distinct phosphoinositide 3-kinases mediate mast cell degranulation in response to G-protein-coupled versus FcepsilonRI receptors. J Biol Chem 2003; 278:11874–11878.
57. Miura K, Lavens-Phillips S, MacGlashan DW Jr. Localizing a control region in the pathway to LTC4 secretion following stimulation of human basophils with anti-IgE antibody. J Immunol 2001; 167:7027–7037.
58. Giorgino F, Pedrini MT, Matera L, et al. Specific increase in p85alpha expression in response to dexamethasone is associated with inhibition of insulin-like growth factor-I stimulated phosphatidylinositol 3-kinase activity in cultured muscle cells. J Biol Chem 1997; 272:7455–7463.

59. Barbour LA, Shao J, Qiao L, et al. Human placental growth hormone increases expression of the p85 regulatory unit of phosphatidylinositol 3-kinase and triggers severe insulin resistance in skeletal muscle. Endocrinology 2004; 145:1144–1150.
60. Miura K, MacGlashan DW Jr. Phosphatidylinositol-3 kinase regulates p21ras activation during IgE-mediated stimulation of human basophils. Blood 2000; 96:2199–2205.
61. Tkaczyk C, Beaven MA, Brachman SM, et al. The phospholipase C gamma 1-dependent pathway of Fc epsilon RI-mediated mast cell activation is regulated independently of phosphatidylinositol 3-kinase. J Biol Chem 2003; 278:48474–48484.
62. Manetz TS, Gonzalez-Espinosa C, Arudchandran R, et al. Vav1 regulates phospholipase cgamma activation and calcium responses in mast cells. Mol Cell Biol 2001; 21:3763–3774.
63. Hata D, Kawakami Y, Inagaki N, et al. Involvement of Bruton's tyrosine kinase in FcepsilonRI-dependent mast cell degranulation and cytokine production. J Exp Med 1998; 187:1235–1247.
64. Kawakami Y, Kitaura J, Hartman SE, et al. Regulation of protein kinase CbetaI by two protein-tyrosine kinases, Btk and Syk. Proc Natl Acad Sci U S A 2000; 97:7423–7428.
65. Iwaki S, Tkaczyk C, Satterthwaite AB, et al. Btk plays a crucial role in the amplification of Fc epsilonRI-mediated mast cell activation by kit. J Biol Chem 2005; 280:40261–40270.
66. Roos J, DiGregorio PJ, Yeromin AV, et al. STIM1, an essential and conserved component of store-operated Ca^{2+} channel function. J Cell Biol 2005; 169:435–445.
67. Vig M, Peinelt C, Beck A, et al. CRACM1 is a plasma membrane protein essential for store-operated Ca^{2+} entry. Science 2006; 312:1220–1223.
68. Feske S, Gwack Y, Prakriya M, et al. A mutation in Orai1 causes immune deficiency by abrogating CRAC channel function. Nature 2006; 441:179–185.
69. Peinelt C, Vig M, Koomoa DL, et al. Amplification of CRAC current by STIM1 and CRACM1 (Orai1). Nat Cell Biol 2006; 8:771–773.
70. Mercer JC, Dehaven WI, Smyth JT, et al. Large store-operated calcium selective currents due to co-expression of Orai1 or Orai2 with the intracellular calcium sensor, Stim1. J Biol Chem 2006; 281:24979–24990.
71. Soboloff J, Spassova MA, Tang XD, et al. Orai1 and STIM reconstitute store-operated calcium channel function. J Biol Chem 2006; 281:20661–20665.
72. Choi OH, Kim JH, Kinet JP. Calcium mobilization via sphingosine kinase in signaling by the FcεRI antigen receptor. Nature 1996; 380:634–636.
73. Miura K, MacGlashan DW Jr. Dual phase priming by interleukin-3 for leukotriene C4 generation in human basophils. J Immunol 2000; 164:3026–3034.
74. Millard PJ, Ryan TA, Webb WW, et al. Immunoglobulin E receptor cross-linking induces oscillations in intracellular free ionized calcium in individual tumor mast cells. J Biol Chem 1989; 264:19730–19739.
75. Duffy SM, Berger P, Cruse G, et al. The K^+ channel iKCA1 potentiates Ca^{2+} influx and degranulation in human lung mast cells. J Allergy Clin Immunol 2004; 114:66–72.
76. Bradding P, Okayama Y, Kambe N, et al. Ion channel gene expression in human lung, skin, and cord blood-derived mast cells. J Leukoc Biol 2003; 73:614–620.
77. Warner JA, Peters SP, Lichtenstein LM, et al. Differential release of mediators from human basophils: differences in arachidonic acid metabolism following activation by unrelated stimuli. J Leukoc Biol 1989; 45:558–571.
78. MacGlashan DW Jr, Botana L. Biphasic Ca^{++} responses in human basophils: evidence that the initial transient elevation associated with mobilization of intracellular calcium is an insufficient signal for degranulation. J Immunol 1993; 150:980–991.
79. Rivera J, Beaven MA. Regulation of secretion from secretory cells by protein kinase C. In: Parker P, Dekker L, eds. Protein kinase C. Austin: Landes Company; 1997:131–164.
80. Chang EY, Szallasi Z, Acs P, et al. Functional effects of overexpression of protein kinase C alpha, beta, delta, epsilon, and eta in the mast cell line RBL 2H3. J Immunol 1997; 159:2624–2632.
81. Song JS, Haleem-Smith H, Arudchandran R, et al. Tyrosine phosphorylation of Vav stimulates IL-6 production in mast cells by a Rac/c-Jun N-terminal kinase-dependent pathway. J Immunol 1999; 163:802–810.
82. Li G, Lucas JJ, Gelfand EW. Protein kinase C alpha, betaI, and betaII isozymes regulate cytokine production in mast cells through MEKK2/ERK5-dependent and -independent pathways. Cell Immunol 2005; 238:10–18.
83. Massey WA, Cohen VL, MacGlashan DW Jr, et al. Protein kinase C modulates IgE-mediated activation of human mast cells from lung and skin. I. Pharmacologic inhibition. J Pharm Exp Ther 1991; 258:824–829.
84. Miura K, MacGlashan DW Jr. Expression of protein kinase C isozymes in human basophils: regulation by physiological and non-physiological stimuli. Blood 1998; 92:1206–1218.
85. Vilarino N, Miura K, MacGlashan DW Jr. Acute IL-3 priming up-regulates the stimulus-induced Raf-1-Mek-ERK cascade independently of IL-3-induced activation of ERK. J Immunol 2005; 175:3006–3014.
86. Lessmann E, Leitges M, Huber M. A redundant role for PKC-epsilon in mast cell signaling and effector function. Int Immunol 2006; 18:767–773.
87. Cho SH, Woo CH, Yoon SB, et al. Protein kinase Cdelta functions downstream of Ca^{2+} mobilization in FcepsilonRI signaling to degranulation in mast cells. J Allergy Clin Immunol 2004; 114:1085–1092.
88. Leitges M, Gimborn K, Elis W, et al. Protein kinase C-delta is a negative regulator of antigen-induced mast cell degranulation. Mol Cell Biol 2002; 22:3970–3980.
89. Peng Z, Beaven MA. An essential role for phospholipase D in the activation of protein kinase C and degranulation in mast cells. J Immunol 2005; 174:5201–5208.
90. Kitatani K, Akiba S, Sato T. Role of phospholipase D-derived phosphatidic acid as a substrate for phospholipase A2 in RBL-2H3 cells. Biol Pharm Bull 2000; 23:1430–1433.
91. Choi WS, Kim YM, Combs C, et al. Phospholipases D1 and D2 regulate different phases of exocytosis in mast cells. J Immunol 2002; 168:5682–5689.
92. Sarri E, Pardo R, Fensome-Green A, et al. Endogenous phospholipase D2 localizes to the plasma membrane of RBL-2H3 mast cells and can be distinguished from ADP ribosylation factor-stimulated phospholipase D1 activity by its specific sensitivity to oleic acid. Biochem J 2003; 369:319–329.
93. Choi WS, Hiragun T, Lee JH, et al. Activation of RBL-2H3 mast cells is dependent on tyrosine phosphorylation of phospholipase D2 by Fyn and Fgr. Mol Cell Biol 2004; 24:6980–6992.
94. Lee JH, Kim YM, Kim NW, et al. Phospholipase D2 acts as an essential adaptor protein in the activation of Syk in antigen-stimulated mast cells. Blood 2006; 108:956–964.
95. Fonteh AN, Bass DA, Marshall LA, et al. Evidence that secretory phospholipase A2 plays a role in arachidonic acid release and eicosanoid biosynthesis by mast cells. J Immunol 1994; 152: 5438–5446.
96. Hundley TR, Marshall L, Hubbard WC, et al. Characteristics of arachidonic acid generation in human basophils: relationship between the effects of inhibitors of secretory phospholipase A2 activity and leukotriene C4 release. J Pharmacol Exp Ther 1998; 284:847–857.
97. Silliman CC, Moore EE, Zallen G, et al. Presence of the M-type sPLA(2) receptor on neutrophils and its role in elastase release and adhesion. Am J Physiol Cell Physiol 2002; 283: C1102–C1113.
98. Granata F, Petraroli A, Boilard E, et al. Activation of cytokine production by secreted phospholipase A2 in human lung macrophages expressing the M-type receptor. J Immunol 2005; 174:464–474.
99. Norman JC, Price LS, Ridley AJ, et al. The small GTP-binding proteins, Rac and Rho, regulate cytoskeletal organization and exocytosis in mast cells by parallel pathways. Mol Biol Cell 1996; 7:1429–1442.
100. Castellano F, Le Clainche C, Patin D, et al. A WASp-VASP complex regulates actin polymerization at the plasma membrane. EMBO J 2001; 20:5603–5614.
101. Labno CM, Lewis CM, You D, et al. Itk functions to control actin polymerization at the immune synapse through localized activation of Cdc42 and WASP. Curr Biol 2003; 13: 1619–1624.
102. Song JS, Gomez J, Stancato LF, et al. Association of a p95 Vav-containing signaling complex with the FcepsilonRI gamma chain in the RBL-2H3 mast cell line. Evidence for a constitutive in vivo association of Vav with Grb2, Raf-1, and ERK2 in an active complex. J Biol Chem 1996; 271:26962–26970.
103. Miller WE, Lefkowitz RJ. Expanding roles for beta-arrestins as scaffolds and adapters in GPCR signaling and trafficking. Curr Opin Cell Biol 2001; 13:139–145.
104. Vazquez F, Devreotes P. Regulation of PTEN function as a PIP3 gatekeeper through membrane interaction. Cell Cycle 2006; 5:1523–1527.
105. Kimura T, Sakamoto H, Appella E, et al. The negative signaling molecule SH2 domain-containing inositol-polyphosphate 5-phosphatase (SHIP) binds to the tyrosine-phosphorylated beta subunit of the high affinity IgE receptor. J Biol Chem 1997; 272: 13991–13996.
106. Rauh MJ, Kalesnikoff J, Hughes M, et al. Role of Src homology 2-containing-inositol 5'-phosphatase (SHIP) in mast cells and macrophages. Biochem Soc Trans 2003; 31:286–291.
107. Huber M, Helgason CD, Damen JE, et al. The Src homology 2-containing inositol phosphatase (SHIP) is the gatekeeper of mast cell degranulation. Proc Natl Acad Sci U S A 1998; 95:11330–11335.
108. Vonakis BM, Gibbons S Jr, Sora R, et al. Src homology 2 domain-containing inositol 5'-phosphatase is negatively associated with histamine release to human recombinant histamine- releasing factor in human basophils. J Allergy Clin Immunol 2001; 108:822–831.
109. Xie ZH, Zhang J, Siraganian RP. Positive regulation of c-Jun N-terminal kinase and TNF-alpha production but not histamine release by SHP-1 in RBL-2H3 mast cells. J Immunol 2000; 164:1521–1528.
110. Hook WA, Berenstein EH, Zinsser FU, et al. Monoclonal antibodies to the leukocyte common antigen (CD45) inhibit IgE-mediated histamine release from human basophils. J Immunol 1991; 147:2670–2676.
111. Berger SA, Mak TW, Paige CJ. Leukocyte common antigen (CD45) is required for immunoglobulin E-mediated degranulation of mast cells. J Exp Med 1994; 180:471–476.
112. Zhang J, Siraganian RP. CD45 is essential for Fc epsilon RI signaling by ZAP70, but not Syk, in Syk-negative mast cells. J Immunol 1999; 163:2508–2516.
113. Murakami K, Sato S, Nagasawa S, et al. Regulation of mast cell signaling through high-affinity IgE receptor by CD45 protein tyrosine phosphatase. Int Immunol 2000; 12:169–176.
114. Lemay S, Davidson D, Latour S, et al. Dok-3, a novel adapter molecule involved in the negative regulation of immunoreceptor signaling. Mol Cell Biol 2000; 20:2743–2754.
115. Honma M, Higuchi O, Shirakata M, et al. Dok-3 sequesters Grb2 and inhibits the Ras-ERK pathway downstream of protein-tyrosine kinases. Genes Cells 2006; 11:143–151.
116. Abramson J, Rozenblum G, Pecht I. Dok protein family members are involved in signaling mediated by the type 1 Fcepsilon receptor. Eur J Immunol 2003; 33:85–91.
117. Abramson J, Pecht I. Clustering the mast cell function-associated antigen (MAFA) leads to tyrosine phosphorylation of p62Dok and SHIP and affects RBL-2H3 cell cycle. Immunol Lett 2002; 82:23–28.
118. Fong DC, Malbec O, Arock M, et al. Selective in vivo recruitment of the phosphatidylinositol phosphatase SHIP by phosphorylated Fc gammaRIIB during negative regulation of IgE-dependent mouse mast cell activation. Immunol Lett 1996; 54:83–91.
119. Malbec O, Fong DC, Turner M, et al. Fc epsilon receptor I-associated Lyn-dependent phosphorylation of Fc gamma receptor IIB during negative regulation of mast cell activation. J Immunol 1998; 160:1647–1658.
120. Kepley CL, Cambier JC, Morel PA, et al. Negative regulation of FcepsilonRI signaling by FcgammaRII costimulation in human blood basophils. J Allergy Clin Immunol 2000; 106: 337–348.
121. Daheshia M, Friend DS, Grusby MJ, et al. Increased severity of local and systemic anaphylactic reactions in gp49B1-deficient mice. J Exp Med 2001; 194:227–234.
122. Castells MC, Klickstein LB, Hassani K, et al. gp49B1-alpha(v)beta3 interaction inhibits antigen-induced mast cell activation. Nat Immunol 2001; 2:436–442.
123. Abramson J, Xu R, Pecht I. An unusual inhibitory receptor – the mast cell function-associated antigen (MAFA). Mol Immunol 2002; 38:1307–1313.
124. Cherwinski HM, Murphy CA, Joyce BL, et al. The CD200 receptor is a novel and potent regulator of murine and human mast cell function. J Immunol 2005; 174:1348–1356.
125. Kumagai H, Oki T, Tamitsu K, et al. Identification and characterization of a new pair of immunoglobulin-like receptors LMIR1 and 2 derived from murine bone marrow-derived mast cells. Biochem Biophys Res Commun 2003; 307:719–729.
126. Yokoi H, Myers A, Matsumoto K, et al. Alteration and acquisition of Siglecs during in vitro maturation of $CD34^+$ progenitors into human mast cells. Allergy 2006; 61:769–776.

127. Zhang J, Chiang YJ, Hodes RJ, et al. Inactivation of c-Cbl or Cbl-b differentially affects signaling from the high affinity IgE receptor. J Immunol 2004; 173:1811–1818.
128. Paolini R, Molfetta R, Beitz LO, et al. Activation of Syk tyrosine kinase is required for c-Cbl-mediated ubiquitination of Fcepsilon RI and Syk in RBL cells. J Biol Chem 2002; 277:36940–36947.
129. Qu X, Sada K, Kyo S, et al. Negative regulation of FcepsilonRI-mediated mast cell activation by a ubiquitin-protein ligase Cbl-b. Blood 2004; 103:1779–1786.
130. Gustin SE, Thien CB, Langdon WY. Cbl-b is a negative regulator of inflammatory cytokines produced by IgE-activated mast cells. J Immunol 2006; 177:5980–5989.
131. MacGlashan D, Miura K. Loss of Syk kinase during IgE-mediated stimulation of human basophils. J Allergy Clin Immunol 2004; 114:1317–1324.
132. Kyo S, Sada K, Qu X, et al. Negative regulation of Lyn protein-tyrosine kinase by c-Cbl ubiquitin-protein ligase in Fc varepsilon RI-mediated mast cell activation. Genes Cells 2003; 8:825–836.
133. Faeder JR, Hlavacek WS, Reischl I, et al. Investigation of early events in Fc epsilon RI-mediated signaling using a detailed mathematical model. J Immunol 2003; 170:3769–3781.
134. Hlavacek WS, Faeder JR, Blinov ML, et al. The complexity of complexes in signal transduction. Biotechnol Bioeng 2003; 84:783–794.
135. MacGlashan DW Jr. Relationship between Syk and SHIP expression and secretion from human basophils in the general population. J Allergy Clin Immunol 2007; 119:626–633.
136. Liu ZJ, Haleem-Smith H, Chen H, et al. Unexpected signals in a system subject to kinetic proofreading. Proc Natl Acad Sci U S A 2001; 98:7289–7294.
137. Hlavacek WS, Redondo A, Metzger H, et al. Kinetic proofreading models for cell signaling predict ways to escape kinetic proofreading. Proc Natl Acad Sci U S A 2001; 98:7295–7300.
138. Kitaura J, Kinoshita T, Matsumoto M, et al. IgE- and IgE+Ag-mediated mast cell migration in an autocrine/paracrine fashion. Blood 2005; 105:3222–3229.
139. Peachell PT, MacGlashan DW Jr, Lichtenstein LM, et al. Regulation of human basophil and lung mast cell function by cyclic adenosine monophosphate. J Immunol 1988; 140:571–579.
140. Gauvreau GM, Plitt JR, Baatjes A, et al. Expression of functional cysteinyl leukotriene receptors by human basophils. J Allergy Clin Immunol 2005; 116:80–87.
141. Jolly PS, Bektas M, Olivera A, et al. Transactivation of sphingosine-1-phosphate receptors by FcepsilonRI triggering is required for normal mast cell degranulation and chemotaxis. J Exp Med 2004; 199:959–970.
142. Jolly PS, Bektas M, Watterson KR, et al. Expression of SphK1 impairs degranulation and motility of RBL-2H3 mast cells by desensitizing S1P receptors. Blood 2005; 105:4736–4742.
143. Dvorak AM. Basophils and mast cells: piecemeal degranulation in situ and ex vivo: a possible mechanism for cytokine-induced function in disease. In: Coffey RG, ed. Granulocyte responses to cytokines, New York: Marcel Dekker, 1992; 169–271.
144. Dvorak AM, Warner JA, Kissell S, et al. F-met peptide-induced degranulation of human basophils. Lab Invest 1991; 64:234–253.
145. Paumet F, Le Mao J, Martin S, et al. Soluble NSF attachment protein receptors (SNAREs) in RBL-2H3 mast cells: functional role of syntaxin 4 in exocytosis and identification of a vesicle-associated membrane protein 8-containing secretory compartment. J Immunol 2000; 164:5850–5857.
146. Puri N, Kruhlak MJ, Whiteheart SW, et al. Mast cell degranulation requires N-ethylmaleimide-sensitive factor-mediated SNARE disassembly. J Immunol 2003; 171:5345–5352.
147. Pombo I, Martin-Verdeaux S, Iannascoli B, et al. IgE receptor type I-dependent regulation of a Rab3D-associated kinase: a possible link in the calcium-dependent assembly of SNARE complexes. J Biol Chem 2001; 276:42893–42900.
148. Hepp R, Puri N, Hohenstein AC, et al. Phosphorylation of SNAP-23 regulates exocytosis from mast cells. J Biol Chem 2005; 280:6610–6620.

149. Puri N, Roche PA. Ternary SNARE complexes are enriched in lipid rafts during mast cell exocytosis. Traffic 2006; 7:1482–1494.
150. Hirasawa N, Santini F, Beaven MA. Activation of the mitogen-activated protein kinase/cytosolic phospholipase A2 pathway in a rat mast cell line. J Immunol 1995; 154:5391–5402.
151. Miura K, Schroeder JT, Hubbard WC, et al. Extracellular signal-regulated kinases regulate leukotriene C4 generation, but not histamine release or IL-4 production from human basophils. J Immunol 1999; 162:4198–4206.
152. Chang WC, Nelson C, Parekh AB. Ca^{2+} influx through CRAC channels activates cytosolic phospholipase A2, leukotriene C4 secretion, and expression of c-fos through ERK-dependent and -independent pathways in mast cells. FASEB J 2006; 20:2381–2383.
153. Fujishima H, Sanchez Mejia RO, Bingham CO, et al. Cytosolic phospholipase A2 is essential for both the immediate and the delayed phases of eicosanoid generation in mouse bone marrow-derived mast cells. Proc Natl Acad Sci U S A 1999; 96:4803–4807.
154. Huang CY, Ferrell JE Jr. Ultrasensitivity in the mitogen-activated protein kinase cascade. Proc Natl Acad Sci U S A 1996; 93:10078–10083.
155. Jabril-Cuenod B, Zhang C, Scharenberg AM, et al. Syk-dependent phosphorylation of Shc. A potential link between FcepsilonRI and the Ras/mitogen-activated protein kinase signaling pathway through SOS and Grb2. J Biol Chem 1996; 271:16268–16272.
156. Klemm S, Ruland J. Inflammatory signal transduction from the Fc epsilon RI to NF-kappaB. Immunobiology 2006; 211:815–820.
157. Klemm S, Gutermuth J, Hultner L, et al. The Bcl10-Malt1 complex segregates Fc epsilon RI-mediated nuclear factor kappa B activation and cytokine production from mast cell degranulation. J Exp Med 2006; 203:337–347.
158. Nguyen KL, Gillis S, MacGlashan DW Jr. A comparative study of releasing and nonreleasing human basophils: nonreleasing basophils lack an early component of the signal transduction pathway that follows IgE cross-linking. J Allergy Clin Immunol 1990; 85: 1020–1029.
159. Kepley CL, Youssef L, Andrews RP, et al. Syk deficiency in nonreleaser basophils. J Allergy Clin Immunol 1999; 104:279–284.
160. Lavens-Phillips SE, MacGlashan DW Jr. The tyrosine kinases, p53/56Lyn and p72Syk are differentially expressed at the protein level but not at the mRNA level in non-releasing human basophils. Am J Resp Cell Mol Biol 2000; 23:566–571.
161. MacDonald SM, Schroeder JT, MacGlashan DW Jr, et al. Human recombinant HRF: a unique cytokine. J Invest Med 1996; 44:222a.
162. Yamaguchi M, Hirai K, Ohta K, et al. Culturing in the presence of IL-3 converts anti-IgE nonresponding basophils into responding basophils. J Allergy Clin Immunol 1996; 97: 1279–1287.
163. Kepley CL, Youssef L, Andrews RP, et al. Multiple defects in Fc epsilon RI signaling in Syk-deficient nonreleaser basophils and IL-3-induced recovery of Syk expression and secretion. J Immunol 2000; 165:5913–5920.
164. Tschopp CM, Spiegl N, Didichenko S, et al. Granzyme B, a novel mediator of allergic inflammation: its induction and release in blood basophils and human asthma. Blood 2006; 108:2290–2299.
165. Kepley CL. Antigen-induced reduction in mast cell and basophil functional responses due to reduced Syk protein levels. Int Arch Allergy Immunol 2005; 138:29–39.
166. Green LJ, Marder P, Ray C, et al. Development and validation of a drug activity biomarker that shows target inhibition in cancer patients receiving enzastaurin, a novel protein kinase C-beta inhibitor. Clin Cancer Res 2006; 12:3408–3415.
167. Burkey JL, Campanale KM, Barbuch R, et al. Disposition of [^{14}C]ruboxistaurin in humans. Drug Metab Dispos 2006; 34:1909–1917.

Stem Cells: What Are They and Why Do We Need Them?

Leah Bellehsen, Arnon Nagler, and Francesca Levi-Schaffer

15

CONTENTS

SUMMARY OF IMPORTANT CONCEPTS

>> Stem cells (SC) are clonogenic multipotential unspecialized cells capable of: (1) prolonged self-renewal; (2) differentiation along many lineages giving rise to or replenishing cells of the various tissues and organs

>> There are embryonic (ESC) and adult SC (ASC). The first are totipotent, while the second (present in almost every tissue) are more restricted in their capacity to differentiate and may be somatic or organ-specific. ASC also display age- and health-related changes

>> Hematopoietic SC (HSC) are found in the bone marrow and peripheral blood

>> The SC niche is a defined microenvironment that allows molecular interaction and signals that are crucial for regulating SC quiescence, self-renewal, differentiation and proliferation, mobilization and homing

>> SC (from adult blood or cord blood) with their self-renewal capacity and pluripotency are a potential therapy for a number of diseases such as tumor and immunodeficiencies or in reconstitutive therapy of damaged tissues

STEM CELLS: DEFINITION AND GENERAL CHARACTERISTICS

Stem cells (SC) are clonogenic multipotent unspecialized cells capable of prolonged or long-term self-renewal that have the capacity to differentiate along many lineages, giving rise to or replenishing cells of the various tissues and organ systems of the body.[1] The SC concept arose four decades ago with the discovery by Till and McCulloch[2] that the bone marrow of adult animals contains a single precursor cell capable of both extensive self-renewal and multilineage differentiation.

The overall aim of this chapter is to summarize what is known about embryonic and adult SC in general and in particular about the hematopoietic SC (HSC), their biological characteristics, how they are maintained in tissue niches, the principal factors and signal transduction mechanisms involved in their fate, and their clinical applications.

EMBRYONIC AND ADULT STEM CELLS

SC may be primarily categorized into embryonic and adult SC.[3] Embryonic SC (ESC), which originate from the first two divisions of the zygote, give rise to the embryo and its supporting tissues are totipotent (Fig. 15.1, Table 15.1) in their capacity to differentiate into almost every cell type present in the body.[4] While ESC have the capacity to grow to large numbers and for lengthy periods of time in culture, their differentiation is difficult to control. Cells forming the inner cell mass of the blastocyst are considered more restricted (pluripotent) as they may give rise to somatic SC destined to become either ectoderm (skin, neural tissue), or mesoderm (blood, adipose tissue, cartilage, bone, or muscle), or endoderm (cells of the digestive and respiratory systems) (Fig. 15.1). SC that have totipotency similar or equal to ESC may also be derived from germ cells, i.e., embryonic germ cells, embryonal carcinoma cells (from adult testicular tumors), and germ line cells derived from spermatogonial SC or surface cells from adult ovaries. Beyond this stage, SC persist into adulthood but

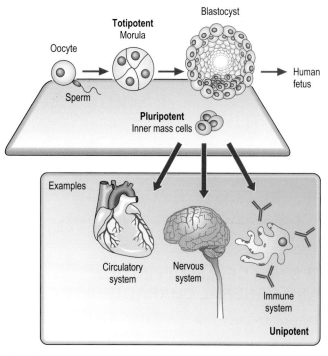

Fig. 15.1. Derivation of embryonic stem cells. Totipotent embryonic stem cells (ESC) are derived from the inner cell mass of the blastocyst, 4–5 days after fusion of the egg and sperm. These cells have the potential to give rise to all cell types in the body.

Table 15.1 Defining stem cell potential

Potential	Definition
Totipotent	SC arising from the fusion of egg and sperm, arising from the inner cell mass at the blastocyst stage, that are capable of differentiating into all embryonic and extraembryonic cell types.
Pluripotent	SC that are descendants of totipotent cells which can differentiate into cells derived from the three germ layers – i.e., ectoderm, mesoderm, or endoderm.
Multipotent	SC that show more restricted differentiation capacity and can produce only cells of a closely related family (e.g., HSC which can give rise to blood elements such as erythrocytes, lymphocytes, granulocytes, megakaryocytes, etc.).
Oligopotent	SC with even more restricted differentiation capacity that can give rise to a particular lineage of cells (e.g., CLP (common lymphoid progenitor) which gives rise to T lymphocytes, B lymphocytes, and NK cells).
Unipotent	SC that can give rise to only one cell type but have the property of self-renewal which distinguishes them from non-stem cells.

the dogma has been that these adult stem cells (ASC) are more restricted in their capacity to differentiate and may be somatic or organ-specific. Diaz-Flores et al[3] define ASC as small subpopulations of quiescent, slow-cycling, undifferentiated resident cells with high proliferative and pluripotent potential (Table 15.1). ASC also have the ability to self-renew and to give rise to cells which may undergo structural and functional differentiation into mature cells, thus regenerating all cell types characteristic of the tissue where they are located.[3]

ESC present an attractive potential for cell-based therapy in reconstituting and repairing every tissue of the body. Human ESC have the additional advantage in that they express low levels of MHC class I and II antigens and co-stimulatory molecules, are not recognized by NK cells, and are inhibitory for T cells. However, several important issues concerning their use remain unresolved. These include: ethical issues pertaining to the use of human embryos; epigenetic problems arising from IVF and other assisted reproduction techniques or long-term culture that lead to abnormal DNA and/or histone methylation and genomic imprinting; the requirement for feeder layers and potential problems arising from the use of heterologous feeder cells; difficulties in balancing ESC proliferation and differentiation; the need to develop better methods to ensure accurate homing and establishment of ESC; and still undiscovered issues pertaining to tissue matching, graft rejection or GVHD, etc.

■ ADULT STEM CELLS (ASC) ■

LOCATION, CHARACTERISTICS, AND ROLE

The principal role of ASC is in regenerating and repair of the tissue in which they reside. They have been described in almost every tissue including skeletal muscle, mammary gland, skin, hair follicle, gut, kidney, liver, pancreas, brain, and inner ear, as well as in the bone marrow, peripheral blood, and cord blood. During physiological growth or after tissue trauma and disease, ASC may replicate and participate in replenishing the damaged organ (intrinsic regeneration). SC from the bone marrow or peripheral blood may also be mobilized and home into the damaged organ where they contribute to regeneration (extrinsic regeneration).

ASC have a few distinguishing morphologic and biochemical characteristics. They demonstrate large nuclear:cytoplasmic ratios and a paucity of cytoplasmic organelles. They may also express certain markers (such as CD34, Sca-1, integrins, c-kit [CD117], Oct-4 [Oct-3, NFA-3, Pou5fl], Nanog, nestin, Bml-1, bcl-2, and CD133 [AC133], prominin-1, and HoxB4, and utilize certain signaling pathways (Notch, Wnt, and sonic hedgehog [Shh]) in maintaining their self-renewal in an undifferentiated state.[3,5]

DIFFERENTIATION AND PLASTICITY

ASC usually differentiate along pathways that result in regeneration of the tissues in which they reside.[3,4] The high plasticity of ASC was first revealed in bone marrow (BM) HSC, which were shown to be not only capable of replenishing all blood cellular elements but also to differentiate into non-hematopoietic cell types. Other examples of ASC plasticity include: liver SC that proliferate and regenerate tissue after partial hepatectomy; satellite cells that are involved in repair of damaged skeletal muscle; skin SC that are located in the basal epidermis and hair follicles which participate in skin renewal, wound healing and which may give rise to other cells such as chondrocytes, osteoblasts, myocytes, and adipocytes, etc.[3,4]

Moreover, there is increasing documentation of 'reversed' differentiation or transdifferentiation, with reports of highly differentiated cells such as muscle or neural cells giving rise to blood cells.[4] Thus, there are ASC that are not tissue-specific and are capable of repopulating and differentiating into various phenotypes. In fact, Blau and colleagues[4] have redefined the SC as 'a biological function that can be induced in many distinct types of cells, even differentiated cells', making the SC

a concept rather than a cellular entity. Thus, while ASC demonstrate high plasticity (differentiation capacity, see Fig. 15.2), the outcome of their differentiation is highly dependent upon interactions with other cells and factors present in their microenvironment or 'niche' (see 'The Stem Cell Niche').

AGE- AND HEALTH-RELATED CHANGES

Differentiated somatic cells have limited replication capacity and undergo senescence. In contrast, both ESC and ASC show longevity and self-renewal capacity that is dependent upon unique mechanisms for preventing senescence and subsequent apoptosis and for maintaining cell division at slow and sustained rates. A unique feature of SC which retards their senescence is that they have abundant telomerase activity which enables them to maintain telomere lengths.[3]

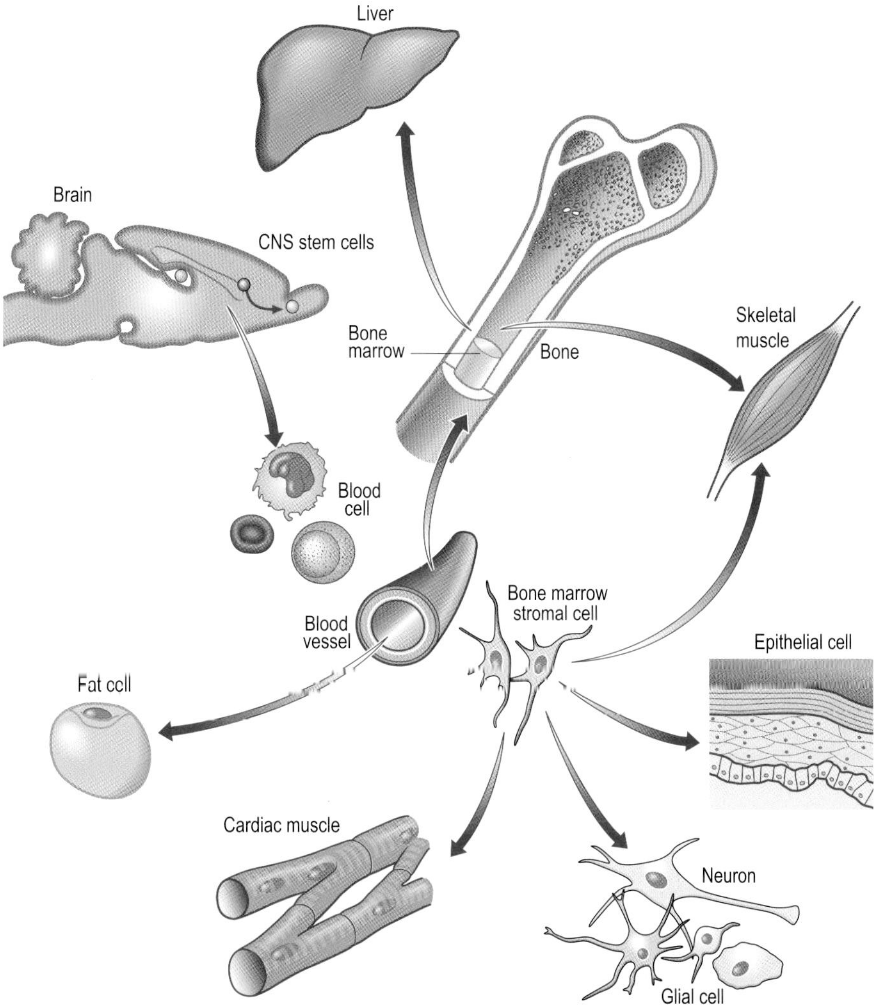

Fig. 15.2. Stem cell plasticity. Adult stem cells originating from the bone marrow have the capacity to differentiate into all blood elements as well as other cells including hepatocytes in the liver, skeletal and cardiac muscle, adipocytes in fatty tissue, neural cells, etc. Reverse or transdifferentiation may also occur with differentiated cells reverting to other phenotypes.

ADULT STEM CELLS (ASC)

Nevertheless, in humans, ASC number and functional characteristics deteriorate with increasing age and in some diseases. In HSC populations significant functional decline such as in the mobilization response to G-CSF and colony forming capacity, ability to give rise to differentiated progeny, and higher senescence are observed with increasing age.[6]

Last, but not least, age-associated alterations of HSC may result in loss of immune functions and in an increase of many genes involved in leukemic transformation.[7]

Health and other physiologic factors influencing release of progenitors from bone marrow also affect HSC frequencies in peripheral blood and may impact on the ability of tissues to undergo regeneration and repair. Some examples of such changes include: observation of high in vitro senescence of SC in patients with high cardiovascular disease risk;[8] and decreased absolute numbers, functional differentiation, and homing of endothelial cell progenitors in patients with chronic renal failure[9] and in pulmonary disease.[10]

◼ HEMATOPOIETIC STEM CELLS ◼

GENERAL FEATURES

Hematopoietic stem cells (HSC) were discovered by Till and McCulloch who found that bone marrow (BM) contained a small population of cells capable on transplantation of forming macroscopic colonies in the spleens of lethally-irradiated sheep.[2] These were termed colony forming units-spleen (CFU-S) and were found to contain the differentiated progeny of the various hematopoietic lineages; they also formed secondary colonies when transplanted into new hosts. Functionally defined, HSC should be able to engraft a myeloablated recipient and reconstitute long-term, multi-lineage hematopoiesis.[11] HSC are currently the only SC routinely used in transplantation therapy. Advancement of technologies for the expansion of HSC, monoclonal antibodies for characterizing lineage markers, flow cytometric techniques for purification and concentration, and in vitro assays for determining their lineage potential have enabled better molecular characterization of HSC and their progeny.[12]

HSC may be found in the mid-gestational placenta, fetal liver after 6 weeks' of gestation, adult bone marrow (BM) and in peripheral blood (including adult blood and cord blood). In the BM, their estimated frequency is one HSC in 10^5–10^6 BM cells.[11,13] By extrapolation from animal studies, the surface phenotype of human HSC is believed to be: $CD34^+$ $CD38$;[14] Kit^+ Thy^+ and Lin^-;[15] and $CD133^+$.[16] Upon differentiation, the CD34 antigen is downregulated and CD133 is considered to be a more definitive marker for primitive HSC.[17] In the course of their development HSC give rise to progressively more oligopotent and lineage-restricted progenitors with lesser self-renewal capacity and greater proliferative potential[12] (Table 15.1), culminating in the differentiation of the various hematopoietic lineages (Fig. 15.3). This multi-tiered differentiation scheme has many advantages. It permits extensive clonal amplification of differentiated cells from a single precursor and thus fine-tunes effector cell supply according to homeostatic demands. It also allows more pluripotent HSC to maintain self-renewal by cycling slowly. This protects the HSC from potentially mutagenic factors associated with DNA replication, cell division, and enhanced metabolic activity.[12] Both primitive and mature HSC express the tyrosine kinase receptor c-Kit, the ligand for stem cell factor (SCF) which influences their entry into the cell cycle, proliferation, and subsequent differentiation.[18] Nerve growth factor (NGF) a cytokine affecting neuronal development, also appears to be important and synergizes with other cytokines (G-CSF, M-CSF, IL-1, IL-3, IL-5, and SCF) in promoting HSC differentiation into the various lineages including the myeloid/granulocytic lineages.[19]

DEVELOPMENTAL REGULATION

HSC numbers, self-renewal, differentiation state, and trafficking are tightly regulated by the BM milieu, extracellular matrix and niches as well as by early- and late-acting cytokines (see Fig. 15.3).[20] Early-acting cytokines include: stem cell factor (SCF); thrombopoietin (TPO); interleukin (IL)-3, IL-7, and granulocyte-monocyte colony stimulating factor (GM-CSF).

HSC express a great variety of gene transcripts, many of which are characteristic of more differentiated progeny. Such global transcription may afford a mechanism for priming of HSC for differentiation, or it may be that progressive differentiation along certain lineages comes as a result of step-wise restriction of locus specificity.[12] Gene regulation is very important for maintaining the balance between quiescence and proliferation/activation. It was recently reported that PTEN (phosphatase and tensin homologue) a negative regulator of the phosphatidylinositol-3-OH kinase (PI3k)/Akt pathway (which plays a crucial role in cell proliferation, survival, differentiation, and migration) prevents HSC proliferation, thus supporting quiescence.[21]

Late-acting developmental forces (Fig. 15.3) include lineage-specific hematopoietic growth factors such as: erythropoietin (EPO), which promotes proliferation of erythroid progenitors by reducing levels of cell cycle inhibitors, augmenting cyclins, and inducing anti-apoptotic proteins such as Bclx; G-CSF, which supports survival, stimulates proliferation, and promotes morphologic and functional maturation of neutrophil progenitors and HSC mobilization from the BM; GM-CSF, which stimulates production of neutrophils, eosinophils, basophils, monocytes, and dendritic cells; and TPO, which is the primary regulator of megakaryocyte proliferation, differentiation, and platelet production.[20] EPO, G-CSF, and TPO have been used clinically for in vitro expansion of hematopoietic progenitors prior to transplantation. Interaction of these growth factors with specific receptors on various progenitors results in recruitment and activation of Janus kinase (JAK) kinases which secondarily activate signaling pathways involving: signal transducer and activator of transcription factors (STAT3, STAT5), phosphoinositol-3 kinase (PI-3K), and mitogen-activated protein kinase (MAPK), each of which activate a tertiary cascade of signaling molecules (Fig. 15.4).[20] Growth arrest is brought about by internalization of receptors, activation of phosphatases, and production of cytokine signaling suppressor molecules. Dysregulation of hematopoietic growth has been associated with genetic mutations, over expression or failure to deactivate specific growth factors, receptors, or signaling pathways.[20]

Finally, there is increasing evidence that HSC self-renewal and differentiation is not predictable (stochastic) or inducible (deterministic) but may also be epigenetically regulated in that the adult HSC compartment consists of a limited number of SC subsets which undergo clonal diversity by epigenetically preprogrammed behavior.[22] It has also been considered that epigenetic programming may influence SC development

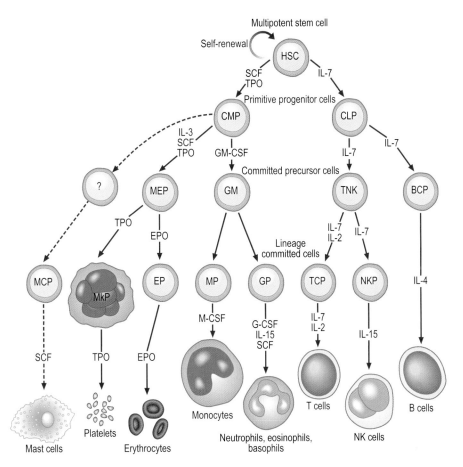

Fig. 15.3. Hematopoietic stem cell differentiation. Multipotent hematopoietic stem cells (HSC) in the bone marrow and other hematopoietic tissues may self-renew or undergo proliferation and differentiation to progenitors which become progressively more committed to various lineages, including lymphocytic, granulocytic, and myelocytic ones. This occurs under the influence of various cytokines and growth factors which are also shown in the scheme. CMP, common myeloid progenitor; CLP, common lymphoid progenitor; MEP, megakaryocytes and erythroid cells; GM, granulocytes and macrophages; TNK, T cells and natural killer cells; BCP, committed progenitors for B cells; MCP, mast cell progenitors; MkP, megakaryocytes; EP, erythrocytes; MP, monocytes; GP, granulocytes; TCP, T cells; NKP, NK cells. (Adapted, with permission, from Kaushansky K. Lineage–specific hematopoietic growth factors. N Engl J Med 2006; 354 (19): 2035 (Figure 1). Copyright, Massachusetts Medical Society.)

during embryogenesis. This may partially explain why the HSC compartment contains (myeloid and lymphoid) lineage-biased SC, in addition to HSC with fully-balanced pluripotential, and why HSC division is asymmetric (see 'Choice between self-renewal and differentiation'). It may also explain the shifts in pluripotency of the HSC compartment that are induced by disease, chemotherapy, transplantation, cytokine treatment, and aging.

HEMATOPOIETIC STEM CELL PLASTICITY

The high plasticity of SC has been described above and there are numerous reports of the ability of these cells to transdifferentiate into non-hematopoietic cell types such as hepatocytes, skeletal muscle cells, cardiomyocytes, neurons, and various epithelial cells; however, experimental evidence has not been entirely supportive of this concept.[12] Parabiotic experiments in mice have revealed that circulating HSC in

peripheral blood may re-enter the BM to resume their primitive HSC function.[12]

BONE MARROW-DERIVED AND PERIPHERAL BLOOD HEMATOPOIETIC STEM CELLS

Hematopoietic SC (HSC) which have the capacity to give rise to all blood cell types are present in the adult bone marrow (BM) (Fig. 15.2). Mesenchymal SC (multipotent adult progenitor cells, MAPC) are located in the BM stroma. MAPC are Stro-1$^+$ cells, show a high degree of plasticity and can differentiate along various mesenchymal lineages or de-differentiate into embryonic cells capable of giving rise to all cell lineages depending upon their microenvironment.[3,4] Gene expression is regulated by local tissue environmental or microenvironmental factors. For example, in the presence of c/EBP and PPAR-γ MAPC will undergo differentiation into either adipocytes or osteocytes.[3]

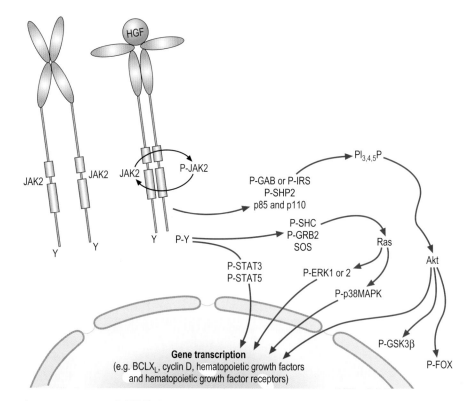

Fig. 15.4. Signaling in hematopoietic stem cell (HSC) development. Hematopoietic growth factor receptor signaling occurs at three levels progressively involving the activation of JAK2, STATs, Erk 1/2, and Akt. This results in nuclear activation of gene transcription of hematopoietic growth factors, cyclins, and regulators of apoptosis. (Reproduced with permission from Kaushansky K. Lineage-specific Hematopoietic Growth Factors. N Engl J Med 2006; 354 (19):2039 (Figure 3). Copyright, Massachusetts Medical Society. All rights reserved.)

Normal human peripheral blood also contains a small population of CD34+ primitive HSC capable of differentiating along either the myeloid or lymphoid lineage under the influence of specific growth factors. For example, the addition of IL-5 in combination with GM-CSF and IL-3 (or GM-CSF or IL-3 alone) to cultures containing such CD34+ SC gave rise to a large proportion of colonies with eosinophilic phenotype and characteristic gene expression.[23] ASC are also present in a CD34+ CD45+ CD14+ monocytic subset in peripheral blood.[3,24] Depending upon microenvironmental factors, these cells have been shown to undergo morphologic and/or functional differentiation along many lineages including: macrophages, T lymphocytes, endothelial cells, epithelial cells, etc.[20,25]

▌ THE STEM CELL NICHE ▌

DEFINITION AND GENERAL FEATURES

The concept of a SC niche was first proposed by Schofield[26] who hypothesized that in the proximity of SC there are heterologous cell types that have the ability to influence SC behavior. The first niches characterized were the ovarian and testicular niches controlling germline SC maintenance and differentiation in *Drosophila melanogaster*.[27,28] A hematopoietic niche controlling HSC maintenance and differentiation was only recently identified in mice.[29,30] Three niches have now been extensively characterized (although not as yet, at the ultrastructural level): the intestinal

epithelial niche; the epidermal niche; and the bone marrow niche. The notion that heterologous cell types compose the niche was supported by the early work in *Drosophila* and by more recent discoveries.[29-31]

A SC niche can be defined as a specific site or defined microenvironment composed of not only supporting cells but also matrix glycoproteins organized into a functional three-dimensional matrix. The contact between these elements allows molecular interactions and signals that are crucial for regulating SC quiescence, self-renewal, differentiation, and proliferation, as well as factors influencing mobilization and homing of progeny. The regulation of self-renewal and differentiation of ASC is crucial for maintaining tissue homeostasis. Therefore, the structure of the niche not only provides a nurturing environment for SC but also, in a dynamic way, determines the SC state in a proper spatiotemporal manner regulated by intrinsic mechanisms and molecular cross-talk. This chapter focuses on hematopoietic SC niches which regulate HSC fate.

CHOICE BETWEEN SELF-RENEWAL AND DIFFERENTIATION

The choice between cell divisions in which SC progeny retain parental cell properties, and differentiation in which the daughter cells become more oligopotent with lesser capacity for self-renewal, determines SC fate. The dynamic balance between SC self-renewal/quiescence and proliferation/

differentiation is regulated at increasing levels of complexity: cellular, microenvironmental (niche), macroenvironmental (i.e., responsiveness to factors emanating from surrounding tissues), systemic, and external environmental. One mechanism that ensures this balance is the control of asymmetric/symmetric SC division.[5] In asymmetric division, the SC divides into two daughter cells, one of which remains in the niche as a pluripotent SC, while the other leaves the niche to produce a large number of lineage-restricted progeny. In symmetric division, the SC divides into two identical daughter cells, both of which remain in the niche as SC. In the hematopoietic system under normal physiological conditions asymmetric division is likely the favored mechanism. Two types of HSC have been described: long-term (LT) HSC which contribute to hematopoiesis for months or even a lifetime that are kept as quiescent or slow cycling cells, and short term (ST) actively cycling HSC that have reconstitution capabilities limited to several weeks. In normal hematopoiesis SC must periodically divide to produce transit amplifying cells (TAC) that become progressively committed to various blood cell lineages. For the most part the niche microenvironment keeps the SC in a quiescent state, maintaining self-renewal, and activates SC proliferation only under conditions of tissue turnover and/or injury response.

While it appears that cytokines in the niche are involved, it is unclear whether this choice between self-renewal is a stochastic event in which cytokines are involved only in SC survival, or whether certain cytokines influence or instruct SC differentiation.[5]

HEMATOPOIETIC STEM CELL NICHES

At the present time, two hematopoietic niches have been characterized: the osteoblastic BM niche and the vascular niche.

Osteoblastic niche

The link between hematopoiesis and bone development (osteogenesis) was first recognized in the 1970s. More recently, the identification of several mutant mouse strains in which hematopoiesis is defective as a consequence of primary defects in bone development or remodeling, have revealed that osteoblasts or osteoclasts are important functional components of the BM niche.[32] In transgenic mice where osteoblasts have been genetically ablated, the marrow is aplastic and extensive extramedullary hematopoiesis occurs. Nagayoshi et al,[33] employing a cell implantation based strategy with a unique osteoblast cell line that resulted in the generation of ectopic bones, showed that transplanted osteoblasts were responsible for the increase in HSC observed in the transplant recipients. An accumulating body of evidence supports the model that HSC adjacent to the endosteum produce progenitors that migrate to blood vessels at the center of the BM cavity as they mature and differentiate. The BM consists of a hematopoietic portion which is surrounded by mesenchymal cells containing pluripotential mesenchymal SC. Postnatally, hematopoiesis occurs almost solely in the BM close to or on endosteum which is lined primarily by osteoblasts, osteoclasts, and stromal fibroblasts, and it has been shown that many of the cytokines that are critical for normal hematopoiesis and megakaryopoiesis are produced by osteoblasts.[34]

Vascular niche

The identity of a hematopoietic vascular niche was discovered only very recently.[31,35,36] Indeed, hematopoiesis and vascularization occur concurrently during development as HSC and endothelial cells are derived from the same progenitor cells (hemangioblasts) at the embryonic stage. Moreover, postnatal hematopoiesis occurring in the BM recapitulates the ontogeny of hematopoiesis that occurs in the yolk sac, aorta-gonad-mesonephros, placenta, fetal liver, and spleen. Vascular endothelial cells maintain HSC in vitro and are required for hematopoiesis in vivo. Applying single combinations of SLAM receptors HSC (CD150+ CD244- CD48- or CD150+ CD48- CD41-) have been distinguished from non-self-renewing multipotent hematopoietic progenitors (MPP)-more committed progenitors (CD244+ CD150- CD48-).[37] These are located not only adjacent to osteoblasts but also near sinusoidal endothelium in both the BM and extramedullary spleen, thus establishing a vascular niche for HSC. The vascular niche constitutes a more dynamic location in that it provides a more nutrient-rich microenvironment, with higher concentration of oxygen and growth factors from which mature blood cells may be ultimately released into the peripheral circulation. Hence, the vascular niche also functions in transendothelial migration important during homing and mobilization of hematopoietic cells. However, both the osteoblastic and vascular niches regulate HSC mobilization that includes HSC exodus from the osteoblastic niche, mobilization to the vascular niche, endothelial transmigration, and circulation in the vascular system. Thus, the currently accepted operational model of the BM niche is that HSC may utilize either osteoblast or endothelial cells for niche function under different circumstances for maintaining quiescence/self-renewal, or for inducing proliferation and further differentiation and mobilization of HSC to the circulation, respectively.

INTRINSIC vs EXTRINSIC FACTORS INFLUENCING HEMATOPOIETIC STEM CELL FATE

Only recently has it become evident that niche regulators are not only heterologous cells but also extracellular matrix (ECM) proteins and other inorganic components. Molecular intrinsic and extrinsic mechanisms regulating SC fate, i.e., self-renewal and quiescence, competence, propagation and differentiation of progenitors, and trafficking, have been the subject of intensive investigations (Fig. 15.5) Much of what we know of these mechanisms comes from studies of embryonic SC (ESC) lines and from studies in murine HSC.

Factors influencing self-renewal/quiescence, competence, and proliferation

In both ESC and HSC, increased self-renewal and retention of pluripotency appears to be associated with elements of the canonical Wnt (Wingless-related protein)/β-catenin signaling pathway,[5,38] soluble Notch modulators, fibroblast growth factors (FGFs), and sonic Hedgehog (Shh) which contribute in a paracrine manner to mammalian SC maintenance and development demonstrating varying capacity to induce proliferation or to impair differentiation.[5] Notch signaling seems to inhibit differentiation mechanisms that accompany Wnt-induced proliferation and therefore, expansion of the HSC pools. In the case of ESC both Wnt and TGFβ signaling appear to be important requirements for maintaining pluripotency and the undifferentiated state.[39] Studies with mouse ESC have shown that Wnt5A and Wnt6 produced by feeder cells and factors present in serum present in the culture medium were potent inhibitors of differentiation.[40] However, direct activation of the Wnt/β-catenin signaling pathway upregulated mRNA for STAT3 (signal transducer and activator of transcription-3),

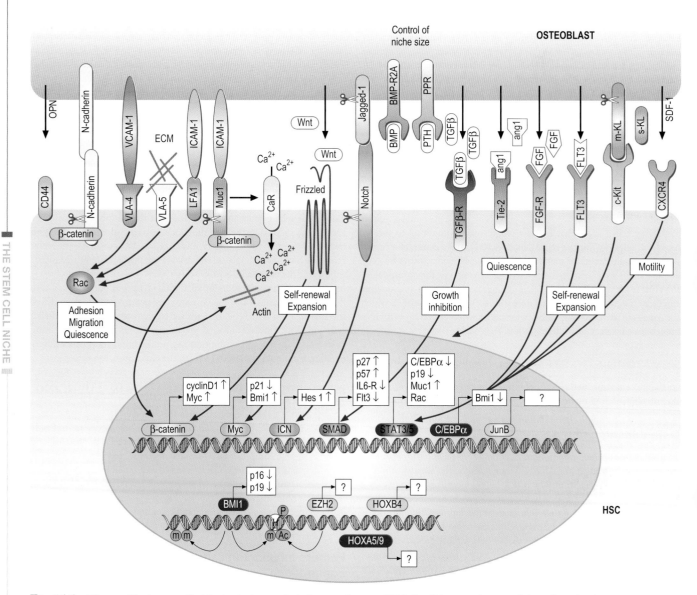

Fig. 15.5. The osteoblastic stem cell niche: intrinsic vs extrinsic factors influencing HSC fate. Schematic diagram of the endosteal niche–stem cell synapse showing ligand–receptor interactions and adhesion molecules, as well as some of the intracellular pathways that are activated following signaling. For abbreviations in the figure, see the text. (Modified from Rizo A, Vellenga E, de Haan G, Schuringa JJ. Signaling pathways in self-renewing hematopoietic and leukemic stem cells: do all stem cells need a niche? Hum Mol Genet 2006; IS: R210–R219. By permission of Oxford University Press.)

an established regulator for ESC self-renewal in the mouse, recapitulating the effects of Wnt5A and Wnt6. An additional role for phosphoinositide 3-kinase (Pi3Ks) in positively regulating mouse ESC self-renewal has recently been proposed.[41] In these studies it was also demonstrated that the anti-apoptotic effect of Wnt proteins (specifically, Wnt3A) was associated with increased ERK-dependent expression of Bcl-2 and phosphorylation of GSK-3β, downstream activation of β-catenin mediated transcription that required ERK, PI3K and Akt signaling. In more differentiated SC lines such as human osteoblast progenitors, Wnt proteins are likely to be involved in growth and survival,

and apoptosis induced by serum withdrawal may be prevented by addition of Wnt proteins (which induce transient phosphorylation of Src and Akt and nuclear accumulation of phosphorylated ERKs).[42] Another mechanism by which osteoblasts might negatively regulate the number of HSC and maintain their quiescence is by secreting osteopontin (OPN, Fig. 15.5) which functions like angiopoietin-1 (ang1) as a potent constraining factor on HSC proliferation.[43]

BMP signaling via an as yet, undefined receptor, inhibits cell proliferation while FGF promotes proliferation (Fig. 15.5). A recent study demonstrated that the inhibition of glycogen synthase kinase 3 (GSK-3) modulates Wnt, Notch and Shh signaling, and enhances HSC progenitor activity and also maintains (but does not expand) the SC pool.[44]

On the other hand, Calvi[45] established that parathyroid hormone (PTH) through activation of its receptor (PPR) on osteoblasts could alter the niche resulting in HSC expansion via the Jagged-1/Notch signaling pathway.

Membrane-bound SCF and its receptor c-Kit (Fig. 15.5) may also have a role to play in SC homeostasis. Studies in mutant mice have shown that both are important for long-term maintenance and self-renewal of adult HSC, raising the possibility that the SCF-Kit pathway mediates endosteal bone marrow HSC niche activity.[46] Loss of SCF from supporting cells in Sl/Sl mice or of the receptor in HSC in W^v/W^v mice leads to hematopoietic failure.[47] Finally, lipid raft clustering induced by cytokines also appears to be essential for HSC re-entry into the cell cycle.[48]

Factors influencing stem cell trafficking and adherence

The ability of HSC to mobilize or to home to the niche relies on specific molecular recognition, cell–cell adhesion or disengagement, transendothelial migration, and anchoring to the BM niche. The chemokine SDF-1 (stromal cell derived factor 1, CXCL12, Fig. 15.5) is one of the most important molecules in this regard. Endothelial cells, osteoblasts and stromal cells constitutively express SDF-1 while HSC express the SDF-1 receptor, CXCR4. These are involved in the regulation of migration, survival and development of HSC.[49] SDF-1 released from endothelial cells promotes transendothelial migration of HSC and high levels of SDF-1 on osteoblastic cell surfaces guide HSC homing to the niche. G-CSF, widely used clinically, induces HSC mobilization by decreasing SDF-1 in osteoblasts and increasing its concentration in the blood.[50]

In the case of megakaryocyte progenitors, FGF-4 (Fig. 15.5) augments their adhesion to the vascular niche while SDF-1 acts as a trigger for the transendothelial migration of $CD41^+$ megakaryocytes.[51] Both FGF-4 and SDF-1 enhance the expression of the adhesion molecule VLA-4 on megakaryocytes as well as VCAM-1 on endothelial cells.

The adhesion molecules and ligands important in niche function include: N-cadherin/β-catenin, VCAM/integrin, and osteopontin/$β_1$-integrin (Fig. 15.5). They play a role in either SC attachment to, or migration from, the niche. N-cadherin-expressing osteoblasts that form an N-cadherin/β-catenin adherens complex with HSC likely mediate the attachment or adhesion or retention of HSC within the BM niche. N-cadherin is negatively regulated by c-Myc in differentiating HSC, perhaps by promoting their displacement from the endosteum. c-Myc upregulation is required to release HSC from the niche. Myc activity in HSC represses the expression of N-cadherin and of several integrins. Most importantly, HSC overexpressing Myc are lost over time because of differentiation, presumably owing to their failure to be retained in the niche. These data indicate that the balance between self-renewal and differentiation might be controlled by Myc-dependent retention or exit of HSC from the niche.[52,53]

Osteopontin expressed on endosteal osteoblasts was found to contribute to HSC migration toward the endosteal region through interaction with β-integrin. Integrin $α_4β_1$ is involved in the mobilization and migration of HSC or progenitor cells. It has been demonstrated that maintenance of HSC quiescence and anchorage is also dependent on angiopoietin-1 (ang1) signaling from the osteoblastic niche through the receptor tyrosine kinase, Tie-2 (Fig. 15.5) expressed on HSC and endothelial cells.[54] The identification of N-cadherin as a target in ang1 signaling suggests an interesting link between adhesion molecules and cell-cycle regulators in modulating HSC–niche interaction.

In addition to other secreted proteins such as VEGF (vascular endothelial growth factor) and PLGF (platelet-derived growth factor) involved in HSC mobilization/recruitment, non-protein components such as Ca^{2+} ions, or ROS or other products of oxidative stress present in the microenvironment may also affect SC function. High Ca^{2+} concentrations that exist near active osteoclasts might influence SC and, indeed, a G-protein calcium sensing receptor is expressed on HSC and SC. Ca^{2+} receptor knockout mice demonstrated markedly abnormal ability to undergo BM engraftment and readily released HSC into the blood. HSC express Ca^{2+} sensing receptors that would help them to localize to the endosteal niche by promoting HSC adhesion to collagen.[55]

■ STEM CELL CLINICAL APPLICATIONS ■

The use of living cells as therapeutic agents is an alternative approach to traditional medicine and is presently being used in several clinical settings including treatment of injured joints, chronic ulcers, corneal damage, large burns, neural damage and others. SC with their self-renewal capacity and pluripotency are of special interest as potential therapy for a number of diseases. While considerable effort is being made to develop tissue reconstitutive therapy using ESC, we are considerably far from practical application and in many jurisdictions legal issues concerning their use still need to be resolved. However, as described above, BM and adult peripheral blood contains various populations of ASC including HSC giving rise to all blood elements and mesenchymal SC which have more diverse potential. Cord blood is a good source of pluripotential SC and these populations have been exploited with a good measure of success in reconstitutive therapy[56] and other applications such as antitumor therapy.[57] However, success is limited by the frequencies of SC in these populations as well as issues pertaining to engraftment.

THERAPY USING BONE MARROW-DERIVED STEM CELLS

Bone marrow transplantation (BMT) was the first stem cell therapy that utilized adult HSC to replenish ablated bone marrow in malignant, genetic or autoimmune diseases and to reconstitute the hematopoietic system. Under various conditions, BM-derived ASC can give rise to additional tissues such as blood vessels, liver, nerve cells as well as insulin-secreting Langerhans cells. Bone marrow, cord and peripheral blood also contain endothelial progenitor cells (EPC) that can form new blood vessels (neo-vascularization) or replenish existing blood vessels (re-endothelialization).

THERAPY USING ADULT PERIPHERAL BLOOD STEM CELLS

SC present in adult blood have also been employed in clinical therapy. Pluripotent SC are found among the HSC compartment, but also among the mononuclear cell (MNC) compartment of peripheral blood.[58] Co-expression of hematopoietic, endothelial, and mesenchymal markers was reported in those progenitor populations, and it is apparent that the adherent CD14+ (monocytic) compartment in the normal peripheral blood is a major source of mesenchymal SC as well as endothelial progenitor cells. It is not clear whether committed precursors exist for each cell lineage, or most of the monocytic SC are truly pluripotent, giving rise to various lineages under different culture conditions and combinations of growth factors.

Nonetheless, it seems that the monocytic compartment represents a rich source of ASC and thus, the proportion of potential ASC in the peripheral blood may be much higher than previously expected.

The frequency of CD34+ SC in peripheral blood of normal healthy individuals is estimated to be $1-2 \times 10^3$ per ml (or about $0.45-1.35 \times 10^6$ cells per unit of blood)[59] but may be improved by more sophisticated extraction techniques.[60] Monocytes constitute approx. 10% of the peripheral blood mononuclear (MNC) cell population. Attempts to isolate monocytic SC have provided some estimates of their frequency in blood. About 0.18% of MNC isolated from peripheral blood are CD133+ or CD34+ SC.[61] The number of SC in 1 ml of blood is about 3×10^3 cells. Yields of CD34+ cells recovered from one unit of cord blood are similar to that in adult blood ($1-5 \times 10^6$ cells). It is not clear, however, how similar these two cell populations are, and functional studies are still required to clarify their regenerative potential.

Peripheral blood HSC derived from healthy donors treated with G-CSF (to induce SC mobilization) is widely used in transplantation. Clinical scientists have already started to explore the therapeutic potential of non-mobilized and mobilized circulating SC in clinical trials for non-hematopoietic tissue regeneration.

The success of HSC transplantation depends upon several factors including the ability of the SC to respond to migration and growth/differentiation factors in the target tissue. Negative issues limiting the use of HSC in tissue repair and reconstitution include: the low frequency of SC in donor tissue which is age-dependent; difficulties in isolating and expanding HSC prior to transplantation; the extent of tissue damage; the occurrence of graft-vs-host disease (GVHD) in allogeneic partially-matched transplantation; and potential premature fusion of donor SC cells with mature cells in tissue which circumvents SC expansion and functional differentiation. However, when transplantation of autologous mobilized HSC is possible, GVHD is ruled out.

THERAPY USING CORD BLOOD-DERIVED STEM CELLS

Human umbilical cord blood (CB) has established itself as a legitimate source for HSC transplantation. Since the first transplantation was performed in 1988, it is estimated that approximately 7000 patients with malignant and non-malignant diseases have been successfully transplanted with CB-derived SC.[11] The main advantage of using CB as a source of HSC rather than BM is its relative ease of collection from the umbilical vein, before, or after the expulsion of the placenta Another advantage is the naivety of newborn's immune system. This permits transplantations under less stringency for HLA matching and lesser risk of GVHD.[11,14,15] A disadvantage of using CB-derived SC for transplantation is the observed slow rate of engraftment. However, their high proliferation capacity and excellent response to exogenous cytokines makes up for this deficiency. The main strategies aimed at solving this problem are based on expansion of the number of the stem cells in CB grafts, induction of a temporary engraftment with other SC sources, and reduction of the toxicity of the conditioning regimens.

▮ FUTURE DIRECTIONS ▮

While much progress has been made in defining SC populations and understanding their role in tissue homeostasis and repair, there remains much to be discovered. Future research will focus on unraveling the complex cellular interactions within tissue niche, particularly those outside of the BM. An exciting area for discovery will include investigations into epigenetic effects regulating SC gene expression during self-renewal/quiescence and proliferation/differentiation. Novel epigenetic approaches will include gene silencing involving promoter methylation or histone deacetylation.

Continued efforts to develop better methods of identifying unique markers useful in purification of SC from complex cellular mixtures, and methods for expanding SC and their progenitors in vitro will bring better therapeutic success. In vitro studies revealed that SC proliferate with the addition of cytokines.[62–64] However, care must be exercised as extensive proliferation may have the undesired effect of reducing SC competence and long-term self-renewal capacity.

Techniques to improve homing of injected SC to the desired tissue site must also be improved. For example, in vivo manipulation of CBSC with all-trans retinoic acid to upregulate the expression of the adhesion molecules ICAM-1 and VCAM-1 is under experimentation as well as intra-osseous transplantation that has been suggested as a way to shorten the SC homing process.

In the future CB stem cell transplantation may also be exploited for gene transfer (in the treatment of primary immune or other genetic deficiencies) and as a source of regenerative cells in non-hematopoietic injured tissues. In an era in which 20% of patients requiring transplants will not find a matched related or unrelated BM or peripheral HSC donor, CB transplantation is an attractive alternative to achieving a cure for a wide variety of diseases. Clinical trials in which the missing adenosine deaminase gene was transferred into children with severe combined immunodeficiency disease (SCID) employed BM and CB SC as vehicles for gene transfer. Another, as yet only investigational, field has focused on the ability of HSC to differentiate into or form heterokaryons with cells of other tissues in regeneration or repair of damaged tissues.[65,66]

Understanding cancer SC and their contribution to minimal residual disease (MRD), and continued efforts to define useful markers to serve as targets for cancer cell elimination will be an important direction in future research.[67–69]

Finally, ESC with their totipotency show the greatest potential for reconstitutive therapy. Nevertheless, there are many obstacles to be overcome in addition to the ethical ones concerning the use of human embryos. Arriving at this point, scientists will be faced with additional challenges which will include: issues pertaining to the homing of donor ESC populations to the appropriate tissues; whether they will fuse with host cells or establish chimeric populations; and immunologic issues pertaining to graft rejection.

All the issues relating to stem cells and therapy constitute one of the hottest topics in the biomedical field because they open opportunities for nearly limitless new therapeutic frontiers.

References

Stem cells: definition and general characteristics

1. Weissman IL. Stem cells: units of development, units of regeneration, and units in evolution. Cell 2000; 100:157–168.
2. Till J, McCulloch EA. A direct measurement of the radiation sensitivity of normal mouse bone marrow cells. Radiat Res 1961; 14:213–222.

Embryonic and adult stem cells

3. Diaz-Flores L Jr, Madrid JF, Gutierrez R, et al. Adult stem and transit-amplifying cell location. Histol Histopatol 2006; 21:995–1027.
4. Blau HM, Brazelton TR, Weimann JM. The evolving concept of a stem cell: entity or function? Cell 2001; 105:829–841.

Adult stem cells

5. Wagers AJ, Christensen JL, Weissman IL. Review. Cell fate determination from stem cells. Gene Therapy 2002; 9:606–612.
6. Chen J. Senescence and functional failure in hematopoietic stem cells. Exp Hematol 2004; 32:1025–1032.
7. Rossi DJ, Bryder D, Zahn JM, et al. Cell intrinsic alterations underlie hematopoietic stem cell aging. PNAS 2005; 102:9194–9199.
8. Hill JM, Zalos G, Halcox JP, et al. Circulating endothelial progenitor cells, vascular function, and cardiovascular risk. N Engl J Med 2003; 348:593–600.
9. Choi JH, Kim KL, Huh W, et al. Decreased number and impaired angiogenic function of endothelial progenitor cells in patients with chronic renal failure. Arterioscler Thromb Vasc Biol 2004; 24:1246–1252.
10. Palange P, Testa U, Huertas A, et al. Circulating haemopoietic and endothelial progenitor cells are decreased in COPD. Eur Res J 2006; 27:529–541.

Hematopoietic stem cells

11. Cohen Y, Nagler A. Umbilical cord blood transplantation – how, when and for whom? Blood Rev 2004; 18:167–79.
12. Bryder D, Rossi DJ, Weissman IL. Hematopoietic stem cells. The paradigmatic tissue-specific stem cell. Am J Pathol 2006; 169:338–346.
13. Weissman IL. Translating stem and progenitor cell biology to the clinic: barriers and opportunities. Science 2000; 287:1442–1446.
14. Rocha V, Cornish J, Sievers EL, et al. Comparison of outcomes of unrelated bone marrow and umbilical cord blood transplants in children with acute leukemia. Blood 2001; 97:2962–2971.
15. Rocha V, Wagner JE, Sobocinski KA, et al. Graft-versus-host disease in children who have received a cord-blood or bone marrow transplant from HLA-identical sibling. N Engl J Med 2000; 342:1846–1854.
16. Elchalal U, Fasouliotis SJ, Shtockheim D, et al. Postpartum umbilical cord blood collection for transplantation: a comparison of three methods. Am J Obstet Gynecol 2000; 182:227–232.
17. Handgretinger R, Gordon PR, Leimig T, et al. Biology and plasticity of CD133+ hematopoietic stem cells. Ann N Y Acad Sci 2003; 996:141–151.
18. McNiece IK, Briddell RA. Stem cell factor. J Leukoc Biol 1995; 58:14–22.
19. Simone MD, De Santis S, Vigneti F, et al. Nerve growth factor: a survey of activity on immune and hematopoietic cells. Hematol Oncol 1999; 17:1–10.
20. Kaushansky K. Lineage-specific hematopoietic growth factors. N Engl J Med 2006; 354:2034–2045.
21. Zhang J, Grindley JC, Yin T, et al. PTEN maintains haematopoietic stem cells and acts in lineage choice and leukaemia prevention. Nature 2006; 441:518–522.
22. Muller-Sieburg CE, Sieburg HB. The GOD of hematopoietic stem cells: a clonal diversity model of the stem cell compartment. Cell Cycle 2006; 5:394–398.
23. Shalit M. Growth and differentiation of eosinophils from peripheral blood CD34+ cells. Allerg Immunol (Paris) 1997; 29:7–10.
24. Kodama H, Inoue T, Watanabe R, et al. Neurogenic potential of progenitors derived from human circulating CD14 monocytes. Immunol Cell Biol 2006; 84:209–217.
25. Rohde E, Malischnik C, Thaler D, et al. Blood monocytes mimic endothelial progenitor cells. Stem Cells 2006; 24:357–367.

The stem cell niche

26. Schofield R. The relationship between the spleen colony-forming cell and the haemopoietic stem cell. Blood Cells 1978; 4:7–25.
27. Xie T, Spradling AC. A niche maintaining germ line stem cells in the Drosophila ovary. Science 2000; 290:328–330.
28. Kiger AA, White-Cooper H, Fuller MT. Somatic support cells restrict germline stem cell self-renewal and promote differentiation. Nature 2000; 407:750–754.
29. Calvi LM, Adams GB, Weibrecht KW, et al. Osteoblastic cells regulate the haematopoietic stem cell niche. Nature 2003; 425:841–846.
30. Zhang J, Niu C, Ye L, et al. Identification of the haematopoietic stem cell niche and control of the niche size. Nature 2003; 425:836–841.

31. Kiel MJ, Iwashita T, Yilmaz OH, et al. Spatial differences in hematopoiesis but not in stem cells indicate a lack of regional patterning in definitive hematopoietic stem cells. Dev Biol 2005; 283:29–39.
32. Visnjic D, Kalajzic Z, Rowe DW, et al. Hematopoiesis is severely altered in mice with an induced osteoblast deficiency. Blood 2004; 103:3258–3264.
33. Nagayoshi K, Ohkawa H, Yorozu K, et al. Increased mobilization of c-kit(+) Sca-1(+) Lin(-) (KSL) cells and colony-forming units in spleen (CFU-S) following de novo formation of a stem cell niche depends on dynamic, but not stable, membranous ossification. Cell Physiol 2006; 208(1):188–194.
34. Kacena MA, Gundberg CM, Horowitz MC. A reciprocal regulatory interaction between megakaryocytes, bone cells, and hemopoietic stem cells. Bone 2006; 39:978–984.
35. Heissig B, Hattori K, Dias S, et al. Recruitment of stem and progenitor cells from the bone marrow niche requires MMP-9 mediated release of kit-ligand. Cell 2002; 109:625–637.
36. Kiel MJ, Morrison SJ. Maintaining hematopoietic stem cells in the vascular niche. Immunity 2006; 25:862–864.
37. Kiel MJ, Yilmaz OH, Iwashita T, et al. SLAM family receptors distinguish hematopoietic stem and progenitor cells and reveal endothelial niches for stem cells. Cell 2005; 121:1109–1121. Comment in: Cell 2005; 121:967–970.
38. Sato N, Meijer L, Skaltsounis L, et al. Maintenance of pluripotency in human and mouse embryonic stem cells through activation of Wnt signaling by a pharmacologic GSK-specific inhibitor. Nat Med 2004; 10:55–63.
39. Noggle SA, James D, Brivanlou AH. A molecular basis for human embryonic stem cell pluripotency. Stem Cell Rev 2005; 1:111–118.
40. Hao J, Li TG, Qi X, et al. WNT/beta catenin pathway up-regulates Stat3 and converges on LIF to prevent differentiation of embryonic stem cells. Devel Biol 2006; 290:81–91.
41. Paling NR, Wheadon H, Bone HK, et al. Regulation of embryonic stem cell self-renewal by phosphoinositide 3-kinase-dependent signaling. J Biol Chem 2004; 279:48063–48070.
42. Almeida M, Han L, Bellido T, et al. Wnt proteins prevent apoptosis of both uncommitted osteoblast progenitors and differentiated osteoblasts by beta-catenin-dependent and -independent signaling cascades involving Src/ERK and phosphatidylinositol 3-kinase/AKT. J Biol Chem 2005; 280:41342–41351.
43. Haylock DN, Nilsson SK. Osteopontin: a bridge between bone and blood. Br J Haematol 2006; 134:467–474.
44. Trowbridge JJ, Xenacostas Am, Moon RT, et al. Glycogen synthase kinase-3 is an in vivo regulator of hematopoietic stem cell repopulation. Nat Med 2006; 12:89–98.
45. Calvi LM. Osteoblastic activation in the hematopoietic stem cell niche. Ann NY Acad Sci 2006; 1068:477–488.
46. Driessen RL, Johnston HM, Nilsson SK. Membrane-bound stem cell factor is a key regulator in the initial lodgment of stem cells within the endosteal marrow region. Exp Hematol 2003; 31:1284–1291.
47. Bernstein A, Forrester L, Reith AD, et al. The murine W/c-kit and Steel loci and the control of hematopoiesis. Semin Hematol 1991; 28:138–142.
48. Yamazaki S, Iwama A, Takayanagi S, et al. Cytokine signals modulated via lipid rafts mimic niche signals and induce hibernation in hematopoietic stem cells. EMBO J 2006; 25:3515–3523.
49. Dar A, Kollet O, Lapidot T. Mutual, reciprocal SDF-1/CXCR4 interactions between hematopoietic and bone marrow stromal cells regulate human stem cell migration and development in NOD/SCID chimeric mice. Exp Hematol 2006; 34:967–975.
50. Petit I, Szyper-Kravitz M, Nagler A, et al. G-CSF induces stem cell mobilization by decreasing bone marrow SDF-1 and upregulating CXCR4. Nat Immunol 2002; 3:687–694. Erratum in: Nat Immunol 2002; 3:787.
51. Avecilla ST, Hattori K, Heissig B, et al. Chemokine-mediated interaction of hematopoietic progenitors with the bone marrow vascular niche is required for thrombopoiesis. Nat Med 2004; 10:64–71.
52. Wilson A, Murphy MJ, Oskarsson T, et al. c-Myc controls the balance between hematopoietic stem cell self-renewal and differentiation. Genes Dev 2004, 18:2747–2763.
53. Murphy MJ, Wilson A, Trumpp A. More than just proliferation: Myc function in stem cells. Trends Cell Biol 2005; 15:128–137.
54. Arai F, Hirao A, Ohmura M, et al. Tie2/angiopoietin-1 signaling regulates hematopoietic stem cell quiescence in the bone marrow niche. Cell 2004; 118:149–161. Comment in: Cell 2004; 118:139–140.
55. Adams GB, Chabner KT, Alley IR, et al. Stem cell engraftment at the endosteal niche is specified by the calcium-sensing receptor. Nature 2006; 439:599–603.

Stem cell clinical applications

56. Takahashi S, Ooi J, Tomonari J, et al. Comparative single-institute analysis of cord blood transplantation from unrelated donors with bone marrow or peripheral blood stem cell transplantation from related donors in adult patients with hematological malignancies after myeloablative conditioning regimen. Blood 2007; 109:1322–1330.
57. Condiotti R, Nagler A. Effect of interleukin-12 on antitumor activity of human umbilical cord blood and bone marrow cytotoxic cells. Exp Hematol 1998; 26:571–579.
58. Porat Y, Porozov S, Belkin D, et al. Isolation of an adult blood-derived progenitor cell population capable of differentiation into angiogenic, myocardial and neural lineages. Br J Haematol 2006; 135:703–714.
59. Taguchi A, Matsuyama T, Moriwaki H, et al. Circulating CD34-positive cells provide an index of cerebrovascular function. Circulation 2004; 109:2972–2975.
60. Ivanovic Z, Duchez P, Morgan MA, et al. Whole-blood leukodepletion filters as a source of CD34+ progenitors potentially usable in cell therapy. Transfusion 2006; 46:118–125.
61. Walenta K, Friedrich EB, Sehnert F, et al. In vitro differentiation characteristics of cultured human mononuclear cells – implications for endothelial progenitor cell biology. Biochem Biophys Res Commun 2005; 333:476–482.

REFERENCES

Future directions

62. Pick M, Nagler A, Grisaru D, et al. Expansion of megakaryocyte progenitors from human umbilical cord using a new two-step separation procedure. Br J Haematol 1998; 103:639–650.
63. Peled T, Landau E, Mandel J, et al. Linear polyamine copper chelator tetraethylenepentamine augments long-term ex vivo expansion of cord blood-derived $CD34^+$ cells and increases their engraftment potential in NOD/SCID mice. Exp Hematol 2004; 32:547–555.
64. Peled T, Mandel J, Goudsmid RN, et al. Pre-clinical development of cord blood-derived progenitor cell graft expanded ex vivo with cytokines and the polyamine copper chelator tetraethylenepentamine. Cytotherapy 2004; 6:344–355.
65. Leor J, Guetta E, Chouraqui P, et al. Human umbilical cord blood cells: a new alternative for myocardial repair? Cytotherapy 2005; 7:251–257.
66. Leor J, Guetta E, Feinberg MS, et al. Human umbilical cord blood-derived $CD133^+$ cells enhance function and repair of the infarcted myocardium. Stem Cells 2006; 24:772–780. Erratum in: Stem Cells 2006; 24:1627–1627.
67. Nagler A, Condiotti R, Rabinowitz R, et al. Detection of minimal residual disease (MRD) after bone marrow transplantation (BMT) by multi-parameter flow cytometry (MPFC). Med Oncol 1999; 16:177–187.
68. Schulenburg A, Ulrich-Pur H, Thurnher D, et al. Neoplastic stem cells: a novel therapeutic target in clinical oncology. Cancer 2006; 107:2512–2520.
69. Kim JJ, Tannock IF. Repopulation of cancer cells during therapy: an important cause of treatment failure. Nat Rev Cancer 2005; 5:516–525.

Biology of Lymphocytes

16

Lauren Cohn and Anuradha Ray

CONTENTS

SUMMARY OF IMPORTANT CONCEPTS

>> Adaptive immune responses depend on activation of naïve CD4 T cells and differentiation into effector cells

>> Multiple signals coordinate differentiation into specific CD4 T effector cell subsets, Th1, Th2, Th17

>> Each effector subset has a specific influence on inflammation, including activation of B lymphocytes and mobilization of leukocytes to sites of inflammation

>> CD4Th2 cells are critical mediators of inflammation in asthma

>> Many other cell types, Th1, Th17, CD8, NK T γ/δ, NK, and B cells, have been shown to promote allergic airway inflammation

>> Regulatory T cells may play a role in protection from asthma development

INTRODUCTION

Lymphocytes are central to the development of immune responses, either in allergy or in host defense to pathogens. Although allergy is an inappropriate response to environmental antigens that leads to an injurious response, whereas host defense is an essential protective response, the same principles apply. The immune system is made up of adaptive and innate elements of the immune response. A specific response that occurs as an adaptation to encountering a new antigen, such as an inflammatory response to contact with poison ivy, is one of the many types of adaptive immune responses that often confer immunity to a specific antigen for the life of the host.

Adaptive immune responses depend on lymphocytes. Innate immune responses largely take advantage of the immediate and non-specific responses of neutrophils and macrophages, although other inflammatory cells, including lymphocytes, have been shown to respond early to various foreign antigens. Innate immune responses appear to be less critical in the outcomes of allergic diseases compared with their protective role against pathogens. The presumed sites of exposure to allergens, including skin, respiratory tract, and gut, are under surveillance by cells of the innate limb of the immune response. The interaction of the innate response to allergens may have an important influence on the development of adaptive immune responses. This chapter focuses on T and B lymphocytes, how these cells respond to protein antigens such as allergens, and how T and B cells contribute to allergic inflammation in asthma.

T LYMPHOCYTES

Adaptive immune responses are initiated by T cells bearing alpha-beta (α/β) T cell antigen receptors (TCRs), which make up a majority of T cells. The TCR comprises two polypeptide chains and has an antigen-binding or variable region, a constant region, and a region that anchors TCR to the cell membrane (hinge, transmembrane, and cytoplasmic tail regions). During development in the thymus, T cells undergo TCR rearrangement, which creates unique antigen-binding domains, and positive selection, which permits maturation of T cells that will recognize antigens in the context of self-major histocompatibility complex (MHC) antigens. Once released into the bloodstream, a mature T cell bears a single TCR with unique antigen specificity. An estimated 10^6 different TCRs exist in an individual. This extraordinary diversity of TCRs allows the individual to respond to a vast range of antigens throughout life.

Two classes of α/β T lymphocytes, CD4 and CD8, are involved in adaptive immune responses and they are distinguished by the expression of this cell surface co-receptor, their interaction with different MHC molecules and by their different functions. $CD4^+$ T cells are traditionally called T helper (Th) cells. They recognize antigen presented by class II MHC molecules, which are present only on antigen-presenting cells (APCs), including B cells, macrophages, and dendritic cells. Protein antigens are taken up by APCs and processed into peptides in endocytic vesicles, which are presented on the cell surface bound to class II MHC molecules. CD8 cytotoxic T (Tc) cells recognize antigen presented by class I MHC molecules. Class I MHC is present on the surface of all nucleated cells. CD8$^+$ T cells are typically activated by pathogens, especially viruses, which may infect any cell. Therefore, CD8$^+$ T cells are not induced in response to allergens, but, as discussed later, they may enhance airway inflammation in allergic diseases.

CD4$^+$ T CELL ACTIVATION

When a mature CD4$^+$ T cell is released from the thymus into the circulation, it is considered naive, having never come into contact with its specific antigen. The T cell circulates from the bloodstream into peripheral lymphoid tissue, entering the lymph node by way of specialized blood vessels, the high endothelial venules (HEVs). Naive T cells express L-selectin, which binds to vascular addressin expressed on the HEVs and in turn allows for specific homing into the lymphoid tissue.[1] The chemokine CCL21, produced by both the HEVs and stromal cells within the lymphoid tissue, binds to its receptor (CCR7) on naive T cells and promotes T cell recruitment into the lymph node.[2]

In the peripheral lymphoid tissues (lymph nodes, spleen, mucosal lymphoid tissues), T cells come into contact with APCs that bear foreign antigens. Dendritic cells (DCs) are the primary APCs that activate naive T cells.[3] At mucosal sites, DCs form a dense network to catch antigens that penetrate the surfaces. DCs take up antigen when it binds specifically to DC surface receptors or by non-specific macropinocytosis. B cells take up antigen by specific binding to cell surface immunoglobulin, and macrophages engulf large particles and pathogens. APCs break down antigens into peptide fragments in endocytic vesicles, where the peptides are loaded onto class II proteins and then transported to the cell surface.[3] The act of processing antigen leads to maturation of immature DCs to mature DCs, which then leave the mucosal surface and migrate to local lymphoid tissues.

In the peripheral lymphoid tissues, naive CD4$^+$ T cells pass by APCs, sampling by cell contact, causing the TCR to interact with class II MHC and its bound peptide. If specific antigen is not encountered, the CD4$^+$ T cell passes back into the bloodstream and continues recirculating until it contacts its antigen. When a CD4$^+$ T cell contacts its specific antigen on an APC, it migrates no farther. For T cell activation to be initiated, two signals are required: (1) TCR recognition of MHC class II peptide and (2) a simultaneous co-stimulatory signal delivered by the same APC. If both these signals are received, the T cell goes in G1 phase of the cell cycle and begins to produce interleukin-2 (IL-2). IL-2 is an essential T cell autocrine growth factor that stimulates the T cell to progress though the cell cycle and undergo clonal expansion, giving rise to a population of effector cells with the identical TCR specificity to the parental cell (Fig. 16.1).

The principal co-stimulatory molecules expressed on the surface of APCs are CD80 (B7–1) and CD86 (B7–2) which both interact with CD28 on the T cell.[4–6] Although other co-stimulatory molecules have been described, only these B7 molecules have been definitively proven to activate naive T cells. Co-stimulation is responsible for inducing high levels of IL-2 production, which is essential for the T cell to proliferate and become an effector cell. The CD28-B7 interaction has been shown to enhance IL-2 transcription by inducing expression of the transcription factors activator protein-1 (AP-1) and nuclear factor kappa B (NF-κB) and by stabilizing IL-2 messenger ribonucleic acid (mRNA).[7] The co-stimulatory signal also increases the affinity of the IL-2 receptor

for its ligand.[8] Under some conditions, when there is potent local production of IL-2, the co-stimulatory signal between the APC and T cell may be less critical for T cell activation.[8]

Other co-stimulatory molecules have been described, the effects of which become important once T cell activation has been initiated. Activated CD4$^+$ T cells express CD40-ligand (CD40L) that binds CD40 on APCs, leading to increased expression of B7 and further enhancing T cell activation.[9] As described later, CD40 signaling is also essential for B cell activation. Inducible co-stimulator (ICOS), a CD28-related molecule, is expressed on activated T cells in response to TCR and CD28 signaling.[10] ICOS binds to its receptor, B7RP-1, on B cells and macrophages, stimulating those effector cells, but does not appear to be critical for initiating T cell activation.[11] Activated T cells also express the CD28-related molecule, cytotoxic T lymphocyte antigen-4 (CTLA-4, CD152), which binds to the B7 molecules, but with a much higher affinity.[12] CTLA-4 is only induced 48 h after T cell activation and delivers an inhibitory signal to the T cell, blocking IL-2 production and limiting T cell growth and thus serves to downregulate T cell responses once initiated.[13]

If a CD4$^+$ T cell recognizes its specific antigen on an APC (signal 1) in the absence of a co-stimulatory signal, the cell will become anergic or unresponsive because it is unable to proliferate due to a lack of IL-2 production.[14]

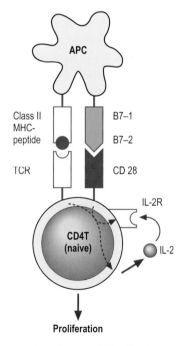

Fig. 16.1. Two-signal mechanism of CD4 T cell activation. Antigen-presenting cell (APC) takes up a protein antigen and processes it into peptide fragments that are presented by class II major histocompatibility complex (MHC) molecules. The first signal required for CD4 T cell activation is recognition by the T cell antigen receptor (TCR) of the class II MHC–peptide complex. The second, co-stimulatory signal is an interaction of CD28 on the T cell with B7–1 or B7–2 on the APC. These signals stimulate interleukin-2 (IL-2) production and induce CD4 T cell proliferation. IL-2R, IL-2 receptor.

CD4 T HELPER DIFFERENTIATION

Cellular mechanisms

Antigen-activated CD4+ T cells have the potential to differentiate into effector cells, each with distinct functional properties conferred by the pattern of cytokines they secrete (Fig. 16.2).[15,16] *T helper type 1* (Th1) cells are a subset of CD4+ T cells that secrete the macrophage activating factor, interferon gamma (IFN-γ), and lymphotoxin (LT), whereas *T helper type 2* (Th2) cells produce interleukin-4 (IL-4), IL-5, IL-9, IL-10, and IL-13.[17,18] *T helper type 17* (Th17) cells produce IL-17A, IL-17F, IL-6, and tumor necrosis factor.[19] Regulatory T cells, which are both naturally occurring and induced, have a suppressive function and are not considered effector cells. Their role in controlling allergic airway inflammation is discussed below. Th1 cells stimulate strong cell-mediated immune responses, particularly against intracellular pathogens. Th2 cells, through the production of IL-4 and IL-13, are potent activators of B cell antibody production, particularly immunoglobulin E (IgE).[20] IL-5 secretion by Th2 cells is critical for eosinophil differentiation and maturation.[21] Th2 cells are elicited in immune responses that require a strong humoral component and in antiparasitic responses. Th17 cells stimulate neutrophil mobilization and may function in host defense against bacteria. Th17 cells promote chronic inflammation dominated by IL-17, IL-6, IL-8 and tumor necrosis factor as well as

neutrophils and monocytes. Additional effects of Th17 cells are being elucidated, as they have only recently been identified. Some have suggested that Th17 cells may work at the interface of innate and adaptive immunity, promoting early neutrophil recruitment, yet avoiding tissue necrosis and sepsis.[22] Most of what we know about Th cell differentiation centers on Th1 and Th2 cells, since they have been studied over the past 20 years.

Effective responses to many foreign antigens result in the induction of both Th1 and Th2 cells to provide strong cellular and humoral immunity. However, some diseases are associated with a skewing toward one subset or the other. In humans, chronic skin infection with *Mycobacterium leprae* results in one of two forms of leprosy. Tuberculoid leprosy, which is the resistant form with few lesions and few bacilli, is characterized by a strong delayed-type hypersensitivity response and Th1 cells producing high levels of IFN-γ.[23] Resistance is conferred by activated macrophages that can kill intracellular bacteria. The susceptible, lepromatous form has multiple skin lesions, large numbers of bacilli, high antibody levels, and weak cell-mediated immunity to leprosy antigens; mRNAs for IL-4, IL-5, and IL-10 predominate in these skin lesions. Therefore, the type of immune response elicited to *M. leprae* determines the course of the disease. Atopic individuals have developed an abnormal immune response to allergens, resulting in allergen-specific Th2 cells in the peripheral blood and at sites of inflammation.[24]

A variety of different factors have been shown to influence Th1 or Th2 cell generation, with *cytokines* the major variable and most studied. IFN-γ and IL-12 stimulate the induction of Th1 cells. Developing Th1 cells acquire expression of interleukin-12 β-2-chain receptor (IL-12Rβ_2),[25] thus enhancing their ability to respond to IL-12. Whereas IL-12 directly induces Th1 cell development, IFN-γ appears to enhance Th1 induction indirectly by inhibiting the generation of Th2 cells.[26] IL-4 drives Th2 cell generation by direct action on CD4+ T cells.[27] IL-13 is involved in the induction of Th2 cells by an unknown mechanism, but not through direct effects on CD4+ T cells.[28] IL-10 enhances Th2 cell development by inhibiting Th1 cell induction.[29] In addition, developing Th2 cells lose IL-12Rβ_2 expression,[25] further helping to polarize a Th2 response.

Within days of activation, Th cell differentiation has begun. Therefore, it is likely that sources of these cytokines are present at the time of T cell activation, either by cells activated in the local environment in the innate immune response or by APC populations in the local lymphoid tissue. The Th1-inducing cytokine, IL-12, is produced by APCs, including macrophages and DCs.[30] IFN-γ is produced at high levels by natural killer (NK) cells that are activated in viral infections. IL-4 and IL-13 can be produced by mast cells and basophils activated by antigen cross-linking of cell surface IgE.[31,32] NK1.1 T cells produce high levels of IL-4 and have been shown to be critical for the development of Th2 cells.[33] Gamma-delta (γ/δ) T cells can produce IFN-γ and IL-4 and may skew CD4+ Th cell differentiation either direction.[34] In addition, antigen-experienced effector or memory T cells, which may have been previously activated locally, produce cytokines that can also affect new CD4+ Th cell generation.

DCs have been shown to influence Th1/Th2 cell generation through the cytokines they produce and by expression of cell surface receptors. Although DCs share many phenotypic and functional properties, including their ability to take up and process antigen and move to the local lymphoid tissue, heterogeneity exists among the population. Differences in the ability to stimulate Th1 or Th2 have been attributed to different cell lineages and to different stages in DC maturation.[30] Early studies

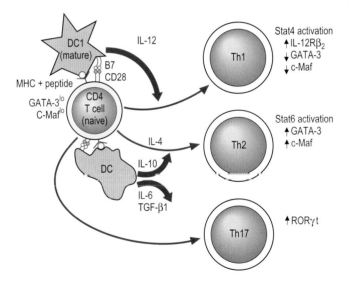

Fig. 16.2. Generation of T helper types 1, 2, and 17 (Th1, Th2, Th17) cells from a naive CD4+ T cell. A naive CD4+ T cell does not secrete cytokines and has low levels of GATA-3 and c-Maf expression. Differentiation along the Th1, Th2, or Th17 pathway is triggered by stimulation by antigen presented to the T cell receptor in the context of the major histocompatibility complex (MHC) by the appropriate antigen-presenting cell (APC) and a second signal imparted by ligation of co-stimulatory molecules B7–1/B7–2 and CD28. Dendritic cells (DCs) represent the key APCs for naive T cells. Those that produce interleukin-10 (IL-10) favor Th2 differentiation, while those that produce interleukin-12 (IL-12) stimulate Th1 differentiation. Th17 cells can be generated in the presence of interleukin-6 (IL-6) and transforming growth factor-β1 (TGF-β1) produced presumably by DC.

showed that Th1-stimulating dendritic cells produced IL-12, tended to express a mature phenotype, and were isolated from peripheral lymphoid organs and the spleen.[35] Mucosal surface DCs promoted Th2 induction and expressed low levels of surface MHC class II, produced IL-10 and minimal IL-12.[36,37] These classifications have not proven to be so distinct as the heterogeneity of DC populations has been revealed, yet DC control of CD4 Th1 or Th2 bias is based on DC cytokine production, the cytokine milieu in the local environment, co-stimulatory signals and chemokines.[38]

The dose and form of the antigen can also influence Th1/Th2 cell generation. The antigenic peptide sequence has been shown to modulate Th1/Th2 induction. If the peptide–MHC class II complex on the APC has a high-affinity interaction with the TCR, Th1-predominant responses are induced, whereas weaker-affinity interactions lead to Th2-like responses.[39] Very low doses of soluble protein antigens tend to stimulate Th2-predominant responses and at higher antigen doses Th1 responses. This finding may result from low doses of antigen causing fewer MHC–peptide complexes to interact with TCRs, resulting in a lower-affinity APC–T cell interaction. This may have important implications in allergy, since it has been estimated that exposure to common allergens is so small that it does not exceed 1 microgram per year. Another line of investigation suggests that high-affinity interactions lead to preferential generation of Th2 cells.[40] Ultimately, the quality of the signal delivered to the T cell in a low-affinity versus high-affinity interaction may influence whether Th1 or Th2 cells are induced.

The co-stimulatory molecules CD28 and B7 have been shown to effect Th1/Th2 cell generation, presumably because they draw T cells and APCs close and influence the signals delivered to the T cell. Blockade of CD28, which binds both B7–1 and B7–2, inhibits Th2 more than Th1 responses, indicating that CD28 signaling is more critical for Th2 cell development.[41] In some cases, blockade of B7–2 alone also inhibits Th2 responses. The variable effects of B7–1 and B7–2 signaling on Th1/Th2 induction may be caused by the different kinetics and distribution of these molecules on different APC populations. Blockade of ICOS on T cells preferentially blocks Th2 responses, possibly from the higher expression of ICOS on Th2 cells compared with Th1 cells.[42] ICOS, through interactions with B7RP-1, enhances Th2 cytokine production and increases expression of cell surface chemokine receptors, leading to enhanced Th2 inflammatory responses.

Chemokines have also been shown to influence Th1/Th2 cell generation. *Monocyte chemoattractant protein-1* (MCP-1) may directly stimulate Th2 cell development.[43] Other MCPs at least can induce Th2 cells indirectly by reducing IL-12 production by monocytes.[44] Th1 cells are enhanced by macrophage inflammatory protein-1-alpha (MIP-1α), MIP-1β, and regulated on activation, normal T cells expressed and secreted (RANTES), although it is not clear if these chemokines directly affect the naive T cells or alter local cytokine production that skews toward Th1 development.[44]

In response to inhaled allergens, some individuals develop Th2-dominated inflammatory responses in the respiratory tract. Th1 induction is the more typical response to respiratory pathogens. A number of factors explain how the respiratory tract promotes Th2 generation in response to inhaled protein antigens.[36] Mast cells, NK T and γ/δ T cells, which line the airways and offer early protective immunity, have been shown to secrete IL-4 and may contribute to the cytokine environment that leads to the development of Th2 immune responses.[31,34] The biochemical properties of some aeroallergens have been shown to

shift responses toward Th2. The major dust mite antigen, Der p 1, has cysteine protease activity that stimulates mast cell and basophil degranulation and IL-4 production and cleaves B cell surface CD23,[45] possibly reducing its inhibitory effects on IgE production. In addition, Der p 1 has been shown to cleave the α subunit of the IL-2R on T cells, reducing proliferation, IL-2 production, and IFN-γ secretion[46] and to condition DCs to generate Th2 responses.[47] All of these actions may be responsible for the tendency of Der p 1 to stimulate Th2 responses. Other allergens have been shown to possess similar structural components, which may explain their allergenicity and Th2-biasing nature.[48] Thus, the respiratory tract has evolved to regulate immune responses through the induction of Treg or bias immune responses towards Th2. This effect may limit inflammation by avoiding robust cell-mediated immunity, such as occurs in Th1 responses, thus protecting the lungs for gas exchange.

Molecular mechanisms of Th1/Th2/Th17 differentiation

The ultimate outcome, whether a naive $CD4^+$ T cell becomes Th1 or Th2, is determined by the coordinate action of multiple signals induced by stimulation of the TCR, co-stimulatory molecules, and cytokine receptors. It is becoming increasingly clear that just as the induction of critical lineage-determining molecules is important for stimulation of T cell differentiation, the concomitant inhibition of the opposing phenotype is equally critical to seal the fate of the differentiating cell. The process of differentiation involves T cell proliferation, epigenetic remodeling involving alteration of chromatin structure and cytosine methylation, activation/upregulation of expression of key transcription factors, and the simultaneous inhibition/downregulation of signaling pathways that induce the opposing phenotype.

By all accounts, the transcription factor GATA-3, previously shown to be essential for T cell development, is a master regulator of Th2 differentiation. Naive $CD4^+$ T cells express low levels of GATA-3.[49] The expression of GATA-3 is, however, markedly upregulated in cells differentiating along the Th2 lineage and is downregulated in cells differentiating along the Th1 pathway.[49] It appears that GATA-3 may be the critical downstream regulator of chromatin remodeling around the IL-4 locus. The differentiation of a naive $CD4^+$ T cell along the Th1 or Th2 pathway is accompanied by extensive reorganization of chromatin structure around the IFN-γ or IL-4/IL-5/IL-13 locus, respectively.[50] Under Th2 differentiating conditions, the IL-4 locus, has been shown to undergo extensive demethylation with concomitant acquisition of DNaseI hypersensitive (HS) sites which is an indicator of chromosome accessibility to regulatory factors.[50,51] Interestingly, although Th2-inducing conditions are generally unable to stimulate Th2-type gene expression in committed Th1 cells, ectopic expression of GATA-3 in fully differentiated Th1 cells was shown to induce Th2 cytokine production.[52] GATA-3 has been shown to bind a distal enhancer within an antigen-inducible DNaseI HS site in the 3' flanking region of the IL-4 gene, suggesting the involvement of GATA-3 in active transcription of the IL-4/IL-13 genes.[53] Possibly, this site and other potential GATA-3 binding elements dispersed throughout the IL-4 locus mediate antigen-induced IL-4 and IL-13 gene expression.[54] Additionally, GATA-3 directly activates the IL-5 promoter.[49] GATA-3 appears to function in a feedback positive autoregulatory loop in an IL-4/STAT6-independent fashion to upregulate its own expression, thus stabilizing the Th2 phenotype.[55] The TCR–NF-κB axis, critical for GATA-3, but not STAT6, function may be a key cytokine (IL-4)-independent step in the initiation of Th2 differentiation.[56] Analysis of conditional *Gata3* knockout mice has confirmed a critical role for GATA-3 in Th2 cell differentiation (both IL-4 dependent and IL-4 independent) and has also showed the importance of basal GATA-3 expression in inhibiting Th1 differentiation.[57] While Th2-specific factors such as GATA-3 are essential and determine the tissue specificity of gene expression, the concomitant activation of more general factors such as NF-κB, AP-1, NF-AT, and C/EBPβ is required for high-level expression of the Th2 cytokine genes (Fig. 16.3).[58]

A considerable advancement in our understanding of Th1 lineage commitment and IFN-γ gene expression was made with the identification of a novel protein T-bet (*T-box expressed in T cells*).[59] T-bet belongs to the T-box family of transcription factors that regulate several developmental processes. T-bet expression was found to be specifically upregulated in Th1 cells but not in Th2 cells. Ectopic expression of T-bet in vitro was shown to induce transactivation of an IFN-γ gene-reporter construct and also introduction of T-bet into primary developing T cells by retroviral gene transfer techniques induced a high level of IFN-γ production.[59] Like GATA-3-induced Th2 cytokine production in fully committed Th1 cells, expression of T-bet in already differentiated Th2 cells was shown to induce IFN-γ gene expression.[59] Interestingly, IL-12/STAT4 signaling

has been shown to be not critical for T-bet expression but to stabilize the commitment to the Th1 lineage by acting as a growth signal and sustaining IFN-γ expression through interactions of STAT4 with the co-activator CREB-binding protein.[60] T-bet knockout mice have impaired IFN-γ production primarily in CD4 and γ/δ T cells and develop spontaneous Th2-mediated allergic airways disease.[61] Also, in an interesting study, the Tec kinase Itk-mediated phosphorylation of T-bet was shown to result in interaction between T-bet and GATA-3, which prevented the DNA-binding activity of GATA-3.[62]

The orphan nuclear receptor RORγt was recently shown to induce differentiation of naive CD4+ T cells to Th17 cells.[22] RORγt is required for the expression of IL-17 and the related gene IL-17F in response to IL-6 and TGF-β. Th17 cells, constitutively present throughout intestinal lamina propria, were found to express RORγt, and were absent in mice deficient for RORγt or IL-6. RORγt-deficient mice displayed attenuated autoimmune disease and lacked tissue-infiltrating Th17 cells. The role of RORγt in allergic disease has not yet been defined.

An important consideration in discussions of Th differentiation is cross-regulation between the subsets, which results in apparent exclusivity of one type of immune response during infection or in disease. For example, during the course of differentiation, IFN-γ produced by Th1 cells facilitates Th1 development but inhibits Th2 cell proliferation

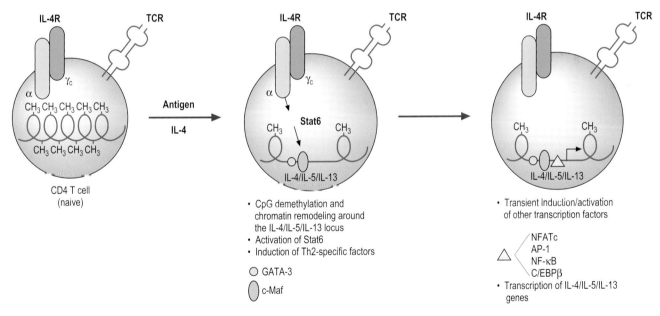

Fig. 16.3. Molecular mechanisms of differentiation of a naive CD4+ T cell into Th2 cells. A naive CD4+ T cell contains a condensed chromatin structure with extensive methylation. Stimulation by antigen together with engagement of the interleukin-4 receptor (IL-4R) results in activation of signal transducer and activator of transcription-6 (STAT-6, Stat6), which in turn causes specific demethylation around the IL-4/IL-5/IL-13 locus (similarly, antigen plus IL-12 causes demethylation around the IFN-γ locus). Chromatin remodeling is accompanied by induction of Th2-specific transcription factors (e.g., GATA-3, c-Maf), which bind to target sequences in the IL-4/IL-5/IL-13 locus. The chromatin, rendered accessible by demethylation and perhaps by binding of c-Maf, and other as yet undiscovered Th2-specific transcription factors, is next bound by more widely expressed and transiently induced transcription factors (e.g., AP-1, NF-κB, NF-Atc, C/EBPβ). This may allow synergistic interactions between the tissue-specific and general transcription factors, resulting in the active transcription of the IL-4, IL-5, and IL-13 genes. Effector/memory cells are postulated to be in a state of suspended animation with an open chromatin structure and high levels of GATA-3 and c-Maf expression. Restimulation of these cells by antigen would result in transient induction of the general factors, leading to rapid induction of Th2 gene expression. Like GATA-3 for Th2 cells, T-bet and RORγt are transcription factors that function as master regulators of Th1 and Th17 generation, respectively. TCR, T cell antigen receptor.

whereas IL-4 and IL-10 produced by Th2 cells amplify the Th2 pathway but inhibit Th1 differentiation. To determine the functional significance of GATA-3 downregulation in Th1 cells, GATA-3 was forcibly over-expressed in Th1 cells using retroviral gene transfer methods.[63] These studies showed that overexpression of GATA-3 in developing but not committed Th1 cells results in inhibition of IFN-γ production and ex-tinction of IL-12Rβ2 expression.[63] The lack of any effect of GATA-3 in already differentiated Th1 cells argues against direct effects of GATA-3 on the IFN-γ promoter.[63] Similarly, overexpression of T-bet, both in developing and in committed Th2 cells, not only induces IFN-γ gene expression but also inhibits the production of the Th2 cytokines IL-4 and IL-5. Overall, it is likely that T-bet and GATA-3 not only induce Th1 and Th2 differentiation, respectively, but also serve to stabilize the differentiated phenotype by inhibiting the development of the oppos-ing phenotype. Recently, the signaling lymphocyte activation molecule (SLAM)-associated protein (SAP), which associates with the cyto-plasmic tail of SLAM family members and prevents interactions with SHP-2, was shown to play an important role in Th2 differentiation.[64] Mice deficient in SAP displayed excessive IFN-γ production by CD4+ and CD8+ T cells during infections with lymphocytic choriomeningi-tis virus and SAP-deficient BALB/c mice were resistant to *Leishmania major* infection. These results suggest that the exaggerated Th1 response resulting from SAP-1-deficiency is a consequence of defective Th2 re-sponses in these animals. Similar to cross-regulation between Th1 and Th2 cells, negative regulation of IL-17 production by IL-4 and IFN-γ from effector cells has been also described.[65]

Effector/memory cells

After 4–5 days of proliferation induced by IL-2, a naive T cell differenti-ates into an effector cell. These changes are associated with the acquisi-tion of different cell adhesion molecules. Effector cells no longer express L-selectin but do express very late antigen-4 (VLA-4), which allows the T cell to bind to the vascular endothelium and home to sites of tissue inflammation.[1] Effector T cells express high levels of the adhesion mol-ecules lymphocyte function-associated antigen-1 (LFA-1) and CD2, enhancing non-specific binding to its target cells, including B cells and macrophages. Compared with naive T cells, effector cells do not require co-stimulation, allowing them to respond to antigen with 'hair trigger' rapidity to produce high levels of cytokines and chemokines, which then direct the immune response. Chemokine receptor expression also distin-guishes naive from effector CD4+ T cells, with naive cells expressing re-ceptors for chemokines that direct them to peripheral lymphoid organs, as described earlier, and effector cells being directed to inflammatory tis-sues. Some of the receptors, including CXCR5 and CCR2, are expressed on both Th1 and Th2 cells.[66] To direct specific immune responses in dif-ferent tissues or in response to different insults, Th1 from Th2 express different chemokine receptors. Th1 cells express CCR5 and CXCR3, while Th2 cells express CCR4 and CCR8. CCR3 and CXCR4 may also be preferentially expressed on Th2 cells, but this more controversial.[67] The chemokines that stimulate Th1 cells are induced by IFN-γ and sup-pressed by IL-4, resulting in a chemokine milieu that attracts Th1 cells; therefore once initiated, augmentation of specific immunity is insured.

Most activated effector CD4+ T cells die subsequent to an immune response through the process of activation-induced cell death, but a sub-set of CD4+ T cells will persist as memory cells for the life of the host. IL-7 is required for CD4+ memory T cell generation and maintenance.[68]

When reactivated, these cells will initiate and coordinate a quicker, more effective, stronger, and longer duration response. CD4+ memory T cells persist in non-lymphoid organs as a central memory cells (T_{CM}) and in non-lymphoid tissues as effector memory cells (T_{EM}).[69] T_{EM} respond rapidly to re-exposure to antigen, while T_{CM} are slower to be mobi-lized.[69] Among these memory populations there is both overlap and het-erogeneity in their phenotypic markers, yet T_{EM} cells isolated from lung home back to the lung on adoptive transfer.[70] Thus, CD4+ memory T cell subsets appear to be adapted to function at the site in which they reside.

■ B LYMPHOCYTES ■

The humoral immune response is generated by B cells. A mature B cell expresses immunoglobulin on its cell surface, which is its antigen-specific B cell receptor (BCR). As with the TCR, the BCR is a molecular com-plex made up of antigen-binding or variable (V) regions. This region of the protein is so different among immunoglobulins as to allow each antibody in an individual to bind to any foreign structure that the indi-vidual might encounter. To generate this diverse immunoglobulin reper-toire, during development in the bone marrow, B cells undergo somatic deoxyribonucleic acid (DNA) recombination of the V, diversity (D), and joining (J) regions of the immunoglobulin heavy and light chains, termed VDJ recombination. This process is similar to the recombination events that occur in developing T cells in the thymus, which results in the extensive repertoire of TCRs. The invariant or constant region of the antibody is specialized for different effector functions in the immune system once antibody is secreted. There are five main constant-region forms: IgM, IgD, IgG, IgE, and IgA. Naive B cells that have not yet encountered antigen express IgM and IgD on their surface. The BCR in the membrane-bound form serves to recognize and bind antigen and transmit activation signals into the cell.

A naive B cell recirculates through peripheral lymphoid tissues until it binds specific antigen through surface immunoglobulin and is activated (signal 1). Certain microbial antigens, including bacterial polysaccha-rides, can stimulate B cells to produce antibody in the absence of helper T cells. Most antibody responses, including antibody responses to protein antigens, require antigen-specific T cell help. Antigen bound to surface immunoglobulin is internalized, processed, complexed with-MHC class II, and displayed on the cell surface. This encounter with specific anti-gen stimulates changes in B cell adhesion molecules and responsiveness to chemokines such that the B cells are trapped in T cell zones in the peripheral lymphoid tissues, thus promoting T-B interactions.[71] A pre-viously primed CD4+ T cell that recognizes the peptide–MHC class II complex on the B cell provides the second signal for activation. CD40L on the activated T cell interacts with CD40 on the B cell and provides a critical stimulus for the B cell to enter the cell cycle.[72] The interac-tion with CD4+ T cells also provides signals for proliferation, the most important being secreted IL-4. B cells proliferate in germinal centers, where they undergo a number of important changes, including somatic hypermutation, in which the V regions undergo point mutations that enhance their diversity; affinity maturation, which selects for B cells with higher affinity for their antigen; and heavy-chain class switching, a proc-ess by which the V region of the immunoglobulin becomes associated with different constant regions. The cytokines secreted by CD4+ T cells during B cell activation regulate which immunoglobulin heavy-chain constant regions will be selected during class-switch recombination.[73]

LYMPHOCYTES IN ASTHMA

T HELPER TYPE 2 CELLS

$CD4^+$ T cells are believed to play a crucial role in controlling inflammation in asthma. They make up the predominant lymphocyte population that infiltrates the airways in asthmatic patients and are activated in these sites, expressing the surface activation markers, class II MHC and CD25 (IL-2R).[74,75] $CD4^+$ T cells make up only a small fraction of leukocytes in the lung, but they have been implicated as important in asthma because they regulate the adaptive immune response in normal individuals, can rapidly expand in response to specific stimuli, and communicate with other cells by initiating cascades of inflammatory mediators.

In asthmatic patients, $CD4^+$ T cells producing IL-4, IL-5, and IL-13 have been identified in bronchoalveolar lavage (BAL) and airway biopsies and are secreted in the airways of patients with mild or asymptomatic disease.[75,76] A significant increase in GATA-3 expression was also demonstrated in airways of asthmatic patients compared with those in control subjects,[77] indicating the presence of Th2 cells. After antigen challenge in allergic asthmatic patients, Th2 lymphocytes were increased in the airways.[75,76,78,79] In asthmatic patients, airway hyperreactivity (AHR) and airway eosinophilia correlate with airway CD4 T cells that produce IL-4 or IL-5 or express GATA-3.[77,80–82] Thus the association of Th2 cells with their effects in the respiratory tract has led to the theory that Th2 cells orchestrate the characteristic inflammatory response that results in asthma.

Animal studies show that Th2 cells cause the pathophysiologic changes seen in asthma. Eosinophilic airway inflammation and AHR have both been shown to be dependent on $CD4^+$ T cells.[83,84] Studies that employed adoptive transfer of $CD4^+$ T cells from animals with antigen-induced AHR resulted in airway inflammation and hyperresponsiveness in aerosol-challenged recipient mice,[84,85] indicating that $CD4^+$ T cells could control many aspects of the disease. $CD4^+$ Th2 cells were shown to induce many of the characteristic features of asthma in mice. Th2 cells induced airway eosinophilia, mucus hypersecretion, and AHR, whereas Th1 cells caused a neutrophil-predominant inflammatory response without any of these features of asthma.[86,87] Inhibition of GATA-3 activity caused a severe blunting of Th2 effects both locally in the lung (eosinophil influx, mucus production) as well as systemically (IgE production),[88] confirming the necessity of Th2 cells in allergic airway inflammation. Individual Th2 cytokines, when constitutively produced in the respiratory tract, have also been found to induce an asthma-like syndrome. Transgenic mice that overexpress the Th2 cytokines IL-4, IL-5, IL-13, and IL-9 in the airway epithelium exhibit characteristic allergic inflammatory features in the airways, including eosinophilia and mucus overproduction.[89–92] Transgenic mice that overexpress IL-13, IL-9, and IL-5 showed AHR and collagen deposition in the airways, indicating that chronic exposure to Th2 cytokines can also induce airway remodeling. Therefore, activation of Th2 cells is sufficient for the induction of inflammation, the physiology, and the chronic pathologic changes associated with asthma.

When Th2 cells are generated and recruited to the respiratory tract in asthmatics, individual Th2 cytokines control different aspects of the characteristic pathophysiology. Of all of the Th2 cytokines, IL-13 appears to have the most profound effector role in asthma.[93] In allergic airway inflammation in mice, IL-13 is required for AHR.[94,95] The precise mechanisms by which IL-13 leads to AHR are unknown, yet IL-13 receptors on the airway epithelium mediate this physiological effect.[96]

Mucus hypersecretion in animal models of asthma requires IL-13. IL-13 stimulates the generation of goblet cells, followed by the induction of mucin genes and mucus production.[97] IL-13 and IL-4 both promote eosinophilia by stimulating Stat6-dependent eotaxins.[98] IL-13 also promotes airway remodeling through effects on matrix metalloproteases and activation of TGF-β1.[99] Airway eosinophilia also depends on IL-5, which controls eosinophil maturation in the bone marrow and recruitment and activation in the respiratory tract.[100] IL-4 remains an essential factor for Th2 cell differentiation, but compared with IL-13, has a limited role in driving the pulmonary inflammatory response in asthma.

CD4 lymphocytes likely produce a majority of the Th2 cytokines in the respiratory tract in asthma. In airway biopsies and BAL cells from asthmatics, IL-4, IL-5 and IL-13 co-localize with T cell markers in a majority of BAL cells.[93] Yet, Th2 cytokine production has been identified in eosinophils, mast cells, basophils, NK cells, and subsets of class II MHC-expressing accessory cells.[93] It is becoming clear that Th2 cytokines, IL-4, IL-5, IL-13, produced by these non-CD4 Th2 cells may be critical in the development and perpetuation of asthma. The period of cytokine secretion from this array of cells will vary; thus, as lymphocytes die or cease production of cytokines after their activation, waves of cytokines produced by non-CD4 Th2 cells may follow.

Genetics of the individual may also play a role in biasing immune responses toward Th2 in allergic diseases. This is reflected in the hereditary nature of asthma and atopy and is detailed in Chapter 4. Strong linkages have been identified to flanking markers of the human cytokine gene cluster on chromosomes 5q31 and 16p12, which include genes for IL-4, IL-13, and IL-4Rα.[101] Variants in the IL-4 promoter region are associated with atopy. Some of these nucleotide polymorphisms lead to increased binding of transcription factors (e.g., NFAT-1, AP-1) and enhanced IL-4 transcription.[102–104] Two variants of IL-13 have been identified and are associated with asthma; the variant in the promoter region affects production of the cytokine, and the second variant alters the cytokine charge and may ultimately increase IL-13 signaling.[105,106] In addition, polymorphisms of IL-4Rα, which is a component of both the IL-4 and IL-13 receptors, have been linked to atopy.[107] A variant IL-13R that is associated with atopy and asthma was tested in vitro and found to promote increased Stat6 phosphorylation, thus resulting in increased IL-13 effects.[108] The MHC region on chromosome 6 has also been linked to asthma in several studies, suggesting that MHC molecule polymorphisms may influence T cell responses to allergens.[109–113]

While some of the Th2-biasing components of the immune system are encoded in DNA, other hereditary effects may be present, but these are still poorly understood. Animal studies show that female mice with allergic airways disease transmit the propensity for disease to their offspring.[114] Offspring of affected mothers developed airway disease with low-dose stimuli that did not cause disease in offspring from normal mothers. This suggests that the maternal–fetal interaction can transmit a risk to develop of asthma.

T HELPER TYPE 1 CELLS

Th1 cells have also been identified in the airways of asthmatic patients, but it is still not clear if they protect from or augment allergic airway disease. Some studies show that Th1 cell activation inhibits allergic airway inflammation, whereas other studies suggest that Th1 cells potentiate the inflammatory response in asthma due to the proinflammatory effects of Th1 cytokines.[115,116]

Human and animal studies suggest that enhancing Th1 cytokines in the lung before or early in the generation of a Th2 response may protect against the development of asthma. IFN-γ-dominated immune responses to viral or mycobacterial infection in childhood are associated with a reduced incidence of asthma.[117,118] Attendance at day care and exposure to other siblings, presumably increasing their viral respiratory infections, was protective against wheezing later in childhood.[119] Also, mice immunized in the presence of a Th1-stimulating environment exhibited a reduction in antigen-induced eosinophilic airway inflammation and AHR.[120] Thus, reducing the generation of Th2 cells appears to decrease allergic inflammation.

Th1 cells can also inhibit the effects of ongoing Th2 cell responses. Th1 cells, through the production of IFN-γ, have been shown to inhibit Th2 cell cytokine production and Th2 cell proliferation in vitro.[121] In mice the Th1 cytokine IFN-γ has inhibitory effects on Th2-induced airway eosinophilia and AHR. When administered before inhaled antigen challenge, IFN-γ reduced the number of CD4+ T cells in the respiratory tract[122,123] or reduced Th2 cytokine secretion.[122] These effects may result from inhibition of Th2 cell recruitment by IFN-γ. Once Th2 cells are present in the respiratory tract, IFN-γ promotes the resolution of airway eosinophilia and suppresses Th2 cytokine production.[124] Th1 cells, through the production of IFN-γ, can inhibit airway eosinophilia, mucus production, and AHR without an increase in airway inflammation.[125] Although many studies support Th1 cells and IFN-γ as inhibitors of Th2-type responses, other studies show that Th1 cells enhance inflammation and do not ameliorate disease.[126] The proinflammatory effects of Th1 cells are supported by the association of viral respiratory infections, which tend to induce Th1 responses, and exacerbation of symptoms in asthmatic patients.[127] Ultimately, Th1 cell influence on allergic airway inflammation may depend on the site and timing of Th1 relative to Th2 cell activation.

T HELPER TYPE 17 CELLS

The concentration of IL-17A was found to be increased in the airways, sputum, and blood from patients with asthma.[128,129] In sputum, IL-17A mRNA expression correlated with CD3δ showing an association of CD3+ cells and IL-17. Other studies indicate that allergen-specific Th17 cells contribute to IL-17 production in the respiratory tract.[128,130] In animals studied after the induction of an antigen-specific immune response, IL-17 had an inhibitory effect on allergic airway inflammation and enhanced neutrophil recruitment,[131,132] thus suggesting IL-17 might downregulate inflammation in asthma. The precise function of Th17 cells in respiratory tract is still unclear, since in these studies IL-17 was either delivered intranasally or blocked in all cells by antibody or gene deletion. Thus, Th17 cell-specific effects cannot be determined. This work is still evolving and future studies will clarify if Th17 cells are pathogenic or regulatory in asthma.

CD8 T CELLS

In atopic asthmatics with stable disease, CD8 T cells in airway biopsies are increased compared to non-asthmatic, atopic, and normal patients.[133] The function of CD8 T cells in asthma, though, remains complex. Since CD8 T cells recognize endogenous antigens, such as self and viral peptides, it is unlikely that they are allergen-specific. Thus, it is unclear if CD8 T cells are recruited non-specifically to the respiratory tract or have a specific antiviral function, and if CD8+ T cells protect or promote disease. During asthma exacerbations, which are commonly caused by viral respiratory infections, there are increased CD8+ T cells in the respiratory tract.[134] Activated CD8+ cells have been identified in patients who die from asthma [135] and this may reflect a virus-specific CD8 T cell response. Like CD4 T cells, CD8 cytotoxic T cells can be polarized into subsets. Cytotoxic T cell-Type 1 (Tc1) cells are activated in viral infections and generally produce IFN-γ and lymphotoxin. When activated in the presence of IL-4, CD8 T cytotoxic-Type 2 (Tc2) cells can be induced to produce IL-4, IL-5, and IL-13. Animal studies show that Tc2 cells retain their cytotoxic function, stimulate recruitment of eosinophils, provide B cell help for IgE production, and promote airways hyperresponsiveness.[136-138] CD8 T cells worsen CD4 Th2-mediated allergic airway disease.[139] Because of the association of childhood respiratory infection with asthma, it has been theorized that some viral respiratory infections may stimulate CD8 Tc2 responses, thus initiating or exacerbating local allergic responses. CD8+ T cells may also contribute to airway remodeling as suggested by an inverse correlation of CD8+ T cells and FEV1 in airway biopsies of asthmatics.[140]

NATURAL KILLER T CELLS

NK T cells are a small population of lymphocytes that respond to glycolipid antigens. NK T cells respond rapidly by secreting preformed cytokines, such as IL-4, IL-10, and IFN-γ, early in the development of an immune response. NK T cells are, thus, believed to be an important regulatory component in the innate immune response that helps to model the development of the local adaptive immune response. NK T cells can promote IgE production and have been theorized to contribute to the early cytokine environment that influences Th2 differentiation in the respiratory tract.[33] In moderate to severe asthmatics, CD4+ NK T cells make up a majority of CD4 T cells in the bronchoalveolar lavage.[141] The glycolipid antigen to which these cells are responding is unknown, as is the function of the NK T cell in ongoing asthma. Additional studies are necessary to define the mechanisms by which NK T cells influence disease. In animal models, some studies have shown that NK T cells are important in the generation of Th2 responses,[142,143] while others have observed no effect on allergic airway inflammation.[144]

GAMMA/DELTA T CELLS

Gamma/delta (γ/δ) cells are a subset of T cells that have a TCR with γ and δ chains, rather than the more common alpha/beta (α/β) TCR. γ/δ T cells develop earlier than α/β T cells and, once released from the thymus, are found in lymphoid tissue and in intraepithelial regions in the skin and mucosal surfaces. Intraepithelial γ/δ T cells express a restricted repertoire of TCRs. They respond to non-peptide and non-processed bacterial and environmental antigens, including mycobacterial lipids and heat shock proteins.[145] They do not appear to recognize antigens in the context of class I or II MHC; rather, they may recognize their target antigens directly. Their presence at epithelial barriers suggests that γ/δ T cells play a role in surveillance and protection from infection, possibly bridging innate and adaptive immune responses. γ/δ T cells elaborate chemokines to recruit inflammatory cells and secrete cytokines. γ/δ T cells produce IFN-γ and IL-4 in vivo in response to Th1-stimulating or Th2-stimulating pathogens, respectively.[34] In asthmatic patients,

γ/δ T cells that produce IL-4, IL-5, and IL-13 cytokines have been isolated from the airways [146,147] and were increased after antigen challenge.[146] The presence of Th2-like γ/δ T cells in the airways suggests that they can amplify the local immune response by increasing disease-causing Th2 cytokines. In mice, the γ/δ T cells have been shown to be critical to both generate Th2 cells and to protect from Th2-mediated disease.[148,149] These animal studies highlight the multifunctional nature of γ/δ T cells, making it unclear what function they might serve in the airways of asthmatics.

NATURAL KILLER CELLS

Natural killer (NK) cells are not lymphocytes but represent another cellular component of innate immunity. NK cells are best known for their ability to produce high levels of IFN-γ very early after infection and to kill virally infected cells. However, NK cells also can be induced to produce IL-5 when stimulated in the presence of Th2 cytokines and may contribute to eosinophilic inflammation.[150,151] In mice, NK cells appear to play an important role in generating CD4 T cell responses to protein antigens.[144] In rats, NK cells control a strain-related difference in susceptibility to a postviral asthma-like syndrome.[152] Mice that developed allergic airway inflammation after viral infection had reduced production of IFN-γ by NK cells compared with unaffected mice, suggesting that the level of IFN-γ produced by NK cells may confer protection from the development of asthma. NK cells appear to have the potential to enhance or protect animals from airway inflammation. Their role in the development or provocation of allergic airway disease in humans is not known.

B CELLS AND IMMUNOGLOBULIN E

Th2 responses to allergens give rise to elevated levels of allergen-specific IgE. When IgE binds to its high-affinity receptor (FcϵRI) on mast cells, basophils, or eosinophils, and IgE is cross-linked by polyvalent antigen, immediate hypersensitivity reactions are induced by the release of preformed vasoactive mediators. IgE cross-linking leads to production of cytokines, leukotrienes, and other inflammatory mediators. If IgE cross-linking leads to production of IL-4 and induction of surface expression of CD40L on T lymphocytes, then this further enhances IgE production.[153,154] The importance of IgE in allergic asthma was controversial, until studies of therapeutic anti-IgE showed efficacy in the treatment of severe asthma. Anti-IgE binds to circulating free IgE, reduced serum IgE levels, and decreases both early and late asthmatic responses.[155,156] In a multicenter randomized placebo-controlled trial, anti-IgE treatment in patients with moderate to severe allergic asthma improved symptoms and allowed patients to reduce their use of corticosteroids.[157] Airway biopsies from patients treated with anti-IgE showed fewer eosinophils, CD4+ CD8+, and B lymphocytes and fewer cells staining for IL-4,[158] thus confirming that IgE augments airway inflammation. Animal studies show that IgE can induce eosinophilia and AHR.[159,160] Yet, there are non-IgE-mediated pathways that enhance Th2 cytokine production. Eosinophilia and AHR can be induced as effectively in the absence of B cells and IgE as compared with mice with B lymphocytes.[161,162] The ability of IgE to activate Th2-mediated pathways may depend on the experimental methods used. In humans with IgE-low, non-atopic asthma, IgE-independent pathways are likely to stimulate disease.

IgE also binds to its low-affinity receptor (FcϵRII, or CD23), which is found on B cells, activated T cells, monocytes, eosinophils, platelets, follicular DCs, and thymic epithelial cells. Cell surface CD23 fluctuates with IgE levels and flares of disease.[163] Ligation of CD23 downregulates IgE synthesis.[164] In a model of allergic airway inflammation, mice deficient in CD23 showed increased levels of IgE, eosinophilia, and AHR compared with CD23-expressing mice.[165] B cell surface CD23 is cleaved by the protease activity of the allergen Der p1.[45] Destruction of this inhibitory feedback loop regulating IgE production may explain, in part, how allergens stimulate Th2 responses.

ANTIGEN-INDUCED IMMUNOSUPPRESSION OF ALLERGIC AIRWAYS DISEASE

It is evident from both murine and human studies that allergic airway disease can be regulated by active mechanisms of immunosuppression and cytokines play an integral role in this process. Not only do cytokines play a critical role in shaping T helper differentiation along different pathways, Th1, Th2, or Th17, they also serve equally important functions in inhibiting the development of the Th subsets. For example, T cells engineered to secrete TGF-β were found to inhibit airway inflammation and AHR.[166] Like TGF-β, IL-10 was also shown to inhibit the development of the asthma phenotype.[167] The importance of TGF-β as a key immunoregulatory molecule in mucosal inflammation was first described in the form of TGF-β-secreting Th3 cells in studies of oral tolerance in mice.[168] Later, both TGF-β and IL-10 were implicated in regulatory function of T cells in a murine model of allergic airways disease.[169] TGF-β has been shown to induce Foxp3 mRNA expression in activated CD4+CD25- T cells resulting in the accumulation of CD4+CD25+ Tregs.[170,171] When adoptively transferred to mice, these Tregs block antigen-induced airway inflammation.[170] In a reciprocal fashion, expression of a negative regulator of TGF-β signaling, Smad7, in T cells enhanced airway inflammation and AHR.[172]

Murine models of airway tolerance have been developed using inhaled or intranasally (i.n.) delivered antigen. In a model of tolerance, involving delivery of ovalbumin (OVA) i.n. consecutively for 3 days, regulatory T cells secreting IL-10 were implicated in the development of tolerance in the respiratory tract.[173] In the same system, ICOS–ICOS ligand interaction has been shown to be important for the generation of IL-10-secreting Tregs.[171] In a different study, when antigen-pulsed APCs overexpressing the Notch ligand Jagged-1 were introduced into mice, subsequent challenge with the same antigen profoundly inhibited immune responses as measured in vitro.[175] Adoptive transfer of CD4+ T cells, but not CD8+ T cells, transferred tolerance to recipient mice and the tolerance was shown to be antigen-specific.[175] Using repeated exposure to inhaled antigen as the model of tolerance induction,[176] a role for CD4+CD25+ T regulatory cells (Tregs) has been identified.[177,178] In these studies, CD4+CD25+ Tregs expressing Foxp3 and membrane-bound TGF-β were shown to be induced by inhaled antigen and mediate immunosuppressive functions by engaging the Notch1-Hes1 axis in target T helper cells. Interestingly, cross-talk between the TGF-β and Notch pathways has been recently shown to induce inhibitory mechanisms in other systems ranging from inhibition of endothelial cell migration to myogenesis.[179] Several other studies published recently have also implicated CD4+CD25+ Tregs in suppression of allergic airways disease in murine models.[180–184]

Since the identification of Tregs and description of their characteristics in mice, there has been a surge of interest to identify these cells in humans. $CD4^+CD25^+$ T cells from atopic individuals were found to have defective suppressive effects on autologous $CD4^+CD25^-$ T cells stimulated with allergens, compared with similar cells from non-atopics and this defect was found to be specific to allergen-stimulated cells and not a general effect on anti-CD3/anti-CD28-stimulated $CD4^+$ T cells.[185] In other studies, both $CD4^+CD25^+$ TGF-β^+[186] and IL-10$^+$ Tregs[187] were shown to be important for the development of tolerance to allergens since children with proper function of these Tregs outgrew allergic responses to allergens from cows' milk. In other disease settings, dysfunctional $CD4^+CD25^+$ Tregs have been identified in patients with multiple sclerosis.[188] Changes in regulatory capacity of $CD4^+CD25^+$ Tregs have been also noted in other diseases such as rheumatoid arthritis[189] and idiopathic arthritis.[190]

References

T lymphocytes

1. Picker LJ. Control of lymphocyte homing. Curr Opin Immunol 1994; 6:394–406.
2. Cyster JG. Chemokines and cell migration in secondary lymphoid organs. Science 1999; 286:2098–2102.
3. Banchereau J, Steinman RM. Dendritic cells and the control of immunity. Nature 1998; 392:245–252.
4. Harding FA, McArthur JG, Gross JA, et al. CD28-mediated signalling co-stimulates murine T cells and prevents induction of anergy in T-cell clones. Nature 1992; 356:607–609.
5. Jenkins MK, Taylor PS, Norton SD, et al. CD28 delivers a costimulatory signal involved in antigen-specific IL-2 production by human T cells. J Immunol 1991; 147:2461–2466.
6. Azuma M, Ito D, Yagita H, et al. B70 antigen is a second ligand for CTLA-4 and CD28. Nature 1993; 366:76–79.
7. Jain J, Loh C, Rao A. Transcriptional regulation of the IL-2 gene. Curr Opin Immunol 1995; 7:333–342.
8. Cerdan C, Martin Y, Courcoul M, et al. CD28 costimulation regulates long-term expression of the three genes (alpha, beta, gamma) encoding the high-affinity IL2 receptor. Res Immunol 1995; 146:164–168.
9. Van Gool SW, Vandenberghe P, de Boer M, et al. CD80, CD86 and CD40 provide accessory signals in a multiple-step T-cell activation model. Immunol Rev 1996; 153:47–83.
10. Hutloff A, Dittrich AM, Beier KC, et al. ICOS is an inducible T-cell co-stimulator structurally and functionally related to CD28. Nature 1999; 397:263–266.
11. Coyle AJ, Lehar S, Lloyd C, et al. The CD28-related molecule ICOS is required for effective T cell-dependent immune responses. Immunity 2000; 13:95–105.
12. Linsley PS, Brady W, Urnes M, et al. CTLA-4 is a second receptor for the B cell activation antigen B7. J Exp Med 1991; 174:561–569.
13. Walunas TL, Bakker CY, Bluestone JA. CTLA-4 ligation blocks CD28-dependent T cell activation. J Exp Med 1996; 183:2541–2550.
14. DeSilva DR, Urdahl KB, Jenkins MK. Clonal anergy is induced in vitro by T cell receptor occupancy in the absence of proliferation. J Immunol 1991; 147:3261–3267.
15. Cher D, Mosmann T. Two types of murine helper T cell clone: II. Delayed type hypersensitivity is mediated by Th1 clones. J Immunol 1987; 138:3688–3694.
16. Kim J, Woods A, Becker-Dunn E, et al. Distinct functional phenotypes of cloned Ia-restricted helper T cells. J Exp Med 1985; 162:188–201.
17. Killar L, MacDonald G, West J, et al. Cloned Ia restricted T cells that do not produce IL4/BSF-1 fail to help antigen specific B cells. J Immunol 1987; 138:1674–1679.
18. Mosmann TR, Cherwinski H, Bond MW, et al. Two types of murine helper T cell clone. I. Definition according to profiles of lymphokine activities and secreted proteins. J Immunol 1986; 136:2348–2357.
19. Langrish CL, Chen Y, Blumenschein WM, et al. IL-23 drives a pathogenic T cell population that induces autoimmune inflammation. J Exp Med 2005; 201:233–240.
20. Barner M, Mohrs M, Brombacher F, et al. Differences between IL-4R alpha-deficient and IL-4-deficient mice reveal a role for IL-13 in the regulation of Th2 responses. Curr Biol 1998; 8:669–672.
21. Coffman RL, Seymour BW, Hudak S, et al. Antibody to interleukin-5 inhibits helminth-induced eosinophilia in mice. Science 1989; 245:308–310.
22. Ivanov, II, McKenzie BS, et al. The orphan nuclear receptor RORgammat directs the differentiation program of proinflammatory IL-17+ T helper cells. Cell 2006; 126:1121–1133.
23. Yamamura M, Uyemura K, Deans RJ, et al. Defining protective responses to pathogen: cytokine profiles in leprosy lesions. Science 1992; 254:277–279.
24. Wierenga EA, Snoek M, de Groot C, et al. Evidence for compartmentalization of functional subsets of CD4+ T lymphocytes in atopic patients. J Immunol 1990; 144:4651–4656.
25. Szabo SJ, Dighe AS, Gubler U, et al. Regulation of the interleukin (IL)-12R beta 2 subunit expression in developing T helper 1 (Th1) and Th2 cells. J Exp Med 1997; 185:817–824.
26. Seder RA, Gazzinelli R, Sher A, et al. Interleukin 12 acts directly on CD4+ T cells to enhance priming for interferon gamma production and diminishes interleukin 4 inhibition of such priming. Proc Natl Acad Sci U S A 1993; 90:10188–10192.
27. Swain SL, Weinberg AD, English M, et al. IL4 directs the development of Th2 like helper effectors. J Immunol 1990; 145:3796–3806.
28. McKenzie GJ, Emson CL, Bell SE, et al. Impaired development of Th2 cells in IL-13-deficient mice. Immunity 1998; 9:423–432.
29. Hsieh C, Heimberger A, Gold J, et al. Differential regulation of T helper phenotype development by IL-4 and IL-10 in α-β T-cell receptor transgenic system. Proc Natl Acad Sci USA 1992; 89:6065–6069.
30. Moser M, Murphy KM. Dendritic cell regulation of TH1-TH2 development. Nat Immunol 2000; 1:199–205.
31. Bradding P, Feather IH, Howarth PH, et al. Interleukin 4 is localized to and released by human mast cells. J Exp Med 1992; 176:1381–1386.
32. Brunner T, Heusser CH, Dahinden CA. Human peripheral blood basophils primed by interleukin 3 (IL-3) produce IL-4 in response to immunoglobulin E receptor stimulation. J Exp Med 1993; 177:605–611.
33. Yoshimoto T, Bendelac A, Watson C, et al. Role of NK1.1+ T cells in a TH2 response and in immunoglobulin E production. Science 1995; 270:1845–1847.
34. Ferrick DA, Schrenzel MD, Mulvania T, et al. Differential production of interferon-gamma and interleukin 4 in response to Th1- and Th2-stimulating pathogens by gamma-delta T cells. Nature 1995; 373:255–257.
35. Rissoan MC, Soumelis V, Kadowaki N, et al. Reciprocal control of T helper cell and dendritic cell differentiation. Science 1999; 283:1183–1186.
36. Stumbles PA, Thomas JA, Pimm CL, et al. Resting respiratory tract dendritic cells preferentially stimulate T helper cell type 2 (Th2) responses and require obligatory cytokine signals for induction of Th1 immunity. J Exp Med 1998; 188:2019–2031.
37. Iwasaki A, Kelsall BL. Freshly isolated Peyer's patch, but not spleen, dendritic cells produce interleukin 10 and induce the differentiation of T helper type 2 cells. J Exp Med 1999; 190:229–239.
38. de Jong EC, Smits HH, Kapsenberg ML. Dendritic cell-mediated T cell polarization. Springer Semin Immunopathol 2005; 26:289–307.
39. Constant SL, Bottomly K. Induction of Th1 and Th2 CD4+ T cell responses: the alternative approaches. Annu Rev Immunol 1997; 15:297–322.
40. Sperling AI, Bluestone JA. The complexities of T-cell co-stimulation: CD28 and beyond. Immunol Rev 1996; 153:155–182.
41. Rulifson IC, Sperling AI, Fields PE, et al. CD28 costimulation promotes the production of Th2 cytokines. J Immunol 1997; 158:658–665.
42. Gonzalo JA, Tian J, Delaney T, et al. ICOS is critical for T helper cell-mediated lung mucosal inflammatory responses. Nat Immunol 2001; 2:597–604.
43. Gu L, Tseng S, Horner RM, et al. Control of TH2 polarization by the chemokine monocyte chemoattractant protein-1. Nature 2000; 404:407–411.
44. Luther SA, Cyster JG. Chemokines as regulators of T cell differentiation. Nat Immunol 2001; 2:102–107.
45. Hewitt CR, Brown AP, Hart BJ, et al. A major house dust mite allergen disrupts the immunoglobulin E network by selectively cleaving CD23: innate protection by antiproteases. J Exp Med 1995; 182:1537–1544.
46. Schulz O, Sewell HF, Shakib F. Proteolytic cleavage of CD25, the alpha subunit of the human T cell interleukin 2 receptor, by Der p 1, a major mite allergen with cysteine protease activity. J Exp Med 1998; 187:271–275.
47. Ghaemmaghami AM, Gough L, Sewell HF, et al. The proteolytic activity of the major dust mite allergen Der p 1 conditions dendritic cells to produce less interleukin-12: allergen-induced Th2 bias determined at the dendritic cell level. Clin Exp Allergy 2002; 32:1468–1475.
48. Furmonaviciene R, Shakib F. The molecular basis of allergenicity: comparative analysis of the three dimensional structures of diverse allergens reveals a common structural motif. Mol Pathol 2001; 54:155–159.
49. Zhang D-H, Cohn L, Ray P, et al. Transcription factor GATA-3 is differentially expressed in Th1 and Th2 cells and controls Th2-specific expression of the interleukin-5 gene. J Biol Chem 1997; 272:21597–21603.
50. Agarwal S, Rao A. Modulation of chromatin structure regulates cytokine gene expression during T cell differentiation. Immunity 1998; 9:765–775.
51. Takemoto N, Koyano-Nakagawa N, Yokota T, et al. Th2-specific DNase I-hypersensitive sites in the murine IL-13 and IL-4 intergenic region. Int Immunol 1998; 10:1981–1985.
52. Lee HJ, Takemoto N, Kurata H, et al. GATA-3 induces T helper cell type 2 (Th2) cytokine expression and chromatin remodeling in committed Th1 cells. J Exp Med 2000; 192:105–115.
53. Agarwal S, Avni O, Rao A. Cell-type-restricted binding of the transcription factor NFAT to a distal IL-4 enhancer in vivo. Immunity 2000; 12:643–652.
54. Lee GR, Fields PE, Flavell RA. Regulation of IL-4 gene expression by distal regulatory elements and GATA-3 at the chromatin level. Immunity 2001; 14:447–459.
55. Ouyang W, Lohning M, Gao Z, et al. Stat6-independent GATA-3 autoactivation directs IL-4-independent Th2 development and commitment. Immunity 2000; 12:27–37.
56. Das J, Chen C-H, Yang L, et al. A critical role for NF-kB in Gata3 expression and Th2 differentiation in allergic airway inflammation. Nat Immunol 2001; 2:45–50.
57. Zhu J, Yamane H, Cote-Sierra J, et al. GATA-3 promotes Th2 responses through three different mechanisms: induction of Th2 cytokine production, selective growth of Th2 cells and inhibition of Th1 cell-specific factors. Cell Res 2006; 16:3–10.
58. Glimcher LH, Singh H. Transcription factors in lymphocyte development-T and B cells get together. Cell 1999; 96:13–23.
59. Szabo SJ, Kim ST, Costa GL, et al. A novel transcription factor, T-bet, directs Th1 lineage commitment. Cell 2000; 100:655–669.
60. Mullen AC, High FA, Hutchins AS, et al. Role of T-bet in commitment of TH1 cells before IL-12-dependent selection. Science 2001; 292:1907–1910.
61. Szabo SJ, Sullivan BM, Stemmann C, et al. Distinct effects of T-bet in TH1 lineage commitment and IFN-gamma production in CD4 and CD8 T cells. Science 2002; 295:338–342.

62. Hwang ES, Szabo SJ, Schwartzberg PL, et al. T helper cell fate specified by kinase-mediated interaction of T-bet with GATA-3. Science 2005; 307:430–433.
63. Ouyang W, Ranganath SH, Weindel K, et al. Inhibition of Th1 development mediated by GATA-3 through an IL-4-independent mechanism. Immunity 1998; 9:745–755.
64. Wu C, Nguyen KB, Pien GC, et al. SAP controls T cell responses to virus and terminal differentiation of TH2 cells. Nat Immunol 2001; 2:410–414.
65. Park H, Li Z, Yang XO, et al. A distinct lineage of CD4 T cells regulates tissue inflammation by producing interleukin 17. Nat Immunol 2005; 6:1133–1141.
66. Sallusto F, Lanzavecchia A, Mackay CR. Chemokines and chemokine receptors in T-cell priming and Th1/Th2- mediated responses. Immunol Today 1998; 19:568–574.
67. Rot A, von Andrian UH. Chemokines in innate and adaptive host defense: basic chemokinese grammar for immune cells. Annu Rev Immunol 2004; 22:891–928.
68. Bradley LM, Haynes L, Swain SL. IL-7: maintaining T-cell memory and achieving homeostasis. Trends Immunol 2005; 26:172–176.
69. Sallusto F, Lenig D, Forster R, et al. Two subsets of memory T lymphocytes with distinct homing potentials and effector functions. Nature 1999; 401:708–712.
70. Bingaman AW, Patke DS, Mane VR, et al. Novel phenotypes and migratory properties distinguish memory CD4 T cell subsets in lymphoid and lung tissue. Eur J Immunol 2005; 35:3173–3186.

B lymphocytes

71. Garside P, Ingulli E, Merica RR, et al. Visualization of specific B and T lymphocyte interactions in the lymph node. Science 1998; 281:96–99.
72. Valle A, Zuber CE, Defrance T, et al. Activation of human B lymphocytes through CD40 and interleukin 4. Eur J Immunol 1989; 19:1463–1467.
73. Stavnezer J. Immunoglobulin class switching. Curr Opin Immunol 1996; 8:199–205.

Lymphocytes in asthma

74. Corrigan CJ, Hartnell A, Kay AB. T lymphocyte activation in acute severe asthma. Lancet 1988; 1:1129–1132.
75. Walker C, Bode E, Boer L, et al. Allergic and nonallergic asthmatics have distinct patterns of T-cell activation and cytokine production in peripheral blood and bronchoalveolar lavage. Am Rev Respir Dis 1992; 146:109–115.
76. Robinson DS, Hamid Q, Ying S, et al. Predominant TH2-like bronchoalveolar T-lymphocyte population in atopic asthma. N Engl J Med 1992; 326:298–304.
77. Nakamura Y, Ghaffar O, Olivenstein R, et al. Gene expression of the GATA-3 transcription factor is increased in atopic asthma. J Allergy Clin Immunol 1999; 103:215–222.
78. Huang SK, Xiao HQ, Kleine-Tebbe J, et al. IL-13 expression at the sites of allergen challenge in patients with asthma. J Immunol 1995; 155:2688–2694.
79. Robinson D, Hamid Q, Bentley A, et al. Activation of CD4+ T cells, increased Th2-type cytokine mRNA expression, and eosinophil recruitment in bronchoalveolar lavage after allergen inhalation challenge in patients with atopic asthma. J Allergy Clin Immunol 1993; 92:313–324.
80. Bradley BL, Azzawi M, Jacobson M, et al. Eosinophils, T-lymphocytes, mast cells, neutrophils, and macrophages in bronchial biopsy specimens from atopic subjects with asthma: comparison with biopsy specimens from atopic subjects without asthma and normal control subjects and relationship to bronchial hyperresponsiveness. J Allergy Clin Immunol 1991; 88:661–674.
81. Robinson D, Hamid Q, Ying S, et al. Prednisolone treatment in asthma is associated with modulation of bronchoalveolar lavage cell interleukin-4, interleukin-5, and interferon-gamma cytokine gene expression. Am Rev Respir Dis 1993; 148:401–406.
82. Walker C, Kaegi MK, Braun P, et al. Activated T cells and eosinophilia in bronchoalveolar lavages from subjects with asthma correlated with disease severity. J Allergy Clin Immunol 1991; 88:935–942.
83. Nakajima H, Iwamoto I, Tomoe S, et al. CD4+ T-lymphocytes and interleukin-5 mediate antigen-induced eosinophil infiltration into mouse trachea. Am Rev Respir Dis 1992; 146:374–377.
84. Wills-Karp M. Immunologic basis of antigen-induced airway induced hyperresponsiveness. Ann Rev Immunol 1999; 17:255–281.
85. Renz H, Saloga J, Bradley KL, et al. Specific V beta T cell subsets mediate the immediate hypersensitivity response to ragweed allergen. J Immunol 1993; 151:1907–1917.
86. Cohn L, Homer RJ, Marinov A, et al. Induction of airway mucus production By T helper 2 (Th2) cells: a critical role for interleukin 4 in cell recruitment but not mucus production. J Exp Med 1997; 186:1737–1747.
87. Cohn L, Tepper JS, Bottomly K. IL-4-independent induction of airway hyperresponsiveness by Th2, but not Th1, cells. J Immunol 1998; 161:3813–3816.
88. Zhang DH, Yang L, Cohn L, et al. Inhibition of allergic inflammation in a murine model of asthma by expression of a dominant-negative mutant of GATA-3. Immunity 1999; 11:473–482.
89. Lee JJ, McGarry MP, Farmer SC, et al. Interleukin-5 expression in the lung epithelium of transgenic mice leads to pulmonary changes pathognomonic of asthma. J Exp Med 1997; 185:2143–2156.
90. Rankin JA, Picarella D, Tarallo A, et al. In vivo effects of the overexpression of IL-4 in the lungs of transgenic mice. Am J Resp Crit Care Med 1994; 149:1071a.
91. Temann UA, Geba GP, Rankin JA, et al. Expression of interleukin 9 in the lungs of transgenic mice causes airway inflammation, mast cell hyperplasia, and bronchial hyperresponsiveness. J Exp Med 1998; 188:1307–1320.
92. Zhu Z, Homer R, Wang Z, et al. Transgenic expression of IL-13 in murine lung causes airway inflammation, mucus hypersecretion, subendothelial fibrosis, eotaxin production and airways hyperresponsiveness to methacholine. J Clin Invest 1999; 103:779–788.
93. Cohn L, Elias JA, Chupp GL. Asthma: mechanisms of disease persistence and progression. Annu Rev Immunol 2004; 22:789–815.
94. Grunig G, Warnock M, Wakil AE, et al. Requirement for IL-13 independently of IL-4 in experimental asthma [see comments]. Science 1998; 282:2261–2263.
95. Wills-Karp M, Luyimbazi J, Xu X, et al. Interleukin-13: central mediator of allergic asthma. Science 1998; 282:2258–2261.
96. Kuperman DA, Huang X, Koth LL, et al. Direct effects of interleukin-13 on epithelial cells cause airway hyperreactivity and mucus overproduction in asthma. Nat Med 2002; 8:885–889.
97. Cohn L. Mucus in chronic airway diseases: sorting out the sticky details. J Clin Invest 2006; 116:306–308.
98. Zimmermann N, Hershey GK, Foster PS, et al. Chemokines in asthma: cooperative interaction between chemokines and IL-13. J Allergy Clin Immunol 2003; 111:227–242; quiz 243.
99. Lee CG, Homer RJ, Zhu Z, et al. Interleukin-13 induces tissue fibrosis by selectively stimulating and activating transforming growth factor beta(1). J Exp Med 2001; 194:809–821.
100. Rothenberg ME, Hogan SP. The eosinophil. Annu Rev Immunol 2006; 24:147–174.
101. Ober C, Hoffjan S. Asthma genetics 2006: the long and winding road to gene discovery. Genes Immun 2006; 7:95–100.
102. Kawashima T, Noguchi E, Arinami T, et al. Linkage and association of an interleukin 4 gene polymorphism with atopic dermatitis in Japanese families. J Med Genet 1998; 35:502–504.
103. Song Z, Casolaro V, Chen R, et al. Polymorphic nucleotides within the human IL-4 promoter that mediate overexpression of the gene. J Immunol 1996; 156:424–429.
104. Rosenwasser LJ, Borish L. Genetics of atopy and asthma: the rationale behind promoter-based candidate gene studies (IL-4 and IL-10). Am J Respir Crit Care Med 1997; 156: S152–155.
105. Heinzmann A, Mao XQ, Akaiwa M, et al. Genetic variants of IL-13 signalling and human asthma and atopy. Hum Mol Genet 2000; 9:549–559.
106. van der Pouw Kraan TC, van Veen A, Boeije LC, et al. An IL-13 promoter polymorphism associated with increased risk of allergic asthma. Genes Immun 1999; 1:61–65.
107. Deichmann KA, Heinzmann A, Forster J, et al. Linkage and allelic association of atopy and markers flanking the IL4- receptor gene. Clin Exp Allergy 1998; 28:151–155.
108. Vladich FD, Brazille SM, Stern D, et al. IL-13 R130Q, a common variant associated with allergy and asthma, enhances effector mechanisms essential for human allergic inflammation. J Clin Invest 2005; 115:747–754.
109. A genome-wide search for asthma susceptibility loci in ethnically diverse populations. The Collaborative Study on the Genetics of Asthma (CSGA). Nat Genet 1997; 15:389–392.
110. Daniels SE, Bhattacharrya S, James A, et al. A genome-wide search for quantitative trait loci underlying asthma. Nature 1996; 383:247–250.
111. Hizawa N, Freidhoff LR, Chiu YF, et al. Genetic regulation of Dermatophagoides pteronyssinus-specific IgE responsiveness: a genome-wide multipoint linkage analysis in families recruited through 2 asthmatic sibs. Collaborative Study on the Genetics of Asthma (CSGA). J Allergy Clin Immunol 1998; 102:436–442.
112. Ober C, Cox NJ, Abney M, et al. Genome-wide search for asthma susceptibility loci in a founder population. The Collaborative Study on the Genetics of Asthma. Hum Mol Genet 1998; 7:1393–1398.
113. Wjst M, Fischer G, Immervoll T, et al. A genome-wide search for linkage to asthma. German Asthma Genetics Group. Genomics 1999; 58:1–8.
114. Hubeau C, Apostolou I, Kobzik L. Adoptively transferred allergen-specific T cells cause maternal transmission of asthma risk. Am J Pathol 2006; 168:1931–1939.
115. Holtzman MJ, Sampath D, Castro M, et al. The one-two of T helper cells: does interferon-gamma knock out the Th2 hypothesis for asthma? [comment]. Am J Respir Cell Mol Biol 1996; 14:316–318.
116. Krug N, Madden J, Redington AE, et al. T cell cytokine profile evaluated at the single cells level in BAL and blood in allergic asthma. Am J Respir Cell Mol Biol 1996; 14:319–326.
117. Shaheen SO, Aaby P, Hall AJ, et al. Measles and atopy in Guinea-Bissau [see comments]. Lancet 1996; 347:1792–1796.
118. Shirakawa T, Enomoto T, Shimazu S, et al. The inverse association between tuberculin responses and atopic disorder [see comments]. Science 1997; 275:77–79.
119. Ball TM, Castro-Rodriguez JA, Griffith KA, et al. Siblings, day-care attendance, and the risk of asthma and wheezing during childhood. N Engl J Med 2000; 343:538–543.
120. Erb KJ, Holloway JW, Sobeck A, et al. Infection of mice with Mycobacterium bovis-Bacillus Calmette-Guerin (BCG) suppresses allergen-induced airway eosinophilia. J Exp Med 1998; 187:561–569.
121. Fernandez Botran R, Sanders VM, Mosmann TR, et al. Lymphokine-mediated regulation of the proliferative response of clones of T helper 1 and T helper 2 cells. J Exp Med 1988; 168:543–558.
122. Iwamoto I, Nakajima H, Endo H, et al. Interferon γ regulates antigen-induced eosinophil recruitment into the mouse airways by inhibiting the infiltration of CD4+ T cells. J Exp Med 1993; 177:573–576.
123. Li XM, Chopra RK, Chou TY, et al. Mucosal IFN-γ gene transfer inhibits pulmonary allergic responses in mice. J Immunol 1996; 157:3216–3219.
124. Coyle AJ, Tsuyuki S, Bertrand C, et al. Mice lacking the IFN-γ receptor have an impaired ability to resolve a lung eosinophilic inflammatory response associated with a prolonged capacity of T cells to exhibit a Th2 cytokine profile. J Immunol 1996; 156:2680–2685.
125. Cohn L, Homer RJ, Niu N, et al. T helper 1 cells and interferon gamma regulate allergic airway inflammation and mucus production. J Exp Med 1999; 190:1309–1318.
126. Hansen G, Berry G, DeKruyff RH, et al. Allergen-specific Th1 cells fail to counterbalance Th2 cell-induced airway hyperreactivity but cause severe airway inflammation. J Clin Invest 1999; 103:175–183.
127. Busse WW, Gern JE, Dick EC. The role of respiratory viruses in asthma. Ciba Found Symp 1997; 206:208–213.
128. Molet S, Hamid Q, Davoine F, et al. IL-17 is increased in asthmatic airways and induces human bronchial fibroblasts to produce cytokines. J Allergy Clin Immunol 2001; 108:430–438.
129. Chakir J, Shannon J, Molet S, et al. Airway remodeling-associated mediators in moderate to severe asthma: effect of steroids on TGF-beta, IL-11, IL-17, and type I and type III collagen expression. J Allergy Clin Immunol 2003; 111:1293–1298.
130. Hashimoto T, Akiyama K, Kobayashi N, et al. Comparison of IL-17 production by helper T cells among atopic and nonatopic asthmatics and control subjects. Int Arch Allergy Immunol 2005; 137(Suppl 1):51–54.

131. Schnyder-Candrian S, Togbe D, Couillin I, et al. Interleukin-17 is a negative regulator of established allergic asthma. J Exp Med 2006; 203:2715–2725.

132. Hellings PW, Kasran A, Liu Z, et al. Interleukin-17 orchestrates the granulocyte influx into airways after allergen inhalation in a mouse model of allergic asthma. Am J Respir Cell Mol Biol 2003; 28:42–50.

133. Azzawi M, Bradley B, Jeffery PK, et al. Identification of activated T lymphocytes and eosinophils in bronchial biopsies in stable atopic asthma. Am Rev Respir Dis 1990; 142:1407–1413.

134. Marsland BJ, Le Gros G. CD8+ T cells and immunoregulatory networks in asthma. Springer Semin Immunopathol 2004; 25:311–323.

135. O'Sullivan SM. Asthma death, CD8+ T cells, and viruses. Proc Am Thorac Soc 2005; 2:162–165.

136. Coyle AJ, Erard F, Bertrand C, et al. Virus-specific CD8+ cells can switch to interleukin 5 production and induce airway eosinophilia. J Exp Med 1995; 181:1229–1233.

137. Croft M, Carter L, Swain SL, et al. Generation of polarized antigen-specific CD8 effector populations: reciprocal action of interleukin (IL)-4 and IL-12 in promoting type 2 versus type 1 cytokine profiles. J Exp Med 1994; 180:1715–1728.

138. Seder RA, Boulay JL, Finkelman F, et al. CD8+ T cells can be primed in vitro to produce IL-4. J Immunol 1992; 148:1652–1656.

139. Hamelmann E, Oshiba A, Paluh J, et al. Requirement for CD8+ T cells in the development of airway hyperresponsiveness in a marine model of airway sensitization. J Exp Med 1996; 183:1719–1729.

140. van Rensen EL, Sont JK, Evertse CE, et al. Bronchial CD8 cell infiltrate and lung function decline in asthma. Am J Respir Crit Care Med 2005; 172:837–841.

141. Akbari O, Faul JL, Hoyte EG, et al. CD4+ invariant T-cell-receptor+ natural killer T cells in bronchial asthma. N Engl J Med 2006; 354:1117–1129.

142. Akbari O, Stock P, Meyer E, et al. Essential role of NKT cells producing IL-4 and IL-13 in the development of allergen-induced airway hyperreactivity. Nat Med 2003; 9:582–588.

143. Lisbonne M, Diem S, de Castro Keller A, et al. Cutting edge: invariant V alpha 14 NKT cells are required for allergen-induced airway inflammation and hyperreactivity in an experimental asthma model. J Immunol 2003; 171:1637–1641.

144. Korsgren M, Persson CG, Sundler F, et al. Natural killer cells determine development of allergen-induced eosinophilic airway inflammation in mice. J Exp Med 1999; 189:553–562.

145. Hayday AC. [gamma][delta] cells: a right time and a right place for a conserved third way of protection. Annu Rev Immunol 2000; 18:975–1026.

146. Krug N, Erpenbeck VJ, Balke K, et al. Cytokine profile of bronchoalveolar lavage-derived CD4(+), CD8(+), and gammadelta T cells in people with asthma after segmental allergen challenge. Am J Respir Cell Mol Biol 2001; 25:125–131.

147. Spinozzi F, Agea E, Bistoni O, et al. Local expansion of allergen-specific CD30+Th2-type gamma delta T cells in bronchial asthma. Mol Med 1995; 1:821–826.

148. Lahn M, Kanehiro A, Takeda K, et al. Negative regulation of airway responsiveness that is dependent on gammadelta T cells and independent of alphabeta T cells. Nat Med 1999; 5:1150–1156.

149. Zuany-Amorim C, Ruffie C, Haile S, et al. Requirement for gammadelta T cells in allergic airway inflammation. Science 1998; 280:1265–1267.

150. Warren HS, Kinnear BF, Phillips JH, et al. Production of IL-5 by human NK cells and regulation of IL-5 secretion by IL-4, IL-10, and IL-12. J Immunol 1995; 154:5144–5152.

151. Walker C, Checkel J, Cammisuli S, et al. IL-5 production by NK cells contributes to eosinophil infiltration in a mouse model of allergic inflammation. J Immunol 1998; 161:1962–1969.

152. Mikus LD, Rosenthal LA, Sorkness RL, et al. Reduced interferon-gamma secretion by natural killer cells from rats susceptible to postviral chronic airway dysfunction. Am J Respir Cell Mol Biol 2001; 24:74–82.

153. Gauchat JF, Henchoz S, Fattah D, et al. CD40 ligand is functionally expressed on human eosinophils. Eur J Immunol 1995; 25:863–865.

154. Gauchat JF, Henchoz S, Mazzei G, et al. Induction of human IgE synthesis in B cells by mast cells and basophils. Nature 1993; 365:340–343.

155. Boulet LP, Chapman KR, Cote J, et al. Inhibitory effects of an anti-IgE antibody E25 on allergen-induced early asthmatic response. Am J Respir Crit Care Med 1997; 155:1835–1840.

156. Fahy JV, Fleming HE, Wong HH, et al. The effect of an anti-IgE monoclonal antibody on the early- and late- phase responses to allergen inhalation in asthmatic subjects. Am J Respir Crit Care Med 1997; 155:1828–1834.

157. Milgrom H, Fick RB, Jr., Su JQ, Reimann JD, Bush RK, et al. Treatment of allergic asthma with monoclonal anti-IgE antibody. rhuMAb- E25 Study Group. N Engl J Med 1999; 341:1966–1973.

158. Djukanovic R, Wilson SJ, Kraft M, et al. Effects of treatment with anti-immunoglobulin E antibody omalizumab on airway inflammation in allergic asthma. Am J Respir Crit Care Med 2004; 170:583–593.

159. Coyle AJ, Wagner K, Bertrand C, et al. Central role of immunoglobulin (Ig) E in the induction of lung eosinophil infiltration and T helper 2 cell cytokine production: inhibition by a non-anaphylactogenic anti-IgE antibody. J Exp Med 1996; 183:1303–1310.

160. Lack G, Oshiba A, Bradley KL, et al. Transfer of immediate hypersensitivity and airway hyperresponsiveness by IgE-positive B cells. Am J Respir Crit Care Med 1994; 152:1765–1773.

161. Korsgren M, Erjefalt JS, Korsgren O, et al. Allergic eosinophil-rich inflammation develops in lungs and airways of B cell-deficient mice. J Exp Med 1997; 185:885–892.

162. Mehlhop PD, van de Rijn M, Goldberg AB, et al. Allergen-induced bronchial hyperreactivity and eosinophilic inflammation occur in the absence of IgE in a mouse model of asthma. Proc Natl Acad Sci U S A 1997; 94:1344–1349.

163. Muller KM, Rocken M, Joel D, et al. Mononuclear cell-bound CD23 is elevated in both atopic dermatitis and psoriasis. J Dermatol Sci 1991; 2:125–133.

164. Yu P, Kosco-Vilbois M, Richards M, et al. Negative feedback regulation of IgE synthesis by murine CD23. Nature 1994; 369:753–756.

165. Haczku A, Takeda K, Hamelmann E, et al. CD23 exhibits negative regulatory effects on allergic sensitization and airway hyperresponsiveness. Am J Respir Crit Care Med 2000; 161:952–960.

166. Hansen G, McIntire JJ, Yeung VP, et al. CD4(+) T helper cells engineered to produce latent TGF-beta1 reverse allergen-induced airway hyperreactivity and inflammation. J Clin Invest 2000; 105:61–70.

167. Oh JW, Seroogy CM, Meyer EH, et al. CD4 T-helper cells engineered to produce IL-10 prevent allergen-induced airway hyperreactivity and inflammation. J Allergy Clin Immunol 2002; 110:460–468.

168. Chen Y, Kuchroo VK, Inobe J, et al. Regulatory T cell clones induced by oral tolerance: suppression of autoimmune encephalomyelitis. Science 1994; 265:1237–1240.

169. Zuany-Amorim C, Sawicka E, Manlius C, et al. Suppression of airway eosinophilia by killed Mycobacterium vaccae-induced allergen-specific regulatory T cells. Nature Med 2002; 8:625–629.

170. Chen W, Jin W, Hardegen N, et al. Conversion of peripheral CD4+CD25- naive T cells to CD4+CD25+ regulatory T cells by TGF-beta induction of transcription factor Foxp3. J Exp Med 2003; 198:1875–1886.

171. Fantini MC, Becker C, Monteleone G, et al. Cutting edge: TGF-beta induces a regulatory phenotype in CD4+CD25- T cells through Foxp3 induction and down-regulation of Smad7. J Immunol 2004; 172:5149–5153.

172. Nakao A, Miike S, Hatano M, et al. Blockade of transforming growth factor beta/Smad signaling in T cells by overexpression of Smad7 enhances antigen-induced airway inflammation and airway reactivity. J Exp Med 2000; 192:151–158.

173. Akbari O, DeKruyff RH, Umetsu DT. Pulmonary dendritic cells producing IL-10 mediate tolerance induced by respiratory exposure to antigen. Nat Immunol 2001; 2:725–731.

174. Akbari O, Freeman GJ, Meyer EH, et al. Antigen-specific regulatory T cells develop via the ICOS-ICOS-ligand pathway and inhibit allergen-induced airway hyperreactivity. Nat Med 2002; 8:1024–1032.

175. Hoyne GF, Le Roux I, Corsin-Jimenez M, et al. Serrate1-induced notch signalling regulates the decision between immunity and tolerance made by peripheral CD4(+) T cells. Int Immunol 2000; 12:177–185.

176. McMenamin C, Pimm C, McKersey M, et al. Regulation of IgE responses to inhaled antigen in mice by antigen-specific gamma delta T cells. Science 1994; 265:1869–1871.

177. Ostroukhova M, Seguin-Devaux C, Oriss TB, et al. Tolerance induced by inhaled antigen involves CD4(+) T cells expressing membrane-bound TGF-beta and FOXP3. J Clin Invest 2004; 114:28–38.

178. Ostroukhova M, Qi Z, Oriss TB, et al. Treg-mediated immunosuppression involves activation of the Notch-HES1 axis by membrane-bound TGF-beta. J Clin Invest 2006; 116:996–1004.

179. Soares R, Alcada MN, Azevedo I. Triggering TGFbeta and notch signalling cross-talk. Bioessays 2005; 27:763.

180. Kearley J, Barker JE, Robinson DS, et al. Resolution of airway inflammation and hyperreactivity after in vivo transfer of CD4+CD25+ regulatory T cells is interleukin 10 dependent. J Exp Med 2005; 202:1539–1547.

181. Lewkowich IP, Herman NS, Schleifer KW, et al. CD4+CD25+ T cells protect against experimentally induced asthma and alter pulmonary dendritic cell phenotype and function. J Exp Med 2005; 202:1549–1561.

182. Mucida D, Kutchukhidze N, Erazo A, et al. Oral tolerance in the absence of naturally occurring Tregs. J Clin Invest 2005; 115:1923–1933.

183. Wilson MS, Taylor MD, Balic A, et al. Suppression of allergic airway inflammation by helminth-induced regulatory T cells. J Exp Med 2005; 202:1199–1212.

184. Strickland DH, Stumbles PA, Zosky GR, et al. Reversal of airway hyperresponsiveness by induction of airway mucosal CD4+CD25+ regulatory T cells. J Exp Med 2006; 2649–2660.

185. Ling EM, Smith T, Nguyen XD, et al. Relation of CD4+CD25+ regulatory T-cell suppression of allergen-driven T-cell activation to atopic status and expression of allergic disease. Lancet 2004; 363:608–615.

186. Karlsson MR, Rugtveit J, Brandtzaeg P. Allergen-responsive CD4+CD25+ regulatory T cells in children who have outgrown cow's milk allergy. J Exp Med 2004; 199:1679–1688.

187. Tiemessen MM, Van Ieperen-Van Dijk AG, Bruijnzeel-Koomen CA, et al. Cow's milk-specific T-cell reactivity of children with and without persistent cow's milk allergy: key role for IL-10. J Allergy Clin Immunol 2004; 113:932–939.

188. Viglietta V, Baecher-Allan C, Weiner HL, et al. Loss of functional suppression by CD4+CD25+ regulatory T cells in patients with multiple sclerosis. J Exp Med 2004; 199:971–979.

189. Cao D, Malmstrom V, Baecher-Allan C, et al. Isolation and functional characterization of regulatory CD25brightCD4+ T cells from the target organ of patients with rheumatoid arthritis. Eur J Immunol 2003; 33:215–223.

190. Prakken BJ, Samodal R, Le TD, et al. Epitope-specific immunotherapy induces immune deviation of proinflammatory T cells in rheumatoid arthritis. Proc Natl Acad Sci U S A 2004; 101:4228–4233.

Biology of Neutrophils

Jodie L Simpson, Katherine J Baines and Peter G Gibson

17

CONTENTS

- Introduction 283
- Neutrophil migration 283
- Mediators released by activated neutrophils 286
- Neutrophil clearance and death 287
- Neutrophils in asthma 288
- Conclusion 293

SUMMARY OF IMPORTANT CONCEPTS

>> Neutrophils play a key role in innate immune defenses

>> Respiratory triggers and insults (shown in Box 17.2) result in neutrophil accumulation in the airways (neutrophilic bronchitis)

>> Airway neutrophils can release newly synthesized and preformed inflammatory mediators which are toxic and can support angiogenesis and remodeling processes

>> Inappropriate or uncontrolled neutrophil responses contribute to airway disease pathogenesis

INTRODUCTION

Neutrophils play an important role in inflammatory responses that are critical for host defense against infection, contribute to the pathogenesis of chronic inflammatory conditions that involve the sinuses and respiratory tract, and comprise 50–75% of circulating leukocytes in humans. They are the first circulating cells to migrate to the site of infection. Through phagocytosis, the production of reactive oxygen intermediates (ROI), and the release of cytotoxic granule contents, these cells function to contain and eliminate invading microorganisms. Representing a major mechanism of innate immunity, neutrophils also release cytokines and chemokines that initiate and amplify inflammation, as well as contribute to the development of the acquired immune response.

Given the toxic nature of an activated neutrophil, these cells are associated with the pathogenesis of inflammatory airway diseases, including chronic obstructive pulmonary disease (COPD) and asthma, as well as acute parenchymal lung conditions such as pneumonia and acute lung injury. This chapter examines the biology of the neutrophil, with a focus on its contribution to inflammation in asthma.

NEUTROPHIL MIGRATION

Neutrophils migrate from the blood to the airways, where they play an important role during infection and inflammation. This complex process requires the maturation of neutrophils in the bone marrow and their release into the bloodstream, from where they migrate to the airways under the influence of chemotactic factors and adhesion molecules. Mature neutrophils do not undergo cell division. They are generated continuously from the bone marrow ($\sim 10^{11}$ cells/day), and their numbers, although tightly regulated, can be greatly amplified in times of stress, e.g., infection. The maturation of neutrophils in the bone marrow involves the highly controlled process of myelopoiesis, where pluripotent stem cells divide and differentiate into myeloid precursors that follow a specific differentiation program. During maturation, neutrophil granules are formed, which contribute to the inflammatory response in the fight against microorganisms.

A variety of preformed compounds exist in neutrophil granules including serine and metalloproteinases, reactive oxygen species, lipid mediators, and defensins (Fig. 17.1). These toxic molecules are released from activated neutrophils, and have the ability to cause significant tissue damage to the lung and airways in asthma. This damage occurs when neutrophils accumulate in large numbers, and their activation is inappropriate or uncontrolled.

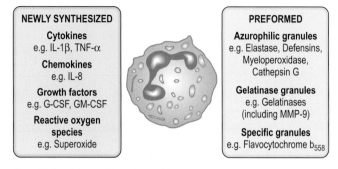

Fig. 17.1. Neutrophil mediators. The neutrophil is a source of a range of preformed and newly synthesized mediators.

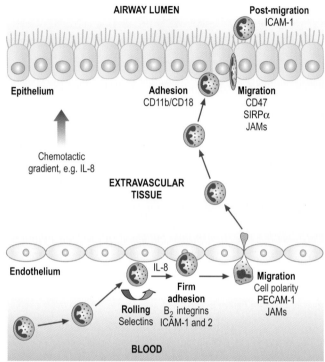

Fig. 17.2. Neutrophil migration to the airways. The migration of neutrophils from the blood stream requires neutrophil rolling, activation and firm adhesion to endothelial cells, and this is followed by migration through the endothelial layer, the basement membrane and the epithelial interface where the cells accumulate in the airway lumen.

MYELOID DEVELOPMENT

Neutrophils are generated continuously from hematopoietic stem cells of the bone marrow, and this process is referred to as myelopoiesis. Myelopoiesis begins with the differentiation of pluripotent stem cells into myeloid progenitors, which then develop into myeloid precursors that under certain conditions result in the development of neutrophils. Developing neutrophils can be divided into six subtypes, including the myeloblast, the promyelocyte where primary (azurophilic) granules appear, the myelocyte where cell division ceases and secondary (specific) granules appear, the metamyelocyte where tertiary (gelatinase) granules appear, followed by band cells and finally mature neutrophils, characterized by their multilobed nucleus and cytoplasm containing granules.[1]

Many factors influence the development of neutrophils in the bone marrow. These include stromal cells such as fibroblastoid cells, endothelial cells, adipocytes, reticular cells and macrophages; components of the extracellular matrix such as collagens, glycoproteins, and proteoglycans; as well as adhesion molecules such as CD11b/CD18, and growth factors such as G-CSF and GM-CSF. Important also in this process are specific changes in gene expression patterns controlled by transcription factors such as C/EBPs and PU.1.[2] During maturation, neutrophils increase their mobility, deformability, and responsiveness to chemokines.

Neutrophil maturation in the bone marrow takes approximately 10–15 days, and depends on the detachment of the cells from the marrow microenvironment, and the mechanical 'pumping' of the cells into the bone marrow sinuses. Immature neutrophils can be released prematurely into the circulation in times of infection or inflammation, and these cells preferentially sequester into the lung microvessels.[3] Exposure to inhalants, such as cigarette smoke, can decrease the transit time of neutrophils through the bone marrow, and cause the release of immature neutrophils into the bloodstream.[4] Contact with cytokines (e.g., G-CSF, GM-CSF, IL-1) and chemokines (e.g., IL-8) can influence this process through the release of proteases (e.g., MMP-9) and the shedding of L-selectin.[5] Once released into the bloodstream, neutrophils have a half-life of 4–10 h, and can migrate into the tissues.

NEUTROPHIL TRAFFICKING AND MARGINATION

Peripheral blood neutrophils are divided between a circulating pool, present in large and small blood vessels, and a marginating pool that is arrested in capillaries. Margination in the systemic circulation is regulated by selectin-mediated capture from the bloodstream. Rolling adhesion of neutrophils to the endothelium is mediated by L-selectin on the neutrophil and P- and E-selectin on the endothelium. The pulmonary capillary bed is the main site containing marginating neutrophils and measuring 20–60 times that of the concentration of large systemic blood vessels.[6] Most neutrophils have to deform and elongate to travel through the pulmonary capillaries due to the vast network of the capillary bed, and the vessels being of a smaller diameter in comparison to spheric neutrophils. The requirement of neutrophils to deform to travel through the pulmonary capillaries increases their transit time, resulting in a higher concentration of neutrophils in this space.[7]

Normal margination should not be confused with neutrophil sequestration, which is defined as amplified intravascular neutrophil numbers induced by inflammatory mediators and complement factors. Initial stages of sequestration are thought to involve cytoskeletal rearrangements such as increases in F actin at the periphery of the cell to reduce neutrophil deformability. Prolonged sequestration of neutrophils requires CD11b/CD18.[6] The migration of neutrophils into tissues involves neutrophil rolling, activation and firm adhesion to endothelial cells, followed by migration through the endothelial cell layer, the basement membrane and the epithelial interface and accumulation in the airway lumen (Fig. 17.2). These events involve complex interactions between neutrophils and the endothelium, extracellular matrix, and epithelium, and are largely mediated by cellular adhesion molecules (CAMs) such as the β_2 integrins. This process gradually changes the functional state of the neutrophil from a passive circulating cell into a highly activated effector cell of innate immunity.

CELLULAR ADHESION MOLECULES

Neutrophil adherence to the endothelium involves cellular adhesion molecules on the neutrophil and endothelial cell, whose expression is tightly regulated. Rolling adhesion of neutrophils to the endothelium is mediated by L-selectin on the neutrophil and P- and E-selectin on the endothelium. Rolling allows interaction between CXC chemokines such as IL-8 presented on the surface of endothelial cells, which activates β_2 integrin expression. Interaction between the integrins CD11a/CD18 and CD11b/CD18 and the endothelial immunoglobulin (Ig) superfamily members, intercellular adhesion molecule (ICAM)-1 and ICAM-2, are required for effective neutrophil transmigration and firm adhesion to the endothelium.[8]

Integrins

The integrins are a family of heterodimeric transmembrane glycoproteins that mediate direct cell–cell, cell–extracellular matrix, and cell–pathogen interactions. They contain two functional units: α and β chains. The β_2 integrins are expressed on neutrophils and consist of four different heterodimers: CD11a/CD18 or leukocyte function associated antigen-1 (LFA-1); CD11b/CD18 or Mac-1; CD11c/CD18 or p150,95; and CD11d/CD18. Leukocyte adhesion deficiency (LAD) results from a mutation in the gene for CD18 and is associated with recurrent bacterial infections due to an inability to recruit these cells to a site of infection.

The functional state and presence of integrins on neutrophils is regulated by lipid, cytokine, and chemokine signaling molecules as well as 'cross talk' from other adhesion molecules. Integrins exist in predominately inactive states on circulating immune cells. Multiple mechanisms, including conformational change (affinity regulation) and clustering associated with the cytoskeleton (avidity regulation), are responsible for integrin activation, arising from or caused by ligand binding. Interestingly, the ability of the extracellular domains of integrins to bind ligands can be activated in <1 s via signals from within the cell (inside-out signaling).[9]

Inflammatory stimulus

In the pulmonary circulation, neutrophil migration occurs through at least two pathways: CD11b/CD18-dependent and -independent, and dependent on the inflammatory stimulus. Inflammatory stimuli that invoke CD18-dependent neutrophil migration include *Escherichia coli* lipopolysaccharide (*E. coli* LPS), *Pseudomonas aeruginosa* immunoglobulin G (IgG), IL-1, immune complexes, and phorbol myristate acetate (PMA). Stimuli that induce CD11b/CD18-independent neutrophil migration include *Streptococcus pneumoniae;* group B streptococcus, *Staphylococcus aureus,* hydrochloric acid, hypoxia, and C5a.[6] In vitro models have demonstrated that the bacterial-derived chemoattractant fMLP stimulates CD18-dependent neutrophil migration, whereas the host-derived chemoattractants IL-8 and LTB_4 stimulate CD18-independent neutrophil migration. It is unclear if one pathway is preferentially used over another in relation to neutrophil influx into the lung. However,

a recent study adding cystic fibrosis sputum, which is a cocktail of both bacterial- and host-derived chemoattractants, to neutrophils in vitro preferentially induced CD18-independent migration.[10]

Endothelial cell interactions

Although a significant amount of information is known about the first three steps of neutrophil migration (rolling, activation, and adhesion), the mechanisms that underlie transendothelial migration remain unclear. Generally, leukocytes traverse the endothelial barrier through the cleft between two to three adjacent cells. Transendothelial migration, but also acquisition of cell polarity of the neutrophil, is thought to be mediated by platelet/endothelial cell adhesion molecule (PECAM)-1 and junction adhesion molecules (JAMs) expressed at intercellular tight junctions of endothelial and epithelial cells.[11] Recently, the binding of JAM-C to Mac-1 was found to be of importance in neutrophil transendothelial migration.

Epithelial cell interactions

Mechanisms underlying neutrophil migration through the epithelium are only beginning to emerge. This process involves three stages, which are epithelial adhesion, migration and post-migration. Initially neutrophil firm adherence to the basolateral epithelial membrane is mediated exclusively by Mac-1. Transepithelial migration of neutrophils involves both cell–cell interactions that include adhesion molecules and signaling events to open the epithelial tight junctions, allowing the passage of cells without disturbance of the epithelial barrier. The interaction between CD47 and signal regulatory protein-a (SIRPa) enhances the migration rate of neutrophils through the epithelium.[12] Further to this, JAMs are likely to be important in the migratory process, as well as the formation of a seal around migrating cells to preserve barrier function. After migration through the epithelium, neutrophils can adhere to ICAM-1 present on the apical surface of the epithelial cells.

CHEMOTACTIC MEDIATORS

Once through the endothelial basement membrane, neutrophils migrate along a chemotactic gradient. Neutrophil chemotactic proteins include chemokines (e.g., IL-8), bacterial products (e.g., N-formyl methionyl peptides), lipid mediators (e.g., LTB_4) and complement split products (e.g., C5a).

Chemokines

The chemokine family constitutes about 50 low molecular weight proteins that exert their effects through activation of one of 19 G-protein coupled chemokine receptors. There are two main subfamilies of chemokines, CXC and CC, which are classified according to the position of the first two cysteines in their amino acid sequence (separated by one amino acid – CXC, or adjacent CC). Many chemokines can bind to more than one receptor and most chemokine receptors can bind more than one chemokine. Chemokines are produced by inflamed tissues and activate signal cascades in the neutrophil that lead to increase in cell motility, adhesion and survival.

IL-8 is a potent chemotactic factor for neutrophils. It is the main chemoattractant in the lung, since blocking of IL-8 with a neutralizing antibody resulted in a 75–98% inhibition of its chemotactic activity.[13] IL-8 is a member of the CXC subfamily, is produced by several cell types, in particular epithelial cells, macrophages and neutrophils themselves, and is released upon proinflammatory stimulation. Other members of this family include epithelial cell-derived neutrophil activator-78 (ENA-78), growth regulatory gene (Gro)-α, Gro-β; neutrophil-activating peptide-2 (NAP-2), and granulocyte chemotactic protein-2 (GCP-2).

Leukotriene B$_4$

Leukotrienes (LTs) are potent lipid mediators that have been implicated in the pathogenesis of airway diseases including asthma.[14] LTs are synthesized from arachidonic acid via the actions of 5-lipooxygenase (5-LO), along with 5-LO-activating protein and terminal LTA$_4$ hydrolase. They are classified into two classes; leukotriene B$_4$ (LTB$_4$) and the cysteinyl LTs. LTB$_4$ is a potent chemoattractant and activator as well as enhances neutrophil adhesion and migration. LTB$_4$ exerts its action through two seven-transmembrane G-protein receptors: the high-affinity BLT-1 and the low-affinity BLT-2. Pretreatment with the LTB$_4$ receptor antagonist SC-53228 in dogs had no significant effect on neutrophil numbers in the bronchoalveolar lavage (BAL) but significantly reduced the oxygen radical release of BAL neutrophils as well as ozone-induced airway hyperresponsiveness (AHR).

Innate immune activation

Activation of the innate immune system involves the detection of pathogen associated molecular patterns (PAMPs) by pattern recognition receptors (PRRs) including the toll-like receptor (TLR) family. Activation of TLRs results in an activation of a signalling cascade involving MyD88 and NF-κB that results in the release of chemokines and cytokines to further recruit neutrophils (Fig. 17.3).

Toll-like receptors (TLRs)

TLRs play a crucial role in the detection of invading microorganisms and the initiation of host defenses. Currently the TLR family contains 10 members, and at the mRNA level, neutrophils appear to express all of these receptors except for TLR3.[15] TLR4 is the major endotoxin receptor, and TLR2 recognizes PAMPs from Gram-positive organisms. TLR2 agonists include lipoteichoic acids (LTAs) and peptidoglycans. TLR2 combines TLR1 or TLR6 to initiate a signaling cascade. Activation of both TLR2 and TLR4 regulates several important proinflammatory neutrophil functions through the activation of the NF-κB pathway, and these include neutrophil activation, migration, and survival.[16]

Exposure to LPS increases neutrophil expression of TLR2 and CD14 but does not change expression of TLR4. Upon stimulation with PAMPs including peptidoglycan, zymosan and araLAM (a component of *Mycobacterium tuberculosis*) neutrophils produce IL-8 and superoxide and also have increased phagocytosis.[15]

The rate of neutrophil apoptosis is delayed by the presence of bacterial lipoprotein and LPS to result in the augmentation of neutrophilic inflammation. The presence of an anti-TLR2 monoclonal antibody prevents the delay in apoptosis in peripheral blood neutrophils and suggests a role for TLR2 in this process.[17]

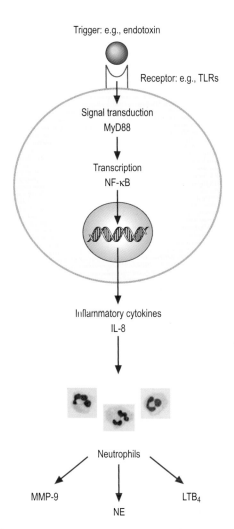

Fig. 17.3. Innate immune activation pathway leading to accumulation of neutrophils and neutrophil activation.

■ MEDIATORS RELEASED BY ACTIVATED NEUTROPHILS ■

PROTEASES

Proteolytic enzymes play an important role in tissue remodeling and repair in the airways. Levels of proteolytic enzymes, including active neutrophil elastase (NE)[18] and matrix metalloproteinase-9 (MMP-9),[19] are increased in asthma and thought to indicate an imbalance in the protease/antiprotease system.

Neutrophil elastase (NE) is a 30 kDa serine protease, which can attack a number of proteins including lung elastin. It is present in high concentrations within the azurophilic granules of neutrophils and is important in host defence, specifically for the intracellular killing of Gram-negative infections. The presence of extracellular active NE results in tissue destruction and is also a potent secretagogue, contributing to increased mucus production. The presence of extracellular active NE may indicate a protease/antiprotease imbalance where the protease is present in excess compared with the antiprotease. However, the presence of free active enzyme can also represent the inability of the antiprotease defenses to inactivate the protease. The latter can occur when the antiprotease is altered, for example, by oxidation or inhibited by other proteases such as MMPs. When inhibition is deficient or the enzyme load exceeds an inhibitor's capacity to inactivate, proteolytic lung degradation occurs. Neutrophil elastase can upregulate IL-8 gene expression and protein production in bronchial epithelial cells via a MyD88-dependent NF-κB signalling pathway.[20] This upregulation is inhibited when cells are pretreated with a TLR4 neutralizing antibody,[21] indicating that upregulation of IL-8 production is via an innate immune pathway (Fig. 17.3). Neutrophil elastase is increased in asthma[18] and also prominent in other airway diseases including COPD, cystic fibrosis, and bronchiectasis.

Secretory leucocyte protease inhibitor (SLPI) is a broad-spectrum inhibitor of mast cell and leukocyte serine proteases and produced by epithelial cells and submucosal glands. SLPI levels are increased in pneumonia and in the peripheral airways of subjects with emphysema, but decreased in chronic diseases such as diffuse pan-bronchiolitis and in COPD subjects with frequent exacerbations. SLPI inhibits NF-κB activation and LPS-induced TNF-α and IL-6 production in monocytes and macrophages. In vitro experiments have shown that once SLPI is inactivated, either by oxidation or complexed by NE, both antiprotease activity and antiinflammatory capacity are lost.[22] α_1-Antitrypsin (α1AT) is the major endogenous serine protease inhibitor produced by hepatocytes and is also expressed by neutrophils, epithelial cells, and macrophages. Both α1AT and SLPI counterbalance NE activity. Airway levels of α1AT are increased in the sputum of subjects with asthma[18] and are related to the duration of the asthma and lung function.[19] While levels of active NE are increased in asthma, so is the inhibitor α1AT, suggesting that the presence of antiproteases either are not sufficient or not functionally capable of inactivating the free enzyme.

MMP-9 is a member of a family of zinc-containing enzymes that degrade extracellular matrix, modulate cytokine activity, and alter the activity of other proteases. MMP-9 has been identified in cells such as bronchial epithelial cells, neutrophils, mast cells, eosinophils, and macrophages,[23] and is released as a pro-enzyme that can then be activated by a number of mechanisms including other MMPs, bacterial proteases, reactive oxygen species,[24] and neutrophil proteins such as lipocalin.[25] Tissue inhibitor of metalloproteinase (TIMP-1) is the major tissue inhibitor of MMP-9, secreted in association with MMP-9, and binds with both the pro- and active-forms of MMP-9 to cause inactivation. Levels of MMP-9 are increased in asthma compared to healthy controls and also in severe asthma compared to mild asthma.[26]

MMP-9 is expressed in the sub-basement membrane (SBM) in asthma and increased with increasing severity. The presence of MMP-9 in the SBM has been associated with the presence of neutrophils in the submucosa and also TGF-β positive cells. BAL levels of MMP-9 are also inversely related to FEV_1 suggesting a relationship between this mediator and airflow obstruction.[27]

MMP-9 can inactivate α1AT to further NE-mediated tissue destruction.[28] Once degraded, α1AT is a potent activator of neutrophils. Oxidant radicals, including the hydroxyl radical, peroxide, and hypochloride, can modify α1AT to a form that has no inhibitory capacity against proteases. Similarly, TIMP-1 can be inactivated upon exposure to hypochlorous acid, which is released by activated neutrophils.

REACTIVE OXYGEN SPECIES (ROS)

The respiratory burst involves the activation of NADPH oxidase, which is an enzymatic complex composed of cytosolic ($p40^{phox}$, $p47^{phox}$, and $p67^{phox}$) and flavocytochrome b_{558} which is composed of membrane proteins ($p22^{phox}$ and $gp91^{phox}$). Flavocytochrome b_{558} is located between the plasma membrane and the membrane of the specific granules, and is incorporated into the phagocytic vacuole, where it pumps electrons from NADPH in the cytosol to oxygen in the vacuole.[29] When neutrophils are activated, $p47^{phox}$ is phosphorylated to cause cytosolic components to migrate to the plasma membrane, where they are able to associate with flavocytochrome b_{558}, assembling the active oxidase. Reactive oxygen species (ROS) are generated as a result of NADPH oxidase activity to produce superoxide (O_2^-). Superoxide can be rapidly converted into hydrogen peroxide (H_2O_2) by the enzyme superoxide dismutase. Superoxide and hydrogen peroxide can also form to create the highly reactive hydroxyl radical (HO^-). In addition, myeloperoxidase (MPO), a constituent of the azurophilic granules, generates hyperchlorous acid (HOCl) from hydrogen peroxide.[29]

Exposure to ROS can result in pulmonary injury. Recent findings demonstrate an expanded role for ROS, in that they can activate granule proteins, interact with various signaling cascades, and modulate neutrophil functions. Superoxide can activate granule proteins through the recruitment of K^+ to the phagosome, thus allowing cationic proteases of the azurophilic granules such as neutrophil elastase (NE) and cathepsin G (CG) to go from a highly organized intragranule structures into solution where they can kill ingested microbes.[30] ROS can inhibit a variety of protein tyrosine phosphatases through oxidation of key residues, allowing the phosphorylation of other molecules to proceed. ROS can disrupt intercellular tight junctions, increase the permeability of the endothelial barrier via the phosphorylation of focal adhesion kinase in endothelial cells, and modulate neutrophil function by inducing apoptosis through a caspase-8 dependent manner.

DEFENSINS

There are six identified human defensins. These small, arginine-rich peptides play an important role in host defense to infections. Four defensins that are present in neutrophils are the human neutrophil peptides (HNP-1 to HNP-4). These peptides kill pathogens by causing permeabilization of the bacterial membrane.[31] Mature defensins are present in high concentration in the azurophilic granules and constitute 5–7% of the neutrophil's total protein.[32] Defensins also modulate the inflammatory response, as they can bind to protease inhibitors such as α_1-antitrypsin.

■ NEUTROPHIL CLEARANCE AND DEATH ■

After killing and digesting invading microbes, neutrophils at the inflammatory site undergo programmed cell death (apoptosis) and are cleared by macrophages (efferocytosis).[33] The regulation of neutrophil apoptosis is crucial to maintain neutrophil numbers in the blood, as well as for the effective removal of invading pathogens, the resolution of inflammation, and the prevention of a necrotic cell death resulting in the release of the neutrophil's toxic cellular contents.

In vivo, this process may limit neutrophils, destructive capability. Within a few minutes, neutrophil apoptosis results in irreversible chromatin condensation, nuclear collapse, cytosolic vacuolation, and cell shrinkage. During this time the cell is unable to respond to agonists, is immobilized and inert. Apoptotic neutrophils become instantly recognizable to alveolar macrophages, which result in cell removal via efferocytosis.[34] This process can also induce changes in the activation phenotype of lung macrophages, suppressing the release of proinflammatory mediators.

Neutrophil apoptosis is an active process that can be modulated by various mediators. Defined inflammatory stimuli, such as growth factors (e.g. GM-CSF and G-CSF), cytokines (e.g. IL-1 and IL-6), chemokines (e.g. IL-8), and even bacterial products (e.g. LPS), can delay neutrophil apoptosis. Conversely, TNF-α and Fas-ligand (Fas-L) can increase the rate of neutrophil apoptosis. Interestingly, certain pathogenic bacteria and viruses have strong effects on inducing neutrophil apoptosis, increasing the likelihood of these organisms to evade intracellular killing and inhibiting neutrophil functions. Corticosteroids delay neutrophil apoptosis, thus increasing their survival time, and influencing the persistence of neutrophilic inflammation.[35]

Neutrophil apoptosis is induced by activation of cellular caspases and can occur through two main pathways. The first is the death receptor (DR) pathway, where the clustering of TNF and Fas-receptors activates the caspase cascade beginning with cleavage of pro-caspase 8. The second is an intrinsic pathway consisting of mitochondrial cytochrome c and members of the Bcl-2 family that forms an apoptosome activating caspase 9. Cell stress due to exposure to ROS, DNA damage, or lack of growth factors can result in apoptosis, induced by the release of cytochrome c.[36] Activated caspase 8 and 9 can then activate caspase 3 to cleave proteins essential for cell survival. Cross-talk exists between the two apoptosis pathways; for example, activation of caspase 8 by ligation of DRs is not enough to trigger caspase 3 activation, and activation of caspase 8, through this mechanism cleaves Bid, a protein of the Bcl-2 family to amplify cytochrome c release from the mitochondria.

CYTOKINE SYNTHESIS

The neutrophil is both a target and source of various proinflammatory cytokines (e.g., TNF-α and IL-1), chemokines (e.g., IL-8), and growth factors (e.g., GM-CSF and G-CSF), and hence has the ability to create a positive feedback loop on its own proinflammatory functions. These cytokines can amplify several neutrophil functions, including the ROS generation. Chemokines can promote neutrophil migration to the inflammatory site. Finally, both cytokines and chemokines can prime neutrophils.

Neutrophils were always thought to be devoid of transcriptional activity or protein synthesis. Recent evidence, however, indicates that neutrophils are an important source of newly synthesized cytokines and growth factors. Cytokine synthesis by neutrophils occurs to a lesser degree than monocytes;[37] however, this is overshadowed in vivo by both the number of circulating neutrophils being 20 times that of monocytes, and neutrophils are the first cell to arrive at sites of inflammation. Cytokine production by neutrophils is increased by inflammatory stimuli, bacterial endotoxin (LPS) being the most potent. The secretion of cytokines is varied and dependent on the agonist, and for some cytokine production, stimulation with more than one agonist is required, such as stimulation with IFN and LPS is needed for IL-12 production.[37] Neutrophil cytokine expression can be modulated by T cell-derived

cytokines: positively by Th1 cytokines (e.g., IFN) and negatively by Th2 cytokines (e.g., IL-4 and IL-13).

■ NEUTROPHILS IN ASTHMA ■

Neutrophils are commonly found in the airway lumen in healthy people and are in increased numbers of subgroups with stable asthma (neutrophilic asthma), during exacerbations and also in cases of fatal asthma. The precise role of neutrophils in the pathogenesis of asthma remains unclear.

Recruitment of neutrophils to the airways is orchestrated, in part, by the potent chemokine IL-8 (CXCL8). Epithelial cells release IL-8 on exposure, to a variety of stimuli, to promote their movement to the airways. Neutrophils themselves are a source of IL-8 and, in this way, may influence their own activation and sequestration from the circulation. Once activated, neutrophils release a variety of proinflammatory proteins, which induce further inflammatory processes and have the potential to induce remodeling of the airways. Proteolytic enzymes also influence the chemotaxis and activation of neutrophils. NE can induce IL-8 production and MMP-9 can enhance IL-8 potency by augmenting amino terminal processing of IL-8.[38]

The role of neutrophils in asthma is unclear, but increases in neutrophils have been reported in severe asthma requiring intubation,[39] sudden-onset fatal asthma, and life-threatening asthma,[40,41] suggesting a role for these cells in the most severe forms of disease. Neutrophils are increased in a number of airway compartments, including the lumen[42] and submucosa.[43] Neutrophil numbers increase with increasing severity of asthma.[44] Neutrophil numbers and products are increased during exacerbations in both adults[45] and children with asthma[46,47] and have been associated with damaged epithelium.[48] Neutrophilic inflammation is a feature of respiratory viral infections in both healthy subjects and those with asthma.[49] While generally overlooked in less severe forms of asthma, increased neutrophils are also present in milder forms of asthma. More recently there have been reports of subgroups of patients with stable asthma who have a persistent neutrophilic bronchitis.[50–52] Subjects with neutrophilic asthma have a number of unique inflammatory abnormalities to distinguish them from typical eosinophilic asthma (where sputum eosinophils are outside the normal range) and paucigranulocytic asthma (where sputum granulocytes are within normal ranges).

NEUTROPHILIC ASTHMA

Neutrophilic asthma is defined as symptomatic asthma and airway hyperresponsiveness in the presence of a neutrophilic bronchitis (Fig. 17.4, sputum neutrophils >60%). Neutrophilic asthma represents between 10 and 30% of stable asthma in adults.[53–55] Subjects with neutrophilic asthma are older[53–55] than subjects with normal levels of neutrophils and tend to have less severe airway hyperresponsiveness. However, they are similar in terms of gender, atopy, smoking, and lung function.[54]

Neutrophilic airway inflammation asthma is not restricted to adults. In a study of difficult asthma in children, both eosinophils and neutrophils were significantly elevated in the epithelium.[56] Another study found increased neutrophils and neutrophil proteases in children with mild-to-moderate asthma compared to intermittent asthma,[57] indicating a similar increase in neutrophils with greater severity as observed in adults. It has been recently postulated that a significant proportion of asthma

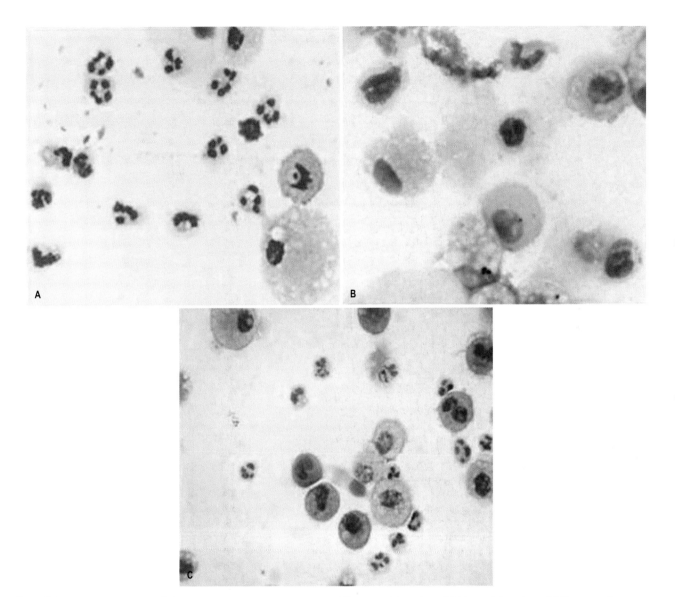

Fig. 17.4. Sputum cytospins in different asthma inflammatory phenotypes. (A) Neutrophilic asthma. (B) Eosinophilic asthma. (C) Paucigranulocytic asthma. (Reproduced from Simpson JL, Scott R, Boyle M, et al. Inflammatory subtypes in asthma: assesment and identification using induced sputum Respirology 2006; 11:54–61,[54] with permission.)

is the result of neutrophilic airway inflammation in childhood. A group of children with autoimmune neutropenia were studied and a very low prevalence of asthma was found compared with control children; thus the hypothesis for a pivotal role for neutrophils in asthma development.[58]

PATHOPHYSIOLOGY AND MECHANISMS OF NEUTROPHILIC ASTHMA

There is evidence of innate immune activation in neutrophilic asthma, representing an important mechanism of inflammation. Several key steps in the innate immune activation pathway (Fig. 17.5) are upregulated in

neutrophilic asthma. First, there is increased expression of key innate immune receptors such as TLR2, TLR4, CD14, and surfactant protein A, as well as proinflammatory cytokines IL-8 and IL-1β. Second, high levels of airway endotoxin and colonization with bacteria, particularly *Haemophilus influenzae*, are noted[53] and may represent key stimuli to potentiate innate immune activation in neutrophilic asthma. In addition, airway endotoxin levels in subjects with asthma showed a significant negative correlation with airway obstruction (FEV_1% predicted and FEV_1/FVC) and positively correlated with sputum neutrophils and sputum IL-8 protein levels, indicating a role for endotoxin stimulating a neutrophilic inflammation and worsening airway disease (Fig. 17.5).

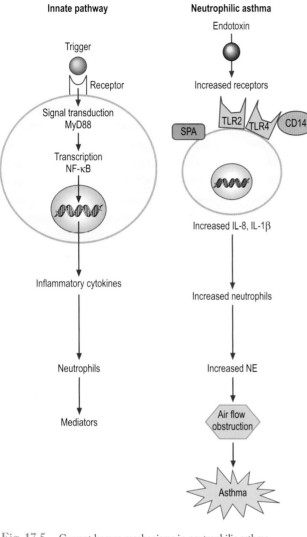

Fig. 17.5. Current known mechanisms in neutrophilic asthma.

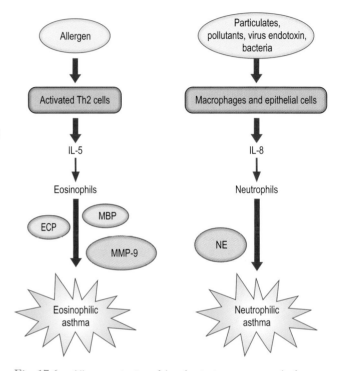

Fig. 17.6. Allergen activation of the adaptive immune system leads to the accumulation of eosinophils and eosinophilic asthma while non-allergic triggers can stimulate an innate immune response leading to the accumulation of neutrophils and neutrophilic asthma. (Reproduced from Simpson JL, Scott RJ, Boyle MJ, et al. Differential proteolytic enzyme activity in eosinophilic and neutrophilic asthma. Am J Resp Crit Care 2005; 172:559–565,[59] with permission.)

Proteolytic enzymes show specific changes in neutrophilic asthma. Levels of active NE are highest in neutrophilic asthma and more than 40% of subjects have evidence of elastase activity compared with just 5% of those with eosinophilic asthma; no activity has been found in paucigranulocytic asthma.[59] The primary inhibitor of NE, α1AT, is increased in the airways of those with neutrophilic asthma compared with healthy controls and the other asthma subtypes and appears insufficient to control NE.

Total MMP-9 levels (active and/or pro-MMP-9) in induced sputum are elevated in neutrophilic asthma and correlate significantly with neutrophilia.[19,59] However, active MMP-9 levels are low in neutrophilic asthma, representing only 0.4% of total MMP-9, whereas, in eosinophilic asthma there are higher levels of active MMP-9. The primary inhibitor of MMP-9, TIMP-1 is increased in the airways in neutrophilic asthma compared to other asthma subtypes. Thus, although there is increased MMP-9 release in neutrophilic asthma, it is inhibited by complexing with TIMP-1 (Fig. 17.6).

Persistent neutrophilic bronchitis in asthma (neutrophilic asthma) may represent a chronic condition that is driven by distinct immune and inflammatory mechanisms involving innate immune dysfunction. Generally, on exposure to pathogens, the respiratory epithelium controls microbial invasion by innate defenses including mucociliary clearance. In some situations, a controlled inflammatory response may be required, which involves movement of leukocytes into the bronchial lumen. If this response is insufficient to eliminate the invading pathogen, the resulting inflammation may become chronic and damage host tissue (see Box 17.1).

Neutrophils accumulate in the airway lumen in response to epithelial release of IL-8. Neutrophil proteinases, including NE, damage airway cilia and reduce ciliary beat frequency. In addition to host proteinases, bacterial toxins and proteinases are released from invading pathogens including *Pseudomonas aeruginosa* and *Haemophilus influenzae*. These toxins can inhibit ciliary beat frequency and disrupt the respiratory epithelium.[60] In asthma, airway epithelium is abnormal, with structural damage that may reduce or impair epithelial defense responses and interfere with an effective response to microbial exposure.

Asthma, which is complicated by allergic bronchopulmonary aspergillosis (ABPA), is associated with increased neutrophils and neutrophil activation in the airways. This occurs together with eosinophil influx, leading to a mixed granulocytic response. The neutrophil influx into the airways of patients with ABPA is associated with IL-8 gene expression and results in protease release (MMP-9) and airflow obstruction (FEV_1).[61]

BOX 17.1 NEUTROPHILIC BRONCHITIS IN ASTHMA

>> Persistent
- Neutrophilic asthma
- Allergic bronchopulmonary aspergillosis
- Smoking

>> Transient
- Viral exacerbations
- Bacterial bronchitis
- Pollutants
- Occupational settings

BOX 17.2 TRIGGERS OF NEUTROPHILIC ASTHMA

>> Endotoxin
>> Particulate matter
>> Respiratory viruses
>> Smoking

TRIGGERS OF NEUTROPHILIC ASTHMA

There are several triggers that induce neutrophilic inflammation in the airways, including endotoxin, particulate air pollution, and respiratory viruses (Box 17.2).

Endotoxin (or LPS) is a component of household dusts and grain dusts and has been implicated in occupational respiratory disease. Endotoxins are found in the outer membrane of Gram-negative bacteria and consist of a hydrophilic polysaccharide region and a hydrophobic lipid region (lipid A). Inflammatory responses to LPS require accessory proteins, which include LPS binding protein (LBP) and CD14. LBP binds to the lipid A region of LPS to form a complex which is then recognized by CD14 and subsequently TLR4, and results in signal transduction and cellular activation. Exposure to LPS can cause fever, coughing, dyspnea, and a reduced FEV_1. In response to an LPS exposure, mediators are released from macrophages, including TNF-α, IL-6, IL-1, IL-8, reactive oxygen species, and platelet activating factor. In addition, the neutrophil response to endotoxin is associated with increased phagocytosis and release of chemokines such as IL-8. T-lymphocytes also proliferate and secrete Th1 cytokines. These mediators stimulate host cells to initiate an acute phase response and remove the invading bacteria.[62] In very high concentrations endotoxin is lethal, resulting in septic shock;[62] however, only small quantities are required to stimulate an immune response.

Inhalation of particulate matter from air pollution can cause exacerbations of asthma in both adults and children. Inhalation of larger size particles ($PM_{2.5-10}$) can cause airway inflammation. This particulate matter contains both bacteria and fungi in addition to their degradation products such as LPS. It is believed that it is the bacterial component of pollutants that cause the inflammatory response. Cytokine production in response to exposure to bacteria found in particulate matter was inhibited by blocking CD14, an essential protein required for responses

to LPS. In addition, both TLR2 and TLR4 were activated in response to exposure to particulate matter that was contaminated by bacteria.[63]

Respiratory viruses are an important trigger of asthma exacerbations. The viruses have been implicated in these asthma exacerbations, including influenza, RSV, and rhinovirus. In children, exacerbations are caused by viruses in 85% of cases, with the most common viruses isolated being rhinovirus and RSV.[64] RSV is an important respiratory tract infection in infants, accounting for more than 70% of all cases of infantile bronchiolitis and may be linked to the development of asthma.[65] The rate of viral identification is higher in asthmatic compared to non-asthmatic children,[66] suggesting either a greater susceptibility of children with asthma to viral infection or greater viral load.

In addition to their links with asthma exacerbations and development of asthma, many respiratory viruses stimulate immune and inflammatory responses via the innate immune pathway to provide a mechanistic link between the trigger (virus), inflammation, and resulting asthma. RSV proteins can stimulate an innate immune response through TLR4 and CD14, leading to an increased production of the proinflammatory cytokine, IL-6.[67] When TLR4-deficient mice are exposed to RSV, there is a decreased infiltration of CD14 positive cells and both a reduced infiltration into the BAL and cytotoxicity of natural killer cells. In addition, there were lower BAL IL-12 levels in TLR-4-deficient mice compared with wild-type animals. Combined with an impairment of the innate immune response, this can also result in a delayed clearance of RSV from the airways.[68] SP-A deficient mice also have an impaired clearance of RSV infection and, in addition, have increased BAL neutrophils, and proinflammatory cytokines TNF-α, IL-6, and IL-8 in BAL compared with wild mice. These findings suggest that a deficient innate immune response may contribute to a heightened granulocytic infiltration and airway inflammation. Antiviral responses to influenza virus utilize TLR7[69] and may involve CD14 and TLR2 or TLR4.[70] Human rhinovirus induce epithelial cell production of beta defensins-2, an innate antimicrobial peptide.[71]

NEUTROPHILS AND AHR

Airways hyperresponsiveness (AHR) is considered a hallmark feature of asthma. Neutrophils and their products can induce AHR in a number of animal and human studies. Inhalation of a variety of triggers, ozone,[72] infection,[73] endotoxin,[74] smoking,[75] and dust,[76] are associated with neutrophil accumulation and AHR. These triggers have also been implicated in the activation of the innate airway immune response (Fig. 17.3). The role of neutrophils in the induction of AHR is further strengthened by several studies showing neutrophil depletion reducing the resulting hyperresponsiveness or normal responsiveness.[72,77] Cytokines involved in neutrophil accumulation such as LTB_4, IL-17, and IL-8 have also been associated with AHR.[78]

NEUTROPHILS AND AIRWAY REMODELING

Remodeling is a normal process of wound repair but can also result in permanent airway changes that result in fixed airflow obstruction. Airway remodeling can include alterations in the basement membrane, interstitial matrix, and angiogenesis.[79]

Fibrogenic growth factors such as transforming growth factor are increased in asthma, especially severe asthma, and are associated with the thickness of the basement membrane.[43] Neutrophils express TGF-β, and neutrophils isolated from patients with asthma release more TGF-β than control neutrophils.[80] Increased TGF-β release and expression may lead to activation of fibroblasts and alterations in extracellular matrix turnover, leading to airway remodeling.

Angiogenesis refers to the growth of new blood vessels, which is an important process in remodeling in the airways. Vascular endothelial growth factor (VEGF) can regulate vascular permeability. VEGF is increased in the airways of patients with stable asthma[81] and also with an acute asthma exacerbation.[82] In asthma, there is a positive association between the number of cells staining positive for VEGF and both the number of vessels and the thickness of the basement membrane.[83] Neutrophils are an important source of angiogenic factors and release VEGF upon stimulation with bacterial products; the released VEGF can then activate endothelial cells to induce angiogenesis.[84] The potent neutrophil chemoattractant IL-8 is another multifunctional cytokine involved in both inflammation and angiogenesis.

Airway neutrophils have been associated with fixed airflow obstruction in a number of studies.[51,85] In addition, products of neutrophil activation have also been associated with airflow obstruction. As outlined in the previous section, airway proteases by themselves can restructure the airways.

NEUTROPHILS AND CORTICOSTEROIDS

The response to corticosteroids in asthma is variable. Recent investigations into the non-eosinophilic forms of asthma clearly show that the best responses to corticosteroids are largely limited to patients with an eosinophilic bronchitis.[54,86] In fact, a recent study found that baseline FEV_1 and sputum eosinophils significantly correlated with changes in FEV_1 after corticosteroid treatment. Only in those patients with sputum eosinophilia were significant improvements experienced with treatment.[87]

The importance of recognizing the heterogeneity of airway inflammation in asthma was highlighted in a recent randomized controlled trial of asthma management conducted by Green and co-workers. She and her co-workers demonstrated that asthma management based upon reducing sputum eosinophils was superior to traditional guideline-based management.[50] There was a subgroup of subjects who maintained normal sputum eosinophil levels throughout the 12-month study. Of these subjects, those who were randomized to sputum-based management had their inhaled dose of corticosteroids reduced by approximately 960 μg daily. In subjects randomized to guideline-based management, the daily dose of inhaled corticosteroid treatment was increased by around 460 μg daily. This suggests that the recognition of non-eosinophilic asthma by sputum cell counts can assist in preventing overtreatment of asthma.

Neutrophils also influence the effectiveness of ICS. Neutrophil numbers have been shown to predict the ICS's ability to reduce allergen-induced eosinophilic inflammation,[88] suggesting that in those with asthma and a neutrophilic bronchitis, corticosteroid therapy will be less effective for the treatment of allergen-induced eosinophilia. It is also possible that corticosteroid treatment may enhance neutrophilic inflammation through delaying neutrophil apoptosis.[89]

NEUTROPHILS AND SMOKING

More than one-third of asthmatic patients actively smoke and more have a past history of smoking. Active smoking in asthma results in an increase in symptoms, decreasing lung function,[90] and an impaired response to both inhaled[91] and oral[92] corticosteroids. While the mechanisms of these effects remain unclear, they appear closely linked with the neutrophilic airway inflammation induced by cigarette smoking. Smokers with asthma have increased neutrophils and IL-8 in their airways compared to non-smoking controls. The airway neutrophilia and IL-8 are inversely associated with FEV_1 values, highlighting the relationship of neutrophils with airflow obstruction.[93] When smoking stops, there is an improvement in FEV_1 and less neutrophilia within 6 weeks,[94] suggesting that alterations in airway obstruction can be reversed by improving neutrophilia.

OPTIONS FOR THERAPY IN NEUTROPHILIC ASTHMA

Macrolide antibiotics have been widely used in the treatment of infection, and are particularly effective in the eradication of Gram-positive bacteria as well as intracellular pathogens such as *Chlamydia pneumoniae*. In addition, these antibiotics are also capable of inducing a therapeutic antiinflammatory effect independently of their antimicrobial activity. The mechanisms behind this antiinflammatory action are still unclear but are likely to be associated with an ability of macrolides to accumulate in host cells such as macrophages and neutrophils (Fig. 17.7). In low doses, macrolide antibiotics are reported be effective in patients with chronic neutrophilic diseases such as diffuse panbronchiolitis[95] and sinusitis[96] and leading to a significant reduction in neutrophil counts and IL-8 concentrations.[96] In both cystic fibrosis and bronchiectasis, lung function values improve with macrolides; in asthma, airway hyperresponsiveness may improve with macrolide therapy.[97,98] The role of macrolide antibiotics in

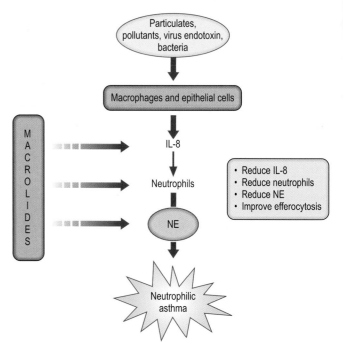

Fig. 17.7. Potential mechanism for the action of macrolide antibiotic therapy in the reduction of neutrophilic airway inflammation.

BOX 17.3 OPTIONS FOR THERAPY IN NEUTROPHILIC ASTHMA

1. Reduce inhaled corticosteroid therapy
2. Bacterial eradication
3. Macrolide antibiotics
4. Anti-interleukin-8 antibodies
5. Anti α_1-antitrypsin antibodies
6. PPAR agonists

the treatment of non-eosinophilic, and specifically neutrophilic asthma, requires further investigation but may be a practical way to reduce airway inflammation in these subjects.

Several other treatment strategies have emerged and could be applied to subjects with neutrophilic asthma. In COPD, improvements in dyspnea followed treatment with a human monoclonal IL-8 antibody. Anti-IL-8 treatment was safe over a 3-month period and provided a potentially useful insight into the possible applications of such treatments in other airway diseases where IL-8 is implicated.[99] Similarly, a purified α1AT treatment (prolastin) reduces endotoxin-induced cytokine release from neutrophils and monocytes in vitro and also reduced nasal IL-8 release following LPS challenge.[100] Finally, the role of peroxisome proliferator-activated receptor (PPAR) agonists in the inhibition of LPS-induced airway neutrophilia in mice provides valuable in vitro evidence suggesting further investigation in the role of these agonists in human disease is required.[101] Therapeutic options for neutrophilic asthma are summarized in Box 17.3.

■ CONCLUSION ■

It is clear that neutrophils are an important part of innate immune defense against infections; however, uncontrolled or inappropriate neutrophil responses contribute extensively to the pathogenesis of a number of inflammatory lung diseases including neutrophilic asthma. Neutrophils are a source of both preformed and newly synthesized inflammatory mediators, and are recruited to the lungs after exposure to respiratory triggers such as viruses, endotoxin, particulate air pollution, and cigarette smoke. Current asthma treatments, in particular corticosteroids, are not effective at treating neutrophilic inflammation in asthma and potentially promote this type of inflammation through delaying neutrophil apoptosis. A better understanding of the mechanisms modulating the recruitment and activation of neutrophils in neutrophilic asthma will impact on future therapeutic strategies, which may include macrolide antibiotics.

References

Neutrophil migration

1. Bainton DF, Ullyot JL, Farquhar MG. The development of neutrophilic polymorphonuclear leukocytes in human bone marrow. J Exp Med 1971; 134:907–934.
2. Bjerregaard MD, Jurlander J, Kausen P, et al. The in vivo profile of transcription factors during neutrophil differentiation in human bone marrow. Blood 2003; 101:4322–4332.
3. van Eeden SF, Kitagawa Y, Klut ME, et al. Polymorphonuclear leukocytes released from the bone marrow preferentially sequester in lung microvessels. Microcirculation 1997; 4:369.
4. Terashima T, Wiggs B, English D, et al. The effect of cigarette smoking on the bone marrow. Am J Respir Crit Care Med 1997; 155:1021–1026.
5. Terashima T, English D, Hogg JC, et al. Release of polymorphonuclear leukocytes from the bone marrow by interleukin-8. Am Soc Hematol 1998; 92:1062–1069.
6. Doerschuk CM. Leukocyte trafficking in alveoli and airway passages. Resp Res 2000; 1: 136–140.
7. Gebb SA, Graham JA, Hanger CC, et al. Sites of leukocyte sequestration in the pulmonary microcirculation. J Appl Physiol 1995; 79:493–497.
8. Issekutz AC, Rowter D, Springer TA. Role for ICAM-1 and ICAM-2 and alternate CD11/CD18 ligands in neutrophil transendothelial migration. J Leukoc Biol 1999; 65:117–126.
9. Harris ES, McIntyre TM, Prescott SM, et al. The leukocyte integrins. J Biol Chem 2000; 275:23409–23412.
10. Mackarel AJ, Plant BJ, Fitzgerald MX, et al. Cystic fibrosis sputum stimulates CD18-independent neutrophil migration across endothelial cells. Exp Lung Res 2005; 31:377–390.
11. Ebnet K, Suzuki A, Ohno S, et al. Junctional adhesion molecules (JAMs): more molecules with dual functions. J Cell Sci 2004; 117:19–29.
12. Liu Y, Merlin D, Burst SL, et al. The role of CD47 in neutrophil transmigration. Increased rate of migration correlates with increased cell surface expression of CD47. J Biol Chem 2001; 276:40156–40166.
13. Richman-Einstat JB, Jorens PG, Hebert CA, et al. Interleukin-8: an important chemoattractant in sputum of patients with chronic inflammatory airway diseases. Am J Physiol 1993; 264:L413–L418.
14. Wenzel SE. The role of leukotrienes in asthma. Prostaglandins Leukot Essent Fatty Acids 2003; 69:145–155.
15. Hayashi F, Means TK, Luster AD. Toll-like receptors stimulate human neutrophil function. Blood 2003; 102:2660–2669.
16. Sabroe I, Jones EC, Whyte MK, et al. Regulation of human neutrophil chemokine receptor expression and function by activating Toll-like receptors 2 and 4. Immunology 2005; 115:90–98.
17. Power CP, Wang JH, Manning B, et al. Bacterial lipoprotein delays apoptosis in human neutrophils through inhibition of caspase-3 activity: regulatory roles for CD14 and TLR2. J Immunol 2004; 173:5229–5237.

Mediators released by activated neutrophils

18. Vignola AM, Bonanno A, Mirabella A, et al. Increased levels of elastase and α1-antitrypsin in sputum of asthmatic patients. Am J Respir Crit Care Med 1998; 157:505–511.
19. Vignola AM, Bonanno A, Profita M, et al. Effect of age and asthma duration upon elastase and α1-antitrypsin levels in adult asthmatics. Eur Resp J 2003; 22:795–801.
20. Walsh DE, Greene CM, Carroll TP, et al. Interleukin-8 up-regulation by neutrophil elastase is mediated my My88/IRAK/TRAF-6 in human bronchial epithelium. J Biol Chem 2001; 276:35494–35499.
21. Devaney JM, Greene CM, Taggart CC, et al. Neutrophil elastase up-regulates interleukin-8 via toll-like receptor 4. FEBS Lett 2003; 544:129–132.
22. Greene CM, McElvaney NG, O'Neill SJ, et al. Secretory leucoprotease inhibitor impairs toll-like receptor 2- and 4-mediated responses in monocytic cells. Infect Immun 2004; 72:3684–3687.
23. Dahlen B, Shute J, Howarth P. Immunohistochemical localisation of the matrix metalloproteinases MMP-3 and MMP-9 within the airways in asthma. Thorax 1999; 54: 590–596.
24. Siwik DA, Pagano PJ, Colucci WS. Oxidative stress regulates collagen synthesis and matrix metalloproteinase activity in cardiac fibroblasts. Am J Physiol Cell Physiol 2001; 280: c53–c60.
25. Tschesche H, Zolzer V, Triebel S, et al. The human neutrophil lipocalin supports the allosteric activation of matrix metalloproteinases. Eur J Biochem 2001; 268:1918–1928.
26. Mattos W, Lim S, Russell R, et al. Matrix metalloproteinase-9 expression in asthma: effect of asthma severity, allergen challenge, and inhaled corticosteroids. Chest 2002; 122:1543–1552.
27. Cundall M, Sun Y, Miranda C, et al. Neutrophil-derived matrix metalloproteinase-9 is increased in severe asthma and poorly inhibited by glucocorticoids. J Allergy Clin Immunol 2003; 112:1064–1071.
28. Liu Z, Zhou X, Shapiro SD, et al. The serpin alpha 1-proteinase inhibitor is a critical substrate for gelatinase B/MMP-9 in vivo. Cell 2000; 102:647–655.
29. Segal AW. How neutrophils kill microbes. Ann Rev Immunol 2005; 23:197–223.
30. Reeves EP, Lu H, Jacobs HL, et al. Killing activity of neutrophils is mediated through activation of proteases by K⁺ flux. Nature 2002; 416:291–297.
31. Scheel-Toellner D, Wang K, Assi LK. Clustering of death receptors in lipid rafts initiates neutrophil spontaneous apoptosis. Biochem Soc Trans 2004; 32:679–681.
32. Lehrer RI. Defensins: antimicrobial and cytotoxic peptides of mammalian cells. Annu Rev Immunol 1993; 11:105–128.

Neutrophil clearance and death

33. Savill JS, Wyllie AH, Henson JE, et al. Macrophage phagocytosis of aging neutrophils in inflammation. Programmed cell death in the neutrophil leads to its recognition by macrophages. J Clin Invest 1989; 83:865–875.
34. Savill J, Fadok V. Corpse clearance defines the meaning of cell death. Nature 2000; 407:784–788.
35. Cox G. Glucocorticoid treatment inhibits apoptosis in human neutrophils. J Immunol 1995; 154:4719–4725.
36. Scheel-Toellner D, Wang KQ, Webb PR, et al. Early events in spontaneous neutrophil apoptosis. Biochem Soc 2004; 32:461–464.
37. Cassatella MA. The production of cytokines by polymorphonuclear neutrophils. Immunol Today 1995; 16:21–26.

Neutrophils in asthma

38. Van Den Steen PE, Proost P, Wuyts A, et al. Neutrophil gelatinase B potentiates interleukin-8 tenfold by aminoterminal processing, whereas it degrades CTAP-III, PF-4, and GRO-α and leaves RANTES and MCP-2 intact. Blood 2000; 96:2673–2681.

39. Ordonez CL, Shaughnessy TE, Matthay MA, et al. Increased neutrophil numbers and IL-8 levels in airway secretions in acute severe asthma. Am J Respir Crit Care Med 2000; 161:1185–1190.

40. Lamblin C, Gosset P, Tillie-Lebond I, et al. Bronchial neutrophilia in patients with noninfectious status asthmaticus. Am J Respir Crit Care Med 1998; 157:394–402.

41. Chilmonczyk BA, Salmun LM, Megathlin KN, et al. Association between exposure to environmental tobacco smoke and exacerbations of asthma in children. New Engl J Med 1993; 328:1665–1669.

42. Wenzel SE, Szefler SJ, Leung DY, et al. Bronchoscopic evaluation of severe asthma. Persistent inflammation associated with high dose glucocorticoids. Am J Resp Crit Care Med 1997; 156:737–743.

43. Wenzel SE, Schwartz LB, Largmack EL, et al. Evidence that severe asthma can be divided pathologically into two inflammatory subtypes with distinct physiologic and clinical characteristics. Am J Respir Crit Care Med 1999; 160:1001–1008.

44. Jatakanon A, Lalloo UG, Lim S, et al. Increased neutrophils and cytokines, TNF-α and IL-8, in induced sputum of non-asthmatic patients with chronic dry cough. Thorax 1999; 54:234–237.

45. Wark PA, Johnston SL, Moric I, et al. Neutrophil degranulation and cell lysis is associated with clinical severity in virus-induced asthma. Eur Resp J 2002; 19:68–75.

46. Norzila MZ, Fakes K, Henry RL, et al. Interleukin-8 and neutrophil recruitment accompanies induced sputum eosinophil activation in children with acute asthma. Am J Respir Crit Care Med 2000; 161:769–774.

47. Teran LM, Johnston SL, Schroeder JM, et al. Role of nasal interleukin-8 in neutrophil recruitment and activation in children with virus induced asthma. Am J Respir Crit Care Med 1997; 155:1362–1366.

48. Yoshihara S, Yamada Y, Abe T, et al. Association of epithelial damage and signs of neutrophil mobilization in the airways during acute exacerbations of pediatric asthma. Clin Exp Allergy 2006; 144:212–216.

49. Grissell TV, Powell H, Shafren DR, et al. Interleukin-10 gene expression in acute virus-induced asthma. Am J Respir Crit Care Med 2005; 172:433–439.

50. Green RH, Brightling CE, McKenna S, et al. Asthma exacerbations and sputum eosinophil counts: a randomised controlled trial. Lancet 2002; 30:1715–1721.

51. Baines KJ, Simpson JL, Scott RJ, et al. Enhanced IL-8 release from neutrophils in non-eosinophilic asthma. Respirology 2006; 11:A29.

52. Lex C, Payne DN, Zacharasiewicz A, et al. Sputum induction in children with difficult asthma: safety, feasibility, and inflammatory cell pattern. Pediatr Pulmonol 2005; 39:318–324.

53. Simpson JL, Grissell TV, Douwes J, et al. Innate immune activation in neutrophilic asthma and bronchiectasis. Thorax 2007; 62:211–218.

54. Simpson JL, Scott R, Boyle M, et al. Inflammatory subtypes in asthma: assessment and identification using induced sputum. Respirology 2006; 11:54–61.

55. Green RH, Brightling CE, Woltmann G, et al. Analysis of induced sputum in adults with asthma: identification of subgroup with isolated sputum neutrophilia and poor response to inhaled corticosteroids. Thorax 2002; 57:875–879.

56. de Blic J, Tillie-Leblond I, Tonnel AB, et al. Difficult asthma in children: an analysis of airway inflammation. J Allergy Clin Immunol 2004; 113:94–100.

57. Barbato A, Panizzolo C, Gheno M, et al. Bronchoalveolar lavage in asthmatic children: evidence of neutrophil activation in mild to moderate persistent asthma. Pediatr Allergy Immunol 2001; 12:73–77.

58. Yasui K, Kobayashi N, Tamazaki T, et al. Neutrophilic inflammation in childhood asthma. Thorax 2005; 60:704–705.

59. Simpson JL, Scott RJ, Boyle MJ, et al. Differential proteolytic enzyme activity in eosinophilic and neutrophilic asthma. Am J Resp Crit Care Med 2005; 172:559–565.

60. Cole JP. Inflammation: a two-edged sword – the model of bronchiectasis. Eur J Respir Dis Suppl 1986; 147:6–15.

61. Gibson PG, Wark PAB, Simpson JL, et al. Induced Sputum IL-8 gene expression, neutrophil influx and MMP-9 in allergic bronchopulmonary aspergillosis. Eur Resp J 2003; 21:582–588.

62. Heine H, Rietschel ET, Ulmer AJ. The biology of endotoxin. Mol Biotech 2001; 19:279–296.

63. Becker S, Fenton MJ, Soukup JM. Involvement of microbial components and toll-like receptors 2 and 4 in cytokine response to air pollution particles. Am J Respir Cell Mol Biol 2002; 27:611–618.

64. Message SD, Johnston SL. Viruses in asthma. Br Med Bull 2002; 61:29–43.

65. Openshaw PJ, Dean GS, Culley FJ. Links between respiratory syncytial virus bronchiolitis and childhood asthma: clinical and research approaches. Pediatr Infect Dis 2003; 22:S58–S64.

66. Azevedo AM, Durigon EL, Okasima V, et al. Detection of influenza, parainfluenza, adenovirus and respiratory syncytial virus during asthma attacks in children older than 2 years old. Allergol Immunopathol 2003; 31:311–317.

67. Kurt-Jones EA, Popova L, Kwinn L, et al. Pattern recognition receptors TLR4 and CD14 mediate response to respiratory syncytial virus. Nat Immunol 2000; 1:398–401.

68. Haynes LM, Moore DD, Kurt-Jones EA, et al. Involvement of Toll-like receptor 4 in innate immunity to respiratory syncytial virus. J Virol 2001; 75:10730–10737.

69. Diebold SS, Kaisho T, Hemmi H, et al. Innate antiviral responses by means of TLR7-mediated recognition of single-stranded RNA. Science 2004; 303:1529–1531.

70. Pauligk C, Nain M, Reiling N, et al. CD14 is required for influenza A virus-induced cytokine and chemokine production. Immunobiology 2004; 209:3–10.

71. Proud D, Sanders SP, Wiehler S. Human rhinovirus infection induces epithelial cell production of human β-defensin 2 both in vitro and in vivo. J Immunol 2004; 172:4637–4645.

72. DeLorme MP, Yang H, Elbon-Copp C, et al. Hyperresponsive airways correlate with lung tissue inflammatory cell changes in ozone-exposed rats. J Toxicol Environ Health A 2002; 65:1453–1470.

73. Makela MJ, Tripp R, Dakhama A, et al. Prior airway exposure to allergen increases virus-induced airway hyperresponsiveness. J Allergy Clin Immunol 2003; 112:861–869.

74. Brass DM, Savov JD, Whitehead GS, et al. LPS binding protein is important in the airway response to inhaled endotoxin. J Allergy Clin Immunol 2004; 114:586–592.

75. Nishikawa M, Ikeda H, Fukuda T, et al. Acute exposure to cigarette smoke induces airway hyperresponsiveness without airway inflammation in guinea pigs. Dose-response characteristics. Am Rev Resp Dis 1990; 142:177–183.

76. Vogelzang PF, van der Gulden JW, Folgering H, et al. Longitudinal changes in bronchial responsiveness associated with swine confinement dust exposure. Chest 2000; 117:1488–1495.

77. Park SJ, Wiekowski MT, Lira SA, et al. Neutrophils regulate airway responses in a model of fungal allergic disease. J Immunol 2006; 176:2538–2545.

78. Barczyk A, Pierzchala W, Sozanska E. Interleukin-17 in sputum correlates with airway hyperresponsiveness to methacholine. Respir Med 2003; 97:726–733.

79. Vignola AM, Bonanno A, Profita M, et al. Effect of age and asthma duration upon elastase and α1-antitrypsin levels in adult asthmatics. Eur Resp J 2003; 22:795–801.

80. Chu HW, Trudeau JB, Balzar S, et al. Peripheral blood and airway tissue expression of transforming growth factor beta by neutrophils in asthmatic subjects and normal control subjects. J Allergy Clin Immunol 2000; 106:1115–1123.

81. Feltis BN, Wignarajah D, Zheng L, et al. Increased vascular endothelial growth factor and receptors: relationship to angiogenesis in asthma. Am J Resp Crit Care Med 2006; 173:1201–1207.

82. Abdel-Rahman AM, el-Sahrigy SA, Bakr SI. A comparative study of two angiogenic factors: vascular endothelial growth factor and angiogenin in induced sputum from asthmatic children in acute attack. Chest 2006; 129:266–271.

83. Chetta A, Zanini A, Foresi A, et al. Vascular endothelial growth factor up-regulation and bronchial wall remodelling in asthma. Clin Exp Allergy 2005; 35:1437–1442.

84. van Der Flier M, Coenjaerts F, Kimpen JL, et al. Streptococcus pneumoniae induces secretion of vascular endothelial growth factor by human neutrophils. Infect Immun 2000; 68:4792–4794.

85. Woodruff PG, Khashayar R, Lazarus SC, et al. Relationship between airway inflammation, hyperresponsiveness, and obstruction in asthma. J Allergy Clin Immunol 2001; 108:753–758.

86. Meijer RJ, Postma DS, Kauffman HF, et al. Accuracy of eosinophils and eosinophilic cationic protein to predict steroid improvement in asthma. Clin Exp Allergy 2002; 32:1096–1103.

87. Bacci E, Cianchetti S, Bartoli M, et al. Low sputum eosinophils predict the lack of response to beclomethasone in symptomatic asthmatic patients. Chest 2006; 129:503–504.

88. Gauvreau GM, Inman MD, Kelly M, et al. Increased levels of airway neutrophils reduce the inhibitory effects of inhaled glucocorticoids on allergen-induced airway eosinophils. Can Resp J 2002; 9:26–32.

89. Meagher LC, Cousin JM, Seckl JR, et al. Opposing effects of glucocorticoids on the rate of apoptosis in neutrophilic and eosinophilic granules. J Immunol 1996; 156:4422–4428.

90. Boulet LP, Lemiere C, Archambault F, et al. Smoking and asthma: clinical and radiologic features, lung function, and airway inflammation. Chest 2006; 129:661–668.

91. Chalmers GW, Macleod KJ, Little SA, et al. Influence of cigarette smoking on inhaled corticosteroid treatment in mild asthma. Thorax 2002; 57:226–230.

92. Chaudhuri R, Livingston E, McMahon AD, et al. Cigarette smoking impairs the therapeutic response to oral corticosteroids in chronic asthma. Am J Respir Crit Care Med 2003; 168:1308–1311.

93. Chalmers GW, MacLeod KJ, Thomson L, et al. Smoking and airway inflammation in patients with mild asthma. Chest 2001; 120:1917–1922.

94. Chaudhuri R, Livingston E, McMahon AD, et al. Effects of smoking cessation on lung function and airway inflammation in smokers with asthma. Am J Resp Crit Care Med 2006; 174:127–133.

95. Kadota J, Mukae H, Ishii H, et al. Long-term efficacy and safety of clarithromycin treatment in patients with diffuse panbronchiolitis. Respir Med 2003; 97:844–850.

96. Yamada T, Fujieda S, Mori S, et al. Macrolide treatment decreased the size of nasal polyps and IL-8 levels in nasal lavage. Am J Rhinol 2000; 14:143–148.

97. Equi A, Balfour-Lynn IM, Bush A, et al. Long term azithromycin in children with cystic fibrosis: a randomised, placebo-controlled crossover trial. Lancet 2002; 360:978–984.

98. Kostadima E, Tsiodras S, Alexopoulos EI, et al. Clarithromycin reduces the severity of bronchial hyperresponsiveness in patients with asthma. Eur Resp J 2004; 23:714–717.

99. Mahler D, Huang S, Tabrizi M, et al. Efficacy and safety of a monoclonal antibody recognizing interleukin-8 in COPD. Chest 2004; 126:926–934.

100. Nita I, Hollander C, Westin U, et al. Prolastin, a pharmaceutical preparation of purified human alpha-1 antitrypsin, blocks endotoxin-mediated cytokine release. Respir Med 2005; 6:12.

101. Birrell BA, Patel HJ, McCluskie K, et al. PPAR-gamma agonists as therapy for diseases involving airway neutrophilia. Eur Resp J 2004; 24:18–23.

Biology of Eosinophils

18

Redwan Moqbel, Paige Lacy, Darryl J Adamko, and Solomon O Odemuyiwa

CONTENTS

- Introduction 295
- Eosinophil differentiation and tissue recruitment 295
- Surface markers in eosinophils 298
- Eosinophil-derived mediators 299
- Eosinophil as effector cells in worm infections 307
- Conclusions 308

SUMMARY OF IMPORTANT CONCEPTS

>> Eosinophils are important inflammatory leukocytes in asthma and related allergic diseases, eosinophilic esophagitis, hypereosinophilic syndromes, and parasitic helminth infections

>> The blood and bone marrow eosinophil counts are low in normal healthy individuals, but are significantly elevated in disease

>> Maturation of eosinophils in the bone marrow is dependent on the eosinophil-specific cytokine, interleukin-5, while egression from the bone marrow requires eotaxin

>> Eosinophils are morphologically characterized by an abundance of unique crystalloid granules in the cytoplasm, which are highly enriched in major basic protein and other cationic molecules

>> Activated eosinophils generate a plethora of mediators, including lipid messengers, reactive oxygen species, granule-derived enzymes and proteins, and a wide range of immunomodulatory cytokines and chemokines

>> Eosinophils have a range of roles in immune and inflammatory responses associated with their tissue presence ranging from effector to immune regulator

■ INTRODUCTION ■

The eosinophil is a bone-marrow-derived, peripheral blood and tissue granulocyte prominent in allergic,[1–3] and inflammatory responses against metazoan helminthic parasites but rare in otherwise healthy individuals.[4,5] It is strongly associated with disorders of the respiratory tract, particularly allergic asthma and rhinitis that exhibit a significant correlation with the number as well as activation status of infiltrating tissue eosinophils. As well, many disorders of the gastrointestinal system exhibit prominent eosinophilic inflammation in the mucosa. The presence of eosinophils in the airway and gut mucosa has been associated with both IgE-dependent (allergic) and IgE-independent (non-allergic) manifestations of disease. Although clinically these conditions have been characterized as either allergic or non-allergic, it appears that the mechanisms underlying recruitment and activation of eosinophils in both types of disease are similar. This chapter will concentrate mainly on aspects of the biology and function of the human eosinophil.

■ EOSINOPHIL DIFFERENTIATION AND TISSUE RECRUITMENT ■

Eosinophils are terminally differentiated granulocytes that arise principally from the bone marrow.[6] Morphologically, they are approximately 8 μm in diameter with usually bilobed nuclei, although three or more lobes are also observed (Fig. 18.1). The eosinophil is characterized by five different types of secretory granules and vesicles, the most prominent being the unique crystalloid granule which is the site of storage of the highly cationic major basic protein (MBP; Fig. 18.2).

Allergen and parasite-induced eosinophilia have been shown to be T cell-dependent, and are mediated by soluble factors (cytokines) released from sensitized lymphocytes.[7] Thus, eosinophil infiltration into the tissue is regulated by biological events which include a complex interplay between immunological and inflammatory mechanisms including cytokines and chemokines that may also be derived from eosinophils themselves (see below).[8,9]

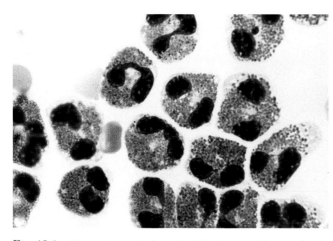

Fig. 18.1. Photomicrograph of peripheral blood eosinophils stained with Romanowski stain (Diff-Quick).

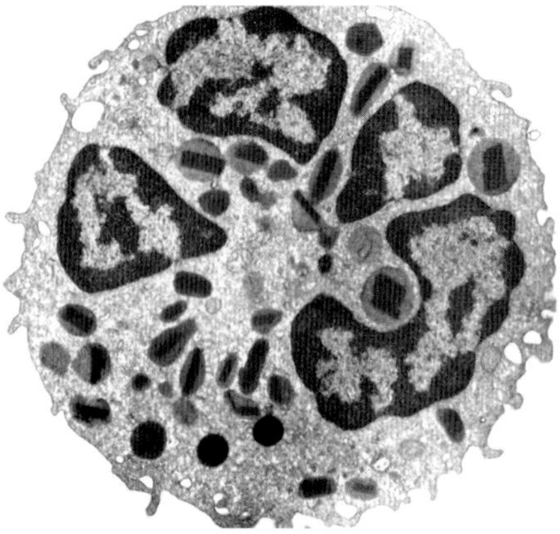

Fig. 18.2. Electron photomicrograph of a peripheral blood eosinophil (×7000). MBP is evident in the electron-dense crystalline cores of the secretory granules.

Peripheral blood and tissue eosinophils are derived by hematopoiesis from $CD34^+$ myelocytic progenitors found in the bone marrow and in inflamed tissues. Eosinophils make up approximately 3% of the bone marrow from healthy individuals. About 37% of these bone marrow eosinophils are fully differentiated while the remainder are promyelocytes/myelocytes and metamyelocytes.[6,10] The appearance of newly matured cells in the blood occurs approximately 2.5 days from the time of the last mitotic division.[6] The turnover of eosinophils is approximately 2.2×10^8 cells/kg per day. The bone marrow possesses the largest end-differentiated eosinophil reservoir in the healthy body ($9–14 \times 10^8$ cells/kg).[11]

The half-life of eosinophils in the circulation is approximately 18 h, with a mean blood transit time of 26 h.[12] This time is extended in eosinophilic conditions, possibly due to the elevation of systemic eosinophil-activating cytokines that promote eosinophil survival. The normal range of blood eosinophils is 0 to $0.5 \times 10^3/mm^3$, with counts ranging 0.015 to $0.65 \times 10^3/mm^3$.[13] Circulating eosinophil counts exhibit diurnal variation in humans; the lowest and highest levels are seen in the morning and evening, respectively. There is often more than 40% variation in counts within a day.[14,15] Mild eosinophilia is generally considered to be $0.5–1.5 \times 10^3/mm^3$, moderate eosinophilia as $1.5–5.0 \times 10^3/mm^3$, and marked eosinophilia $>5.0 \times 10^3/mm^3$. Allergy is commonly associated with eosinophilia in the mild range, whereas parasitic infestation is often characterized by a marked eosinophilia.

Progenitors differentiate upon exposure to a network of cytokines and chemokines to become committed to the eosinophil/basophil (Eo/B) lineage.[16] Eosinophils are more closely related to basophils than neutrophils and monocytes due to lineage differentiation at this stage.[17] In addition, eosinophils retain elements of expression of basophil/mast cell-specific high-affinity Fcε receptor (α subunit),[18] while basophils express small amounts of the eosinophil granule protein MBP.[19] The key cytokines that are critical for stimulation of bone marrow production of eosinophils include interleukin-3 (IL-3), IL-5, and granulocyte/macrophage colony-stimulating factor (GM-CSF).[20,21] These three cytokines are also produced by $CD4^+$ and $CD8^+$ T lymphocytes from peripheral blood as well as inflamed tissues.[22] In bone marrow samples, committed eosinophil precursors can be recognized by their expression of the IL-5 receptor (IL-5R) and the C-C chemokine receptor, CCR3, in addition to CD34.[23]

It is now well recognized that IL-5 is a key cytokine in terminal differentiation of eosinophils,[24] and expression of the IL-5R on the progenitor cell is one of the first signs of commitment to the eosinophil lineage. The expression of IL-5R is almost exclusively limited to eosinophil progenitors and mature peripheral blood eosinophils, with some expression on basophils but not neutrophils or monocytes. This selectivity in receptor distribution indicates that IL-5 acts primarily as an eosinophilopoietic cytokine.

The obligatory role of IL-5 in the differentiation of the eosinophil has been confirmed by numerous studies on transgenic mice in which the expression of the gene for IL-5 caused marked eosinophilia and increased numbers of eosinophil precursors in the bone marrow.[25,26] Interestingly, eosinophil differentiation in this transgenic model appeared to be completely independent of IL-3 and GM-CSF, suggesting that IL-5 alone may be sufficient to generate an eosinophilia from stem cell precursors. However, although IL-5 gene-deficient mice exhibit almost no eosinophils in their blood, a small pool of apparently IL-5-independent eosinophils persist in the mucosal tissues of these animals. Tissue eosinophils appear to sustain their survival through autocrine release of GM-CSF. Additional eosinophilopoietic factors may assist in inducing the differentiation of Eo/B progenitors in the bone marrow, including IL-4, IL-6, IL-11, IL-12, SCF, and others.[27] In addition, C-C chemokines, named for their adjacent cysteine residues in the C-terminus amino acid sequence as distinct from CXC chemokines, including CCL11 (eotaxin) and CCL5 (RANTES), are important in the development of eosinophils.[28] Overall, at the level of the bone marrow, the early development of Eo/B progenitors is driven by IL-3 and GM-CSF, among other factors, while at later stages, IL-5 regulates the terminal differentiation of eosinophils. CCL11 may facilitate the efflux of fully mature eosinophils into the peripheral circulation and, ultimately, inflamed tissue.

Eosinophils are predominantly tissue cells, and their major target organ for homing in the healthy individual is the gastrointestinal tract,[29,30] possibly in response to environmental factors as part of a role in innate defense against parasites. In disease states, eosinophils also home to other tissues including the lungs, the skin, and the brain (e.g., during strokes). Once they enter target tissues, eosinophils do not return to the blood circulation. Eosinophil numbers can remain high in tissues even when peripheral numbers are low, suggesting that their survival is enhanced upon extravasation. Curiously, pathogen-free laboratory animals have no eosinophils in their blood, while tissue eosinophils are difficult to find, suggesting that the appearance of eosinophils may be related to microbial colonization.[10]

EOSINOPHIL PRODUCTION AND SURVIVAL IN PERIPHERAL TISSUE

Eosinophil development and maturation may also occur in situ in peripheral (extramedullary) sites outside of the bone marrow. In this case, Eo/B precursors released into the bloodstream from the bone marrow circulate to sites where they specifically transmigrate in response to locally produced cytokines and chemokines. This may provide an alternative mechanism for the persistence or accumulation of tissue eosinophils. Mature peripheral blood eosinophils are non-dividing end-stage cells, which, in culture, rapidly undergo cell death by either apoptosis or necrosis. However, activated eosinophils synthesize, store, and release a number of cytokines, in vitro. Cytokines, such as IL-3, IL-5, and GM-CSF, as well as interferon-γ (IFN-γ) prolong eosinophil survival in culture for up to 2 weeks.[31-33] This may lead to autocrine prolongation of eosinophil maturation and survival in tissues.[34] Such cytokines enhance receptor expression and cell function including cytotoxicity against metazoan targets. Other tissue cells such as endothelial cells, fibroblasts, and epithelial cells may also contribute to the production of IL-5 and GM-CSF for in situ eosinophil maturation and differentiation. In situ IL-5 and GM-CSF delay eosinophil apoptosis and promote eosinophil priming and activation.[35] In addition, IL-5 production by airway CD4+ T cells may be directly stimulated by eosinophils in a paracrine manner to enhance survival of tissue eosinophils.[36] Eosinophil progenitors in nasal explants from atopic patients survive and develop into fully mature eosinophils ex vivo using similar mechanisms.[37] Allergen challenge of these explants, as well as lung explants of Brown–Norway rats, was shown to evoke a rapid (6 h) accumulation of MBP-positive cells after allergen challenge.[38] This was dependent on IL-5 production within the explant, a key cytokine in eosinophil survival.

IL-5 exerts its biological effects through its receptor (IL-5R). IL-5R consists of two subunits, an α subunit of 60–80 kDa, and a common βc subunit of between 120 and 140 kDa, which is shared with IL-3R and GM-CSFR. IL-5 interacts with its α subunit specifically but at a lower affinity than the βc subunit.[39] IL-5 stimulation through the βc subunit leads to phosphorylation of the tyrosine kinases, Jak2, Lyn, and Syk. While Jak2 signals through the nuclear translocation factor STAT1, Lyn, and Syk signal through the mitogenic Ras-Raf1-MEK-ERK pathway (Fig. 18.3). Tyrosine phosphorylation enhances the expression of the antiapoptotic protein Bcl-xL in eosinophils, and decreases translocation of the proapoptotic signaling molecule Bax, resulting in decreased activation of apoptotic signaling through the caspase family.[40,41]

Similarly, extracellular matrix proteins have been shown to modulate eosinophil responses to physiological soluble stimuli.[42] Eosinophils adhere to fibronectin,[43] an abundant extracellular matrix protein, likely through VLA-4.[44] Similarly, VLA-6 expressed on eosinophils interacts with the connective tissue protein laminin. In addition, binding of eosinophils to tissue sites via α_4 integrin promotes eosinophil survival for up to 2 weeks through a GM-CSF-dependent mechanism.[43]

EOSINOPHIL TISSUE ACCUMULATION

The selective tissue recruitment of eosinophils occurs across the vascular endothelium and into tissues (Fig. 18.4). Most migration through endothelium occurs at post-capillary venules. Each of these steps is

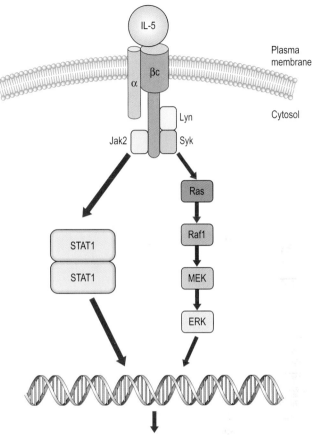

Transcriptional activation leading to antiapoptotic effects

Fig. 18.3. Signaling pathway leading from binding of IL-5 to its receptor in the membrane to transcriptional activation in the cell nucleus via the Ras-Raf1-MEK-ERK pathway. The β subunit of the receptor is also able to activate the Jak2-STAT1 pathway. Transcriptional activation is proposed to generate antiapoptotic effects in eosinophils. Reproduced from Lacy P, Becker AC, Moqbel R. The human eosinophil, In: Wintrobe's Clinical Hematology, 11th edn, 2004 (Vol 1, Ch.11) with permission. Copyright, Lippincott, Williams and Wilkins.

controlled by a complex network of chemotactic factors and adhesion molecules, which collectively directs the movement of the eosinophil into the tissues. Selectins and α_4 integrins are thought to be important in tethering and rolling, while α_4 and β_2 (CD18) integrins mediate firm adhesion. The transmigration step is primarily regulated by β_2 integrins as well as C-C chemokines such as CCL11/eotaxin. Cytokines and chemokines are elaborated by surrounding tissues to modulate the transmigration of eosinophils into tissues. Many of these mechanisms appear to be controlled at the level of the T cell response to antigen (allergen)-presenting cells, and the subsequent release of cytokines and chemokines, which in turn regulate the activity of eosinophils. For example, IL-4 and IL-13 may be involved in upregulating eosinophil adhesion, primarily through VCAM-1 on endothelial cells.[45,46] IL-5 also upregulates eosinophil, but not neutrophil, adhesion to unstimulated endothelium.[47] IL-5 has been shown to activate transendothelial migration of eosinophils through ICAM-1 via decreased β_1 and increased

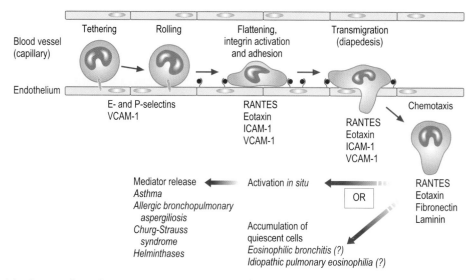

Fig. 18.4. Eosinophil tethering, rolling, adhesion, transmigration and chemotaxis in response to inflammatory signals in tissues. During chemotaxis, eosinophils may either become activated in response to local inflammation and release mediators, as in asthma and other related conditions, or they accumulate in tissues in the apparent absence of mediator release. Reproduced from Lacy P, Becker AC, Moqbel R. The human eosinophil. In: Wintrobe's Clinical Hematology, 11th edn 2004 (Vol. 1 Ch11) with permission. Copyright, Lippincott, Willams and Wilkins.

β_2 integrin function and/or expression.[48] Similarly, stimulation of eosinophil CCR3 with a chemokine such as CCL11, which can be released from endothelial cells, also increases β_2 integrin expression, resulting in preferential binding to ICAM-1.[49] Complement-mediated inflammation is associated with the release of C3a and C5a. C3a increases binding of eosinophils to endothelium but does not increase migration, while C5a increases both adhesion and migration.[50] IL-1 and TNF are also released during inflammation with significant effects on eosinophil migration.[51]

Upon adherence to vascular endothelium, eosinophils commence diapedesis, emerge out of the capillaries, and traverse the adjacent connective tissue. These cells move by extending lamellipodia using a uropod, leading to lamellar motion.[45] Changes in the binding affinity for adhesion molecules and extracellular matrix proteins are thought to contribute to cell movement on a substratum. A gradient in eosinophil VLA-4 binding affinity to fibronectin has been demonstrated,[52] where increased adherence at the leading edge of the cell is followed by a rear de-adherence, allowing the cell to move forward. Cytokines and chemokines also influence the binding of eosinophils to tissue surfaces. For example, GM-CSF increases the binding affinity of VLA-4 to VCAM-1 or CS-1[53] while CCL11 stimulates the reverse reaction.[49] CCL11 may also induce cytoskeletal changes via mitogen-activated protein kinases (MAPK).[51] Other chemotactic factors, such as CCL5, CCL7, and C5a, may also alter β_1 integrin affinity.[53,54] The balance of these factors determines the rate of eosinophil migration.

The most potent eosinophil chemoattractants include the phospholipid-derived mediators, platelet activating factor (PAF; 1-O-alkyl-2-acetyl-sn-glycerol-3-phosphocholine), LTD$_4$, C5a, IL-2, and C-C chemokines such as CCL11/Eotaxin and CCL5/RANTES.[55,56] C-C chemokines appear to be essential for inducing the specific migration of eosinophils to inflamed sites due to the nearly exclusive expression of CCR3 in eosinophils.[28] This family of chemokines consists of CCL11/Eotaxin-1, CCL24/Eotaxin-2, CCL26/Eotaxin-3, CCL5/RANTES, CCL8/MCP-2, CCL7/MCP-3, murine CCL12/MCP-5, and CCL3/MIP-1a. Chemokines binding CCR3 may be selective for eosinophils and basophils, as neutrophils do not

express this receptor. Eotaxin is the only chemokine specific to eosinophils, making it a key member of the CCR3 family.[55,57] CCR3 chemokines are produced by endothelial cells, epithelial cells, parasympathetic nerves, T cells, macrophages, fibroblasts, and eosinophils, among other tissue sources.[34,58,59] Basal expression of CCL11 in the gut is elevated compared with other tissues in the normal animal.[60] CCL11 expression during allergen-induced eosinophilia is increased within affected tissues.[61] Some synergism exists between IL-5 and CCL11, as IL-5 stimulation enhances the eosinophil response to CCL11 both in vitro and in vivo.[62,63]

Eosinophils also express a range of receptors for immunoglobulins that contribute to chemotactic and activation responses in tissues. These include receptors for IgA, IgD, IgE, IgG, and IgM. There has been controversy around the existence of the high-affinity receptor for IgE (FcϵRI) on the eosinophil. Studies have shown that the α subunit of FcϵRI in eosinophils is expressed intracellularly rather than on the cell surface in resting cells, which, in turn, may be mobilized to the cell surface and released during activation.[64,65] Eosinophils also express an IgE-binding protein, galectin-3 (Mac-2/ϵ binding protein), which may explain the high-affinity binding for IgE in earlier studies. Cross-linking of immunoglobulin receptors on eosinophils has been shown to be highly effective at inducing respiratory burst and degranulation in eosinophils. The hierarchy of effectiveness in degranulation has been shown to be in the order of secretory IgA (sIgA) = IgA > IgG >> IgE.[66] IL-3, IL-5, and GM-CSF were shown to enhance immunoglobulin-mediated degranulation.[67]

■ SURFACE MARKERS IN EOSINOPHILS ■

Eosinophils express a substantial array of surface markers, such as Fc receptors, CD11a-c, CD18, CystLT1/2 receptors, and PAF receptor, among many others, which are generally based on evidence of their expression as determined by flow cytometry analysis or inferred by cellular responsiveness to specific stimuli. These are grouped into immunoglobulin receptors and members of the immunoglobulin superfamily, cytokine receptors, adhesion molecules, chemotactic factors, enzymes, and molecules associated with apoptosis and cellular signalling.[68] Eosinophils do not express unique, cell-specific markers that distinguish them from other hematopoietic cells; however, they can be isolated from peripheral blood by immunomagnetically based negative selection for CD16, which is usually expressed at relatively low levels in normal eosinophils compared with neutrophils, the other major CD16-expressing leukocyte present in circulation.

■ EOSINOPHIL-DERIVED MEDIATORS ■

The eosinophil is both a factory and a store for a large array of mediators. These are released upon activation and thought to be important in various inflammatory reactions associated with this cell type (Fig. 18.5).

MEMBRANE-DERIVED MEDIATORS

Eosinophils produce a wide variety of lipid-derived mediators, which have profound biological activity. The more important products are eicosanoid lipid mediators, which include leukotrienes (especially LTC_4), prostaglandins (particularly PGE_2), thromboxane, lipoxins (especially LXA_4), and PAF. The main substrate for these mediators is arachidonic acid (AA), which is specifically liberated from membrane phospholipids at the sn-2 position by phospholipase A_2 (PLA_2) during receptor stimulation. Of the nine known families of PLA_2, two families are expressed in eosinophils, the type IIA and type IV enzymes. These enzymes are commonly known as secretory and cytosolic PLA_2, respectively.[69,70] They are distinguished by their distribution, size, and sensitivity to Ca^{2+},

where granule-stored $sPLA_2$ (13–15 kDa) requires millimolar amounts of Ca^{2+} for activity while cytosolically localized $cPLA_2$ (85 kDa) is catalytically active in the presence of micromolar amounts of Ca^{2+}. Interestingly, eosinophils express 20–100-fold higher levels of secretory PLA_2 in their granules than other circulating leukocytes, suggesting a functional role in inflammatory processes involving eosinophil degranulation.

Eosinophils are a rich source of LTC_4 (5S-hydroxy-6R,S-glutathionyl-7,9,-$trans$-11,14-cis-eicosatetraenoic acid).[71,72] Stimulation with the calcium ionophore A23187 generates between 40–70 ng/10^6 cells of LTC_4 from human eosinophils. Eosinophils produce negligible amounts of LTB_4 (5S-12R-dihydroxy-6,14-cis-8,10-$trans$-eicosatetraenoic acid) compared with neutrophils. LTC_4 generation by human eosinophils occurs following stimulation with opsonized zymosan and via an FcγRII-dependent mechanism using IgG-coated Sepharose beads.[73] The production of LTC_4 is critically dependent upon the activation of 5-lipoxygenase, an enzyme which resides in the euchromatin region of the nucleus and translocates to the nuclear membrane upon cell activation where it activates an 18 kDa protein called 5-lipoxygenase activating protein (FLAP).[74] The substrate for 5-lipoxygenase is AA, which is thought to be released from the membrane phospholipids by PLA_2. The first product of this enzyme is an intermediary compound, 5-HPETE, which is transformed into the unstable epoxide LTA_4. At this point, human eosinophils predominantly generate LTC_4 through the action of LTC_4 synthetase.[71,72] Eosinophils are particularly rich in LTC_4 synthetase, and account for 70% of all LTC_4 synthetase-positive cells in the airway mucosa of normal and asthmatic individuals.[75] LTC_4 is generated intracellularly in human eosinophils and later exported from the cell in a regulated manner.[76] Activated eosinophils produce 15-HETE, a lipid mediator generated via the 15-lipoxygenase pathway, which is pro-inflammatory and can modulate the chemotactic effects of LTB_4 on neutrophils.[77] Unlike 5-lipoxygenase, the enzyme 15-lipoxygenase can modify a larger pool of fatty acid substrates and will oxygenate fatty acids that are esterified in phospholipids. Substrates include

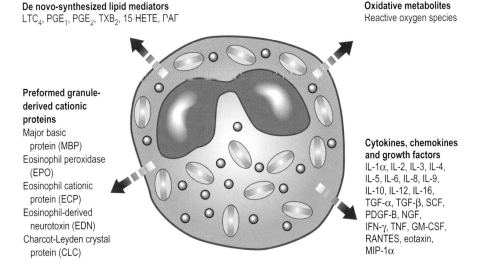

Fig. 18.5. Mediators released by activated eosinophils. De novo-synthesized lipid mediators and oxidative metabolites are elaborated directly from the cell membrane or lipid bodies following enzyme activation, while granule-derived cationic proteins and cytokines, chemokines, and growth factors are released following granule-plasma membrane fusion during degranulation. Reproduced from Lacy P, Becker AC, Moqbel R. The human eosinophil. In: Wintrobe's Clinical Hematology, 11th edn 2004 (Vol 1, Ch11) with permission. Copyright, Lippincott Williams and Wilkins.

arachidonic acid, linoleic acid, polyenoic acids, and more complex lipids, such as lipoproteins. Eosinophils are the major cellular source of elevated 15-HETE in asthmatic airways and are capable of generating 100–300 times more 15-HETE than neutrophils, endothelial cells, and fibroblasts.[78] Eosinophils also account for 85% of cells positive for 15-lipoxygenase in the airway submucosa of normal and asthmatic subjects.[79,80]

Eosinophils generate large amounts of PAF in response to a variety of stimuli.[81,82] PAF, a potent phospholipid mediator, induces leukocyte activation. Much of the eosinophil-derived PAF remains cell-associated, possibly acting as an intracellular messenger, or alternatively binding to PAF receptors on adjacent eosinophils, thus acting as an autocrine agent. Interestingly, stimulation of eosinophils with fMLF does not augment PAF release.

The cyclooxygenase pathway is also prominent in eosinophils, and eosinophils are capable of producing PGE_1, PGE_2, and thromboxane B_2 from cyclooxygenase acting on free AA. In studies with guinea pig eosinophils, thromboxane B_2 and PGE_2 were shown to be generated following PAF or A23187 stimulation.[83] Many of the enzymes associated with membrane-derived mediator release from eosinophils, including cyclooxygenase and 5-lipoxygenase, are found stored in association with lipid bodies (Table 18.1).[84,85]

GRANULE-DERIVED PROTEINS

Eosinophils contain large crystalloid granules, also known as secondary or specific granules, which have been shown by light microscopy to stain bright orange red with the dye, eosin (Fig. 18.1). In electron micrographs, crystalloid granules appear to contain electron-dense crystalline cores surrounded by an electron-lucent granule matrix (Fig. 18.2). Eosinophils contain up to four other 'granule' types, namely: primary granules, small granules, lipid bodies, and small secretory vesicles.

Eosinophils contain at least five different populations of phospholipid bilayer membrane-bound granules.

1. Crystalloid granules: these specialized and unique granules measure between 0.5 and 0.8 μm in diameter, contain crystalline electron-dense cores (internum) surrounded by an electron-lucent matrix, and can take up acidic dyes avidly due to their cationic nature.[86] They are mainly present in mature eosinophils, although coreless granules have been observed in immature eosinophils. These granules contain the bulk of highly charged cationic proteins present in eosinophils, including MBP, eosinophil peroxidase (EPO), eosinophil cationic protein (ECP), and eosinophil-derived neurotoxin (EDN). These proteins are implicated in tissue damage in allergic inflammatory conditions including asthma. There are approximately 200 crystalloid granules in each cell. The core is predominantly composed of crystallized MBP (Fig. 18.6).

2. Primary granules: these coreless granules are enriched with Charcot–Leyden crystal protein (CLC), and are present in immature as well as mature eosinophils. Some authors refer to immature crystalloid granules as primary granules in eosinophil promyelocytes. Primary granules measure between 0.1 and 0.5 μm in diameter and are less abundant than crystalloid granules.

3. Small granules: these granules are also free of cores and contain acid phosphatase, arylsulfatase B, catalase, and cytochrome b_{558}.

4. Lipid bodies: there are around five lipid bodies per mature eosinophil, the number of which increase in certain eosinophilic disorders, especially in idiopathic hypereosinophilia. Lipid bodies are enriched in arachidonic acid esterified into glycerophospholipids.

5. Secretory vesicles: eosinophils are densely packed with small secretory vesicles in their cytoplasm. These vesicles appear as dumbbell-shaped structures in cross-sections, and contain albumin, suggesting an endocytotic origin. These structures are also known as microgranules or tubulo-vesicular structures.

EOSINOPHIL MBP

MBP (13.8 kDa) is an arginine-rich 117 amino acid protein that constitutes a significant proportion of total cell protein in human eosinophils (5–10 pg/cell). MBP is abundant in eosinophils, which contain as much as 250 pg/cell, making up 50% of the total cellular protein.[86] The high isoelectric point of $MBP^{10.9}$ cannot be measured accurately due to the extremely basic nature of the protein.[87] MBP is synthesized during the promyelocytic stage of eosinophil development, characterized by the presence of message encoding this protein, in a neutral prepro-form, which is later processed to form pro-MBP and subsequently transported to the immature crystalloid granule and cleaved to form MBP.[88,89] Mature MBP undergoes condensation from the periphery of immature crystalloid granules to the internum, where it develops a crystalline core as its concentration is increased.[89] Once eosinophils have reached full maturity, MBP is no longer synthesized and MBP-encoding messenger RNA disappears from the cell.[89,90] MBP acts on other inflammatory cells, including neutrophils and eosinophils, to induce degranulation and lipid mediator release.[91–94]

Basophils also synthesize and store MBP (as well as ECP and EDN) but at a much lower concentration than eosinophils, which may reflect the common differentiation path shared between these two cell phenotypes.[19]

MBP has been shown to be cytotoxic to airway tissues, including bronchial epithelial cells and pneumocytes. Airway smooth muscle is controlled largely by parasympathetic nerves. Neural dysfunction is associated with eosinophil infiltration into the bronchial mucosa in asthma.[2,95,96] Indeed, airway sections from patients with status asthmaticus exhibit intense MBP-specific immunofluorescence, suggesting that infiltrated eosinophils were fully activated, undergoing extracellular secretion of their contents of MBP.[97] The position of eosinophils within the airway may also be important. While patients with eosinophilic bronchitis have increased sputum and tissue eosinophils, they do not develop asthma.[98] From histopathological samples of patients with asthma, eosinophils can be found clustered around the vagal nerve ganglia in the lung.[96] In guinea pig models of asthma, antigen sensitization followed by challenge[99] and antigen sensitization followed by virus infection,[95] the release of MBP from eosinophils causes M2 receptor dysfunction and vagal nerve hyperreactivity. The development of airway hyperreactivity may be related to the increased number of eosinophils found in closer proximity to the parasympathetic nerves.[100]

MBP is also cytotoxic to metazoan parasitic targets in the absence of opsonization, thought to result from increased membrane permeability through surface charge interactions leading to perturbation of the lipid bilayer.[101]

EPO, ECP, AND EDN

Other eosinophil basic proteins include EPO, ECP, and EDN, which reside in the matrix compartment of the crystalloid granule. EPO is a highly basic (pI of 10.9) heme-containing protein composed of two subunits, a heavy chain of 50–57 kDa and a light chain of 11–15 kDa. EPO is a unique protein synthesized by and stored in eosinophils,

Table 18.1 Content of human eosinophil granules and secretory vesicles. Reproduced from Lacy P, Becker AC, Moqbel R. The human eosinophil. In: Wintrobe's Clinical Hematology, 11th edn. 2004 (Vol.1. Ch.11), with permission. Copyright, Lippincott, Williams and Wilkins.

Crystalloid granules	Primary granules	Small granules	Lipid bodies	Secretory vesicles
Core				
Catalase				
Cathepsin D				
Enoyl-CoA-hydrolase				
β-Glucuronidase				
Major basic protein				
Matrix				
Acid phosphatase	Charcot-Leyden crystal protein (galectin-10)	Acid phosphatase	Arachidonic acid	Plasma proteins (Albumin)
Acyl-CoA oxidase		Aryl-sulfatase B (active)	Cyclooxygenase	
Arylsulfatase B (inactive)		Catalase Eosinophil peroxidase		
Acid β-glycerophosphatase		Elastase	Esterase	
Bactericidal/permeability-increasing protein		Eosinophil cationic protein	5-Lipoxygenase	
Catalase			15-Lipoxygenase	
Cathepsin D			LTC_4 synthase	
Collagenase				
Elastase				
Enoyl-CoA-hydrolase (also in core)				
Eosinophil cationic protein				
Eosinophil-derived neurotoxin				
Eosinophil peroxidase				
Flavin adenine dinucleotide (FAD)				
β-Glucuronidase				
β-Hexosaminidase				
3 Ketoacyl-CoA thiolase				
Lysozyme				
Major basic protein				
Phospholipase A_2 (Type II)				
Non-specific esterases				
Membrane				
CD63		VAMP-7		Cytochrome b_{558} (p22*phox*)
V-type H+-ATPase		VAMP-8		VAMP-2
VAMP-7				VAMP-7
VAMP-8				VAMP-8

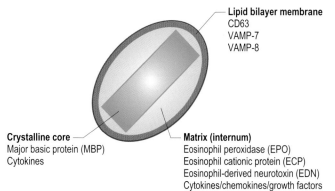

Lipid bilayer membrane
CD63
VAMP-7
VAMP-8

Crystalline core
Major basic protein (MBP)
Cytokines

Matrix (internum)
Eosinophil peroxidase (EPO)
Eosinophil cationic protein (ECP)
Eosinophil-derived neurotoxin (EDN)
Cytokines/chemokines/growth factors

Fig. 18.6. Structure of the eosinophil crystalloid granule. This membrane-bound organelle is a major site of storage of eosinophil cationic granule proteins as well as a number of cytokines, chemokines, and growth factors. Reproduced from Lacy P, Becker AC, Moqbel R. The human eosinophil. In: Wintrobe's Clinical Hematology, 11th edn. 2004 (Vol.1. Ch.11), with permission. Copyright, Lippincott, Williams and Wilkins.

a fact which was exploited to produce an eosinophil-deficient mouse (PHIL).[102] It is a haloperoxidase that shares 68% sequence identity with neutrophil myeloperoxidase, suggesting that a peroxidase multigene family may have developed through gene duplication.[87,103] Eosinophils store approximately 15 pg/cell of EPO, which is important in catalyzing the peroxidative oxidation of halides and pseudohalides, leading to the formation of bactericidal hypohalous acids in reaction with hydrogen peroxide generated during respiratory burst.[104,105]

The molecular mass of ECP is between 16 and 21 kDa, with approximately 15 pg/cell expressed in human eosinophils. The pI of ECP[10.8] is identical to that of MBP due to a similar arginine-rich sequence. Early studies have demonstrated that ECP, a member of a subfamily of RNase A multigenes and which possesses intrinsic ribonuclease (RNase) activity, is bactericidal, promotes degranulation of mast cells, and is toxic to helminthic parasites on its own.[106,107] The mechanism of action of ECP is thought to involve the formation of pores or channels in the target membrane, which is apparently not dependent on its reversible RNase activity.[108] ECP is perhaps most well-known for its ability to elicit the Gordon phenomenon when it was injected into the cranial ventricles of rabbits, causing the destruction of Purkinje cells and leading to spongiform changes in the cerebellum, pons, and spinal cord.[109,110]

EDN, another member of the RNase A multigene family of 18.5 kDa with approximately 100-fold higher RNase activity than ECP, is less basic than MBP or ECP with a pI of 8.9 due to a relatively smaller number of arginine resides in its sequence.

ECP and EDN share a remarkable sequence homology of 70% at the amino acid level for the pre-form of both proteins, suggesting that evolutionarily, these proteins are derived from the same gene.[111,112] Eosinophils express approximately 10 pg/cell of EDN, but there is marked variation between individuals. EDN similarly induces the Gordon phenomenon when injected intracranially in laboratory animals.[109,110] Messenger RNA encoding EPO, ECP, and EDN are detectable in mature eosinophils, suggesting that eosinophils have the capacity to continue to synthesize these proteins.[90]

The gene family expressing ECP and EDN has among the highest rates of mutation in the primate genome, ranking with those of immunoglobulins, T cell receptors, and major histocompatibility complex (MHC) classes.[112] These genes effectively comprise a superfamily of RNases expressed in the mammalian genome. Such an extreme rate of mutation suggests that the evolutionary constraints acting on the ECP/EDN superfamily have promoted the acquisition of a specialized antiviral activity. This may be inferred from the high mutation rates of other genes commonly associated with host protection against viral infection. Whether ECP or EDN possess any antiviral activity has yet to be demonstrated, although some studies have indicated that EDN may be potent antiviral factor in respiratory infections.[113]

CHARCOT-LEYDEN CRYSTAL PROTEIN

The CLC protein (17.4 kDa) is produced in eosinophils at very high levels (accounting for 10% of the total cellular protein) although its functional role is still obscure. CLC is a hydrophobic protein with strong sequence homology to the carbohydrate-binding galectin family of proteins, and has been designated galectin-10.[114] CLC is released in large quantities in the tissues in eosinophilic disorders, resulting in the formation of distinct, needle-shaped structures which are colorless and measure 20–40 μm in length and 2–4 μm across. CLC crystals are abundant in the sputum and feces of patients with severe respiratory and gastrointestinal eosinophilia, which were first observed by Charcot and Robin in 1853.

A list of these and other granule proteins synthesized and stored in eosinophils is presented in Table 18.1 and published elsewhere.[27,115]

EOSINOPHIL-DERIVED CYTOKINES

Human eosinophils have been shown to synthesize, store, and release over 29 different cytokines, chemokines, and growth factors (Table 18.2) with the potential to participate in the regulation of various immune responses. These cytokines have been identified in eosinophils by detecting mRNA and/or protein using RT-PCR, in situ hybridization, and immunocytochemical staining.[116–118] In addition, picogram amounts of cytokines, chemokines, and growth factors were measured in supernatants of stimulated eosinophils.[117,119] These cytokines are likely to act in an autocrine, paracrine, or juxtacrine manner, thereby regulating local inflammatory events. Studies have demonstrated that the production of eosinophil-activating cytokines (e.g., IL-3, IL-5, and GM-CSF) by eosinophils may be important in prolonging the survival of these cells by a putative autocrine loop.[43,117] For instance, adherence of highly purified eosinophils to the extracellular matrix protein, fibronectin, resulted in prolongation of survival of these cells in the absence of exogenous cytokines.[43] Fibronectin-induced eosinophil survival was inhibitable by antibodies against fibronectin and VLA-4 and upregulated by picogram amounts of IL-3 and GM-CSF derived from eosinophils.[43] Observations on eosinophil cytokine release have been mainly studied in vitro, and confirmed in vivo.[120–123]

A major distinction in cytokine production between eosinophils and T cells is that the former store their cytokines intracellularly as pre-formed mediators, while the latter produce and release cytokines only following activation. Although most eosinophil-derived cytokines are elaborated at lower concentrations than other leukocytes, eosinophils possess the ability to release these cytokines immediately (within minutes) following stimulation. Stored cytokines include IL-2, IL-4, IL-5, IL-6, IL-10, IL-13, IL-16, GM-CSF, TNF, NGF, and TGF, as well as the chemokines CCL5/RANTES, CCL11/Eostaxin, and CXCL8/IL-8.[34] Studies

Table 18.2 Cytokines, chemokines, and growth factors produced by human eosinophils (Reproduced from Lacy P, Becker AC, Moqbel R. The human eosinophil. In: Wintrabe's Clinical Hematology, 11th edn. 2004 (Vol.1. Ch.11), with permission. Copyright, Lippincott, Williams and Wilkins).

Cytokine	Products	Stored protein in resting cells (per 10^6 cells)	Intracellular site of storage
Interleukins			
Interleukin-1	mRNA protein	–	–
Interleukin-2	mRNA protein	6 ± 2 pg	Crystalloid granules (core)
Interleukin-3	mRNA protein	–	–
Interleukin-4	mRNA protein	≈75 ± 20 pg	Crystalloid granules (core)
Interleukin-5	mRNA protein	–	Crystalloid granules (core/matrix)
Interleukin-6	mRNA protein	25 ± 6 pg	Crystalloid granules (matrix)
Interleukin-9	mRNA protein	–	–
Interleukin-10	mRNA protein	≈25 pg	–
Interleukin-11	mRNA	–	–
Interleukin-12	mRNA protein	–	–
Interleukin-13	mRNA protein	–	–
Interleukin-16	mRNA protein	1.6 ± 0.8 ng	–
Leukemia inhibitory factor (LIF)	mRNA protein	–	–
Interferons and others			
Interferon-γ (IFN-γ)	mRNA protein	–	–
Tumor necrosis factor (TNF)	mRNA protein	–	Crystalloid granules (matrix)
Granulocyte/macrophage colony-stimulating factor (GM-CSF)	mRNA protein	15.1 ± 0.3 pg	Crystalloid granules (core)
Chemokines			
CXCL8 (Interleukin-8)	mRNA protein	72 ± 15 pg	Crystalloid granules (matrix) and small secretory vesicles
CCL2 (MCP-1)	mRNA protein	19 ± 4 pg	Crystalloid granules
CCL3 (MIP-1α)	mRNA protein	140 pg	Cytoplasmic
CCL5 (RANTES)	mRNA protein	–	
CCL7 (MCP-3)	Protein	–	–
CCL11 (Eotaxin)	mRNA	–	–
CCL13 (MCP-4)	mRNA	–	–
Growth factors			
Heparin-binding epidermal growth factor-like binding protein (HB-EGF-LBP)	mRNA	–	–
Nerve growth factor (NGF)	mRNA protein	4 ± 2 pg	–
Platelet-derived growth factor, β-chain (PDGF-B)	mRNA	–	–
Stem cell factor (SCF)	mRNA protein	–	Membrane, cytoplasm
Transforming growth factor-α (TGF-α)	mRNA protein	22 ± 6 pg	Crystalloid granules (matrix) and small secretory vesicles
Transforming growth factor-β_1 (TGF-β_1)	mRNA protein	–	–

using immunogold electron microscopic analysis or confocal laser scanning microscopy coupled with double immunofluorescence labeling have indicated that several of these cytokines are found in close association with either the crystalline core or matrix of the crystalloid specific granules of the cell (Table 18.2).[124–129] For example, CCL5/RANTES was found to be associated predominantly with the matrix compartment of the crystalloid granule in eosinophils (Fig. 18.7).

Developing eosinophils possess the ability to express cytokine message and protein at early stages of maturation. Eosinophils generated from semi-solid culture of cord blood-derived CD34+ cells in the presence of IL-3 and IL-5 were shown to express IL-5 and GM-CSF mRNA after 10 days of culture.[130] Freshly purified CD34+ cells expressed IL-4 and CCL5 mRNA, but not IL-4 and CCL5 protein. On day 23 of culture, IL-4 and CCL5 localized to the matrix of MBP+ crystalloid granules as determined by immunofluorescence.[131] In addition, IL-6 protein expression was found in cells after day 16 of culture.[132]

Another site of storage of cytokines and chemokines is within the small secretory vesicle. At least two such proteins were shown to be associated with these vesicles, namely CCL5 and TGF.[118,133] These organelles belong to the same group of secretory vesicles identified by electron microscopy analysis as tubulovesicular structures. CCL5-positive vesicles are highly sensitive to stimulation by IFN-γ and are rapidly mobilized (within 10 min of stimulation) to secrete CCL5 extracellularly.[118,134] Crystalloid granules, which also contain CCL5 within their matrix compartment, were found to release this chemokine more slowly in response to IFN-γ (1 h), while the majority of MBP remained associated with the core of these granules. These observations suggest that eosinophils have the ability to 'shuttle' CCL5 from the crystalloid granules to the cell exterior, and may provide an important in vitro model for eosinophil piecemeal degranulation (see Degranulation mechanisms, below).

RESPIRATORY BURST

Respiratory burst is defined as the increase in cell metabolism (measured by the elevated activity of the hexose monophosphate shunt) and oxygen consumption, coupled with the release of reactive oxygen species (ROS). The principal product of respiratory burst is superoxide (O_2^-), the function of which is thought to reside in its ability to dismutate into more reactive ROS, including hydrogen peroxide (H_2O_2), the hydroxyl radical (OH^-), and formation of hypohalous acids (HOBr) upon reaction with EPO produced following eosinophil degranulation. O_2^- is also able to react with nitric oxide (NO) produced from nitric oxide synthase enzymes (e.g., iNOS, eNOS) to form the highly reactive peroxynitrite (ONOO-), which has been shown to alter cell function.

The regulated burst of O_2^- production is largely mediated through the activation of NADPH oxidase, which is crucial for maintenance of host defense (Fig. 18.8). Overactivation of the NADPH oxidase is cytotoxic to tissues, and has been implicated in the pathogenesis of many eosinophil-related disorders including allergic asthma.[135] Interestingly, eosinophils possess the ability to generate up to 10-fold more superoxide than other phagocytes, including neutrophils.[136] The ability of the eosinophil to release more O_2^- is thought to be the result of higher levels of expression of the protein components that make up the NADPH oxidase complex.[137,138] In addition, preferential assembly of NADPH oxidase occurs at the cell membrane in eosinophils, eliciting a predominantly extracellular form of O_2^- release.[139] This was in contrast to neutrophils, which showed intracellular NADPH oxidase assembly

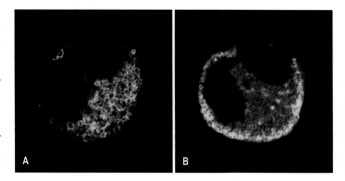

Fig. 18.7. Translocation of the chemokine CCL5/RANTES in human eosinophils activated by IFN-γ in vitro. Immunoreactivities for CCL5/RANTES (green fluorescence) and eosinophil MBP (red fluorescence) are shown in control (A) and IFN-γ-stimulated (10 min, 500 U/ml) (B) cells. The yellow color in (B) resulted from colocalization of green and red immunofluorescence stains. Note that immunoreactivity for MBP remained associated with the cores of the crystalloid granules in both cells, while the green label for CCL5/RANTES translocated towards the cell membrane. CCL5/RANTES was proposed to be released from eosinophils by piecemeal degranulation. Experimental conditions described in Lacy et al.[118] Reproduced from Lacy P, Becker AC, Moqbel R. The human eosinophil. In: Wintrobe's Clinical Hematology, 11th edn. 2004 (Vol.1 Ch.11), with permission. Copyright, Lippincott, Williams and Wilkins.

during respiratory burst stimulation and bacterial infection.[139,140] NADPH oxidase is a complex of at least five subunits, of which two (p22phox and gp91phox) reside in the membrane as part of the cytochrome b_{558} protein, and the remaining three (p47phox, p67phox, and Rac1 or Rac2) are cytosolic in resting states.[136] The release of O_2^- from eosinophils is likely to be a crucial component of the pathophysiological processes underlying eosinophilic inflammation in mucosal tissues.

MECHANISMS OF EOSINOPHIL EXOCYTOSIS

Degranulation is defined as the exocytotic fusion of granules with the plasma membrane during receptor-mediated secretion. During exocytosis, the outer leaflet of the lipid bilayer membrane surrounding the granule encounters the inner leaflet of the plasma membrane, a process known as 'docking' The docking step is hypothesized to be regulated by intracellular membrane-associated proteins which act as receptors directing the specificity of granule targeting. After docking, the granule and plasma membrane fuse together and form a reversible structure called the fusion pore, which is also thought to be regulated by similar, or the same, membrane-associated proteins regulating granule docking. Depending on the intensity of the stimulus, the fusion pore may either retreat, leading to re-separation of the granule from the plasma membrane, or it may expand and allow complete integration of the granule membrane into the plasma membrane as a continuous sheet. The inner leaflet of the granule membrane becomes outwardly exposed, and the granule contents are subsequently expelled to the exterior of the cell.[141]

The eosinophil exhibits one of four main forms of granule release observed both in vitro and in vivo (Fig. 18.9). The first is the classical sequential release of single crystalloid granules, which was the original hypothesis suggested for a predominant route of degranulation in eosinophils. This type of release is typically seen in vitro and can be

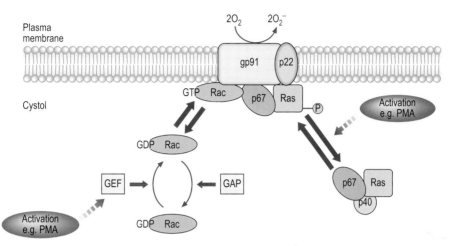

Fig. 18.8. Assembly and activation of the NADPH oxidase complex during respiratory burst. This complex is essential for the inducible release of superoxide for microbicidal reactions and is also present in neutrophils. During cell activation, the GTPase Rac, normally bound to GDP in the resting cell, is activated by a guanine exchange factor (GEF) to bind to GTP. This results in translocation of Rac-GTP to the cell membrane, where other cytosolic proteins p67$phox$ and p47$phox$ have also translocated, to bind to the two subunits of cytochrome b_{558} (gp91$phox$ and p22$phox$). Following the assembly of the oxidase, electrons are transferred from NADPH in the cytosol via flavin adenine dinucleotide (a co-factor) to oxygen molecules to form the highly reactive oxygen intermediate, superoxide. Assembly of this complex is reversed by GTPase-activating protein (GAP), which hydrolyzes GTP on Rac to GDP, and by the dissociation of the $phox$ subunits. Reproduced from Lacy P, Becker AC, Moqbel R. The human eosinophil. In: Wintrobe's Clinical Hematology, 11th edn. 2004 (Vol.1 Ch.11), with permission. Copyright, Lippincott, Williams and Wilkins.

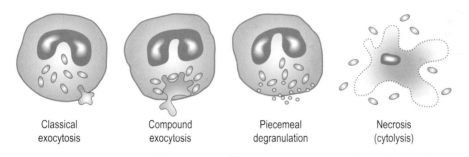

| Classical exocytosis | Compound exocytosis | Piecemeal degranulation | Necrosis (cytolysis) |

Fig. 18.9. Four putative physiological modes of eosinophil degranulation. The most commonly observed forms of degranulation in allergic disease are piecemeal degranulation and necrosis (cytolysis). Parasitic and fungal diseases typically exhibit eosinophils undergoing compound exocytosis. (Reproduced from Lacy P, Becker AC, Moqbel R. The human eosinophil. In: Wintrobe's Clinical Hematology, 11th edn. 2004 (Vol.1 Ch.11), with permission. Copyright, Lippincott, Williams and Wilkins).

elegantly demonstrated electrophysiologically using patch-clamp procedures that measure changes in membrane capacitance. The latter are directly proportional to increases in the surface area of the cell membrane. During the sequential release of individual crystalloid granules, a stepwise increment in capacitance may be observed as their membranes fuse with that of the cell membrane.[142] The second mode of granule release is compound exocytosis, also demonstrated by patch-clamp analysis, in which sudden, very large increments in whole cell capacitance occur resulting from individual granules fusing with the cell membrane.[143]

Ultrastructural studies of guinea pig eosinophils have also demonstrated evidence for compound exocytosis[144] similar to that observed in rat eosinophils adhering to the outer surface of opsonized parasitic larvae.[143,145] Additional evidence for compound exocytosis was suggested in eosinophils stimulated with a cocktail of IL-3, IL-5, and GM-CSF, which were observed to fuse their granules following activation as determined by immunofluorescence for CD63, a marker for crystalloid granules.[146]

The third manner in which eosinophils degranulate is by piecemeal degranulation (PMD). PMD was first characterized by Dvorak and colleagues for the appearance of numerous small vesicles in the cytoplasm coupled with the apparent loss of crystalloid granule core and matrix components, creating a 'mottled' appearance in electron microscopy analysis.[147] This was thought to be due to small vesicles budding off from the larger secondary granules and moving to the plasma membrane for fusion, thereby causing gradual emptying of the crystalloid granules to the outside of the cell. PMD was the most commonly observed pattern of degranulation seen in situ in biopsy samples from the upper airways of allergic individuals,[148] and is likely to be physiologically the most important mechanism for eosinophil mediator release in allergic disease. A few years ago, an in vitro model for PMD was developed using IFN-γ-stimulated eosinophils, in which a piecemeal manner of CCL5 release was detected by a combination of confocal laser scanning microscopy, immunogold labeling, and subcellular fractionation.[118]

Airway tissue eosinophils not undergoing PMD appeared necrotic, which is a fourth pattern of granule release, also termed 'cytolysis'.[149] This type of release has been previously observed to occur following in vitro stimulation of human eosinophils with the calcium ionophore A23187,[150] and appears to be a physiologically relevant granule release event.

THE EOSINOPHIL SNARE COMPLEX

The mechanisms associated with classical exocytosis, compound exocytosis, and PMD, but not cytolysis, are thought to require specific intracellular membrane-associated proteins acting as receptors for granule docking and fusion. These proteins include a family of molecules known as SNAREs (an acronym for *SNA*P *re*ceptors). The paradigm associated with SNARE molecule function predicts that these proteins are essential for exocytosis. SNAREs were originally described in neuronal tissues and were found to group themselves into two distinct locations, the granule-associated SNAREs (the so-called vesicular SNAREs or v-SNAREs) and the plasma membrane-associated SNAREs (target SNAREs or t-SNAREs).[151] In order for a functional SNARE complex to form, allowing the granule to dock with the plasma membrane, the model for this predicts that one v-SNARE binds to two t-SNARE molecules. In neuronal cells, a commonly observed v-SNARE is vesicle-associated membrane protein (VAMP)-1 or its isoforms, VAMP-2. In these cells, the t-SNAREs associating with VAMP-2 that were originally described were synaptosome-associated protein of 25 kDa (SNAP-25) and syntaxin-1A. These three molecules form a stable detergent-resistant four-helix coiled-coil bundle, which may be regulated by protein phosphorylation. The precise mechanisms regulating SNARE binding and activation are not yet known.

Non-neuronal cells also express SNAREs, although some isoforms have been identified with high sequence homology to the neuronal SNAREs. Up to three SNAP-25 isoforms and approximately 16 syntaxin-1 isoforms have been characterized based on detection of homologous SNARE motif messenger RNA sequences. Interestingly, most non-neuronal secretory cells appear to require SNAP-23 and syntaxin-3, syntaxin-4, or syntaxin-6[152] for control of exocytosis. Eosinophils have

been shown to express the v-SNARE, VAMP-2, in their small secretory vesicles containing CCL5, but not their crystalloid granules.[153] Crystalloid granules express mainly VAMP-7 and VAMP-8, the former being important in regulation of crystalloid granule secretion during degranulation responses from permeabilized eosinophils.[154] The t-SNARE isoforms syntaxin-4 and SNAP-23 are expressed in the cell membrane of eosinophils, and these have the potential to act as cognate membrane binding partners for VAMP-2 and VAMP-7 degranulation.[155] The SNARE molecules VAMP-2, SNAP-23, and syntaxin-4 identified in eosinophils are proposed to regulate docking and fusion of CCL5-containing small secretory vesicles during piecemeal degranulation (Fig. 18.10).

Mechanisms associated with granule release in eosinophils are critical for the effector function of eosinophils. Without degranulation and mediator secretion, the eosinophil is a relatively inert cell, and does not affect the surrounding tissues, as seen in cases of idiopathic pulmonary eosinophilia and eosinophilic pneumonia. In these conditions, eosinophil numbers are increased in the capillaries and tissues of the lung, with no cellular or evident structural damage, probably because of the absence of eosinophil degranulation. In contrast, asthmatic patients show profound eosinophilia in the airways combined with significant tissue destruction, suggesting that, in addition to eosinophilic infiltration, their undergoing degranulation may contribute to mucosal damage in the airways and related symptoms of asthma.

THE HUMAN EOSINOPHIL AS AN IMMUNE REGULATORY CELL

To determine the involvement of eosinophil-derived factors in modulating the immune response, the bioactivity of cytokines released from eosinophils has been explored for their potential physiological effects in immune regulation. Allergy is characterized by a polarization towards enhanced production of Th2 cytokines and a dramatic increase in allergen-specific and total immunoglobulin E (IgE) levels. Since eosinophils generate both bioactive Th1 and Th2 cytokines (Table 18.2) they have

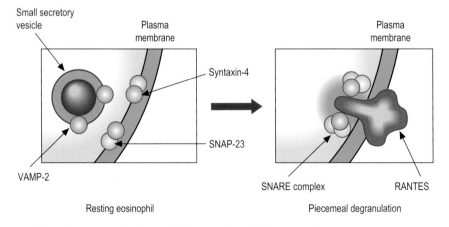

Resting eosinophil

Piecemeal degranulation

Fig. 18.10. Schematic model for molecular regulation of granule-plasma membrane fusion proposed to occur in piecemeal degranulation in eosinophils. In this model, the v-SNARE VAMP-2 is expressed on small secretory vesicles which store CCL5/RANTES as a preformed mediator, while t-SNAREs, SNAP-23 and syntaxin-4, reside on the inside of the plasma membrane. Following cell activation, v- and t-SNAREs bind together to form a SNARE complex, resulting in fusion and release of vesicular contents including CCL5/RANTES (see Lacy et al;[153] Logan et al;[155]). Reproduced from Lacy P, Becker AC, Moqbel R. The human eosinophil. In: Wintrobe's Clinical Hematology, 11th edn. 2004 (Vol.1 Ch.11), with permission. Copyright, Lippincott, Williams and Wilkins.

been implicated as active components of the immune allergic reaction, rather than as bystander cells.[34,115]

On the whole, eosinophils produce significantly smaller amounts of cytokines than T cells, B cells, and other cells in the immune system. However, in eosinophilic inflammation, eosinophils outnumber T cells in the tissues by as much as a hundred-fold. As such, the magnitude of the presence of eosinophils may be a determining factor in regulating immune responses at a local level. The release of eosinophil cytokines often takes place within a much shorter period than cytokines released by T cells (which may be several hours), as eosinophil-derived cytokines are stored as preformed mediators in crystalloid granules and may be secreted in response to stimuli in a matter of minutes.

The release of IL-4 from eosinophils is important in driving the initiation of a Th2-type response in *Schistosoma mansoni* infection in mice.[156] IL-2 and IFN-γ from CD28-stimulated eosinophils were shown to stimulate proliferation in an IL-2-dependent cell line and MHC class II expression on Colo 205 cells, respectively.[157] These studies have demonstrated that eosinophil-derived cytokines and chemokines have the ability to at least regulate local inflammatory responses.

It is paradoxical that eosinophils, a Th2-type response marker cell type for allergic diseases or helminthic infections, generate both Th1 and Th2 cytokines. For example, binding of CD28 on human eosinophils induced the release of bioactive IL-2 and IFN-γ,[157] both of which are Th1 cytokines, and IL-13, a Th2 cytokine.[158] Since Th1 and Th2 responses are mutually inhibitory, it has been very difficult to dissect the specific roles of eosinophil-derived cytokines in the initiation and effector phases of the allergic immune response. The role of eosinophil-derived Th1 or Th2 cytokines may, therefore, depend on the timing of eosinophil infiltration into sites of allergic inflammation. Indeed, recent studies using a mouse model of *Nippostrongylus brasiliensis* infection have shown that while eosinophils may be crucial for secondary Th2 polarized immune response against this parasite, the primary response does not require eosinophil-derived IL-4 or IL-13.[159]

The implications of eosinophil cytokine production are extensive, such as in the case of IL-4, where this cytokine may be released from eosinophils to direct Th2 cell differentiation in local lymph nodes in allergy. In support of this possibility, eosinophils have been shown to traffic to paratracheal draining lymph nodes (in a mouse model of asthma), where they were demonstrated to function as antigen-presenting cells expressing MHC class II and co-stimulatory CD80 and CD86 to stimulate CD4+ T cells.[160] During intimate cell-cell contact, the production of IL-4 and IL-13 is not required in abundance to effect important immunoregulatory events, such as enhanced switching of T cells to Th2 phenotype and increased IgE synthesis, both of which are hallmarks of allergic disorders.[161,162] Under such conditions, antigen-loaded eosinophils acting as antigen-presenting cells were found to preferentially initiate the generation of a Th2 response to ovalbumin in an experimental mouse model.[36,163] These studies have confirmed the ability of eosinophils to participate in the generation of allergic immune response through the secretion of immunomodulatory cytokines.

INDOLEAMINE 2,3-DIOXYGENASE (IDO), EOSINOPHILS, AND TH2 POLARIZATION

Apart from cytokine production, other eosinophil-derived immunoregulatory factors have been recently recognized. Based on initial data showing that its inhibition resulted in an immune-mediated abortion

in mice,[164] recent studies have shown that indoleamine 2,3-dioxygenase (IDO), the rate-limiting enzyme in the oxidative catabolism of tryptophan, may play a central role in immune regulation.[165] Subsequent studies have associated tryptophan catabolism with mechanisms of tumor escape from T cells,[166] dysfunctional tolerance in autoimmune diabetes mellitus in NOD mice,[167] and protective negative regulation of trinitrozobenzene-induced (Th1) model of colitis in the mouse.[168] According to this mechanism, a discrete population of dendritic cells (DCs) that express functional IDO in lymphoid tissues is able to inhibit T cell proliferation and induce T cell apoptosis.[169] The presence of this minority population of inhibitory DCs in lymphoid tissue can override the activating properties of other DCs and, therefore, act as a strong negative feedback mechanism on immune activation.[170] Further studies have shown that regulatory T cells (Tregs) that constitutively express cytotoxic T-lymphocyte antigen-4 (CTLA-4), the so-called central Tregs, downregulate the immune response using this mechanism.[171,172]

Human eosinophils constitutively express the enzyme IDO,[173] in contrast to DCs where IDO is inducible. Furthermore, co-culture of IDO-expressing eosinophils with T lymphocytes selectively inhibited the proliferation of Th1 cells while having no effect on Th2 cells. Immunostaining of histological sections of human lymphoid tissues and those from ovalbumin-sensitized and -challenged mice also showed the presence of IDO-expressing eosinophils. Similarly, a study investigating the expression of IDO in tumor biopsies from 25 cases of non-small cell lung cancer showed that eosinophils were the only IDO-expressing cells in these tissues, and concluded that eosinophil-derived IDO may play a significant role in the escape of non-small cell lung cancer from immune surveillance.[174] In this study, the presence of IDO-expressing tumor-infiltrating eosinophils was strongly correlated with poor survival. When these findings are juxtaposed with previous studies investigating the prognostic value of tumor-associated tissue eosinophilia, it becomes apparent that eosinophil-derived IDO may be a major immunoregulatory mechanism in several eosinophil-associated conditions.[174,175]

EOSINOPHIL AS EFFECTOR CELLS IN WORM INFECTIONS

Infection with helminths is the most common cause of moderate to marked eosinophilia. Studies in the late 1970s demonstrated that eosinophils had the capacity to kill parasitic targets and led to the concept that eosinophils were immunoprotective.[135] As in allergic inflammation, the precise role of eosinophils in the immunopathological changes associated with helminth infections remains ill-understood and rather controversial. Increases in the number of tissue and peripheral blood eosinophils, together with a rise in the levels of total and parasite-specific IgE and mastocytosis, have been considered for a long time to be hallmarks of infection with parasitic worms,[4] particularly during their tissue migratory phases. Much has been published about the inimical role this cell may play in protection against helminths, but there is equally important evidence to suggest that their presence may be a reflection of their participation in the pathology of the disease rather than immunity to the parasitic metazoa. The original observation of Basten and Beeson[7] that helminth-associated eosinophilia is T cell-dependent was an important turning point in our current understanding of eosinophil-mediated inflammation in worm infections. The identification and subsequent cloning of GM-CSF, IL-3, and particularly IL-5 helped to explain the T cell control of eosinophilic response both in terms of eosinophilopoiesis and differentiation as well as priming and activation of the mature cell. The question, however, remains as to why there is a selective increase of eosinophils and what is their function, both locally, and systematically, in infected subjects.

■ CONCLUSIONS ■

The eosinophil is an enigmatic and fascinating cell that has continued to intrigue biomedical scientists for more than a century. The precise function of this cell in allergic inflammation and asthma remains a matter of debate and requires further study in appropriately designed research projects. However, it is vital to accept that no single cell type, whether the eosinophil, T or B cell, mast cell, neutrophil, or other lung cell, can be responsible for all aspects of the immunopathology and clinical sequelae of airway inflammation in asthma and related allergic diseases. In recognition of this fact, the attention currently focused on the eosinophil is warranted and timely. This relates partially to the overwhelming evidence in favor of a potential effector role of the eosinophil in parasitic helminthic and allergic diseases, including asthma.

While the mechanisms of eosinophilia in association with allergic disease are not yet fully understood, they seem likely to be controlled at the level of the interactions between the innate and adaptive immune response and the subsequent elaboration of cytokines which exert both direct and indirect effect on these inflammatory cells. It seems inevitable that a complex biological system that includes eosinophils and their cytokine products may participate in a cascade of events leading to allergic inflammation and ultimately manifesting as asthma.

References

Introduction

1. Gleich GJ, Adolphson CR, Leiferman KM. The biology of the eosinophilic leukocyte. Annu Rev Med 1993; 44:85–101.
2. Wardlaw AJ, Moqbel R, Kay AB. Eosinophils: biology and role in disease. Adv Immunol 1995; 60:151–266.
3. Wardlaw AJ, Moqbel R, Kay AB. Eosinophils and the allergic inflammatory response. In: Kay AB, ed. Allergy and allergic diseases. Oxford: Blackwell, 1997:171–197.
4. Kay AB, Moqbel R, Durham SR, et al. Leucocyte activation initiated by IgE-dependent mechanisms in relation to helminthic parasitic disease and clinical models of asthma. Int Arch Allergy Appl Immunol 1985; 77:69–72.
5. Wardlaw AJ, Moqbel R. The eosinophil in allergic and helminth-related inflammatory responses. In: Moqbel R, ed. Allergy and immunity to helminths. Common mechanisms or divergent pathways? London: Taylor & Francis; 1992:154–186.

Eosinophil differentiation and tissue recruitment

6. Spry CJF. Eosinophils. A comprehensive review and guide to the scientific and medical literature. Oxford: Oxford University Press, 1988:1–484.
7. Basten A, Beeson PB. Mechanism of eosinophilia. II. Role of the lymphocyte. J Exp Med 1970; 131:1288–1305.
8. Kay A, B. Asthma and inflammation. J Allergy Clin Immunol 1991; 87:893–910.
9. Corrigan CJ, Kay AB. T cells and eosinophils in the pathogenesis of asthma. Immunol Today 1992; 13:501–507.
10. Spry CJ. The natural history of eosinophils. In: Smith H, Cook RM, eds. Immunopharmacology of eosinophils. London: Academic Press, 1993:241–243.
11. Walle AJ, Parwaresch MR. Estimation of effective eosinopoiesis and bone marrow eosinophil reserve capacity in normal man. Cell Tissue Kinet 1979; 12:249–255.
12. Steinbach KH, Schick P, Trepel F, et al. Estimation of kinetic parameters of neutrophilic, eosinophilic, and basophilic granulocytes in human blood. Blut 1979; 39:27–38.

13. Krause JR, Boggs DR. Search for eosinopenia in hospitalized patients with normal blood leukocyte concentration. Am J Hematol 1987; 24:55–63.
14. Horn BR, Robin ED, Theodore J, et al. Total eosinophil counts in the management of bronchial asthma. N Engl J Med 1975; 292:1152–1155.
15. Winkel P, Statland BE, Saunders AM, et al. Within-day physiologic variation of leukocyte types in healthy subjects as assayed by two automated leukocyte differential analyzers. Am J Clin Pathol 1981; 75:693–700.
16. Denburg JA, Sehmi R, Saito H, et al. Systemic aspects of allergic disease: bone marrow responses. J Allergy Clin Immunol 2000; 106:S242–S246.
17. Inman MD, Sehmi R,O'Byrne P, et al. The role of the bone marrow in allergic disease. In: Denburg JA, ed. Allergy and allergic diseases: the new mechanisms and therapeutics. Totowa: Humana Press, 1998:85–102.
18. Dombrowicz D, Woerly G, Capron M. IgE receptors on human eosinophils. Chem Immunol 2000; 76:63–76.
19. Ackerman SJ, Kephart GM, Habermann TM, et al. Localization of eosinophil granule major basic protein in human basophils. J Exp Med 1983; 158:946–961.
20. Denburg JA. Bone marrow in atopy and asthma: hematopoietic mechanisms in allergic inflammation. Immunol Today 1999; 20:111–113.
21. Foster PS. Allergic networks regulating eosinophilia. Am J Respir Cell Mol Biol 1999; 21:451–454.
22. Hamelmann E, Gelfand EW. IL-5-induced airway eosinophilia – the key to asthma? Immunol Rev 2001; 179:182–191.
23. Sutherland DR, Stewart AK, Keating A. CD34 antigen: molecular features and potential clinical applications. Stem Cells 1993; 11:50–57.
24. Clutterbuck EJ, Hirst EM, Sanderson CJ. Human interleukin-5 (IL-5) regulates the production of eosinophils in human bone marrow cultures: comparison and interaction with IL-1, IL-3, IL-6, and GMCSF. Blood 1989; 73:1504–1512.
25. Dent LA, Strath M, Mellor AL, et al. Eosinophilia in transgenic mice expressing interleukin 5. J Exp Med 1990; 172:1425–1431.
26. Tominaga A, Takaki S, Koyama N, et al. Transgenic mice expressing a B cell growth and differentiation factor gene (interleukin 5) develop eosinophilia and autoantibody production. J Exp Med 1991; 173:429–437.
27. Giembycz MA, Lindsay MA. Pharmacology of the eosinophil. Pharmacol Rev 1999; 51:213–339.
28. Bochner BS, Schleimer RP. Mast cells, basophils, and eosinophils: distinct but overlapping pathways for recruitment. Immunol Rev 2001; 179:5–15.
29. Mishra A, Hogan SP, Lee JJ, et al. Fundamental signals that regulate eosinophil homing to the gastrointestinal tract. J Clin Invest 1999; 103:1719–1727.
30. Rothenberg ME, Mishra A, Brandt EB, et al. Gastrointestinal eosinophils. Immunol Rev 2001; 179:139–155.
31. Rothenberg ME, Owen WF Jr, Silberstein DS, et al. Eosinophils cocultured with endothelial cells have increased survival and functional properties. Science 1987; 237:645–647.
32. Rothenberg ME, Owen WF Jr, Silberstein DS, et al. Human eosinophils have prolonged survival, enhanced functional properties, and become hypodense when exposed to human interleukin 3. J Clin Invest 1988; 81:1986–1992.
33. Silberstein DS, Austen KF, Owen WF Jr. Hemopoietins for eosinophils. Glycoprotein hormones that regulate the development of inflammation in eosinophilia-associated disease. Hematol Oncol Clin North Am 1989; 3:511–533.
34. Lacy P Moqbel R. Eosinophil cytokines. Chem Immunol 2000; 76:134–155.
35. Simon HU, Yousefi S, Schranz C, et al. Direct demonstration of delayed eosinophil apoptosis as a mechanism causing tissue eosinophilia. J Immunol 1997; 158:3902–3908.
36. Foster PS, Mould AW, Yang M, et al. Elemental signals regulating eosinophil accumulation in the lung. Immunol Rev 2001; 179:173–181.
37. Cameron L, Christodoulopoulos P, Lavigne F, et al. Evidence for local eosinophil differentiation within allergic nasal mucosa: inhibition with soluble IL-5 receptor. J Immunol 2000; 164:1538–1545.
38. Eidelman DH, Minshall E, Dandurand RJ, et al. Evidence for major basic protein immunoreactivity and interleukin 5 gene activation during the late phase response in explanted airways. Am J Respir Cell Mol Biol 1996; 15:582–589.
39. Miyajima A, Kitamura T, Harada N, et al. Cytokine receptors and signal transduction. Annu Rev Immunol 1992; 10:295–331.
40. Pazdrak K, Olszewska-Pazdrak B, Stafford S, et al. Lyn, Jak2, and Raf-1 kinases are critical for the antiapoptotic effect of interleukin 5, whereas only Raf-1 kinase is essential for eosinophil activation and degranulation. J Exp Med 1998; 188:421–429.
41. Wardlaw AJ, Brightling C, Green R, et al. Eosinophils in asthma and other allergic diseases. Br Med Bull 2000; 56:985–1003.
42. Dri P, Cramer R, Spessotto P, et al. Eosinophil activation on biologic surfaces. Production of O_2- in response to physiologic soluble stimuli is differentially modulated by extracellular matrix components and endothelial cells. J Immunol 1991; 147:613–620.
43. Anwar AR, Moqbel R, Walsh GM, et al. Adhesion to fibronectin prolongs eosinophil survival. J Exp Med 1993; 177:839–843.
44. Mould AP, Wheldon LA, Komoriya A, et al. Affinity chromatographic isolation of the melanoma adhesion receptor for the IIICS region of fibronectin and its identification as the integrin alpha 4 beta 1. J Biol Chem 1990; 265:4020–4024.
45. Schleimer RP, Sterbinsky SA, Kaiser J, et al. IL-4 induces adherence of human eosinophils and basophils but not neutrophils to endothelium. Association with expression of VCAM-1. J Immunol 1992; 148:1086–1092.
46. Bochner BS, Klunk DA, Sterbinsky SA, et al. IL-13 selectively induces vascular cell adhesion molecule-1 expression in human endothelial cells. J Immunol 1995; 154:799–803.
47. Walsh GM, Mermod JJ, Hartnell A, et al. Human eosinophil, but not neutrophil, adherence to IL-1-stimulated human umbilical vascular endothelial cells is alpha 4 beta 1 (very late antigen-4) dependent. J Immunol 1991; 146:3419–3423.
48. Werfel SJ, Yednock TA, Matsumoto K, et al. Functional regulation of β_1 integrins on human eosinophils by divalent cations and cytokines. Am J Respir Cell Mol Biol 1996; 14:44–52.

49. Tachimoto H, Burdick MM, Hudson SA, et al. CCR3-active chemokines promote rapid detachment of eosinophils from VCAM-1 in vitro. J Immunol 2000; 165:2748–2754.
50. DiScipio RG, Daffern PJ, Jagels MA, et al. A comparison of C3a and C5a-mediated stable adhesion of rolling eosinophils in postcapillary venules and transendothelial migration in vitro and in vivo. J Immunol 1999; 162:1127–1136.
51. Broide D, Sriramarao P. Eosinophil trafficking to sites of allergic inflammation. Immunol Rev 2001; 179:163–172.
52. Masumoto A, Hemler ME. Multiple activation states of VLA-4. Mechanistic differences between adhesion to CS1/fibronectin and to vascular cell adhesion molecule-1. J Biol Chem 1993; 268:228–234.
53. Kitayama J, Mackay CR, Ponath PD, et al. The C-C chemokine receptor CCR3 participates in stimulation of eosinophil arrest on inflammatory endothelium in shear flow. J Clin Invest 1998; 101:2017–2024.
54. Shahabuddin S, Ponath P, Schleimer RP. Migration of eosinophils across endothelial cell monolayers: interactions among IL-5, endothelial-activating cytokines, and C-C chemokines. J Immunol 2000; 164:3847–3854.
55. Jose PJ, Griffiths-Johnson DA, Collins PD, et al. Eotaxin: a potent eosinophil chemoattractant cytokine detected in a guinea pig model of allergic airways inflammation. J Exp Med 1994; 179:881–887.
56. Alam R, Stafford S, Forsythe P, et al. RANTES is a chemotactic and activating factor for human eosinophils. J Immunol 1993; 150:3442–3448.
57. Rothenberg ME. Eotaxin. An essential mediator of eosinophil trafficking into mucosal tissues. Am J Respir Cell Mol Biol 1999; 21:291–295.
58. Schall TJ. Biology of the RANTES/SIS cytokine family. Cytokine 1991; 3:165–183.
59. Fryer AD, Stein LH, Nie Z, et al. Neuronal eotaxin and the effects of CCR3 antagonist on airway hyperreactivity and M2 receptor dysfunction. J Clin Invest 2006; 116:228–236.
60. Zimmermann N, Hogan SP, Mishra A, et al. Murine eotaxin-2: a constitutive eosinophil chemokine induced by allergen challenge and IL-4 overexpression. J Immunol 2000; 165:5839–5846.
61. Rothenberg ME, Luster AD, Lilly CM, et al. Constitutive and allergen-induced expression of eotaxin mRNA in the guinea pig lung. J Exp Med 1995; 181:1211–1216.
62. Collins PD, Marleau S, Griffiths-Johnson DA, et al. Cooperation between interleukin-5 and the chemokine eotaxin to induce eosinophil accumulation in vivo. J Exp Med 1995; 182:1169–1174.
63. Mould AW, Ramsay AJ, Matthaei KI, et al. The effect of IL-5 and eotaxin expression in the lung on eosinophil trafficking and degranulation and the induction of bronchial hyperreactivity. J Immunol 2000; 164:2142–2150.
64. Kita H, Kaneko M, Bartemes KR, et al. Does IgE bind to and activate eosinophils from patients with allergy? J Immunol 1999; 162:6901–6911.
65. Seminario MC, Saini SS, MacGlashan DW Jr, et al. Intracellular expression and release of Fc epsilon RI alpha by human eosinophils. J Immunol 1999; 162:6893–6900.
66. Abu-Ghazaleh RI, Fujisawa T, Mestecky J, et al. IgA-induced eosinophil degranulation. J Immunol 1989; 142:2393–2400.
67. Kita H, Abu-Ghazaleh RI, Gleich GJ, et al. Regulation of Ig-induced eosinophil degranulation by adenosine 3',5'- cyclic monophosphate. J Immunol 1991; 146:2712–2718.

Surface markers in eosinophils

68. Rothenberg ME, Hogan SP. The eosinophil. Annu Rev Immunol 2006; 24:147–174.

Eosinophil-derived mediators

69. Zhu X, Munoz NM, Rubio N, et al. Quantitation of the cytosolic phospholipase A2 (type IV) in isolated human peripheral blood eosinophils by sandwich-ELISA. J Immunol Methods 1996; 199:119–126.
70. Blom M, Tool AT, Wever PC, et al. Human eosinophils express, relative to other circulating leukocytes, large amounts of secretory 14-kD phospholipase A2. Blood 1998; 91:3037–3043.
71. Weller PF, Lee CW, Foster DW, et al. Generation and metabolism of 5-lipoxygenase pathway leukotrienes by human eosinophils: predominant production of leukotriene C4. Proc Natl Acad Sci U S A 1983; 80:7626–7630.
72. Shaw RJ, Cromwell O, Kay AB. Preferential generation of leukotriene C4 by human eosinophils. Clin Exp Immunol 1984; 56:716–722.
73. Shaw RJ, Walsh GM, Cromwell O, et al. Activated human eosinophils generate SRS-A leukotrienes following IgG-dependent stimulation. Nature 1985; 316:150–152.
74. Cowburn AS, Holgate ST, Sampson AP. IL-5 increases expression of 5-lipoxygenase-activating protein and translocates 5-lipoxygenase to the nucleus in human blood eosinophils. J Immunol 1999; 163:456–465.
75. Cowburn AS, Sladek K, Soja J, et al. Overexpression of leukotriene C4 synthase in bronchial biopsies from patients with aspirin-intolerant asthma. J Clin Invest 1998; 101:834–846.
76. Lam BK, Owen WF Jr, Austen KF, et al. The identification of a distinct export step following the biosynthesis of leukotriene C4 by human eosinophils. J Biol Chem 1989; 264:12885–12889.
77. Nasser SM, Lee TH. Products of 15-lipoxygenase: are they important in asthma? Clin Exp Allergy 2002; 32:1540–1542.
78. Holtzman MJ, Pentland A, Baenziger NL, et al. Heterogeneity of cellular expression of arachidonate 15-lipoxygenase: implications for biological activity. Biochim Biophys Acta 1989; 1003:204–208.
79. Bradding P, Redington AE, Djukanovic R, et al. 15-lipoxygenase immunoreactivity in normal and in asthmatic airways. Am J Respir Crit Care Med 1995; 151:1201–1204.
80. Chu HW, Balzar S, Westcott JY, et al. Expression and activation of 15-lipoxygenase pathway in severe asthma: relationship to eosinophilic phenotype and collagen deposition. Clin Exp Allergy 2002; 32:1558–1565.
81. Lee T, Lenihan DJ, Malone B, et al. Increased biosynthesis of platelet-activating factor in activated human eosinophils. J Biol Chem 1984; 259:5526–5530.
82. Cromwell O, Wardlaw AJ, Champion A, et al. IgG-dependent generation of platelet-activating factor by normal and low density human eosinophils. J Immunol 1990; 145:3862–3868.
83. Giembycz MA, Kroegel C, Barnes PJ. Platelet activating factor stimulates cyclo-oxygenase activity in guinea pig eosinophils. Concerted biosynthesis of thromboxane A2 and E- series prostaglandins. J Immunol 1990; 144:3489–3497.
84. Dvorak AM, Morgan E, Schleimer RP, et al. Ultrastructural immunogold localization of prostaglandin endoperoxide synthase (cyclooxygenase) to non-membrane-bound cytoplasmic lipid bodies in human lung mast cells, alveolar macrophages, type II pneumocytes, and neutrophils. J Histochem Cytochem 1992; 40:759–769.
85. Bozza PT, Yu W, Penrose JF, et al. Eosinophil lipid bodies: specific, inducible intracellular sites for enhanced eicosanoid formation. J Exp Med 1997; 186:909–920.
86. Gleich GJ, Loegering DA, Maldonado JE. Identification of a major basic protein in guinea pig eosinophil granules. J Exp Med 1973; 137:1459–1471.
87. Hamann KJ, Barker RL, Ten RM, et al. The molecular biology of eosinophil granule proteins. Int Arch Allergy Appl Immunol 1991; 94:202–209.
88. Popken-Harris P, McGrogan M, Loegering DA, et al. Expression, purification, and characterization of the recombinant proform of eosinophil granule major basic protein. J Immunol 1995; 155:1472–1480.
89. Popken-Harris P, Checkel J, Loegering D, et al. Regulation and processing of a precursor form of eosinophil granule major basic protein (ProMBP) in differentiating eosinophils. Blood 1998; 92:623–631.
90. Shalit M, Sekhsaria S, Mauhorter S, et al. Early commitment to the eosinophil lineage by cultured human peripheral blood CD34+ cells: messenger RNA analysis. J Allergy Clin Immunol 1996; 98:344–354.
91. Moy JN, Gleich GJ, Thomas LL. Noncytotoxic activation of neutrophils by eosinophil granule major basic protein. Effect on superoxide anion generation and lysosomal enzyme release. J Immunol 1990; 145:2626–2632.
92. Kita H, Abu-Ghazaleh RI, Sur S, et al. Eosinophil major basic protein induces degranulation and IL-8 production by human eosinophils. J Immunol 1995; 154:4749–4758.
93. Page SM, Gleich GJ, Roebuck KA, et al. Stimulation of neutrophil interleukin-8 production by eosinophil granule major basic protein. Am J Respir Cell Mol Biol 1999; 21:230–237.
94. O'Donnell MC, Ackerman SJ, Gleich GJ, et al. Activation of basophil and mast cell histamine release by eosinophil granule major basic protein. J Exp Med 1983; 157:1981–1991.
95. Adamko DJ, Yost BL, Gleich GJ, et al. Ovalbumin sensitization changes the inflammatory response to subsequent parainfluenza infection. Eosinophils mediate airway hyperresponsiveness, M2 muscarinic receptor dysfunction, and antiviral effects. J Exp Med 1999; 190:1465–1478.
96. Costello RW, Schofield BH, Kephart GM, et al. Localization of eosinophils to airway nerves and effect on neuronal M2 muscarinic receptor function. Am J Physiol 1997; 273:L93–103.
97. Filley WV, Holley KE, Kephart GM, et al. Identification by immunofluorescence of eosinophil granule major basic protein in lung tissues of patients with bronchial asthma. Lancet 1982; 2:11–16.
98. Brightling CE, Bradding P, Symon FA, et al. Mast-cell infiltration of airway smooth muscle in asthma. N Engl J Med 2002; 346:1699–1705.
99. Evans CM, Fryer AD, Jacoby DB, et al. Pretreatment with antibody to eosinophil major basic protein prevents hyperresponsiveness by protecting neuronal M2 muscarinic receptors in antigen-challenged guinea pigs. J Clin Invest 1997; 100:2254–2262.
100. Adamko DJ, Fryer AD, Bochner BS, et al. CD8+ T lymphocytes in viral hyperreactivity and M2 muscarinic receptor dysfunction. Am J Respir Crit Care Med 2003; 167:550–556.
101. Wasmoen TL, Bell MP, Loegering DA, et al. Biochemical and amino acid sequence analysis of human eosinophil granule major basic protein. J Biol Chem 1988; 263:12559–12563.
102. Lee JJ, Dimina D, Macias MP, et al. Defining a link with asthma in mice congenitally deficient in eosinophils. Science 2004; 305:1773–1776.
103. Ten RM, Pease LR, McKean DJ, et al. Molecular cloning of the human eosinophil peroxidase. Evidence for the existence of a peroxidase multigene family. J Exp Med 1989; 169:1757–1769.
104. Weiss SJ, Test ST, Eckmann CM, et al. Brominating oxidants generated by human eosinophils. Science 1986; 234:200–203.
105. Mayeno AN, Curran AJ, Roberts RL, et al. Eosinophils preferentially use bromide to generate halogenating agents. J Biol Chem 1989; 264:5660–5668.
106. Gleich GJ, Loegering DA, Bell MP, et al. Biochemical and functional similarities between human eosinophil-derived neurotoxin and eosinophil cationic protein: homology with ribonuclease. Proc Natl Acad Sci U S A 1986; 83:3146–3150.
107. Lehrer RI, Szklarek D, Barton A, et al. Antibacterial properties of eosinophil major basic protein and eosinophil cationic protein. J Immunol 1989; 142:4428–4434.
108. Young JD, Peterson CG, Venge P, et al. Mechanism of membrane damage mediated by human eosinophil cationic protein. Nature 1986; 321:613–616.
109. Durack DT, Sumi SM, Klebanoff SJ. Neurotoxicity of human eosinophils. Proc Natl Acad Sci U S A 1979; 76:1443–1447.
110. Fredens K, Dahl R, Venge P. The Gordon phenomenon induced by the eosinophil cationic protein and eosinophil protein X. J Allergy Clin Immunol 1982; 70:361–366.
111. Hamann KJ, Ten RM, Loegering DA, et al. Structure and chromosome localization of the human eosinophil-derived neurotoxin and eosinophil cationic protein genes: evidence for intronless coding sequences in the ribonuclease gene superfamily. Genomics 1990; 7:535–546.
112. Rosenberg HF, Dyer KD, Tiffany HL, et al. Rapid evolution of a unique family of primate ribonuclease genes. Nat Genet 1995; 10:219–223.
113. Rosenberg HF, Domachowske JB. Eosinophils, eosinophil ribonucleases, and their role in host defense against respiratory virus pathogens. J Leukoc Biol 2001; 70:691–698.
114. Ackerman SJ, Liu L, Kwatia MA, et al. Charcot-Leyden crystal protein (galectin-10) is not a dual function galectin with lysophospholipase activity but binds a lysophospholipase inhibitor in a novel structural fashion. J Biol Chem 2002; 277:14859–14868.
115. Lacy P, Moqbel R. Immune effector functions of eosinophils in allergic airway inflammation. Curr Opin Allergy Clin Immunol 2001; 1:79–84.

116. Moqbel R, Hamid Q, Ying S, et al. Expression of mRNA and immunoreactivity for the granulocyte/macrophage colony-stimulating factor in activated human eosinophils. J Exp Med 1991; 174:749–752.

117. Kita H, Ohnishi T, Okubo Y, et al. Granulocyte/macrophage colony-stimulating factor and interleukin 3 release from human peripheral blood eosinophils and neutrophils. J Exp Med 1991; 174:745–748.

118. Lacy P, Mahmudi-Azer S, Bablitz B, et al. Rapid mobilization of intracellularly stored RANTES in response to interferon-γ in human eosinophils. Blood 1999; 94:23–32.

119. Hamid Q, Barkans J, Meng Q, et al. Human eosinophils synthesize and secrete interleukin-6, in vitro. Blood 1992; 80:1496–1501.

120. Wong DT, Weller PF, Galli SJ, et al. Human eosinophils express transforming growth factor α. J Exp Med 1990; 172:673–681.

121. Wong DT, Elovic A, Matossian K, et al. Eosinophils from patients with blood eosinophilia express transforming growth factor β1. Blood 1991; 78:2702–2707.

122. Desreumaux P, Janin A, Colombel JF, et al. Interleukin 5 messenger RNA expression by eosinophils in the intestinal mucosa of patients with coeliac disease. J Exp Med 1992; 175:293–296.

123. Broide DH, Paine MM, Firestein GS. Eosinophils express interleukin 5 and granulocyte macrophage-colony- stimulating factor mRNA at sites of allergic inflammation in asthmatics. J Clin Invest 1992; 90:1414–1424.

124. Beil WJ, Weller PF, Tzizik DM, et al. Ultrastructural immunogold localization of tumor necrosis factor-α to the matrix compartment of eosinophil secondary granules in patients with idiopathic hypereosinophilic syndrome. J Histochem Cytochem 1993; 41:1611–1615.

125. Dubucquoi S, Desreumaux P, Janin A, et al. Interleukin 5 synthesis by eosinophils: association with granules and immunoglobulin-dependent secretion. J Exp Med 1994; 179:703–708.

126. Levi-Schaffer F, Lacy P, Severs NJ, et al. Association of granulocyte-macrophage colony-stimulating factor with the crystalloid granules of human eosinophils. Blood 1995; 85:2579–2586.

127. Moqbel R, Ying S, Barkans J, et al. Identification of messenger RNA for IL-4 in human eosinophils with granule localization and release of the translated product. J Immunol 1995; 155:4939–4947.

128. Levi-Schaffer F, Barkans J, Newman TM, et al. Identification of interleukin-2 in human peripheral blood eosinophils. Immunology 1996; 87:155–161.

129. Lacy P, Levi-Schaffer F, Mahmudi-Azer S, et al. Intracellular localization of interleukin-6 in eosinophils from atopic asthmatics and effects of interferon γ. Blood 1998; 91:2508–2516.

130. Gauvreau GM, O'Byrne PM, Moqbel R, et al. Enhanced expression of GM-CSF in differentiating eosinophils of atopic and atopic asthmatic subjects. Am J Respir Cell Mol Biol 1998; 19:55–62.

131. Velazquez JR, Lacy P, Mahmudi-Azer S, et al. Interleukin-4 and RANTES expression in maturing eosinophils derived from human cord blood CD34+ progenitors. Immunology 2000; 101:419–425.

132. Mahmudi-Azer S, Velazquez JR, Lacy P, et al. Immunofluorescence analysis of cytokine and granule protein expression during eosinophil maturation from cord blood-derived CD34 progenitors. J Allergy Clin Immunol 2000; 105:1178–1184.

133. Egesten A, Calafat J, Knol EF, et al. Subcellular localization of transforming growth factor-α in human eosinophil granulocytes. Blood 1996; 87:3910–3918.

134. Bandeira-Melo C, Gillard G, Ghiran I, et al. EliCell: a gel-phase dual antibody capture and detection assay to measure cytokine release from eosinophils. J Immunol Methods 2000; 244:105–115.

135. Butterworth AE, Thorne KJ. Eosinophils and parasitic diseases. In: Smith H, Cook RM, eds. Immunopharmacology of eosinophils. London: Academic Press, 1993:119–150.

136. DeLeo FR, Quinn MT. Assembly of the phagocyte NADPH oxidase: molecular interaction of oxidase proteins. J Leukoc Biol 1996; 60:677–691.

137. Bolscher BG, Koenderman L, Tool AT, et al. NADPH:O₂ oxidoreductase of human eosinophils in the cell-free system. FEBS Lett 1990; 268:269–273.

138. DeChatelet LR, Shirley PS, McPhail LC, et al. Oxidative metabolism of the human eosinophil. Blood 1977; 50:525–535.

139. Lacy P, Abdel Latif D, Steward M, et al. Divergence of mechanisms regulating respiratory burst in blood and sputum eosinophils and neutrophils from atopic subjects. J Immunol 2003; 170:2670–2679.

140. Carlyon JA, Abdel-Latif D, Pypaert M, et al. Anaplasma phagocytophilum utilizes multiple host evasion mechanisms to thwart NADPH oxidase-mediated killing during neutrophil infection. Infect Immun 2004; 72:4772–4783.

141. Moqbel R, Lacy P. Exocytotic events in eosinophils and mast cells. Clin Exp Allergy 1999; 29:1017–1022.

142. Hartmann J, Scepek S, Lindau M. Regulation of granule size in human and horse eosinophils by number of fusion events among unit granules. J Physiol (Lond) 1995; 483:201–209.

143. Scepek S, Moqbel R, Lindau M. Compound exocytosis and cumulative degranulation by eosinophils and its role in parasitic killing. Parasitol Today 1994; 10:276–278.

144. Newman TM, Tian M, Gomperts BD. Ultrastructural characterization of tannic acid-arrested degranulation of permeabilized guinea pig eosinophils stimulated with GTP-γ-S. Eur J Cell Biol 1996; 70:209–220.

145. McLaren DJ, Mackenzie CD, Ramalho-Pinto FJ. Ultrastructural observations on the in vitro interaction between rat eosinophils and some parasitic helminths (Schistosoma mansoni, Trichinella spiralis and Nippostrongylus brasiliensis). Clin Exp Immunol 1977; 30:105–118.

146. Mahmudi-Azer S, Downey GP, Moqbel R. Translocation of the tetraspanin CD63 in association with human eosinophil mediator release. Blood 2002; 99:4039–4047.

147. Dvorak AM, Furitsu T, Letourneau L, et al. Mature eosinophils stimulated to develop in human cord blood mononuclear cell cultures supplemented with recombinant human interleukin-5. Part I. Piecemeal degranulation of specific granules and distribution of Charcot-Leyden crystal protein. Am J Pathol 1991; 138:69–82.

148. Erjefält JS, Andersson M, Greiff L, et al. Cytolysis and piecemeal degranulation as distinct modes of activation of airway mucosal eosinophils. J Allergy Clin Immunol 1998; 102:286–294.

149. Persson CG, Erjefält JS. Eosinophil lysis and free granules: an in vivo paradigm for cell activation and drug development. Trends Pharmacol Sci 1997; 18:117–123.

150. Fukuda T, Ackerman SJ, Reed CE, et al. Calcium ionophore A23187 calcium-dependent cytolytic degranulation in human eosinophils. J Immunol 1985; 135:1349–1356.

151. Söllner T, Whiteheart SW, Brunner M, et al. SNAP receptors implicated in vesicle targeting and fusion. Nature 1993; 362:318–324.

152. Ravichandran V, Chawla A, Roche PA. Identification of a novel syntaxin- and synaptobrevin/VAMP- binding protein, SNAP-23, expressed in non-neuronal tissues. J Biol Chem 1996; 271:13300–13303.

153. Lacy P, Logan MR, Bablitz B, et al. Fusion protein vesicle-associated membrane protein 2 is implicated in IFN-γ-induced piecemeal degranulation in human eosinophils from atopic individuals. J Allergy Clin Immunol 2001; 107:671–678.

154. Logan MR, Lacy P, Odemuyiwa SO, et al. A critical role for vesicle-associated membrane protein-7 in exocytosis from human eosinophils and neutrophils. Allergy 2006; 61:777–784.

155. Logan MR, Lacy P, Bablitz B, et al. Expression of eosinophil target SNAREs as potential cognate receptors for vesicle-associated membrane protein-2 in exocytosis. J Allergy Clin Immunol 2002; 109:299–306.

156. Sabin EA, Kopf MA, Pearce EJ. Schistosoma mansoni egg-induced early IL-4 production is dependent upon IL-5 and eosinophils. J Exp Med 1996; 184:1871–1878.

157. Woerly G, Roger N, Loiseau S, et al. Expression of CD28 and CD86 by human eosinophils and role in the secretion of type 1 cytokines (interleukin 2 and interferon γ): inhibition by immunoglobulin a complexes. J Exp Med 1999; 190:487–495.

158. Woerly G, Lacy P, Younes AB, et al. Human eosinophils express and release IL-13 following CD28-dependent activation. J Leukoc Biol 2002; 72:769–779.

159. Voehringer D, Reese TA, Huang X, et al. Type 2 immunity is controlled by IL-4/IL-13 expression in hematopoietic non-eosinophil cells of the innate immune system. J Exp Med 2006; 203:1435–1446.

160. Shi HZ, Humbles A, Gerard C, et al. Lymph node trafficking and antigen presentation by endobronchial eosinophils. J Clin Invest 2000; 105:945–953.

161. Corrigan CJ. T cells in asthma. In: Holgate ST, Busse WW, eds. Inflammatory mechanisms in asthma. New York: Marcel Dekker, 1998:343–359.

162. Wills-Karp M, Luyimbazi J, Xu X, et al. Interleukin-13: central mediator of allergic asthma. Science 1998; 282:2258–2261.

163. Shi HZ, Xiao CQ, Li CQ, et al. Endobronchial eosinophils preferentially stimulate T helper cell type 2 responses. Allergy 2004; 59:428–435.

164. Munn DH, Zhou M, Attwood JT, et al. Prevention of allogeneic fetal rejection by tryptophan catabolism. Science 1998; 281:1191–1193.

165. Mellor AL, Munn DH. IDO expression by dendritic cells: tolerance and tryptophan catabolism. Nat Rev Immunol 2004; 4:762–774.

166. Uyttenhove C, Pilotte L, Theate I, et al. Evidence for a tumoral immune resistance mechanism based on tryptophan degradation by indoleamine 2,3-dioxygenase. Nat Med 2003; 9:1269–1274.

167. Grohmann U, Fallarino F, Bianchi R, et al. A defect in tryptophan catabolism impairs tolerance in nonobese diabetic mice. J Exp Med 2003; 198:153–160.

168. Gurtner GJ, Newberry RD, Schloemann SR, et al. Inhibition of indoleamine 2,3-dioxygenase augments trinitrobenzene sulfonic acid colitis in mice. Gastroenterology 2003; 125:1762–1773.

169. Mellor AL, Chandler P, Baban B, et al. Specific subsets of murine dendritic cells acquire potent T cell regulatory functions following CTLA4-mediated induction of indoleamine 2,3 dioxygenase. Int Immunol 2004; 16:1391–1401.

170. Baban B, Hansen AM, Chandler PR, et al. A minor population of splenic dendritic cells expressing CD19 mediates IDO-dependent T cell suppression via type I IFN signaling following B7 ligation. Int Immunol 2005; 17:909–919.

171. Munn DH, Sharma MD, Mellor AL. Ligation of B7–1/B7–2 by human CD4+ T cells triggers indoleamine 2,3-dioxygenase activity in dendritic cells. J Immunol 2004; 172:4100–4110.

172. Grohmann U, Orabona C, Fallarino F, et al. CTLA-4-Ig regulates tryptophan catabolism in vivo. Nat Immunol 2002; 3:1097–1101.

173. Odemuyiwa SO, Ghahary A, Li Y, et al. Cutting edge: human eosinophils regulate T cell subset selection through indoleamine 2,3-dioxygenase. J Immunol 2004; 173:5909–5913.

174. Astigiano S, Morandi B, Costa R, et al. Eosinophil granulocytes account for indoleamine 2,3-dioxygenase-mediated immune escape in human non-small cell lung cancer. Neoplasia 2005; 7:390–396.

175. Finkelman FD, Pearce EJ, Urban JF Jr et al. Regulation and biological function of helminth-induced cytokine responses. Immunol Today 1991; 12:A62–A66.

Biology of Mast Cells and Their Mediators

19

F Ida Hsu and Joshua A Boyce

CONTENTS

- Introduction 311
- Histologic identification of mast cells 311
- Morphology of mast cells 312
- Mast cell growth and development 315
- Activating and inhibitory receptors of mast cells 318
- Mast cell-derived mediators 319
- Mast cell pathobiology 323
- Summary 325

SUMMARY OF IMPORTANT CONCEPTS

>> Besides their role in IgE-mediated responses, mast cells are sentinels of innate immune responses and can be activated by a wide range of pathogens

>> Normal mast cell development depends on the interaction of the c-Kit tyrosine kinase and membrane-bound stem cell factor

>> Deficient c-Kit signaling results in mast cell deficiency (W/Wv mice). Gain-of-function mutations in c-Kit result in mastocytosis in humans

>> Mast cell hyperplasia in mucosal epithelial surfaces is T cell-dependent, reflecting functions of IL-3, IL-4, and IL-9

>> Mast cell activation results in both immediate (degranulation, lipid mediator production) and late (cytokine secretion) mediator release

INTRODUCTION

Mast cells are potent tissue-dwelling effector cells of hematopoietic origin. In addition to their role in allergy, they are implicated in innate immunity to bacterial and parasitic infections on the basis of animal

studies. They are particularly abundant in a perivascular distribution in connective tissues and at mucosal surfaces. Classic mast cell-mediated hypersensitivity (allergic) reactions are initiated by the binding of multivalent allergen to membrane-bound IgE that is coupled to the tetrameric high-affinity Fc receptor for IgE (FcεRI) on mast cells. IgE-dependent activation of mast cells results in their release of preformed inflammatory mediators that are stored in their secretory granules, including histamine, neutral proteases, preformed cytokines, and proteoglycans (Table 19.1). Additionally, mast cells activated via FcεRI secrete newly synthesized lipid mediators that are the products of endogenous arachidonic acid metabolism, such as prostaglandin (PG) D_2, leukotriene (LT) B_4, and LTC_4, the parent molecule of the cysteinyl leukotrienes (cys-LTs). Finally, activated mast cells synthesize and secrete a host of proinflammatory cytokines. The net result of tissue mast cell activation thus includes the rapid development of plasma extravasation, tissue edema, bronchoconstriction, leukocyte recruitment, and persistent inflammation, with the clinically recognizable syndromes of anaphylaxis, urticaria, angioedema, and acute exacerbations of asthma. The importance of mast cells and their products in allergic diseases is supported by the fact that pharmacologic pretreatment of susceptible humans with cromolyn, an inhibitor of mast cell exocytosis, attenuates symptoms in response to allergen challenge.[1] Recent advances in the developmental biology of mast cells and the use of mast cell-deficient mice in an array of experimental disease models have tremendously expanded the scope of mast cell biology and its implications for disease treatment. This chapter deals with the current understanding of mast cell development, the effector capabilities of mast cells, the mediators released, and the relevance of these findings to disease and immunity.

HISTOLOGIC IDENTIFICATION OF MAST CELLS

Mast cells were originally identified in 1878 by Paul Ehrlich in his doctoral thesis presented at Leipzig University, Germany. Ehrlich described them as granular cells in connective tissue that stained purple with aniline dyes, a property known as 'metachromasia'.[2] He noted that these

Table 19.1 Preformed mediators of mast cells

Type	Mediator	Major functions
Biogenic amine	Histamine	Vasopermeability; vasodilation; smooth muscle contraction; secretion of gastric acid; pruritus through actions on endothelial cells, smooth muscle, and nerve endings
Neutral proteases	Tryptase	Degrades fibrinogen; attracts neutrophils through induction of IL-8; stimulates angiogenesis, fibroblast and epithelial proliferation; cleaves complement factors C3 and C3a; degrades VIP and CGRP; kallikrein-like activity
	Chymase	Converts angiotensin to angiotensin II; degrades extracellular matrix; affects endothelin and lipoprotein metabolism; activates matrix metalloproteinases; stimulates angiogenesis; degrades C3a, VIP, substance P, SCF, procollagen, and cytokines including IL-6 and TNF-α; stimulates bronchial mucus secretion; chemoattractant for monocytes, neutrophils
	Carboxypeptidase	Carboxypeptidase-A-like activity, acts in concert with other proteases, may protect against venoms
Acid hydrolases	β-hexosaminidase	Cleavage of β-linked hexosamines from complex carbohydrates and glycoproteins, used experimentally as an easily quantifiable marker of in vitro mast cell activation
	β-glucuronidase, β-D-galactosidase	Removes β-linked glucuronic acid or galactose from complex carbohydrate chains
	Arylsulfatase	Hydrolyzes sulfate esters of aromatic compounds
Proteoglycans	Heparin	Anticoagulant, necessary for granule storage and substrate specificity of proteases and histamine
	Chondroitin sulfate	Unknown – probably protease storage function
Preformed cytokine	TNF-α	Leukocyte recruitment, effects on dendritic cell and lymphocyte functions

VIP, vasoactive intestinal peptide; CGRP, calcitonin gene-related peptide; SCF, stem cell factor.

cells had 'a tendency to collect around developing preformed structures in the connective tissue', such as blood vessels, nerves, secretory ducts, sites of inflammation, and neoplastic foci. Metachromatic staining of granules with toluidine blue remains a classic feature by which mast cells are identified (Fig. 19.1) and is a property that they share with basophils (further discussed in Chapter 20).

MORPHOLOGY OF MAST CELLS

Mature human mast cells range from 7 to 20 μm in diameter and appear as round, spindle-shaped, or spiderlike cells in tissues with round or oval nuclei. They have thin 1–2 μm processes (microplicae) emanating from their plasma membranes (Fig. 19.2A). The most notable feature of mature tissue mast cells is their abundant cytoplasmic secretory granules that constitute about half of their volume. The metachromatic staining of mast cell granules reflects their content of sulfated proteoglycans that bind mediators such as histamine and proteases. Reagents that detect mast cell-specific proteases, such as chloroacetate esterase activity (an indicator of chymotryptic proteases), or immunoreactivity for their trypsin-like proteases (tryptases) (Fig. 19.1) also provide reliable markers of mature mast cells.

Mast cells in different tissue locations vary in their granule content. In human tissues, mast cell granules may contain either tryptase alone (designated MC_T) or a combination of tryptase, mast cell-specific chymase, carboxypeptidase A, and cathepsin G (designated MC_{TC}). Each of these

granule types predominates in the mast cells of particular locations. MC_T are the primary type of mast cell in lung alveoli, the mucosa of the small intestine, and the mucosa in allergic eye disease. MC_{TC} predominate in normal skin, blood vessels, the submucosa, and synovium. With mucosal inflammation, a selective increase in MC_T occurs in the involved epithelial surface. At the ultrastructural level, the secretory granules of human mast cells contain electron-dense material with crystalline features. With IgE-dependent stimulation, the crystalline structures become amorphous, and only amorphous material is discharged as the granules fuse with the plasma membrane. The crystalline granules contain one of three structural arrangements: scrolls (Fig. 19.2B); gratings (parallel electron-dense lines separated by lucent areas) (Fig. 19.2C); and lattices (two sets of parallel, electron-dense lines running in different directions) (Fig. 19.2D). All three crystal patterns may be present in a single granule. The relative amounts of these granule structures differ among the mast cells at different tissue locations in humans and likely reflect corresponding differences in protease and proteoglycan content. The granules of mast cells in breast parenchyma, skin, axillary lymph nodes, and bowel submucosa contain relatively few scrolls ('scroll-poor' granules) but are rich in gratings and lattices, indicating the presence of chymase, whereas mast cells in the lung alveoli and in the bowel mucosa contain many scrolls ('scroll-rich') but relatively few gratings and lattices.[3] These scroll-rich cells tend to lack chymase. Studies of human mast cells developing in the tissues of immunodeficient mice that received infusions of umbilical cord blood CD34+ progenitor cells indicate that protease content is determined by the specific tissue microenvironment rather than by the characteristics

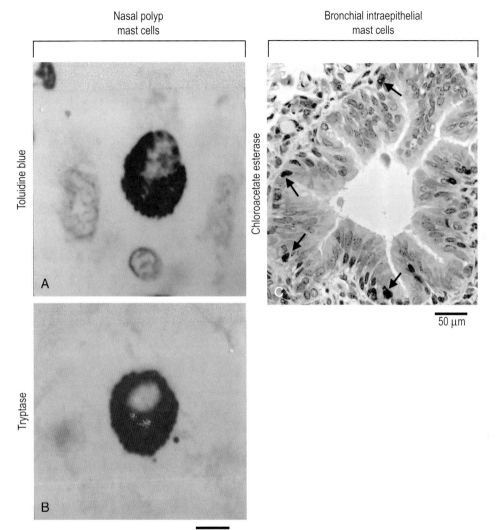

Nasal polyp mast cells

Bronchial intraepithelial mast cells

Toluidine blue

Chloroacetate esterase

Tryptase

50 μm

10 μm

Fig. 19.1. Staining and immunohistochemical features of mast cells. (A,B) Sections of an excised human nasal polyp show prominent granule metachromasia with toluidine blue and immunoreactivity with an antitryptase antibody. (C) Section of a mouse bronchus with red staining of mast cells (arrows) indicative of chloroacetate esterase activity. (Photomicrograph courtesy of Daniel S Friend, MD, Harvard Medical School.)

of the progenitor cell per se.[4] The distribution of MC_T and MC_{TC} in normal human tissue sections is summarized in Table 19.2.

In rodents, the heterogeneity of mast cell granules is defined by their distinctive responses to fixation and histochemical staining. Rodent *mucosal mast cells* (MMCs) contain chondroitin sulfate as their dominant proteoglycan, whereas *connective tissue mast cells* (CTMCs) contain heparin proteoglycan as well as chondroitin sulfate. MMCs in the gastrointestinal mucosa stain metachromatically with Alcian blue but not safranin, and they are rendered invisible by formalin fixation and hence are referred to as formalin-sensitive.[5] CTMCs in the mesentery and submucosa of the intestine and in the skin are formalin-tolerant and safranin-positive. Rodent MMCs and CTMCs can also be distinguished

by their expression patterns of mast cell-specific proteases (Table 19.2). Rat MMCs contain chymase II, while CTMCs contain chymase I and carboxypeptidase A.[6] Mouse mast cells express at least seven different chymases (MMCP-1 through 5, 8, and 9) and two tryptases (MMCP-6 and 7). MMCP-1 is unique to MMCs, and MMCP-5 is expressed only in CTMCs. Unlike human mast cells, which almost all express tryptase, the mouse tryptases (MMCP-6 and 7) are primarily limited to CTMCs.[7]

Mast cell heterogeneity extends to their content of histamine and other biogenic amines, capacity for arachidonic acid metabolism, and functional responses to immunologic and pharmacologic stimuli. These features are summarized in Table 19.2.

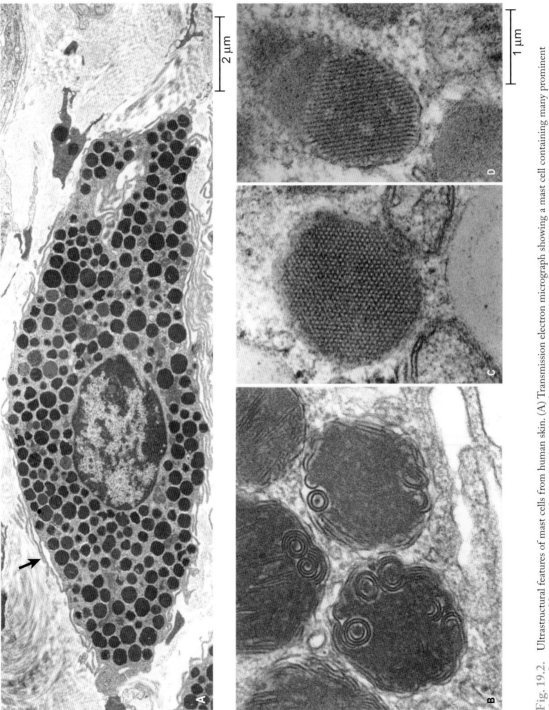

Fig. 19.2. Ultrastructural features of mast cells from human skin. (A) Transmission electron micrograph showing a mast cell containing many prominent electron-dense granules. Note 1–2 μm processes (microplicae) emanating from the plasma membrane (arrow). Higher magnification of electron-dense granule crystals shows three structural arrangements: scrolls (B), gratings (C), and lattices (D). (Photomicrograph courtesy of Daniel S Friend, MD, Harvard Medical School.)

Table 19.2 Mast cell heterogeneity

Cell type	Human mast cells		Mouse mast cells	
	MC$_T$	**MC$_{TC}$**	**MMCs**	**CTMCs**
Biogenic amine	Histamine	Histamine	Histamine	Histamine, serotonin
Granule proteases	Tryptase	Tryptase, chymase, carboxypeptidase, cathepsin-G	Chymases, MMCP-1,2,4,9	Chymases, MMCP-3,4,5,8, tryptases MMCP-6,7
Proteoglycans	Heparin, chondroitin sulfate	Heparin, chondroitin sulfate	Chondroitin sulfate	Heparin, chondroitin sulfate
Granule ultrastructure	Scroll-rich	Gratings/lattices, 'scroll-poor'		
Tissue distribution	Mucosal surfaces, alveoli, bronchi allergic conjunctiva	Skin, submucosa, normal conjunctiva, synovium heart vascular wall	Mucosal surfaces	Connective tissues, peritoneal cavity
T-cell dependency	Yes	No	Yes	No
Staining	Metachromatic	Metachromatic	Formalin-sensitive, safranin-negative	Formalin-tolerant, safranin-positive
Arachidonic acid metabolism	PGD$_2$, LTC$_4$	PGD$_2$ (skin MCs)		
Responses to stimuli	Antigen, anti-IgE, calcium ionophore	Antigen, anti-IgE, calcium ionophore, compound 40/80 basic polypeptides, morphine sulfate fMLP peptides substance P VIP, somatostatin C5a		
Pharmacologic inhibition	Release inhibited by chromones	Chromones not effective		

MMCP, mouse mast cell protease; MC, mast cell; PGD$_2$, prostaglandin D$_2$, LTC$_4$, leukotriene C$_4$, VIP, vasoactive intestinal peptide.

MAST CELL GROWTH AND DEVELOPMENT

ORIGINS OF MAST CELLS

The receptor protein-tyrosine kinase Kit (CD117) is encoded by the proto-oncogene c-*kit*. Mice with loss-of-function mutations in c-*kit* (W/W^v; W=white spotting locus) or inversion mutations in upstream transcriptional regulatory elements (W^{sh}/W^{sh}) are deficient in mast cells. The ligand for Kit, stem cell factor (SCF) is encoded by the Steel (Sl) locus. Mice with a mutant Sl locus (Sl/Sl^d) are unable to produce a membrane-bound isoform of SCF and are similarly deficient in mast cells. Kitamura and colleagues reported that transplantation of bone marrow cells from wild-type mice could restore mast cells to the tissues of W/W^v mice, but not Sl/Sl^d mice.[8,9] These experiments established that mast cells derive from cells of bone marrow origin that require expression of c-*kit*, as well as the presence of membrane-bound SCF in the tissues. The constitutive and abundant expression of membrane-bound SCF on the surface of fibroblasts, stromal cells, and endothelial cells likely explains the juxtaposition of mast cells to these cell types in tissues.

Early studies by Schrader and colleagues revealed that the intestinal mucosa of mice contain lymphocyte-like cells that are Thy-1 negative and capable of mast cell differentiation, in retrospect providing the first identification of committed mast cell progenitors.[10] Later, a population of cells isolated from fetal mouse blood that expressed high levels of Kit and low levels of Thy-1, called *promastocytes*, was found to give rise to pure colonies of FcεRI-positive mast cells when cultured with a combination of SCF and interleukin (IL)-3. These cells lacked developmental potential for other hematopoietic lineages.[11] Intraperitoneal injection of purified promastocytes reconstituted the intraperitoneal population of CTMCs in genetically mast cell-deficient W/Wv mice. More recently, committed mast cell progenitors, marked by their expression of CD34, FcεRI, and β_7 integrin, were identified in the intestine of adult mice.[12]

Recombinant human SCF, like its mouse homologue, supports mast cell growth in vitro.[13] Furthermore, a gain-of-function mutation in the c-*kit* receptor gene is associated with an aggressive form of systemic mastocytosis (see Chapter 60), and the injection of SCF into humans with advanced breast cancer results in mast cell hyperplasia.[14] Thus, as in the mouse, SCF and *kit* are important for mast cell development in humans. As in rodents, human mast cell progenitors exhibit bone marrow and peripheral phases of development. The mast cell progenitor in human bone marrow and circulation appears to be CD34+/Kit+ and is clearly distinct from the basophil lineage (Fig. 19.3). Cells isolated from human blood that are CD34+/Kit+ and also positive for CD13 (aminopeptidase N) give

rise to only mast cells and monocytes in culture under a variety of conditions.[15] While entirely 'committed', mast cell progenitors have not yet been identified in the human; they are probably a subpopulation of the CD34+Kit+CD13+ population of cells in peripheral blood and in tissues.

HOMING OF MAST CELLS AND THEIR PROGENITORS

The mechanisms involved in the recruitment and distribution of the circulating pool of committed mast cell progenitors, and the movement of mast cells in tissues, have only been recently explored. In mice, the small intestine contains an especially rich supply of mast cell progenitors, which constitutively traffic to this organ, likely ensuring the capacity for a rapid expansion of the mast cell population in the intestinal epithelium during the effector response to helminth infection. Mast cell progenitor trafficking to the intestine depends on the expression of the α chemokine receptor CXCR2 (CD182)[16] and the β_7 integrin subunit.[17] The $\alpha_4\beta_7$ integrin (LPAM-1) interacts with vascular cell adhesion molecule 1 (VCAM-1, CD106) and mucosal addressin cell adhesion molecule 1 (MAdCAM-1) for tissue-specific homing. Additionally, blockade

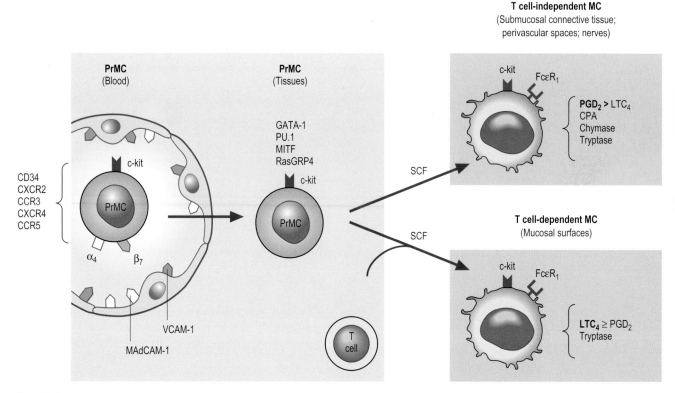

Fig. 19.3. Divergent pathways of mast cell development. CD34+Kit+ mast cell progenitors (PrMC) circulate from the bone marrow to tissues, where $\alpha_4\beta_7$ integrin binding to vascular cell adhesion molecule 1 (VCAM-1) and mucosal addressin cell adhesion molecule 1 (MAdCAM-1), and chemokine receptors such as CXCR2 mediate homing to tissues such as the intestine. PrMC express the transcription factors GATA-1, MITF, PU.1, and the guanine nucleotide exchange factor RasGRP4, and require the Kit ligand, stem cell factor (SCF), for development and maturation. Mast cell development in submucosal connective tissues is independent of T cell-derived growth factors. These T cell-independent mast cells express multiple granule-associated proteases and produce more prostaglandin D_2 (PGD_2) than leukotriene C_4 (LTC_4). With the influence of T cell cytokines such as IL-3, IL-4, IL-5, and IL-9, mast cells that develop in the mucosa contain tryptase and produce more cysteinyl leukotrienes.

of either α_4 (CD49d) or β_7 integrins inhibits the increase in mucosal mast cells in the intestinal mucosa of rats infected with *Nippo Strongylus brasiliensis.*[18] Although normal mouse lung tissue contains few mast cell progenitors (and few mast cells), these cells are recruited to the lung in substantial numbers in response to allergen-induced pulmonary inflammation. This inflammatory recruitment pathway requires $\alpha_4\beta_7$ and $\alpha_4\beta_1$ (VLA-4, CD49d/CD29) integrins as counter-ligands for inducible VCAM-1, whereas MAdCAM-1 is not expressed in the lung.[19]

Several additional homing receptors have been reported on mast cells and/or their progenitors in humans and mice (Table 19.3).[20] In rats but not humans, the intramuscular injection of CCL5 (RANTES) resulted in the accumulation of mast cells at the injection site.[21] Mast cells of both humans and mice express several integrins, many of which are counter-ligands for extracellular matrix proteins such as fibronectin ($\alpha_5\beta_1$), laminin ($\alpha_3\beta_1$ and $\alpha_6\beta_1$), and vitronectin ($\alpha_V\beta_3$).[22] Additional integrins such as $\alpha_L\beta_2$ (also known as lymphocyte function antigen

Table 19.3 Mast cell chemoattractants

Mast cell chemotactic factors	Receptors demonstrated	Cell types
Chemotaxis shown in vitro		
Stem cell factor	Kit	HMC-1, cord blood-derived human MC
C3a, C5a	PTX-sensitive pathway	HMC-1
Serum amyloid A	PTX-sensitive pathway	HMC-1, cord blood-derived human MC
IL-8	CXCR1, CXCR2	HMC-1, cord blood-derived human MC
Platelet-activating factor	PTX-sensitive pathway	HMC-1, cord blood-derived human MC
TGF-β	TGF-β serine/threonine type I and II receptors	HMC-1, cord blood-derived human MC
CCL5 (RANTES)	CCR1, CCR4	Cord blood-derived human MC
TNF-α, IL-4		HMC-1
5-HT (serotonin)	5-HT(1A) receptor	Mouse BMMC, human PBMC
LTB$_4$	BLT$_1$, BLT$_2$	Mouse BMMC, HMC-1
Fractalkine/CX3CL1 (+VIP)	CX3CR1	HMC-1, mouse BMMC, human dermal MC
CXCL10 (IP-10)	CXCR3	Human lung MC
CXCL9 (mig), CXCL10 (IP-10), CXCL11 (I-TAC)	CXCR3, CCR3, CXCR1, CXCR4	Human lung MC (but not human BMMC)
CCL5 (RANTES), CCL11 (eotaxin)	CCR3	Human lung MC (chemotaxis), skin, gut, lung, cardiac MC$_{TC}$ (receptor expression)
CXCL8 (IL-8), CCL3 (MIP-1α), CCL11 (eotaxin), CXCL12 (SDF-1α)	CXCR2, CCR3, CXCR4, CCR5	Human MC progenitors (cord blood)
CCL11, CCL3, CXCL12	CCR3, CCR5, CXCR4	HIV-susceptible peripheral blood MC progenitors
C1q	C1q receptor	Mouse BMMC
IL-3	CD129	Mouse BMMC
CCL2 (MCP-1), CCL3 (MIP-1α)		Mouse BMMC
CCL2 (MCP-1)	CCR2	Mouse BMMC
CCL3 (MIP-1α)	CCR1	Mouse BMMC
CCL4 (MIP-1β)	CCR5	Mouse BMMC, cord blood-derived human MC
CCL11 (eotaxin)	CCR3	Mouse BMMC, cord blood-derived human MC
Role demonstrated in vivo		
CCL2 (MCP-1)	Increase in human wounds precedes MC infiltrate	
CCL5 (RANTES)	Injection into rat paw, but not human skin, caused accumulation of MC	

HMC-1, human mast cell line; MC, mast cell; BMMC, bone marrow-derived mast cells; PBMC, peripheral blood-derived mast cells; PTX, pertussis toxin; VIP, vasoactive intestinal peptide.

(LFA)-1 or CD11a/CD18) and $\alpha_E\beta_7$ may be induced by inflammatory cytokines for interaction with their ligands on epithelial cells (intercellular adhesion molecule (ICAM)-1 (CD54) and E-cadherin, respectively).[23, 24] It seems likely that the process of mast cell homing and localization is regulated in a coordinated fashion in vivo, with each set of determinants acting in a tissue-specific and context-specific fashion.

ACCESSORY GROWTH FACTORS

Although mast cells absolutely require SCF and Kit for their development in vivo, cytokines derived from T cells are required to induce MMC hyperplasia in mucosal inflammation. Helminth-induced MMC hyperplasia is severely blunted or absent in athymic nude (T-cell deficient) mice, as well as in mice deficient in IL-3 or IL-4.[25–27] These same mice have normal numbers of CTMCs in intestinal submucosa. In vitro studies indicate that several T cell-derived cytokines control the rate of SCF-driven mast cell proliferation (comitogenesis), rate of apoptosis, or expression of certain key genes. IL-3 is a powerful comitogen for mouse mast cells and can substitute for SCF for mast cell growth in vitro (although it lacks this activity in cultures of human bone marrow or cord blood). Culturing mouse bone marrow-derived mast cells (BMMCs) in SCF induces certain features of a CTMC phenotype that can be prevented by including IL-3 in the culture medium.[28] Peritoneal mast cells also change from the CTMC to the MMC phenotype when cultured ex vivo in IL-3 plus IL-4; this change is reversible with reinjection of the cells into mouse peritoneal cavities.[29] Mice with tissue-specific overexpression of an IL-9 transgene display hyperplasia of both CTMCs and MMCs in the intestine and lung.[30] Moreover, both IL-9 and IL-10 can induce the expression of MMCP-1 and MMCP-2 by mouse mast cells in vitro.[31] These studies confirm the dynamic nature of mast cell phenotype and its dependency on tissue-specific determinants such as local cytokines.

The selective lack of MC_T in the intestinal epithelium of humans with CD4 lymphopenia (in the face of normal numbers of MC_{TC} in the submucosa)[32] indicates that T cell-dependent and -independent pathways for mast cell development are conserved across species. Although human IL-3 fails to promote mast cell growth by itself, the IL-3 receptor is constitutively expressed by human mast cell progenitors, is inducible on mature mast cells, and mediates an SCF-driven comitogenic effect on human mast cells and their progenitors in vitro. In the absence of SCF, IL-3 also sustains the survival of human mast cells derived from cord blood or isolated from surgically resected intestinal tissue. More recently, IL-9 was shown to selectively enhance SCF-dependent mast cell development from cultures of human CD34+ cells from both cord blood and peripheral blood.[33] Human mast cell progenitors also exhibit SCF-dependent comitogenic responses to IL-5.[15] IL-4 is a powerful comitogen for mature human mast cells derived from peripheral blood[34] or isolated from intestinal tissue.[35] Furthermore, many of the same T cell-derived cytokines that support comitogenic responses from human mast cells, such as IL-3, IL-4, IL-5, and IL-6, also attenuate their apoptosis in vitro independently of SCF.[36] A transcriptional profiling study revealed that IL-4, IL-5, and IL-9 can each induce a distinctive signature of gene expression by cultured human mast cells, including several genes involved in cell cycle progression.[37] Thus, the activity of T cell-derived cytokines as cofactors for mast cell development and viability may help to explain the prominence of mast cells at sites of allergic inflammation, where these cytokines are abundant. Moreover, regional differences in mast cell subpopulation characteristics and numbers may reflect regional differences in the local repertoire of T cell-derived cytokines.

TRANSCRIPTION FACTORS AND SIGNALING MOLECULES

The microphthalmia (Mi) locus-encoded transcription factor (MITF) is a basic helix-loop-helix leucine zipper-type transcription factor. Mice with a mutation at this locus are mast cell deficient, although not as severely as mice with the W or Sl mutations. MITF controls c-*kit* transcription in mast cells. It also regulates the expression of MMCP-4 and -5, the tryptase MMCP-6 (the earliest protease expressed during mouse mast cell development), plus the mast cell adhesion molecule spermatogenic immunoglobulin superfamily (SgIGSF), which is necessary for mast cell adhesion to fibroblasts.[38] MITF also regulates the expression of hematopoietic PGD_2 synthase (H-PGDS), the terminal enzyme in the synthesis of PGD_2 by all tissue mast cell subsets.[39] RasGRP4 is a guanine nucleotide exchange factor that is restricted to mast cells in its expression. Like MITF, RasGRP4 is necessary for the normal expression of H-PGDS,[40] suggesting that both may be part of a coordinated transcriptional system.

The GATA family of transcription factors is a group of highly conserved zinc finger proteins. GATA-1 may control differentiation and apoptosis of mast cell precursors.[41] GATA-1 also promotes expression of the α- and β-chains of the FcεRI receptor.[42] GATA-2 is important for the differentiation of yolk sac cells to mast cells.[43] The GATA consensus sequence is found in the promoter region of genes expressed by the mast cell such as carboxypeptidase A, IL-4, IL-13, several proteases, as well as the high-affinity IgE receptor.[42] PU.1, an Ets family transcription factor, may also play a role in regulating mast cell development, possibly in cooperation with GATA-2.[42]

APOPTOSIS

The removal of SCF or IL-3 from mast cell cultures leads to rapid onset of apoptosis. SCF regulates the expression of antiapoptotic molecules Bcl-2 and Bcl-x_L in human mast cell cultures, but not in SCF-independent mast cell lines.[44] IL-15 may also block mast cell apoptosis, through regulation of Bcl-x_L.[45] Mastocytosis (see section below) is often associated with expression of a constitutively active c-*kit* mutation in these cells, resulting in independence from SCF for their development, proliferation, and survival. In mouse BMMCs, the combination of IL-4 with the regulatory cytokine IL-10 inhibits Kit expression and induces apoptosis after several days in culture.[46] A gain-of-function mutation in the IL-4 receptor correlates with a better prognosis in human mastocytosis.[47] The evident dichotomy of functions served by IL-4 (i.e. comitogenic and proapoptotic) may ensure that mast cell hyperplasia in helminth infection is self-limited.

ACTIVATING AND INHIBITORY RECEPTORS OF MAST CELLS

FcεRI

When occupied by monomeric allergen-specific IgE and cross-linked by a multivalent allergen, FcεRI transduces signals that result in immediate granule fusion and exocytosis, arachidonic acid metabolism, and induction of cytokine and chemokine gene transcription. IgE-mediated activation of mast cells occurs exclusively via FcεRI and is thought to account for the clinical manifestations of rhinitis, conjunctivitis, urticaria, angioedema, and bronchoconstriction that immediately follow allergen challenge in susceptible hosts.

It is not clear what physiologic role requires such high expression of FcεRI on mast cells. Mice genetically deficient in FcεRI are developmentally and immunologically normal and normally eliminate *Schistosoma mansoni* from the intestine after experimental infection, although they do develop increased hepatic granulomas and hepatic fibrosis.[48] Deficiencies in mast cells or IgE impair the ability of mice to eliminate *Haemaphysalis longicornis* ticks,[49] suggesting a role for IgE-mediated hypersensitivity in resistance against this parasite.

Regulation of mast cell FcεRI expression and function

FcεRI expression on the surface of mast cells and basophils is regulated by the level of circulating IgE, due to stabilization of receptors at the cell membrane.[50] Thus, decreased IgE concentrations in vivo lead to decreased levels of membrane expression of FcεRI. The administration of a humanized monoclonal anti-human IgE antibody to atopic individuals decreases the levels of FcεRI on the surfaces of their circulating basophils,[51] skin mast cells,[52] and lung mast cells.[53] The deficiency of mast cell surface FcεRI in an IgE-deficient mouse strain was corrected by injecting the mice with exogenous IgE, and the incubation of in vitro BMMCs with IgE enhanced not only their FcεRI expression but also signal transduction and mediator release in response to FcεRI cross-linking.[54]

Locally derived cytokines may also regulate FcεRI expression and signaling. Human mast cells derived in vitro from cord blood mononuclear cells cultured in the presence of SCF plus IL-6 respond to the addition of exogenous IL-4 with dose-and time-dependent enhancement of their surface FcεRI expression.[55] Similarly, human mast cells purified from dispersed intestinal tissue respond to recombinant IL-4 ex vivo with upregulated FcεRI expression and priming for IgE-dependent activation.[56] Unlike the effect of IgE, IL-4 causes an increase of mRNA encoding FcεRIα.[55] Given that they act by separate mechanisms, it is not surprising that IL-4 and IgE are synergistic for FcεRI expression and FcεRI-mediated mast cell activation in vitro.[57] The structure and signaling mechanisms of FcεRI are comprehensively reviewed in Chapter 14.

Fcγ RECEPTORS

While IgE-dependent mast cell activation and anaphylaxis require the intact FcεRI,[58] anaphylaxis can also occur in rodents through IgG-dependent activation of the low-affinity receptor for IgG, FcγRIII (CD16).[59] This receptor shares β and γ subunits with the FcεRI but has not been identified on human mast cells. When ligated in vitro by antibody, FcγRIII induces mouse mast cells to degranulate and release LTC$_4$, similar to their responses via FcεRI,[59] and mast cell activation by FcγRIII in vivo can mediate anaphylaxis in mice.[60] Human mast cells exposed ex vivo to interferon-gamma (IFN-γ) inducibly express high-affinity FcγRI receptors (CD64),[61] and FcγRIIa receptors (CD32) have been detected on skin-derived human mast cells.[62] In these studies, cross-linkage of either receptor

resulted in generation of similar mediator profiles as did cross-linkage of FcεRI.

NON-Fc ACTIVATING RECEPTORS

Mast cells also undergo exocytosis and generate arachidonic acid metabolites via activation of Kit by soluble SCF, with kinetics that are similar to IgE-dependent activation.[63] Mast cells release histamine in response to the anaphylatoxin complement fragments, C3a and C5a.[64] Mast cells may also play a protective role against bacteria through the production of tumor necrosis factor alpha (TNF-α) and other cytokines due to Toll-like receptor-2 (TLR2) or TLR4-mediated activation.[65] Human mast cells stimulated by exogenous cys-LTs secrete cytokines and chemokines but do not release histamine.[66] It is likely that these non-Fc receptor-dependent mechanisms for mast cell activation can elicit or modify mediator release in non-allergic diseases and host defense responses that involve contributions from mast cells (see below).

INHIBITORY RECEPTORS

Mast cells express several receptors that inhibit their activation, potentially contributing to homeostasis in mast cell-dependent inflammatory responses. Mouse mast cells possess at least four inhibitory receptors that contain an immunoreceptor tyrosine-like inhibitory motif (ITIM). These include the closely related low-affinity Fc receptors for IgG, FcγRIIb1, and FcγRIIb2,[67] leukocyte immunoglobulin-like receptor B4 (LILRB4, previously called GP49B1),[68] and CD300a.[69] When coligated with FcεRI, each of these receptors inhibits mast cell exocytosis,[69-71] as well as LTC$_4$ generation.[72] Mice deficient in the FcγRIIB or LILRB4 genes exhibit an augmented experimentally induced IgE-dependent anaphylactic response in vivo.[73,74] Inhibitory Fc receptors have not yet been reported for human mast cells.[62] RNA transcripts for LILRB4 have been detected in human mast cells, but their function has not been confirmed.[75] Unlike FcγRII, the natural counter-ligands for LILRB4 and CD300a are not known. Members of the Sialic acid-binding immunoglobulin-like lectin (Siglec) family that contain ITIMs have also been recently identified on mast cells.[76]

Mast cell activation can also be downregulated by G-protein coupled receptors (GPCRs) that couple to G$_s$ proteins and adenylyl cyclase (AC). These include the β$_2$ adrenergic receptor, the A2B receptor for adenosine, and the EP$_2$ receptor for PGE$_2$, an eicosanoid generated in abundance by epithelial and other cell types. Inhalation of PGE$_2$ by individuals with asthma prevents both early and late asthmatic responses. A recent study revealed that the A2B receptor for adenosine plays a major role in regulating endogenous levels of cyclic AMP in mouse mast cells, and A2B knockout mice display exaggerated IgE-dependent anaphylactic responses.[77]

■ MAST CELL-DERIVED MEDIATORS ■

Upon activation, mast cells immediately release a host of preformed mediators from storage in secretory granules via exocytosis. Concomitantly, lipid mediators of inflammation are generated from arachidonic acid, and further cytokine production is induced (Fig. 19.4).

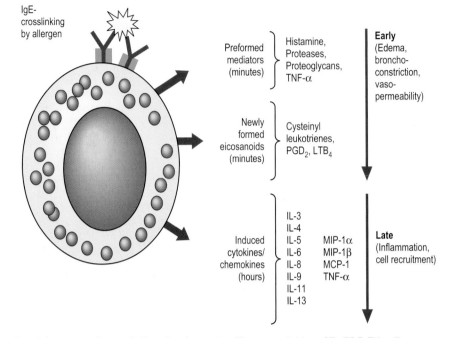

Fig. 19.4. Mediators released from mast cells upon IgE-mediated activation. Upon cross-linking of FcεRI-IgE by allergen, mast cells immediately release a host of preformed mediators from storage in secretory granules via exocytosis. Concomitantly, leukotrienes and PGD_2 are generated from arachidonic acid, and cytokine and chemokine production is induced.

PREFORMED MEDIATORS

Histamine

Human mast cells contain 1–10 pg of histamine per cell, depending on their size and location.[78] Histamine is synthesized in the Golgi apparatus by decarboxylation of the amino acid histidine by the enzyme histidine decarboxylase (HDC). Histamine has a positive charge and associates with carboxyl groups of proteoglycans in mast cell granules. After exocytosis, histamine dissociates from the mast cell proteoglycans at neutral pH (see below). HDC-deficient mice have fewer mast cells than wild-type mice, with abnormal morphology and decreased granular proteoglycan and protease content.[79] Once released into the extracellular environment, histamine is rapidly metabolized (half-life ≈1 min) by methylation or oxidation. Methylation, catalyzed by histamine N-methyltransferase, is the primary route of metabolism in the airways.[80] The initial product, N-methylhistamine (MHA), can be excreted by the kidney or deaminated by monoamine oxidase to be excreted as N-methylimidazoleacetic acid (MIAA). Histamine may also be oxidized by diamine oxidase (histaminase) to imidazoleacetic acid (IAA). Although the measurement of histamine release in the plasma is challenging due to its rapid metabolism, histamine and its metabolites can be measured in the urine.[81]

Histamine acts through four different GPCRs, H_1 through H_4, to mediate effects that include vasodilation and vasopermeability, bronchial and gastrointestinal smooth muscle contraction, secretion of gastric acid, and induction of pruritus.[82] The majority of effects associated with histamine in allergic responses, such as the pruritus, vascular effects, and smooth muscle contraction (bronchospasm), are mediated by the H_1 receptor, accounting for the efficacy of H_1 antagonists for symptomatic treatment of allergic disease. Histamine also exerts both stimulatory and inhibitory effects on immune cells, including enhancement of antigen presentation by dendritic cells; suppression of TNF-α and IL-12, and increase in IL-10 production by monocytes and dendritic cells; regulation of Th1, Th2, and T regulatory cell balance; and chemotactic activity for T cells and eosinophils. Most recently, a key role for H_1 receptors in T cell chemotaxis was recognized in a mouse model of allergen-induced pulmonary inflammation.[83] H_2 receptors are best known for their role in potentiating gastric acid secretion. They also play a role in the allergic immune response, by mediating mucus production in the airway, vasodilation, and bronchial smooth muscle relaxation,[84] as well immunoregulatory effects.[85] H_3 receptors are found mainly in the central and peripheral nervous systems as presynaptic receptors controlling the release of histamine and other neurotransmitters.[85] H_4 receptors are highly expressed by leukocytes, including mast cells, and mediate mast cell chemotaxis in vivo. H_4 receptors influence dendritic cell induction of Th2 responses in a mouse model of asthma,[86] and may play a role in mediating pruritus.[87]

Neutral proteases

Mast cell granules are rich in the neutral serine proteases which fall into two major families: tryptases (named because its members have trypsin-like activity) and chymases (which have chymotrypsin-like activity). The MC_{TC} subset contains two additional proteases based on immunolocalization: a carboxypeptidase and a chymotryptic protease with similarities to neutrophil cathepsin G. The existence of other mast cell proteases with elastase-like and kallikrein-like activity has been proposed but not confirmed.

Tryptase

Antibody reagents specific for α- and β-tryptases have been useful as immunohistochemical markers of mast cells in tissue as well as biochemical indicators of mast cell activation in vivo. Tryptase is also expressed by basophils, but at levels <1% of levels in mast cells.[88] In biologic fluids and in mast cell granules, human tryptases exist as tetramers of non-covalently linked subunits each 31–38 kDa in size, with enzymatic preference similar to pancreatic trypsin for cleaving substrates at the C-terminal side of Arg and Lys (basic) residues. The major forms of human tryptase, all encoded by genes on chromosome 16, are α-tryptase, of which 2 alleles have been identified (αI and αII), and β-tryptase, of which there are three alleles (βI, βII, and βIII). Notably, the α allele shares a locus with one of the β alleles.[89] Thus, the haploid genotype for tryptase is $\alpha\beta$ or $\beta\beta$, and 25% of individuals may be α-tryptase deficient.[90] Mast cells also express δ- and γ-tryptases. The former appears to be C-terminally truncated. The latter is a transmembrane protein.[91] Each of these tryptase genes likely arose from a single ancestral gene to encode enzymes with distinct functions, but full characterization of the expression patterns and functions of these additional human tryptases is pending.

There is 90% sequence identity between α- and β-tryptases, but the differences impact the secretion and activity of the enzymes. β-Protryptase is processed by autocatalytic cleavage at acidic pH in the presence of heparin, followed by removal of a final dipeptide by dipeptidyl peptidase I (DPPI) to generate a mature monomer.[92] The assembly of active tetramer then follows at acidic pH with stabilization by heparin or another negatively charged polysaccharide.[93] The crystal structure of the human β-tryptase tetramer has revealed orientation of the active site of each monomer towards a central pore, thereby explaining its limited substrate specificity and resistance to endogenous serine protease inhibitors.[94] α-Tryptase appears to have a propeptide mutation that hinders removal and activation, and as a consequence it is continuously secreted as an inactive proenzyme along with unprocessed β-protryptase, rather than directed to accumulate in the secretory granules. α-Tryptase has additional differences in its substrate binding and catalytic domains, limiting its potential enzymatic activity even after propeptide removal.[95]

Most monoclonal antibodies prepared against tryptase detect both the α and β forms, except for one clone, G5, which binds to mature β-tryptase with much higher affinity. Using these antibodies, it has been found that most tryptase in the circulation of normal individuals (about 5 ng/ml) is composed of the α and pro-β forms and that it is these forms that are elevated in patients with systemic mastocytosis and mature β-tryptase that can be increased in anaphylaxis. α- and pro-β tryptases, released constitutively, can thus be a marker for total body mast cell burden, whereas mature β-tryptase, the form stored in secretory granules and released on activation, is a marker for mast cell activation. It has also been found that mast cells in different locations differ in their quantities of stored tryptase. For example, the mast cells dispersed from the epithelial layer of nasal polyps contained five-fold less tryptase than submucosal mast cells from the same specimens.[96] In another study, dispersed human lung mucosal mast cells contained three-fold less tryptase than dispersed skin mast cells.[78]

On mast cell activation, tryptase is exocytosed in association with proteoglycans in complexes of 200–250 kDa.[97] In the absence of stabilizing polyanions such as heparin, active tryptase tetramers quickly dissociate into inactive monomers at neutral pH, with a half-life of 6–8 min.[98] Tryptase activity may thus be regulated by the limited diffusing capacity of the proteoglycan complexes or by the pH of the microenvironment into which it is secreted.

One mouse tryptase, MMCP-7, potently and selectively degrades plasma fibrinogen, even in the presence of plasma protease inhibitors.[99] Another mouse tryptase, MMCP-6, is retained along with the exocytosed secretory granule core in connective tissues, where it can elicit a selective and sustained influx of neutrophils that is attributed to induction of IL-8 expression by endothelial cells.[100] Purified human β-tryptase also induces the expression of IL-8 and IL-1β by endothelial cells.[101] The stimulation of vascular tube formation by β-tryptase in vitro suggests a role for it in angiogenesis, and the stimulation of fibroblast, airway smooth muscle, and epithelial cell proliferation in vitro implies a role for β-tryptase in remodeling and repair. Human α- and β-tryptases both activate protease-activated receptor (PAR) 2,[102] a GPCR expressed by several stromal cell types that requires proteolytic modification of its extracellular domain for its activation. Finally, human tryptases have been proposed to potentiate bronchoconstriction in response to histamine,[103] an effect ascribed to the enzymatic cleavage of inhibitory airway neuropeptides. Instillation of soluble recombinant human tryptase-γ into the tracheas of naive mice elicits airway hyperresponsiveness and IL-13 production.[91] Pretreatment of sensitized sheep with tryptase inhibitors attenuates allergen-induced airway inflammation, reflecting inhibition of the above actions in vivo.[104]

Chymase

Only one mast cell-specific chymase gene has been identified in humans, in contrast to the mouse, where at least nine mast cell chymase genes exist. Human chymase is a 30-kDa serine protease with chymotryptic activity, i.e. a preference for cleaving peptide bonds on the carboxyl side of aromatic side chains such as phenylalanine. After removal of a dipeptide pro-region, positively charged chymase is stored in its active form in mast cell granules bound to negatively charged heparin proteoglycans but has little activity in the granules' acidic environment.[105] While stored in the same granules as tryptase, chymase is released with carboxypeptidase and proteoglycans in complexes larger and distinct from those containing tryptase.[106] After release, chymase may remain bound to the granule heparin proteoglycan but is also able to bind proteoglycans of the extracellular matrix and basement membrane. Chymases are susceptible to endogenous circulating inhibitors such as α_1-antitrypsin, α_1-antichymotrypsin, α_2-macroglobulin, as well as locally secreted inhibitors such as secretory leukocyte protease inhibitor (SLPI); but they may be resistant to, and even degrade, these inhibitors while bound to heparin.[97] Chymase has also been identified in cardiac endothelial and mesenchymal cells,[107] and pineal and pituitary gland parenchyma.[108] It is found in tissues throughout the body but is not active in human serum.[109]

All chymases cleave angiotensin I to form angiotensin II. In humans, α-chymase is the major non-angiotensin-converting enzyme (ACE), angiotensin II-generating enzyme in human tissues. It may contribute to ACE-resistant ventricular hypertrophy, vascular restenosis due to lipid deposition and intimal hyperplasia, and hypertension. Chymases can also degrade extracellular matrix directly or activate matrix metalloproteinases; they activate TGF-β_1 and IL-1β, affect remodeling of atherosclerotic lesions, promote angiogenesis and synthesis of endothelins, and are involved in lipoprotein metabolism.[107] Other chymase-associated functions are listed in Table 19.1.

Carboxypeptidase

Carboxypeptidases are enzymes that act at the free C-terminus of polypeptides to liberate single amino acid residues. Mast cell carboxypeptidase A (MC-CPA) has substrate specificity similar to that of pancreatic CPA, with preference for C-terminal phenylalanine and leucine, but not arginine or lysine residues.[110] Structurally, however, it resembles carboxypeptidase B. Evolutionary trees constructed from carboxypeptidase sequences suggested that MC-CPA evolved from a carboxypeptidase B-like enzyme, but with resultant substrate specificity similar to pancreatic CPA.[110] Heparin is likely required for processing of the proenzyme in the secretory granules, as mice deficient in heparin due to mutation in N-deacetylase/N-sulphotransferase-2 (NDST-2) are also deficient in mature CPA but contain normal levels of pro-CPA.[111] MC-CPA colocalizes with chymase to proteoglycan complexes in the granules of MC_{TC},[112] and may cooperate with chymase to degrade apolipoprotein B and form angiotensin II.[113] A potential protective role for CPA in enhancing resistance to snake venom has also been demonstrated.[114]

Proteoglycans

Proteoglycans are macromolecules comprising a protein core to which glycosaminoglycan (GAG) side chains are covalently bound. They are a major component of all mast cell granules and account for some of the granules' staining characteristics, and they play a major role in the storage and stability of histamine, proteases, and other granule constituents. All mast cell proteoglycans have a common peptide core, termed 'serglycin' for its repetitive serine and glycine residues, to which GAG side chains are covalently bound to every second and third serine residue.[115] The GAG side chains primarily contain heparin and chondroitin sulfate, the relative content of which depends on species, tissue distribution, and maturity of the cell, and which is a determinant of the staining characteristics of mast cell subsets. Mast cells are the exclusive cellular source of heparin, and all human mast cells contain heparin. Chondroitin sulfate is also present in human mast cells, with the relative content of each likely mediated by microenvironmental factors, and heparin content reflected by safranin-positive staining. In rodents, heparin is found primarily in connective tissue and peritoneal mast cells, whereas chondroitin sulfate is the primary proteoglycan in mucosal mast cells. These differences correspond to differences in protease composition and histamine content. Bone marrow-derived mast cells from both mice[116] and humans[117] cocultured with skin-derived fibroblasts dramatically increased their heparin content, an effect possibly mediated through SCF, resembling the biochemical and functional phenotype of mast cells in connective tissues. Knockout mice lacking serglycin or lacking the heparin-synthesizing enzyme mice NDST-2 show profoundly abnormal mast cell granule development and cannot store proteases, thereby confirming the key role of proteoglycans in mast cell function.[93]

NEWLY GENERATED MEDIATORS

Arachidonic acid metabolites

Both rodent and human mast cells rapidly synthesize the eicosanoid inflammatory mediators, LTC_4, LTB_4, and PGD_2 from endogenous membrane arachidonic stores when stimulated via FcεRI or Kit.

Arachidonic acid released from cell membrane phospholipids by cytosolic PLA_2 ($cPLA_2$) is largely converted either to prostaglandins by cyclooxygenase (COX) enzymes or to leukotrienes by the 5-lipoxygenase (5-LO) pathway. 5-LO, in cooperation with 5-lipoxygenase activating protein (FLAP), produces LTA_4, which is then either converted by an LTA_4 hydrolase to LTB_4 or conjugated to reduced glutathione by LTC_4 synthase (LTC_4S) to form LTC_4, the parent compound of the cysteinyl leukotrienes. Both LTB_4 and LTC_4 are exported to the extracellular space by distinct, energy-dependent steps. LTB_4 is a potent chemotactic mediator for neutrophils and effector T cells via at least two specific GPCRs, termed BLT_1 and BLT_2. LTC_4 is sequentially converted extracellularly to LTD_4 and LTE_4. These mediators also act through at least two GPCRs, termed $CysLT_1$ and $CysLT_2$. In humans, cys-LTs are potent bronchoconstrictors and mediators of vascular permeability, induce mucus secretion, and recruit eosinophils. PGD_2, which is not produced by basophils, is generated by the conversion of arachidonic acid through the sequential actions of COX-1 or -2, prostaglandin endoperoxide synthase (PGHS)-1 or -2, and hematopoietic PGD_2 synthase. PGD_2, like the cys-LTs, is a bronchoconstrictor, and its active metabolite, $9\alpha,11\beta$-PGF_2, is a potent constrictor of coronary arteries. PGD_2 also attracts Th2 cells, eosinophils, and basophils through the DP_2 receptor, and induces migrational arrest of dendritic cells through actions at the DP_1 receptor. Thus, the lipid mediators of mast cells are likely involved in several aspects of allergic responses, including airflow obstruction, alterations in vascular caliber and tone, leukocyte recruitment, and antigen presentation.[118]

As with the profile of mast cell granule constituents, mast cell subpopulations differ in their patterns of arachidonic acid metabolism. Rat peritoneal mast cells respond to IgE-dependent activation with preferred generation of PGD_2, whereas mast cells from rat intestinal mucosa generate PGD_2 and LTC_4. Mast cells isolated from various human tissues generate abundant PGD_2 but widely variable amounts of LTC_4. The pattern of inter-tissue heterogeneity of arachidonic acid metabolism exhibited by human mast cell subsets does not parallel their pattern of protease composition, indicating that these features are regulated differently. Th2 cytokines (IL-3 and IL-4 in particular) figure prominently in the regulation of synthetic steps in the cys-LT-generating pathways of mast cells,[119] which likely explains the tendency for cys-LT generation to be amplified in mucosal inflammation concomitantly with mast cell hyperplasia. In contrast, PGDS expression is controlled by the requisite mast cell growth factor, SCF, which may account for the fact that virtually all recognized mast cell subsets generate at least some PGD_2.

MAST CELL-DERIVED CYTOKINES

Early-acting cytokines

Mouse mast cells produce a number of cytokines in response to IgE-dependent stimulation, including cytokines that are associated with the early phases of an inflammatory response, such as TNF-α, IL-1, and IL-6. Such early-acting cytokines initiate hepatic acute-phase protein production, endothelial cell adhesion molecule expression, and leukocyte recruitment. TNF-α immunolocalization to mast cells in human skin, nasal mucosa, and intestine, and its release within 2 minutes of allergen challenge,[120] confirm that TNF-α also is synthesized and stored by human mast cells. The finding of a greater number of TNF-α-positive mast cells in bronchial biopsy specimens from patients with asthma compared to non-asthmatic control subjects supports a role for IgE-dependent TNF-α release by mast cells in leukocyte recruitment to the bronchial wall in asthma.[121] The secretion of TNF-α by mast cells also mediates their protective role in a mouse model of septic peritonitis.[122] In this model, mast cell activation for TNF-α generation is initiated by a bacterial cell wall constituent, indicating a role for mast cells and TNF-α in innate immunity. Mast cell-derived TNF-α plays an important role in regulating dendritic cell[123] and lymphocyte function[124] in certain mouse models. Anti-TNF-α therapy holds promise in the treatment of refractory asthma.[125]

Allergy-associated cytokines

In various contexts, mast cells generate a wide range of cytokines that are associated with allergen-induced inflammatory responses and allergic disease. IL-4 and IL-5 proteins localize to mast cells in the lung tissue of patients with asthma[121] and in the nasal mucosa of patients with allergic rhinitis.[126] Mast cells express various Th2-associated cytokines upon IgE-dependent activation, including IL-3, IL-4, IL-5, IL-6, IL-10, IL-13, and granulocyte/macrophage colony-stimulating factor (GM-CSF).[127] Thus, de novo production of cytokines occurs downstream of FcεRI-mediated mast cell activation, with potential relevance to asthma and allergic inflammation. When cord blood-derived human mast cells are primed with IL-4, not only are FcεRI, LTC$_4$ synthase, and cysteinyl leukotriene receptor expression induced, but IgE-dependent transcription and release of IL-13 can be induced. Human intestinal mast cells also respond to IL-4 priming with augmented IgE-dependent production of IL-3, IL-5, and IL-13, but decreased release of IL-6.[128] The process of Th2 cytokine generation in mast cells therefore bears similarity to the same process in T cells, where IL-4 is required for optimal production of the Th2 cytokines IL-13 and IL-5. In this way, mast cells are a source of both proinflammatory and Th2-type cytokines, and their IgE-dependent release serves as a potential amplifying mechanism for allergic inflammation.

Chemokines

The mast cells of both mice and humans generate several members of the CC and CXC chemokine families. Human mast cells produce CXCL8 (IL-8), a potent neutrophil-active chemokine, and the closely related CXCL5 (ENA-78) after IgE-dependent activation. Human cord blood-derived mast cells also generate CCL3 (MIP-1α) in response to IgE-dependent activation, whereas the production of CCL2 (MCP-1) by human lung mast cells is enhanced by SCF and anti-IgE in vitro. Contact between mouse mast cells and fibroblasts induces the production of CCL11 (eotaxin) by mast cells. Other chemokines expressed in transcriptional profiling studies with IgE-receptor cross-linkage include CCL1 (I-309), CCL4 (MIP-1β), CCL7 (MCP-3), CCL8 (MCP-2), CCL15 (MCP-1γ), and CXCL1, 2, and 3 (GROα, β, and γ).[128] Thus, mast cells are a potential source of several chemotactic mediators involved in inflammation-based leukocyte recruitment.

Fibrogenic and angiogenic growth factors

Mast cells generate factors that are involved in fibroblast proliferation, extracellular matrix deposition, and angiogenesis, including vascular permeability factor/vascular endothelial cell growth factor, TGF-β, and basic fibroblast growth factor. The latter property supports the role of mast cells as modulators of tissue repair, fibrosis, and remodeling. Finally, the fact that mast cells store and secrete SCF illustrates a potential autocrine capability.

■ MAST CELL PATHOBIOLOGY ■

ROLES IN HUMAN DISEASE

Anaphylaxis

Mast cells, along with basophils, play a fundamental role in the pathology of anaphylaxis. The mediators derived from such cells produce hypotension, urticaria and angioedema, bronchospasm, rhinorrhea, and/or abdominal symptoms. The role for mast cells is supported by the observation that serum or plasma levels of mature β-tryptase are elevated in most individuals with systemic anaphylaxis of sufficient severity to result in hypotension.[129] β-Tryptase released from mast cells diffuses more slowly than histamine, presumably because of its association with proteoglycans. During bee sting-induced anaphylaxis, β-tryptase levels in the circulation peak 1–2 h after the sting and have a half-life of about 2 h, whereas histamine levels peak 5–10 min after the sting and decline to baseline by 15–60 min.[130] β-Tryptase levels are thus a more practical indicator of anaphylaxis in the clinical setting, as they may be obtained up to several hours after a reaction. Although anaphylactic reactions to cyclooxygenase inhibitors and radiocontrast media generally are not mediated by IgE, elevated levels of β-tryptase are observed in these circumstances, implicating mast cell involvement. β-Tryptase levels are often higher with parenteral than with oral allergen, despite equal severity of anaphylaxis. This finding may indicate a principal role for basophils versus mast cells in situations where β-tryptase is low, but such a conclusion is difficult to verify in the absence of basophil-specific markers of activation. In serum and plasma, reference ranges of normal values have been established. Lavage fluid levels, however, are dependent on technique and dilutional factors, so corresponding control fluid must be obtained for comparative assessment.

Measurement of other mast cell mediators has not proven to be as clinically useful, as lipid mediators such as LTC$_4$ and PGD$_2$ and their metabolites lack sufficient cell specificity or are rapidly metabolized. Histamine is also rapidly metabolized in the circulation, is released from basophils as well as mast cells, and may be ingested in certain foods. Nonetheless, elevated levels of histamine along with either tryptase or PGD$_2$ suggest mast cell activation, whereas elevated histamine levels in the absence of tryptase and PGD$_2$ suggest basophil activation.

Role in mastocytosis

Humans can develop a hyperplasia of mast cells that is isolated to one location *(mastocytoma)*, is limited to the skin *(cutaneous mastocytosis, also known as urticaria pigmentosa)*, or is more widely distributed *(systemic mastocytosis)*. Systemic mastocytosis is a rare condition that generally involves mast cell hyperplasia in organs such as the skin, gastrointestinal mucosa, liver, spleen, and bone marrow. It is usually indolent and non-neoplastic, although more aggressive variants may lead to a poorer prognosis. Symptoms such as flushing, pruritus, headache, diarrhea and abdominal pain, and hypotension are attributable to non-specific mast cell mediator release. Total tryptase levels, as mentioned above, are generally elevated in systemic, but not cutaneous, mastocytosis. The most common cause of systemic mastocytosis is a somatic activating mutation in c-*kit* (A816V) that leads to dysregulated (constitutive, SCF-independent) proliferation. The clinical features, diagnostic criteria, classification, and management of patients with mastocytosis are discussed in Chapter 60.

Role in asthma

Mounting evidence from human studies supports a pivotal role for mast cells and their mediators in asthma. Bronchial biopsy specimens obtained from patients with asthma contain increased numbers of mast cells in the mucosal epithelium compared with biopsy specimens obtained from non-asthmatic control individuals, irrespective of whether the asthmatic patients are atopic or non-atopic. Mast cells are rarely found in the bronchial smooth muscle layer in non-asthmatics or in patients with eosinophilic bronchitis (a syndrome of bronchial mucosal inflammation without airway hyperreactivity (AHR) or airflow obstruction). In contrast, substantial numbers of mast cells are found at this tissue site in patients with asthma.[131] These data implicate a complex bilateral interaction between mast cells and smooth muscle that may lead to AHR and bronchoconstriction. The numbers of mast cells in bronchial biopsy specimens from asthmatic individuals also predict treatment failure during weaning of these patients from glucocorticoid treatment.[132] Mast cell degranulation is a prominent feature of postmortem bronchial tissues from patients who die from asthma and also is observed in bronchial biopsy specimens from living patients with asthma. Relative to non-asthmatic individuals, the levels of tryptase and other mast cell mediators often are markedly increased in the bronchoalveolar lavage fluid of asthmatic patients, even without allergen provocation. Thus, it is now apparent that the process of chronic mast cell activation and degranulation is a common feature of asthma. Supporting this conclusion is the finding that anti-IgE therapy is relatively effective in controlling exacerbations of atopic asthma. The clinical efficacy of $CysLT_1$ receptor antagonists and 5-LO inhibitors validate the importance of the cys-LT pathway in this disease as well.

Role in other allergic conditions

Mast cell activation and mediator release are implicated in all conditions involving IgE-mediated responses to antigen. Whereas systemic responses to allergen lead to anaphylaxis, local allergen challenge can lead to symptoms of allergic rhinitis and rhinosinusitis, allergic conjunctivitis, oral allergy syndrome, urticaria, angioedema, and atopic dermatitis, in addition to asthma. Release of granule contents such as histamine leads to symptoms of itching and sneezing, bronchoconstriction, local edema (in the form of rhinorrhea, congestion, or angioedema) due to increased vascular permeability, erythema due to vascular dilation, mucus production, and cellular infiltration. Urticaria and angioedema are common cutaneous responses to allergen, but idiopathic urticaria and angioedema are also be caused by mast cell activation, leading to degranulation. Further information about the role of the mast cell in the pathophysiology of individual allergic diseases may be found in the chapters that discuss these diseases in the clinical science portion of this text.

ROLES IMPLICATED BY ANIMAL MODELS

Responses to pathogens

The distribution of mast cells in and near epithelial surfaces, around blood vessels, and in potential spaces such as the peritoneum is consistent with a role in immune surveillance. Mast cells have long been linked to antihelminthic host defense. More recently, they have been linked to protective innate and adaptive immunity against bacteria, parasites, and toxins.

Parasites

Mast cells are important in mice for control of several infectious helminths, such as *Trichinella spiralis*.[133] However, studies with mast-cell deficient mice have not found mast cells to be critical in immunity to expulsion of other nematodes, such as *Nippostrongylus brasiliensis*.[134] Rather, they may help boost the Th2-type immunity that is important to parasite immunity. Thus, while mucosal mast cell hyperplasia is a consistent feature of antihelminthic host responses, the specific function served by the mast cell depends on the nature of the parasite.

Bacteria

Mouse models of bacterial peritonitis and pneumonia reveal clear-cut functions of mast cells in the recruitment of neutrophils and subsequent clearance of bacterial infection.[122] Mouse and human mast cells are endowed with a broad range of receptors for pathogen-associated molecular patterns (PAMPS), including various members of the toll-like receptors (TLRs). In vitro, mast cells respond to stimulation with various PAMPs by generating cytokines and chemokines and, in the case of the staphylococcal peptidoglycan, LTC_4. In vivo, the protective effects of mast cells involve contributions from TNF-α, LTs, and proteases. The range of receptors for PAMPs and the biological responses of mast cells to stimulation through these receptors suggests that they may participate in antiviral, antifungal, and antimycobacterial host defense as well. These observations in animals await translation into humans, as no immunodeficiency has been attributed to mast cells.

Role in adaptive immunity

Mast cells, IgE, and mast cell-derived mediators play a role in the development of experimentally induced contact hypersentivitiy,[135] and may augment migration of dendritic cells to local lymph nodes for presentation of antigen.[123] The latter involves a prominent contribution from TNF-α. The results of another study suggest a role for mast cells in sensitization via TLR-4 via the airways.[136] Mast cell degranulation may also influence dendritic cell activation of T cells away from a Th1, and towards a Th2 response.[137] Potential mechanisms for this function include PGD_2 or histamine suppression of IL-12 release by dendritic cells.

Mast cell mediators also play a role in T cell responses. Histamine can be chemotactic for T cells via the H_1 receptor[83] and can regulate the production of Th1 and Th2 cytokines via the H_1 and H_2 receptors.[138] Mast cells and IL-9 may play an important role in skin allograft tolerance mediated by regulatory T cells.[139] It has been reported that mast cell-derived LTB_4 controls the selective recruitment of $CD8^+$ effector memory T cells through the GPCR, BLT_1 receptor[140] and that mast cell-derived TNF-α and surface expression of OX40 ligand enhance T cell proliferation and activation.[124] Mast cells also produce chemokines that may play a role in T cell recruitment.

Role in autoimmune diseases

Inflammatory arthritis

Mast cells accumulate at sites of chronic inflammation, not just in allergic conditions, but also in settings such as the synovium of patients with rheumatoid arthritis. Whether they play a pathogenic role, are protective (immunoregulating), or are innocent bystanders has recently been clarified by investigators who found that mast cell-deficient mice are resistant to mouse models of antibody-mediated arthritis.[141] FcγRIII and complement-dependent mechanisms account for mast cell activation in this context, contributing to arthritis pathogenesis through neutrophil recruitment when exposed to immune complexes.

Multiple sclerosis

Mast cells have been identified in the brains of patients with multiple sclerosis within and around plaques of demyelination,[142] and tryptase levels are elevated in cerebrospinal fluid in these patients.[143] It is not clear if mast cells play a causative role or appear as a result of inflammation. Mast cells may contribute to the increased permeability of the blood–brain barrier that develops in multiple sclerosis through secretion of vasoactive and proinflammatory molecules. Although mast cells contribute to the severity of disease in a mouse model of multiple sclerosis, experimental autoimmune encephalomyelitis, no mast cells are found in the mouse brain.[144]

Bullous pemphigoid

Alterations in mast cell morphology and degranulation are present in early lesions of bullous pemphigoid, followed by infiltration with lymphocytes, eosinophils, and basophils.[145] In a mouse experimental model of bullous pemphigoid, mast cell degranulation was necessary for the influx of neutrophils and subsequent development of subepidermal blistering.[146]

Glomerulonephritis

Mast cell numbers are increased in the renal cortical tubulointerstitium in chronic glomerulonephritis, but reports differ about whether the presence of mast cells is protective or pathogenic in experimentally induced immune complex glomerulonephritis. Indeed, the presence of mast cells and SCF in the interstitium correlates with fibrosis in human biopsy specimens regardless of underlying pathology, and SCF immunostaining is correlated with proteinuria and lower creatinine clearance in patients with crescentic glomerulonephritis.[147–149]

Other potential roles

Wound healing, fibrosis, and angiogenesis

Cutaneous wound closure is impaired in mast cell-deficient mice.[150] The remodeling effects of proteases on extracellular matrix may play a role in wound healing, and through released factors such as VEGF growth factor (VEGF), FGF, PGE_2, and IL-8, mast cells can also stimulate angiogenesis. Mast cells are also implicated in the development of fibrosis in the context of chronic inflammation. While fibroblasts affect mast cell differentiation, survival, and activation through signals such as stem cell factor, mast cells are also able to enhance in vitro proliferation of human skin, lung and intestinal fibroblasts, collagen production, matrix metalloproteinase activity, and myofibroblast differentiation through mediators such as histamine, tryptase, carboxypeptidase A, PGD_2, LTD_4, and growth factors such as TGF-β. Mast cell hyperplasia and degranulation have been observed in various conditions such as idiopathic pulmonary fibrosis, bleomycin- or radiation-induced fibrosis, chronic asthma, scleroderma, keloid formation, neurofibromatosis, chronic graft-versus-host disease, liver cirrhosis, peritoneal adhesions, and fibrotic lesions of Crohn's disease. Mast cells are also a source of plasminogen activator inhibitor (PAI)-1, an inhibitor of the fibrinolytic cascade associated with tissue/airway remodeling in asthma.[151]

Atherosclerosis

Degranulated mast cells are present in atherosclerotic plaques and sites of plaque rupture. Granule contents such as heparin and neutral proteases contribute to foam cell formation and cholesterol accumulation through effects on lipoproteins and to plaque instability through effects on the extracellular matrix and inhibition of smooth muscle proliferation.[152] Chymase, in turn, facilitates angiotensin-II formation and endothelin metabolism.[109]

Ischemic tissue injury

Mast cell proteases appear to contribute to the muscle injury that occurs after ischemia and reperfusion of skeletal muscle.[153] Cerebral mast cells have been implicated in early ischemic brain swelling and neutrophil accumulation.[154]

▦ SUMMARY ▦

The broad range of functions served by mast cells fits with their wide distribution, strong evolutionary conservation, and potent effector systems. The application of therapy directed against mast cell-associated mediators will continue to be a staple of allergic disease treatment, and the repertoire of such treatments will likely extend to additional mediators and strategies. At the same time, the discovery of mast cell contributions to autoimmunity and cardiovascular disease in animal models will likely prompt extension of treatments into areas beyond allergy. Research into the activation mechanisms and mediators that are essential to these processes continues to develop. Finally, the role of mast cells as initiators and effectors of host defense presents a challenge for therapeutic development, so as to maintain these benefits without sacrificing efficacy.

References

Introduction

1. Cockcroft DW, Murdock KY. Comparative effects of inhaled salbutamol, sodium cromoglycate, and beclomethasone dipropionate on allergen-induced early asthmatic responses, late asthmatic responses, and increased bronchial responsiveness to histamine. J Allergy Clin Immunol 1987; 79:734–740.

Histologic identification of mast cells

2. Vyas H, Krishnaswamy G. Paul Ehrlich's 'Mastzellen' – from aniline dyes to DNA chip arrays: a historical review of developments in mast cell research. Methods Mol Biol 2006; 315:3–11.

Morphology of mast cells

3. Weidner N, Austen KF. Ultrastructural and immunohistochemical characterization of normal mast cells at multiple body sites. J Invest Dermatol 1991; 96:26S–31S.
4. Kambe N, Hiramatsu H, Shimonaka M, et al. Development of both human connective tissue-type and mucosal-type mast cells in mice from hematopoietic stem cells with identical distribution pattern to human body. Blood 2004; 103:860–867.
5. Enerback L. Mast cells in rat gastrointestinal mucosa. I. Effects of fixation. Acta Pathol Microbiol Scand 1966; 66:289–302.
6. Gibson S, Miller HR. Mast cell subsets in the rat distinguished immunohistochemically by their content of serine proteinases. Immunology 1986; 58:101–104.
7. Reynolds DS, Stevens RL, Lane WS, et al. Different mouse mast cell populations express various combinations of at least six distinct mast cell serine proteases. Proc Natl Acad Sci U S A 1990; 87:3230–3234.

Mast cell growth and development

8. Kitamura Y, Go S. Decreased production of mast cells in S1/S1d anemic mice. Blood 1979; 53:492–497.
9. Kitamura Y, Go S, Hatanaka K. Decrease of mast cells in W/Wv mice and their increase by bone marrow transplantation. Blood 1978; 52:447–452.
10. Schrader JW, Scollay R, Battye F. Intramucosal lymphocytes of the gut: Lyt-2 and thy-1 phenotype of the granulated cells and evidence for the presence of both T cells and mast cell precursors. J Immunol 1983; 130:558–564.
11. Rodewald HR, Dessing M, Dvorak AM, et al. Identification of a committed precursor for the mast cell lineage. Science 1996; 271:818–822.
12. Gurish MF, Boyce JA. Mast cells: ontogeny, homing, and recruitment of a unique innate effector cell. J Allergy Clin Immunol 2006; 117:1285–1291.
13. Valent P, Spanblochl E, Sperr WR, et al. Induction of differentiation of human mast cells from bone marrow and peripheral blood mononuclear cells by recombinant human stem cell factor/kit-ligand in long-term culture. Blood 1992; 80:2237–2245.
14. Costa JJ, Demetri GD, Harrist TJ, et al. Recombinant human stem cell factor (kit ligand) promotes human mast cell and melanocyte hyperplasia and functional activation in vivo. J Exp Med 1996; 183:2681–2686.
15. Kirshenbaum AS, Goff JP, Semere T, et al. Demonstration that human mast cells arise from a progenitor cell population that is CD34(+), c-kit(+), and expresses aminopeptidase N (CD13). Blood 1999; 94:2333–2342.
16. Abonia JP, Austen KF, Rollins BJ, et al. Constitutive homing of mast cell progenitors to the intestine depends on autologous expression of the chemokine receptor CXCR2. Blood 2005; 105:4308–4313.
17. Gurish MF, Tao H, Abonia JP, et al. Intestinal mast cell progenitors require CD49dbeta7 (alpha4beta7 integrin) for tissue-specific homing. J Exp Med 2001; 194:1243–1252.
18. Issekutz TB, Palecanda A, Kadela-Stolarz U, et al. Blockade of either alpha-4 or beta-7 integrins selectively inhibits intestinal mast cell hyperplasia and worm expulsion in response to Nippostrongylus brasiliensis infection. Eur J Immunol 2001; 31:860–868.
19. Abonia JP, Hallgren J, Jones T, et al. Alpha-4 integrins and VCAM-1, but not MAdCAM-1, are essential for recruitment of mast cell progenitors to the inflamed lung. Blood 2006; 108:1588–1594.
20. Juremalm M, Nilsson G. Chemokine receptor expression by mast cells. Chem Immunol Allergy 2005; 87:130–144.
21. Conti P, Reale M, Barbacane RC, et al. Mast cell recruitment after subcutaneous injection of RANTES in the sole of the rat paw. Br J Haematol 1998; 103:798–803.
22. Columbo M, Bochner BS, Marone G. Human skin mast cells express functional beta 1 integrins that mediate adhesion to extracellular matrix proteins. J Immunol 1995; 154:6058–6064.
23. Toru H, Kinashi T, Ra C, et al. Interleukin-4 induces homotypic aggregation of human mast cells by promoting LFA-1/ICAM-1 adhesion molecules. Blood 1997; 89:3296–3302.
24. Smith TJ, Ducharme LA, Shaw SK, et al. Murine M290 integrin expression modulated by mast cell activation. Immunity 1994; 1:393–403.
25. Ruitenberg EJ, Elgersma A. Absence of intestinal mast cell response in congenitally athymic mice during Trichinella spiralis infection. Nature 1976; 264:258–260.
26. Madden KB, Urban JF Jr, Ziltener HJ, et al. Antibodies to IL-3 and IL-4 suppress helminth-induced intestinal mastocytosis. J Immunol 1991; 147:1387–1391.
27. Lantz CS, Boesiger J, Song CH, et al. Role for interleukin-3 in mast-cell and basophil development and in immunity to parasites. Nature 1998; 392:90–93.
28. Gurish MF, Ghildyal N, McNeil HP, et al. Differential expression of secretory granule proteases in mouse mast cells exposed to interleukin 3 and c-kit ligand. J Exp Med 1992; 175:1003–1012.
29. Kanakura Y, Thompson H, Nakano T, et al. Multiple bidirectional alterations of phenotype and changes in proliferative potential during the in vitro and in vivo passage of clonal mast cell populations derived from mouse peritoneal mast cells. Blood 1988; 72:877–885.
30. Godfraind C, Louahed J, Faulkner H, et al. Intraepithelial infiltration by mast cells with both connective tissue-type and mucosal-type characteristics in gut, trachea, and kidneys of IL-9 transgenic mice. J Immunol 1998; 160:3989–3996.
31. Eklund KK, Ghildyal N, Austen KF, et al. Induction by IL-9 and suppression by IL-3 and IL-4 of the levels of chromosome 14-derived transcripts that encode late-expressed mouse mast cell proteases. J Immunol 1993; 151:4266–4273.
32. Irani AM, Craig SS, DeBlois G, et al. Deficiency of the tryptase-positive, chymase-negative mast cell type in gastrointestinal mucosa of patients with defective T lymphocyte function. J Immunol 1987; 138:4381–4386.
33. Matsuzawa S, Sakashita K, Kinoshita T, et al. IL-9 enhances the growth of human mast cell progenitors under stimulation with stem cell factor. J Immunol 2003; 170:3461–3467.
34. Kulka M, Metcalfe DD. High-resolution tracking of cell division demonstrates differential effects of TH1 and TH2 cytokines on SCF-dependent human mast cell production in vitro: correlation with apoptosis and Kit expression. Blood 2005; 105:592–599.
35. Lorentz A, Wilke M, Sellge G, et al. IL-4-induced priming of human intestinal mast cells for enhanced survival and Th2 cytokine generation is reversible and associated with increased activity of ERK1/2 and c-Fos. J Immunol 2005; 174:6751–6756.
36. Yanagida M, Fukamachi H, Ohgami K, et al. Effects of T-helper 2-type cytokines, interleukin-3 (IL-3), IL-4, IL-5, and IL-6 on the survival of cultured human mast cells. Blood 1995; 86:3705–3714.
37. Lora JM, Al-Garawi A, Pickard MD, et al. Fc epsilon RI-dependent gene expression in human mast cells is differentially controlled by T helper type 2 cytokines. J Allergy Clin Immunol 2003; 112:1119–1126.
38. Kitamura Y, Oboki K, Ito A. Molecular mechanisms of mast cell development. Immunol Allergy Clin North Am 2006; 26:387–405; v.
39. Morii E, Oboki K. MITF is necessary for generation of prostaglandin D2 in mouse mast cells. J Biol Chem 2004; 279:48923–48929.
40. Li L, Yang Y, Stevens RL. RasGRP4 regulates the expression of prostaglandin D2 in human and rat mast cell lines. J Biol Chem 2003; 278:4725–4729.
41. Migliaccio AR, Rana RA, Sanchez M, et al. GATA-1 as a regulator of mast cell differentiation revealed by the phenotype of the GATA-1low mouse mutant. J Exp Med 2003; 197:281–296.
42. Nishiyama C, Ito T, Nishiyama M, et al. GATA-1 is required for expression of Fc{epsilon}RI on mast cells: analysis of mast cells derived from GATA-1 knockdown mouse bone marrow. Int Immunol 2005; 17:847–856.
43. Tsai FY, Orkin SH. Transcription factor GATA-2 is required for proliferation/survival of early hematopoietic cells and mast cell formation, but not for erythroid and myeloid terminal differentiation. Blood 1997; 89:3636–3643.
44. Mekori YA, Oh CK, Metcalfe DD. The role of c-Kit and its ligand, stem cell factor, in mast cell apoptosis. Int Arch Allergy Immunol 1995; 107:136–138.
45. Masuda A, Matsuguchi T, Yamaki K, et al. Interleukin-15 prevents mouse mast cell apoptosis through STAT6-mediated Bcl-xL expression. J Biol Chem 2001; 276:26107–26113.
46. Yeatman CF 2nd, Jacobs-Helber SM, Mirmonsef P, et al. Combined stimulation with the T helper cell type 2 cytokines interleukin (IL)-4 and IL-10 induces mouse mast cell apoptosis. J Exp Med 2000; 192:1093–1103.
47. Daley T, Metcalfe DD, Akin C. Association of the Q576R polymorphism in the interleukin-4 receptor alpha chain with indolent mastocytosis limited to the skin. Blood 2001; 98:880–882.

Activating and inhibitory receptors of mast cells

48. Jankovic D, Kullberg MC, Dombrowicz D, et al. FcepsilonRI-deficient mice infected with Schistosoma mansoni mount normal Th2-type responses while displaying enhanced liver pathology. J Immunol 1997; 159:1868–1875.
49. Matsuda H, Watanabe N, Kiso Y, et al. Necessity of IgE antibodies and mast cells for manifestation of resistance against larval Haemaphysalis longicornis ticks in mice. J Immunol 1990; 144:259–262.
50. MacGlashan DW Jr, Bochner BS, Adelman DC, et al. Serum IgE level drives basophil and mast cell IgE receptor display. Int Arch Allergy Immunol 1997; 113:45–47.
51. MacGlashan DW Jr, Bochner BS, Adelman DC, et al. Down-regulation of Fc(epsilon)RI expression on human basophils during in vivo treatment of atopic patients with anti-IgE antibody. J Immunol 1997; 158:1438–1445.
52. Beck LA, Marcotte GV, MacGlashan D, et al. Omalizumab-induced reductions in mast cell Fc epsilon RI expression and function. J Allergy Clin Immunol 2004; 114:527–530.
53. Djukanovic R, Wilson SJ, Kraft M, et al. Effects of treatment with anti-immunoglobulin E antibody omalizumab on airway inflammation in allergic asthma. Am J Respir Crit Care Med 2004; 170:583–593.
54. Yamaguchi M, Lantz CS, Oettgen HC, et al. IgE enhances mouse mast cell Fc(epsilon)RI expression in vitro and in vivo: evidence for a novel amplification mechanism in IgE-dependent reactions. J Exp Med 1997; 185:663–672.
55. Toru H, Ra C, Nonoyama S, et al. Induction of the high-affinity IgE receptor (Fc epsilon RI) on human mast cells by IL-4. Int Immunol 1996; 8:1367–1373.
56. Bischoff SC, Sellge G, Lorentz A, et al. IL-4 enhances proliferation and mediator release in mature human mast cells. Proc Natl Acad Sci U S A 1999; 96:8080–8085.
57. Yamaguchi M, Sayama K, Yano K, et al. IgE enhances Fc epsilon receptor I expression and IgE-dependent release of histamine and lipid mediators from human umbilical cord blood-derived mast cells: synergistic effect of IL-4 and IgE on human mast cell Fc epsilon receptor I expression and mediator release. J Immunol 1999; 162:5455–5465.
58. Dombrowicz D, Flamand V, Brigman KK, et al. Abolition of anaphylaxis by targeted disruption of the high affinity immunoglobulin E receptor alpha chain gene. Cell 1993; 75:969–976.
59. Katz HR, Raizman MB, Gartner CS, et al. Secretory granule mediator release and generation of oxidative metabolites of arachidonic acid via Fc-IgG receptor bridging in mouse mast cells. J Immunol 1992; 148:868–871.
60. Miyajima I, Dombrowicz D, Martin TR, et al. Systemic anaphylaxis in the mouse can be mediated largely through IgG1 and Fc gamma RIII. Assessment of the cardiopulmonary changes, mast cell degranulation, and death associated with active or IgE- or IgG1-dependent passive anaphylaxis. J Clin Invest 1997; 99:901–914.
61. Okayama Y, Kirshenbaum AS, Metcalfe DD. Expression of a functional high-affinity IgG receptor, Fc gamma RI, on human mast cells: Up-regulation by IFN-gamma. J Immunol 2000; 164:4332–4339.

62. Zhao W, Kepley CL, Morel PA, et al. Fc gamma RIIa, not Fc gamma RIIb, is constitutively and functionally expressed on skin-derived human mast cells. J Immunol 2006; 177:694–701.
63. Columbo M, Horowitz EM, Botana LM, et al. The human recombinant c-kit receptor ligand, rhSCF, induces mediator release from human cutaneous mast cells and enhances IgE-dependent mediator release from both skin mast cells and peripheral blood basophils. J Immunol 1992; 149:599–608.
64. el-Lati SG, Dahinden CA, Church MK. Complement peptides C3a- and C5a-induced mediator release from dissociated human skin mast cells. J Invest Dermatol 1994; 102:803–806.
65. Okayama Y. Mast cell-derived cytokine expression induced via Fc receptors and Toll-like receptors. Chem Immunol Allergy 2005; 87:101–110.
66. Mellor EA, Austen KF, Boyce JA. Cysteinyl leukotrienes and uridine diphosphate induce cytokine generation by human mast cells through an interleukin 4-regulated pathway that is inhibited by leukotriene receptor antagonists. J Exp Med 2002; 195:583–592.
67. Benhamou M, Bonnerot C, Fridman WH, et al. Molecular heterogeneity of murine mast cell Fc gamma receptors. J Immunol 1990; 144:3071–3077.
68. Castells MC, Wu X, Arm JP, et al. Cloning of the gp49B gene of the immunoglobulin superfamily and demonstration that one of its two products is an early-expressed mast cell surface protein originally described as gp49. J Biol Chem 1994; 269:8393–8401.
69. Bachelet I, Munitz A, Moretta A, et al. The inhibitory receptor IRp60 (CD300a) is expressed and functional on human mast cells. J Immunol 2005; 175:7989–7995.
70. Kepley CL, Taghavi S, Mackay G, et al. Co-aggregation of FcgammaRII with FcepsilonRI on human mast cells inhibits antigen-induced secretion and involves SHIP-Grb2-Dok complexes. J Biol Chem 2004; 279:35139–35149.
71. Ono M, Bolland S, Tempst P, et al. Role of the inositol phosphatase SHIP in negative regulation of the immune system by the receptor Fc(gamma)RIIB. Nature 1996; 383:263–266.
72. Katz HR, Vivier E, Castells MC, et al. Mouse mast cell gp49B1 contains two immunoreceptor tyrosine-based inhibition motifs and suppresses mast cell activation when coligated with the high-affinity Fc receptor for IgE. Proc Natl Acad Sci U S A 1996; 93:10809–10814.
73. Ujike A, Ishikawa Y, Ono M, et al. Modulation of immunoglobulin (Ig)E-mediated systemic anaphylaxis by low-affinity Fc receptors for IgG. J Exp Med 1999; 189:1573–1579.
74. Daheshia M, Friend DS, Grusby MJ, et al. Increased severity of local and systemic anaphylactic reactions in gp49B1-deficient mice. J Exp Med 2001; 194:227–234.
75. Arm JP, Nwankwo C, Austen KF. Molecular identification of a novel family of human Ig superfamily members that possess immunoreceptor tyrosine-based inhibition motifs and homology to the mouse gp49B1 inhibitory receptor. J Immunol 1997; 159:2342–2349.
76. Yokoi H, Myers A, Matsumoto K, et al. Alteration and acquisition of Siglecs during in vitro maturation of CD34+ progenitors into human mast cells. Allergy 2006; 61:769–776.
77. Hua X, Kovarova M, Chason KD, et al. Enhanced mast cell activation in mice deficient in the A2b adenosine receptor. J Exp Med 2007; 204:117–128.

Mast cell-derived mediators

78. Schwartz LB, Irani AM, Roller K, et al. Quantitation of histamine, tryptase, and chymase in dispersed human T and TC mast cells. J Immunol 1987; 138:2611–2615.
79. Ohtsu H, Tanaka S, Terui T, et al. Mice lacking histidine decarboxylase exhibit abnormal mast cells. FEBS Lett 2001; 502:53–56.
80. Okinaga S, Ohrui T, Nakazawa H, et al. The role of HMT (histamine N-methyltransferase) in airways: a review. Methods Find Exp Clin Pharmacol 1995; 17(Suppl C):16–20.
81. Keyzer JJ, de Monchy JG, van Doormaal JJ, et al. Improved diagnosis of mastocytosis by measurement of urinary histamine metabolites. N Engl J Med 1983; 309:1603–1605.
82. Jutel M, Blaser K, Akdis CA. Histamine in allergic inflammation and immune modulation. Int Arch Allergy Immunol 2005; 137:82–92.
83. Bryce PJ, Mathias CB, Harrison KL, et al. The H1 histamine receptor regulates allergic lung responses. J Clin Invest 2006; 116:1624–1632.
84. Parsons ME, Ganellin CR. Histamine and its receptors. Br J Pharmacol 2006; 147(Suppl 1): S127–S135.
85. Akdis CA, Simons FE. Histamine receptors are hot in immunopharmacology. Eur J Pharmacol 2006; 533:69–76.
86. Dunford PJ, O'Donnell N, Riley JP, et al. The histamine H4 receptor mediates allergic airway inflammation by regulating the activation of CD4+ T cells. J Immunol 2006; 176:7062–7070.
87. Dunford PJ, Williams KN, Desai PJ, et al. Histamine H4 receptor antagonists are superior to traditional antihistamines in the attenuation of experimental pruritus. J Allergy Clin Immunol 2007; 119:176–183.
88. Castells MC, Irani AM, Schwartz LB. Evaluation of human peripheral blood leukocytes for mast cell tryptase. J Immunol 1987; 138:2184–2189.
89. Pallaoro M, Fejzo MS, Shayesteh L, et al. Characterization of genes encoding known and novel human mast cell tryptases on chromosome 16p13.3. J Biol Chem 1999; 274:3355–3362.
90. Schwartz LB. Diagnostic value of tryptase in anaphylaxis and mastocytosis. Immunol Allergy Clin North Am 2006; 26:451–463.
91. Wong GW, Foster PS, Yasuda S, et al. Biochemical and functional characterization of human transmembrane tryptase (TMT)/tryptase gamma. TMT is an exocytosed mast cell protease that induces airway hyperresponsiveness in vivo via an interleukin-13/interleukin-4 receptor alpha/signal transducer and activator of transcription (STAT) 6-dependent pathway. J Biol Chem 2002; 277:41906–41915.
92. Sakai K, Ren S, Schwartz LB. A novel heparin-dependent processing pathway for human tryptase. Autocatalysis followed by activation with dipeptidyl peptidase I. J Clin Invest 1996; 97:988–995.
93. Hallgren J, Pejler G. Biology of mast cell tryptase. An inflammatory mediator. FEBS J 2006; 273:1871–1895.
94. Pereira PJ, Bergner A, Macedo-Ribeiro S, et al. Human beta-tryptase is a ring-like tetramer with active sites facing a central pore. Nature 1998; 392:306–311.
95. Marquardt U, Zettl F, Huber R, et al. The crystal structure of human alpha1-tryptase reveals a blocked substrate-binding region. J Mol Biol 2002; 321:491–502.
96. Finotto S, Dolovich J, Denburg JA, et al. Functional heterogeneity of mast cells isolated from different microenvironments within nasal polyp tissue. Clin Exp Immunol 1994; 95:343–350.
97. Goldstein SM, Leong J, Schwartz LB, et al. Protease composition of exocytosed human skin mast cell protease-proteoglycan complexes. Tryptase resides in a complex distinct from chymase and carboxypeptidase. J Immunol 1992; 148:2475–2482.
98. Schwartz LB, Bradford TR. Regulation of tryptase from human lung mast cells by heparin. Stabilization of the active tetramer. J Biol Chem 1986; 261:7372–7379.
99. Huang C, Wong GW, Ghildyal N, et al. The tryptase, mouse mast cell protease 7, exhibits anticoagulant activity in vivo and in vitro due to its ability to degrade fibrinogen in the presence of the diverse array of protease inhibitors in plasma. J Biol Chem 1997; 272:31885–31893.
100. Huang C, Friend DS, Qiu WT, et al. Induction of a selective and persistent extravasation of neutrophils into the peritoneal cavity by tryptase mouse mast cell protease 6. J Immunol 1998; 160:1910–1919.
101. Compton SJ, Cairns JA, Holgate ST, et al. The role of mast cell tryptase in regulating endothelial cell proliferation, cytokine release, and adhesion molecule expression: tryptase induces expression of mRNA for IL-1 beta and IL-8 and stimulates the selective release of IL-8 from human umbilical vein endothelial cells. J Immunol 1998; 161:1939–1946.
102. Molino M, Barnathan ES, Numerof R, et al. Interactions of mast cell tryptase with thrombin receptors and PAR-2. J Biol Chem 1997; 272:4043–4049.
103. Caughey GH. Roles of mast cell tryptase and chymase in airway function. Am J Physiol 1989; 257(2 Pt 1):L39–46.
104. Clark JM, Abraham WM, Fishman CE, et al. Tryptase inhibitors block allergen-induced airway and inflammatory responses in allergic sheep. Am J Respir Crit Care Med 1995; 152(6 Pt 1): 2076–2083.
105. McEuen AR, Sharma B, Walls AF. Regulation of the activity of human chymase during storage and release from mast cells: the contributions of inorganic cations, pH, heparin and histamine. Biochim Biophys Acta 1995; 1267:115–121.
106. Lindstedt L, Lee M, Kovanen PT. Chymase bound to heparin is resistant to its natural inhibitors and capable of proteolyzing high density lipoproteins in aortic intimal fluid. Atherosclerosis 2001; 155:87–97.
107. Doggrell SA, Wanstall JC. Cardiac chymase: pathophysiological role and therapeutic potential of chymase inhibitors. Can J Physiol Pharmacol 2005; 83:123–130.
108. Baltatu O, Nishimura H, Hoffmann S, et al. High levels of human chymase expression in the pineal and pituitary glands. Brain Res 1997; 752:269–278.
109. Doggrell SA, Wanstall JC. Vascular chymase: pathophysiological role and therapeutic potential of inhibition. Cardiovasc Res 2004; 61:653–662.
110. Reynolds DS, Gurley DS, Austen KF. Cloning and characterization of the novel gene for mast cell carboxypeptidase A. J Clin Invest 1992; 89:273–282.
111. Henningsson F, Ledin J, Lunderius C, et al. Altered storage of proteases in mast cells from mice lacking heparin: a possible role for heparin in carboxypeptidase A processing. Biol Chem 2002; 383:793–801.
112. Irani AM, Goldstein SM, Wintroub BU, et al. Human mast cell carboxypeptidase. Selective localization to MCTC cells. J Immunol 1991; 147:247–253.
113. Lundequist A, Tchougounova E, Abrink M, et al. Cooperation between mast cell carboxypeptidase A and the chymase mouse mast cell protease 4 in the formation and degradation of angiotensin II. J Biol Chem 2004; 279:32339–32344.
114. Metz M, Piliponsky AM, Chen CC, et al. Mast cells can enhance resistance to snake and honeybee venoms. Science 2006; 313:526–530.
115. Tantravahi RV, Stevens RL, Austen KF, et al. A single gene in mast cells encodes the core peptides of heparin and chondroitin sulfate proteoglycans. Proc Natl Acad Sci U S A 1986; 83:9207–9210.
116. Levi-Schaffer F, Austen KF, Gravallese PM, et al. Coculture of interleukin 3-dependent mouse mast cells with fibroblasts results in a phenotypic change of the mast cells. Proc Natl Acad Sci U S A 1986; 83:6485–6488.
117. Gilead L, Bibi O, Razin E. Fibroblasts induce heparin synthesis in chondroitin sulfate E containing human bone marrow-derived mast cells. Blood 1990; 76:1188–1195.
118. Boyce JA. Eicosanoid mediators of mast cells: receptors, regulation of synthesis, and pathobiologic implications. Chem Immunol Allergy 2005; 87:59–79.
119. Hsieh FH, Lam BK, Penrose JF, et al. T helper cell type 2 cytokines coordinately regulate immunoglobulin E-dependent cysteinyl leukotriene production by human cord blood-derived mast cells: profound induction of leukotriene C(4) synthase expression by interleukin 4. J Exp Med 2001; 193:123–133.
120. Bradding P, Mediwake R, Feather IH, et al. TNF alpha is localized to nasal mucosal mast cells and is released in acute allergic rhinitis. Clin Exp Allergy 1995; 25:406–415.
121. Bradding P, Roberts JA, Britten KM, et al. Interleukin-4, -5, and -6 and tumor necrosis factor-alpha in normal and asthmatic airways: evidence for the human mast cell as a source of these cytokines. Am J Respir Cell Mol Biol 1994; 10:471–480.
122. Echtenacher B, Mannel DN, Hultner L. Critical protective role of mast cells in a model of acute septic peritonitis. Nature 1996; 381:75–77.
123. Suto H, Nakae S, Kakurai M, et al. Mast cell-associated TNF promotes dendritic cell migration. J Immunol 2006; 176:4102–4112.
124. Nakae S, Suto H, Iikura M, et al. Mast cells enhance T cell activation: importance of mast cell costimulatory molecules and secreted TNF. J Immunol 2006; 176:2238–2248.
125. Berry MA, Hargadon B, Shelley M, et al. Evidence of a role of tumor necrosis factor alpha in refractory asthma. N Engl J Med 2006; 354:697–708.
126. Bradding P, Feather IH, Wilson S, et al. Immunolocalization of cytokines in the nasal mucosa of normal and perennial rhinitic subjects. The mast cell as a source of IL-4, IL-5, and IL-6 in human allergic mucosal inflammation. J Immunol 1993; 151:3853–3865.
127. Bischoff SC, Sellge G, Manns MP, et al. Interleukin-4 induces a switch of human intestinal mast cells from proinflammatory cells to Th2-type cells. Int Arch Allergy Immunol 2001; 124:151–154.

128. Okumura S, Kashiwakura J, Tomita H, et al. Identification of specific gene expression profiles in human mast cells mediated by Toll-like receptor 4 and Fc epsilon RI. Blood 2003; 102: 2547–2554.

Mast cell pathobiology

129. Schwartz LB, Metcalfe DD, Miller JS, et al. Tryptase levels as an indicator of mast-cell activation in systemic anaphylaxis and mastocytosis. N Engl J Med 1987; 316:1622–1626.
130. Schwartz LB, Yunginger JW, Miller J, et al. Time course of appearance and disappearance of human mast cell tryptase in the circulation after anaphylaxis. J Clin Invest 1989; 83:1551–1555.
131. Brightling CE, Bradding P, Symon FA, et al. Mast-cell infiltration of airway smooth muscle in asthma. N Engl J Med 2002; 346:1699–1705.
132. Kraft M, Martin RJ, Lazarus SC, et al. Airway tissue mast cells in persistent asthma: predictor of treatment failure when patients discontinue inhaled corticosteroids. Chest 2003; 124:42–50.
133. Knight PA, Wright SH, Lawrence CE, et al. Delayed expulsion of the nematode Trichinella spiralis in mice lacking the mucosal mast cell-specific granule chymase, mouse mast cell protease-1. J Exp Med 2000; 192:1849–1856.
134. Ishikawa N, Horii Y, Nawa Y. Reconstitution by bone marrow grafting of the defective protective capacity at the migratory phase but not at the intestinal phase of Nippostrongylus brasiliensis infection in W/Wv mice. Parasite Immunol 1994; 16:181–186.
135. Bryce PJ, Miller ML, Miyajima I, et al. Immune sensitization in the skin is enhanced by antigen-independent effects of IgE. Immunity 2004; 20:381–392.
136. Nigo YI, Yamashita M, Hirahara K, et al. Regulation of allergic airway inflammation through Toll-like receptor 4-mediated modification of mast cell function. Proc Natl Acad Sci U S A 2006; 103:2286–2291.
137. Mazzoni A, Siraganian RP, Leifer CA, et al. Dendritic cell modulation by mast cells controls the Th1/Th2 balance in responding T cells. J Immunol 2006; 177:3577–3581.
138. Jutel M, Watanabe T, Klunker S, et al. Histamine regulates T-cell and antibody responses by differential expression of H1 and H2 receptors. Nature 2001; 413:420–425.
139. Lu LF, Lind EF, Gondek DC, et al. Mast cells are essential intermediaries in regulatory T-cell tolerance. Nature 2006; 442:997–1002.

140. Taube C, Miyahara N, Ott V, et al. The leukotriene B4 receptor (BLT1) is required for effector CD8+ T cell-mediated, mast cell-dependent airway hyperresponsiveness. J Immunol 2006; 176:3157–3164.
141. Lee DM, Friend DS, Gurish MF, et al. Mast cells: a cellular link between autoantibodies and inflammatory arthritis. Science 2002; 297:1689–1692.
142. Olsson Y. Mast cells in plaques of multiple sclerosis. Acta Neurol Scand 1974; 50:611–618.
143. Rozniecki JJ, Hauser SL, Stein M, et al. Elevated mast cell tryptase in cerebrospinal fluid of multiple sclerosis patients. Ann Neurol 1995; 37:63–66.
144. Tanzola MB, Robbie-Ryan M, Gutekunst CA, et al. Mast cells exert effects outside the central nervous system to influence experimental allergic encephalomyelitis disease course. J Immunol 2003; 171:4385–4391.
145. Dvorak AM, Mihm MC Jr, Osage JE, et al. Bullous pemphigoid, an ultrastructural study of the inflammatory response: eosinophil, basophil and mast cell granule changes in multiple biopsies from one patient. J Invest Dermatol 1982; 78:91–101.
146. Chen R, Ning G, Zhao ML, et al. Mast cells play a key role in neutrophil recruitment in experimental bullous pemphigoid. J Clin Invest 2001; 108:1151–1158.
147. Hochegger K, Siebenhaar F, Vielhauer V, et al. Role of mast cells in experimental anti-glomerular basement membrane glomerulonephritis. Eur J Immunol 2005; 35:3074–3082.
148. Kanamaru Y, Scandiuzzi L, Essig M, et al. Mast cell-mediated remodeling and fibrinolytic activity protect against fatal glomerulonephritis. J Immunol 2006; 176:5607–5615.
149. Timoshanko JR, Kitching R, Semple TJ, et al. A pathogenetic role for mast cells in experimental crescentic glomerulonephritis. J Am Soc Nephrol 2006; 17:150–159.
150. Weller K, Foitzik K, Paus R, et al. Mast cells are required for normal healing of skin wounds in mice. FASEB J 2006; 20:2366–2368.
151. Oh CK. Mast cell mediators in airway remodeling. Chem Immunol Allergy 2005; 87:85–100.
152. Lindstedt KA, Kovanen PT. Mast cells in vulnerable coronary plaques: potential mechanisms linking mast cell activation to plaque erosion and rupture. Curr Opin Lipidol 2004; 15: 567–573.
153. Abonia JP, Friend DS, Austen WG Jr, et al. Mast cell protease 5 mediates ischemia-reperfusion injury of mouse skeletal muscle. J Immunol 2005; 174:7285–7291.
154. Strbian D, Karjalainen-Lindsberg ML, Tatlisumak T, et al. Cerebral mast cells regulate early ischemic brain swelling and neutrophil accumulation. J Cereb Blood Flow Metab 2006; 26:605–612.

Biology of Basophils

20

John T Schroeder

CONTENTS

- Introduction 329
- Development and morphology 329
- Functional and phenotypic markers 330
- Inflammatory mediators 332
- Basophil activation 333
- Pharmacological modulation of secretion 336
- Basophil involvement in disease 337
- Summary 338

SUMMARY OF IMPORTANT CONCEPTS

>> Basophil granulocytes develop in the bone marrow and are released into circulation as mature end-stage cells that represent <1% of the leukocytes in blood

>> While their exact role in in vivo processes remains an enigma, basophils secrete a variety of mediators and cytokines that are central in allergic disease

>> Evidence indicates that basophils are particularly capable of generating IL-4 and IL-13, cytokines that promote IgE synthesis

>> While having a role in IgE-dependent reactions, basophils also express receptors specific for microbial products that indicate a role in innate immunity

>> Immunohistochemistry has confirmed evidence that basophils selectively migrate into sites of allergic inflammation in the skin, nose, and lung

■ INTRODUCTION ■

Paul Ehrlich first identified basophil granulocytes in 1879, at which time he noted their distinctive cytoplasmic granules that bore remarkable similarity to those in tissue mast cells, which he had described a year

earlier.[1,2] Nearly 100 years were to pass before it was discovered that basophils, which constitute only ~1% of the circulating blood leukocytes, account for essentially all of the histamine released by blood cells in a reaction requiring immunoglobulin E (IgE).[3] While this observation initially prompted the notion that basophils might represent a surrogate with which to study the more elusive tissue mast cell, this belief has since been abandoned, as studies have demonstrated that the two cell types differ more than they are alike. Nonetheless, even though the basophil response has been extensively studied in vitro, the exact role for this cell in in vivo processes remains an enigma. However, there is renewed appreciation, more so now than ever, that basophils selectively infiltrate allergic lesions hours after allergen exposure, thereby releasing mediators and cytokines that perpetuate allergic inflammation and disease.

Symptoms that are the hallmark of immediate hypersensitivity reactions (see Chapter 29) begin when preformed (e.g., histamine) and newly synthesized (e.g., leukotrienes) mediators are released from basophils and mast cells. Degranulation events resulting in the release of these mediators are preceded by a cascade of intricate intracellular signals resulting from the interaction of allergen with specific IgE molecules bound to the high-affinity IgE receptors on the surface of these cells (see Chapter 14). This IgE-mediated activation also leads to the production of immunomodulatory cytokines. In particular, basophils have the capacity to produce more IL-4 and IL-13 in response to allergen than any other cell type found in blood. Since these two cytokines are critical for the development of atopy and, in fact, are found in high levels in allergic lesions, the role of basophils in allergic diseases takes on a whole new significance. Therefore, this chapter, while providing an overview, will focus on some of the more recent developments pertaining to the biology of basophils.

■ DEVELOPMENT AND MORPHOLOGY ■

Like all granulocytes, basophils (Fig. 20.1) are of myeloid origin developing from pluripotent stem cell precursors found in the bone marrow. While the exact factors important in this differentiation remain

329

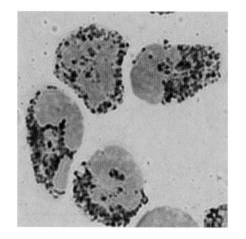

Fig. 20.1.   Human basophils purified from blood (Wright's stain, ×1000).

Table 20.1 General properties of human basophils

Origin	Bone marrow
Lineage	Myeloid
Frequency in circulation	<1% of WBCs
Size (μm)	5–8
Nucleus	Lobed
Chromatin appearance	Condensed
Metachromatic granules	Yes, (but less than in mast cells)
Granule glycosaminoglycan	Chondroitin sulfate
Proliferative capacity	None
Survival in circulation (days)	~3–7

WBCs, white blood cells.

unknown, the cytokine interleukin-3 (IL-3), likely plays a critical role. This belief is supported by in vitro studies showing that $CD34^+$ precursor cells, when cultured in the presence of IL-3, differentiate into cells that morphologically and functionally resemble basophils. As will become apparent in discussions below, IL-3 also plays a significant role in the survival and activation of mature basophils, which are functional consequences of these cells retaining the expression of IL-3 receptors at remarkably high levels. However, upon being released from the marrow as mature cells, basophils have little capacity (if any) for further development and are thought to survive for only days. For comparison, mast cell development involves the release of intermediate precursors from the bone marrow that are capable of targeting specific tissue sites for maturation where their survival has been estimated on the order of months. A recent study in mice has shown compelling evidence that mast cells and basophils are derived from a common precursor.[4] And while recurrent proposals suggesting that human basophils and mast cells are also of the same lineage,[5] the general consensus at this time is that the two cell types are unrelated developmentally. In fact, basophils are more closely related to eosinophils than they are to mast cells.[6] Precursor cells giving rise to cells possessing characteristics of basophils and eosinophils have been identified in bone marrow, cord blood, and whole blood. The frequencies of these precursor cells are increased in asthmatics and in subjects who have undergone experimental allergen provocation, suggesting a positive feedback mechanism by which exposure to allergen results in bone marrow activation and increased production of both basophils and eosinophils.

A vast amount of information regarding the morphology of basophils has come from the work of Ann Dvorak and her colleagues using electron microscopy to probe ultrastructural features found in both normal and activated cells.[7] For the purpose of brevity, only a few properties of human basophils are listed in Table 20.1.

Since the 1970s, Dvorak and her colleagues have also described, at the subcellular level, at least two major non-cytotoxic degranulation patterns that occur in basophils depending on the type of stimulus used. Anaphylactic degranulation is a very rapid and 'explosive' event that is characterized by a regulated granule extrusion by exocytosis that can ultimately result in an intact cell that is completely degranulated. As expected, this pattern is common with IgE-mediated degranulation resulting from the binding of specific antigen or anti-IgE antibody. Piecemeal degranulation was initially used to describe the pattern of degranulation observed in basophils found in certain cell-mediated pathological conditions, including contact dermatitis, skin graft rejection, Crohn's disease, and ulcerative colitis. It is characterized by an induced vesicular transport of granular content that does not involve direct granule extrusion. Various cytokines and chemokines that modulate basophil activity (see below) are believed to induce this type of degranulation.

■ FUNCTIONAL AND PHENOTYPIC MARKERS ■

ADHESION

Basophils possess the ability to selectively infiltrate into tissue sites, particularly in the skin, nose, and lung (see below). They are thought to achieve this through the timely expression of various molecules that enable their migration from the circulation across the endothelial barrier through a complex series of adhesion-deadhesion events. Specific selectins, integrins, and members belonging to the immunoglobulin (Ig) family have all been identified on basophils. As for other leukocytes, the initial steps of basophil attachment to endothelium occur during the so-called 'rolling' events where selectins play a critical role for basophils; this is done through the expression of L-selectin (CD62L), which attaches to the ligands CD34 and MAdCAM-1.[8] In contrast, the β1- and β2-integrins, along with intracellular adhesion molecules (ICAMs) (or Ig-like molecules) are all thought to mediate the firm attachment of cells to the endothelium, which is ultimately necessary for transmigration through this barrier. Basophils, along with eosinophils and certain lymphocytes, are all thought to achieve this, in part, through their expression of the β1-integrin, very late antigen (VLA)-4 (α4β1). The ligand for VLA-4, vascular cell adhesion molecule (VCAM)-1, has been shown to play an integral role in the selective trafficking of all three cell types into allergic lesions. In fact, the expression of VCAM-1 on endothelium is specifically upregulated by exposure to IL-4 and IL-13.[9] Therefore, by producing these cytokines, basophils (see below) could potentially facilitate their own migration into tissue as well as that of eosinophils and lymphocytes.

CYTOKINE RECEPTORS

Efforts to determine the cytokine receptors expressed by basophils initiated with studies by Thueson et al describing basophil histamine releasing activity in the supernatants of mitogen-activated peripheral blood mononuclear cells (PBMCs).[10] Since that time, receptors for several of the interleukins have been identified on basophils, including IL-2, IL-3, IL-4, IL-5, and IL-8. The physiologic significance of the expression of many, particularly the IL-2 and IL-4 receptors, remains a mystery. In fact, high-affinity receptors have only been identified for IL-3, IL-4, and IL-8. As noted above, high levels of the IL-3 receptor (CD123) are retained on mature basophils.[11,12] Interestingly, plasmacytoid dendritic cells (pDC) are the only other circulating leukocyte that expresses an equivalent amount of CD123, suggesting some level of crosstalk between these two cell types. Recent evidence also supports this belief. First, pDC are the major source of Type I interferons (e.g., IFN-α/β), which are innate immunity-associated cytokines known not only for their antiviral properties but more recently for possessing pro-Th1 activity. Basophils express the major receptor (IFNαR1) that binds these cytokines, and both IFN-α and IFN-β inhibit the priming effects that IL-3 has on basophil function.[13] While the hypothetical consequences for this innate immune regulation are discussed in sections below, by secreting Type I IFNs, pDC may play an important role in suppressing basophil activity. This is despite the fact that IL-3 plays an important role in augmenting the responses of both cell types. Other cytokine receptors found on basophils include those for GM-CSF, interferon (IFN)-γ, tumor necrosis factor (TNF), and the high-affinity receptor for nerve growth factor (NGF), also known as TrkA.[14,15] There is some evidence that the stem cell factor (SCF) receptor (or CD117) is found on basophils, but its levels are significantly lower than those found on mast cells.[16]

Basophils also express a variety of chemokine receptors, particularly those belonging to the so-called CC or β-family, which have no intervening amino acids between their conserved cysteine residues. Of these, CCR3 is the most prominently expressed on basophils, and it likely accounts for the overlapping activity mediated by several of the CC chemokines.[17] The monocyte chemotactic protein (MCP) subfamily, RANTES (CCL5), and eotaxin-1, 2, 3 (CCL11, 24, 26), all bind this receptor and all are reported to possess potent chemotactic activity for basophils. Until recently, CXCR2 was thought to be the only non-CC chemokine receptor found on basophils, its expression accounting for the histamine-releasing activity described for IL-8 (CXCL8), one of its ligands. However, basophils also express CXCR4 for which stromal cell-derived factor (SDF)-1 (CXCL12) is an important ligand capable of activating basophils for chemotaxis in addition to causing mediator release.[18,19] This receptor is found on lymphocytes and is a cofactor necessary for infection by the human immunodeficiency virus (HIV). Whether it also facilitates HIV's infection of basophils remains unknown.

The recently described chemoattractant receptor-homologous molecule expressed on T helper (Th)2 cells (CRTH2) is a newly described receptor for prostaglandin (PG) D2 that, like the chemokine receptors, is important for cell trafficking. It is expressed at high levels on basophils, eosinophils, and Th2 cells, suggesting that it is a key player in allergic inflammation.[20]

ACTIVATION-LINKED MARKERS

The most distinguishing functional characteristic of basophils (and mast cells) is their ability to bind IgE immunoglobulin with high affinity. This interaction is mediated through the α-subunit of FcϵRI, the entire receptor being composed of three subunits organized in the cell membrane as an $\alpha\beta\gamma_2$ tetramer. The structure for the α-subunit has been resolved by X-ray crystallography, revealing an unusual ringed-like structure within the subunit that consist of four tryptophan residues.[21,22] The unique orientation of these very hydrophobic amino acids is believed to confer the high affinity for IgE (Ka >10^{10}). Human basophils may express between 5000 and 1 million FcϵRI sites per cell, depending on the donor, and it is now well accepted that serum IgE levels regulate this expression. For instance, FcϵRI levels increase with higher serum IgE concentrations through a mechanism where the receptor half-life on the cell surface is stabilized when occupied by the immunoglobulin.[23] This is an important aspect to consider in light of anti-IgE therapy for the prevention of allergic disease. With just an estimated ~200 IgE/receptor cross-links being required to initiate mediator release from basophils (and presumably from mast cells), a minimum reduction in allergen-specific IgE of ~96% is required to achieve clinical efficacy. Thus, both the amount of drug and the duration that it is given become very important parameters in achieving this efficacy. Finally, it is also important to note that all IgE-binding to basophils is mediated through FcϵRIα, as these cells do not express FcϵRII (CD23) which is the low-affinity IgE receptor more commonly expressed on B lymphocytes.

Cell types other than basophils and mast cells are also reported to express FcϵRI, including Langerhan cells,[24,25] monocytes,[26] and dendritic cells (DC).[27,28] Eosinophils have high levels of intracellular FcϵRIα.[29] All of these cells lack mRNA and protein for the β-subunit and therefore do not appear to express the full tetrameric form of the receptor. While this has made it difficult to interpret the function of FcϵRI expression on the surface of these cells, a role in allergen presentation (DCs) and parasitic immunity (eosinophils) have been suggested. FcϵRI cross-linking has also been shown to induce pro-inflammatory cytokines (TNF-α, IL-6) from pDCs yet simultaneously suppresses their capacity to secrete IFN-α. This finding suggests one potential mechanism for dysregulation between adaptive (IgE-dependent) vs innate immune responses.[30]

The only other immunoglobulin receptor identified on basophils is FcγRII (CD32), which binds various subclasses of IgG antibody. It is suggested that the function of FcγRII on basophils is to induce intracellular signals that oppose those mediated through FcϵRI, thereby downregulating IgE-mediated responses in basophil and mast cells. Studies have shown that FcγRII/FcϵRI co-stimulation attenuates mediator release and cytokine production by basophils.[31] A reagent seemingly capable of this co-stimulation has been synthesized and shown to possess clinical efficacy in an animal model.[32]

Basophils are one of just a few cell types that express the cell surface ligand for CD40 (CD40L);[33] others include mast cells, activated T cells, platelets, and endothelial cells. Cells expressing CD40L, by interacting with CD40 on the surface of B lymphocytes, can relay signals necessary for the latter cell type to develop into immunoglobulin-producing cells. By expressing CD40L and secreting IL-4 and IL-13, basophils have long been shown to provide the two necessary signals for B cells to produce IgE.[33]

In recent years, there has been rationale for using the increased expression of specific surface activation markers readily detected by flow cytometry as a clinical means to determine basophil activation. In particular, both CD63 and CD203c are rapidly expressed (within minutes) on the basophil surface following FcεRI-dependent activation, such as that occurring with allergen. CD69 also increases with this mode of activation but the kinetics are slower (hours) and it is more readily induced following prolonged exposure to IL-3. A variety of issues relating to specificity and concentration of stimulus required for inducing these activation markers has raised concern regarding their diagnostic utility. [34]

RECEPTORS ASSOCIATED WITH INNATE IMMUNITY

Basophils express a number of receptors associated with innate immunity. Receptors for complement (CR) are found on basophils including CR1, CR3, CR4, and the receptor for the anaphylatoxin C5a (C5aR). At this time, only C5aR seems to be of functional consequence; it mediates degranulation induced by C5a (see below). The bacterial peptide, fMLP, binds a seven-membrane transverse receptor that structurally resembles those that bind chemokines. It too mediates basophil degranulation (see below). Basophils have more recently been found to express two additional types of innate immunity-associated receptors: (1) Toll-like receptors (e.g., TLR1, 2, 4, 6, and 9),[35] which bind a variety of microbial products; (2) leukocyte immunoglobulin-like receptors (e.g., LIR3, 7),[36] for which the natural ligands have not yet been identified. Receptors in both families, when ligated using natural ligands or receptor-specific antibodies, have been shown to mediate either inhibitory or stimulatory activity (see below).

OTHER RECEPTORS/SPECIFIC MARKERS

Many other markers and receptors have been characterized or identified on basophils. Receptors for prostacyclin, platelet-activating factor (PAF), adenosine, and histamine have all been detected on basophils. At least three monoclonal antibodies have been described that immunologically detect proteins unique to basophils and/or their progenitors. Two such antibodies, 2D7 and BB1, have specificity for proteins found within the cytoplasmic granules. The monoclonal antibody, 2D7, recognizes a 72 kDa protein that is released upon degranulation,[37] while BB1 is specific for a large (MW = 5×10^6 Da) complex referred to as basogranulin.[38] A third antibody, 97A6, detects protein found on the surface of basophil progenitors as well as mature cells.[39] All three antibodies have utility in identifying basophils in allergic lesions. However, there is presently no known role or function for the proteins they detect. Finally, there has been recent evidence that an antibody targeting pro-major basic protein-1 (J175–7D4) specifically recognizes basophils, suggesting that it too may have potential use in identifying basophil involvement in allergic and non-allergic lesion sites.[40]

■ INFLAMMATORY MEDIATORS ■

HISTAMINE

Basophils constitutively store, on average, approximately 1 pg of histamine per cell, and this amount is remarkably consistent among allergic and non-allergic donor populations. Histamine is synthesized by

the actions of histidine decarboxylase, which removes a carboxyl group from L-histidine. Its storage in basophils is mediated through ionic interactions with the highly charged proteoglycan, chondroitin sulfate, as opposed to heparin sulfate in the mast cell. These complexes dissociate with changes in pH and ionic strength that occur during the process of degranulation, thus resulting in the release of histamine. The physiological consequences of histamine on smooth muscle, the vasculature, and neural tissues are well documented. As a spasmogen, it is capable of smooth muscle contraction; it causes vascular leakage by its ability to dilate terminal arterioles. The clinical efficacy of H_1-receptor antagonists in the treatment of allergic symptoms is partially mediated by their ability to prevent histamine from binding H_1 receptors in the airways and vasculature.

Through its interaction with H_2-receptor sites found on various leukocytes, histamine has also been shown to modulate specific immune responses. Most recently, pro-Th1 cytokines secreted by dendritic cell subtypes are reportedly inhibited following histamine exposure,[41,42] thus indicating that histamine modulates immune reactions by polarizing for Th2-like responses.

OTHER PREFORMED MEDIATORS

Although tryptase and major basic protein (MBP) have long been considered mast cell- and eosinophil-specific mediators, respectively, small quantities of these proteins are also stored in basophils. In fact, one study has shown that the tryptase levels detected in basophils of some donors may reach those found in mast cells.[43] While the significance of these findings are unclear at this time, it does raise caution in evaluating studies that use tryptase as the sole specific marker for identifying the presence of mast cells in tissue using immunohistochemistry.

LEUKOTRIENE C4

Upon activation with various stimuli, basophils rapidly metabolize arachidonic acid (AA) through the lipoxygenase pathway to generate leukotriene C4 (LTC4). Thus, unlike histamine, this mediator is not stored in the cytoplasmic granules, but its rate of secretion (i.e., min) is only slightly slower than that of histamine, suggesting that it also contributes the acute symptoms associated with allergic reactions. The levels of LTC4 generated by both basophils and mast cells (i.e., 10^{-14} to 10^{-13}g per cell) are far less than the amounts of histamine stored in these cell types (i.e., 10^{-12} g per cell). However, on a molar basis, LTC4 is some 6000 times more potent than histamine in contracting airway smooth muscle. Studies in various animal models have shown that LTC4 and its products D4 and E4 can account for profound bronchoconstrictive and mucus-producing effects when released in the airways. In the skin, these leukotrienes produce a prolonged wheal and flare. As a result, LTC4, LTD4, and LTE4 are all thought to play a significant role in late phase responses (LPRs) following allergen exposure. Studies investigating the clinical efficacy of leukotriene blockers have supported this belief.[44,45]

CYTOKINES

Cytokines represent a third class of mediator released by basophils. In particular, basophils are a significant source of IL-4 and IL-13, two of the so-called Th2 cytokines, whose expression is characteristic of allergic lesions and which are now considered critical components in the pathogenesis of allergic disease. Most importantly, isotype-switching in B cells, from IgM to IgE, is absolutely dependent on the biological activities of either IL-4 or IL-13. Subsequently, when CD40 on the surface of B cells is engaged with cells expressing CD40L, including basophils themselves, then synthesis of IgE occurs. Both IL-4 and IL-13 upregulate VCAM-1 expression on endothelium, thus playing an important role in the selective recruitment of eosinophils, basophils, and lymphocytes into sites of allergic inflammation.[9] Class II major histocompatibility (MHC) antigens, such as human leukocyte antigen (HLA)-DR, are also upregulated on cells exposed to IL-4 or IL-13. Only IL-4, however, is thought to promote the Th2 phenotype. This immunomodulatory effect of IL-4 is of great importance because it implies that in order for T cells to produce Th2 cytokines (e.g., IL-4, IL-5, IL-13), they must first encounter IL-4. As a result, it has been suggested that several non-T lymphocyte cell types, including basophils, might provide the IL-4 necessary for amplifying Th2 responses.[46]

The belief that a non-T cell source of IL-4 might amplify Th2 responses and therefore promote allergic disease has sparked considerable debate among investigators as to the cell type(s) capable of such a feat. At this time, the volume of evidence indicates that basophils are a primary source of IL-4. Early studies revealed that both mRNA and protein for this cytokine correlated with the presence of basophils.[47] In peripheral blood mononuclear cell (PBMC) cultures, which have been traditionally used to demonstrate T-cell cytokine production, the 1–2% basophils typically found in these suspensions accounted for essentially all of the IL-4 secreted in response to allergen stimulation.[48] This finding has a simple explanation: the frequency of antigen-specific basophils (i.e., those expressing antigen-specific IgE) far out-numbers the antigen-specific T cells, which at best, are estimated at 1 in 3000–5000. Table 20.2 lists the relative amounts of IL-4 produced by basophils, mast cells, and eosinophils.

Recently developed IL-4 reporter mice strains (i.e., G4 and 4get mice) have substantiated the importance of IL-4 production by basophils by providing direct in vivo evidence for these cells driving Th2 polarization. Interestingly, these animals all have eosinophils, mast cells, and basophils that are positive for IL 4 mRNA, but only the basophils in these animals secrete significant levels of IL-4 protein.[49] Moreover, the evidence emerging from studies using these mice is showing that the basophil may very well provide the initial source of IL-4 responsible for amplifying Th2 responses. Animals depleted of mast cells, eosinophils, and T cells still mount a Th2 inflammatory response, which, by all accounts, is dependent on granulocytes resembling basophils.[50]

The evidence at this time indicates that basophils produce only Th2-like cytokines. There are no reports of basophils secreting Th1-like cytokines. In addition to producing IL-4 and IL-13, basophils have been shown to express mRNA for an IL-17 family cytokine, referred to as ML-1.[51] Furthermore, Li et al have reported the production of MIP-1α by basophils and it seems likely that other chemokines are made by these cells, with implications that basophils may modulate cell trafficking into lesion sites.[52]

A recent study has shown that basophils synthesize and release granzyme B, perhaps suggesting yet another class of mediator produced by these cells.[53] While generally considered to be a NK cell product, large quantities of granzyme B were made by basophils in response to IL-3 stimulation, but not in response to IgE receptor activation. The significance for such a finding remains undetermined.

■ BASOPHIL ACTIVATION ■

IgE-DEPENDENT

When allergen interacts with specific IgE occupying FcεRI receptors on the surface of basophils a succession of intracellular events is initiated that culminate in the secretion of mediators and cytokines. Mediator release induced by antigen has often been depicted as the simple cross-linking of at least two IgE/receptor complexes. In reality, the interaction is far more complex with the overall response being dependent on the sensitivity of the cell, or the number of receptors needed for aggregation in order to achieve 50% of maximal release.[54] This is further complicated by the fact that basophils can express many different IgE specificities that potentially affect sensitivity by creating changes in spatial availability for antigen binding. As it stands, sensitivities vary significantly among the basophils of different donors, with the number of aggregates required for histamine release ranging from as few as 200 to as many as 30 000. It is not fully understood at this time whether the numbers of aggregates for LTC4 release and cytokine secretion differ significantly from those optimal for histamine release. However, it has been shown that only subtle differences exist in the sensitivities for the three classes of mediators, despite clear differences in the general parameters important for their release.[55]

Under optimal conditions, which include an absolute requirement for calcium, basophils will release histamine, LTC4, and cytokines over a wide range of antigen concentrations, with the dose–response curves for all three classes of mediators following a typical bell-shaped curve. Because of their ability to interact indiscriminately with the IgE and FcεRIα on basophils of both allergic and non-allergic subjects, investigators often rely on the use of anti-IgE and anti-FcεRIα antibodies, respectively, to activate cells from both donor populations in responses that mimic that occurring with specific antigen. These stimuli also produce classic bell-shaped dose–response curves with regard to the release of these mediators, although generally over a much narrower range of concentrations.

While all three classes of mediators are released from basophils upon IgE-mediated stimulation, there are considerable differences in the rates at which they are secreted. Maximum release of preformed histamine, with either anti-IgE or antigen, is nearly complete within 20 min. As noted earlier, LTC4 is not stored as a preformed mediator, but its synthesis and release is also nearly complete within minutes following IgE-mediated stimulation. In contrast, the time course for cytokine generation is very different and appears dependent on signals that initiate transcription and translation for de novo synthesis. For example, increased levels of IL-4 protein are secreted within 1 h following IgE-mediated activation, are half maximal at 2 h, and peak after 4–6 h incubation.[56,57] Cycloheximide, an inhibitor of protein synthesis, will ablate any further increases in IL-4 secretion if added at any time during the culture incubation. Increases in mRNA for IL-4 are detected within 30 min following activation, with levels peaking at about 2 h.[47,58] Message levels are back near baseline by 3–4 h, which likely accounts for the waning in the secretion of IL-4 protein at this time. The generation of IL-13 also involves de novo synthesis, but the general consensus at this time is that it begins minutes to hours after IL-4 secretion is initiated and peaks some 18–20 h later. Despite an apparent longer duration in IL-13 secretion, basophils from most

Table 20.2 Reported levels of IL-4 and IL-13 secreted by human basophils in response to selected stimuli: comparison with those reported for human mast cells, eosinophils, and lymphocytes[a]

		(pg/10^6 cells)		Stimulus	References
		IL-4	IL-13		
Basophils		20–1200	<10–500	Antigen, anti-IgE, anti-FcεRI	47,56,57
		<100	50–1000	IL-3	56,57,59,60,71
		20–500	nr	HRF[b]	56
		<10	10–120	NGF	15
		500–2000	~250–1500	Ca^{2+} ionophores	38,56
		<50	~100–700	PMA	59
Mast cells	(isolated from lung) (culture-derived)	~5–10	nr	SCF/anti-IgE	53a
		nr	42–240	SCF+IL-4+anti-IgE	53b
Eosinophils		0–45	nr	sonicated cells, Ca^{2+} ionophore	53c
Blood lymphocytes[c]		50–150	nt	PMA+Ca^{2+} ionophore	58
T-cell clones	(culture-derived)	~10,000	~10,000	Antigen	Many

nr, no report found; nt, not tested.
[a]Cytokine protein levels determined by ELISA.
[b]Using HRF-responder cells.
[c]Mixed lymphocyte suspensions depleted of basophils.

donors consistently produce more IL-4 than IL-13 following IgE-mediated activation.

Several laboratories have shown that mRNA for IL-4 is constitutively expressed (at about ~10 copies per cell) in unstimulated or 'resting' basophils.[47,58] While this is also true for IL-13 mRNA expression,[59,60] it seems to be more consistent with IL-4. In agreement with these findings, others have shown that small quantities of IL-4 protein are secreted within 5–10 min following activation, and that, with time, gradual accumulations are seen when cells are simply placed in medium alone.[57] While the significance of these findings are unclear at this time, the low levels of IL-4 that are constitutively expressed may simply represent a small percentage of basophils that have either been activated while in the donor prior to blood drawing or during their preparation ex vivo.

While IgE-dependent mediator release and cytokine secretion follow bell–shaped dose–response curves, they do so using very different concentration gradients. Optimal levels of IL-4 and IL-13 are produced when concentrations of the cross-linking stimulus are 10-fold less than those required for optimal release of histamine and LTC4. This is particularly true with anti-IgE stimulation, but also with antigen challenge.[61] It seems probable that this dissociation in cytokine secretion and mediator release may mean that basophils play a dual role in allergic inflammation, depending on antigen concentrations within the microenvironment. At low concentrations of antigen, basophils may modulate the immune responses of B cells, T cells, and eosinophils through the production of IL-4 and IL-13. As they infiltrate the lesion site, and the concentration of antigen increases,

basophils may take on more of an effector role by secreting the two substances (i.e., histamine and LTC4) most responsible for the acute symptoms of allergic reactions.

The IgE-dependent release of mediators and cytokines discussed thus far refer to interactions between antigen and the variable light regions of specific IgE. However, Marone and colleagues have described an IgE-dependent activation of basophils mediated by the gp120 glycoprotein of the human immunodeficiency antigen (HIV), which apparently acts as a superantigen.[62] Gp120 non-specifically binds to the variable heavy domain (VHD)-3 of IgE. The production of IL-4 and IL-13, which results from this interaction, has been hypothesized as playing an important role in regulating the high IgE levels often observed in HIV-infected patients.

IgE-INDEPENDENT

Studies have long demonstrated that basophils are more reactive than are mast cells to a greater number of substances that induce histamine release independently of IgE/FcεRI cross-linking.[10] This is particularly true of products generated during immune reactions, such as cytokines and complement factors, but more recently has included agonists of specific innate immune responses (see below). Early studies collectively group such substance as histamine-releasing factors (HRFs). However, the development of recombinant DNA technology helped facilitate in identifying many HRFs as known proteins (e.g., chemotactic factors). While their exact significance in the pathogenesis of allergic disease remain unknown, these substances likely play a role in amplifying allergic reactions by inducing mediator release from basophils as they infiltrate allergic lesions during LPRs.

Specific chemokines are capable of activating basophils, particularly when using cells from allergic subjects. Members of the monocyte chemotactic protein (MCP) family (e.g., MCP-1,-3, and -4) have all been reported to cause degranulation when used at nanomolar concentrations.[17,63] They mediate this activity by interacting through several CCR receptors. Other CC chemokines, like RANTES/CCL5, MIP-1α/CCL3, and the eotaxins (I/CCL11 and II/CCL24), have more limited potential at inducing histamine release, mostly from cells obtained from allergic subjects or from cells primed first in IL-3. These chemokines interact with the CCR3 receptor, and appear to have a greater role in the selective recruitment of eosinophils, basophils, and lymphocytes into allergic lesions. As noted above, stromal cell-derived factor (SDF)-1/CXCL12 is a potent chemoattractant for basophils and is also capable of inducing histamine release from these cells.[18] This activity is mediated through the CXCR4 receptor that is reported to be inducible on basophils under certain culture conditions.[19] To date, there have been no reports of any of these chemokines directly inducing the secretion of IL-4 or IL-13 from basophils. However, Devouassoux et al have shown evidence that eotaxin/CCL11 enhances the production of IL-4 in response to IgE-mediated secretion.[64]

Early studies also showed evidence for the existence of a factor(s) that activated basophils of certain allergic subjects in a reaction that was very much dependent on the type of IgE expressed. This so-called IgE-dependent HRF was often found in lavage fluids taken from allergic lesions, and defined by its ability to induce histamine release from cells expressing an immunoglobulin referred to as IgE+.[65] Basophils not directly responding to this protein were said to express IgE−. MacDonald and colleagues eventually succeeded in subcloning and characterizing such a protein referred to as human recombinant HRF (HrHRF). It was subsequently determined that an intracellular protein referred to as translationally controlled tumor protein (TCTP) is identical to HrHRF, suggesting both extra- and intracellular functions for this protein. HrHRF induces histamine release only from basophils expressing IgE+, however, it seemingly does so through a specific, yet elusive, receptor that remains unidentified. It's also active on other cell types, including eosinophils and lymphocytes.[66,67] Therefore, insight into the significance of the IgE heterogeneity, which initially defined HrHRF activity, remains a mystery. Nonetheless, there has been no evidence of HrHRF interacting directly with IgE+, suggesting that it is not simply acting as an antigen.[68] Studies using electron microscopy have also supported this belief by demonstrating that HrHRF does not induce the classical anaphylactic degranulation typically observed in basophils undergoing activation with IgE-cross-linking stimuli.[69]

HrHRF not only induces histamine release but also can stimulate IL-4 secretion from basophils expressing IgE+. In cells expressing IgE−, HrHRF has been shown to act much like IL-3 (see below) in that it too is capable of priming for enhanced secretion of IL-4, IL-13, and histamine in response to FcεRI-mediated activation. This information first suggested that HrHRF activity is mediated through a specific receptor rather than IgE+, since it clearly showed that this protein exerted activity on basophils from all donors (i.e., those also expressing IgE−).

Several other cytokines play a role in enhancing basophil responses, in particular, IL-3, IL-5, GM-CSF, and NGF. These cytokines,

however, appear to play more of a role in modulating basophil secretion in response to other substances rather than acting as complete secretagogues. For example, all four cytokines possess some ability to acutely prime basophils for enhanced histamine release in response to IgE-dependent activation. At relatively high concentrations (~300 nM), IL-3 acts as a complete stimulus for histamine release. IL-3 by itself has essentially no ability to induce LTC4 synthesis and is generally a poor activator of IL-4. However, these products are also released to a greater extent following IgE-mediated activation of cells primed in IL-3. Studies have shown that IL-3 and IL-5 have late priming effects on LTC4 secretion, which are related to intracellular events involving the activation of cytosolic phospholipase A2 (cPLA2).[70] Perhaps the most striking activity mediated by IL-3 is its ability to activate basophils for IL-13 secretion directly.[59,60,71] In fact, studies have indicated that IL-3 is more potent in stimulating IL-13 secretion than is antigen or anti-IgE, which likely reflects difference in the mechanisms utilized by the two types of stimuli. The secretion of IL-13 in response to IL-3 is relatively slow to start, beginning after 4 h incubation; however, it remains ongoing beyond 20 h in culture. Interestingly, NGF possesses similar activity in that it, too, will stimulate IL-13 secretion, although at levels ~5–10-fold less than those produced by IL-3. Both cytokines induce ~2–3-fold more IL-13 from basophils obtained from allergic compared to normal subjects.[15] While the significance of this finding is unclear at this time, it does suggest an in vivo priming event occurring in allergic subjects, perhaps following allergen challenge, which causes their cells to be more responsive to IL-3 and NGF. Several other studies support this hypothesis.[72,73] Overall, it is becoming apparent that IL-3 affects essentially every aspect of basophil biology, including development and maturation, survival, acute/late effects on mediator release, and direct stimulation of IL-13 production. Studies continue to unravel some of the intracellular signaling pathways occurring in basophils following treatment with this cytokine.[74–76] Table 20.3 summarizes some of the effects IL-3 and other cytokines have on basophil function.

To date, only Type I interferons (IFN) such as IFN-α and IFN-β have been shown to negatively regulate basophil function.[13] However, these cytokines were shown not to affect FcεRI responses, but only those involving cytokine secretion in response either to IL-3 priming of IgE receptor activation or to the IL-13 secreted in direct response to IL-3.

The anaphylatoxins C5a and C3a and the bacterial-derived peptide f-Met-Leu-Phe (fMLP) are some of the most potent basophil secretogogues. Unlike the chemokines and cytokines described above, these are not necessarily linked to allergic inflammation, suggesting that basophil involvement in immune responses likely extends beyond that associated with immediate hypersensitivity reactions (see below). fMLP is a particularly active and rapid inducer of basophil histamine release, and mediates degranulation through a G protein-coupled receptor that is structurally related to the 7-membrane transversing chemokine receptors. As a result, the intracellular pathways utilized by fMLP during degranulation are very different from those culminating after FcεRI-mediated activation using antigen or anti-IgE. This is important to consider because neither fMLP, nor the chemokines that activate basophils for histamine release, when used alone, typically induce IL-4 and IL-13 secretion.[77] These findings support the belief that cytokine generation (particularly IL-4) is primarily a response mediated through FcεRI. As noted above, the exception to this is the stimulation of IL-13 in response to IL-3 or NGF, and, in fact, there is evidence that either C5a or fMLP,

Table 20.3 Selected cytokines and chemokines affecting basophil development and survival, chemotaxis, and secretion

	Receptor	Dev./survival	Chemotaxis	Activation[a]	Secreted products			
					HR	LTC4	IL-4	IL-13
Cytokine								
IL-3	(CD123)	Potent	–	Alone	±	±	+	+++
				Priming	+++	+++	+++	+
HRF	(Unknown)	nr	–	Alone[b]	++	nr	++	–
				Priming[c]	++	nr	++	++
IL-5	(CD125)	Weak	–	Alone	–	–	–	–
				Priming	+	+	nr	nr
GM-CSF	(CD-116)	Moderate	–	Alone	–	–	–	–
				Priming	+	+	nr	nr
NGF	(TrkA)	Weak	–	Alone	–	–	–	+
				Priming	+	+	++	+++
Chemokine								
MCP-1,2,3,4	CCR2, CCR3	–	Potent	Alone[b]	+	±	–	–
				With IL-3	+	+	±	±
Eotaxins, RANTES	CCR3	–	Potent	Alone[b]	+	±	–	–
				With IL-3	++	±	±	±
SDF-1	CXCR4	–	Potent	Alone	+	±	nr	nr

+, Relative in vitro response; ±, positive responses rarely observed; TrkA, tyrosine-kinase associated; nr, no reports; –, no activity.
[a]Used alone or for priming of FcεRI-mediated activation.
[b]Cells from selected allergic donors.
[c]Cells from most donors.

when combined with IL-3, can stimulate the generation of IL-4 and IL-13 in basophils.[78] Like fMLP, C5a does not normally activate basophils for cytokine secretion. Both of these stimuli are, however, capable of promoting LTC4 synthesis; the amount generated in response to C5a is greatly augmented in IL-3-primed basophils.

As noted above there is now evidence that basophils, like many other leukocytes, express various receptors associated with innate immunity and are responsive to specific agonists known to bind these receptors. In particular, TLR2 ligands, such as peptidoglycan (PGN), a major constituent of the cell wall of Gram-positive bacteria, have been shown to directly induce IL-4 and IL-13 from human basophils albeit at levels approximately one-tenth of what are typically induced upon IgE receptor stimulation.[35] Moreover, PGN and a synthetic TLR2 agonist, Pam$_3$Cys, were shown to markedly augment mediator release and/or cytokine secretion when combined with other stimuli, both IgE-dependent and -independent. In contrast, the same study indicated that basophils were unresponsive to TLR4 agonists such as LPS, a major constituent of Gram-negative bacteria, despite expressing mRNA and protein for this receptor. Other observations indicate that basophils express relatively high levels of TLR9, with evidence that ligands binding this receptor (i.e., CpG-DNA) inhibit rather

than augment IgE-dependent cytokine responses (JTS, unpublished observations). In related studies, the LIR family of receptors mediated similar differential effects on basophil function. Antibodies directed at LIR3 mediated inhibitory activity on basophil secretion whereas those that cross-linked LIR7 actually caused mediator release and cytokine secretion.[36]

PHARMACOLOGICAL MODULATION OF SECRETION

The relative ease of using washed leukocyte suspensions to investigate basophil histamine release has long made it possible for investigators to study the effects of various therapeutic drugs or inhibitors on both IgE-dependent and -independent responses. With the added knowledge that basophils secrete IL-4 and IL-13, and under conditions that differ dramatically from those important for histamine release, it is now possible to investigate whether certain drugs differentially affect these responses. It is important to note here that many such studies have also investigated the signal transduction events involved in these responses. This section will briefly focus on those therapeutic agents that are currently in use for the treatment of allergic conditions and how they affect mediator release by basophils challenged in vitro.

Many recent studies have found that drugs long known for inhibiting the release of preformed histamine from basophils are more effective at preventing the generation and secretion of cytokines from these cells. For instance, it has long been known that increases in cytosolic levels of cAMP negatively affect the IgE-mediated release of histamine.[79] Thus, substances that either stimulate cAMP synthesis through receptor-mediated activation of adenylate cyclase (i.e., β_2-agonists, PGE_2, histamine) or prevent its metabolism by inhibiting phosphodiesterases (theophylline) have been shown to inhibit, with varying potencies, the histamine released in response to anti-IgE stimulation (reviewed in reference 80). Gibbs and colleagues have shown that the β_2-agonist salmeterol is some 2–9 times more potent at inhibiting IL-4 and IL-13 secretion from basophils than it is at blocking histamine release.[81] In the same study, theophylline was found to be nearly 10-fold more active at inhibiting IL-4 than either histamine or IL-13. Like the cAMP-enhancing agents, various H_1-receptor antagonists have also long been known to inhibit IgE-mediated histamine release by basophils in vitro. In comparing the inhibitory effects on mediator release vs cytokine secretion, desloratadine was some ~7-fold more potent at inhibiting IL-4 than inhibiting either histamine or LTC4.[82] Terfenadine has also been shown to inhibit mediator release and cytokine secretion, but with similar potencies.[81] Interestingly, cetirizine was shown to have a slight enhancing effect on cytokine secretion in this study. Whether the clinical efficacy of these drugs in vivo is due, in part, to their ability to inhibit the basophil response is not currently known. Their relatively greater potency on cytokine secretion compared with mediator release has, however, renewed this debate.[83] In contrast, glucocorticosteroids have proven efficacy in the treatment of allergic disease by inhibiting many factors contributing to inflammation. These drugs were shown to inhibit in vitro histamine release from basophils some 20 years ago.[84] However, they did so only after an 8–20 h pre-incubation before activating the basophils with anti-IgE. Studies have since shown that anti-inflammatory steroids are far more effective in blocking basophil cytokine secretion; there is an immediate inhibition and at concentrations much lower than those required for the inhibition of mediator release.[85] Finally, the most potent inhibitors of IgE-mediated cytokine secretion are those agents that block Ca^{2+}-dependent calcineurin activity, such as tacrolimus and cyclosporin A (CsA). This has implied that the nuclear factor of activated T-cell (NFAT) family of transcription factors are involved in the transcription of IL-4 and IL-13 initiated with FcεRI activation. Interestingly, basophils have been shown to selectively and constitutively express high levels of NFAT2, with evidence that this transcription factor is important for the generation of IL-4 in these cells.[86] While NFAT2 is also believed to play a role in IL-4 transcription in T cells, its expression must first be induced. This may account for the somewhat delayed time course for IL-4 production by T cells compared to basophils. Unlike most leukocytes and lymphocytes, basophils appear to lack NFAT1 expression – a transcription factor believed to play an important role in the transcription of Th1 cytokines. Both tacrolimus and CsA have long been known to inhibit mediator release from basophils.[87,88] However, they do so at concentrations nearly 100-fold greater than those required to inhibit IgE-mediated cytokine secretion. Interestingly, tacrolimus has no effect on the IL-13 mRNA and protein produced by basophils in response to

IL-3 stimulation, suggesting that NFAT molecules are not involved in the signaling occurring with this mode of activation.[59]

▪ BASOPHIL INVOLVEMENT IN DISEASE ▪

CORRELATES OF ALLERGIC DISEASE

By the mid 1960s it was demonstrated that the histamine released by a patient's basophils challenged in vitro with ragweed allergen could predict the severity of the respiratory symptoms that the individual would experience during the ragweed season.[89] Other clinical correlates have since linked the basophil response to disease severity, particularly in conditions such as urticaria and asthma (reviewed in references 90 and 91). For instance, the basophils of some asthmatic subjects have been reported to spontaneously secrete histamine in vitro, and to possess an overall increased releasability to various substances, both physiological and non-physiological. Studies have indicated similar releasability phenomena observed for basophil cytokines. In this context, at least one report has demonstrated a 2- to 3-fold increase in the levels of IL-13 secreted from the basophils of allergic subjects compared to non-allergic controls, following exposure to IL-3 or NGF.[15] Likewise, it was recently suggested that repeated nasal allergen challenge induced changes in circulating basophils that are consistent with priming.[73] In this study, basophils spontaneously secreted IL-13 and expressed greater levels of FcεRIβ mRNA 4–24 h following a 3rd consecutive-day challenge, both of which had waned when examined 1 week later. The numbers of basophils and their progenitors are also often increased in the blood of asthmatics and in allergic individuals having been experimentally challenged with allergen.[92] From these studies, it does seem evident that there is a systemic activation or 'priming' of basophils in individuals presenting with clinical inflammatory disease. While this increased responsiveness of the basophil is likely a manifestation rather than a cause, the release of mediators and cytokines that result are thought to play an important role in the perpetuation of the inflammatory process and overall pathogenesis of the disease itself.

IN ALLERGIC DISEASE

The development of monoclonal antibodies that specifically detect human basophils in tissue have provided direct evidence that this once elusive cell is, indeed, found within sites of allergic inflammation and in naturally occurring diseases. By using the 2D7 basophil-specific antibody, Kepley et al confirmed earlier reports that indicated large numbers of basophils in the lungs of asthmatics, particularly from those individuals having died from severe asthma compared to those dying from non-asthmatic deaths.[93] Basophil-specific antibodies have also confirmed basophil involvement in chronic idiopathic urticaria and atopic dermatitis.[40,94]

LATE PHASE RESPONSES

The evidence that best supports the involvement of basophils in allergic inflammatory reactions has come from studies investigating the cellular inflammation, mediators, and parameters associated with the LPR following experimental allergen challenge. These reactions typically occur several hours (6–12 h) after attenuation of the immediate response and are manifested not only by symptoms that resemble those occurring during the early response but also by a selective recruitment of inflammatory cells from the circulation that accumulate at the lesion site. It has long been acknowledged that infiltrating eosinophils and, to a lesser extent, lymphocytes, are hallmark in these reactions. However, Lichtenstein and colleagues beginning in the early 1980s conducted numerous studies in the skin as well as in the upper and lower airways to demonstrate that basophils also selectively infiltrate these lesion sites and thus contribute to mediator release. As a result, their findings played an important role in establishing the belief that the LPR is largely mediated by basophils, while the immediate response is orchestrated by mast cells.[90]

There has since been a renewed appreciation of the participation of basophils in the LPR. This interest has evolved from knowledge that these cells secrete cytokines in addition to mediators, and that their identification in tissue has been made easier with the development of specific antibodies suitable for immunohistochemistry. Most interestingly, both 2D7 and BB1 have detected basophils infiltrating LPR lesions at frequencies significantly higher than those reported in earlier studies. This is particularly true in the skin where the frequency of basophils have approached 50% of that observed for eosinophils infiltrating these lesions.[95] Although the presence of basophils infiltrating the lung was somewhat less than that described in the skin, they still accounted for approximately 10% of the eosinophil infiltrate.[96,97] The sensitivity achieved using these antibodies has further indicated that basophil influx into reaction sites of the lung and skin is occurring within 6–7h and persisting for at least 24h. In the nose, the numbers of basophils were higher after 1h, rather than 24h, post-allergen challenge.[98] As a result of these findings, it is clear that the involvement of basophils in the LPR has been somewhat underestimated.

At least two independent studies indicate that basophils found in the LPR of the lung may also be a significant source of IL-4. In recovering BAL cells 18–24h following segmental allergen challenge, ongoing or spontaneous secretion of IL-4 ex vivo was detected only in the basophil suspensions, suggesting that these cells had been activated in vivo.[99] In sharp contrast, the lymphocytes and eosinophils that were also recovered from these lesions did not secrete detectable levels of this cytokine. Using dual immunohistochemical staining, Nouri-Aria et al showed that basophils detected by the 2D7 antibody in bronchial biopsies taken 24h after SAC accounted for over 70% of the cells co-staining for IL-4 protein and 25% of the cells expressing mRNA for this cytokine.[100] It seems probable that these results will prompt further studies evaluating the cells responsible for IL-4, given that most previous reports have emphasized lymphocytes as the primary source of this cytokine in allergic lesions.

DELAYED-TYPE HYPERSENSITIVITY

It has been known since the early 1970s that basophils participate in specific delayed-type hypersensitivity reactions that are apparent manifestations of cellular immunity. For instance, the Dvoraks and colleagues described the selective recruitment of basophils into sites of allergic contact dermatitis in humans that resembled the so-called cutaneous basophilic hypersensitivity reactions originally reported in the guinea-pig model.[101] When given rhus toxoid (the active agent in poison ivy) or dinitrochlorobenzene in a patch test, sensitized subjects developed skin reactions that were characterized by a cellular infiltrate into the dermis consisting of up to ~16% basophils by 3–6 days after

application of the antigen.[102] It was often noted that basophils were the only granulocytes found in these lesions. However, mononuclear cells accounted for most of the cells infiltrating these lesions, which led to the hypothesis that the selective recruitment of basophils resulted from the secretion of some factor(s) released by T cells. To date, there has been no description of a known chemokine or cytokine that is responsible for the recruitment of basophils in these reactions. The profound changes in the dermal microvasculature that often accompanied these CBH reactions suggested the release of inflammatory mediators. It remains unknown whether the basophils migrating into these reaction sites are secreting cytokines, although, it is intriguing to think that they may be producing IL-13, since the synthesis of this cytokine (unlike IL-4) seems less dependent on signals generated through FcεRI. Ultrastructural analysis of the cells recovered in biopsies taken from lesion sites showed basophils undergoing 'piecemeal' degranulation. Interestingly, an increased number of basophils showing an identical morphology have also been described in many other conditions involving a cellular immune component, including skin allograft and tumor rejection, viral hypersensitivity, and Crohn's disease.[103–106]

Finally, there is mounting evidence to support a relatively novel belief that human basophils play a role in impaired immunity to parasitic infections, which is completely opposite from the original theory that basophils are involved in natural immunity to parasites. First, there is a striking relationship between immediate hypersensitivity reactions and parasitic infections in that increased IgE, eosinophils, basophils, and mast cells are often associated with both immune responses. However, parasite antigens seldom, if ever, induce the clinical manifestations typically seen in immediate hypersensitivity reactions, despite high levels of antigen-specific IgE that is capable of sensitizing basophils and mast cells. It has been shown that basophils from patients with helminth infections secrete IL-4 and IL-13 in response to antigens derived from specific life stages of parasites.[107–110] The production of these cytokines by basophils is hypothesized in 'driving' the Th2 response seen in helminth infections, much like that proposed in immediate hypersensitivity. Interestingly, this apparent favoring of Th2-like responses is associated with impaired immunity to the parasite, suggesting that the production of IL-4 and IL-13 by basophils may create conditions that favor the survival of the organism.[107] In agreement with this belief, the translationally controlled tumor protein (TCTP) of *Plasmodium falciparum*, the organism responsible for malaria, is homologous to the HRF that causes histamine release and IL-4 secretion described above.[111] This form of immune mimicry by the organism, which is well known among certain viruses, is thought to benefit the organism by modifying the immune response that normally removes it from the host.

SUMMARY

Basophils have long been seen has a surrogate with which to study the more elusive mast cell. This view, however, is no longer valid, since there is substantial developmental and physiological evidence that these two cell types differ from one another more than they are alike. Once thought to do little other than secrete histamine and leukotriene C4, there is now firm evidence that basophils are the predominant cellular source of IL-4 and IL-13, perhaps the two most important cytokines having a role in the pathogenesis of allergic disease. This information, along with evidence that these cells infiltrate allergic lesions and are capable of responding to variety of stimuli, has sparked a renewed interest in them and in their role in allergic inflammation and disease.

References

Introduction

1. Ehrlich P. Beitrage zur kenntnis der granuliertan bindegewebszellen und der eosinophilen leukocyten. Arch Anat Physiol 1879; 3:166–169.
2. Ehrlich P. Beitrage zur kenntnis der anilinfarbungen und ihrer verwendung in der mikroskopischen technik. Arch Mikrosk Anat 1877; 13:263–277.
3. Ishizaka T, DeBernardo R, Tomioka H, et al. Identification of basophil granulocytes as a site of allergic histamine release. J Immunol 1972; 108:1000–1008.

Development and morphology

4. Arinobu Y, Iwasaki H, Gurish MF, et al. Developmental checkpoints of the basophil/mast cell lineages in adult murine hematopoiesis. Proc Natl Acad Sci USA 2005; 102:18105–18110.
5. Li L, Li Y, Reddel SW, et al. Identification of basophilic cells that express mast cell granule proteases in the peripheral blood of asthma, allergy, and drug-reactive patients. J Immunol 1998; 161:5079–5086.
6. Denburg J. The origins of basophils and eosinophils in allergic inflammation. J Allergy Clin Immunol; 102:S74–S6, 1998.
7. Dvorak A. Ultrastructural studies of human basophils and mast cells. J Histochem Cytochem 2005; 53:1043–1070.

Functional and phenotypic markers

8. Wimazal F, Ghannadan M, Muller M, et al. Expression of homing receptors and related molecules on human mast cells and basophils: a comparative analysis using multi-color flow cytometry and toluidine blue/immunofluorescence staining techniques. Tissue Antigens 1999; 54:599–507.
9. Bochner B, Klunk D, Sterbinsky S, et al. IL-13 selectively induces vascular cell adhesion molecule-1 expression in human endothelial cells. J Immunol 1995; 154:799–803.
10. Thueson D, Speck L, Lett-Brown M, et al. Histamine-releasing activity (HRF). I. Production by mitogen- or antigen-stimulated human mononuclear cells. J Immunol 1979; 123:626–631.
11. Sarmiento E, Espiritu B, Gleich G, et al. IL-3, IL-5, and granulocyte-macrophage colony-stimulating factor potentiates basophil mediator release stimulated by eosinophil granule major basic protein. J Immunol 1995; 155:2211–2221.
12. Yamada T, Sun Q, Zeibecoglou K, et al. IL-3, IL-5, granulocyte-macrophage colony-stimulating factor receptor alpha-subunit, and common beta-subunit expression by peripheral leukocytes and blood dendritic cells. J Allergy Clin Immunol 1998; 101:677–682.
13. Chen Y-H, Bieneman AP, Creticos PS, et al. IFN-alpha inhibits IL-3 priming of human basophil cytokine secretion but not leukotriene C4 and histamine release. J Allergy Clin Immunol 2003; 112:944–950.
14. Burgi B, Otten U, Ochensberger B, et al. Basophil priming by neurotrophic factors. Activation through the trk receptors. J Immunol 1996; 157:5582–5588.
15. Sin A, Roche E, Togias A, et al. Nerve growth factor or IL-3 induces more IL-13 production from basophils of allergic subjects than from basophils of nonallergic subjects. J Allergy Clin Immunol 2001; 108:387–393.
16. Columbo M, Horowitz EM, Botana LM, et al. The human recombinant c-kit receptor ligand, rhSCF, induces mediator release from human cutaneous mast cells and enhances IgE-dependent mediator release from both skin mast cells and peripheral blood basophils. J Immunol 1992; 149:599–608.
17. Uguccioni M, Mackay C, Ochensberger B, et al. High expression of the chemokine receptor CCR3 in human blood basophils. Role in activation by eotaxin, MCP-4, and other chemokines. J Clin Invest 1997; 100:1137–1143.
18. Jinquan T, Jacobi H, Jing C, et al. Chemokine stromal cell-derived factor 1α activates basophils by means of CXCR4. J Allergy Clin Immunol 2000; 106:313–320.
19. Iikura M, Miyamasu M, Yamaguchi M, et al. Chemokine receptors in human basophils: inducible expression of functional CXCR4. J Leukoc Biol 2001; 70:113–120.
20. Hirai H, Tanaka K, Yoshie O, et al. Prostaglandin D2 selectively induces chemotaxis in T helper 2 cells, eosinophils, and basophils via seven-transmembrane receptor CRTH2. J Exp Med 2001; 193:255–261.
21. Garman S, Kinet J, Jardetzky T. The crystal structure of the high-affinity IgE receptor (Fc epsilon RI alpha). Annu Rev Immunol 1997; 1:973–976.
22. Hulett M, Brinkworth R, McKenzie I, et al. Fine structure analysis of interaction of FcepsilonRI with IgE. J Biol Chem 1999; 274:13345–13352.
23. MacGlashan DW. IgE and Fc{epsilon}RI regulation. Ann NY Acad Sci 2005; 1050:73–88.
24. Bieber T, de la Salle H, Wollenberg A, et al. Human epidermal Langerhans cells express the high affinity receptor for immunoglobulin E (FceRI). J Exp Med 1992; 175:1285–1290.
25. Wang B, Rieger A, Kilgus O, et al. Epidermal Langerhans cells from normal human skin bind monomeric IgE via Fc epsilon RI. J Exp Med 1992; 175:1353–1365.
26. Maurer D, Fiebiger E, Reininger B, et al. Expression of functional high affinity immunoglobulin E receptors (FceRI) on monocytes of atopic individuals. J Exp Med 1994; 179:745–750.
27. Maurer D, Fiebiger S, Ebner C, et al. Peripheral blood dendritic cells express Fc epsilon RI as a complex composed of Fc epsilon RI alpha- and Fc epsilon RI gamma-chains and can use this receptor for IgE-mediated allergen presentation. J Immunol 1996; 157:607–616.

28. Foster B, Metcalfe D, Prussin C. Human dendritic cell 1 and dendritic cell 2 subsets express FcepsilonRI: correlation with serum IgE and allergic asthma. J Allergy Clin Immunol 2003; 112:1132–1138.
29. Seminario M, Saini S, MacGlashan DW Jr, et al. Intracellular expression and release of Fc epsilon RI alpha by human eosinophils. J Immunol 1999; 162:6893–6900.
30. Schroeder JT, Bieneman AP, Xiao H, et al. Toll-like receptor 9- and FcepsilonRI-mediated responses oppose one another in plasmacytoid DC by down-regulating receptor expression. J Immunol 2005; 175:5724–5731.
31. Kepley C, Cambier J, Morel P, et al. Negative regulation of FcepsilonRI signaling by FcgammaRII costimulation in human blood basophils. J Allergy Clin Immunol 2000; 106:337–348.
32. Zhu D, Kepley CL, Zhang M, et al. A novel human immunoglobulin Fc gamma Fc epsilon bifunctional fusion protein inhibits Fc epsilon RI-mediated degranulation. Nat Med 2002; 8:518–521.
33. Gauchat J-F, Henchoz S, Mazzel G, et al. Induction of human IgE synthesis in B cells by mast cells and basophils. Nature 1993; 365:340–343.
34. Kleine-Tebbe J, Erdmann S, Knol EF, et al. Diagnostic tests based on human basophils: potentials, pitfalls and perspectives. Int Arch Allergy Immunol 2006; 141:79–90.
35. Bieneman AP, Chichester KL, Chen Y-H, et al. Toll-like receptor 2 ligands activate human basophils for both IgE-dependent and IgE-independent secretion. J Allergy Clin Immunol 2005; 115:295–301.
36. Sloane DE, Tedla N, Awoniyi M, et al. Leukocyte immunoglobulin-like receptors: novel innate receptors for human basophil activation and inhibition. Blood 2004; 104:2832–2839.
37. Kepley C, Craig S, Schwartz LB. Identification and partial characterization of a unique marker for human basophils. J Immunol 1995; 154:6548–6555.
38. McEuen A, Buckley M, Compton S, et al. Development and characterization of a monoclonal antibody specific for human basophils and the identification of a unique secretory product of basophil activation. Lab Invest 1999; 79:27–38.
39. Buhring H, Simmons P, Pudney M, et al. The monoclonal antibody 97A6 defines a novel surface antigen expressed on human basophils and their multipotent and unipotent progenitors. Blood 1999; 94:2343–2356.
40. Plager DA, Weiss EA, Kephart GM, et al. Identification of basophils by a mAb directed against pro-major basic protein 1. J Allergy Clin Immunol 2006; 117:626–634.

Inflammatory mediators

41. Mazzoni A, Leifer CA, Mullen GE, et al. Cutting edge: histamine inhibits IFN-alpha release from plasmacytoid dendritic cells. J Immunol 2003; 170:2269–2273.
42. Mazzoni A, Young H, Spitzer J, et al. Histamine regulates cytokine production in maturing dendritic cells, resulting in altered T cell polarization. J Clin Invest 2001; 108:1865–1873.
43. Foster B, Schwartz L, Metcalfe D, et al. Characterization of mast-cell tryptase-expressing peripheral blood cells as basophils. J Allergy Clin Immunol 2002; 109:287–293.
44. Calhoun W, Lavins B, Minkwitz M, et al. The effect of Accolate (zafirlukast) on cellular mediators of inflammation: BAL findings after segmental allergen challenge. Am J Respir Crit Care Med 1998; 157:1381–1389.
45. Kane GC, Pollice M, Kim C-J, et al. A controlled trial of the 5-lipoxygenase inhibitor, zileuton, on lung inflammation produced by segmental antigen challenge in human beings. J Allergy Clin Immunol 1996; 97:646–654.
46. Romagnani S. The Th2 hypothesis in allergy – 'Eppur si muove!'. Allergy Clin Immunol Int 1998; 10:158–164.
47. MacGlashan DW, White JM, Huang SK, et al. Secretion of interleukin-4 from human basophils: the relationship between IL-4 mRNA and protein in resting and stimulated basophils. J Immunol 1994; 152:3006–3016.
48. Devouassoux G, Foster G, Scott LM, et al. Frequency and characterization of antigen-specific IL-4- and IL-13- producing basophils and T cells in peripheral blood of healthy and asthmatic subjects. J Allergy Clin Immunol 1999; 104:811–819.
49. Min B, Prout M, Hu-Li J, et al. Basophils produce IL-4 and accumulate in tissues after infection with a Th2-inducing parasite. J Exp Med 2004; 200:507–517.
50. Voehringer D, Reese TA, Huang X, et al. Type 2 immunity is controlled by IL-4/IL-13 expression in hematopoietic non-eosinophil cells of the innate immune system. J Exp Med 2006; 203:1435–1446.
51. Kawaguchi M, Onuchic L, Li X-D, et al. Identification of a novel cytokine, ML-1, and its expression in subjects with asthma. J Immunol 2001; 167:4430–4435.
52. Li H, Sim T, Grant J, et al. The production of macrophage inflammatory protein-a by human basophils. J Immunol 1996; 157:1207–1212.
53. Tschoop CM, Spiegl N, Didichenko S, et al. Granzyme B, a novel mediator of allergic inflammation: its induction and release in blood basophils and human asthma. Blood 2006; 108:2290–2299.
53a. Gibbs BF, Arm JP, Gibson K, et al. Human lung mast cells release small amounts of interleukin-4 and tumor necrosis factor-alpha in response to stimulation by anti-IgE and stem cell factor. Eur J Pharmacol 1997; 327:73–78.
53b. Ochi H, De Jesus NN, Hsieh FH, et al. IL-4 and -5 prime human mast cells for different profiles of IgE-dependent cytokine production. Proc Natl Acad Sci U S A 2000; 97:10509.
53c. Moqbel R, Ying S, Barkans J, et al. Identification of messenger RNA for IL-4 in human eosinophils with granule localization and release of the translated product. J Immunol 1995; 55:4939.

Basophil activation

54. MacGlashan DW Jr. Releasability of human basophils: cellular sensitivity and maximal histamine release are independent variables. J Allergy Clin Immunol 1993; 91:605–615.
55. MacGlashan DW Jr, Schroeder JT. Functional consequences of FceRIa up-regulation by IgE in human basophils. J Leuk Biol 68:479–486.

56. Schroeder JT, MacGlashan DW Jr, Lichtenstein LM. Human basophils: mediator release and cytokine production. Adv Immunol 2001; 77:93–122.
57. Falcone F, Zillikens D, Gibbs BF. The 21st century renaissance of the basophils? Current insights into its role in allergic responses and innate immunity. Exp Dermatol 2006; 15:855–864.
58. Schroeder JT, Howard BP, Jenkens MK, et al. IL-4 secretion and histamine release by human basophils are differentially regulated by protein kinase C activation. J Leuk Biol 1998; 63:692–698.
59. Redrup AC, Howard BP, MacGlashan DW Jr, et al. Differential regulation of IL-4 and IL-13 secretion by human basophils: their relationship to histamine release in mixed leukocyte cultures. J Immunol 1998; 160:1957–1964.
60. Ochensberger B, Daepp G-C, Rihs S, et al. Human blood basophils produce interleukin-13 in response to IgE-receptor-dependent and -independent activation. Blood 1996; 88:3028–3037.
61. Schroeder JT, MacGlashan DW Jr, Kagey-Sobotka A, et al. IgE-dependent IL-4 secretion by human basophils: the relationship between cytokine production and histamine release in mixed leukocyte cultures. J Immunol 1994; 153:1808–1818.
62. Marone G, Florio G, Triggiani M, et al. Mechanisms of IgE elevation in HIV-1 infection. Crit Rev Immunol 2000; 20:477–496.
63. Stellato C, Collins P, Ponath P, et al. Production of the novel C-C chemokine MCP-4 by airway cells and comparison of its biological activity to other C-C chemokines. J Clin Invest 1997; 99:926–936.
64. Devouassoux G, Metcalfe DD, Prussin C. Eotaxin potentiates antigen-dependent basophil IL-4 production. J Immunol 1999; 163:2877–2882.
65. MacDonald SM. Human recombinant histamine-releasing factor. Int. Arch Allergy Appl Asthma Rep 1997; 113:187–189.
66. Bheekha-Escura R, Schroeder JT, MacDonald SM. HrHRF: function and regulation. Drug News Perspect 1998; 11:223–229.
67. Bheekha-Escura R, MacGlashan DW Jr, Langdon J, et al. Human recombinant histamine-releasing factor activates human eosinophils and the eosinophilic cell line, AML14–A3D10. Blood 2000; 96:2191–2198.
68. Wantke F, MacGlashan DW Jr, Langdon JM, et al. The human recombinant histamine releasing factor: functional evidence that it does not bind to the IgE molecule. J Allergy Clin Immunol 1999; 103:642–648.
69. Dvorak AM, Schroeder JT, MacGlashan DW Jr, et al. Comparative ultrastructural morphology of human basophils stimulated to release histamine by anti-IgE, recombinant IgE-dependent histamine-releasing factor, or monocyte chemotactic protein-1. J Allergy Clin Immunol 1996; 98:355–370.
70. Miura K, Saini SS, Gauvreau G, et al. Differences in functional consequences and signal transduction induced by IL-3, IL-5, and nerve growth factor in human basophils. J Immunol 2001; 167:2282–2291.
71. Li H, Sim T, Alam R. IL-13 released by and localized in human basophils. J Immunol 1996; 156:4833–4838.
72. Lie W, Knol E, Mul F, et al. Basophils from patients with allergic asthma show a primed phenotype. J Allergy Clin Immunol 1999; 104:1000–1007.
73. Saini SS, Bloom DC, Bieneman A, et al. Systemic effects of allergen exposure on blood basophil IL-13 secretion and FceRIb expression. J Allergy Clin Immunol 2004; 114:768–774.
74. Miura K, MacGlashan DW Jr. Dual phase priming by IL-3 for leukotriene C4 generation in human basophils: differences in characteristics between acute and late priming effects. J Immunol 2000; 164:3026–3034.
75. Muira K, Saini SS, Gauvreau G, et al. Differences in functional consequences and signal transduction induced by IL-3, IL-5, and nerve growth factor in human basophils. J Immunol 2001; 167:2282–2291.
76. Vilarino N, Miura K, MacGlashan DW Jr. Acute IL-3 priming up-regulates the stimulus-induced Raf-1-Mek-Erk cascade independently of IL-3-induced activation of Erk. J Immunol 2005; 175:3006–3014.
77. Schroeder JT, MacGlashan DW Jr, Kagey-Sobotka A, et al. Cytokine generation by human basophils. J Allergy Clin Immunol 1994; 94:1189–1195.
78. Ochensberger B, Tassera L, Bifrare D, et al. Regulation of cytokine expression and leukotriene formation in human basophils by growth factors, chemokines and chemotactic agonists. Eur J Immunol 1999; 29:11–22.

Pharmacological modulation of secretion

79. Lichtenstein LM, Margolis S. Histamine release in vitro: inhibition by catecholamines and methylxanthines. Science 1968; 161:902–903.
80. Weston M, Peachell P. Regulation of human mast cell and basophil function by cAMP. Gen Pharmacol 1998; 31:715–719.
81. Gibbs B, Vollrath I, Albrecht C, et al. Inhibition of interleukin-4 and interleukin-13 release from immunologically activated basophils due to the actions of anti-allergic drugs. Naunyn Schmiedebergs Arch Pharmacol 1998; 57:573–578.
82. Schroeder JT, Schleimer RP, Lichtenstein LM, et al. Inhibition of cytokine generation and mediator release by human basophils treated with desloratadine. Clin Exp Allergy 2001; 31:1369–1377.
83. Church M. H1-antihistamines and inflammation. Clin Exp Allergy 2001; 31:1341–1343.
84. Schleimer RP, Lichtenstein LM, Gillespie E. Inhibition of basophil histamine release by anti-inflammatory steroids. Nature 1981; 292:454–455.
85. Schroeder JT, MacGlashan DW Jr, MacDonald SM, et al. Regulation of IgE-dependent IL-4 generation by human basophils treated with glucocorticoids. J Immunol 1997; 158:5448–5454.
86. Schroeder JT, Miura K, Cianferoni A, et al. Selective expression of nuclear factor of activated T cells 2/c1 in human basophils: evidence for NFAT2 involvement in IgE-mediated IL-4 generation. J Allergy Clin Immunol 2002; 109:507–513.
87. De Paulis A, Cirillo R, Ciccarelli A, et al. FK-506, a potent novel inhibitor of the release of proinflammatory mediators from human FceRI+ cells. J Immunol 1991; 146:2374–2381.
88. Cirillo R, Triggiani M, Siri L, et al. Cyclosporin A rapidly inhibits mediator release from human basophils presumably by interacting with cyclophilin. J Immunol 1990; 144:3891–3897.

Basophil involvement in disease

89. Lichtenstein LM, Norman PS, Winkenwerder WL. Clinical and in vitro studies on the role of immunotherapy in ragweed hay fever. Am J Med 1968; 44:514–524.
90. Schroeder JT, Kagey-Sobotka A, Lichtenstein LM. The role of the basophil in allergic inflammation. Allergy 1995; 50:452–463.
91. MacGlashan DW Jr, Gauvreau G, Schroeder JT. Basophils in airway disease. Curr Allergy Asthma Rep 2002; 2:126–132.
92. Cyr MM, Denburg JA. Systemic aspects of allergic disease: the role of the bone marrow. Curr Opin Immunol 2001; 13:727–732.
93. Kepley CL, McFeely PJ, et al. Immunohistochemical detection of human basophils in postmortem cases of fatal asthma. Am J Respir Crit. Care Med 2001; 164:1053–1058.
94. Ying S, Kikuchi Y, Meng Q, et al. TH1/TH2 cytokines and inflammatory cells in skin biopsy specimens from patients with chronic idiopathic urticaria: comparison with the allergen-induced late-phase cutaneous reaction. J Allergy Clin Immunol 2002; 109:694–700.
95. Irani A-M, Huang C, Han-Zhang X, et al. Immunohistochemical detection of human basophils in late-phase skin reactions. J Allergy Clin Immunol 1998; 101:354–362.
96. Macfarlane AJ, Kon OM, Smith SJ, et al. Basophils, eosinophils, and mast cells in atopic and nonatopic asthma and in late-phase allergic reactions in the lung and skin. J Allergy Clin Immunol 1999; 105:99–107.
97. Gauvreau G, Lee J, Watson R, et al. Increased numbers of both airway basophils and mast cells in sputum after allergen inhalation challenge of atopic asthmatics. Am J Respir Crit Care Med 2000; 161:1473–1478.
98. KleinJan A, McEuen A, Dijkstra M, et al. Basophil and eosinophil accumulation and mast cell degranulation in the nasal mucosa of patients with hay fever after local allergen challenge. J Allergy Clin Immunol 2000; 106:677–686.
99. Schroeder JT, Lichtenstein LM, Roche EM, et al. IL-4 production by human basophils found in the lung following segmental allergen challenge. J Allergy Clin Immunol 2001; 107:265–271.
100. Nouri-Aria K, Irani A-M, Jacobson M, et al. Basophil recruitment and IL-4 production during human allergen-induced late asthma. J Allergy Clin Immunol 2001; 108:205–211.
101. Richerson H. Cutaneous basophil (Jones-Mote) hypersensitivity after 'tolerogenic' doses of intravenous ovalbumin in the guinea pig. J Exp Med 1971; 34:630.
102. Dvorak HF, Dvorak AM, Simpson BA, et al. Cutaneous basophil hypersensitivity. II. A light and electron microscopic description. J Exp Med 1970; 132:558.
103. Dvorak AM, Mihm MC Jr, Dvorak HF. Degranulation of basophilic leukocytes in allergic contact dermatitis reactions in man. J Immunol 1976; 116:687–694.
104. Dvorak HF. Role of basophil leukocytes in allograft reactions. J Immunol 1971; 106:279.
105. Dvorak A, McLeod R, Onderdonk A, et al. Ultrastructural evidence for piecemeal and anaphylactic degranulation of human gut mucosal mast cells in vivo. Int Arch Allergy Immunol 1992; 99:74–83.
106. Dvorak H, Mihm MJ, Dvorak A, et al. Rejection of first-set skin allografts in man. The microvasculature is the critical target of the immune response. J Exp Med 1979; 150:322–337.
107. King C. Transmission intensity and human immune responses to lymphatic filariasis. Parasite Immunol 2001; 23:363–371.
108. Haisch K, Schramm G, Falcone F, et al. A glycoprotein from Schistosoma mansoni eggs binds non-antigen-specific immunoglobulin E and releases interleukin-4 from human basophils. Parasite Immunol 2001; 23:427–434.
109. Mitre E, Nutman TB. Basophils, basophilia and helminth infections. Chem Immunol Allergy 2006; 90:141–156.
110. Aumuller E, Schramm G, Gronow A, et al. Echinococcus multilocularis metacestode extract triggers human basophils to release Interleukin-4. Parasite Immunol 2004; 26:387–395.
111. MacDonald S M, Bhisutthibhan J, Shapiro A, et al. Immune mimicry in malaria: Plasmodium falciparum secretes a functional histamine-releasing factor homolog in vitro and in vivo. Proc Natl Acad Sci USA 2001; 98:10829–10832.

Antigen-Presenting Dendritic Cells

Bart N Lambrecht and Hamida Hammad

21

CONTENTS

- Introduction 341
- Dendritic cell terminology and heterogeneity 341
- Antigen uptake 342
- Antigen presentation 342
- Integrated function of dendritic cells in the immune response 344
- Role for dendritic cells in allergic sensitization in humans 350
- Dendritic cells in allergic asthma 350
- Dendritic cells in atopic dermatitis 352
- Role of dendritic cells in allergic rhinitis 352
- Dendritic cells as drug targets in allergic diseases 352
- Conclusion 353

SUMMARY OF IMPORTANT CONCEPTS

>> Dendritic cells are the most important antigen-presenting cells that are responsible for allergic Th2 sensitization to inhaled allergens

>> Allergens are not recognized directly by T cells, but rather are digested into immunogenic peptides for presentation onto MHCI and MHCII to CD8 and CD4 T cells, respectively

>> Tolerance is the usual outcome of allergen exposure. Sensitization occurs when dendritic cells become activated by adjuvants like cigarette smoke, diesel exhaust particles or by enzymatically active allergens

>> Dendritic cells determine the T cell polarization process into Th1 (producing mainly IFNγ), Th2 (producing mainly IL-4, IL-5, and IL-13), Th17 (producing mainly IFNγ and IL-17), and Treg (producing mainly IL-10 and/or TGFβ)

>> Dendritic cells are recruited into inflamed sites in allergic disease. They are crucial in mounting a Th2 effector response in already established disease

>> Dendritic cells are ideal targets for developing new treatments against allergic disease, because they control so many aspects of the allergic cascade

INTRODUCTION

The prevalence of sensitization to allergens and allergic diseases has reached epidemic proportions in Western societies. Allergic sensitization is the presence of IgE antibody to common environmental allergens, and is controlled by Th2 cells that provide help for IgE synthesis by B cells. In addition, many of the inflammatory cell types found within sites of allergic inflammation, such as eosinophils and mast cells, depend on Th2 cells for their development and function. Th2 cells will only react to allergen when it is presented in the context of MHC molecules by professional antigen-presenting cells such as dendritic cells, macrophages, and B cells. Dendritic cells (DCs) are the most important antigen-presenting cells found throughout the body and are mainly recognized for their exceptional potential to generate a primary immune response and sensitization to (aero)allergens. Increasingly, these cells are also recognized for their potential to maintain ongoing effector responses and therefore they might be crucial in maintaining allergic inflammation. B cells present

allergen to T cells mainly in the context of immunoglobulin synthesis, for which they need T cell help. Macrophages are seen as scavenger cells that can also regulate the function of DCs. They are equally important in controlling pathogen clearance and tissue remodeling.

DENDRITIC CELL TERMINOLOGY AND HETEROGENEITY

Dendritic cells (DCs) were originally described by their capacity to efficiently process and present antigens and to prime naive T cells. Over the last three decades, multiple DC subtypes have been defined, differing in phenotype, localization, and immune function.[1] Myeloid DCs, Langerhans cells (LC) as well as natural type I interferon-producing cells (IPCs, also called plasmacytoid DCs, pDCs) are part of the hematopoietic system and have a relatively short half life in tissues. To maintain DC numbers in the tissues, there is a continuous renewal of DCs from hematopoietic precursors residing in the bone marrow or within the skin (for LC in steady-state conditions). A universal feature of DCs in tissues is their typical morphology with long dendrite-like extensions (hence their name) that can be beautifully demonstrated by staining for MHC class II (Fig. 21.1). Myeloid DCs in humans express markers shared with monocytes/macrophages such as CD33, CD4, and CD11c, whereas in the mouse, they typically express CD11c and CD11b. In humans, pDCs were described in the bloodstream, lungs, and lymph nodes as lineage^{neg} CD11c^{lo} CD123^{+} BDCA2^{+} cells.[1] In the mouse, pDCs express specific markers (120G8, PDCA-1) as well as cell markers shared with myeloid DCs (MHCI and II, CD11c) but also with granulocytes (Gr1) and B cells (B220).[1] Langerhans cells express CD1a, Langerin and intracellularly demonstrate so-called Birbeck granules, tennis racket shaped organelles. Recently, another DC subset sharing marker expression with NK cells was identified as 'natural killer DC'. These DCs originate as cells with NK function, upon which killed material is taken up and presented to T cells.

Dendritic cells originate in the bone marrow from a CD34^{+} precursor and circulate in the bloodstream as a monocyte-like precursor before entering peripheral tissues.[2] The exact nature of the precursor DC cell type is currently unknown (Fig. 21.2), and could vary for myeloid versus

plasmacytoid DC, inflammation versus steady state, or for lymphoid organ versus peripheral tissues.[3]

■ ANTIGEN UPTAKE ■

There are various ways by which an antigen-presenting cell can acquire foreign antigen. A first mechanism is via receptor-mediated endocytosis involving clathrin-coated pits. Immature DCs express a plethora of specialized cell receptors for patterns associated with foreign antigens, such as the C-type lectin carbohydrate receptors (Langerin, DC-SIGN, Dectin, BDCA-2, macrophage mannose receptor, and the unique carbohydrate receptor DEC-205).[4] Lectin-receptor-mediated uptake by DCs results in a ~100-fold more efficient presentation to T cells, as compared with antigens internalized via fluid phase. Interestingly, Langerin is a C-type lectin displaying mannose-binding specificity and is exclusively expressed by DCs that display Birbeck granules (BG), such as lung DCs and skin Langerhans cells, but seems to be functionally irrelevant.[5] Pollen starch granules were shown to bind to C-type lectin receptors on AMs and DCs, although internalization occurred only in macrophages.[6] Also, Pestel demonstrated that Der p 1 uptake into cultured DCs involves mannose-receptor-mediated endocytosis, a process that is more efficient in DCs obtained from allergic donors.[7] In allergic individuals, DCs are furthermore loaded with allergen-specific IgE binding to the high-affinity IgE receptor (FcεRI), thus leading to efficient receptor-mediated endocytosis of the allergen.

A second mechanism of antigen uptake is constitutive macropinocytosis that involves the actin skeleton-driven engulfment of large amounts of fluid and solutes (~one cell volume/h) by the ruffling membrane of the DC followed by concentration of soluble antigen in the endocytic compartment. Macropinocytosis seems to be a dominant mechanism involved in the uptake of recombinant Bet v 1 and Phl p 1 pollen allergens by LCs and of Der p 1 by cultured DCs, and can be inhibited by cytochalasin D and amiloride.[8] Third, immature LCs, cultured DCs, plasmacytoid DC, and macrophages have been shown to phagocytose particulate antigens such as latex beads and even whole bacteria, as well as apoptotic cells, and this could be the dominant mechanism of uptake of particulate allergens.[9]

The extracellular antigens that are taken up by any of these mechanisms accumulate in the endocytic compartment, where they are loaded on newly synthesized and recycling MHC class II molecules but may also be transported into the cytosol, where they become accessible to the class I antigen presentation pathway, a process called cross-presentation.

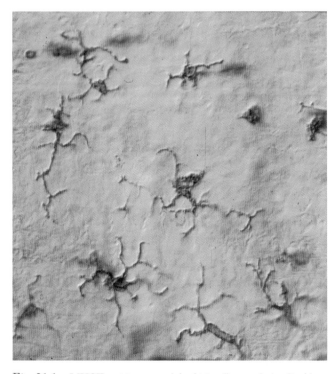

Fig. 21.1. MHCII positive mucosal dendritic cell network visualized by MHCII staining on a murine tracheal wholemount. Trachea was taken from a naive unimmunized mouse.

■ ANTIGEN PRESENTATION ■

PRESENTATION OF EXOGENOUS ANTIGENS ON MHC CLASS II TO CD4^{+} T CELLS

Allergens are extracellular antigens, and like most extracellular antigens they are processed for presentation onto MHC class II molecules. The T-cell receptor of CD4 T lymphocytes will respond only to processed antigen in the context of MHC class II, a process called MHC restriction. In contrast to MHCI, which is expressed on all nucleated cells types, MHC class II is mainly expressed by professional antigen-presenting cells, but also to a lesser extent by epithelial cells, mast cells, and eosinophils.

Within the endocytic compartment, antigen is cleaved into short immunogenic peptides by proteolytic enzymes of the cathepsin family.

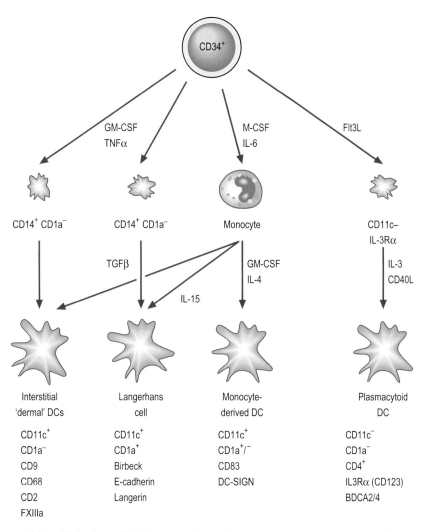

Fig. 21.2. Different origins and fate of DC subsets. All DCs originate from a CD34+ precursor in the bone marrow. These cells then further differentiate under the influence of various cytokines into Langerhans cells of the skin, interstitial DCs of tissues, monocyte-derived DCs or plasmacytoid DCs, each expressing specific markers. Certain cytokines like IL-6 amd M-CSF inhibit DC development when precursors are continuously exposed to them.

Antigen loading on MHC class II molecules occurs in an acidic cellular compartment rich in newly synthesized MHC class II molecules, called the MIIC compartment.[10] This multivesicular complex is located at the intersection of the biosynthetic (ER, Golgi complex, secretory granules) and endocytic pathway of vesicle transport within the cell and contains the MHC II-related HLA-DM peptide exchanger that is essential for loading high-affinity antigenic peptides on MHC II.[11] Alternatively, there is a pathway of peptide loading onto pre-formed MHC II molecules that have been internalized into mildly acidic endosomal vesicles after being expressed on the cell surface.

At present, it is unclear how allergens are loaded onto MHC class II molecules by DCs. In sensitized individuals, internalization of allergens via receptor-mediated endocytosis by multivalent crosslinking of the high-affinity IgE receptor (FcεRI) on immature DCs targets the antigen to the MIIC compartment.[12] In contrast, the generation of peptide-MHC complexes derived from macropinocytosis of Bet v 1 and Phl p 1 pollen allergens was only partly inhibited when the pH of the endosomes was altered, suggesting that part of the molecules were not metabolized in the lysosomal MIIC compartment.

ANTIGEN PRESENTATION ON MHC CLASS I TO CD8+ T CELLS

After a virus enters a host and infects cells, the major adaptive immune response that clears the infection is mediated by CD8+ cytotoxic T lymphocytes (CTLs). These cells also provide the major defense against cancers. CD8+ lymphocytes recognize infected cells that display on their surface major histocompatibility complex (MHC) class I molecules presenting antigenic peptides derived from viral proteins or tumor antigens expressed in the cytoplasm. All nucleated cells have the capacity to present peptides derived from the cytoplasm onto MHC class I molecules.

A second, less well-defined, approach to load peptides on MHCI molecules is for the DCs to capture extracellular antigens and to process these captured exogenous antigens into the MHC class I pathway. This form of presentation is referred to as cross-presentation. In the field of experimental allergy, evidence is present for this cross-priming. Aerosolization of OVA in OVA-sensitized mice leads to the generation of class I-restricted $CD8^+$ T cells that can regulate the magnitude and duration of IgE responses and suppress airway inflammation.[13]

■ INTEGRATED FUNCTION OF DENDRITIC CELLS IN THE IMMUNE RESPONSE ■

DENDRITIC CELL ACTIVATION

Dendritic cells originate in the bone marrow and circulate in the bloodstream as a monocyte-like precursor before entering peripheral tissues.[2] Dendritic cell migration is a tightly regulated process in which many chemokines and other factors are involved (Table 21.1, Fig. 21.3). Myeloid DC are attracted to peripheral tissues by a specific set of chemokines such as MIP3α (CCL20), MCP-1, and epithelial β-defensins acting on CCR2 and CCR6.[14] Plasmacytoid DCs respond preferentially to SDF1 (CXCL12) and CXCL9–11 and the newly described chemerin, a ligand for ChemR23.[15] Once DCs extravasate, they form a network in the upper layers of the epithelium and lamina propria of the airways (Fig. 21.1), gut, and skin. Here, DCs are said to be in an immature state, specialized for internalizing foreign antigens but not yet able to activate naïve T cells.[16] The DC network serves a patrolling function, continuously scanning the environment for foreign antigens. The dendritic cell is endowed with numerous ancient receptors for foreign antigenic signature molecules such as bacterial cell walls, viral and bacterial DNA, and foreign sugar molecules (Fig. 21.4). These so-called pathogen associated molecular patterns (PAMPs) are recognized by toll-like receptors (TLR1–10) and C-type lectin receptors, which are abundantly expressed on the surface of DCs.[4] The expression of various TLRs varies between DC subsets, particularly in human DCs. In the human and mouse, pDCs preferentially express the TLR7 and TLR9 and thus respond to the corresponding ligands (imidazoquinolines and single-stranded RNA vs CpG motif bacterial DNA) but not to ligands for TLR2, 3, 4 or 5. In contrast, in vitro generated conventional monocyte-derived DCs or ex vivo isolated mDCs express all TLRs except TLR9.

In addition to the direct molecular recognition of foreign antigenic structures, exposure to foreign antigens or necrotic cell death leads to tissue damage and this by itself can activate the DC system (Fig. 21.3). DCs express a plethora of receptors for these so-called damage associated molecular patterns (DAMPs), including high mobility group box 1 (HMGB1) protein, heat shock proteins, uric acid, adenosine triphosphate (ATP), complement cascade fragments, neuropeptides, prostaglandins, etc. (Fig. 21.4). Many of these compounds not only activate the already residing DCs but also attract new waves of cells to the periphery.[17] DC activation and maturation in the periphery can occur directly by ligation of DAMP or PAMP receptors and can occur indirectly through activation of the same receptors on the surrounding structural cells such as keratinocytes, epithelial cells or fibroblasts.[18] Keratinocytes and lung epithelial cells make granulocyte–macrophage colony-stimulating factor (GM-CSF) and thymic stromal lymphopoietin (TSLP) that activate the underlying

Table 21.1 Chemokines and other factors involved in the dendritic cell migration process

	Chemokine receptors/ molecules controlling migration	Ligands
mDCs	CCR1	CCL5, CCL3, CCL7
	CCR2	CCL2, CCL7, CCL8, CCL13
	CCR4	CCL17, CCL22
	CCR5	CCL3, CCL4, CCL5, CCL8
	CCR6	CCL20
	CCR7	CCL19, CCL21
	CCR8	CCL1
	CXCR3	CXCL9, CXCL10, CXCL11
	CXCR4	CXCL12
	PAFR	PAF
	S1PR	Sphingosine 1-phosphate
	EP4	Prostaglandin E_2
	CD38	CD31
	CystLT1	Cysteinyl leukotrienes
	ChemR23	Chemerin
	DP1	Prostaglandin D_2
	IP	Prostaglandin I_2
	ChemR23	Resolvin E1
	FPRL1	Lipoxin A4
pDCs	CCR7	CCL19, CCL21
	CXCR3	CXCL9, CXCL10, CXCL11
	CXCR4	CXCL12
	ChemR23	Chemerin

mDCs, myeloid dendritic cells; pDCs, plasmacytoid dendritic cells.

DC network (Fig. 21.3).[19] These cytokines are regarded as the principal maturation inducing factors that can also be used to mature DCs in vitro.

DENDRITIC CELL MIGRATION TO THE DRAINING LYMPH NODES

The recognition of danger (PAMPs or DAMPs) by peripheral dendritic cells dramatically alters the migration behavior of DCs and thus induces the surface expression of CCR7 on peripheral DCs (Fig. 21.3). The ligands

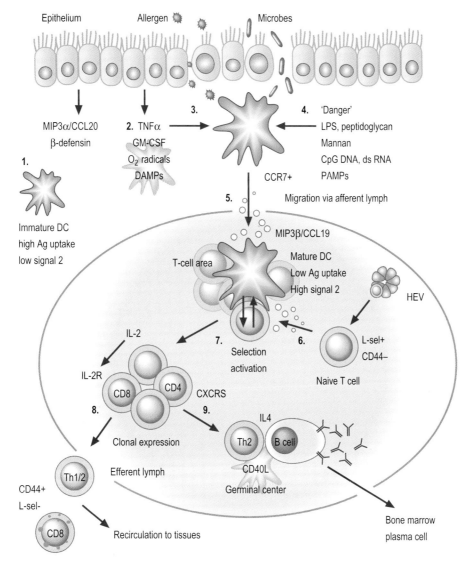

Fig. 21.3. Induction of the primary immune response by DCs. (1) Under baseline conditions and upon exposure to foreign antigens, epithelia produce macrophage inflammatory protein (MIP)3α (CCL20) and β-defensin to attract CCR6+ immature DCs from the bloodstream. (2) Resident cell types produce inflammatory mediators and growth factors that attract and activate the recently recruited DC. (3) DCs capture allergens and other foreign antigens such as bacteria and viruses. (4) DCs can discriminate between 'dangerous' antigens, and non-pathogenic antigens such as self-antigens and probably most allergens, by recognizing certain viral and bacterial patterns. (5) The recognition of infection and tissue damage upregulates the CCR7 and CXCR4 and DCs migrate to the T-cell area of draining lymph nodes where the ligand MIP3β and SDF-1 is constitutively expressed. During this migration, DCs lose the capacity to take up antigen, but become strong stimulators of naive T cells by their strong expression of co-stimulatory molecules (signal 2). (6) In the T-cell area, DCs produce chemokines to attract naive T cells that continuously leave the bloodstream via the high endothelial venules (HEV). (7) Naive T cells are first arrested and then selected for antigen specificity. The recognition of the correct peptide-MHC induces the activation of naive T cell, which will lead to further terminal differentiation of DC function. (8) The activation of T cells leads to autocrine production of IL-2 and to clonal expansion of Ag specific CD4+ and CD8+ T cells. These cells differentiate into effector cells that leave the lymph node via the efferent lymphatic. These effector cells are poised to migrate to peripheral tissues, especially to inflamed areas. (9) Upon contact with DCs, some Ag specific CD4+ T cells upregulate CXCR5 receptor and migrate to the B-cell follicles of the draining lymph node. Here, they further interact with germinal center DCs to induce CD40L-dependent B-cell immunoglobulin switching and affinity maturation (germinal center reaction). Most high-affinity B cells go to the bone marrow to become Ig-producing plasma cells.

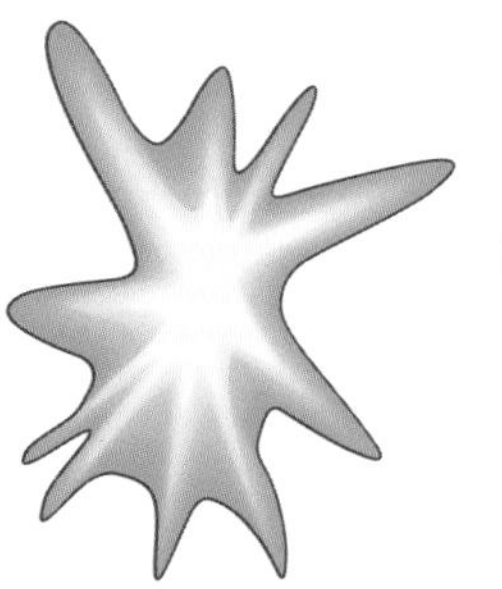

Toll-like receptors 1–10

Intracellular receptors
NOD1/2
TLR7,9
PKB

C-type lectin receptors
Dectin
Macrophage mannose receptor
DEC205
BDCA-2

Protease activated receptors

Complement receptors

Prostanoid receptors
DP1, EP4, IP

Neuropeptide receptors
NK1, CGRPR

Purinergic receptors
P2X, P2Y

Receptors for
Uric acid,
HMGB1
Heat shock proteins

Fig. 21.4. Expression of 'danger' receptors by dendritic cells. Dendritic cells express the ancient receptors of the innate immune system also expressed by macrophages, such as the toll-like receptors (TLRs) and C-type lectin receptors. These receptors react to foreign pathogen associated molecular patterns (PAMPs). In addition, DCs express numerous receptors for inflammatory mediators and necrotic cell debris, the so-called damage associated molecular patterns (DAMPs). The exact receptors for uric acid, high mobility group box 1 (HMGB1) protein and heat shock proteins are not yet known.

for CCR7 are secondary lymphoid chemokine (SLC, now known as CCL21) and MIP3β (CCL19), which are expressed at the luminal side of afferent lymph vessels and by the T-cell area of draining lymph nodes. Another factor attracting DCs to the lymph node is the lipid mediator sphingosine-1-P. Blocking the S1P type receptor dramatically reduces the migration of lung DCs to the mediastinal LNs.[20] The responsiveness of CCR7 to CCL19 and CCL21 and the consequent lymph node migration of DCs are controlled by lipid mediators such as the leukotrienes and prostaglandins. Prostaglandin D_2 acts on the DP1 receptor expressed by lung DCs and suppresses the migration of lung DCs.[21] The downstream metabolite, 15-deoxy(δ)12–14PGJ2, could also slow down the migration of DCs, by acting on the nuclear PPARγ receptor.[22] Leukotriene B_4 is exported from the cytoplasm of the DC by the multi drug resistance (MDR) protein, where it is metabolized into LTC_4, which regulates the CCR7 responsiveness.[23] In contrast to skin DCs, it was recently shown that lung DC migration is less dependent on the export of leukotriene B_4 by the MDR.[24] For emigration of DCs from the skin, the CCR8 receptor for the chemokine CCL-1 (also known as I-309 in humans and TCA-3 in mice) acts in concert with CCR7.[25] Whether this is also true for lung DC migration remains to be shown. It is clear that the regulation of DC migration by arachidonic acid metabolites is a very amenable to modification by various drugs already being developed for allergy treatment.

Just as in the gut, airway DCs extend long dendrites to the lumen of the airways, forming bud-like extensions at the border of the air interface. Within a few hours after inhalation, airway myeloid DCs (mDCs) and plasmacytoid DCs (pDCs) have taken up fluorescently labeled antigen within the draining mediastinal LNs.[21,26,27] After 24 h, both mDCs and pDCs in the mediastinal LNs contain antigen inside vesicles of the cytoplasm. What is unclear at present is whether pDCs take-up antigen in the periphery of the lung and subsequently migrate to the nodes, or whether antigen is being transported to them by migratory mDCs or even a specific

subset of CD8α⁻ CD11b⁻ migratory DCs recently described by Belz et al.[28] Transport of immunogenic material from one non-migratory DC to another is certainly a possibility, as CD8α⁺ DCs injected into the lung induce an immune response in the mediastinal node without migrating into it.[29] Under steady-state conditions, mDCs continuously migrate to draining LNs and present either (self)-auto antigens or harmless antigen in a tolerogenic form. Once they have reached the draining LNs, mDCs express intermediate levels of co-stimulatory molecules and MHCII.

T-CELL ACTIVATION BY DENDRITIC CELLS

By upregulating the lymph node homing chemokine receptors, DCs that have seen foreign antigen thus direct their interest to the regional draining LN T-cell area where they interact with recirculating T cells and B cells (Fig. 21.5). Dendritic cells that have arrived in the lymph node undergo short-lived interactions with T cells in the paracortical region and during this initial antigen-independent event, individual T cells are scanned for specificity for antigen. When antigen is being recognized, there is formation of a more long-term immunological synapse (Fig. 21.6), leading to full blown T-cell activation, after which the T cell detaches, divides, and differentiates into an effector and possibly memory T cell. Dendritic cells also transport antigen without degrading it and thus offer intact protein to B cells at the interface between paracortex and B-cell follicle.[30] Dendritic cells that have reached the T-cell area have lost the capacity to take up antigen, and now express a plethora of cell adhesion and surface molecules interacting with T cells, not previously expressed on peripheral based DCs. This phenotype is called 'mature dendritic cell' implying that functionally these cells are now fully adapted to induce naive T-cell responses. DCs express the antigen on MHC molecules, and provide so called co-stimulatory molecules (CD80/CD86 family; TNF/TNFR family, Fig. 21.6) together with cytokines to optimally expand and differentiate T cells for the particular job that needs to be done to clear the foreign antigen. Initially, T cells are stimulated in the draining lymph node, but after a cell few divisions they acquire effector potential,[31] start expressing chemokine receptors for inflammatory chemokines expressed at sites of pathogen entry, and lose the expression of CD69, thus rendering them insensitive to the lymph node retention signal S1P (Fig. 21.5).

Th POLARIZATION BY DENDRITIC CELLS

Dendritic cells (DCs) are crucial in regulating the immune response by bridging innate and adaptive immunity. Signals from the type of antigen and the response of the innate immune system to it are translated by DCs into a signal that can be read by the cells of the adaptive immune response leading to an optimal response for a particular insult (Fig. 21.7). Together, these signals consist of provision of a particular density of peptide-MHC, the expression of co-stimulatory or Th polarizing cell-surface molecules, and the expression of soluble cytokines and chemokines that polarize T cells or enhance their survival. At the same time, DCs also control the function and expansion of regulatory T (Treg) cells that tightly control overzealous inflammatory T-cell responses. Although controversial, it has been suggested over recent years that particular functions of DCs, such as tolerance or immunity or Th1/Th2 differentiation, might be a specialized function of defined subtypes of DCs. Others have refuted this idea and have claimed that DCs are very versatile cells, and can virtually induce any type of response depending on the need of the moment.[32]

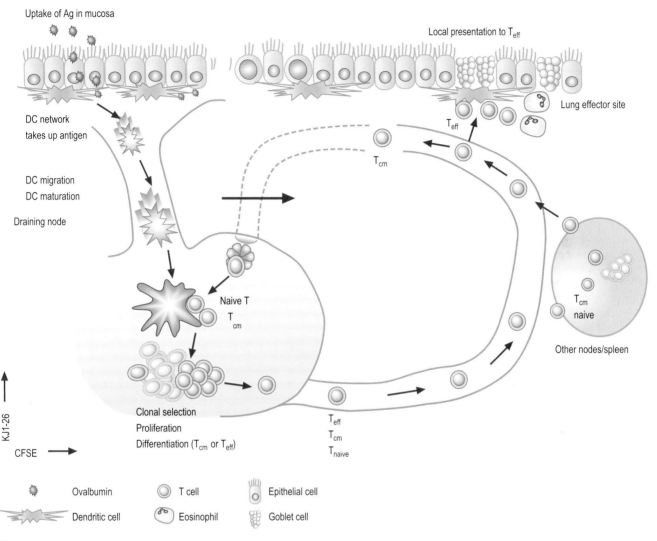

Fig. 21.5. An integrated overview of DCs and CD4[+] T-cell migration during primary and secondary immune responses. Antigen is taken up by dendritic cells (DCs) across the mucosal impermeable barrier. Mucosal DCs continuously migrate from the lungs to the T-cell area of mediastinal lymph nodes (MLNs). In the presence of inflammation, this process is amplified, increasing the possibility that pathogenic substances will be presented to recirculating naive T cells or central memory T (TCM) cells. At the same time, DC maturation will be fully induced. When mature DCs arrive in the MLNs, they select specific T cells from the polyclonal repertoire of cells that migrates through the high endothelial venules and T-cell area. Within 4 days, this will lead to clonal expansion of antigen-specific T cells. This is illustrated in the FACS plot where antigen-specific T cells, identified by staining with a specific KJ1–26 antibody for the OVA T-cell receptor dilute the CFSE signal. When a T cell has acquired a certain threshold number of divisions (usually four or more), it will leave the MLN, to become either a TCM cell or an effector T cell. This is where migration pathways separate, and consequently the anatomical requirements for reactivation diverge. The TCM cells will extravasate in other non-draining nodes and spleen, and will eventually accumulate in the spleen over time (see FACS plot for non-lung-draining lymphoid tissue where both divided TCMs and naive T cells can be found). Reactivation of these cells will, therefore, only occur in central lymphoid organs. By contrast, effector T cells will extravasate in peripheral sites of inflammation (see FACS plot for lungs, where only divided cells can be found), including the lung when the original inflammation is still present. In contrast to naive T cells, which are excluded from lung tissues, these effector T cells can be stimulated by local airway DCs to mediate their effector function. In this scenario, alternative antigen-presenting cells might be eosinophils or even epithelial cells, expressing MHC molecules.

Recent studies have suggested that myeloid lung DCs mediate protective immunity to inhaled antigens only when properly activated by innate immune system activating immune signals, acting through toll-like receptors or other pattern recognition receptors. Under inflammatory conditions such as those provided by LPS or virus infection, the expansion of T cells induced by myeloid DCs leads to the generation of Th1 or Th2 effector cells in the mediastinal nodes.[33] The signals that determine the type of response after encountering a pathogen in the lung are delivered by DCs in the lymph node. Sporri and Reis e Sousa recently

INTEGRATED FUNCTION OF DENDRITIC CELLS IN THE IMMUNE RESPONSE

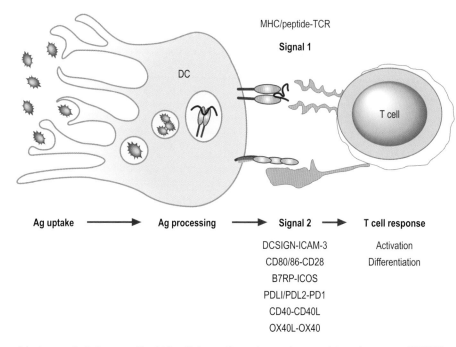

Fig. 21.6 Formation of the immunological synapse Dendritic cells internalize antigen and present it into the groove of MHCI and MHCII molecules to, respectively, CD8 and CD4 T lymphocytes (signal 1). In the process of recognizing foreign antigen, they are induced to express some co-stimulatory molecules for naive T cells (signal 2). The T cell bearing a specific receptor upregulates CD40L that induces the terminal differentiation of DCs through CD40 signaling, inducing the full expression of all co-stimulatory molecules like CD80, CD86, ICOSL, etc. that further polarize the immune response. In addition, DCs produce cytokines to expand and differentiate the T-cell response (signal 3).

suggested that DC maturation and provision of peptide-MHC to T cells is not sufficient to generate effector cells.[34] Cytokines are dominant signals that determine the quality and quantity of an effector immune response. During generation of an efficient effector immune response, DCs also have to overcome suppression by Treg cells, and the dominant way by which they seem to do this is by producing IL-6, that releases the suppression by naturally occurring Tregs.[35] Certain pathogens or pathogen-derived products induce the direct secretion of Th1 polarizing cytokines by DCs and thus instruct the type of immune response generated. Alternatively, it was shown that tissue environment can also determine Th differentiation. Stumbles et al showed that resting respiratory tract DCs mainly induced Th2 responses.[36] As a direct proof that myeloid DCs can induce Th2 sensitization in the lung, it was shown that intratracheal injection of bone marrow-derived mDCs pulsed with OVA induced a Th2 response to OVA and subsequently led to severe features of asthma when mice were rechallenged with OVA aerosol.[37] Recently, much information has been gathered how exactly Th2 polarization is controlled by DCs. Mice that conditionally overexpress thymic stromal lymphopoietin (TSLP) in the lungs mount vigorous Th2 responses in the airways, in a process driven by DCs.[19] TSLP is increased in the airways of asthmatic patients[38] and it can activate mDCs to prime naive CD4+ T cells to differentiate into pro-inflammatory Th2 cells. The Th2 skewing effect induced by TSLP-activated DCs was found to be dependent on OX40-ligand, a co-stimulatory molecule shown to play a critical role in the development of allergic lung inflammation.[39] As TSLP is such an important

factor in the sensitization process, it will be very important to study how its release by epithelial cells and other inflammatory cells is regulated in response to natural allergen exposure.

The type of immune response induced by mDCs also depends on the strength of the activating innate immune system stimulus. Elegant studies by Eisenbarth showed that low-level TLR4 agonists prime mDCs to induce a Th2 response, by inducing their full maturation, yet not their production of IL-12.[33] High-level LPS administration induced high-level IL-12. These findings might help to explain the effects of environmental exposure to LPS on the reduced incidence of allergic sensitization. IL-12 seems to be a dominant cytokine for Th1 responses in the lung, yet the LPS-induced Th1 response induced by myeloid DCs in the lung was not dependent on IL-12.[40] Although IL-12 may be redundant for some Th1-inducing stimuli, it is certainly sufficient as retroviral overexpression of this cytokine in myeloid DCs in the lung induced strongly polarized Th1 responses.[41] The transcription factor T-bet is a master controller of Th1 development and was recently found to be expressed in DCs in addition to T cells. Tbet[-/-] DCs were less potent in inducing Th1 responses and produced less pro-inflammatory cytokines.[42] The exact role of IL-23 and IL-27, as well as surface expression of the notch ligands Delta/Jagged in DC-driven Th1 development in the lung remains to be studied.[43] Cells of the innate immune system such as NK cells are recruited to the draining nodes by DCs and could also be an early source of Th1 polarizing cytokines.[44]

Recently, Th17 cells that produce IL-17 and regulate autoimmune inflammation have been identified. They are induced by a cytokine cocktail of TGFβ and IL-6, and their numbers are expanded by IL-23.[45]

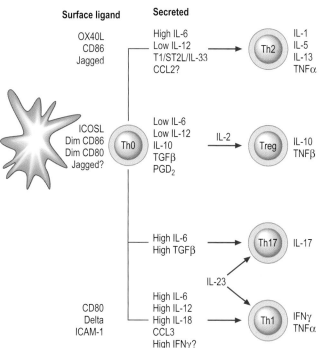

Fig. 21.7. T-helper cell polarization by DCs. Depending on the type of antigen, the dose, the genetic background, and the tissue environment where antigen is first introduced, DCs can induce various types of Th response, tailor-made to protect the host, while avoiding autoimmunity. Often the response is extremely well balanced, to avoid tissue damage, while allowing clearance of the threat. The various cytokines and co-stimulatory molecules that favor a particular direction are indicated.

DCs can produce all these factors, and have been shown to induce Th17 cells in a model of EAE.[45] In view of the fact that IL-17 also plays a crucial role in regulating allergic airway inflammation, the involvement of the DC-Th17 axis in allergy will have to be ascertained.[46]

TOLERANCE INDUCTION BY DCs

Immature DCs are distributed throughout the lung and are at the focal control point determining the induction of pulmonary immunity or tolerance.[47-49] Airway DCs form a dense network in the lung where they are ideally placed to sample inhaled antigens and these cells migrate to draining lymph nodes (LNs) to stimulate naive T cells.[27] As most allergens are immunologically inert proteins, the usual outcome of their inhalation is tolerance and inflammation does not develop upon chronic exposure.[26] This is best shown for the model antigen ovalbumin (OVA). When given to the airways of naive mice via aerosolization, nasal droplet aspiration or intratracheal injection, it renders mice tolerant to a subsequent immunization with OVA in adjuvant, and effectively inhibits the development of airway inflammation, a feature of true immunological tolerance.[26] It was therefore long enigmatic how sensitization to natural allergens occurred. An important discovery was the fact that most clinically important allergens, such as the major Der p 1 allergen from HDM, are proteolytic enzymes that can directly activate

DCs or epithelial cells to break the process of tolerance and promote Th2 responses.[50,51] However, other allergens such as the experimental allergen OVA do not have any intrinsic activating properties. For these antigens, contaminating molecules or environmental exposures (respiratory viruses, air pollution) might pull the trigger on DC activation. Eisenbarth showed that low-level TLR4 agonists admixed with harmless OVA prime DCs to induce a Th2 response, by inducing their full maturation, yet not their production of IL-12. This process has been recently described as being dependent on the activation of the adapter molecule MyD88 in pulmonary DCs.[52] This is clinically important information as most natural allergens, such as HDM, cockroach, and animal dander, contain endotoxin and undoubtedly other TLR agonists.

From the above discussion, is seems that the decision between tolerance or immunity (in the lungs) is controlled by the degree of maturity of mDCs interacting with naive T cells, a process driven by signals from the innate immune system.[53] It has indeed been shown that immature mDCs induce abortive T-cell proliferation in responding T cells and induce regulatory T cells (Tregs).[47] Another level of complexity arose when it was shown that (respiratory) tolerance might be a function of a subset of plasmacytoid DCs.[26,54] Removal of pDCs from mice using depleting antibodies led to a break in inhalational tolerance to OVA and the development of 'asthmatic' inflammation.[26] The precise mechanisms by which pDCs promote tolerance are unknown, but in the absence of pDCs, mDCs become more immunogenic and induce the formation of effector cytokines from dividing T cells.[53] The negative signal that is delivered by pDCs has not been elucidated, but could be the high-level expression of programmed death ligand (PDL)-1, delivering a negative signal to T cells or to mDCs directly.[26,55] Additionally, pDCs can produce the tryptophan-metabolizing enzyme indoleamine 2,3-dioxygenase (IDO), which has a strong inhibitory activity on T-cell proliferation,[56] and inhibits inflammatory airway disease. Interestingly, IDO expression has been demonstrated recently in pulmonary CD11c+ cells although the exact cell type involved has not clearly been identified. Another explanation to the tolerogenic properties of pDCs is related to their immature phenotype, as it has been demonstrated that immature DCs can induce regulatory T cells. Ex vivo at least, lung-derived pDCs promoted formation of Treg cells that were specific for OVA.[26]

CONTROL OF LUNG DC FUNCTION BY REGULATORY T CELLS

The signals that determine the type of response after encountering a pathogen in the lung are delivered by DCs in the lymph node. Induction of DC maturation and provision of peptide-MHC to T cells is not sufficient to generate effector cells.[34] During generation of an efficient effector immune response, DCs have to overcome suppression by regulatory T (Treg) cells, and the dominant way by which they seem to do this is by producing the cytokine IL-6, that counteracts the suppression by naturally occurring CD4+CD25+ Tregs.[57] Established airway inflammation seems to be regulated by Tregs expressing membrane TGFβ or secreting bioactive TGFβ and possibly IL-10.[58] This is a pleiotropic cytokine with significant antiinflammatory and immunosuppressive properties in the lungs, as reduced expression of this cytokine exacerbates airway pathology in an asthma model. Several papers now support the concept that Tregs alter airway DC function. Mice lacking the transcription factor RunX3, involved in downstream TGFβ signaling, spontaneously develop asthma features.[59] In the lungs of these mice, there is

INTEGRATED FUNCTION OF DENDRITIC CELLS IN THE IMMUNE RESPONSE a strong increase in the number of alveolar myeloid DCs, displaying a mature phenotype with increased expression of MHC II, OX40 ligand, and CCR7 and demonstrating an increased immunostimulatory capacity. Moreover, RunX3$^{-/-}$ DCs are able to mount inflammatory responses to otherwise harmless inhaled antigens, possibly through their lack of responsiveness to locally secreted TGFβ.[59] In mice normally resistant to HDM-induced asthma and AHR (C3H mice), Treg cell depletion using the CD25 depleting Ab similarly led to increased numbers of pulmonary myeloid DCs with elevated expression of MHCII, CD80, and CD86 and an increased capacity to stimulate T-cell proliferation and Th2 cytokine production. In normally susceptible A/J mice, Tregs did not suppress inflammation and AHR. These data suggest that resistance to allergen-driven AHR is mediated in part by CD4$^+$CD25$^+$ Treg cell suppression of DC activation and that the absence of this regulatory pathway contributes to susceptibility.[60] In the rat it was shown that Tregs also control the level of CD86 expression on lung DCs and are responsible for the tolerance to inhaled allergen that occurs upon repeated exposure to allergens.[61] In humans with allergy, there is a reduction in the number and possibly function of Tregs,[62] but it is unclear at present whether this would also lead to altered function of DCs in these patients.

■ ROLE FOR DENDRITIC CELLS IN ALLERGIC SENSITIZATION IN HUMANS ■

Although it has not been proven directly in humans that DCs are responsible for the Th2 sensitization process, some in vitro findings strongly imply these cells. The way in which allergens are handled by DCs is fundamentally different between atopic and non-atopic individuals.[63,64] When DCs obtained from house dust mite (HDM)-sensitive asthmatic subjects were exposed to the endotoxin-free major allergen component Der p1 in vitro, they mainly produced IL-10, but little IL-12. They expressed the co-stimulatory molecules CD86 and PDL1.[50] When monocyte-derived DCs from non-HDM-allergic donors or non-allergic donors were exposed to Der p1, they produced mainly IL-12, expressed CD80 and generated the Th1-cell specific chemokine CXCL10. Not surprisingly, monocyte-derived DCs from allergic patients induced Th2-cell responses of naive alloreactive T cells in vitro, whereas those DCs from non-allergic individuals induced Th1 responses. Therefore, the way HDM is handled by DCs is crucial to the generation of Th2-cell sensitization, and is clearly different in patients with allergy to HDM. The cysteine protease activity of Der p1 induced these changes in the DCs of allergic individuals, indicating that the activation of a protease-activated receptor on DCs leads to aberrant cellular activation in patients with asthma.[50] The enzyme activity of Der p1 could also indirectly facilitate antigen presentation by DCs in vivo by allowing access to intraepithelial DCs through cleavage of epithelial tight junctions and by locally activating the release of epithelial GM-CSF.[65] In this way, the epithelial response to allergens might also determine the type of adaptive immune response induced by DCs. Supporting this idea, DCs treated with lipase (an industrial allergen displaying an enzymatic activity) have been reported to induce a strong recall CD4$^+$ T cell response associated with a high production of IL-4 and IL-13, and a low production of IFNγ.[66] However, allergens without enzymatic activity can also directly activate DCs to induce Th2 priming. For instance, phytoprostane lipids

contained in pollen allergens can induce DC maturation and inhibit IL-12 production by LPS-activated DCs. When cocultured with allogeneic naive T cells, pollen-treated DCs polarized the immune response towards Th2.[67]

■ DENDRITIC CELLS IN ALLERGIC ASTHMA ■

Not only do DCs play a role in the primary immune response to inhaled allergens but also they are crucial for the outcome of the effector phase in asthma. Indeed, the number of mDCs is increased in the airways of sensitized and challenged mice during the acute phase of the response.[68] However, during the chronic phase of the pulmonary response, induced by prolonged exposure to a large number of aerosols, respiratory tolerance develops through unclear mechanisms. During this regulatory phase, the number of mDCs in the lungs steadily decreased, and this was associated with a reduction of BHR. Inflammation however reappeared when mDCs were given.[69] The role of mDCs in the secondary immune response was further supported by the fact that their depletion at the time of allergen challenge abrogated all the features of asthma, including airway inflammation, goblet cell hyperplasia, and bronchial hyperresponsiveness.[70] Again the defect was restored by intratracheal injection of mDCs. It therefore seems that mDCs are both necessary and sufficient for secondary immune responses to allergen. Co-stimulatory molecules expressed by DCs could play a crucial role in established asthma. Pulmonary DCs upregulate the expression of CD40, CD80, CD86, ICOS-L, PD-L1, and PD-L2 during eosinophilic airway inflammation, particularly upon contact with Th2 cells.[26,70] Co-stimulatory molecules might be involved in activation of effector T cells in the tissues. In allergen-challenged mice, mDCs might also be a prominent source of the chemokines CCL17 and CCL22, involved in attracting CCR4$^+$ Th2 cells to the airways.[55] The pro-allergic cytokine TSLP induces the production of large amounts of CCL17 by mDCs, thus contributing to the recruitment of a large number of Th2 cells to the airways, explaining how it may act to enhance inflammation.[19]

In humans, allergen challenge leads to an accumulation of myeloid, but not plasmacytoid DCs to the airways of asthmatic subjects, concomitantly with a reduction in circulating CD11c$^+$ cells, showing that these cells are recruited from the bloodstream in response to allergen challenge.[71] In stable asthma, the number of CD1a$^+$ DCs is increased in the airway epithelium and lamina propria, and these numbers are reduced by treatment with inhaled corticosteroids.[72] Based on the above argumentation in mice studies of asthma, it is very likely that part of the efficacy of inhaled steroids might be due to their effects in dampening airway DC function. According to current thinking, epithelial dysfunction, either intrinsic to asthma or caused by persistent inflammation, leads to epithelial release of pro-fibrotic cytokines such as epidermal growth factor and transforming growth, factor-β to act on fibroblasts and smooth muscle cells, disturbing the equilibrium between epithelial destruction, growth, and repair. Moreover, asthmatic epithelium might release factors such as GM-CSF, TSLP or chemokines that profoundly influence DC survival and/or function (Fig. 21.8). The exact consequences of this epithelial remodeling on the functioning of the airway DCs are currently unknown. Finally, many inflammatory cell

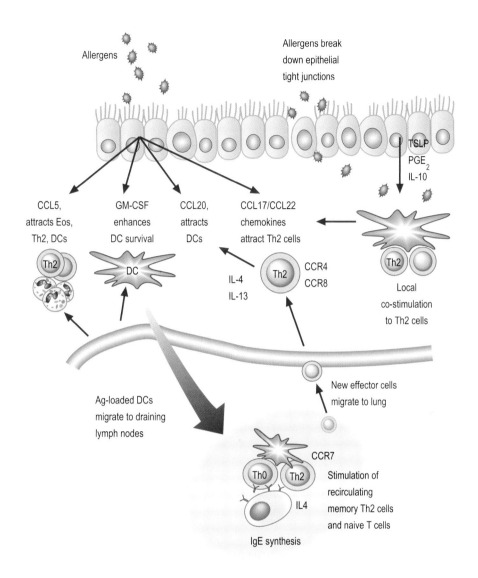

Fig. 21.8. Interaction between epithelial cells and dendritic cells during established inflammation. Allergens stimulate epithelial cells to release chemokines and growth factors for DCs, Th2 cells, and eosinophils. Thymic stromal lymphopoietin (TSLP) and GM-CSF are instrumental in inducing a Th2 prone phenotype in lung DCs. Epithelial cell tight junctions are opened up by protease activity of certain allergens like Der p1 from house-dust mite. In this way, allergens gain access to the DC extensions. The recruited DCs are also stimulated directly by allergen and produce even more chemokines for Th2 cells (TARC and MDC). Locally attracted Th2 cells interact with DCs in the airways, leading to local DC maturation and T-cell co-stimulation of effector cytokine production. These activated Th2 cells eventually control the inflammatory process by activating eosinophils and mast cells and by feeding back on the epithelium and DCs. At the same time, DCs also migrate to the draining lymph nodes where they restimulate recirculating memory Th2 cells to become effector cells, and they recruit new cells into the response. In this way, effector cells are continuously replenished. DCs are also crucial for maintaining IgE synthesis, through their stimulation of IL-4-producing Th2 cells.

types such as mast cells, basophils, and eosinophils are recruited to the airways in chronic asthma. These cells release many mediators such as cytokines, neuropeptides, enzymes, and lipid mediators that may also profoundly influence DC function and in this way might perpetuate ongoing inflammation.[49] As only one example, it is known that histamine and PGD_2, both released by mast cells upon cross-linking, reduce the potential of DCs to produce bioactive IL-12, and thus contribute to Th2 polarization.[21]

The exact role of plasmacytoid DCs in ongoing allergen-specific responses in asthma is currently unknown. It was shown that pDCs accumulate in the nose, but not lungs, of allergen-challenged atopic subjects.[73] When pDCs were pulsed with pollen allergens, they were as efficient as mDCs in inducing Th2 proliferation and effector function.[74] Others have suggested, as in the mouse, that pDCs might also confer protection against allergic responses. In children at high risk of developing atopic disease, the number of circulating pDCs was reduced.[75]

■ DENDRITIC CELLS IN ATOPIC DERMATITIS ■

AD is a chronic inflammatory skin disease that is characterized by eczematous lesions and associated with elevated serum IgE levels, and tissue and blood eosinophilia. AD is characterized by the infiltration of Th2 cells and the increased secretion of Th2-related cytokines (IL-4 and IL-5) and chemokines (TARC) in early lesions. However, Th1 cells also emerge during the chronic phase of the disease. Recent evidence suggests that DCs in the skin and the blood of patients with AD play a pivotal role in the generation and/or control of inflammation.

In patients with AD, DCs highly express FcεRI, the high-affinity receptor for IgE. Two FcεRI$^+$ subsets of myeloid DCs have been identified in skin lesions of AD patients: (1) Langerhans cells expressing CD1a and Birbeck granules found in the epidermis and (2) inflammatory dendritic epidermal cells (IDEC) only found in inflamed skin.[76,77] In AD, FcεRI$^+$ LCs bearing the antigen migrate from the skin to the draining lymph nodes where they activate FcεRI-mediated Th2 immune responses. At the same time, LCs also present allergen-derived peptides locally to transiting T cells and induce a classic secondary immune response. Moreover, the aggregation of FcεRI on LCs stimulates them to release chemokines such as IL-16, TARC, MDC, and monocyte-attracting chemokines.[78] All these molecules contribute to the recruitment of FcεRI^{hi} IDEC into the skin. IDEC are only found under inflammatory conditions, display high stimulatory capacities toward T cells and serve as amplifiers of the allergic-inflammatory immune response. The stimulation of FcεRI on IDEC induces the release of IL-12 and IL-18, leading to the priming of Th1 cells, probably contributing to the Th1 response observed in the chronic phase of AD. In the mouse, overexpression of TSLP under the control of a keratinocyte specific promotor led to an AD-like phenotype. In these mice, skin DCs were likely activated to induce Th2 responses to some self or environmental antigen.

In addition to mDC, pDCs have been found in increased numbers in the blood of AD patients and express FcεRI.[79] pDC can process allergens by FcεRI-IgE and promote Th2-type immune responses. However, in contrast to LC or IDEC, pDCs fail to accumulate in skin lesions of AD patients and seem to be retained in the bloodstream. Whether this is due to a lack of recruitment from the blood to the skin or to the high sensitivity of pDCs to proapoptotic signals present in AD skin remains unclear.

■ ROLE OF DENDRITIC CELLS IN ALLERGIC RHINITIS ■

In allergic rhinitis (AR), CD4$^+$ Th2 cells control inflammation by secreting Th2 cytokines, but little is known how these cells are activated to cause disease. Elevated numbers of CD1a$^+$ Langerhans cells are present in the nasal mucosa of symptomatic grass pollen-sensitive AR patients, and these numbers further increase upon relevant allergen challenge to the nose.[80] In symptomatic AR patients, DCs bearing allergen-specific IgE in the nasal mucosa are present.[81] In house dust mite perennial allergic AR patients, the number of CD1a$^+$ and CD11c$^+$ MHCII$^+$ DCs was higher in the epithelium and lamina propria of the nasal mucosa when compared with healthy controls. In AR, DCs had a more mature

phenotype and were found in close approximation with T cells. Similarly, in a mouse model of ovalbumin-induced AR, CD11c$^+$DCs accumulated in areas of nasal eosinophilic inflammation and clustered with CD4$^+$ T cells. To address the functional role of DCs in maintaining inflammation, CD11c$^+$DCs were conditionally depleted during allergen challenge by systemic administration of diphtheria toxin (DT) to CD11c-DT-receptor-Tg mice. In the absence of CD11c$^+$ DCs, nasal OVA challenge of OVA-sensitized mice did not induce nasal eosinophilia, and did not boost OVA-specific IgE levels or Th2 cytokine production in the cervical lymph nodes. Conversely, when OVA-pulsed DCs were administered intranasally to sensitized mice, they strongly enhanced OVA-induced nasal eosinophilia and Th2 cytokine productions. These data in humans and mice suggest an essential role for nasal DCs in activation of effector Th2 function leading to allergic rhinitis and identify DCs as a novel target for therapeutic intervention.[82] In support of this proposal, treatment of allergic rhinitis patients with intranasal corticosteroids dramatically reduced the numbers of DCs in the nasal mucosa.

■ DENDRITIC CELLS AS DRUG TARGETS IN ALLERGIC DISEASES ■

If dendritic cells are so crucial in mounting immune responses during ongoing inflammation in the lung, nose, and skin, then interfering with their function could constitute a novel form of treatment for allergic diseases. Additionally, pharmacological modification of DCs might fundamentally reset the balance of the allergic immune response in favor of regulatory T cells and thus lead to a more long-lasting effect on the natural course of allergic disease. Steroids are currently the cornerstone of antiinflammatory treatment in allergic disease. Inhaled steroids reduce the number of lung and nose DCs in patients with AA and AD, whereas local application of steroids to the skin of AD patients reduces the influx of IDECs.[72,80] The immunosuppressant drug tacrolimus is currently in use for topical treatment for AD. It suppresses the expression of MHCII and co-stimulatory molecules and FcεRI on LC from AD patients in vitro and reduces the number of IDECs in lesional skin. Recently several other new molecules have surfaced that may alter DC function in allergic inflammation and thus treat disease. In one report, administration of CpG-containing immunostimulatory DNA sequences (ISS) to the lungs of allergen-challenged mice inhibited the upregulation of these co-stimulatory molecules, suggesting that this is one mechanism by which they suppress inflammation.[83] The sphingosine-1-P analogue FTY720 is currently used in clinical trials for multiple sclerosis and transplant rejection. When given to the lungs of mice with established inflammation, it strongly reduced inflammation by suppressing the T-cell stimulatory capacity and migratory behavior of lung DCs.[20] Also selective agonists of particular prostaglandin series receptors might suppress DC function. The DP1 agonist BW245C strongly suppressed airway inflammation and bronchial hyperreactivity when given to allergic mice by inhibiting the maturation of lung DCs. DCs thus exposed to DP1 agonists induced the formation of Foxp3$^+$ Treg cells that suppressed inflammation upon adoptive transfer.[84] A very similar mechanism was described for inhaled iloprost, a prostacyclin analogue acting on the IP receptor expressed by lung DCs.[85] A specific small molecule compound (VAF347) that blocks the function of B cells and DCs was also shown to be effective in suppressing allergic airway inflammation in a mouse model of asthma.[86] Finally, specific inhibitors of *syk* kinase were shown to suppress DC function and cure established inflammation.[87]

■ CONCLUSION ■

Dendritic cells are crucial in determining the functional outcome of an allergen encounter in the lung, nose, and skin. Antigen presentation by myeloid DCs leads to Th2 sensitization typical of allergic disease. It is increasingly clear that DCs have an antigen-presenting function beyond sensitization. DCs therefore constitute a novel target for the development of anti-allergic therapy aimed at the origin of the inflammatory cascade.

References

Dendritic cell terminology and heterogeneity

1. Shortman K, Liu YJ. Mouse and human dendritic cell subtypes. Nat Rev Immunol 2002; 2:151–161.
2. Geissmann F, Jung S, Littman DR. Blood monocytes consist of two principal subsets with distinct migratory properties. Immunity 2003; 19:71–82.
3. Naik SH, Metcalf D, van Nieuwenhuijze A, et al. Intrasplenic steady-state dendritic cell precursors that are distinct from monocytes. Nat Immunol 2006; 7:663–671.

Antigen uptake

4. Figdor CG, van Kooyk Y, Adema GJ. C-type lectin receptors on dendritic cells and Langerhans cells. Nat Rev Immunol 2002; 2:77–84.
5. Kissenpfennig A, Ait-Yahia S, Clair-Moninot V, et al. Disruption of the langerin/CD207 gene abolishes Birbeck granules without a marked loss of Langerhans cell function. Mol Cell Biol 2005; 25:88–99.
6. Currie AJ, Stewart GA, McWilliam AS. Alveolar macrophages bind and phagocytose allergen-containing pollen starch granules via C-type lectin and integrin receptors: implications for airway inflammatory disease. J Immunol 2000; 164:3878–3886.
7. Deslée G, Charbonnier AS, Hammad H, et al. Involvement of the mannose receptor in the uptake of der p 1, a major mite allergen, by human dendritic cells. J Allergy Clin Immunol 2002; 110:763–770.
8. Noirey N, Rougier N, Andre C, et al. Langerhans-like dendritic cells generated from cord blood progenitors internalize pollen allergens by macropinocytosis, and part of the molecules are processed and can activate autologous naive T lymphocytes. J Allergy Clin Immunol 2000; 105:1194–1201.
9. Ochando JC, Homma C, Yang Y, et al. Alloantigen-presenting plasmacytoid dendritic cells mediate tolerance to vascularized grafts. Nat Immunol 2006; 7:652–662.

Antigen presentation

10. Nijman HW, Kleijmeer MJ, Ossevoort MA, et al. Antigen capture and major histocompatibility class II compartments of freshly isolated and cultured human blood dendritic cells. J Exp Med 1995; 182:163–174.
11. Denzin LK, Cresswell P. HLA-DM induces CLIP dissociation from MHC class II alpha beta dimers and facilitates peptide loading. Cell 1995; 82:155–165.
12. Maurer D, Fiebiger E, Reininger B, et al. Fcε receptor I on dendritic cells delivers IgE-bound multivalent antigens into a cathepsin S-dependent pathway of MHC class II presentation. J Immunol 1998; 161:2731–2739.
13. Wells JW, Cowled CJ, Giorgini A, et al. Regulation of allergic airway inflammation by class I-restricted allergen presentation and CD8 T-cell infiltration. J Allergy Clin Immunol 2007; 119:226–234.

Integrated function of dendritic cells

in the immune response

14. Yang D, Chertov O, Bykovskaia SN, et al. Beta-defensins: linking innate and adaptive immunity through dendritic and T cell CCR6. Science 1999; 286:525–528.
15. Vermi W, Riboldi E, Wittamer V, et al. Role of ChemR23 in directing the migration of myeloid and plasmacytoid dendritic cells to lymphoid organs and inflamed skin. J Exp Med 2005; 201:509–515.
16. Bancheureau J, Steinman RM. Dendritic cells and the control of immunity. Nature 1998; 392:245–252.
17. Lotze MT, Tracey KJ. High-mobility group box 1 protein (HMGB1): nuclear weapon in the immune arsenal. Nat Rev Immunol 2005; 5:331–342.
18. Lambrecht BN, Hammad H. The other cells in asthma: dendritic cell and epithelial cell crosstalk. Curr Opin Pulm Med 2003; 9:34–41.
19. Zhou B, Comeau MR, De Smedt T, et al. Thymic stromal lymphopoietin as a key initiator of allergic airway inflammation in mice. Nat Immunol 2005; 6:1047–1053.
20. Idzko M, Hammad H, van Nimwegen M, et al. Local application of FTY720 to the lung abrogates experimental asthma by altering dendritic cell function. J Clin Invest 2006; 116: 2935–2944.
21. Hammad H, de Heer HJ, Souillie T, et al. Prostaglandin D₂ modifies airway dendritic cell migration and function in steady state conditions by selective activation of the DP-receptor. J Immunol 2003; 171:3936–3940.
22. Hammad H, de Heer HJ, Souillie T, et al. Activation of peroxisome proliferator-activated receptor pathway in dendritic cells inhibits development of eosinophilic airway inflammation in a mouse model of asthma. Am J Pathol 2004; 164:263–271.
23. Robbiani F, Finch RA, Jager D, et al. The leukotriene C4 transporter MRP1 regulates CCL19 (MIP-3b, ELC)-dependent mobilization of dendritic cells to lymph nodes. Cell 2000; 103: 757–768.
24. Jakubzick C, Tacke F, Llodra J, et al. Modulation of dendritic cell trafficking to and from the airways. J Immunol 2006; 176:3578–3584.
25. Qu C, Edwards EW, Tacke F, et al. Role of CCR8 and other chemokine pathways in the migration of monocyte-derived dendritic cells to lymph nodes. J Exp Med 2004; 200: 1231–1241.
26. De Heer HJ, Hammad H, Soullie T, et al. Essential role of lung plasmacytoid dendritic cells in preventing asthmatic reactions to harmless inhaled antigen. J Exp Med 2004; 200:89–98.
27. Vermaelen KY, Carro-Muino I, Lambrecht BN, et al. Specific migratory dendritic cells rapidly transport antigen from the airways to the thoracic lymph nodes. J Exp Med 2001; 193:51–60.
28. Belz GT, Smith CM, Kleinert L, et al. Distinct migrating and nonmigrating dendritic cell populations are involved in MHC class I-restricted antigen presentation after lung infection with virus. Proc Natl Acad Sci USA 2004; 101:8670–8675.
29. Hammad H, de Vries VC, Maldonado-Lopez R, et al. Differential capacity of CD8+ alpha or CD8- alpha dendritic cell subsets to prime for eosinophilic airway inflammation in the T-helper type 2-prone milieu of the lung. Clin Exp Allergy 2004; 34:1834–1840.
30. Qi H, Egen JG, Huang AY, et al. Extrafollicular activation of lymph node B cells by antigen-bearing dendritic cells. Science 2006; 312:1672–1676.
31. Lambrecht BN, Pauwels RA, Fazekas De St Groth B. Induction of rapid T cell activation, division, and recirculation by intratracheal injection of dendritic cells in a TCR transgenic model. J Immunol 2000; 164:2937–2946.
32. Kapsenberg ML. Dendritic-cell control of pathogen-driven T-cell polarization. Nat Rev Immunol 2003; 3:984–993.
33. Eisenbarth SC, Piggott DA, Huleatt JW, et al. Lipopolysaccharide-enhanced, toll-like receptor 4-dependent T helper cell type 2 responses to inhaled antigen. J Exp Med 2002; 196: 1645–1651.
34. Sporri R, Reis e Sousa C. Inflammatory mediators are insufficient for full dendritic cell activation and promote expansion of CD4+ T cell populations lacking helper function. Nat Immunol 2005; 6:163–170.
35. Pasare C, Medzhitov R. Toll pathway-dependent blockade of CD4+CD25+ T cell-mediated suppression by dendritic cells. Science 2003; 299:1033–1036.
36. Stumbles PA, Thomas JA, Pimm CL, et al. Resting respiratory tract dendritic cells preferentially stimulate T helper cell type 2 (Th2) responses and require obligatory cytokine signals for induction of Th1 immunity. J Exp Med 1998; 188:2019–2031.
37. Lambrecht BN, De Veerman M, Coyle AJ, et al. Myeloid dendritic cells induce Th2 responses to inhaled antigen, leading to eosinophilic airway inflammation. J Clin Invest 2000; 106:551–559.
38. Ying S, O'Connor B, Ratoff J, et al. Thymic stromal lymphopoietin expression is increased in asthmatic airways and correlates with expression of Th2-attracting chemokines and disease severity. J Immunol 2005; 174:8183–8190.
39. Ito T, Wang YH, Duramad O, et al. TSLP-activated dendritic cells induce an inflammatory T helper type 2 cell response through OX40 ligand. J Exp Med 2005; 202:1213–1223.
40. Kuipers H, Hijdra D, De Vries VC, et al. Lipopolysaccharide-induced suppression of airway Th2 responses does not require IL-12 production by dendritic cells. J Immunol 2003; 171:3645–3654.
41. Kuipers H, Heirman C, Hijdra D, et al. Dendritic cells retrovirally overexpressing IL-12 induce strong Th1 responses to inhaled antigen in the lung but fail to revert established Th2 sensitization. J Leukoc Biol 76:1028–1038.
42. Wang J, Fathman JW, Lugo-Villarino G, et al. Transcription factor T-bet regulates inflammatory arthritis through its function in dendritic cells. J Clin Invest 2006; 116:414–421.
43. Amsen D, Blander JM, Lee GR, et al. Instruction of distinct CD4 T helper cell fates by different notch ligands on antigen-presenting cells. Cell 2004; 117:515–526.
44. Martin-Fontecha A, Thomsen LL, Brett S, et al. Induced recruitment of NK cells to lymph nodes provides IFN-gamma for T(H)1 priming. Nat Immunol 2004; 5:1260–1265.
45. Veldhoen M, Hocking RJ, Atkins CJ, et al. TGFbeta in the context of an inflammatory cytokine milieu supports de novo differentiation of IL-17-producing T cells. Imsmunity 2006; 24:179–189.
46. Schnyder-Candrian S, Togbe D, Couillin I, et al. Interleukin-17 is a negative regulator of established allergic asthma. J Exp Med 2006; 203:2715–2725.
47. Akbari O, DeKruyff RH, Umetsu DT. Pulmonary dendritic cells producing IL-10 mediate tolerance induced by respiratory exposure to antigen. Nat Immunol 2001; 2:725–731.
48. Akbari O, Freeman GJ, Meyer EH, et al. Antigen-specific regulatory T cells develop via the ICOS-ICOS-ligand pathway and inhibit allergen-induced airway hyperreactivity. Nat Med 2002; 8:1024–1032.
49. Lambrecht BN, Hammad H. Taking our breath away: dendritic cells in the pathogenesis of asthma. Nat Rev Immunol 2003; 3:994–1003.
50. Hammad H, Charbonnier AS, Duez C, et al. Th2 polarization by Der p 1-pulsed monocyte-derived dendritic cells is due to the allergic status of the donors. Blood 2001; 98:1135–1141.

51. Kheradmand F, Kiss A, Xu J, et al. A protease-activated pathway underlying Th cell type 2 activation and allergic lung disease. J Immunol 2002; 169:5904–5911.

52. Piggott DA, Eisenbarth SC, Xu L, et al. MyD88-dependent induction of allergic Th2 responses to intranasal antigen. J Clin Invest 2005; 115:459–467.

53. de Heer HJ, Hammad H, Kool M, et al. Dendritic cell subsets and immune regulation in the lung. Semin Immunol 2005; 17:295–303.

54. Oriss TB, Ostroukhova M, Seguin-Devaux C, et al. Dynamics of dendritic cell phenotype and interactions with CD4+ T cells in airway inflammation and tolerance. J Immunol 2005; 174:854–863.

55. Kohl J, Baelder R, Lewkowich IP, et al. A regulatory role for the C5a anaphylatoxin in type 2 immunity in asthma. J Clin Invest 2006; 116:783–796.

56. Fallarino F, Asselin-Paturel C, Vacca C, et al. Murine plasmacytoid dendritic cells initiate the immunosuppressive pathway of tryptophan catabolism in response to CD200 receptor engagement. J Immunol 2004; 173:3748–3754.

57. Doganci A, Eigenbrod T, Krug N, et al. The IL-6R alpha chain controls lung CD4+CD25+ Treg development and function during allergic airway inflammation in vivo. J Clin Invest 2005; 115:313–325.

58. Kearley J, Barker JE, Robinson DS, et al. Resolution of airway inflammation and hyperreactivity after in vivo transfer of CD4+CD25+ regulatory T cells is interleukin 10 dependent. J Exp Med 2005; 202:1539–1547.

59. Fainaru O, Woolf E, Lotem J, et al. Runx3 regulates mouse TGF-beta-mediated dendritic cell function and its absence results in airway inflammation. EMBO J 2004; 23:969–979.

60. Lewkowich IP, Herman NS, Schleifer KW, et al. CD4+CD25+ T cells protect against experimentally induced asthma and alter pulmonary dendritic cell phenotype and function. J Exp Med 2005; 202:1549–1561.

61. Strickland DH, Stumbles PA, Zosky GR, et al. Reversal of airway hyperresponsiveness by induction of airway mucosal CD4+CD25+ regulatory T cells. J Exp Med 2006; 203: 2649–2660.

62. Kuipers H, Lambrecht BN. The interplay of dendritic cells, Th2 cells and regulatory T cells in asthma. Curr Opin Immunol 2004; 16:702–708.

Role for dendritic cells in allergic sensitization

in humans

63. Hammad H, Lambrecht BN, Pochard P, et al. Monocyte-derived dendritic cells induce a house dust mite-specific Th2 allergic inflammation in the lung of humanized SCID mice: involvement of CCR7. J Immunol 2002; 169:1524–1534.

64. De Wit D, Amraoui Z, Vincart B, et al. Helper T-cell responses elicited by Der p 1-pulsed dendritic cells and recombinant IL-12 in atopic and healthy subjects. J Allergy Clin Immunol 2000; 105:346–352.

65. Wan H, Winton HL, Soeller C, et al. Der P 1 facilitates transepithelial allergen delivery by disruption of tight junctions. J Clin Invest 1999; 104:123–133.

66. Lindstedt M, Schiott A, Johnsen CR, et al. Individuals with occupational allergy to detergent enzymes display a differential transcriptional regulation and cellular immune response. Clin Exp Allergy 2005; 35:199–206.

67. Traidl-Hoffmann C, Mariani V, Hochrein H, et al. Pollen-associated phytoprostanes inhibit dendritic cell interleukin-12 production and augment T helper type 2 cell polarization. J Exp Med 2005; 201:627–636.

Dendritic cells in allergic asthma

68. van Rijt LS, Prins JB, deVries VC, et al. Allergen-induced accumulation of airway dendritic cells is supported by an increase in CD31hi Ly-6Cneg hematopoietic precursors. Blood 2002; 100:3663–3671.

69. Koya T, Kodama T, Takeda K, et al. Importance of myeloid dendritic cells in persistent airway disease after repeated allergen exposure. Am J Respir Crit Care Med 2006; 173:42–55.

70. van Rijt LS, Jung S, Kleinjan A, et al. In vivo depletion of lung CD11c+ dendritic cells during allergen challenge abrogates the characteristic features of asthma. J Exp Med 2005; 201: 981–991.

71. Upham JW, Denburg JA, O'Byrne PM. Rapid response of circulating myeloid dendritic cells to inhaled allergen in asthmatic subjects. Clin Exp Allergy 2002; 32:818–823.

72. Moller GM, Overbeek SE, Van Helden-Meeuwsen CG, et al. Increased numbers of dendritic cells in the bronchial mucosa of atopic asthmatic patients: downregulation by inhaled corticosteroids. Clin Exp Allergy 1996; 26:517–524.

73. Jahnsen FL, Lund-Johansen F, Dunne JF, et al. Experimentally induced recruitment of plasmacytoid (CD123high) dendritic cells in human nasal allergy. J Immunol 2000; 165: 4062–4068.

74. Farkas L, Kvale EO, Johansen FE, et al. Plasmacytoid dendritic cells activate allergen-specific TH2 memory cells: modulation by CpG oligodeoxynucleotides. J Allergy Clin Immunol 2004; 114:436–443.

75. Hagendorens MM, Ebo DG, Schuerwegh AJ, et al. Differences in circulating dendritic cell subtypes in cord blood and peripheral blood of healthy and allergic children. Clin Exp Allergy 2003; 33:633–639.

Dendritic cells in atopic dermatitis

76. Wollenberg A, Wen SP, Bieber T. Langerhans cell phenotyping: a new tool for differential diagnosis of inflammatory diseases. Lancet 1995; 346:1626–1627.

77. Wollenberg A, Kraft S, Hanau D, et al. Immunomorphological and ultrastructural characterization of Langerhans cells and a novel, inflammatory dendritic epidermal cell (IDEC) population in lesional skin of atopic eczema. J Invest Dermatol 1996; 106:446–453.

78. Novak N, Valenta R, Bohle B, et al. FcepsilonRI engagement of Langerhans cell-like dendritic cells and inflammatory dendritic epidermal cell-like dendritic cells induces chemotactic signals and different T-cell phenotypes in vitro. J Allergy Clin Immunol 2004; 113:949–957.

79. Novak N, Allam JP, Hagemann T, et al. Characterization of FcepsilonRI-bearing CD123 blood dendritic cell antigen-2 plasmacytoid dendritic cells in atopic dermatitis. J Allergy Clin Immunol 2004; 114:364–370.

Role of dendritic cells in allergic rhinitis

80. Fokkens WJ. Antigen-presenting cells in nasal allergy. Allergy 1999; 54:1130–1141.

81. KleinJan A, Godthelp T, van Toornenenbergen AW, et al. Allergen binding to specific IgE in the nasal mucosa of allergic patients. J Allergy Clin Immunol 1997; 99:515–521.

82. KleinJan A, Willart M, van Rijt LS, et al. An essential role for dendritic cells in human and experimental allergic rhinitis. J Allergy Clin Immunol 2006; 118:1117–1125.

Dendritic cells as drug targets in allergic diseases

83. Hessel EM, Chu M, Lizcano JO, et al. Immunostimulatory oligonucleotides block allergic airway inflammation by inhibiting Th2 cell activation and IgE-mediated cytokine induction. J Exp Med 2005; 202:1563–1573.

84. Hammad H, Kool M, Soullie T, et al. Activation of the D prostanoid 1 receptor suppresses asthma by modulation of lung dendritic cell function and induction of regulatory T cells. J Exp Med 2007; 204:357–367.

85. Idzko M, Hammad H, van Nimwegen M, et al. Extracellular ATP triggers and maintains asthmatic airway inflammation by activating dendritic cells. Nat Med 2007; 13:913–919.

86. Ettmayer P, Mayer P, Kalthoff F, et al. A novel low molecular weight inhibitor of dendritic cells and B cells blocks allergic inflammation. Am J Respir Crit Care Med 2006; 173:599–606.

87. Matsubara S, Koya T, Takeda K, et al. Syk activation in dendritic cells is essential for airway hyperresponsiveness and inflammation. Am J Respir Cell Mol Biol 2006; 34:426–433.

The Biology of Monocytes and Macrophages

William J Calhoun, Shibu Thomas, and Michael C Saavedra

22

CONTENTS

- Introduction 355
- Macrophages and afferent arm immune function 356
- Macrophages and efferent arm immune function – general concepts 364
- Macrophages in asthma 365
- Summary 369

SUMMARY OF IMPORTANT CONCEPTS

>> Macrophages are the first line of defense in the airway, mediate innate immunity, alert the adaptive immune system of the host to new pathogens, and contribute to effector function to kill and clear microorganisms

>> Innate immune function is activated by the family of Toll-like receptors expressed on the surface of macrophages and monocytes

>> Macrophages and monocytes express antigen with MHC class II, and specific co-stimulatory molecules that regulated T lymphocyte development in a Th1 or Th2 direction

>> Macrophages can be activated in an allergen-specific manner to participate in asthma pathogenesis

>> Macrophages may play a key role in the process of airway remodeling, by secreting and regulating protease activity

INTRODUCTION

GENERAL FUNCTIONS OF MONOCYTES AND MACROPHAGES

Monocytes and macrophages serve critical roles in host defense. They are an important component of innate immunity, can function independently of adaptive (acquired) immunity, serve to alert the immune system of new pathogens, can dictate the character of a new immune response by varying the expression of co-stimulatory molecules during antigen presentation, are functionally activated by allergic responses and by mediators released in the context of allergic responses and asthma, and are a rich source of inflammatory mediators, cytokines, and direct inflammogens. Moreover, other mediators released by macrophages may play a key role in suppressing and resolving inflammatory responses after the initial amplification phase has ended. Hence, an understanding of the biology of these important cells is essential for a complete picture of asthma pathogenesis to emerge.[1]

Monocytes are of myeloid origin, derived from bone marrow precursors, and after maturation in the marrow, are released into the circulation. Under the direction of cytokines, chemokines, and adhesion molecules, monocytes emigrate from the circulation to reach the resident site in tissue or anatomic spaces whereupon they differentiate further to become recognizable morphologically as macrophages. These cells are recruited to the sites of inflammation 24h or more after its initiation. However, clinically important inflammation clearly need not be present for this process to occur, as resident peritoneal, pleural, articular, and alveolar macrophages (AM) are present in health as well. Monocytes and macrophages differ both phenotypically and functionally, but share many common features. For this reason, they will be discussed together; relevant and important differences in asthma will be highlighted. Macrophages and monocytes are pluripotent cells, equipped with a wide variety of surface receptors (Table 22.1), which mediate interactions with the microenvironment, and numerous effector mechanisms which subserve the functions of bacterial killing and immune regulation (Table 22.2). The interested reader is referred to a current review of the immune system.[2]

Table 22.1 Selected surface molecule expression by macrophages

Molecule designation	Function/alternate names
CD11a	α_L integrin; LFA-1α
CD11b	α_M integrin; complement receptor 3; MAC-1
CD11c	α_X integrin; complement receptor 4
CD14	Endotoxin response, as part of TLR4
CD16	Fcγ receptor III
CD18	β-subunit for CD11a, CD11b, CD11c
CD23	Low-affinity IgE receptor
CD32	Fcγ receptor II
CD35	Complement receptors
CD40	Co-stimulatory molecule; receptor for CD40 ligand
CD44	Hyaluronic acid receptor
CD54	Intracellular adhesion molecule (ICAM)-1
CD64	Fcγ receptor I
CD68	Macrosialin – relatively specific macrophage marker
CD71	Transferrin receptor
CD80 (B7-1)	Co-stimulatory molecule for T-cell activation
CD86 (B7-2)	Co-stimulatory molecule for T-cell activation, Th2 facilitating
TLR4	Endotoxin response
TLR2	*Mycobacterial* recognition, Gram-positive bacteria

Table 22.2 Selected effector mechanisms of macrophages and monocytes

Proinflammatory
 IL-1β
 TNF-α
 GM-CSF
 IFN-γ
 IL-8
 iNOS
Antiinflammatory
 IL-10
 Hemoxygenase-1
Lysosomal enzymes
Reactive molecules
 Superoxide anion/peroxynitrite
 H_2O_2
 Hypohalous acid
Lipid mediators
 LTC_4
 PGE_2
 Lipoxins
Immune regulation
 MHC II
 MHC I

LOCALIZATION OF MACROPHAGES AND MONOCYTES IN THE LUNG

Monocytes and macrophages in the lung can be divided into three categories: airway and alveolar macrophages, interstitial macrophages and monocytes anatomically within pulmonary blood vessels. If dendritic cells are included as derivatives of monocytes, then they would represent a fourth category. The function of monocytes in pulmonary blood vessels is probably comparable with that of peripheral blood monocytes, and so will not be independently discussed. Pulmonary interstitial macrophages (PIM) are a small numerical component of lung tissue, and their isolation therefore requires considerable tissue; hence, much of the research on PIM has been conducted in animals, rather than in humans. Details of dendritic cells are presented elsewhere in this textbook. Thus, this chapter will focus primarily on airway and alveolar macrophages and their role in allergic inflammation.

LINKS BETWEEN MACROPHAGES AND ASTHMA

In addition to many proximal proinflammatory cytokines, human alveolar macrophages are known to produce the allergic cytokine IL-4,[3] therefore providing direct linkage of the function of this cell to atopic disease and asthma. In addition, the absence of IL-10, as may occur in asthma, permits a positive feedback loop between nitric oxide (NO) and IL-4,[4] which may lead to prodigious IL-4 release by these cells. From an epidemiologic standpoint, the amount of carbon in airway macrophages bears a significant positive relationship to the degree of airway obstruction in children.[5] This remarkable recent observation highlights the important role played by airway macrophages in scavenging foreign particles, and also strongly implicates the central role of their effector functions in regulating airway caliber.

MACROPHAGES AND AFFERENT ARM IMMUNE FUNCTION

Alveolar macrophages are placed precisely at the interface between the host and environment, and serve important functions to promote host defense independent of adaptive immunity, to alert the host of potential pathogens, to regulate the developing immune response, and to participate in effector functions of bacterial killing and elimination coordinately with the adaptive immune system. Accordingly, they contribute to both innate immunity and acquired (or adaptive) immunity. The functions of macrophages are many, complex, and potent; interactions among these processes are necessary for health (Fig. 22.1).[6] Accordingly, these cells can participate in the pathogenesis of inflammatory diseases of the respiratory tract when invoked inappropriately.

MACROPHAGES AND INNATE IMMUNITY

Macrophages participate directly in innate immunity.[7] They express receptors for endotoxin (CD14, a component of the Toll-like receptor type 4, TLR4), other environmental 'danger signals' (other TLRs), mannose, surfactant proteins, NODs, scavenger receptors, and complement. Collectively, these receptors mediate interaction of the naive unprimed macrophage with lipopolysaccharide (LPS), *Mycobacterium tuberculosis*,[8] carbohydrates, nucleic acids, other foreign macromolecules that express pathogen associated molecular patterns (PAMPs), and host complement proteins activated by the alternative pathway, respectively.[6] PAMPs are typically composed of repeating carbohydrate, lipid, or other moieties, and are identified by pattern recognition receptors (PRRs) on the surface of the macrophages that include TLRs, C-type lectins, and scavenger receptors. Thus, macrophages are designed and equipped to respond quickly to potential pathogens, and to do so without the necessity of adaptive immunity (Fig. 22.2).[6,9]

A prototypical family of PRR is represented by the Toll-like receptors (TLRs). A partial catalog of TLRs expressed on macrophages, their putative ligands, and selected known polymorphisms are summarized in Table 22.3.[10–16] TLRs derive their names from *Drosophila* Toll (great, or master) proteins as these proteins were found to mediate dorsal–ventral patterning in *Drosophila* flies. Mutations in these Toll proteins also regulated the immunity of flies to fungal infections.[17] Further studies in mice proved mutations at TLR4 were associated with poor immune and blunted inflammatory responses to endotoxin.[18] TLRs recognize repeating oligo- and polymeric patterns expressed on or by a wide array of organisms from bacteria to fungi to viruses and protozoa. Twelve mammalian TLRs have been identified to date.[19] Of particular note, is TLR4 (the endotoxin receptor) and TLR9 (the CpG oligonucleotide receptor).[20]

After recognizing 'danger signals' in the environment, TLRs then initiate important intracellular signaling functions. Recognition of microbial ligands by TLRs and other PRRs triggers intracellular signaling pathways, leading to production of pro- and antiinflammatory cytokines.[21] TLR signaling is a complex pathway that includes multiple adapter molecules (e.g., MyD88, TRAF3) that ultimately activate NF-κB, mitogen activated protein (MAP) kinase, and other transcription factors which then promote proinflammatory cytokine gene transcription and production (Fig. 22.3).[22] Of note, TLRs can recognize pathogens both at the cell surface (sampling the extracellular environment) and in endosomes (sampling the intracellular compartment).[19,21]

Toll-like receptor activation has been implicated in many inflammatory lung processes. TLR4 and TLR2 are key molecules in recognizing bacterial components. TLR4 recognizes Gram-negative LPS while TLR2 responses to Gram-negative, Gram-positive and products of *Mycobacterium* ligands.[23] Alveolar macrophages mediate many of the initial responses to inhaled LPS.[24] In the lung, the TLRs can be upregulated and downregulated in disease. Such changes have been observed in the settings of infection or inflammation. Droemann et al[25] showed TLR2

expression in alveolar macrophages was decreased in smokers and COPD patients, suggesting impaired host defense. Healthy subjects who were exposed to endotoxin inhalation, had increased expression of mRNA encoding for TLRs 1,2,7,8 and reduced expression of mRNA encoding for TLR4.[26] Shapiro[27] found activation of monocytes and macrophages by LPS which then released metalloproteinases; the authors suggested that these proteolytic factors may have played a role in the development in COPD.

One polymorphism in the TLR4 receptor has been shown to influence atopic severity,[10] but perhaps surprisingly, genetic associations among TLR4 polymorphisms and asthma, IgE elevations, and clinical allergic disease have not been strong. However, a component of the endotoxin signaling pathway, CD14, does appear to regulate the propensity for atopic development. A promoter polymorphism (–159 C/T) have been identified that appears to associate with altered adaptive immunity. The TT genotype at this locus is associated with higher levels of soluble CD14, reduced skin test reactivity to molds, decreased serum IgE, and reduced likelihood of wheezing in infancy.[28–30] In contrast, individuals with the CC genotype may have serum IgE almost twice that of the TT cohort. This effect of increased soluble CD14 may be mediated through enhanced production of interferon-γ, and consequent suppression of Th2 immunity.

Endotoxin can produce airway obstruction and hyperresponsiveness without pre-existing asthma, apparently independent of adaptive immunity. This response occurs presumably via interaction with TLR4 on monocytes, macrophages, and other cells, and consequent activation of inflammatory pathways. Inhalation of endotoxin by healthy volunteers produces chest symptoms and airflow limitation.[31] Endotoxin is implicated in the pathogenesis of organic dust disease due to grain dust, for example.[32] The effect of endotoxin on airway function and inflammation can be reproduced in animal models; further, competitive inhibitors of LPS binding block airway hyperresponsiveness and inflammatory cytokine production.[33] Direct instillation of endotoxin into human volunteers via bronchoscopy results in increases in IL-1β, TNF-α, and striking increases in neutrophils.[34] Clearly, environmental exposure to endotoxin can have important effects on airway function and airway inflammation via activation of innate immune mechanisms, including participation by monocytes and macrophages.

ANTIGEN PRESENTATION AND ADAPTIVE IMMUNITY

Macrophages and monocytes are also important in adaptive immunity. They express receptors for immunoglobulins G and E, and can be activated thereby, for phagocytic and microbicidal function. They respond to IFN-γ with considerable increase in pro-inflammatory function and bacterial killing, particularly of *Mycobacteria*,[35] and dramatically increased surface expression of MHC class II.[36] In fact, the key role of IFN-γ in host defense against *M.tb* is further demonstrated by dramatically increased susceptibility to *M.tb* infection in children with mutations in the IFN-γ receptor, coded on chromosome 6q.[37] However, the magnitude of increased MHC class II expression induced by IFN-γ is less for AM than for blood monocytes.[38] Via MHC class II molecules, AM can present antigen, although in health they do so relatively poorly. In disease states associated with active influx of new monocyte-like macrophages are associated with increased antigen presentation by AM. Antigen presentation by AM in asthma, for example, is significantly

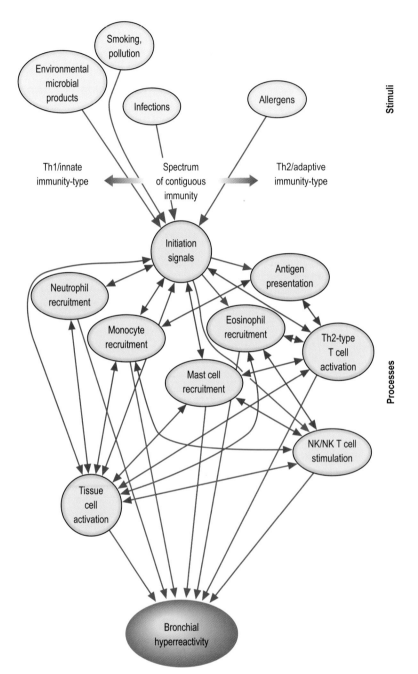

Fig. 22.1. A simplified and conceptualized scheme of key subsystems contributing to contiguous immunity in asthma. Although inflammatory stimuli can be viewed from the position of their bias toward activation of the innate or adaptive systems, or Th1- or Th2-type immunity, in the contiguous immunity of disease, repeated exposures to varying combinations of these immune activators are the norm. Early-response cells contribute upstream signals in the inflammatory response and activate a series of subsystems that together drive pathology (in the case of asthma, summarized as bronchial hyperreactivity). Although some of the connections between subsystems might be more unidirectional (purple arrows), most subsystems probably exist in continual dialog (red arrows). Where cell recruitment or activation is indicated as a system component, both activation and recruitment may be involved, but only one may be specified to simplify the figure. The development of bronchial hyperreactivity and the associated tissue remodeling have the potential to substantially modify the responses to repeated rounds of inflammatory stimuli (dashed arrow). Amelioration of bronchial hyperreactivity might require the targeting of upstream signals, or combinations of subsystems; such targeting may need to be designed on an individual basis according to disease phenotype, patient genotype, and temporal factors (disease duration). NK, natural killer. (Reproduced, with permission, from Sabroe I, Parker LC, Dockrell DH, et al. Pulmonary perspective: targeting the networks that underpin contiguous immunity in asthma and COPD. Am J Respir Crit Care Med 2006; 175:306–311.[6])

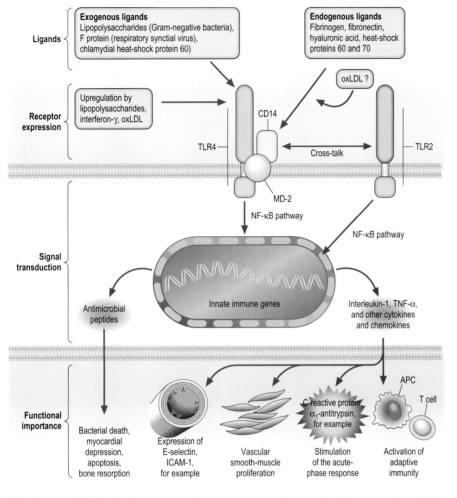

Fig. 22.2. Interaction of endotoxin with TLR4 leads to activation of innate immunity, and serves the afferent arm of acquired immunity. Activation of adaptive immunity includes antigen presentation, and modulation of expression of co-stimulatory molecules and cytokines profiles leading to regulation of T lymphocyte differentiation. (Reproduced, with permission, from Keichl S, Lorenz E, Reindl M, et al. Toll-like receptor 4 polymorphisms and atherogenesis N Engl J Med 2002; 347:185–192.[9])

better than in otherwise healthy individuals,[39] an effect which may be due in part to local airway release of GM-CSF,[38] or IFN-γ[35,36]; either or both of these factors could contribute to enhanced airway immune-inflammatory responses in asthma. Further, endotoxin exposure results in strong upregulation of IL-12 and IL-18,[40] two Th1-like cytokines which influence T cell development.[41,42] Recent evidence shows that MHC class II molecule expression is upregulated by activation of TLRs, and that the mechanism includes activation of the central inflammatory transcription factor NF-κB.[43] Endotoxin also produces dendritic cell maturation.[44]

Regulation of Th1-Th2 differentiation

Dendritic cells, and by inference a subpopulation of macrophages, appear to be key regulators of Th1-Th2 lymphocyte differentiation.[45] However, it is necessary to review briefly some of the mechanisms involved in

order to understand the key role played by macrophages and monocytes in allergic diseases including asthma. Presentation of processed antigen peptide fragments in association with class II MHC molecules to a cognate T cell receptor (TCR) is a function of activated macrophages. However, it is now known that this primary interaction is only one of two signals necessary for regulating T cell activation and maturation (Fig. 22.4).[46] The second signal may be (a) co-stimulatory, leading to activation and maturation (mediated by CD80/86 with CD28; the degree of activation may depend on competitive interaction of CD80/86 with the inhibitor of CD28, CTLA4); (b) apoptosis-inducing, leading to deletion (mediated by Fas ligand/Fas interaction), or (c) absent, leading to anergy to that specific antigen. Thus, the ensemble of molecules expressed by macrophages during antigen presentation plays a central role in determining the T cell response.[46] Moreover, the membrane-bound cognate signals are only one part of the regulatory role played by macrophages. They also have the ability to release IL-12, and thereby

Table 22.3 Innate immunity receptors

TLR	Ligands	Polymorphism	Roles in asthma/atopy
TLR 2	Gram+, Gram−, *Mycobacterium,* others	−16934T allele[12]	Decreased asthma, hay fever, atopy
TLR 3	DS viral RNA	Multiple polymorphism[13]	No change in asthma/atopy
TLR4	LPS/endotoxin	Asp-299–Gly[10]	Airway hyperresponsiveness, increased asthma in Swedish children, and increased atopy in asthmatics[14]
TLR5	Bacterial flagellin		
TLR 6	Heterodimer with TLR2	Ser-249–Pro[15]	Reduced risk of asthma
TLR7/8	Poly I:C/ss RNA		
TLR 9	Bacterial CpG DNA	−1237T–C[14]	Conflicting evidence with asthma; increased protective immunity when given with allergen extracts[11]
TLR 10		1031G–A 2322A–G[16]	Increased asthma
CD 14		Promoter polymorphism − 159 (C/T)[10]	Regulation of IgE and atopy (TT protective)
Mannose	Carbohydrates and microorganisms	Polymorphisms that reduce MBL2 expression	Increased respiratory infections

direct T cell maturation in a Th1 or Th2 direction. Strong induction of IL-12, via activation of TLR4/CD14 by endotoxin, or by CpG oligonucleotides, may favor development of Th1-like responses, and concomitantly, diminish the likelihood of Th2 lymphocyte differentiation[40,47] This pathway may also be abnormal in asthma. Plummeridge and colleagues[48] observed that BAL fluid concentrations of IL-12 were significantly lower in asthma than in controls, and that IL-12 production by AM stimulated with IFN-γ was also significantly blunted. Reduced IL-12 concentration, activity, or receptor signaling would consequently be expected to facilitate lymphocyte differentiation in a Th2-like direction.

AM in asthma appear to mediate immune deviation in a Th2-like direction, facilitating the release of IL-5 and other such cytokines, and producing IL-4.[3] The propensity of AM from asthmatic subjects to induce Th2-like differentiation and T cell activation has been demonstrated repeatedly.[49–53] Although the precise collection of co-stimulatory molecules required have not been entirely defined, it is clear that the effects of AM from asthma to promote Th2-lymphocyte differentiation and activation depend on expression of one or more B7 (B7.1/CD80 and or B7.2/CD86) molecules in physical proximity to antigenic peptide presented by class II MHC molecules. Hence, it is necessary to evaluate the expression of these co-stimulating molecules in asthma, and to determine the functional relevance they have for lymphocyte differentiation.

Mediators produced by AM may also serve to regulate dendritic cell function, and consequently may importantly modify the direction of naïve T cell differentiation. In this regard, products of the 5-LO pathway, abundantly produced by macrophages and monocytes, have been shown to regulate dendritic cell function.[54]

Co-stimulatory molecule expression in asthma

The considerable interest in the possible role of AM in regulating allergic inflammatory responses in asthma has generated a number of important experimental observations, which highlight the phenotypic differences of AM from asthma vs controls, both healthy non-atopic, and atopic subjects without asthma. First, there is increased expression of HLA-DR (class II) molecules in asthma, the signal via which (by virtue of bound peptide) allergen specificity is established, and which is the first interaction needed to begin antigen-specific T cell activation and proliferation.[51,53] Of note, treatment with inhaled corticosteroids significantly reduces the expression of HLA-DR,[53] which likely also reduces antigen presenting activity of AM.

There are minor variations in the literature over the details of expression of B7 molecules in asthma, which likely result from subtle but important differences in the characteristics of patients studied. Some of these characteristics may include the presence or absence of ongoing environmental allergen exposure, recent exacerbations, exposure to environmental irritants or endotoxin, or other factors. However, increased expression of B7 isoforms is a common and replicated thread of this literature. Results from some laboratories suggest that antigen-presenting cells from asthmatic subjects show increased expression of CD86 (B7.2), but not of CD80 (B7.1).[50,55] Of note, the expression of B7.2 can be induced by IL-4.[55] Other investigators have suggested that expression of both B7.1 and B7.2 is increased in allergic subjects, with and without asthma, compared with healthy controls, but that AM from asthmatic patients have less B7.1 expression than non-asthmatics allergic subjects, and consequently show a relative increase in B7.2 vs B7.1. Yet another group found increased CD80 (B7.1), but not CD86 (B7.2)

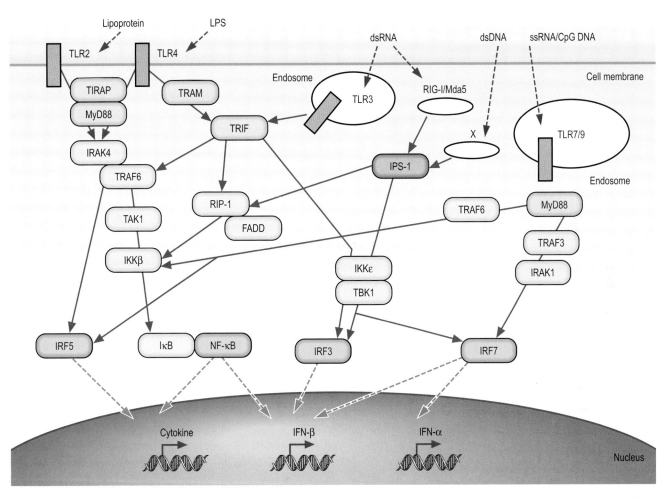

Fig. 22.3. TLR and RIG-1 signaling pathways. TLRs activate the signaling pathways through TIR-domain containing adapters (green). TLR2 and TLR4 trigger the MyD88-dependent pathway, which is dependent also on TIRAP. The TLR9 pathway is MyD88 dependent. TLR3 and TLR4 can stimulate the MyD88-independent, TRIF-dependent pathway. RIG-I/MDA5 activates the IPS-1-dependent (light blue) cytosolic pathway. This pathway is also triggered by another cytosolic PRR (X) that probably recognizes dsDNA. These pathways lead to translocation of various transcription factors (orange) and activation of target genes. (Reproduced from Kaisho T, Akira S. Toll-like receptors function and signaling. J Allergy Clin Immunol 2006; 117:979–987.[22])

in asthmatic compared with atopic non-asthmatic control subjects.[39,52] Despite these small discrepancies in detail, activation of T cells does require interaction of B7 molecules expressed by macrophages with CD28 on T lymphocytes. Collectively, it is clear that increased expression of either of the B7 molecules by AM in asthma is a consistent, reproducible finding.

Another co-stimulatory molecule that influences T cell development is CD40 expressed on AM, which interacts with CD40 ligand (CD154) expressed on T cells. In health, this interaction may suppress T cell activation. Consequently, regulation of expression of CD40 by AM, and its cognate receptor on the T cell, CD40 ligand, is likely to be critically important to a full understanding of T cell activation. Clearly, alterations in this pathway could be a control mechanism in asthma. In this regard, reduced expression of CD40 by AM in asthma has been observed.[51] The loss of inhibition via the CD40/CD154 pathway could contribute to the increased Th2-like lymphocyte activation in asthma (vide infra).

Altered expression of co-stimulatory molecules in asthma

Altered expression of co-stimulatory molecules by AM in asthma appears to lead to significant alteration in the nature of T lymphocyte differentiation. Macrophages from atopic subjects without asthma inhibit the production of IL-5 by T cells. In contrast, AM from atopic asthmatic subjects enhance IL-5 release.[39] This finding is of particular interest in that AM from atopic non-asthmatics do not share this property.[56] Thus, a functional difference in AM differentiates asthma from non-asthma in subjects with atopy. Further, whereas AM from atopic subjects, both with and without asthma, can increase the release of IL-4 and IFN-γ by antigen-specific T cells, only AM from atopic asthmatics support IL-5 release.[57] Release of another key Th2 cytokine, IL-13, is also dependent on expression of B7 molecules.[58] That the AM is involved directly in this effect is suggested by strong correlations between AM release of

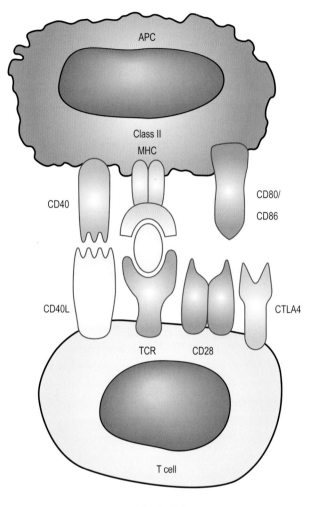

Co-stimulation

Fig. 22.4. Antigen-presenting cells (APC), including macrophages and monocytes, present antigen peptide fragments in the cleft of the MHC class II molecule complex, where it can interact with a cognate T cell receptor (TCR) and thereby generate a first signal for T cell activation. However, the activation response is dependent on the interactions of co-stimulatory molecules to provide a second signal. The second signal is dependent on interaction of CD40 on the APC with CD40 ligand on the T cell, and on the binding of CD80 (B7.1) or CD86 (B7.2) on the APC with CD28 on the T cell. CTLA4 may function as a competitive inhibitor of CD28. Blockade of the co-stimulatory pathways may lead to anergy, whereas MHC II-TCR interaction in the presence of Fas ligand expression by the APC may lead to clonal deletion of the T cell (not shown). (Reprinted with permission from Rotrosen D, Matthews JB, Bluestone JA. The immune tolerance network: a new paradigm for developing tolerance-inducing therapies. J Allergy Clin Immunol 2002; 110:17–23.[46])

IL-6 and IL-1 and the ability of AM to induce IL-5 release; strong inverse correlations between AM production of IL-12 and induction of IL-5 release were also seen.[59] These data link activation of AM, with subsequent cytokine release, to regulatory events controlling T cell differentiation and function. As added functional evidence, the secretion of

IL-12, a potent Th1-inducing cytokine, is significantly reduced in AM populations from asthmatic compared to atopic non-asthmatic subjects.[48,51] Further inhibition of IL-12 effect with neutralizing antibody further increases IL-5 production by cocultured T cells; in contrast, recombinant human IL-12 strongly reduces the stimulating effect of asthmatic AM on IL-5 production.[51] Hence, there are qualitative differences between AM of atopic subjects with and without asthma.

In this regard, the ligation CD28 on the T cell by B7 molecules on the antigen-presenting cell (macrophage) is essential for Th2-like differentiation, as a variety of experimental strategies to block this interaction result in loss of the stimulating effect of asthmatic AM on T cell activation. Moreover, the increased expression of B7 molecules (CD86 and CD80) by AM in asthma,[50,52] may favor development of Th2-like lymphocyte differentiation.[49] Of note, these patients with allergic asthma had ongoing exposure to allergen, and consequent ongoing allergic inflammation. It is of interest and pathogenic importance that alterations in CD86 expression can be replicated in vitro by exposure to IL-13 and IL-4[50] and further upregulation of CD86 can be observed after segmental allergen challenge.[52,60]

Of the two co-stimulatory molecules that interact with CD28 and CTLA-4, CD86 has been suggested to be more important in initiating and maintaining Th2 lymphocyte stimulation. Larche and colleagues evaluated the dependence of human allergen-specific T cell clones on co-stimulation by CD80 or CD86. The release of IL-5, and lymphocyte proliferation were blocked by antibodies that inhibited CD86, but not by antibodies that inhibited CD80. Moreover, they demonstrated that T cell clones derived from peripheral blood were not as dependent for activation on co-stimulation compared to T cell clones derived from BAL cells.[61] This key observation indicates that allergen-specific T lymphocytes differ considerably in their requirement for interactions with APCs, depending on their specific anatomic localization, and is consistent with the broader concept of compartmentalization of immune responses. Further, because airway T cells require such interaction, and airway macrophages in asthma express increased CD86 with antigen and MHC class II molecules, these mechanisms collectively may account for the antigen-specific local activation of Th2 lymphocytes in the lungs of asthmatic patients. However, Th2 cytokine production by airway epithelial biopsies (which contain T cells) does not require CD80/CD86 interaction.[62] This latter observation highlights again the concept of compartmentalization; in addition, it suggests that inflammatory cytokine production by T cells in airway epithelium may be more autonomous than in circulation, or free in the airspace. Similarly, release of T lymphocyte chemotactic activity (TLCA) may be regulated poorly in more severe asthma. Bronchial explants from asthmatic subjects spontaneously release TLCA, whose activity is attributable to IL-16, and release can be further amplified by stimulation with allergen in a CD80/CD86 dependent manner. However, in more severe disease, inhibition of B7/CD28 signaling does not abrogate release of CTLA, and less of the TLCA is attributable to IL-16.[63] The complete implications of the findings are not clear, but one obvious possibility is that autonomous release of Th2 cytokines by epithelial lymphocytes, and autonomous production of chemotactic activity for T cells with their consequent recruitment, could contribute to persistent or increased allergic inflammation in the airway epithelium.

Other investigators have suggested that either CD80 or CD86 expression is sufficient to facilitate IL-5 production by T cells, as blocking antibody against either co-stimulatory molecule reduces the release of IL-5. A specific requirement for CD80 for supporting Th2 responses has been identified.[39] Finally, an important functional role for reduced expression of CD40 was shown by experiments in which neutralizing antibody against CD40 were employed. In this system, inhibition of CD40 reduced the production of IL-12 by AM, and increased the stimulating effect on IL-5 release by T cells.[51]

INTERACTIONS BETWEEN INNATE AND ACQUIRED IMMUNITY

Effects of endotoxin on development of atopy – the 'hygiene hypothesis'

In addition to its ability to augment allergic inflammation in susceptible individuals, endotoxin may also influence the development of adaptive immunity. Given the potent effects of LPS on monocytes and macrophages for IL-12 and IL-18 production, it is perhaps not surprising that endotoxin exposure can alter the development of atopic disease. Evidence in support of this concept exists both at the cellular and clinical levels. First, endotoxin is a potent stimulus for the Th1 signal IL-12,[40] inducing near maximal cytokine release at concentrations as low as 10 pg/mL. Because Th1 and Th2 signals are mutually suppressive, strong Th1 responses block the differentiation of Th2 lymphocytes, and vice versa. Were this Th1-enhancing effect to be operative in vivo, one could reasonably predict that endotoxin exposure early in life might reduce or eliminate the occurrence of atopic diseases. A German group has investigated this question with a series of epidemiologic studies. In a compelling study, performed in over 800 German children, the risks of hay fever, sneezing, and atopic sensitization were found to be reduced by about 50% in children who lived on farms, compared with control children in the same locale who did not live on a farm. Importantly, the controls were drawn in close geographic proximity to the farm group, so that macrogeographic, macroenvironmental, or cultural differences would be minimized. Moreover, the magnitude of the effects appeared to relate to the degree of endotoxin exposure in the home, as measured by several different indices.[42]

An intriguing study by Matricardi and colleagues[64] has demonstrated that patients seropositive for the hepatitis A virus (a presumed surrogate for an unclean environment, and perhaps for endotoxin exposure) had significantly reduced prevalence of both asthma and hay fever. These and other effects on immune development in early childhood have been collectively termed the 'hygiene hypothesis', which argues that early exposure of children to infectious agents or endotoxin may provide benefit to the maturing immune system by encouraging development of Th1 lymphocyte responses.[65,66]

Effects of activation of innate immune mechanisms on existing allergic responses

The adaptive and innate immune systems can and do interact. Following induction of allergic inflammation via segmental allergen challenge (SAC), significant increases in soluble CD14, the endotoxin receptor, are seen; these increases correlate with reductions in surface expression of CD14 by granulocytes but not AM.[67] In fact, other investigators have shown increased expression of CD14 on AM after allergen exposure.[60] These data suggest that AM retain the ability to recognize and respond to LPS even in the face of environmental onslaught by allergen.

Atopy appears to increase the host response to endotoxin. Endotoxin is known to accentuate airway obstruction in asthmatics,[41,68] which may be important in some forms of occupational asthma and in subjects sensitive to indoor air pollution. In fact, in dust mite sensitive subjects, it is the concentration of endotoxin, not the concentration of dust mite antigen, which correlates best with asthma severity.[68] Moreover, expression of CD14, a component of TLR4, is induced by the development of allergic inflammation in atopic subjects; blunting eosinophil recruitment reduces the augmented expression of CD14, and in parallel reduces the responsiveness to LPS.[69] The interaction operates in the opposite direction as well: endotoxin can amplify allergic inflammation. Endotoxin exposure of the nose produces a qualitatively different inflammatory response in atopic and non-atopic individuals: atopic subjects develop eosinophilic inflammation, whereas non-atopic subjects show a neutrophilic response.[70] It has been demonstrated that TLR4 polymorphisms co-segregate with polymorphisms of IL-4.[71] This intriguing observation offers a possible mechanism for some of the linked responses between allergic diseases and reactivity to endotoxin. Certain haplotypes may thus be associated with both increased susceptibility to endotoxin, and an increased likelihood of developing atopic responses. Finally, accumulating evidence suggests that other pathways besides CD14/TLR4 may be important in endotoxin responsiveness,[71] including MHC class II.[72] This latter observation suggests another mechanism by which activation of macrophages via allergic inflammation, with increased expression of MHC class II could lead to exaggerated responsiveness to endotoxin. In short, endotoxin can produce inflammation (non-allergic in character) independent of atopy, and it can amplify allergic inflammatory responses, but only in subjects with pre-existing atopy. In addition, the allergic diathesis may amplify the host response to endotoxin, perhaps resulting in clinically exaggerated sensitivity to endotoxin.

Activation of TLR2 by its synthetic ligand (and presumably its natively occurring ligands) can activate Th2 response and produce experimental asthma.[73] Viral and bacterial infections may play a vital role in asthma exacerbations via innate immune system. One hypothesis holds that Th1 responses are protective against asthma and Th2 bias signals the exaggeration of allergic airway inflammation. Activation of TLR4 in combination to inhaled antigen led to amplified allergic asthma due to overexpression of Th2 immunity.[74] These data suggest that activation of innate immune function via TLRs may amplify existing acquired immune (allergic) responses. This concept is also supported by empiric experimental data.[70] Another piece of evidence of interaction between innate and acquired immunity is the observation that TLRs 2, 3, and 4 were upregulated in subjects who had severe allergic rhinitis.[75] These data suggest that the pathways that mediate activation of innate immunity are heightened in the context of Th2 polarization (atopy). However, others have suggested that the concept of Th2 polarization, and heightened Th2-like activation, does not adequately explain all aspects of allergic inflammation. Of note, Th1 activation can amplify Th2 immunity, particularly in the context of viral infections.[76]

CpG oligonucleotides, macrophages, and regulation of T cell responses

An intriguing application of the interplay between innate and acquired immunity is the deliberate stimulation of both arms of the immune system to promote development of protective, rather than allergic immunity. In this regard, CpG oligonucleotides, the canonical ligand for

TLR9,[20] have received the most attention in the context of allergy immunotherapy. Unmethylated DNA sequences in which cytosine and guanine are in contiguity (via the phosphodeoxyribose bridge) are phylogenetically associated with bacterial genomes, and are recognized as danger signals. These immunostimulatory sequences (ISS) evoke a strong Th1 bias in development of new immunity, and might be expected to reduce allergic sensitization.[77] Parenthetically, this strategy is also being actively pursued in the context of vaccine development for infectious diseases, in which case stimulation of innate immunity serves an adjuvant function.[78]

Human monocytes-derived dendritic cells express TLR9, and consequently express the cellular receptor necessary to recognize and respond to CpG.[79] In fact, CpG oligonucleotides strongly regulate the properties of plasmacytoid dendritic cells, which themselves favor development of Th2-like immune responses.[80] Hence, there is a compelling rationale to combine allergen immunotherapy with TLR9 stimulation by CpG oligonucleotides. The details of the combination appear to be important, as high ratios of CpG to allergen can blunt antibody production altogether, whereas lower ratios favor a strong, presumably protective IgG response.[81]

A large, multicenter trial of the safety and efficacy of a conjugated vaccine containing the major ragweed allergen Amb a 1 and an immunostimulatory DNA sequence (TLR9 agonist) has recently been published.[11] The primary outcome variable was nasal permeability markers following allergen challenge of the nose, and was not significantly affected by vaccine vs placebo. However, compared with placebo, this vaccine was associated with improved nasal symptom scores for 2 years, a small ragweed-specific IgG response, and attenuation of the seasonal rise in ragweed-specific IgE. This small ($n = 25$) study is of particular note because long-lasting (2 year) significant immunologic and clinical changes were noted despite the relatively small group of subjects, and the short duration of immunotherapy.[11]

Additional human studies have further clarified the role of ISS administration in the context of allergic diseases. In patients with established atopic disease, administration of ISS induced strong expression of the cadre of genes inducible by INF-γ, but did not alter allergic inflammation.[82] These data, in combination with other insights, suggest that ISS modulate allergic sensitization and underlying atopy, but may have lesser effects on the development of allergic inflammation. Collectively, the data argue for a strong effect of TLR ligation on the process of allergic sensitization, but a lesser effect on reducing allergic inflammation in response to allergen exposure, and in some cases, TLR activation may actually amplify allergic inflammation. Clearly, timing of the two stimuli, their relative potencies, and other factors appear to be important determinants of the response.

MACROPHAGES AND EFFERENT ARM IMMUNE FUNCTION – GENERAL CONCEPTS

ANTIGEN-DEPENDENT ACTIVATION

AM express receptors for IgE (CD23) and IgG (CD16, 32, 64), as well as receptors for fragments of activated complement (Table 22.1). Via immunoglobulin receptors, antigen-specific antibody is bound, conferring antigen specificity to the AM activation responses. Cross-linking of receptors then leads to AM activation. Secretion of cytokines, lysosomal enzymes, lipid mediators, and reactive oxygen and nitrogen species are all consequences of allergen-specific AM activation.[83] Allergen-dependent activation can also change the morphology and phenotype of AM. Expression of co-stimulatory CD83 molecules is increased by allergen challenge, as is expression of CD14.[60]

MACROPHAGE DIVERSITY

Macrophages are heterogeneous in both phenotype or function. AM range phenotypically from very monocyte-like (small, 12–15 μm, moderate cytoplasm, and few inclusions) to large (30 μm), vacuolated cells with abundant cytoplasm and inclusions. AM with monocytic morphology likely represent cells recently recruited to the airspace from the circulating precursor pool. Moreover, the more recently recruited cells show greater buoyant density (are heavier) than more aged cells.[84] Functional diversity is present as well, as those cells with greater buoyant density have increased production of superoxide anion, more effective antigen presentation, and increased release of IL-1.[83]

More recent observations also support the concept of diversity among AM populations. AM may be separated on the basis of surface molecule expression (RFD1 and RFD7) into stimulatory and suppressive populations. In asthma, the proportion of AM with a suppressive phenotype is smaller than controls. A functional correlate of the phenotypic observation is that AM from asthma demonstrated increased mixed lymphocyte reactions (MLR) compared with AM from healthy controls.[85] Both the phenotypic and functional differences could be reversed by the addition of IL-10 to cultures, suggesting an important consequence of deficient IL-10 release in asthma (vide infra).

Corticosteroids also have an effect on AM populations. In asthma, there is an imbalance in AM populations which facilitate and suppress antigen presentation, with an increased fraction of AM which express high levels of class II MHC molecules, and present antigen well. In culture, fluticasone propionate reduces the expression of RFD1 expressing cells which present antigen well, and these cells in parallel demonstrated reduced MLR reactivity.[86]

In addition to phenotypic diversity in asthma without allergen exposure, further phenotypic changes occur with experimental allergen challenge. AM from asthmatic subjects exposed to repeated, low doses of allergen to which sensitivity had been established showed diminished expression of CD11a, CD16, CD71 and HLA class I antigens. Concomitantly, increased expression of CD11b, CD14, and CD83 was demonstrated.[60] Collectively, the changes in AM surface molecule expression are consistent with an influx of precursor monocytes, which may be associated with increased antigen presentation to T cells, and consequently development and maintenance of airway inflammation in asthma.

DECTIN-1

The pathological effects of *Aspergillus fumigatus* have been well characterized in disease states such as invasive pulmonary aspergillosis (IPA) and allergic bronchopulmonary aspergillosis (ABPA); however, the role of AMs and innate immune mechanisms in defense against this organism has only recently been carefully outlined. In intriguing studies performed by Steele and colleagues[87], the dectin-1 receptor on the surface of resident AMs has been shown to play a critical role in host defense against *Aspergillus fumigatus*. A fungal cell wall component, β-1,3 glucan, is abundantly expressed on the surface of *A. fumigatus,* that binds to dectin-1 expressed on macrophages. Dectin-1 is a C-type, lectin-like, type II transmembrane receptor,[88] which when activated by ligation of *A. fumigatus* (and presumably other organisms expressing β-1,3 glucan), leads to the production of TNF-α, MIP-1α, MIP-2, IL-1β, IL-1α, IL-6, G-CSF, GM-CSF, IL-10, and INF-γ, the latter being critical in enhancing the T helper type-1 response. This vigorous Th1 response is known to be vital in pulmonary host defense to fungal organisms. Hence, this specific PRR appears critically to mediate host defense function. These studies highlight the importance of dectin-1 signaling in the generation of AM-mediated proinflammatory responses to this commonly encountered fungal pathogen in infectious and allergic disease states. However, activation of AM via this pathway may also contribute to ongoing inflammation, and disease in the setting of allergic bronchopulmonary aspergillosis. In this setting, the immunologic response to *A. fumigatus* contributes significantly to the pathogenesis of disease. Interestingly, corticosteroids have been shown to decrease dectin-1 expression on AMs, leading to attenuation of the inflammatory response.[89] This observation may underlie the improved clinical outcomes in some patients with ABPA who receive treatment with corticosteroids. This concept is generalizable: expression of PRRs on the surface of macrophages is essential to host defense, but these same receptors may lead to inappropriately prolonged, or vigorous inflammatory responses that can contribute to disease pathogenesis. As genetic tools advance, it is likely that specific clinical disorders will be linked to abnormalities of these critical surface proteins.

MACROPHAGES IN ASTHMA

RATIONALE FOR INVESTIGATING MACROPHAGES IN ASTHMA

Macrophages are by far the most numerous cells in the airway, both in health, and in the majority of respiratory diseases. Even in asthma, AM generally outnumber airway eosinophils and lymphocytes by 7:1 or more. Moreover, in models of intense allergic inflammation following allergen challenge, the numerical increase in AM exceeds that of eosinophils.[4,84,90] In asthma, AM, but not blood monocytes, show considerable and significant alteration in surface markers of activation.[91] These observations argue that the functional and phenotypic differences between macrophages and monocytes likely have pathogenic importance in asthma, in that the activation markers have demonstrable functional relationship to inflammatory mechanisms in asthma. Because AM have prominent roles in innate immunity, and both the afferent and efferent arms of adaptive immunity, it is not surprising that they have been closely linked to many aspects of asthma pathogenesis. Their interaction with T cells, with focus on the allergic disorders, is the focus of an older but still relevant review.[92] The functional state of AM, as measured by phagocytic ability, is related to airway hyperresponsiveness to methacholine. In a study of 20 asthmatic subjects, impaired phagocytic ability was correlated with both decreased expression of CD64 (FcγR1) and with increased airway responsiveness,[93] suggesting a link between AM function and airway physiology. As noted earlier, a similar relationship has been observed between airway macrophage carbon burden and airflow

limitation.[5] In human asthma, seasonal allergen exposure is associated with significantly increased infiltration of bronchial biopsies with macrophages.[94] Even children can show profound alterations in macrophage products. Such children show reduced MMP-9, and MMP-9/TIMP-1 ratios.[95] Whether or not further changes occur during asthma exacerbation, or allergen challenge was not reported. Finally, nocturnal asthma, associated with more severe clinical disease, is associated with impaired glucocorticoid responses in AM, which is manifest as persistent release of inflammatory cytokines by AM in vitro in the face of steroid treatment.[96] Hew and colleagues[97] have shown that monocytes from patients with severe asthma also share this profound insensitivity to the antiinflammatory effects of steroids. This resistance to steroid activity may relate to the activation of histone acetyl transferases, deactivation of histone deacylases, or both.[98] Moreover, severe asthma has been linked to functional abnormalities of the macrophage.[99] Hence, considerable data link AM with the pathogenesis and clinical manifestations of asthma.

Monocytes and macrophages express CD23, a low-affinity receptor for IgE, and thereby acquire allergen specificity in atopic subjects in whom allergen-specific IgE has been synthesized. Cross-linking of these receptors lead to allergen-dependent release of lysosomal enzymes and superoxide.[83] Interaction of endotoxin with CD14/TLR4 results in brisk production of IL-1β, TNF-α,[100] and IL-12,[40] and delayed release of IL-10.[100] Activation of AM also results in synthesis and release of cysteinyl leukotrienes, key mediators of asthma.[101] As noted above, AM can be activated for inflammatory function by allergen recognized by specific IgE bound to the low-affinity IgE receptor expressed on AM at increased density in allergic diseases.

AM likely suppress immune-inflammatory responses in health. Teleologically, this suppressive function is critical given the ongoing assault on the airway by bacteria, viruses, endotoxin, noxious gases, and other irritants. In health, AM do not present antigen particularly well, but AM from asthmatics are functionally different, and present antigen significantly better than do AM from normals.[38] In addition, AM in health secrete abundant quantities of the potent antiinflammatory cytokine IL-10; in contrast, AM from asthmatic subjects generally produce significantly less IL-10,[102,103] which may contribute to the intensity and persistence of allergic airway inflammation in asthma. Blood monocytes from the same individuals do not show a defect in IL-10 release, suggesting that components in the airspace lead to functional inhibition of IL-10 release, and impaired ability to control inflammation in asthma. Direct experimental evidence also demonstrates this functional suppressive effect of AM in health. Hunt and colleagues[104] showed that airway segments from which the majority of cells had been lavaged developed *increased* inflammation in response to segmental allergen challenge, compared with contralateral segments from which resident cells had not been removed. In addition, surfactant proteins, taken up by AM, may also play a key role in suppressing inflammation, either by promoting resolution of existing inflammation, or by inducing a state of relatively blunted responsiveness to inflammogens.[105–107] AM may serve to suppress inflammation induced by non-allergic triggers as well. The inflammatory response to trimellitic anhydride, an occupational, but non-allergic trigger of airway inflammation, is significantly suppressed by AM.[108] In fact, the AM appear to have a dual role, both amplifying and suppressing the response to trimellitic anhydride.[109] Whether these effects are due to subpopulations of AM, or to a temporal variation in function, is not known. Hence, in health and in stable asthma, AM subserve an antiinflammatory function. In contrast, allergic airway inflammation results in a change in the phenotype and function of resident AM such that proinflammatory functions are enhanced, and antiinflammatory functions are impaired.

Finally, recent provocative evidence suggests that macrophage phenotype may be significantly altered by exposure to mycolic acid. In this model, mycolic acid exposure resulted in a reprogramming of macrophage functions such that tolerance to allergen was enhanced.[110] Modulation of immune responses towards tolerance, if achieved in an antigen-specific manner that preserves specific responses to other antigens, could represent an important advance in the control of allergic diseases including asthma.

PHENOTYPIC AND FUNCTIONAL DIFFERENCES IN ASTHMA OF AM – BASAL DIFFERENCES, AND MODULATION BY ALLERGIC MEDIATORS OR ALLERGEN CHALLENGE

Not only is the phenotype of AM different in asthma compared with normal controls or atopic non-asthmatic subjects but also the quantitative differences are magnified following exposure to allergen, either by natural seasonal means, or via experimental challenge. There are important effects of allergen exposure or challenge on the expression of co-stimulatory B7 molecules (CD80 and CD86). These effects are detailed above.

Activation markers

AM express surface markers of activation relevant to the pathogenesis of allergic diseases and asthma. These include CD23 (low-affinity receptor for IgE), CD14 (LPS receptor), CD35 (complement receptor type 1), HLA class I molecules, and HLA class II (DR and DQ) molecules. In a model of experimental allergic inflammation, Viksman et al[111] showed that expression of CD23, CD14, HLA class I, and HLA-DR were significantly increased following endobronchial allergen challenge. In that macrophages can be activated via CD23, CD14, and other such surface receptors, their heightened expression in the context of allergic inflammation may be a mechanism by which increased inflammation in asthma is maintained.

Peripheral blood monocytes are the progenitors of AM, but are not identical to them in terms of activation and function. Using monocytes and AM from the same individuals, Viksman and colleagues[91] evaluated the expression of a panel of activation markers. CD16, CD18, CD32, CD44, CD71, MHC class I, and MHC class II were higher on AM of asthmatic subjects compared to controls, but with the exception of CD44, those same markers were also elevated on AM from atopic non-asthmatics. Thus, only expression of CD44 differentiated atopic asthmatics from atopic non-asthmatics. Importantly, there were no differences in expression of any marker on peripheral blood monocytes. Additional data to support and expand this idea have recently been published.[112] AM function differs in atopic diseases including asthma, and is further altered by allergen challenge or other triggers of allergic inflammation. Thus, the phenotype of AM is distinct from that of monocytes, and differences in expression of markers on AM is not presaged by equivalent changes on blood monocytes. These data suggest that the environment of the airway plays in important role in the differentiation and maturation of AM.

A comprehensive analysis of the effects of allergen challenge on markers of AM activation has recently been published by the same group. Using the techniques of whole lung allergen challenge (WLAC) and segmental allergen challenge (SAC), allergic inflammation was induced in atopic asthmatic subjects. Expression of the integrins CD11a and CD11b, the TLR4 component CD14, the low-affinity IgE receptor CD23, immunoglobulin receptors CD32 and 64, HLA class I, HLA class II antigens, CD18 (the common β-subunit for CD11 isoforms), and CD63 were increased following SAC. Other surface markers, including HLA-DQ, the transferrin receptor CD71, and the hyaluronic acid receptor CD44, were unchanged by SAC.[111] Of note, many of the activation markers that increased after SAC were positively correlated with the increase in airway responsiveness to methacholine, suggesting their pathogenic importance. More recent data support this concept. Following allergen challenge, there was increased expression of CD14, as was expression of the Th2-biasing B7 species (B7.2) molecule recognized by CD86.[113]

The effects of specific mediators linked to asthma pathogenesis on expression of activation markers have also been investigated. Resident AM increase MHC class II expression in response to IFN-γ, but the response is somewhat blunted relative to that seen with blood monocytes. Caulfield and colleagues[38] evaluated the effects of GM-CSF on MHC class II expression by AM. GM-CSF upregulated expression of HLA-DR, HLA-DP, and HLA-DQ, but curiously did so only in the presence, but not in the absence, of dexamethasone. Further, the optimal dose of dexamethasone required was 1000-fold less for AM (10^{-10}M) compared with blood monocytes (10^{-7}M). The dose required for GM-CSF to upregulate class II molecules in AM is clearly within that achievable with inhaled corticosteroids, whereas that required for blood monocytes (in circulation) is not. The data suggest that GM-CSF may be able to activate AM for class II HLA expression, in an IFN-γ independent manner, and ironically may do so most significantly in those patients being treated with inhaled steroids.

Proinflammatory cytokines, mediators, and mechanisms

Cytokines

Alveolar macrophages from asthma patients, even with mild disease, are functionally activated for increased proinflammatory function. Such AM show heightened release of IL-1β, TNF-α, and IL-8, and in addition, showed markedly increased release of IL-8 on stimulation by either IL-1β or TNF-α, suggesting a significant role of AM in promoting airway inflammation in asthma.[114] In dust mite sensitive asthmatic subjects, the release of IL-1β by blood monocytes is increased; when asthma is in remission, the enhanced IL-1β release is blunted.[115]

Production of the eosinophil chemotactic chemokine RANTES, and the neutrophil chemotactic cytokine IL-8, by AM is increased in atopic asthmatics, compared to controls. Parallel elevations can be seen in BAL fluids. However, AM from non-atopic asthmatic subjects do not share this abnormality.[116] In contrast, non-atopic asthmatics, but not atopic asthmatics, show increased expression of the receptor for GM-CSF on AM.[117] In the same vein, GM-CSF is released spontaneously by AM from asthma,[118] but not by AM from healthy controls, and such release is reduced by inhaled steroid treatment.[119] In addition, AM in asthma show reduced apoptosis which strongly correlates with expression of GM-CSF.[120] Given the abundance of GM-CSF in asthma, and the enhancing effects of GM-CSF on MHC class II molecule expression (vide supra), its potent effects on eosinophil survival,[118] the increased expression of GM-CSF and its receptor are likely of pathogenic importance for AM activation, survival, and antigen presentation.

Activation of AM by allergen or allergic mediators results in prominent activation of the transcription factor NF-κB, which has potent effects on transcription of a variety of proinflammatory cytokine genes, and is strongly expressed in sputum cells from asthmatic patients.[121] Many of these cytokines in turn increase the expression of inducible nitric oxide synthase (iNOS), with resulting increases in the concentration of nitric oxide (NO) in exhaled breath.[122] Subsequently, NO may participate in a homeostatic, negative feedback loop, mechanism to limit further inflammation. Treatment of AM with a synthetic donor of NO results in significant reduction in secretion of TNF-α and GM-CSF; however, cytokine production by blood monocytes under similar conditions was insensitive to suppression by the NO donor, and the different responses of AM and blood monocytes could not be reproduced by in vitro maturation and differentiation;[123] that observation is consistent with functional differentiation of macrophages in the site of inflammation. Activation of NF-κB in AM has been shown to be sensitive to NO. Exposure of AM to LPS in vitro results in activation of NF-κB, and degradation of the chaperone protein IγB. In the presence of synthetic NO donors, in vitro, NF-κB activation is blocked, and IγB levels are preserved, both in NO-dose-dependent manners.[124] Moreover, in asthmatic subjects, activation of NF-κB was low in those with high exhaled NO concentrations, whereas activation of NF-κB was high in those with low NO in exhaled breath. This latter observation argues for a clinical relevance of the previously discussed in vitro findings.

The specific mechanisms, the necessary and sufficient steps, by which monocytes are recruited to the airspace are not entirely clear, but specific monocytes chemotactic factors are known to be involved. Recent evidence now suggests that IL-17 may play a role as well, by promoting the recruitment and survival of macrophages in the context of allergic inflammation.[125]

Reactive oxygen and nitrogen species

AM from asthmatic subjects show increased release of superoxide anion and other reactive oxygen species compared with healthy controls.[84,90] Moreover, this enhanced oxidative stress occurs in relationship to the degree of airway obstruction; ROS production is considerably increased following allergen challenge, either by the aerosol or segmental routes.[84,90] An in vitro observation with possible clinical implications is the finding that thyroxine increases superoxide anion release by AM, suggesting that an enhanced oxidative burden in the airway might develop as a consequence of hyperthyroidism.[126] In addition to important effects on cell function and viability via direct oxidation, ROS have recently been recognized to play a key role in cell signaling. Activation of ROS influences cellular function by at least two mechanisms: (1) via activation of NF-κB and upregulation of inflammatory cytokine transcription, and (2) by oxidative inactivation of protein tyrosine phosphatases (PTP), leading to increased phosphotyrosine signaling.[127] Because inflammatory cytokines generally signal via tyrosine phosphorylation, the inactivation of PTPs leads to increased inflammatory cytokine signaling. Recently, Erdely and colleagues[128] showed that macrophages express arginase. Increased arginase activity lead to reduced arginine concentrations, and can cause iNOS to use an alternative substrate to produce superoxide rather than nitric oxide. Inhibition of PDE4 in this model leads to exaggerated

expression of arginase. Hence, macrophages appear to have a major influence on NO metabolism in the airway.

In asthma, AM demonstrate heightened protein kinase C (PKC) activity. Compared with controls, PKC activity is almost doubled. In addition, the cellular localization may be somewhat different, with a larger fraction of active PKC found in association with cell membrane.[129] PKC has an important regulatory role for (membrane-associated) enzymes responsible for the respiratory burst, suggesting that this abnormal PKC activity could be one mechanisms by which the enhanced respiratory burst of asthmatic AM (both activation and priming) is mediated.

Expression of the inducible form of nitric oxide synthase (iNOS) by AM results in the formation of nitric oxide, a key gaseous signaling molecule. Expression of iNOS is induced by most proinflammatory cytokines, including those involved in allergic inflammation. Nitric oxide is also a component of some types of air pollution. To evaluate the possible effects of exogenous NO exposure on the generation of reactive intermediates of oxygen and nitrogen, mice were exposed to low concentrations of NO.[130] In this model system, AM from animals so exposed expressed iNOS, synthesized NO, and superoxide, and had increased concentrations of peroxynitrite (vide infra), suggesting a priming effect on AM of nitric oxide. Moreover, compelling animal data suggest that deficient production of IL-10 may permit substantial upregulation of iNOS; the NO consequently produced then appears to promote significant upregulation of the allergic Th2 cytokine IL-4.[4] In that allergic cytokines enhance expression of iNOS, these data suggest a positive feedback loop between cytokine signaling and NO pathways that may amplify allergic inflammation.

Oxidants mediate other important functions in inflammation. In the presence of NO, superoxide can react to form the potent nitrosylation moiety peroxynitrite (OONO-). Tyrosine residues appear particularly susceptible to reaction with peroxynitrite, with the formation of nitrotyrosine residues.[131] Peroxynitrite is found abundantly in lungs of patients with acute lung injury, consistent with a pathogenic role.[132] Moreover, increased concentrations of nitrotyrosine are found in breath condensate from asthmatic patients.[133] This finding argues that the peroxynitrite formed via enhanced reactive oxygen and nitrogen species metabolism is reacting and modifying biologically important cellular proteins. Although the functional consequences of such covalent modifications are not known in their entirety, particularly with specific reference to asthma, there are a number of effects of peroxynitrite formation that have relevance to asthma pathogenesis, including DNA fragmentation, inhibition of mitochondrial electron transport and oxidative metabolism, brisk calcium efflux from mitochondria with intracellular calcium overload, and interference with membrane calcium channels.[131] In addition, reactive nitrogen species are known to activate the NF-κB pathway (leading to cell activation and generation of inflammatory cytokines), and the c-Jun N-terminal kinase (JNK), which may be involved in apoptosis of epithelial cells.[134] Hence, the generation of nitric oxide, particularly in concert with superoxide, may lead to stable covalent modification of tyrosine residues, which leads to long-term cell activation and amplification or persistence of inflammation.

Lipid mediators

An important aspect of airway biology in asthma is the activation of the cysteinyl leukotriene pathway, resulting in release of the mediators of bronchoconstriction and mucus secretion, LTC_4 and LTD_4. These enzymes are known to localize in eosinophils and macrophages.[101] In a recent evaluation of the effect of seasonal exposure to birch pollen, 12 atopic asthmatic subjects were studied before and after pollen season. Expression of enzymes involved in the leukotriene pathway (5-lipoxygenase [5-LO], 5-LO activating protein [FLAP], leukotriene A4 hydrolase, and LTC_4 synthase were all significantly increased in post-season biopsies compared to pre-season samples. Moreover, the increased expression of these enzymes was seen primarily in eosinophils and macrophages, and correlated with the magnitude of airflow limitation.[94] Hence, one consequence of allergen exposure is increased expression in AM of enzymes of the leukotriene pathway.

Airway macrophages can produce cysteinyl leukotrienes, due to expression of relevant synthetic enzymes.[101] These key mediators of allergic inflammation interact with a specific G-protein coupled receptor, cys-LT1R, a member of the seven transmembrane receptor family, to produce airway smooth muscle contraction, mucus secretion, and eosinophilic inflammation. Expression and function of cys-LT1R in airway smooth muscle is strongly regulated by IFN-γ,[135] another product of activated AM.[36] It is of note that expression of cys-LT1R on AM and monocytes can also be regulated by mediators of allergic inflammation. Expression of cys-LT1R by AM is significantly increased, both at the mRNA and protein levels, by exposure to IL-13 or IL-4.[136] In this system, IFN-γ did not alter expression of receptor by AM, which contrast to the enhanced expression seen in airway smooth muscle. Chu and colleagues[101] evaluated expression of enzymes involved in leukotriene biosynthesis in AM, and showed significant upregulation of 5-LO and FLAP following ovalbumin sensitization and challenge. The increased expression could be blocked by concomitant treatment with an inhibitor of leukotriene biosynthesis, suggesting that cysteinyl leukotrienes may amplify the expression of enzymes involved in their own biosynthesis.

Supportive evidence of the importance of this pathway is provided by intervention with leukotriene blockers in human asthma. Treatment of asthmatic patients with zafirlukast resulted in significant reductions in measures of allergic inflammation, including basophil accumulation and histamine concentrations in BAL fluid compared to a cross-over placebo arm. In addition, significant reductions in the production of superoxide anion, and the release of TNF-α, by purified AM were seen in the zafirlukast compared with placebo arm.[137] Hence, blockade of the cys-LT1R on AM resulted in reduced proinflammatory functions. Consequently, AM can produce cysteinyl leukotrienes, and via autocrine or paracrine mechanisms become further activated for leukotriene production, inflammatory cytokine release, and reactive oxygen species metabolism. Blockade of the leukotriene pathway may therefore have beneficial effects on inflammation beyond those directly related to cys-LT1R activation.

Antiinflammatory mediators, cytokines, and mechanisms

As noted above, AM are a rich source, and quantitatively the most important source, of the antiinflammatory cytokine IL-10. IL-10 is a member of a family of cytokines, defined by structural homology, which includes IL-19 and IL-20. IL-10 is potently antiinflammatory, reducing release of TNF-α and IFN-γ by activated macrophages, and reducing expression of MHC class II molecules, thereby serving an autocrine regulatory function.[100] However, IL-10 also acts in a paracrine sense, reducing the functional activation of T lymphocytes, particularly the Th1 subset, and

inducing apoptosis of eosinophils.[100] Hence, reduction of IL-10 effect might serve to increase airway inflammation, or to contribute to its persistence.[138]

This hypothesis has been tested in both humans, and in animal models. Two laboratories have evaluated concentrations of IL-10 in BAL fluid from atopic asthmatics compared to healthy controls. In both studies, IL-10 was detectable in all healthy controls, but was significantly lower in atopic asthmatics; moreover, IL-10 was undetectable in BAL fluid from most asthmatic patients.[102,103,119] In addition, BAL IL-10 differentiated atopic subjects with and without asthma, in that subjects with allergies but no asthma had normal levels of IL-10 in BAL fluid.[103] Treatment with inhaled steroids reverses the deficient release of IL-10.[119] Another study replicated the observation that IL-10 release by AM from steroid-treated asthmatic subjects was increased compared with that of untreated patients.[139] It is of interest that blood monocytes from allergic asthmatics show increased expression and release of MIP-1α and IL-10;[140] thus, there is a differentiation between AM, which express and release low levels of IL-10, even after allergen challenge,[103] and monocytes, which appear to be primed for increased cytokine release after allergen challenge.[140] Animal models demonstrate that eliminating IL-10 via genetic knockout results in enhanced allergen-induced airway inflammation, and increased airway responsiveness to methacholine, and increased expression and function of inducible nitric oxide synthase.[141,142] Moreover, IL-10 knockout mice exhibit considerably exaggerated airway IL-4 production, which is dependent on the gaseous signaling molecule nitric oxide.[143]

Hemoxygenase-1 (HO-1) is a stress-inducible protein which catalyzes the conversion of heme to biliverdin, a consequence of which reaction is the release of carbon monoxide (CO). Induction of HO-1 serves a cytoprotective effect against oxidant-induced injury. Asthmatics subjects exhibit increased expression of HO-1 that is localized to AM.[144] Further, increased HO-1 expression was related to both disease activity and treatment, as detectible expression was more frequent in subjects with recently active asthma compared with clinically stable disease. Moreover, corticosteroids appear to inhibit HO-1 expression, as asthmatic subject with recent severe exacerbation requiring oral corticosteroids did not show elevated HO-1 expression.[144]

Increased HO-1 expression might be expected to increase the concentration of CO in exhaled breath. This suggestion has been evaluated in 37 steroid-naive asthmatics, in whom exhaled CO was significantly elevated compared to 37 healthy controls. Of note, 25 asthmatics who were treated with inhaled steroids had exhaled CO levels comparable with the control subjects. It is clear that CO is a potent antiinflammatory molecule, as exogenous CO or HO-1 both suppress TNF-α release, and augment IL-10 release, by cultured monocytes.[145] Thus, induction of HO-1 and release of CO may represent a key endogenous, homeostatic mechanism to limit development of inflammation, or to facilitate its resolution.

MACROPHAGES AND REMODELING

The mechanisms by which airway remodeling in asthma is augmented include TGF-β, metalloproteinase (and inhibitor) release, changes in structural proteins, and participation of cytokines, notably IL-11 and IL-13. Macrophages contribute to may of these mechanisms, principally including protease–antiprotease balance, and expression of TGF-β.

Macrophages from asthmatic subjects express increased concentrations of matrix metalloproteinase 9 (MMP-9), the substrates of which are collagen, elastin, and other structural proteins. The qualitative characteristics of MMP-9 are not different in asthma, compared with bronchitis and healthy controls. However, concentrations of MMP-9, and release of MMP-9 from cultured AM, are significantly greater from asthma than healthy subjects.[146] In addition, in vitro activation of the macrophages resulted in a protein kinase C-dependent, but not protein kinase A-dependent release of MMP-9, but only in AM from asthmatics. AM from control subjects did not show increased stimulated MMP-9 release. Those data suggest that AM from asthma are differentially susceptible to activation for metalloproteinase release, and that such release could be involved in the processes of airway wall remodeling. The same group later reported that AM from untreated asthma patients expressed increased tissue inhibitor of metalloproteinase (TIMP)-1 relative to MMP-9 release. In AM from normal subjects and from asthmatics treated with inhaled steroids, MMP-9 and TIMP-1 were released in coordinate fashion such that the two molecules for complexed with one another. In contrast, AM from untreated asthmatics produced TIMP-1 and MMP-9 in a non-correlated manner.[147] The release of MMP-9 is stimulated by the AM products TNF-α and IL-1β. Hence, AM may serve in an autocrine or paracrine fashion to amplify metalloproteinase release. In an allergen challenge model of human asthma, increased MMP-9 was observed at baseline; following allergen challenge, additional significant increases in this metalloproteinase were seen.[148] As further support of the concept of increased release of proteases, particularly metalloproteinases, as a pathogenic mechanism of remodeling, Vignola and colleagues have suggested that increased MMP-9 relative to TIMP-1 is a feature of asthma, and have shown a correlation between the ratio MMP-9:TIMP-1 and the degree of airflow limitation.[149]

Alveolar macrophages from asthmatic subjects show increased release of fibronectin, and of the key fibrogenic cytokine TGF-β. In culture, these AM from asthmatics further increase the release of TGF-β with endotoxin stimulation, whereas AM from control patients with chronic bronchitis did not release more TGF-β with endotoxin.[150] Recent evidence suggests that TGF-β stimulates remodeling responses by activating the transcription factor Smad2, and phosphorylated Smad2 was correlated both with increased TGF-β, and with histologic quantitation of the subepithelial fibrosis most commonly measured as an index of airway remodeling.[151]

EFFECT OF INTERVENTION ON MACROPHAGE FUNCTION

Corticosteroids

Inhaled corticosteroids are effective therapy for asthma, and are associated with amelioration of some of the exaggerated inflammatory functions of AM in asthma. Faul and colleagues[152] evaluated the effects of fluticasone propionate on markers of inflammation in asthmatic subjects. Reduced eosinophils were observed, but in addition there were significant reductions in inflammation related to macrophages and lymphocytes. As noted above, AM subpopulations in asthma are of a stimulatory, rather than a suppressive phenotype. Inhaled steroids alter these macrophage populations toward normal balance.[86] Similarly, AM in asthma express increased MHC class II molecules, which is normalized by inhaled

steroid treatment.[53] Cytokines relevant to asthma are also altered by steroids. Reduced IL-10, and increased GM-CSF, release by AM in asthma are consistent findings in asthma, and these abnormalities are ameliorated by steroid treatment.[102,103,119,139,153] Comparing asthmatic subjects who were steroid treated and those who were not, Mautino and colleagues[146] found that treated subjects had lower release of MMP-9 by AM. Collectively, these data provide important mechanistic information about the effects of steroids on macrophage functions in asthma.

Particularly in more severe disease, AM may be relatively resistant to the antiinflammatory effects of glucocorticoids,[96] and this insensitivity has been linked to increased GRβ, which binds steroid molecule, but translocates or signals poorly.[154] The degree to which this mechanism is important in the broad context of asthma is not known.

Leukotriene modifiers

Treatment with zafirlukast reduces the influx of lymphocytes and basophils after segmental allergen challenge, reduces superoxide production by AM, and blunts the release of TNF-α by AM. In addition, 5-lipoxygenase inhibitors reduce the expression of 5-LO and FLAP in AM using an ovalbumin sensitization and challenge model.[101]

SUMMARY

Macrophages and monocytes are essential components of both innate and adaptive immune responses. Alveolar macrophages in health subserve a suppressive role in inflammation, but are phenotypically altered in asthma towards a more stimulatory, less suppressive direction. Phenotypic abnormalities in asthma include increased expression of MHC class II molecules and increased antigen presentation, and increased expression of co-stimulatory B7 molecules with consequent bias toward Th2 lymphocyte responses. In addition, increased release of IL-1β, TNF-α, GM-CSF, RANTES, and IL-8, and augmented production of TGF-β and MMP-9 are seen. Reduction of antiinflammatory functions in asthma are also seen, with reduced release of IL-10, and diminished expression of CD40. Alveolar macrophages may also play a role in the process of airway remodeling, via alteration in release of TGF-β, metalloproteinases, and inhibitors thereof. Macrophages and monocytes, using mechanisms of both the innate and acquired immunity, contribute importantly to the pathogenesis of asthma.

References

Introduction

1. Peters-Golden M. The alveolar macrophage: the forgotten cell in asthma. Am J Respir Cell Mol Biol 2004; 31:3–7.
2. Delves PJ, Roitt IM. The immune system. N Engl J Med 2000; 343:37–49.
3. Pouliot P, Turmel V, Gelinas E, et al. Interleukin-4 production by human alveolar macrophages. Clin Exp Allergy 2005; 35:804–810.
4. Ameredes BT, Zamora R, Sethi JM, et al. Alterations in nitric oxide and cytokine production with airway inflammation in the absence of IL-10. J Immunol 2005; 75:1206–1213.
5. Kulkarni N, Pierse N, Rushton L, et al. Carbon in airway macrophages and lung function in children. N Engl J Med 2006; 355:21–30.

Macrophages and afferent arm immune function

6. Sabroe I, Parker LC, Dockrell DH, et al. Pulmonary perspective: targeting the networks that underpin contiguous immunity in asthma and COPD. Am J Respir Crit Care Med 2006; 175:306–311.

7. Gordon SB, Read EC. Macrophage defences against respiratory tract infections. Br Med Bull 2002; 61:45–61.
8. Thoma-Usynski S, Stenger S, Takeuchi O, et al. Induction of direct antimicrobial activity through mammalian toll-like receptors. Science 2001; 291:1544–1547.
9. Keichl S, Lorenz E, Reindl M, et al. Toll-like receptor 4 polymorphisms and atherogenesis. N Engl J Med 2002; 347:185–192.
10. Yang IA, Barton SJ, Rorke S, et al. Toll-like receptor 4 polymorphism and severity of atopy in asthmatics. Genes Immun 2004; 5:41–45.
11. Creticos PS, Schroeder JT, Hamilton RG, et al. and the Immune Tolerance Network Group. Immunotherapy with a ragweed-toll-like receptor 9 agonist vaccine for allergic rhinitis. N Engl J Med 2006; 355:1445–1455.
12. Eder W, Klimecki W, Yu L, et al., ALEX Study Team. Toll-like receptor 2 as a major gene for asthma in children of European farmers. J Allergy Clin Immunol 2004; 113:482–488.
13. Noguchi E, Nishimura F, Fukai H, et al. An association study of asthma and total serum immunoglobin E levels for Toll-like receptor polymorphisms in a Japanese population. Clin Exp Allergy 2004; 34:177–183.
14. Lazarus R, Klimecki WT, Raby BA, et al. Single-nucleotide polymorphisms in the toll-like receptor 9 gene (TLR9): frequencies, pairwise linkage disequilibrium, and haplotypes in three U.S. ethnic groups and exploratory case-control disease association studies. Genomics 2003; 81:85–91.
15. Tantisira K, Klimecki WT, Lazarus R, et al. Toll-like receptor 6 gene (TLR6): single-nucleotide polymorphism frequencies and preliminary association with the diagnosis of asthma. Genes Immun 2004; 5:343–346.
16. Lazarus R, Raby BA, Lange C, et al. TOLL-like receptor 10 genetic variation is associated with asthma in two independent samples. Am J Respir Crit Care Med 2004; 170:594–600.
17. Lemaitre B, Nicolas E, Michaut L, et al. The dorsoventral regulatory gene cassette spatzle/Toll/cactus controls the potent antifungal response in Drosophila adults. Cell 1996; 86: 973–983.
18. Poltorak A, He X, Smirnova I, et al. Defective LPS signaling in C3H/HeJ and C57BL/10ScCr mice: mutations in Tlr4 gene. Science 1998; 282:2085–2088.
19. Uematsu S, Akira S. Toll-like receptors and innate immunity. J Mol Med 2006; 84:712–725.
20. Bauer S, Kirschning CJ, Hacker H, et al. Human TLR9 confers responsiveness to bacterial DNA via species-specific CpG motif recognition. Proc Natl Acad Sci U S A 2001; 98: 9237–9242.
21. Akira S, Uematsu S, Takeuchi O. Pathogen recognition and innate immunity. Cell 2006; 124:783–801.
22. Kaisho T, Akira S. Toll-like receptor function and signaling. J Allergy Clin Immunol 2006; 117:979–987.
23. Means TK, Jones BW, Schromm AB, et al. Differential effects of a Toll-like receptor antagonist on Mycobacterium tuberculosis-induced macrophage responses. J Immunol 2001; 166:4074–4082.
24. Hollingsworth JW, Chen BJ, Brass DM, et al. The critical role of hematopoietic cells in lipopolysaccharide-induced airway inflammation. Am J Respir Crit Care Med 2005; 171: 806–813.
25. Droemann D, Goldmann T, Tiedje T, et al. Toll-like receptor 2 expression is decreased on alveolar macrophages in cigarette smokers and COPD patients. Respir Res 2005; 6:68.
26. Maris NA, Dessing MC, de Vos AF, et al. Toll-like receptor mRNA levels in alveolar macrophages after inhalation of endotoxin. Eur Respir J 2006; 28:622–626.
27. Shapiro SD. The macrophage in chronic obstructive pulmonary disease. Am J Respir Crit Care Med 1999; 160:S29–S32.
28. Leung TF, Tang NL, Sung YM, et al. The C-159T polymorphism in the CD14 promoter is associated with serum total IgE concentration in atopic Chinese children. Pediatr Allergy Immunol 2003; 14:255–260.
29. Leung TF, Tang NL, Wong GW, et al. CD14 and toll-like receptors: potential contribution of genetic factors and mechanisms to inflammation and allergy. Curr Drug Targets Inflamm Allergy 2005; 4:169–175.
30. LeVan TD, Guerra S, Klimecki W, et al. The impact of CD14 polymorphisms on the development of soluble CD14 levels during infancy. Genes Immun 2006; 7:77–80.
31. Rylander R, Bake B, Fischer JJ, et al. Pulmonary function and symptoms after inhalation of endotoxin. Am Rev Respir Dis 1989; 140:981–986.
32. Schwartz DA, Thorne PS, Yagla SJ, et al. The role of endotoxin in grain dust-induced lung disease. Am J Respir Crit Care Med 1995; 152:603–608.
33. Schwartz DA, Christ WJ, Kleeberger SR, et al. Inhibition of LPS-induced airway hyperresponsiveness and airway inflammation by LPS antagonists. Am J Phys Lung Cell Mol Physiol 2001; 280:L771–L778.
34. O'Grady NP, Preas II HL, Pugin J, et al. Local inflammatory responses following endotoxin instillation in humans. Am J Respir Crit Care Med 2001; 163:1591–1598.
35. Lopez-Maderuelo D, Arnalich F, Serantes R, et al. Interferon-γ and interleukin-10 gene polymorphisms in pulmonary tuberculosis. Am J Respir Crit Care Med 2003; 167:970–975.
36. Trinchieri G. Cytokines acting on or secreted by macrophages during intracellular infection (IL-10, IL-12, IFN-γ). Curr Opin Immunol 1997; 9:17–23.
37. Newport MJ, Huxley CM, Huston S, et al. A mutation in the interferon-γ receptor gene and susceptibility to mycobacterial infection. N Engl J Med 1996; 335:1941–1949.
38. Caulfield JJ, Fernandez MH, Sousa AR, et al. Regulation of major histocompatibility complex class II antigens on human alveolar macrophages by granulocyte-macrophage colony-stimulating factor in the presence of glucocorticoids. Immunology 1999; 98:104–110.
39. Burastero SE, Magnani Z, Confetti C, et al. Increased expression of the CD80 accessory molecule by alveolar macrophages in asthmatic subjects and its functional involvement in allergen presentation to autologous Th2 lymphocytes. J Allergy Clin Immunol 1999; 103:1136–1142.
40. Liu AH. Endotoxin exposure in allergy and asthma: reconciling a paradox. J Allergy Clin Immunol 2002; 109:379–392.
41. Reed CE, Milton DK. Endotoxin-stimulated innate immunity: A contributing factor for asthma. J Allergy Clin Immunol 2001; 108:157–166.
42. Braun-Farhlander C, Reidler J, Herz U, et al. Environmental exposure to endotoxin and its relation to asthma in school age children. N Engl J Med 2002; 347:869–877.
43. Lee KW, Lee Y, Kim DS, et al. Direct role of NF-κB activation in Toll-like receptor-triggered HLA-DRA expression. Eur J Immunol 2006; 36:1254–1266.
44. Alexis NE, Lay JC, Almond M, et al. Acute LPS inhalation in healthy volunteers induces dendritic cell maturation in vivo. J Allergy Clin Immunol 2005; 115:345–350.
45. Eisenbarth SC, Piggott DA, Bottomly K. The master regulators of allergic inflammation: dendritic cells in Th2 sensitization. Curr Opin Immunol 2003; 15:620–626.
46. Rotrosen D, Matthews JB, Bluestone JA. The immune tolerance network: a new paradigm for developing tolerance-inducing therapies. J Allergy Clin Immunol 2002; 110:17–23.
47. Wild JS, Sur S. CpG oligonucleotide modulation of allergic inflammation. Allergy 2001; 56:365–376.
48. Plummeridge MJ, Armstrong L, Birchall MA, et al. Reduced production of interleukin 12 by interferon gamma primed alveolar macrophages from atopic asthmatic subjects. Thorax 2000; 55:842–847.
49. Djukanovic R. The role of co-stimulation in airway inflammation. Clin Exp Allergy 2000; 30(Suppl 1):46–50.
50. Hofer MF, Jirapongsananuruk O, Trumble AE, et al. Upregulation of B7.2, but not B7.1, on B cells from patients with allergic asthma. J Allergy Clin Immunol 101:96–102.
51. Tang C, Ward C, Reid D, et al. Normally suppressing CD40 coregulatory signals delivered by airway macrophages to Th2 lymphocytes are defective in patients with atopic asthma. J Allergy Clin Immunol 2001; 107:863–870.
52. Balbo P, Silvestri M, Rossi GA, et al. Differential role of CD80 and CD86 on alveolar macrophages in the presentation of allergen to T lymphocytes in asthma. Clin Exp Allergy 2001; 31:625–636.
53. Bertorelli G, Bocchino V, Zhuo X, et al. Heat shock protein 70 upregulation is related to HLA-DR expression in bronchial asthma. Effects of inhaled glucocorticoids. Clin Exp Allergy 1998; 28:551–560.
54. Hedi H, Norbert G. 5-Lipoxygenase pathway, dendritic cells, and adaptive immunity. J Biomed Biotechnol 2004:99–105.
55. Agea E, Forenza N, Piattoni S, et al. Expression of B7 co-stimulatory molecules and CD1a antigen by alveolar macrophages in allergic bronchial asthma. Clin Exp Allergy 1998; 28: 1359–1367.
56. Tang C, Rolland JM, Li X, et al. Alveolar macrophages from atopic asthmatics, but not atopic nonasthmatics, enhance interleukin-5 production by CD4+ T cells. Am J Respir Crit Care Med 1998; 157:1120–1126.
57. Tang C, Rolland JM, Ward C, et al. Differential regulation of allergen-specific T(H2)- but not T(H1)-type responses by alveolar macrophages in atopic asthma. J Allergy Clin Immunol 1998; 102:368–375.
58. Jaffar Z, Roberts K, Pandit A, et al. B7 costimulation is required for IL-5 and IL-13 secretion by bronchial biopsy tissue of atopic asthmatic subjects in response to allergen stimulation. Am J Respir Cell Mol Biol 1999; 20:153–162.
59. Tang C, Rolland JM, Ward C, et al. Modulatory effects of alveolar macrophages on CD4+ T-cell IL-5 responses correlate with IL-1beta, IL-6, and IL-12 production. Eur Respir J 1999; 14:106–112.
60. Lensmar C, Prieto J, Dahlen B, et al. Airway inflammation and altered alveolar macrophage phenotype pattern after repeated low-dose allergen exposure of atopic asthmatic subjects. Clin Exp Allergy 1999; 29:1632–1640.
61. Larche M, Till SJ, Haselden BM, et al. Costimulation through CD86 is involved in airway antigen-presenting cell and T cell responses to allergen in atopic asthmatics. J Immunol 1998; 161:6375–6382.
62. Lordan JL, Davies DE, Wilson SJ, et al. The role of CD28-B7 costimulation in allergen-induced cytokine release by bronchial mucosa from patients with moderately severe asthma. J Allergy Clin Immunol 2001; 108:976–981.
63. Dent G, Hosking LA, Lordan JL, et al. Differential roles of IL-16 and CD28/B7 costimulation in the generation of T-lymphocyte chemotactic activity in the bronchial mucosa of mild and moderate asthmatic individuals. J Allergy Clin Immunol 2002; 110:906–914.
64. Matricardi PM, Rosmini F, Panetta V, et al. Hay fever and asthma in relation to markers of infection in the United States. J Allergy Clin Immunol 2002; 110:381–387.
65. Holla AD, Roy SR, Liu AH. Endotoxin, atopy and asthma. Curr Opin Allergy Clin Immunol 2002; 2:141–145.
66. Vercelli D. Mechanisms of the hygiene hypothesis – molecular and otherwise. Curr Opin Immunol 2006; 18:733–737.
67. Virchow JC Jr, Julius P, Matthys H, et al. CD14 expression and soluble CD14 after segmental allergen provocation in atopic asthma. Eur Respir J 1998; 11:317–323.
68. Michel O, Kips J, Duchateau J, et al. Severity of asthma is related to endotoxin in house dust. Am J Respir Crit Care Med 1996; 154:1641–1646.
69. Alexis N, Eldridge M, Reed W, et al. CD14-dependent airway neutrophil response to inhaled LPS: role of atopy. J Allergy Clin Immunol 2001; 107:31–35.
70. Peden DB, Tucker K, Murphy P, et al. Eosinophil influx to the nasal airway after local, low-level LPS challenge in humans. J Allergy Clin Immunol 1999; 104:388–394.
71. Schwartz DA. The genetics of innate immunity. Chest 2002; 121:S62–S68.
72. Piani A, Hossle J, Birchler T, et al. Expression of MHC Class II molecules contributes to lipopolysaccharide responsiveness. Eur J Immunol 2000; 30:3140–3146.
73. Redecke V, Hacker H, Datta SK, et al. Cutting edge: activation of Toll-like receptor 2 induces a Th2 immune response and promotes experimental asthma. J Immunol 2004; 172:2739–2743.
74. Eisenbarth SC, Piggott DA, Huleatt JW, et al. Lipopolysaccharide-enhanced, toll-like receptor 4-dependent T helper cell type 2 responses to inhaled antigen. J Exp Med 2002; 196:1645–1651.
75. Fransson M, Adner M, Erjefalt J, et al. Up-regulation of Toll-like receptors 2, 3 and 4 in allergic rhinitis. Respir Res 2005; 6:100–109.
76. Holtzman MJ, Tyner JW, Kim EY, et al. Acute and chronic airway responses to viral infection: implications for asthma and chronic obstructive pulmonary disease. Proc Am Thorac Soc 2005; 2:132–140.

77. Hacker G, Redecke V, Hacker H. Activation of the immune system by bacterial CpG-DNA. Immunology 2002; 105:245–251.
78. Wilson HL, Dar A, Napper SK, et al. Immune mechanisms and therapeutic potential of CpG oligodeoxynucleotides. Int Rev Immunol 2006; 25:183–213.
79. Hoene V, Peiser M, Wanner R. Human monocyte-derived dendritic cells express TLR9 and react directly to the CpG-A oligonucleotide D19. J Leukoc Biol 2006; 80:1328–1336.
80. Guiducci C, Ott G, Chan JH, et al. Properties regulating the nature of the plasmacytoid dendritic cell response to Toll-like receptor 9 activation. J Exp Med 2006; 203:1999–2008.
81. Higgins D, Rodriguez R, Milley R, et al. Modulation of immunogenicity and allergenicity by controlling the number of immunostimulatory oligonucleotides linked to Amb a 1. J Allergy Clin Immunol 2006; 118:504–510.
82. Gauvreau GM, Hessel EM, Boulet LP, et al. Immunostimulatory sequences regulate interferon-inducible genes but not allergic airway responses. Am J Respir Crit Care Med 2006; 174:15–20.

Macrophages and efferent arm immune function – general concepts

83. Daftary SS, Jarjour NN, Calhoun WJ. The role of alveolar macrophages in asthma. In: Beberman S, ed. Inflammatory mechanisms in asthma, New York: Marcel Dekker; 1997: 361–376.
84. Calhoun WJ, Reed HE, Moest DR, et al. Enhanced superoxide production by alveolar macrophages and airspace cells, airway inflammation, and alveolar macrophage density changes follow segmental antigen bronchoprovocation in allergic subjects. Am Rev Respir Dis 1992; 145:317–325.
85. Tormey VJ, Leonard C, Faul J, et al. Dysregulation of monocyte differentiation in asthmatic subjects is reversed by IL-10. Clin Exp Allergy 1998; 28:992–998.
86. Tormey VJ, Bernard S, Ivory K, et al. Fluticasone propionate-induced regulation of the balance within macrophage subpopulations. Clin Exp Immunol 2000; 119:4–10.
87. Steele C, Rapaka RR, Metz A, et al. The beta-glucan receptor dectin-1 recognizes specific morphologies of Aspergillus fumigatus. PLoS Pathog 2005 1:e42.
88. Brown GD. Dectin-1: a signalling non-TLR pattern-recognition receptor. Nat Rev Immunol 2006; 6:33–43.
89. Willment JA, Lin HH, Reid DM, et al. Dectin-1 expression and function are enhanced on alternatively activated and GM-CSF-treated macrophages and are negatively regulated by IL-10, dexamethasone, and lipopolysaccharide. J Immunol 2003; 171:4569–4573.

Macrophages in asthma

90. Calhoun WJ, Bush RK. Enhanced reactive oxygen species metabolism of airspace cells and airway inflammation following antigen challenge in human asthma. J Allergy Clin Immunol 1990; 86:306–313.
91. Viksman MY, Liu MC, Bickel CA, et al. Phenotypic analysis of alveolar macrophages and monocytes in allergic airway inflammation. I. Evidence for activation of alveolar macrophages, but not peripheral blood monocytes, in subjects with allergic rhinitis and asthma. Am J Respir Crit Care Med 1997; 155:858–863.
92. Poulter LW, Burke CM. Macrophages and allergic lung disease. Immunobiology 1996; 195:574–587.
93. Alexis NE, Soukup J, Nierkens S, et al. Association between airway hyperreactivity and bronchial macrophage dysfunction in individuals with mild asthma. Am J Physiol Lung Cell Mol Physiol 2001; 280:L369–L375.
94. Seymour ML, Rak S, Aberg D, et al. Leukotriene and prostanoid pathway enzymes in bronchial biopsies of seasonal allergic asthmatics. Am J Respir Crit Care Med 2001; 164:2051–2056.
95. Doherty GM, Kamath SV, de Courcey F, et al. Children with stable asthma have reduced airway matrix metalloproteinase-9 and matrix metalloproteinase-9/tissue inhibitor of metalloproteinase-1 ratio. Clin Exp Allergy 2005; 35:1168–1174.
96. Kraft M, Hamid Q, Chrousos GP, et al. Decreased steroid responsiveness at night in nocturnal asthma. Is the macrophage responsible? Am J Respir Crit Care Med 2001; 163:1219–1225.
97. Hew M, Bhavsar P, Torrego A, et al. Relative corticosteroid insensitivity of peripheral blood mononuclear cells in severe asthma. Am J Respir Crit Care Med 2006; 174:134–141.
98. Cosio BG, Mann B, Ito K, et al. Histone acetylase and deacetylase activity in alveolar macrophages and blood monocytes in asthma. Am J Respir Crit Care Med 2004; 170:141–147.
99. Kraft M, Hamid Q, Chrousos GP, et al. Decreased steroid responsiveness at night in nocturnal asthma. Is the macrophage responsible? Am J Respir Crit Care Med 2001; 163:1219–1225.
100. de Waal Malefyt R, Yssel H, Roncarolo MG, et al. Interleukin-10. Curr Opin Immunol 1992; 4:314–320.
101. Chu SJ, Tang LO, Watney E, et al. In situ amplification of 5-lipoxygenase and 5-lipoxygenase-activating protein in allergic airway inflammation and inhibition by leukotriene blockade. J Immunol 2000; 165:4640–4648.
102. Borish L, Aarons A, Rumbyrt J, et al. Interleukin-10 regulation in normal subjects and patients with asthma. J Allergy Clin Immunol 1996; 97:1288–1296.
103. Calhoun WJ, Hinton KL, Brick JJ, et al. Spontaneous and stimulated IL-10 release by alveolar macrophages, but not blood monocytes, is reduced in allergic asthmatics. Am J Respir Crit Care Med 1996; 153:A881.
104. Hunt LW, Gleich GJ, Kita H, et al. Removal of bronchoalveolar cells augments the late eosinophilic response to segmental allergen challenge. Clin Exp Allergy 2992; 32:210–216.
105. Haczku A. Role and regulation of lung collectins in allergic airway sensitization. Pharmacol Ther 2006; 110:14–34.
106. Scanlon ST, Milovanova T, Kierstein S, et al. Surfactant protein-A inhibits Aspergillus fumigatus-induced allergic T-cell responses. Respir Res 2005; 6:97–99.
107. Liu CF, Chen YL, Shieh CC, et al. Therapeutic effect of surfactant protein D in allergic inflammation of mite-sensitized mice. Clin Exp Allergy 2005; 35:515–521.

108. Valstar DL, Schijf MA, Arts JH, et al. Alveolar macrophages suppress non-specific inflammation caused by inhalation challenge with trimellitic anhydride conjugated to albumin. Arch Toxicol 2006; 80:561–571.
109. Valstar DL, Schijf MA, Nijkamp FP, et al. Alveolar macrophages have a dual role in a rat model for trimellitic anhydride-induced occupational asthma. Toxicol Appl Pharmacol 2006; 211:20–29.
110. Korf JE, Pynaert G, Tournoy K, et al. Macrophage reprogramming by mycolic acid promotes a tolerogenic response in experimental asthma. Am J Respir Crit Care Med 2006; 174:152–160.
111. Viksman MY, Bochner BS, Peebles RS, et al. Expression of activation markers on alveolar macrophages in allergic asthmatics after endobronchial or whole-lung allergen challenge. Clin Immunol 2002; 104:77–85.
112. Careau E, Proulx LI, Pouliot P, et al. Antigen sensitization modulates alveolar macrophage functions in an asthma model. Am J Physiol Lung Cell Mol Physiol 2006; 290:L871–L879.
113. Lensmar C, Katchar K, Eklund A, et al. Phenotypic analysis of alveolar macrophages and lymphocytes following allergen inhalation by atopic subjects with mild asthma. Respir Med 2006;100:918–925.
114. Mazzarella G, Grella E, D'Auria D, et al. Phenotypic features of alveolar monocytes/macrophages and IL-8 gene activation by IL-1 and TNF-alpha in asthmatic patients. Allergy 2000; 55(Suppl 61):36–41.
115. Noma T, Ichikawa K, Yoshizawa I, et al. Reduced IL-1 production in adolescents with mite antigen asthma in remission. Clin Exp Immunol 1998; 113:10–16.
116. Folkard SG, Westwick J, Millar AB. Production of interleukin-8, RANTES and MCP-1 in intrinsic and extrinsic asthmatics. Eur Respir J 1997; 10:2097–2104.
117. Kotsimbos AT, Humbert M, Minshall E, et al. Upregulation of alpha GM-CSF-receptor in nonatopic asthma but not in atopic asthma. J Allergy Clin Immunol 1997; 99:666–672.
118. Esnault S, Malter JS. Minute quantities of granulocyte-macrophage colony-stimulating factor prolong eosinophil survival. J Interferon Cytokine Res 2001; 21:117–124.
119. John M, Lim S, Seybold J, et al. Inhaled corticosteroids increase interleukin-10 but reduce macrophage inflammatory protein-1alpha, granulocyte-macrophage colony-stimulating factor, and interferon-gamma release from alveolar macrophages in asthma. Am J Respir Crit Care Med 1998; 157:256–262.
120. Vignola AM, Chanez P, Chiappara G, et al. Evaluation of apoptosis of eosinophils, macrophages, and T lymphocytes in mucosal biopsy specimens of patients with asthma and chronic bronchitis. J Allergy Clin Immunol 1999; 103:563–573.
121. Hart LA, Krishnan VL, Adcock IM, et al. Activation and localization of transcription factor, nuclear factor-kappaB, in asthma. Am J Respir Crit Care Med 1998; 158:1585–1592.
122. Marshall HE, Stamler JS. Exhaled nitric oxide (NO), NO synthase activity, and regulation of nuclear factor (NF)-kappaB. Am J Respir Cell Mol Biol 1997; 21:296–297.
123. Dinakar C, Malur A, Raychaudhuri B, et al. Differential regulation of human blood monocyte and alveolar macrophage inflammatory cytokine production by nitric oxide. Ann Allergy Asthma Immunol 1999; 82:217–222.
124. Raychaudhuri B, Dweik R, Connors MJ, et al. Nitric oxide blocks nuclear factor-kappaB activation in alveolar macrophages. Am J Respir Cell Mol Biol 1999; 21:311–316.
125. Sergejeva S, Ivanov S, Lotvall J, et al. Interleukin-17 as a recruitment and survival factor for airway macrophages in allergic airway inflammation. Am J Respir Cell Mol Biol 2005; 33:248–253.
126. Nishizawa Y, Fushiki S, Amakata Y, et al. Thyroxine-induced production of superoxide anion by human alveolar neutrophils and macrophages: a possible mechanism for the exacerbation of bronchial asthma with the development of hyperthyroidism. In Vivo 1998; 12:253–257.
127. Forman HJ, Torres M. Reactive oxygen species and cell signaling. Am J Respir Crit Care Med 2002; 166:S4-S8.
128. Erdely A, Kepka-Lenhart D, Clark M, et al. Inhibition of phosphodiesterase 4 amplifies cytokine-dependent induction of arginase in macrophages. Am J Physiol Lung Cell Mol Physiol 2006; 290:L534–L539.
129. Vachier I, Chanez P, Radeau T, et al. Cellular protein kinase C activity in asthma. Am J Respir Crit Care Med 1997; 155:1211–1216.
130. Weinberger B, Fakhrzadeh L, Heck DE, et al. Inhaled nitric oxide primes lung macrophages to produce reactive oxygen and nitrogen intermediates. Am J Respir Crit Care Med 1998; 158:931–938.
131. Sadeghi-Hashjin G, Folkerts G, Henricks PAJ, et al. Peroxynitrite in airway diseases. Clin Exp Allergy 1998; 28:1464–1473.
132. Sittipunt C, Steinberg KP, Rudzinski JT, et al. Nitric oxide and nitrotyrosine in the lungs of patients with adult respiratory distress syndrome. Am J Respir Crit Care Med 2001; 163:503–510.
133. Hanazawa T, Kharitonov SA, Barnes PJ. Increased nitrotyrosine in exhaled breath condensate of patients with asthma. Am J Respir Crit Care Med 2000; 162:1273–1276.
134. Janssen-Heininger YMW, Persinger RL, Korn SH, et al. Reactive nitrogen species and cell signaling. Am J Respir Crit Care Med 2002; 166; S9–S16.
135. Amrani Y, Moore PE, Hoffman R, et al. Interferon-γ modulates cysteinyl leukotriene receptor 1 expression and function in human airway monocytes. Am J Respir Crit Care Med 2001; 164:2098–2101.
136. Thivierge M, Stankova J, Rola-Pleszczynski M. IL-13 and IL-4 up-regulate cysteinyl leukotriene 1 receptor expression in human monocytes and macrophages. J Immunol 2001; 167:2855–2860.
137. Calhoun WJ, Lavins BJ, Minkwitz MC, et al. Effect of zafirlukast (Accolate) on cellular mediators of inflammation: bronchoalveolar lavage fluid findings after segmental antigen challenge. Am J Respir Crit Care Med 1998; 157:1381–1389.
138. Borish L. IL-10: evolving concepts. J Allergy Clin Immunol 1998; 101:293–297.
139. Magnan A, van Pee D, Bongrand P, et al. Alveolar macrophage interleukin (IL)-10 and IL-12 production in atopic asthma. Allergy 1998; 53:1092–1095.
140. Lim S, John M, Seybold J, et al. Increased interleukin-10 and macrophage inflammatory protein-1 alpha release from blood monocytes ex vivo during late-phase response to allergen in asthma. Allergy 2000; 55:489–495.

REFERENCES

141. Ameredes BT, Sethi J, Otterbein L, et al. Exhaled carbon monoxide and nitric oxide are increased in IL-10-knockout mice. Am J Respir Crit Care Med 2002; 165:A731.

142. Ameredes BT, Zamora R, Gibson KF, et al. Increased nitric oxide production by airway immune cells of sensitized and challenged IL-10 knockout mice. J Leuk Biol 2001; 70: 730–736.

143. Ameredes BT, Zamora R, Gibson KF, et al. IL-18 and IL-4 production by airway cells of allergen-challenged IL-10 knockout mice Am J Physiol 2003 (in press).

144. Harju T, Soini Y, Paakko R, et al. Up-regulation of heme oxygenase-I in alveolar macrophages of newly diagnosed asthmatics. Respir Med 2002; 96:418–423.

145. Otterbein LE, Bach FH, Alam J, et al. Carbon monoxide has anti-inflammatory effects involving the mitogen-activated protein kinase pathway. Nat Med 2000; 6:422–428.

146. Mautino G, Oliver N, Chanez P, et al. Increased release of matrix metalloproteinase-9 in bronchoalveolar lavage fluid and by alveolar macrophages of asthmatics. Am J Respir Cell Mol Biol 1997; 17:583–591.

147. Mautino G, Henriquet C, Gougat C, et al. Increased expression of tissue inhibitor of metalloproteinase-1 and loss of correlation with matrix metalloproteinase-9 by macrophages in asthma. Lab Invest 1999; 79:39–47.

148. Kelly EA, Busse WW, Jarjour NN. Increased matrix metalloproteinase-9 in the airway after allergen challenge. Am J Respir Crit Care Med 2000; 162:1157–1161.

149. Vignola AM, Riccobono L, Mirabella A, et al. Sputum metalloproteinase-9/tissue inhibitor of metalloproteinase-1 ratio correlates with airflow obstruction in asthma and chronic bronchitis. Am J Respir Crit Care Med 1998; 158:1945–1950.

150. Vignola AM, Chanez P, Chiappara G, et al. Release of transforming growth factor-beta (TGF-beta) and fibronectin by alveolar macrophages in airway diseases. Clin Exp Immunol 1996; 106:114–119.

151. Sagara H, Okada T, Okumura K, et al. Activation of TGF-beta/Smad2 signaling is associated with airway remodeling in asthma. J Allergy Clin Immunol 2002; 110:249–254.

152. Faul JL, Demers EA, Burke CM, et al. Alterations in airway inflammation and lung function during corticosteroid therapy for atopic asthma. Chest 2002; 121:1414–1420.

153. Cotter TP, Hood PP, Costello JF, et al. Exposure to systemic prednisolone for 4 hours reduces ex vivo synthesis of GM-CSF by bronchoalveolar lavage cells and blood mononuclear cells of mild allergic asthmatics. Clin Exp Allergy 1999; 29:1655–1662.

154. Sousa AR, Lane SJ, Cidlowski JA, et al. Glucocorticoid resistance in asthma is associated with elevated in vivo expression of the glucocorticoid receptor beta-isoform. J Allergy Clin Immunol 2000; 105:943–950.

Biology of Epithelial Cells

23

David Proud

CONTENTS

- Epithelial anatomy and phenotype 373
- Cell–cell adhesion and communication 374
- Epithelial changes in asthma 376
- Epithelial cells and airway inflammation 376
- Leukocyte–epithelial interactions 379
- Epithelial cells and airway remodeling 379
- Epithelial cells and host defense 380
- Epithelium and innate immunity 381
- Summary 384

SUMMARY OF IMPORTANT CONCEPTS

>> The epithelium is not just a physical barrier but is also an active contributor to responses to inhaled pathogens and irritants

>> The epithelium produces a wide range of mediators that can regulate inflammatory cell recruitment to the airways

>> Epithelial cell function appears to be altered in asthma and epithelial cells contribute to airway remodeling

>> The epithelial cell is an active participant in host innate immune responses, recognizing inhaled pathogens and producing host defense molecules

>> Epithelial cells appear to play an important role in immunoregulation in the airways

EPITHELIAL ANATOMY AND PHENOTYPE

The respiratory epithelium is a complex tissue comprising a variety of cell types with specialized functions. Beginning just distal to the immediate anterior portion of the nasal cavity, the epithelium of the larger proximal airways is characterized by a pseudostratified columnar morphology and contains predominantly three cell types: ciliated cells, secretory cells, and basal cells (Fig. 23.1).

Ciliated cells are columnar in shape, and the apical surface of each cell is covered by ≈250 cilia and numerous microvilli. These cells play a critical role in the body's defense against inhaled pathogens and noxious particles by propelling mucus of the tracheobronchial tree proximally to clear the airway of trapped debris. In the nasal cavity, mucociliary clearance moves irritants to the nasopharynx. In the upper respiratory tract, as much as 80% of the luminal surface of the airway is covered by ciliated cells, which are found in clusters separated by fields of non-ciliated cells and submucosal gland ducts. Effective clearance of the airways by ciliated cells depends on the ability of cilia to beat in synchronous waves

in the low-viscosity sol phase of airway secretions while the claw-like projections on their tips move in the more viscous gel phase, grabbing the mucus and propelling it towards the pharynx. Appropriate viscosity of the sol layer is regulated by active ion transport processes that are coupled to fluid transport across the epithelium.

Goblet cells are much less prevalent than ciliated cells and constitute <1% of total epithelial cell numbers, but their numbers can increase several-fold in airways chronically exposed to irritants, and in patients with asthma. They are metabolically active secretory cells, as evidenced by their extensive rough endoplasmic reticulum, numerous ribosomes, and prominent Golgi apparatus. The mucus granules that are characteristic of these cells contain primarily neutral mucins, sialomucins, and sulfomucins. By contrast, the other major type of secretory cell in the upper airways, serous cells, produce low-viscosity secretions rich in neutral glycoprotein, lysozyme, and the epithelial transfer component of immunoglobulin A (IgA). Serous and mucus cells are also the cell types lining the submucosal glands found throughout the larger airways. As one moves to the more distal airways, submucosal glands are absent, ciliated cells decrease in number

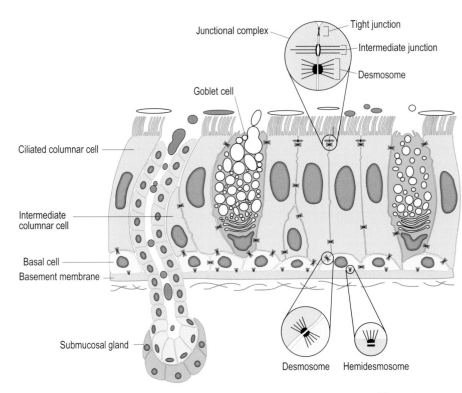

Fig. 23.1. Diagrammatic representation of the pseudostratified columnar epithelium of the proximal airways. Three structures essential for epithelial cell–cell adhesion are shown: the tight junction *(zonula occludens),* the intermediate junction *(zonula adherens),* and the desmosome *(macula adherens).* Note that columnar cells do not form direct junctional attachments to the basement membrane but rely on desmosomal attachments to basal cells, which anchor the epithelium to the basement membrane via hemidesmosomal linkages. (Courtesy of Jacqueline Schaffer, Baltimore.)

and eventually disappear, the epithelium becomes more cuboidal, and basal cells and Clara cells become more prominent. At the bronchiolar level, Clara cells have a major secretory role.

Basal cells are relatively small cells with few mitochondria, scant rough endoplasmic reticulum, a small cytoplasmic-to-nuclear ratio and numerous keratin filaments. As their name indicates, they are found adjacent to the basement membrane of the airways and normally do not reach the luminal surface. They anchor the epithelium by forming hemidesmosomal linkages to the basement membrane. Columnar cells do not form direct junctional attachments to the basement membrane but rely on forming desmosomal attachments to basal cells.

Although the presence of pluripotent stem cell 'niches' within submucosal gland ducts has been reported, recent studies indicate that both basal and secretory cells function as progenitors. Studies using discrete cell populations transplanted into severe combined immunodeficient (SCID) mice have shown that both basal and secretory cells can restore a well-differentiated, pseudostratified epithelium with functional submucosal glands. Secretory cells restored the mucosa more rapidly than basal cells however, implying that secretory cell populations contain more late committed progenitors.[1]

At the alveolar level, epithelial cells are designated as type I and type II cells. Type I cells cover ≈95% of the alveolar surface and have a flattened morphology that permits efficient gas exchange, whereas type II cells are cuboidal and occur at the junction of the alveolar septum.

Even though type II cells cover only 5% of the alveolar surface area, they outnumber type I cells by a ratio of 2:1. Type II cells are highly metabolically active, are the progenitor cell of the alveolar epithelium, and are the major source of surfactant in the lower airways.

■ CELL–CELL ADHESION AND COMMUNICATION ■

Three ultrastructural components are essential for maintaining the integrity of the airway epithelium: the tight junction *(zonula occludens),* the intermediate junction *(zonula adherens),* and the desmosome *(macula adherens)* (Fig. 23.1). The transmembrane proteins that comprise these junctions are linked to components of the cytoskeleton. Moreover, many of the cytoplasmic scaffolding molecules associated with these junctions are involved in regulating a wide array of cellular functions, including transcription and cell proliferation.

Tight junctions seal the apical aspects of the epithelial cell, thereby separating the apical and basolateral membrane domains. In addition, they form a regulated permeability barrier to paracellular fluxes. Ultrastructurally, tight junctions appear as an interconnected belt-like network of linearly arranged strands that encircle the cell. Although it was initially thought that the number of strands correlated with the

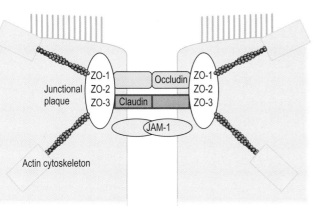

Fig. 23.2. Simplified representation of the molecular architecture of the tight junction. Multiple copies of the integral junctional proteins, occludins, claudins, and junctional adhesion molecule-1 (JAM-1) cross the intrajunctional space between cells. Occludins and claudins bind to the members of the zonula occludens (ZO) family and to other proteins of the junctional plaque. Junctional plaque proteins, such as the ZO proteins, also bind directly to the actin cytoskeleton of the cells.

'tightness' of junctions, more recent data contradict this. In fact, the strands of tight junctions are remarkably dynamic and contain pores that fluctuate between an open and closed confirmation. Almost 40 different proteins now have been identified as components of the tight junction.[2] These include integral junctional proteins that bridge the intercellular space and help to regulate epithelial permeability; plaque proteins that link the integral tight junction proteins to the cytoskeleton and serve as adapters for the recruitment of cytosolic proteins involved in cell signaling; and a group of cytosolic and nuclear proteins that interact, either directly or indirectly, with the junctional plaque proteins to regulate diverse cellular functions (Fig. 23.2). The main integral tight junctional proteins are occludin, junction adhesion molecule (JAM)-1, and the claudins. There are over 20 members of the claudin family, and the expression pattern of these proteins is variable among tissues. While some, such as claudin-1, are ubiquitously expressed, others are very restricted in expression. Claudins play a major role in regulating tight junction permeability, forming size- and charge-selective pores and contain serine/threonine residues that modulate barrier function upon phosphorylation.[3] The C-terminus of claudins contains binding sites for plaque proteins, such as the members of the zona occludens family, ZO-1, ZO-2, and ZO-3. These components of the cytosolic plaque are members of the membrane-associated guanylate kinase superfamily. All three ZO proteins can be co-immunoprecipitated from cultured epithelial cells. They bind directly to the C-terminal region of occludin, linking it to the actin cytoskeleton of the cell (Fig. 23.2). Proteins that are recruited to the junctional plaque to serve as adapters include the dimeric protein cingulin, as well as symplekin, 7H6, and the phosphatase and tensin homolog (PTEN). Interestingly, the cysteine and serine protease components of the house dust mite allergen *Der p 1* have been shown to facilitate penetration of the tight junction barrier via cleavage of junctional proteins including occludin and ZO-1.[4]

Intermediate junctions are adhesive structures that encircle the cell and narrow the intercellular space to 25–35 nm in width. The calcium-dependent adhesion molecule, E-cadherin, which mediates homophilic cell–cell adhesion, is concentrated at the zonula adherens.

The cytoplasmic domain of E-cadherin associates with proteins of the ezrin/radixin/moesin (ERM) family, particularly α-, β-, and γ-catenin, and α-actinin. These proteins all participate, directly or indirectly, in the coupling of E-cadherin to the actin cytoskeleton.

Desmosomes are present along the lateral aspects of columnar epithelial cells, particularly towards the cell apex, and at the junction between columnar and basal cells. Columnar cells do not form adhesive links with the basement membrane but are anchored via their desmosomal attachments to the basal cell layer. Desmosomes measure between 0.1 and 1.5 µmol/L in diameter and are delineated by an electron-dense plaque and electron-dense filaments that span the intercellular space. Anchoring cytokeratin intermediate filaments fan out from the cytoplasmic edge of the plaques into the cytoplasm, looping repeatedly from the cytoplasm to the plaque and back again. A variety of proteins make up the different portions of the desmosome. Membrane glycoproteins known as desmogleins and desmocollins project into the extracellular space to form an intercellular adhesive structure. Desmogleins and desmocollins exist in multiple isoforms that display tissue-specific heterogeneity. Desmoglein and desmocollin proteins are attached to the cytoskeleton via members of the plaque and armadillo protein family, primarily desmoplakins, plakoglobin, and the important stabilizer protein, plakophilin 1.[5]

Hemidesmosomes link basal cells to extracellular matrix in the basement membrane. Binding of epithelial cells to extracellular matrix proteins occurs primarily via integrins, a large family of heterodimeric glycoproteins comprising non-covalently linked α and β subunits, with subfamilies defined on the basis of the common β subunit. Although important in adhesion, the integrins also play a role in a variety of cell signaling pathways that mediate diverse cellular functions (also see Chapter 9). At least seven different integrins are expressed on normal airway epithelium ($\alpha_2\beta_1, \alpha_3\beta_1, \alpha_6\beta_4, \alpha_9\beta_1, \alpha_v\beta_5, \alpha_v\beta_6, \alpha_v\beta_8$).[6] Only three of these integrins are known to interact with normal components of basement membrane. Both $\alpha_3\beta_1$ and $\alpha_6\beta_4$ interact with laminins, and the $\alpha_6\beta_4$ heterodimer has been localized to the hemidesmosome complex, suggesting that it plays an important role in basal cell attachment to the basement membrane. By contrast $\alpha_2\beta_1$ can interact with collagen IV. The epithelium also expresses integrins that interact with matrix proteins that are found only during processes such as inflammation, wound repair, and development. These include $\alpha_v\beta_5$, which binds to vitronectin. Additional integrins include the fibronectin receptor $\alpha_5\beta_1, \alpha_9\beta_1$ which mediates binding to tenascin, and $\alpha_v\beta_6$ that binds to both tenascin and fibronectin. Some integrins, such as $\alpha_5\beta_1$ and $\alpha_v\beta_6$, are expressed at low or undetectable levels on normal epithelium, but expression increases in response to epithelial injury.[6] Other non-integrin molecules that may play a role in adhesion of epithelial cells to extracellular matrix proteins include the family of transmembrane heparan sulfate proteoglycans, called syndecans, which can interact with laminin and fibronectin, and the glycoprotein CD44, which is the major cell surface receptor for hyaluronic acid, as well as being able to interact with collagen and fibronectin. Multiple isoforms of CD44 can be generated by alternative splicing of at least 10 variant exons. Bronchial epithelial cells from normal adult lungs show focal expression of the CD44v6 and CD44v9 isoforms, whereas the so-called standard form of the molecule, CD44s, is observed only on basal cells. Increased epithelial expression of CD44 has been reported in asthmatic subjects.[7]

Gap junctions are channels comprised of homo- or hetero-hexamers of members of the connexin family of proteins. These channels play an important role in the communication between adjacent cells by permitting the reciprocal exchange of ions and small molecules including second messengers, such as cAMP and inositol trisphosphate. Communication through gap junctions plays a crucial role in cell growth and differentiation. Recent studies have found that, as epithelial cells differentiate, small gap junction plaques appear within the network of tight junction strands. Moreover, it has been shown that several connexins can interact with the tight junction plaque protein ZO-1, suggesting that gap junctional proteins also may help regulate the barrier function of tight junctions.[8]

EPITHELIAL CHANGES IN ASTHMA

Epithelial fragility is a characteristic feature of asthma. Although there is some dispute regarding whether the extent of epithelial damage observed upon biopsies of asthmatic subjects is an artifact, it must be noted that such changes are not observed in other inflammatory diseases such as COPD.[9] Moreover, other lines of evidence support increased epithelial damage in asthma. Sloughed clumps of epithelial cells (Creola bodies) are present in sputum from asthmatic subjects and the number of Creola bodies detected increases during disease exacerbations. In addition, increased epithelial desquamation is observed in autopsy specimens from patients who have died of *status asthmaticus*. Although some biopsy specimens show evidence of loss of the epithelium down to the basement membrane, cleavage usually occurs between columnar and basal cells, presumably by disruption of desmosomal linkages. The degree of desquamation in asthma reportedly correlates with bronchial hyperreactivity, and epithelial shedding is reduced with glucocorticoid therapy. It is unclear what predisposes asthmatics to epithelial fragility, but several factors have been implicated as potential causes of damage. Some respiratory viruses cause epithelial damage, as do environmental pollutants, such as ozone. Eosinophil-derived proteins, including major basic protein, eosinophil peroxidase, and eosinophil cationic protein, also cause epithelial damage. Eosinophil peroxidase is particularly potent in the presence of hydrogen peroxide and halide when highly cytotoxic hypothalamus acids are produced.

Goblet cell hyperplasia and metaplasia is a prominent feature in asthma. Given that IL-4 and especially IL-13 have been implicated as playing a significant role in the development of goblet cell hyperplasia, it is of interest that enhanced expression and activation of signal transducer and activator of transcription (STAT)-6 has been reported in asthmatic epithelium. Other biochemical changes are observed in epithelial cells from asthmatic subjects, including constitutive activation of STAT-1. Increased expression of epidermal growth factor receptor is also observed, particularly where basal cells are exposed after loss of columnar cells. This increased expression may play a role in chronic epithelial repair in the asthmatic airways, which, in turn, may contribute to airway remodeling (see below).[9]

EPITHELIAL CELLS AND AIRWAY INFLAMMATION

The unique position of the epithelium at the interface between the host and its environment inevitably means that it will be exposed to a variety of exogenous and endogenous stimuli. The epithelium contributes to the response to such stimuli in a variety of ways. In addition to contributing to host defense (see below), the epithelium can produce a wide array of mediators that can alter the inflammatory status of the airway, and can also regulate the activity of a variety of mediators via catabolic and inhibitory functions.

PRODUCTION OF LIPID MEDIATORS BY EPITHELIAL CELLS

Epithelial cells produce metabolites of arachidonic acid, but considerable species variations exist in terms of products generated. Although 5-lipoxygenase activity is present in canine and ovine epithelial cells, human airway epithelial cells express 15-lipoxygenase. This enzyme converts arachidonic acid to 15-hydroxyeicosatetraenoic acid (15-HETE), as well as a range of hydroperoxy, epoxyhydroxy, keto, and dihydroxy acids. Expression of 15-lipoxygenase is increased in the epithelium of asthmatic subjects, and elevated levels of 15-HETE are found in bronchoalveolar lavage (BAL) fluids of asthmatic subjects after allergen provocation.[10] Production of 15-HETE can enhance epithelial mucus glycoprotein production and augment the acute response to antigen challenge in asthmatic subjects. Another metabolite, 8S,15S- diHETE, induces neutrophil chemotaxis. The recruited neutrophils can then utilize 15-HETE to generate the trihydroxy acid lipoxin A by a transcellular pathway catalyzed by 5-lipoxygenase. Lipoxin A inhibits the cytotoxic activity of human natural killer (NK) cells, causes superoxide generation by neutrophils, and contracts human bronchi.

Epithelial cells also produce mid-chain and ω-terminal HETEs and *cis*-epoxyeicosatrienoic acids (EETs) via the cytochrome P-450 monooxygenase pathway. The CYP2J isoform of P-450 is present in both ciliated and non-ciliated human airway epithelial cells. Metabolites of the P-450 pathway affect epithelial ion transport as well as bronchomotor tone.

Finally, epithelial metabolism of arachidonic acid occurs via the cyclooxygenase (COX) pathway. Epithelial cells express both COX-1 and COX-2, but expression of COX-2 is markedly enhanced in asthmatic subjects. Human epithelial cells generate predominantly prostaglandin E_2 (PGE_2) and $PGF_{2\alpha}$ in response to a variety of inflammatory mediators, including bradykinin, PAF, and histamine.[11] Increased levels of both prostanoids are detected in BAL fluids of asthmatic and atopic subjects, and levels increase further in response to allergen provocation. In vitro, PGE_2 inhibits mast cell degranulation and production of LTB_4 by alveolar macrophages. It also mediates relaxation of airway smooth muscle and regulates mucus glycoprotein secretion. In vivo, PGE_2 increases cough sensitivity and may play a role in the cough associated with angiotensin-converting enzyme-inhibitor therapy. In addition, inhalation of PGE_2 blocks early and late bronchoconstrictor responses to inhaled allergen,[12] abolishes allergen-induced increases in bronchial reactivity, and attenuates exercise-induced bronchoconstriction. By contrast, $PGF_{2\alpha}$, is a potent bronchoconstrictor.

PRODUCTION OF PEPTIDE MEDIATORS BY EPITHELIAL CELLS

Human epithelial cells produce the potent bronchoconstrictors endothelin-1 and endothelin-3. Elevated levels of these peptides are found in BAL fluids from asthmatic patients, and levels of endothelins in BAL correlate with asthma severity. Asthmatic epithelial cells show increased gene expression of pre-proendothelin and produce increased levels of endothelin-1. Production of endothelins can be enhanced by several cytokines, chemokines, and growth factors, while production is inhibited by treatment with glucocorticoids, interferon-γ (IFN-γ), or platelet-derived growth factor. Intranasal administration of endothelin-1 induces sneezing and increased nasal secretion but does not induce increased vascular permeability. Endothelin could exacerbate the asthmatic state not only via direct bronchoconstriction but also by stimulating epithelial production of cyclooxygenase and lipoxygenase products. In addition, endothelin stimulates smooth muscle proliferation and promotes subepithelial fibrosis.[13]

The epithelium also produces antimicrobial peptides, including defensins and cathelicidins, which are discussed below in the section on host defense. In addition, they generate proteases and antiproteases that can modulate inflammation. These are discussed in the section on remodeling.

PRODUCTION OF CYTOKINES AND CHEMOKINES BY EPITHELIAL CELLS

The epithelial cell is a major contributor to the cytokine network in the airways, producing chemoattractant cytokines and chemokines, pleiotropic cytokines, colony-stimulating factors, and growth factors, as well as several cytokine antagonists in response to a wide array of inciting stimuli (Table 23.1). For a more detailed description of the properties of many of these molecules in allergic disorders, the reader is referred to Chapters 10 and 11.

The epithelium can regulate the recruitment of a wide variety of inflammatory cell types into the airways, depending upon the stimuli to which it is exposed, the profile of chemokines produced, and the extent to which selected inflammatory cell populations are primed to respond.

The CXC, or α, chemokine family is subdivided into two classes based on the presence or absence of the amino-terminal sequence Glu-Leu-Arg (ELR). The ELR-containing CXC chemokines are predominantly chemoattractant for neutrophils, while the non-ELR subgroup are chemoattractant for lymphocytes and other cells. Epithelial cells produce both classes of CXC chemokines. The protypical ELR-containing CXC chemokine produced in large quantities by epithelial cells is IL-8 (CXCL8). In vivo, epithelial cell expression of IL-8 is increased in allergic rhinitis and asthma. As shown in Table 23.1, increased epithelial expression of IL-8 occurs in response to a wide variety of stimuli. Given the prominent neutrophilic response upon exposure of the airways to infectious agents, it is of interest that pathogens, particularly respiratory viruses, are potent inducers not only of IL-8 but also of ENA-78 (CXCL5), Gro-α (CXCL1) and Gro-γ (CXCL3). Epithelial cells also make large amounts of the non-ELR CXC chemokines, monokine induced by IFN-γ (Mig, CXCL9), IFN-inducible protein of 10 kDa (IP-10, CXCL10) and IFN-inducible T-cell α-chemoattractant (I-TAC, CXCL11). All of these chemokines are ligands for the CXCR3 receptor found predominantly on type 1 (Th1) lymphocytes and on NK cells. As their names imply, all of these chemokines are induced by type I and type II interferons. Respiratory viral infections also induce expression of non-ELR chemokines. Interestingly, induction of CXCL10 by human rhinovirus occurs independently of interferon

induction.[14] Epithelial expression of most CXC chemokines is not particularly sensitive to inhibition by glucocorticoids.

Epithelial cells also produce members of the CC, or β, chemokine family that function as chemoattractants for eosinophils, basophils, monocytes, dendritic cells, and lymphocytes, depending upon their specific receptor usage. Eotaxin (CCL11) and eotaxin-2 (CCL24) are selective ligands for the CCR3 chemokine receptor. Epithelial expression of CCL11, and gene expression for CCL24, increase in asthmatic epithelium. In cell culture, however, the predominant eosinophil chemoattractant released by epithelial cells is RANTES (regulated on activation, normal T cell expressed and secreted, CCL5). CCL5, together with IL-5, are the major eosinophil chemoattractants in the asthmatic lung.[15] CCL5 levels are increased in the BAL fluids of asthmatic compared with normal subjects, and eosinophil recruitment after allergen challenge is associated with increased levels of CCL5 in BAL fluid. Increased expression of CCL5 also is detected in epithelium of nasal polyps, in the airway secretions of subjects during virally induced asthma exacerbations, and in secretions from allergic subjects after allergen challenge. The epithelium also produces macrophage inflammatory protein (MIP)-1α (CCL3), MIP-3α (CCL20), and monocyte chemoattractant protein (MCP)-1 (CCL2). MCP-4 (CCL13) is induced by inflammatory stimuli and, in vivo, is present in the epithelium of asthmatic patients as well as in patients with sinusitis. Other CC chemokines produced by the epithelium, and overexpressed in asthma, are thymus- and activation-regulated chemokine (TARC, CCL17), which is chemoattractant for T helper type 2 lymphocytes, and mucosae-associated epithelial chemokine (MEC, CCL28).

Interestingly, recent studies have demonstrated the presence of functional chemokine receptors, particularly CCR3 and CXCR3, on epithelial cells, suggesting that epithelial chemokine release can also serve autocrine functions.[16,17]

Fractalkine is the only member of the CX_3C chemokine family. The specific receptor for fractalkine, CX_3CR1, is expressed on monocytes, T lymphocytes and NK cells, and levels of fractalkine in bronchoalveolar lavage fluids from patients with inflammatory airway disease correlate with mononuclear cell counts. IFNγ stimulates epithelial expression of fractalkine, but this chemokine largely remains cell associated. Adhesion of mononuclear cells to IFNγ-stimulated epithelial cells is partially inhibited by antibodies to fractalkine.

Epithelial cells are also capable of releasing numerous multifunctional cytokines and colony-stimulating factors (Table 23.1), several of which are induced in response to proteases from allergens and fungi, or by respiratory virus infection. Among the cytokines produced, IL-6 may modulate allergic diseases because it is known to induce B cell differentiation, T cell proliferation and activation, neural differentiation, and enhanced mucosal IgA production. Transgenic mice that overexpress IL-6 have pronounced peribronchial infiltration of lymphocytes but, interestingly, have reduced airway responsiveness to methacholine.[18] IL-11 is a cytokine with some similarities to IL-6. Epithelial expression of IL-11 is increased in asthma and during respiratory viral infections. Bronchial challenge of mice with IL-11 leads to pronounced airways hyperresponsiveness, and mononuclear cell infiltration, while targeted overexpression of IL-11 in the airways of adult mice induces airway remodeling characterized by subepithelial fibrosis.[19] In addition, IL-11 can activate B cells by means of a mechanism that is T cell-dependent. Epithelial production of thymic

Table 23.1 Some known epithelial cytokines

	Inducing stimuli		Inducing stimuli
Cytokines		Pleiotropic cytokines	
Chemoattractant cytokines		IL-6	IL-1, TNF-α, TGF-β, histamine, ozone, toluene 2,4-diisocyanate, proteases (elastase, dust mite, *Aspergillus*), bacterial products *(Pseudomonas)*, viruses (rhinovirus, RSV)
CXC/α chemokines			
ELR-containing			
IL-8 (CXCL8)	IL-1, TNF-α, ozone, NO_2, asbestos, proteases (elastase, dust mite, aspergillus), viruses (rhinovirus, influenza, RSV), bacterial products *(Pseudomonas)*, neuropeptides, cell deformation	IL-11	IL-1, TNF-α, TGF-β, retinoic acid, viruses (rhinovirus, RSV)
		IL-1	Asbestos, toluene 2,4-diisocyanate, rhinovirus
ENA-78 (CXCL5)	IL-1, rhinovirus	IFNβ	Rhinovirus, dsRNA
Gro-α (CXCL1)	TNF-α, rhinovirus	IFN-λ family	Rhinovirus, LPS
Gro-γ (CXCL3)	TNF-α	IL-10	?
Non-ELR-containing		TNF-α (?)	NO_2
IP-10 (CXCL10)	IFNs, rhinovirus	IL-5 (?)	TNF-α, IFN-γ
I-TAC (CXCL11)	IFNs	TSLP	?
Mig (CXCL9)	IFNs	**Colony-stimulating factors**	
CC/β chemokines		GM-CSF	IL-1, TNF-α, NO_2, elastase, viruses (rhinovirus, RSV), bacterial products *(Pseudomonas)*, house-dust mite proteases
Eotaxin (CCL11)	IL-1, TNF-α, IFN-γ, IL-4, IL-13, rhinovirus		
Eotaxin-2 (CCL24)?	Rhinovirus		
RANTES (CCL5)	IL-1, TNF-α, IFN-γ, viruses (rhinovirus, influenza, RSV)	G-CSF	IL-1, TNF-α, rhinovirus
		CSF-1	?
MCP-1 (CCL2)	TNF-α, RSV infection, fungal proteases	M-CSF	?
		Growth factors	
MCP-4 (CCL13)	IL-1, TNF-α, IL-4	TGF-β	Retinoic acid
MIP-1α (CCL3)	RSV infection	TGF-α	?
MIP-3α (CCL20)	IL-1, TNF-α, IL-4, IL-13, particulates	EGF	?
		HB-EGF	?
TARC (CCL17)	TNF-α, IFN-γ, IL-4, IL-13	Amphiregulin	?
MEC (CCL28)	?	SCF	?
CX$_3$C chemokines		VEGF	Rhinovirus
Fractalkine	IFN-γ		
Other			
IL-16	Histamine		

RSV, respiratory syncytial virus; TSLP, thymic stromal lymphopoietin.

stromal lymphopoietin (TSLP) is discussed in the section on immunoregulation. Increased granulocyte-macrophage colony-stimulating factor (GM-CSF) expression also has been observed in epithelial cells from patients with symptomatic allergic rhinitis, and from bronchial biopsies of asthmatic subjects. Moreover, levels of GM-CSF expression have been reported to correlate with the extent of eosinophil infiltration of the epithelium. GM-CSF could contribute to allergic inflammation via its abilities to prolong eosinophil survival and to activate eosinophils, neutrophils, and macrophages to display enhanced cytotoxic activity, generation of mediators, and phagocytosis. Granulocyte colony-stimulating factor (G-CSF) is also produced by epithelial cells and can enhance the survival and activation of neutrophils. The likely role of other epithelial cytokines and growth factors in allergic diseases is more difficult to predict. Although low levels of IL-1β are secreted, large amounts of IL-1β are seen when cells are exposed to cytotoxic stimuli, or are lysed. Epithelial cells also contain large quantities of intracellular IL-1 receptor antagonist type I (icIL-1ra), however, so the role of epithelial IL-1β may vary depending on conditions. Epithelium from brushings of healthy, normal subjects produce the potent immunoregulatory cytokine IL-10, but production is markedly diminished in cells obtained from patients with cystic fibrosis. The production of interferons by epithelial cells has recently attracted considerable interest. Although it is generally agreed that epithelial cells do not produce the prototypical type II interferon, IFN-γ, there is more controversy regarding type I IFNs. Although mRNA expression of IFN-α and IFN-β have consistently been detected, results on protein release have been more variable, perhaps due to the relative limitations of current ELISAs. While some investigators have failed to detect type I IFNs,[14] it has recently been suggested that impaired epithelial production of IFN-β in response to viral infection may contribute to viral exacerbations of asthma.[20] A recent study also suggests that deficient type III, IFN-λ1 (IL-29) and IFN-λ2/3 (IL-28A/B) production may contribute to asthma exacerbations.[21] Further studies are needed to confirm these important observations. Other cytokines listed in Table 23.1 are either produced in small amounts or require additional studies to confirm their expression.

Epithelial-derived growth factors are discussed below in the section on airway remodeling.

■ LEUKOCYTE–EPITHELIAL INTERACTIONS ■

The mechanisms by which leukocytes interact with, and migrate through, the epithelium remain relatively poorly understood. In terms of adhesion molecules known to interact with leukocyte counter-ligands, epithelial cells do not express E-selectin, and it is controversial whether vascular cell adhesion molecule-1 (VCAM-1) is expressed. The role of epithelial cell adhesion molecule (Ep-CAM), if any, in leukocyte–epithelial interactions is unknown. Airway epithelial cells do express intercellular adhesion molecule-1 (ICAM-1/CD54), and expression is enhanced upon exposure to proinflammatory cytokines, in response to viral infections, and on epithelial cells of asthmatic subjects in vivo. ICAM-1 is a counter-ligand for β2 integrins (CD11/CD18) expressed on leukocytes. These β2 integrins play a central role in leukocyte–epithelial adhesion as preincubation of leukocytes with monoclonal antibodies to CD18 almost totally blocks adhesion. Interestingly, blockade of epithelial ICAM-1 is much less effective in reducing leukocyte adhesion, implying that additional CD18-dependent, ICAM-1-independent, adhesion mechanisms must also exist.[22] Further support for this concept comes from studies with mice in which the genes for both P-selectin and ICAM-1 were mutated, yet neutrophil emigration into the alveolar spaces of these mice during acute *Streptococcus pneumoniae* infection was normal.[23] Recent studies also have examined transepithelial migration of leukocytes in the physiologically relevant basolateral to luminal direction. Again, interactions between epithelial ICAM-1 and β2 integrins contribute to this process but blockade of either ICAM-1 or of β2 integrins does not lead to complete inhibition.[24] Other counter-ligands for β2 integrins on epithelial cells have been sought with mixed success. There is evidence that β2 integrins bind to oligosaccharide determinants on epithelial cells. For example, heparin and heparan sulfate

proteoglycans can bind CD11/CD18, although whether this is a major event on epithelial cells is unclear. Fucosylated proteoglycans also bind to β2 integrins and play a role in neutrophil adhesion to intestinal epithelial cells, but these data have not yet been extended to airway epithelial cells.[25] Interestingly, the junction adhesion molecule, JAM-C, binds specifically to CD11b/CD18 on neutrophils. In contrast to other JAM family proteins, JAM-C is not expressed at the tight junction, but is a component of epithelial desmosomes. Both antibodies against JAM-C and JAM-C fusion proteins were shown to inhibit neutrophil transepithelial migration across intestinal epithelial cells but, again, these studies have not yet been extended to airway epithelium.[26]

■ EPITHELIAL CELLS AND AIRWAY REMODELING ■

Airway remodeling, characterized by increased smooth muscle mass, goblet cell metaplasia, angiogenesis, and increased subepithelial deposition of matrix proteins, is a hallmark of asthma even in relatively young children. Given that marked remodeling is not observed in allergic rhinitis, allergic inflammation per se is clearly not sufficient to trigger these processes. Among possible explanations for the restriction of remodeling to the lower airways is the concept that mechanical strain induced by hyperventilation or bronchoconstriction contributes to changes in the function of epithelial cells and other structural cell types in the lower airways.[27] Aberrant epithelial damage and repair is also a feature of asthma, and it has been suggested that bidirectional communication between regenerating epithelial cells and myofibroblasts plays a major role in the remodeling process.[28] The epithelium is a significant source of a number of growth factors that can act on several cell types within the airways. Bronchial epithelial cells express several members of the epidermal growth factor (EGF) family, including EGF, heparin binding epidermal growth factor (HB-EGF), transforming growth factor-α (TGF-α), and amphiregulin. The epithelium also expresses three members of the epithelial growth factor receptor (EGFR) family (c-erbB1, c-erbB2, and c-erbB3), and members of the EGF family of growth factors are major regulators of epithelial proliferation, differentiation and repair. Interestingly, epithelial expression both of EGF and EGFR is increased in asthma.[9] Stem cell factor (SCF) also is produced by the epithelium, and levels of SCF correlate with numbers of epithelial mast cells in the upper airways. In culture, epithelial cells constitutively produce vascular endothelial growth factor (VEGF) and this is enhanced in response to respiratory viral infections.[29] VEGF production could play a major role in angiogenesis and increased vascular permeability in asthma. Epithelial cells in the process of repair, or in response to other stimuli, elaborate a variety of growth factors that enhance proliferation of fibroblast and differentiation of these cells into activated myofibroblasts. These include several isoforms of transforming growth factor-β (TGF-β), insulin-like growth factor, platelet-derived growth factor, and basic fibroblast growth factor, as well as peptides such as endothelin. It has been reported that TGF-β1, but not other TGF-β isoforms, enhances the speed of epithelial wound repair. Interestingly in a murine model of allergen-induced airway remodeling, the airway epithelium was found to be the main source of TGF-β1 within the airway wall.[30] Epithelial production of endothelin and TGF-β increase in response to mechanical stress.

The epithelium is also a significant source of proteases that can act on airway structural proteins. Although this includes proteinases such as cathepsin B, particular interest is focused on members of the family of zinc-dependent matrix metalloproteinases (MMPs) which, collectively, can degrade all components of the extracellular matrix. Epithelial cells produce MMP-2 (collagenase A), MMP-7 (matrilysin), MMP-9 (gelatinase B), and MMP-12 (metalloelastase). In the context of allergic airway disease, MMP-9 is the dominant MMP in the airways.[31] MMP-9 is strongly expressed in repairing bronchial epithelial cells and can be induced in response to activation of proteinase-activated receptor 2, and by proinflammatory cytokines. Levels of MMP-9 are increased in blood, sputum, BAL fluids and biopsies of asthmatic subjects and in BAL after allergen challenge. Epithelial cells also produce tissue inhibitor of metalloproteinases (TIMP)-1, the major inhibitor of MMP-9, but the ratio of MMP-9 to TIMP-1 is increased by proinflammatory stimuli and also in the airways during acute asthma exacerbations. This increased activity of MMP-9 to TIMP-1 favors airway remodeling. In addition to having direct effects on matrix proteins, MMP-9 activates $TGF-\beta_1$, which, as noted above, is a key regulator of fibrotic processes.

Epithelial cells can also contribute to matrix protein deposition in the airways. They produce both fibronectin and tenascin, and production of these proteins is markedly upregulated at sites of epithelial injury and repair. Epithelial cell expression of tenascin and fibronectin is modulated by cytokine exposure and reduced, if not completely normalized, following anti-IL-5 antibody administration in a clinical trial in asthmatic subjects. Moreover, expression of immunoreactive tenascin increases, and correlates with disease severity, in asthma.[32] Fibronectin serves not only as a substrate for cell adhesion during tissue repair but also is chemotactic for both fibroblasts and epithelial cells.

EPITHELIAL CELLS AND HOST DEFENSE

The epithelium plays a critical role in host defense to inhaled microorganisms. Attachment of pathogens to specific binding sites on the epithelial cell surface is the initiating event for infection of the airways, and the mucosal surface of the normal human airways is highly adapted to prevent, or minimize, such interactions. In addition to producing cytokines and chemokines that regulate the inflammatory response (see above), protective functions include the role of the mucociliary clearance system, as well as the ability of the epithelium to contribute to both innate and specific immune responses to pathogens.

MUCOCILIARY CLEARANCE/BARRIER FUNCTION

An important aspect of the clearance of inhaled pathogens entails the trapping of the microbe in mucus and subsequent clearance of mucus by ciliary movement and by cough. In the more distal airways of the lower respiratory tract, where cilia are absent, clearance occurs primarily by coughing or via phagocytosis by macrophages. In these distal airways, surfactants, produced by both Clara cells and by type II epithelial cells, increase the efficiency of coughing as a clearance mechanism by altering surface charge properties of pathogens, rendering them 'less sticky'. In the upper airways, and in the more proximal airways of the lower respiratory tract, where ciliated cells predominate, mucociliary clearance

moves airway secretions to the nasopharynx or oropharynx where they can be swallowed or expectorated. The importance of mucociliary clearance in removing pathogens is emphasized by conditions in which aspects of this pathway are compromised. For example, patients with primary ciliary dyskinesia experience recurrent upper and lower respiratory infections, chronic bronchitis, and chronic rhinosinusitis. The ability of the gel phase of mucus to capture particulates and pathogens, and the viscoelastic nature of mucus, is due in large part to a high content of mucins. These are heavily glycosylated, high molecular weight, complex glycoproteins. Thus far, 18 different human mucin genes have been cloned and at least 12 of these are expressed at the mRNA level in the human airways.[33] The majority of these mucins contain transmembrane domains and are, therefore, membrane-tethered. In the healthy lung, for example, MUC1 and MUC4 are expressed at the apical portion of the respiratory epithelium. By contrast to these membrane-linked mucins, secreted mucins lack the transmembrane domain. Four of these secreted mucins (MUC2, MUC5AC, MUC5B, and MUC6) contain cysteine-rich domains that facilitate the oligomerization necessary for gel formation. Of these, MUC5AC and MUC5B are the dominant mucins expressed in the airways, with MUC2 being present in lower amounts. In healthy individuals, MUC5AC is the predominant mucin in goblet cells, while MUC5B is present in glandular mucosal cells.[33] Both of these mucins are present in higher levels in sputum from subjects with asthma, chronic bronchitis or cystic fibrosis (CF) compared to normal subjects. Several studies have examined regulation of mRNA for mucins. It must be noted, however, that transcriptional regulation does not always lead to increased levels of mucin proteins. For example, MUC2 gene expression is markedly increased in CF airways, but MUC2 protein is barely detectable.[34] Although various bacteria, viral dsRNA, and numerous cytokines and mediators, including $TNF-\alpha$, $IL-\beta$, IL-9, 15-HETE, and PGE_2, all increase MUC5AC mRNA expression, considerable attention has focused on regulation by Th2 cytokines, particularly IL-13. In murine models, IL-13 increases goblet cell metaplasia and is associated with an increase in Muc5ac (the murine homolog of MUC5AC) mRNA expression, but the main function of IL-13 may be to initiate epithelial differentiation to goblet cells, which then constitutively express Muc5ac as a characteristic product. In cell culture systems, IL-4 does not upregulate MUC5AC/Muc5ac. Although IL-13 did activate a Muc5ac promoter-luciferase construct transfected into a murine Clara cell line, it did not upregulate MUC5AC mRNA expression in either differentiated normal human bronchial epithelial cells or in various cell lines.[33,35]

The carbohydrate components of mucins are diverse in structure. This structural diversity may have arisen as an added host defense mechanism to trap microorganisms in the mucus layer. Thus, recognition sites exist on mucin carbohydrate moieties for adhesins and/or hemagglutinins from several pathogens, including *Haemophilus influenzae, Streptococcus pneumoniae, Staphylococcus aureus, Mycoplasma pneumoniae, Pseudomonas aeruginosa*, and influenza virus.[36,37]

Proteases and peptides derived both from host cells or inhaled pathogens can have profound effects on epithelial function and on airway structural cells. For example, while recruitment and activation of neutrophils and other inflammatory cells is an important component of the host response to inhaled pathogens, overproduction of proteases can have deleterious effects. To protect the airway from excessive protease effects, epithelial cells produce protease inhibitors, including secretory leukocyte protease inhibitor (SLPI), and elafin that regulate the effects of neutrophil elastase on cytokine production, glycoconjugate production, and tissue damage. Administration of SLPI, the major elastase activity in the large airways, to patients with cystic fibrosis (CF) reduces both elastase activity and IL-8 levels in airway secretions.[38] Elafin selectively inhibits elastase and proteinase 3, and is also called elastase-specific inhibitor (ESI). By contrast, SLPI can limit the actions of multiple proteases, including cathepsin G, mast cell chymase, and enzymes with tryptic and chymotryptic specificity. The broad inhibitory function of epithelial cells is further enhanced by production of cystatin C, α_1-antiprotease inhibitor, and α_1-antichymotrypsin. Expression of several of these inhibitors increases in response to proinflammatory cytokines.[39] Epithelial cells also express cell-surface peptidases, such as neutral endopeptidase and aminopeptidase M that can degrade and regulate the actions of several biologically active peptides produced as part of the inflammatory response.[40]

■ EPITHELIUM AND INNATE IMMUNITY ■

PATHOGEN BINDING AND RECOGNITION

As noted above, pathogens must bind to specific sites on epithelial cells to initiate infection. Most viruses accomplish this by using as specific receptors molecules expressed on epithelial cells that serve important roles in host cell biology. A list of some major viral receptors is shown in Table 23.2. They include a variety of cell-surface adhesion molecules, integrins and enzymes, as well as carbohydrates with specific structural properties. In some instances, however, tight junction components can also be utilized. The reovirus attachment protein σ1 interacts with the junctional adhesion molecule JAM-1 to initiate infection, while adenoviruses can interact with the Coxsackie adenovirus receptor (CAR), which is situated basal to the tight junction. Presumably, this latter interaction occurs when there is damage to epithelial integrity.

Table 23.2 Epithelial virus receptors

Receptor	Virus
ICAM-1	Rhinovirus (major group)
LDL/VLDL receptor family	Rhinovirus (minor group)
Aminopeptidase M (CD13)	Coronavirus 229E strain
Angiotensin-converting enzyme-2	SARS coronavirus
9-O-acetylated sialic acid also HLA class I	Coronavirus OC43 strain
Glycans with terminal $\alpha_{2,6}$ or $\alpha_{2,3}$ sialic acid	Influenza
$\alpha_v\beta_5$ integrin/CAR/CD80/CD86 heparan sulfate glycosaminoglycans	Adenoviruses
$\alpha_2\beta_1$ integrin	Echoviruses
Junctional adhesion molecule-1	Reovirus

ICAM-1, intercellular adhesion molecule 1; LDL, low-density lipoprotein; VLDL very-low-density lipoprotein; SARS, severe acute respiratory syndrome; CAR, Coxsackie adenovirus receptor.

The molecular basis by which bacteria attach to epithelial cells is better understood for some strains than for others. In the case of *Pseudomonas aeruginosa*, the major pathogen commonly associated with CF, the bacterium expresses proteins, known as pilins and flagellins that function as ligands for cell attachment. The type-4 pilus protein is a particularly important adhesin for attachment via interaction with asialylated glycosphingolipid receptors, such as asiaoloGM1, on epithelial cells.[41] Epithelial expression of such receptors is increased in CF.[42]

To counteract infections the epithelium must rapidly induce gene products required for host innate immune defense (for more details on innate immunity, see Chapter 2). This is accomplished via the recognition of various pathogen-associated molecular patterns (PAMPS) found in bacteria and viruses. Pattern-recognition receptors can be present in secretions in a soluble form, such as mannan-binding lectin, or can be cell associated, such as the Toll-like receptors (TLR). To date, 10 TLR family members (TLR1-10) have been identified in humans.[43] Epithelial cells express all 10 TLRs at the level of mRNA, but full analysis of protein expression has not yet been conducted.[44] The ability of epithelial cells to respond to a variety of selective bacterial ligands for TLRs, however, has been examined. A range of epithelial responses can be induced upon exposure to a variety of bacterial lipopolysaccharides. Despite the fact that responses to this TLR4 ligand are seen, it must be noted that airway epithelial responses to LPS are generally modest. Epithelial cytokine induction also occurs in response to TLR2 ligands, such as peptidoglycan from *Staphylococcus aureus,* and zymosan from *Saccharomyces cerevisiae*.[44] TLR5 protein is expressed on human tracheal epithelium and binds flagellins from several bacterial strains.[45] Considerable evidence shows that epithelial cells express TLR3, which recognizes viral double-stranded RNA (dsRNA), an intermediate generated during viral replication.[46] Although numerous studies have shown epithelial cell responses to synthetic dsRNA, some controversies exist regarding viral sensing in epithelial cells. This is important considering the major role played by respiratory viruses in inducing exacerbations of asthma and COPD.[47] Although some studies have indicated the presence of cell-surface TLR3,[44] others comparing permeabilized to intact cells suggest that TLR3 is predominantly intracellular.[48] In support of this, transfection of dsRNA is much more potent in inducing cellular responses than extracellular application.[14] Although synthetic dsRNA triggers TLR3-mediated signaling, controversy remains regarding the role of TLR3 in endogenous viral responses. While TLR3 appears to play a role in some aspects of epithelial cell responses to influenza A virus and respiratory syncytial virus,[48] TLR3-deficient mice show no alterations in the host adaptive antiviral responses to several viruses.[49] Moreover, fibroblasts derived from TLR3-deficient mice retain responses to dsRNA.[50] This may be explained by the recent identification of additional intracellular sensors for dsRNA.[51,52] Retinoic acid-inducible gene I (RIG I) and melanoma differentiation-associated gene 5 (mda5) are DExD/H-Box helicases. The helicase domains of these proteins interact with dsRNA, while caspase recruitment and activation domains (CARD) are responsible for activation of downstream signaling processes mediated via a mitochondrial adaptor protein known by four different names: Cardif, VISA, MAVS, and IPS-1 (Fig. 23.3).[53] Human airway epithelial cells not only express TLR3 but also RIG-I and Cardif (S Traves and D Proud, unpublished data). It has been suggested that these helicases may have differential roles in recognizing dsRNA derived from different types of RNA viruses, but additional studies are needed to clarify this.[54]

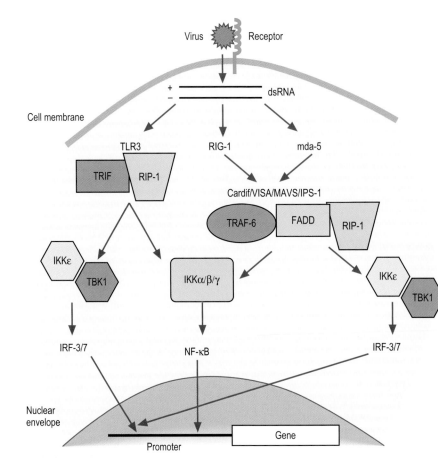

Fig. 23.3. Intracellular recognition pathways for viral double-stranded RNA (dsRNA). After viral entry and uncoating, dsRNA is produced during replication. The molecules capable of interacting with dsRNA are Toll-like receptor 3 (TLR3), retinoic acid-inducible gene-I (RIG-I) and melanoma differentiation antigen-5 (mda-5). Interactions with these molecules may vary depending on cell context and the specific viral type. Interaction with TLR3 leads to upregulation of antiviral genes because TLR3, via the signal adaptor proteins Toll-receptor domain-containing adaptor inducing IFN-β (TRIF) and receptor-interacting protein-1 (RIP-1), can activate both the classical NF-κB pathway, as well as IKK-ε and Tank binding kinase (TBK1). This leads to nuclear translocation of NF-κB and interferon regulatory factors (IRF)-3 and-7. If dsRNA is detected by either RIG-I or mda-5, the adaptor protein known as Cardif, VISA, MAVS or IPS-1 triggers the same transcriptional activation pathways via the downstream signaling proteins TNF receptor-associated factor 6 (TRAF-6), Fas-associated death-domain protein (FADD), and RIP-1.

ANTIMICROBIAL ACTIVITIES

Another aspect of the epithelial contribution to host defense is the production of antimicrobial products, several of which are further induced upon exposure to pathogens (Fig. 23.4).[55] Lysozyme and lactoferrin are derived from serous epithelial cells, are present in high levels in mucosal secretions, and have direct antibacterial activities. Human lysozyme is a 1,4-β-N-acetylmuramidase that kills several Gram-positive microorganisms by enzymatically degrading a glycosidic linkage in the bacterial surface-exposed peptidoglycan. By contrast, many Gram-negative bacteria are resistant to the effects of lysozyme alone because they possess an outer envelope that prevents the enzyme from reaching the peptidoglycan murein sacculus. It is well known that lactoferrin is a high-affinity chelator of iron, depriving bacteria of this essential nutrient, but lactoferrin also has other, direct bactericidal properties, including altering the outer membrane of Gram-negative bacteria.[56] The

combination of lactoferrin and lysozyme, therefore, is more bactericidal than either alone, as the membrane-altering properties of lactoferrin permit lysozyme to penetrate this envelope and cleave the bacterial peptidoglycan.[57] Lactoferrin also enhances the activity of secretory IgA. The protease inhibitors SLPI and elafin display broad-spectrum antimicrobial actions. Lysozyme, lactoferrin, and SLPI are the 3 most abundant antimicrobials in airway lining fluid and display synergistic antimicrobial actions.[58] Among other antimicrobials, secretory phospholipase A2 likely acts via phospholipid degradation within bacterial membranes.[59] In the distal airways, Clara cells and type II cells release surfactant proteins (SP), including SP-A and SP-D, which are members of the collectin family of proteins that have carbohydrate recognition domains (CRD). Both SP-A and SP-D bind, via their CRD regions, to carbohydrates on the surface of a broad range of Gram-positive and Gram-negative bacteria.[60] Depending on the specific carbohydrate interaction and the target bacteria, this leads to killing via permeabilization,

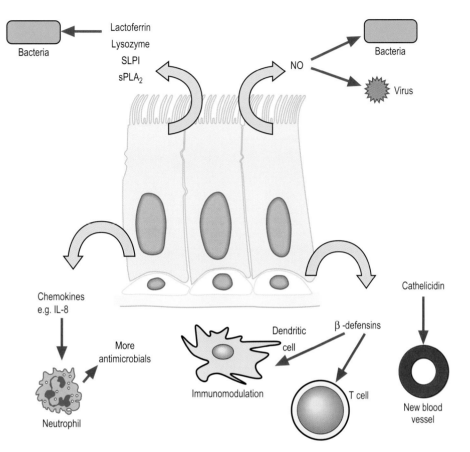

Fig. 23.4. Antimicrobial products of epithelial cells. The epithelium produces a number of proteins, including lysozyme, lactoferrin, secretory leukocyte proteinase inhibitor (SLPI), and soluble phospholipase A_2 ($sPLA_2$) that have broad-ranging antibacterial actions and that function synergistically to kill both Gram-positive and Gram-negative bacteria. Nitric oxide (NO) has both antibacterial and antiviral properties and can directly inhibit the replication of several common respiratory viruses. The release of chemokines, such as IL-8 (CXCL8), will recruit neutrophils that release additional antimicrobials, including α-defensins. The epithelial peptides, β-defensins and cathelicidin, are antibacterial but also exert angiogenic (cathelicidin) and immunomodulatory (β-defensins) properties at lower concentrations. β-Defensins recruit and activate both dendritic cells and memory T cells and can, thereby, link innate and specific immunity.

agglutination, enhanced opsonization by phagocytic cells or increasing the respiratory burst by macrophages and neutrophils. SP-A and SP-D also have antiviral actions. For example, SP-D inhibits influenza virus infection by inducing aggregation of viral particles and inhibiting the activities of the viral hemagglutinin and neuraminidase. SP-A acts as an opsonin for RSV by binding to the F (fusion) and G (attachment) glycoproteins on the virion surface, inhibiting infectivity and enhancing phagocytosis by macrophages.[60]

Epithelial cells also release several antimicrobial peptides, including defensins. Defensins are small (3–6 kDa), cationic antimicrobial peptides characterized structurally by the presence of six cysteine residues that form three intramolecular disulfide bonds. The two main subfamilies of α- and β-defensins are defined based on the pairing of cysteines in these disulfide bridges.[61] Although genomic analysis suggests the presence of a large number of potentially expressed defensin genes, six members of the human α-defensin family and four human β-defensins have, thus far, been characterized at the protein level. While the α-defensins are expressed primarily in neutrophils and intestinal Paneth cells, airway epithelial cells are a rich source of β-defensins.[62] Epithelial expression of β-defensins is increased in response to several cytokines, most notably IL-17, as well as by infection with rhinovirus and exposure to bacterial products. The cationic, amphipathic nature of defensins is critical to microbicidal activity against bacteria and fungi. It is suggested that bacterial membrane depolarization by defensins contributes to rapid killing of bacteria, with additional killing occurring via peptide-mediated activation of cell-wall lytic enzymes.[63] Defensins show synergistic antimicrobial activity with other host defense molecules, including lysozyme and lactoferrin. Human β-defensin-3 inhibits influenza infection by blocking membrane fusion mediated by the viral hemagglutinin.[64] Defensins also have a broad range of immunomodulatory activities,[65] and have been suggested to provide an important link between innate and specific immunity to viral infections, particularly via their ability to recruit immature dendritic cells.[66]

Another low molecular weight antimicrobial with immunomodulatory functions is the cathelicidin LL-37.[65] This peptide is expressed constitutively in airway epithelium but expression is upregulated by inflammatory stimuli. Mice deficient in the murine homolog of this peptide show more prominent bacterial infections.[55] Interestingly, LL-37 binds to formyl-peptide receptor-like 1 on endothelial cells to induce angiogenesis, suggesting this peptide may also contribute to remodeling.[67]

Finally, among the antimicrobial products of epithelial cells, it is important to consider the role of nitric oxide (NO). Epithelial cells express mRNA for all 3 isoforms of the enzyme nitric oxide synthase (NOS), but the inducible enzyme (iNOS) is the predominant form. NO is a potent antibacterial functioning in concert with reactive oxygen species, such as superoxide (which can also be produced by the epithelium), to damage bacterial DNA, protein, and lipids. Viral infection can induce epithelial expression of iNOS and, during experimental rhinovirus infections in vivo, levels of epithelial iNOS induction correlate with levels of exhaled NO.[68] Subjects with the highest levels of exhaled NO cleared virus more rapidly and had fewer symptoms. Consistent with these observations, NO not only exerts direct antiviral activities activity against several common respiratory viruses but also inhibits virally-induced generation of several cytokines/chemokines from epithelial cells.[69] Moreover, inhibition, or genetic inactivation/deletion, of iNOS enhances the susceptibility of experimental animals to microbial infection and leads to a worse outcome to infection. Interestingly, epithelial cells from patients with cystic fibrosis have a markedly impaired capacity to produce iNOS, a defect that has been suggested to contribute to the increased susceptibility of such patients to repeated airway infections.[70]

EPITHELIAL CELLS AND IMMUNOREGULATION

Epithelial cells play a much broader role in immune modulation than previously appreciated. In addition to the innate responses presented above, epithelial cells clearly play a role in mucosal immunity via the production of secretory IgA. Importantly, they play an important role in linking innate and specific immunity via modulation of dendritic cell (DC) function.[71] Both human β-defensins (HBD) and the chemokine CCL20 produced by epithelial cells are ligands for the CCR6 chemokine receptor expressed on immature DC but not on $CD14^+$ DC precursors or mature DC. HBD are chemotactic for immature DCs at concentrations much lower than those needed for antimicrobial activity.[65] Production of HBD and CCL20 in response to pathogens would recruit immature DCs to the airway and enhance antigen capture. Depending on the spectrum of epithelial cell products generated under specific conditions, epithelial cells can differentially regulate DC function. For example, production of $TGF-\beta_1$, IL-10, and/or NO would inhibit antigen presentation and DC activation. PGE_2 also inhibits DC activation while favoring Th2 responses.[71] Particular interest has focused, however, on the role of TSLP in the regulation of DC function.[72] TSLP is an IL-7-like cytokine produced mainly by barrier epithelial cells. Expression of TSLP is increased in the airways of asthmatic subjects and correlates with symptom severity. TSLP not only activates human myeloid DCs but also markedly influences the outcomes of interactions between DCs and $CD4^+$ thymocytes and T cells. Interestingly, TSLP activates DC in a manner that does not induce production of IL-12. As a result of this, TSLP-activated DCs favor a Th2 permissive environment and stimulate $CD4^+$ T cell-mediated allergic inflammation.[73]

In terms of adaptive immunity, epithelial cells display surface expression of several molecules classically associated with antigen presentation, including major histocompatability complex (MHC) class I and class II molecules, and CD40. Class I expression can be enhanced by

viral infections,[74] while epithelial expression of class II MHC is increased in patients with allergic rhinitis or asthma.[75] Epithelial cells also express co-stimulatory molecules associated with optimal T cell activation. There are conflicting reports on whether epithelial cells express B7-1 (CD80) and B7-2 (CD86), but expression of other B7 homologs, B7-H1, B7-H2, B7-H3, and B7-DC, has recently been demonstrated on primary airway epithelial cells and/or on epithelial cell lines.[76] Blockade of B7-H1 enhanced lymphocyte responses in co-culture, suggesting that this B7 homolog inhibits T cell function. By contrast, ICAM-1, which is expressed on the epithelial cell surface in enhanced levels in asthma, can interact with its counter-receptor, LFA-1, on T cells to stimulate lymphocyte proliferation and regulate Th2 cytokine production.[77] Indeed, several studies show that epithelial cells can initiate T cell signaling and proliferation. Airway epithelial cells can internalize antigen and act in the context of class II MHC as antigen-presenting cells in vitro,[78,79] while intestinal epithelial cells have been shown to present influenza virus antigens in the context of class I MHC to antigen-specific $CD8^+$ cytotoxic T cells.[80] Although these studies are intriguing, further work is required to fully define the role of epithelial cells in antigen-specific immune responses.

■ SUMMARY ■

The epithelial cell exhibits a broad range of complex functions. It not only serves an important barrier function but also generates a wide variety of products that can modulate airway tone, vascular permeability, and airway remodeling, regulate the content of airway secretions, control inflammatory cell recruitment to the airways, and contribute to host immune responses. The airway epithelium almost certainly contributes to the pathogenesis of the allergic response and asthma. Given the high metabolic function of the epithelial cell, and the fact that it is the first cell type to be exposed to inhaled medications, the epithelium may be a primary target of such drugs. Thus, a better understanding of the dynamic properties of the airway epithelium during allergic events may provide additional targets for therapeutic interventions.

References

Epithelial anatomy and phenotype

1. Avril-Delplanque A, Casal I, Castillon N, et al. Aquaporin-3 expression in human fetal airway progenitor cells. Stem Cells 2005; 23:992.

Cell–cell adhesion and communication

2. Schneeberger EE, Lynch RD. The tight junction: a multifunctional complex. Am J Physiol Cell Physiol 2004; 286: C1213, 2004.
3. Van Itallie CM, Anderson JM. Claudins and epithelial paracellular transport. Annu Rev Physiol 2006; 68:403.
4. Wan H, Winton HL, Soeller C, et al. The transmembrane protein occludin of epithelial tight junctions is a functional target for serine proteins from faecal pellets of Dermatophagoides pteronyssinus. Clin Exp Allergy 2001; 31:279.
5. South AP. Plakophilin 1: an important stabilizer of desmosomes. Clin Exp Dermatol 2004; 29:161.
6. Sheppard D. Functions of pulmonary epithelial integrins: from development to disease. Physiol Rev 2003; 83:673.
7. Lackie PM, Baker JE, Günthert U, et al. Expression of CD44 isoforms is increased in the airway epithelium of asthmatic subjects. Am J Respir Cell Mol Biol 1997; 16:14.
8. Giepmans BN. Gap junctions and connexin-interacting proteins. Cardiovasc Res 2004; 62:233.

Epithelial changes in asthma

9. Knight DA, Holgate ST. The airway epithelium: structural and functional properties in health and disease. Respirology 2003; 8:432.

Epithelial cells and airway inflammation

10. Kumlin M, Hamberg M, Granström E, et al. 15(S)-hydroxyeicosatetraenoic acid is the major arachidonic acid metabolite in human bronchi: association with airway epithelium. Arch Biochem Biophys 1990; 282:254.
11. Churchill L, Chilton FH, Resau JH, et al. Cyclooxygenase metabolism of endogenous arachidonic acid by cultured human tracheal epithelial cells. Am Rev Respir Dis 1989; 140:449.
12. Pavord ID, Wong CS, Williams J, et al. Effect of inhaled prostaglandin E2 on allergen-induced asthma. Am Rev Respir Dis 1993; 148:87.
13. Goldie RG, Henry PJ. Endothelins and asthma. Life Sci 1999; 65:1.
14. Spurrell JCL, Wiehler S, Zaheer RS, et al. Human airway epithelial cells produce IP-10 (CXCL10) in vitro and in vivo upon rhinovirus infection. Am J Physiol Lung Cell Mol Physiol 289:L85, 2005.
15. Venge J, Lampinen M, Hakansson L, et al. Identification of IL-5 and RANTES as the major eosinophilic chemoattractants in the human lung. J Allergy Clin Immunol 1996; 97:1110.
16. Beck LA, Tancowny B, Brummet ME, et al. Functional analysis of the chemokine receptor CCR3 on airway epithelial cells. J Immunol 2006; 177:3344.
17. Kelsen SG, Aksoy MO, Yang Y, et al. The chemokine receptor CXCR3 and its splice variant are expressed in human airway epithelial cells. Am J Physiol Lung Cell Mol Physiol 2004; 287:L584.
18. DiCosmo BF, Geba GP, Picarella D, et al. Airway epithelial cell expression of interleukin-6 in transgenic mice: uncoupling of airway inflammation and bronchial hyperreactivity. J Clin Invest 1994; 94:2028.
19. Ray P, Tang W, Wang P, et al. Regulated overexpression of interleukin-11 in the lung. Use to dissociate development-dependent and -independent phenotypes. J Clin Invest 1997; 100:2501.
20. Wark PAB, Johnston SL, Bucchieri F, et al. Asthmatic bronchial epithelial cells have a deficient innate immune response to infection with rhinovirus. J Exp Med 2005; 201:937.
21. Contoli M, Message SD, Laza-Stanca V, et al. Role of deficient type-III interferon-lamda production in asthma exacerbations. Nat Med 2006; 12:1023.

Leukocyte–epithelial interactions

22. Tosi MF, Hamedani A, Brosovich J, et al. ICAM-1-independent, CD18-dependent adhesion between neutrophils and human airway epithelial cells exposed in vitro to ozone. J Immunol 1994, 152:1935.
23. Bullard DC, Qin L, Lorenzo I, et al. P-selectin/ICAM-1 double mutant mice: acute emigration of neutrophils into the peritoneum is completely absent but is normal into pulmonary alveoli. J Clin Invest 1995; 95:1782.
24. Kidney JC, Proud D. Neutrophil transmigration across human airway epithelial monolayers; mechanisms and dependence on electrical resistance. Am J Respir Cell Mol Biol 2000; 23:389.
25. Zen K, Parkos CA. Leukocyte-epithelial interactions. Curr Opin Cell Biol 2003; 15:557.
26. Zen K, Babbin BA, Liu Y, et al. JAM-C is a component of desmosomes and a ligand for CD11b/CD18-mediated neutrophil transepithelial migration. Mol Biol Cell 2004; 15:3926.

Epithelial cells and airway remodeling

27. Tschumperlin DJ, Drazen JM. Chronic effects of mechanical force on airways. Annu Rev Physiol 2006; 68:563.
28. Holgate ST, Davies DE, Lackie PM, et al. Epithelial-mesenchymal interactions in the pathogenesis of asthma. J Allergy Clin Immunol 2000; 105:193.
29. Psarras S, Volonaki E, Skevaki CL, et al. Vascular endothelial growth factor-mediated induction of angiogenesis by human rhinovirus. J Allergy Clin Immunol 2006; 117:291.
30. Kelly MM, Leigh R, Bonniaud P, et al. Epithelial expression of profibrotic mediators in a model of allergen-induced airway remodeling. Am J Respir Cell Mol Biol 2005; 32:99.
31. Cohn L, Elias JA, Chupp GL. Asthma: mechanisms of disease persistence and progression. Annu Rev Immunol 2004; 22:789.
32. Laitinen A, Altraja A, Kämpe M, et al. Tenascin is increased in airway basement membrane of asthmatics and decreased by an inhaled steroid. Am J Respir Crit Care Med 1997; 156:951.

Epithelial cells and host defense

33. Rose MC, Voynow JA. Respiratory tract mucin genes and mucin glycoproteins in health and disease. Physiol Rev 2006, 86:2006.
34. Thornton DJ, Sheehan JK. From mucins to mucus. Towards a more coherent understanding of this essential barrier. Proc Am Thorac Soc 2004; 1:54.
35. Chen Y, Thai P, Zhao YH, et al. Stimulation of airway mucin gene expression by interleukin (IL)-17 through IL-6 paracrine/autocrine loop. J Biol Chem 2003; 278:17036.
36. Lamblin G, Aubert JP, Perini JM, et al. Human respiratory mucins. Eur Respir J 1992; 5:247.

37. Plotkowski MC, Bajolet-Laudinet O, Puchelle E. Cellular and molecular mechanisms of bacterial adhesion to respiratory mucosa. Eur Respir J 1993; 6:903.
38. McElvaney NG, Nakamura H, Birrer P, et al. Modulation of airway inflammation in cystic fibrosis. In vivo suppression of interleukin-8 levels on the respiratory epithelial surface by aerosolization of recombinant secretory leukoprotease inhibitor. J Clin Invest 1992; 90:1296.
39. Sallenave J-M, Shulmann J, Crossley J, et al. Regulation of secretory leukocyte proteinase inhibitor (SLPI) and elastase-specific inhibitor (ESI/elafin) in human airway epithelial cells by cytokines and neutrophilic enzymes. Am J Respir Cell Mol Biol 1994; 11:733.
40. Proud D, Subauste MC, Ward PE. Glucocorticoids do not alter peptidase expression on a human bronchial epithelial cell line. Am J Respir Cell Mol Biol 1994; 11:57.

Epithelium and innate immunity

41. Hahn HP. The type-4 pilus is the major virulence-associated adhesin of Pseudomonas aeruginosa – a review. Gene 1997; 192:99.
42. Saiman L, Prince A. Pseudomonas aeruginosa pili bind to asialoGM1 which is increased on the surface of cystic fibrosis epithelial cells. J Clin Invest 1993; 92:1875.
43. Kaisho T, Akira S. Toll-like receptor function and signaling. J Allergy Clin Immunol 2006; 117:979.
44. Sha Q, Truong-Tran AQ, Plitt JR, et al. Activation of airway epithelial cells by Toll-like receptor agonists. Am J Respir Cell Mol Biol 2004; 31:358.
45. Zhang Z, Louboutin JP, Weiner DJ, et al. Human airway epithelial cells sense Pseudomonas aeruginosa infection via recognition of flagellin by Toll-like receptor 5. Infect Immun 2005; 73:7151.
46. Alexopoulou L, Holt AC, Medzhitov R, et al. Recognition of double-stranded RNA and activation of NF-κB by Toll-like receptor 3. Nature 2001; 413:732.
47. Proud D, Chow C-W. Role of viral infections in asthma and COPD. Am J Respir Cell Mol Biol 35:in press, 2006.
48. Guillot L, Le Goffic R, Bloch S, et al. Involvement of Toll-like receptor 3 in the immune response of lung epithelial cells to double-stranded RNA and influenza A virus. J Biol Chem 2005; 280:5571.
49. Edelmann KH, Richardson-Burns S, Alexopoulou L, et al. Does Toll-like receptor 3 play a biological role in virus infections? Virology 2004; 322:231.
50. Hemmi H, Takeuchi O, Sato S, et al. The roles of two IκB kinase-related kinases in lipopolysaccharide and double stranded RNA signaling and viral infection. J Exp Med 2004; 199:1641.
51. Yoneyama M, Kikuchi M, Natsukawa T, et al. The RNA helicase RIG-I has an essential function in double-stranded RNA-induced innate antiviral responses. Nat Immunol 2004; 5:730.
52. Andrejeva J, Childs KS, F YD, et al. The V proteins of paramyxoviruses bind the IFN-inducible RNA helicase, mda-5, and inhibit its activation of the IFN-β promoter. Proc Natl Acad Sci USA 2004; 101:17264.
53. Hiscott J, Lin R, Nakhaei P, et al. MasterCARD. a priceless link to innate immunity. Trends Mol Med 2006; 12:53.
54. Kato H, Takeuchi O, Sato S, et al. Differential roles of MDA5 and RIG-I helicases in the recognition of RNA viruses. Nature 2006; 414:101.
55. Bals R, Hiemstra PS. Innate immunity in the lung; how epithelial cells fight against respiratory pathogens. Eur Respir J 2004; 23:327.
56. Ellison RTI, Giehl TJ, LaForce FM. Damage of the outer membrane of enteric Gram-negative bacteria by lactoferrin and transferrin. Infect Immun 1988; 56:2774.
57. Ellison RTI, Giehl TJ. Killing of Gram-negative bacteria by lactoferrin and lysozyme. J Clin Invest 1991; 88: 1081–1091.
58. Travis SM, Singh PK, Welsh MJ. Antimicrobial peptides and proteins in the innate defense of the airway surface. Curr Opin Immunol 2001; 13:89.
59. Ganz T. Antimicrobial proteins and peptides in host defense. Semin Respir Infect 2001; 16:4.
60. Kishore U, Greenhough TJ, Waters P, et al. Surfactant proteins SP-A and SP-D. Structure, function and receptors. Mol Immunol 2006; 43:1293.
61. Schneider JJ, Unholzer A, Schaller M, et al. Human defensins. J Mol Med 2005; 83:587.
62. Schutte BC, McCray PBJ. [beta]-defensins in lung host defense. Annu Rev Physiol 2002; 64:709.
63. Sahl H-G, Pag U, Bonness S, et al. Mammalian defensins: structures and mechanism of antibiotic activity. J Leukoc Biol 2005; 77:466.
64. Leikina E, Delanoe-Ayari H, Melikov K, et al. Carbohydrate-binding molecules inhibit viral fusion and entry by crosslinking membrane glycoproteins. Nature Immunol 2005; 6:995.
65. Yang D, Biragyn A, Hoover DM, et al. Multiple roles of antimicrobial defensins, cathelicidins, and eosinophil-derived neurotoxin in host defense. Annu Rev Immunol 2004; 22:181.
66. Proud D. The role of defensins in virus-induced asthma. Curr Allergy Asthma Rep 2006; 6:81.
67. Koczulla R, von Degenfeld G, Kupatt C, et al. An angiogenic role for the human peptide antibiotic LL-37/hCAP-18. J Clin Invest 2003; 111:1665.
68. Sanders SP, Proud D, Siekierski ES, et al. Role of nasal nitric oxide in the resolution of experimental rhinovirus infection. J Allergy Clin Immunol 2004; 113:697.
69. Proud D. Nitric oxide and the common cold. Curr Opin Allergy Clin Immunol 2005; 5:37.
70. Zheng S, De BP, Choudhary S, et al. Impaired innate host defense causes susceptibility to respiratory virus infections in cystic fibrosis. Immunity 2003; 18:619.
71. Upham JW, Stick SM. Interactions between airway epithelial cells and dendritic cells: implications for the regulation of airway inflammation. Curr Drug Targets 2006; 7:541.
72. Huston DP, Liu YJ. Thymic stromal lymphopoietin: a potential therapeutic target for allergy and asthma. Curr Allergy Asthma Rep 2006; 6:372.
73. Ziegler SF, Liu Y-J. Thymic stromal lymphopoietin in normal and pathogenic T cell development and function. Nat Immunol 2006; 7:709.
74. Papi A, Stanciu LA, Papadopoulos NG, et al. Rhinovirus infection induces major histo-compatability complex class I and costimulatory molecule upregulation on respiratory epithelial cells. J Infect Dis 2000; 181:1780.

75. Vignola AM, Campbell AM, Chanez P, et al. HLA-DR and ICAM-1 expression on bronchial epithelial cells in asthma and chronic bronchitis. Am Rev Respir Dis 1993; 148:689.
76. Kim J, Myers AC, Chen L, et al. Constitutive and inducible expression of B7 family of ligands by human airway epithelial cells. Am J Respir Cell Mol Biol 2005; 33:280.
77. Salomon B, Bluestone JA. LFA-1 interaction with ICAM-1 and ICAM-2 regulates Th2 cytokine production. J Immunol 1998; 161:5138.
78. Salik E, Tyorkin M, Mohan S, et al. Antigen trafficking and accessory cell function in respiratory epithelial cells. Am J Respir Cell Mol Biol 1999; 21:365.
79. Kalb TH, Chuang MT, Marom Z, et al. Evidence for accessory cell function by class II MHC antigen-expressing airway epithelial cells. Am J Respir Cell Mol Biol 1991; 4:320.
80. Nguyen HH, Boyaka PN, Modoveanu Z, et al. Influenza virus-infected epithelial cells present viral antigens to antigen-specific $CD8^+$ cytotoxic T lymphocytes. J Virol 1998; 72:4534.

Biology of Endothelial Cells

24

Hedwig S Murphy, James Varani, and Peter A Ward

CONTENTS

- Introduction 387
- The endothelium and regulation of the inflammatory response 387
- Endothelial cell injury during acute inflammation 390
- Endothelial cells in allergy and asthma 395
- Conclusions 397

SUMMARY OF IMPORTANT CONCEPTS

>> Vascular endothelium maintains tissue homeostasis by stereotypical responses during coagulation, wound healing, inflammation, and immunity

>> Free radical generation is a final common pathway leading to endothelial cell injury resulting from hypoxia and reoxygenation, exposure to drugs, tobacco smoke, and other injurious agents, and inflammation

>> During acute inflammatory injury, the interaction of neutrophil products with endothelial cells generates free radicals cytotoxic to endothelial cells

>> Acute inflammatory injury to endothelium, especially oxidant-induced injury, initiates cascades of events leading to either protection of tissues or augmentation of the systemic and local inflammatory responses

>> The regulation of the balance of injury, protection, and activation of endothelium involves cytokines, protease inhibitors, endogenous antioxidants, and specific oxygen radicals such as nitric oxide

INTRODUCTION

The intact endothelium is important for the maintenance of tissue homeostasis, regulating such basic biologic processes as coagulation and fibrinolysis, inflammation, wound healing, and immunity. Not surprisingly, therefore, altered endothelial cell function is a component of many disease processes, including cancer, atherosclerosis, stroke, systemic hypertension, renal failure, ischemia-reperfusion injury, and inflammatory diseases.

The microvascular bed of any tissue can be the target of an inflammatory attack, but the pulmonary vasculature in particular is often damaged during the inflammatory process initiated by systemic mediators and local factors generated in other organs. Insults, such as microbial infection, allergic responses, inhalation of toxins, sepsis, burn, and trauma, result in damage to the pulmonary microvasculature and lead to severe lung injury. Inflammatory lung injury, as seen in adult respiratory distress syndrome (ARDS), can be rapidly fatal and is responsible for deaths in a majority of patients in hospital critical care units. Extensive efforts have been made over the past 25 years to understand this disease process. As a result, much is now understood about both the causes and the pathophysiology of acute lung injury.

Although ARDS has been a major focus of much of the inflammatory disease research, recent studies have focused on another common form of lung disease, allergic injury, including asthma. As with ARDS, allergic injury in lung is a manifestation of the inflammatory response, and the endothelium plays an important role in the pathophysiology of the disease process. Thus, much of what has been learned about endothelial cell biology in relation to ARDS is useful in efforts to delineate the events that constitute the allergic lung disease process.

THE ENDOTHELIUM AND REGULATION OF THE INFLAMMATORY RESPONSE

The lung is uniquely specialized for the process of gas exchange between the airway and the vascular compartment. Efficient gas exchange is possible because the lung parenchyma consists of a vast network of alveolar (air) spaces in close contact with an extensive vasculature (Fig. 24.1). Oxygen and carbon dioxide (CO_2) exchange occurs across a single layer of epithelial cells, a single basement membrane, and a single layer of endothelial cells with scant connective tissue and few fibroblasts. The pulmonary vascular tree, from large pulmonary veins through capillaries to pulmonary arteries, is lined by endothelial cells that are heterogenous in their fine structure, cell surface molecule expression, and function.[1,2] Functions are specific to those cells located in particular segments of this vascular tree, including regulation of hemostasis, vascular tone, permeability, leukocyte adhesion and transmigration, transduction of signals, and secretion of soluble molecules.[2,3] Endothelial cells are influenced by, but also contribute to, the inflammatory milieu, playing an important role in acute lung injury and allergic lung disease.

HEMOSTASIS

Hemorrhage is a common feature of inflammatory injury involving the vasculature. Vascular damage occurs in the injured lung, and fibrin, fibrin split products, and red blood cells (RBCs) in the alveolar space act to amplify injury. Fibrin deposited along the alveolar surface interferes with gas exchange, and fibrin and fibrin split products serve as a nidus for the further recruitment and activation of neutrophils and other leukocytes. Iron from hemoglobin is released from damaged RBCs and is a key intermediate in free radical-generating reactions that produce cell injury and extracellular matrix (ECM) degradation.

Endothelial cells are well positioned within the vasculature to influence hemostasis and thrombosis. An intact endothelium provides a protective barrier between platelets and ECM, inhibits platelet aggregation, promotes fibrinolytic activity, and mediates anticoagulant activity. These functions serve to limit clotting, but injury to endothelial cells can alter this role such that the damaged or activated endothelium then promotes thrombosis, decreasing fibrinolytic activity and surface thrombomodulin expression, and promoting adhesion of platelets. Activated or injured endothelial cells release tissue factor, which complexes with factor VII and is central to the coagulation network.[4] Activation of the clotting or fibrinolytic cascades in response to hemorrhage releases a number of potent mediators that participate in inflammatory reactions, but the endothelium, by virtue of its role in limiting hemorrhage, serves to mitigate the proinflammatory consequences of hemorrhage.[5] Anticoagulants released by the endothelium balance this function to prevent excess clotting and thrombosis. For example, the interaction of protein C with the thrombin-thrombomodulin complex on the endothelial cell protein C receptor forms activated protein C (APC), a potent anticoagulant.[6] The uninjured endothelium maintains this balance of pro- and anticoagulative forces, a balance which tips when the endothelium is damaged.

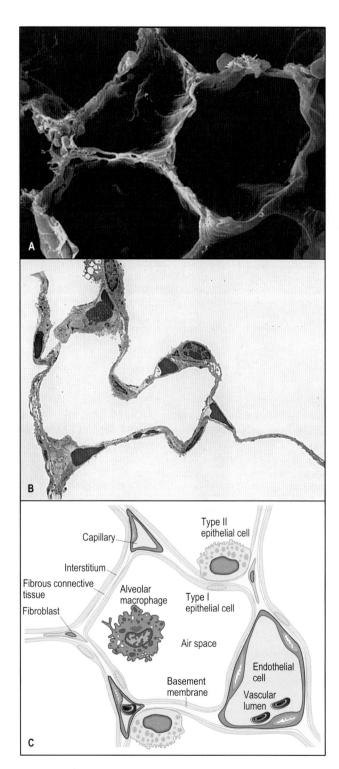

Fig. 24.1. Ultrastructural view of an alveolar unit. (A) Scanning electron micrograph shows expanded alveolar sacs with thin walls separating the air space from the circulation and a paucity of interstitium. Capillary lumen is visible in the alveolar wall. (B) Transmission electron micrograph shows alveoli with type I and type II alveolar epithelial cells and capillaries filled with red blood cells. (C) Alveolar air space is separated from the circulation by a single type I alveolar epithelial cell, single basement membrane, and single endothelial cell.

VASCULAR TONE

Arterial endothelium influences the inflammatory response through its control of vascular tone. The interactions of a complex series of peptides, nitric oxide, and lipid factors promote vessel wall constriction and relaxation. The endothelium is a source of factors that directly or indirectly mediate vasoconstriction, including peptide factors such as platelet-derived growth factor (PDGF) and lipid mediators such as the thromboxanes and platelet-activating factor (PAF). The endothelial cell angiotensin-converting enzyme (ACE) converts angiotensin I to angiotensin II, a potent vasoconstrictor that inactivates the inflammatory mediator and vasodilator bradykinin. Reduction in endothelial cell-derived nitric oxide ($\cdot$NO) activates the renin–angiotensin system as well as increasing levels of vasoconstrictors such as COX-dependent prostaglandins (i.e., thromboxane), and endothelins (ET-1 to ET-4).[7,8] The latter, especially ET-1, promote not only vasoconstriction but mitogenesis and thrombosis as well. Equally important in regulating vascular tone are endothelial cell surface enzymes that metabolize norepinephrine and 5-hydroxytryptamine.

Factors produced by the endothelium are responsible for relaxation of vascular smooth muscle. $\cdot$NO (an endothelium-derived relaxing factor (EDRF), generated by endothelial nitric oxide synthase (eNOS, iNOS) from L-arginine directly acts on smooth muscle cells.[9] It is the intermediate responsible for resting pulmonary vasorelaxation and for mediating the vascular smooth muscle-relaxing activities of acetylcholine and bradykinin.[10,11] The eicosanoid prostacyclin (prostaglandin I_2, PGI_2), increased during the early phase of the acute inflammatory response, has vasorelaxing potential and also has powerful antiaggregation activity for platelets. Under non-injury conditions, the pulmonary vessels maintain a balance among these vasoregulatory forces. The production of factors that counteract vasoconstriction provides a mechanism by which healthy endothelial cells are able to compensate rapidly for excessive constricting activity to 'fine-tune' vascular tone. This balance is often lost during systemic inflammation. The severe hypotension that accompanies the systemic inflammatory response reduces blood flow through the pulmonary capillary network; neutrophil aggregation and neutrophil adhesion to the pulmonary endothelium are promoted. The end result may be non-specific leukocyte accumulation in the lung vasculature, with the potential for pulmonary damage.

PERMEABILITY BARRIER

A major function of the endothelium is to provide a route for normal fluid exchange between intravascular and extravascular spaces. To maintain an osmotic and hydrostatic balance, the endothelium must form a permeability barrier. Alterations in vascular permeability can occur transiently in response to chemical mediators such as histamine and bradykinin, in which case the mechanisms of vascular leakage include endothelial cell contraction, endothelial cell retraction, and alterations in transcytosis. Mechanisms are also in place to stabilize the endothelial cell layer and decrease vascular permeability, including increases in platelet-derived agents such as sphingosine 1-phosphate (SIP), an agent which affects endothelial intercellular adhesion complexes.[12]

Disruption in the permeability barrier is a hallmark of acute inflammation.[13] Inflammatory mediators affect permeability, especially vascular endothelial growth factors (VEGF-A, -B, -C and -D,) which bind to endothelial Flt-1 and Flk-1 receptors; placental growth factor (PIGF), which binds to Flt-1; and tryptase (from mast cells), which activates by binding to PAR-2 on endothelial cells.[14–18] The permeability barrier may also be compromised by agents that either neutralize the anionic charge on the glycocalyx of the endothelium or interfere with cytoskeletal elements to cause endothelial cell shape change and retraction. This non-lethal, reversible 'retraction' of endothelial cells leads to passage of low-molecular-weight moieties and soluble plasma components, but not formed elements (e.g., RBCs), across the cell layer. When the capillary endothelium and the underlying basement membrane have been structurally damaged, RBCs extravasate into the pulmonary interstitium or alveolar space. Damage, either by direct endothelial injury (e.g., from exposure to toxins) or indirectly by leukocyte-mediated injury, leads to loss of the permeability barrier in the lung that may be extensive and life threatening, resulting in exudation of fluid and proteins, extensive pulmonary edema, prevention of normal gas exchange, and ultimately acute lung injury (ALI) or ARDS.[13,19,20]

LEUKOCYTE ADHESION AND TRANSMIGRATION

Recruitment of inflammatory cells from vascular spaces to sites of tissue injury requires adhesion and transmigration of cells across the endothelial cell barrier. The intact vascular endothelium provides a surface that is non-adhesive for leukocytes under normal hemodynamic conditions. The smooth capillary luminal surface and endothelial cell expression of antiadhesive mediators such as PGI_2 and $\cdot$NO combine to prevent leukocytes from adhering to the vascular wall, yet the endothelium must have the capacity to alter its physiology rapidly to facilitate the attachment of leukocytes (see also Chapter 9).[21]

The circulating neutrophil is the primary effector cell responding to acute inflammatory signaling. Under unstimulated conditions, neutrophils circulate in the vasculature, occasionally adhere to the endothelial cell and roll over the cell surface for a limited distance and then are rapidly released back into the flowing blood. The formation of a local inflammatory nidus, however, alters the microenvironment in such a way that nearby endothelial cells (primarily in the postcapillary venules) acquire strong adhesive capacity for neutrophils. Leukocytes that initially roll along the endothelial cells become firmly immobilized on the endothelium and subsequently move out of the circulation and into the extravascular space by diapedesis (Fig. 24.2).

Extravasation of leukocytes across the blood vessel walls requires an elegant cascade of events, including the sequential engagement of reciprocal adhesion molecules on leukocytes and endothelial cells. Inflammatory mediators including cytokines, complement activation products, and VEGF promote the expression of endothelial cell adhesion molecules from a number of gene families on the endothelial cell surface. These include intercellular adhesion molecule-1 and -2 (ICAM-1, ICAM-2), vascular cell adhesion molecule-1 (VCAM-1), and the E- and P-selectins.[21–23] Stimulation of E-selectin and P-selectin on endothelial cells results in the initial slowing of leukocyte flow, loose adhesion, and rolling of the leukocytes along the endothelium. Subsequent interaction between endothelial ICAM-1 and leukocyte β_2 integrins leads to a firm adhesion of the leukocytes to the endothelial cell surface, followed by leukocyte emigration through the vessel wall into the extravascular space. Thus the different families of adhesion receptors play complementary roles in promoting leukocyte accumulation at sites of inflammation.[22,24]

Although adhesion of neutrophils to the endothelium through β_2 integrins is necessary for neutrophil emigration out of the circulation, adhesion is insufficient by itself. Additional chemotactic factors are

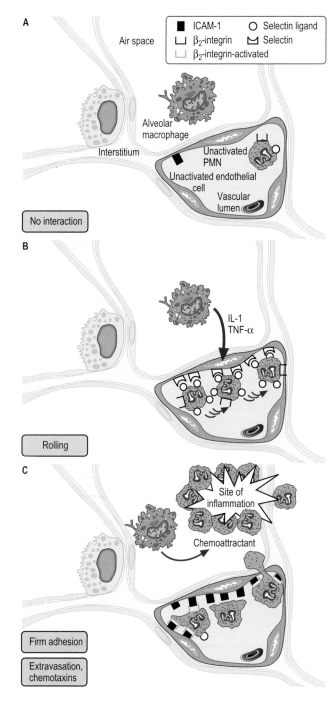

Fig. 24.2. Neutrophil interaction with vascular endothelium. (A) In the absence of inflammatory stimuli, neutrophils circulate in the vasculature, without adhering to the endothelium. (B) In response to cytokines such as tumor necrosis factor alpha (TNF-α) and interleukin-1 (IL-1), endothelial cell selectins are expressed on the cell surface and interact with carbohydrates bearing sialyl LewisX, expressed on neutrophils, resulting in neutrophil rolling on the endothelial cell surface. (C) Stimulation of circulating neutrophils with inflammatory mediators results in increased expression of high-affinity β2 integrins. These integrins on rolling neutrophils contact endothelial cell intercellular adhesion molecule-1 (ICAM-1), resulting in firm adhesion. Chemoattractants generated at the inflammatory nidus serve to attract firmly-adherent neutrophils to migrate out of the vasculature.

involved in the transendothelial migration process. The complement peptide C5a, bacterial peptides such as fMLP, and lipids such as PAF and leukotriene B_4 (LTB$_4$) have potent leukocyte chemotactic activity. More specific are chemokines, cytokines with chemoattractant activity relatively selective for specific populations of inflammatory cells. Several chemokines are found at sites of acute inflammation and are primarily chemotactic for neutrophils, including CXCL1 (Gro-α), CXCL2 (MIP-2α), CXCL3 (MIP-2β), CXCL4 (PF-4), CXCL5 (ENA-78), CXCL7 (NAP-2, CTAP-III), and CXCL8 (interleukin-8, IL-8).

The intact vascular endothelium is an integral component of the normal inflammatory response, and participation in the response results in minimal damage to the endothelial cells themselves. However, if the inflammatory stimulus is too potent, too persistent, or is localized to the vascular wall, the endothelial cell defenses are overwhelmed, the barrier function is lost, and tissue injury occurs.

ENDOTHELIAL CELL INJURY DURING ACUTE INFLAMMATION

Although the inflammatory system is well designed for its function of protecting the body against outside invaders, it is a double-edged sword. Under certain conditions, the same inflammatory effector mechanisms that are used to clear foreign invaders from the body can also produce serious damage to host tissue. Inflammatory injury can be seen in any tissue, but the terminal air spaces of the lung are the areas that frequently undergo severe inflammatory injury. Three major reasons explain this proneness to injury. First, the extensive system of capillaries in lung provides a large surface area for endothelial cell contact with activated inflammatory cells. Second, as noted previously, the lung parenchyma is a very delicate structure and is readily damaged by the products of inflammatory cells. Third, any damage to the lung parenchyma compromises gas exchange, with serious consequences for the host. Thus, any damage to the pulmonary vasculature may lead to serious structural damage (Fig. 24.3).[25]

The events that initiate inflammatory tissue damage in the lung may occur locally, as with microbial infection, or systemically, as in sepsis, ischemia-reperfusion, burn, and trauma. Regardless of the initiating event, there is a rapid accumulation of neutrophils in the lung capillaries. These neutrophils, responding to an inflammatory stimulus, are largely responsible for the damage to host tissue that occurs during acute inflammation. Activated neutrophils generate large amounts of reactive oxygen metabolites that are toxic to virtually all cells of the alveolar unit. Neutrophils also release from intracellular granules a variety of hydrolytic enzymes, including serine proteinases (elastase, cathepsin G, plasminogen

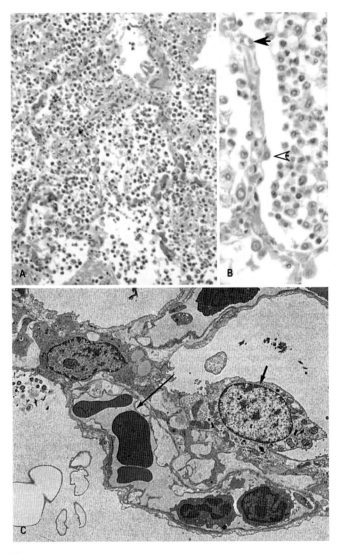

Fig. 24.3. Histologic and ultrastructural appearance of acute inflammatory injury in the lung. (A) Light microscopic view of inflamed lung. Large number of neutrophils and fibrin can be seen in the interstitium and in the alveolar space. (B) High-power light microscopic view of inflamed lung with alveolar space filled with inflammatory cells. Filled arrow indicates congested alveolar capillary. Open arrow indicates type II alveolar cell. (C) Transmission electron micrograph showing a portion of an alveolar unit. Endothelial cell separation from the underlying basement membrane (long arrow) is evident. Neutrophils and red blood cells can be seen within the vascular compartment. The alveolar epithelial cell (short arrow) is also undergoing degeneration (×5000).

activator), matrix metalloproteinases (neutrophil collagenase, 92-kDa gelatinase/type IV collagenase, matrilysin, metalloelastase), and several lipases, phospholipases, and glycolytic enzymes. These enzymes degrade the ECM, which provides the lung with its three-dimensional structure. Along with other granule constituents, these enzymes also can interact with oxidants to injure or kill endothelial cells and lung parenchymal

cells, damaging both the cellular and the structural components of the lung and compromising lung function.

Other inflammatory cells also have a number of effector mechanisms that can contribute to cell injury. Lung macrophages are present in very large numbers and can be activated as the inflammatory process is initiated; eosinophils in particular are highly cytotoxic. As with neutrophils, activated eosinophils generate large amounts of extracellular oxygen radicals. Human eosinophils also contain a number of cationic proteins, including major basic protein (MBP), eosinophil peroxidase (EPO), and eosinophil cationic protein (ECP). Each of these proteins is cytotoxic in its own right, whereas EPO is able to generate hypohalous acids from hydrogen peroxide (H_2O_2). Eosinophils also contain a number of potent proteolytic enzymes in stored granules. Thus, although these cells may not be as highly cytotoxic to endothelial cells, a role in allergic-type inflammatory responses may be critical.[25]

NON-CYTOTOXIC AND CYTOTOXIC CELL INJURY: REVERSIBLE VERSUS IRREVERSIBLE

The vascular endothelium is sensitive to both reversible and irreversible forms of injury. Reversible injury refers to injury that results in the temporary disruption of the intact endothelium rather than the death of individual endothelial cells. This sublethal injury results in a temporary increase in permeability and can trigger tissue damage. Soluble mediators generated during inflammation, such as oxidized lipids, thrombin, histamine, cytokines, arachidonic acid metabolites and serine proteinases (elastase and cathepsin G) from human neutrophils can cause cytoskeletal changes that lead to temporary and reversible retraction of endothelial cells. Cytoskeletal remodeling occurs in response to stress, best documented in states of sustained exposure to sheer stress (flow). Microfilaments containing actin form stress fibers and a dense peripheral band within the cytosol. Tight junctions constructed from occludin and adherens junctions constructed from cadherin associate with the actin microfilaments. This actin cytoskeleton is also structurally and functionally associated with integrins that initiate signaling cascades resulting in cytoskeletal reorganization.[26,27] Endothelial cells are not displaced from the underlying basement membrane, and retracted cells can readily re-form the intact endothelial lining. In the lung, retraction of endothelial cells diminishes the pulmonary barrier function, and the resulting high protein edema interferes with gas exchange giving rise to severe hypoxemia. In vivo the close contact between activated neutrophils and the endothelium provides a 'protective environment' that can exclude serum proteinase inhibitors. In this environment, the neutrophil proteinases, especially elastase and azurocidin, are able to disrupt both the endothelial cell layer and the subendothelial cell matrix. The low-molecular-weight secretory leukocyte protease inhibitor (SLPI) effectively penetrates this neutrophil–endothelial cell interface and prevents neutrophil-mediated endothelial cell retraction in vitro, and is protective against lung injury in vivo. Once endothelial cells have retracted, the extracellular matrix, including the basement membrane and connective tissue, are exposed to neutrophil enzymes.[28–31] Although we normally think of endothelial cell retraction in terms of non-lethal or reversible injury, disruption of cell-substrate adhesive interactions can trigger apoptosis.[32,33] The signaling pathways triggered by cell-substrate disruption are not fully understood. Disruption in the integrin-mediated signals seems to be critical. Possibly, apoptosis is triggered directly in this manner or may reflect a synergy with other effector mechanisms.

A number of physical, chemical, or biologic agents can cause irreversible injury to the endothelium. Many agents produce lethal injury to endothelial cells through the generation of oxygen radicals. These agents include ionizing radiation, hyperoxia, and hypoxia followed by reoxygenation. Chemical agents include bleomycin, paraquat, and menadione, and biologic agents include activated neutrophils and certain cytokines.

Injury induced by activated neutrophils provides a good model of an injury in which oxygen radicals play a central role. Adherence of non-activated neutrophils to endothelial cells (i.e., after endothelial cell activation) does not result in endothelial cell injury, while activated neutrophils induce cytotoxic injury to the endothelium, primarily from oxidant generation.

OXIDANT-INDUCED CELL INJURY

Activation of neutrophils with a variety of agents leads to tight adhesion of the neutrophil to the endothelial cell, creating a microenvironment between the cells. Organization of the components of a reduced form of nicotinamide adenine dinucleotide phosphate (NADPH) oxidase into an active enzyme complex converts molecular oxygen into the superoxide anion radical (O_2^-) in this sequestered space.[34] This radical is then broken down spontaneously or extremely rapidly in the presence of the enzyme superoxide dismutase (SOD) to H_2O_2. H_2O_2 is a central intermediate in a number of different metabolic pathways. In the presence of catalase (a mitochondrial heme enzyme) or glutathione peroxidase (a cytoplasmic selenium-containing enzyme), H_2O_2 can be reduced to molecular oxygen and water. These two enzymes form a major part of the intraendothelial cell antioxidant barrier. Myeloperoxidase, a neutrophil product with a very strong cationic charge, is secreted from granules during exocytosis (in the presence of chloride ion). It catalyzes the conversion of H_2O_2 to hypochlorous acid.

Although a strong oxidant, hypochlorous acid is probably not primarily responsible for cell injury. Rather, iron-catalyzed H_2O_2 reduction, leading to formation of the hydroxyl radical ($^\cdot OH$), is the most injurious pathway (Fenton reaction). H_2O_2 generated extracellularly diffuses freely across the target cell plasma membrane, where it is reduced to $^\cdot OH$ by contact with the transition form of iron (Fe^{2+}) within the endothelial cell (Fig. 24.4). Providing iron to endothelial cells under conditions in which it can be readily taken up increases susceptibility to injury. Deferoxamine and other iron chelators that cross cell membranes are highly effective in protecting endothelial cells from injury.[2] Cells store iron in the ferric

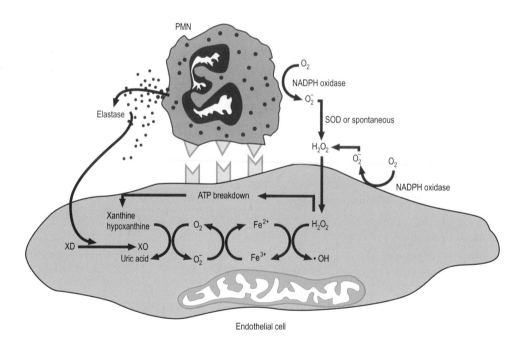

Fig. 24.4. Endothelial cell injury by activated neutrophils. Neutrophil (PMN) NADPH oxidase generates superoxide (O_2^-), which breaks down to hydrogen peroxide (H_2O_2) in the presence of superoxide dismutase (SOD). Endothelial cells produce O_2^- from NADPH oxidase but primarily from the activation and conversion of xanthine dehydrogenase (XD) to xanthine oxidase (XO) in the presence of elastase or inflammatory cytokines. Within the endothelial cells, O_2^- in the presence of reduced iron (Fe^{2+}) and H_2O_2 reacts to form the cytotoxic hydroxyl radical ($^\cdot OH$).

(Fe^{3+}) form complexed with ferritin. To participate in the radical-generating reactions, iron must be freed from ferritin and reduced to ferrous (Fe^{2+}) iron. Intracellular endothelial O_2^- appears to play the critical role in maintaining iron in this transition state. Thus, it appears that the endothelial cell provides both iron and reducing capacity to allow the iron to be used to generate the cytotoxic radical from H_2O_2.

Although vascular endothelial cell O_2^- is generated in 10- to 100-fold lower concentrations than in neutrophils, this radical has a number of important functions. O_2^- is an important modulator of endothelial cell signal transduction elements, specifically nuclear factor kappa B (NF-κB) and activator protein-1 (AP-1). O_2^- interacts with iron and with intracellular and extracellular ·NO to generate toxic radicals, to scavenge superoxide radical, and to modulate the vasomotor response. O_2^- is generated by a number of enzyme systems present within all mammalian cells, including mitochondrial electron transport enzymes; cytochrome P-450 enzymes present in endoplasmic reticulum, as well as in biologic membranes; amino acid oxidases (peroxisomes); and lipid-metabolizing oxidases (e.g., cyclooxygenase, lipoxygenase) in biologic membranes. Two enzyme systems make particularly significant contributions to endothelial cell O_2^-: NAD(P)H oxidase and xanthine oxidase. The multicomponent neutrophil-like NAD(P)H oxidase, responsible for generation of extracellular O_2^- and possibly intracellular O_2^- as well, is involved in pulmonary vasoconstriction and ·NO scavenging.[35,36] Although the exact structure of this enzyme is elusive, the presence of components similar to those found in the neutrophil oxidase suggests that this enzyme may function in a similar manner by an aggregation of components and association with the plasma membrane. The oxidase uses NADH and NADPH as substrates for electron transfer to molecular oxygen and is regulated by angiotensin II as well as by lipopolysaccharide (LPS) and inflammatory cytokines.[36,37] The neutrophil oxidase generates O_2^- extracellularly, predominantly to serve a bactericidal and cytotoxic function. The O_2^- output of the vascular oxidase is significantly lower, but it may generate intracellular as well as extracellular O_2^-, suggesting a role for this oxidant in intracellular signaling as well as ·NO scavenging.[10,38]

The cytosolic purine-metabolizing enzyme xanthine oxidase is a major source of intracellular O_2^-, which under physiologic conditions may be neutralized by intracellular antioxidant systems. Under appropriate conditions, the O_2^- generated by these enzymes may participate in cytotoxic reactions. This may be especially relevant to cell injury in inflammation because the inflammatory nidus can create conditions that increase intracellular O_2^- generation. For example, increased electron transport activity after hypoxia/reoxygenation results in enhanced O_2^- generation in mitochondria. Likewise, excessive adenosine triphosphate (ATP) breakdown can lead to cytoplasmic O_2^- production through xanthine oxidase conversion of xanthine and hypoxanthine to uric acid. Xanthine dehydrogenase and xanthine oxidase have been implicated as a major intracellular source of O_2^- in neutrophil-mediated injury of endothelial cells. Xanthine dehydrogenase uses nicotinamide adenine dinucleotide (NAD) as an electron acceptor. The oxidase transfers a single electron to molecular oxygen to generate O_2^-. Conditions that predispose the endothelial cells to oxidant injury (e.g., hypoxia) appear specifically to upregulate endothelial cell enzyme synthesis. Several factors found in the inflammatory milieu, including leukocyte elastase and certain proinflammatory cytokines, act on the enzyme to convert the dehydrogenase form into the oxidase form. Coordinate with this, H_2O_2 induces rapid breakdown of ATP in endothelial cells. Under conditions of excessive ATP catabolism, the down-stage purine metabolites (xanthine and hypoxanthine) are formed. In the inflammatory milieu, not only does the content of xanthine oxidase increase, concomitant with the appearance of substrate for the enzyme, but xanthine oxidase inhibitors also protect endothelial cells from oxidant injury.

This metabolic scheme summarizes current understanding of at least one sequence of events that leads to endothelial cell injury in acute inflammation (Fig. 24.4). A number of other 'triggers' of endothelial cell injury may act through pathways that at least partially overlap with the mechanism described here. For example, exposure of endothelial cells to hyperoxia results in increased intracellular generation of O_2^-, whereas hypoxic conditions lead to enhanced expression of enzyme systems (e.g., xanthine oxidase) that normally produce intracellular radicals. When reoxygenation suddenly occurs, oxygen radicals are formed. Additionally, as they are metabolized, several drugs, including bleomycin, paraquat, and menadione, produce damage by fostering intracellular free radical formation. Likewise, asbestos and other mineral dusts injure cells, in part by providing a catalytically active surface for the generation of oxygen free radicals. Finally, free radicals are also thought to be involved in lung injury resulting from tobacco smoke and after irradiation.

The formation of free radicals, and particularly ·OH, within endothelial cells is strongly linked with cytotoxic injury; a number of cellular constituents are sensitive to the highly reactive ·OH. Proteins may be inactivated as a result of cross-linking of sulfhydryl (–SH) groups on methionyl residues. Mitochondrial damage with a resultant drop in oxidative phosphorylation is thought to be a primary consequence of protein cross-linking. Cross-linking of deoxyribonucleic acid (DNA) through attack on purine bases can result in mutations, prevention of transcription of critical genes, and activation of apoptotic pathways. In addition to protein and DNA damage, ·OH is also a potent initiator of lipid peroxidation, with resultant damage to biologic membranes and ion imbalances. Ultimately, however, no single target probably accounts for the widespread damage that occurs. On the contrary, ·OH causes such extensive injury because so many target molecules may be damaged.[39]

Although oxygen radicals are thought to account for much of the endothelial cell injury that occurs during acute inflammation, these radicals are not generated in a void. The same stimuli that induce oxygen radical production by neutrophils also stimulate the exocytosis of granules that contain a variety of bioactive materials. Many of these, including proteolytic enzymes, other hydrolases, and cationic peptides, are proinflammatory. Monocytes and tissue macrophages are also found at sites of inflammation, and many of the products of these cells are also proinflammatory. In addition, if the inflammation-inducing stimulus is a microbial infection, products of the inciting cells will be concomitantly present in the nidus. Many of these proinflammatory mediators have little effect by themselves against healthy endothelial cells but are highly cytotoxic against oxidant-stressed cells. Although this interaction is incompletely understood, oxidant damage to cellular proteins may enhance sensitivity to subsequent attack by proteolytic enzymes. Likewise, phospholipid oxidation may render cellular phospholipids more sensitive to phospholipases. Alternatively, oxidant-stressed cells may be less able to repair enzyme-mediated damage than would be reparable in non-stressed cells.[40] Finally, many of the same mediators that increase endothelial cell sensitivity to oxidant injury also act as opsonins, potentiating the respiratory burst in neutrophils. Regardless of molecular mechanism, it appears that lethal injury to the endothelium in acute inflammation is partly a direct consequence of oxidant activity and partly a consequence of a variety of mediators present at the site acting in concert with oxidants.[41]

Intact endothelial cells keep the inflammatory response under control, and injury to these cells leads to widespread tissue damage. In animal models of injury, ultrastructural studies demonstrate early endothelial cell damage, including both separation from the underlying basement membrane and membrane blebbing, indicators of lethal injury. Most importantly, inhibitor studies and studies with blocking antibodies show that agents that prevent endothelial cell injury in vitro also inhibit both endothelial cell damage and acute tissue injury in vivo.

PROTECTION AGAINST INJURY

Inflammation is a regulated process with mechanisms in place to reduce as well as to amplify the tissue response. Protection against inflammatory-mediated injury occurs through a number of endogenous antiinflammatory mediators upregulated during lung inflammation, including cytokines, protease inhibitors, and antioxidants. Cytokines such as interleukin-10 (IL-10) and IL-13 suppress proinflammatory cytokine production, thereby indirectly preventing, among other outcomes, the upregulation of vascular cell adhesion molecules.[19] Protease inhibitors such as SLPI have multiple effects, including reducing pulmonary vascular permeability during acute inflammation.[42] Endothelial cells generate endogenous antioxidants such as superoxide dismutase, reduced glutathione (GSH), and other thiol-containing compounds that affect redox-regulated signal transduction, cell proliferation, apoptosis, and inflammation, presenting a defense against oxidant-mediated injury.[43–45] A number of other factors serve protective functions during inflammation. The anticoagulant APC complex formed on endothelial cells serves to regulate tumor necrosis factor alpha (TNF-α)-mediated endothelial cell injury, and the endothelial cell protein C receptor may directly modulate leukocyte function.[6]

Several molecules serve protective or injurious functions, depending on the milieu. Nitric oxide ($\cdot$NO) plays very diverse roles in the physiology and pathophysiology of the vascular system, earning the conflicting reputation of being both protective and deleterious to vascular function.[10,46] Alterations in $\cdot$NO production and bioavailability occur in human disease and in experimental animal models of hypertension, aging, diabetes, heart failure, pulmonary hypertension, and asthma.[11,47,48] Although $\cdot$NO is increased in exhaled air of patients with untreated asthma, the correlation between changes in exhaled $\cdot$NO concentration and airway inflammation is unclear.[49] The role of $\cdot$NO as a vasodilator and as a cofactor in inflammation, however, is well established, and $\cdot$NO appears to be an important mediator during sepsis.[50]

Nitric oxide synthase (NOS) generates $\cdot$NO by oxidation of a guanidino nitrogen of L-arginine in the presence of molecular oxygen, with L-citrulline as a by-product. Vascular endothelial cells express two NOS isoforms: a constitutively expressed isoform, eNOS, depends on increases in calcium to bind to calmodulin; an inducible form, iNOS, contains calmodulin as a subunit and uses resting levels of calcium. Both forms of the enzyme require the cofactors NADPH, FAD, FMN, heme, and tetrahydrobiopterin.[51,52] Expression and function of eNOS has been predominantly evaluated in large vessel endothelium, where it appears to be the key constitutively expressed enzyme with a role in determining basal vascular wall $\cdot$NO and vascular tone. Under certain pathologic conditions, eNOS gene expression can be modulated; in the context of pulmonary hypertension in hypoxic lung disease, contradictory results support both upregulation and reduced eNOS expression. $\cdot$NO generated by eNOS is a vasoregulatory molecule in these large vessels, while in the microvasculature $\cdot$NO is largely

generated by iNOS and likely serves a very different purpose. Under inflammatory conditions, iNOS is expressed in neutrophils, macrophages, epithelial cells, and endothelial cells. Conflicting experimental studies have demonstrated injurious as well as protective roles for $\cdot$NO.[10,53] In lung sepsis, the iNOS gene has an early response to induction by LPS. The adverse affects of $\cdot$NO include its contribution to septic vascular hypocontractility, organ hypoperfusion, and interaction with superoxide to yield the highly toxic peroxynitrite, as well as ultimately $\cdot$OH. In septic patients, nitrite/nitrate levels correlate with severity of illness.[54,55]

In contrast, chronic overexpression of NOS appears to protect, whereas genetic deficiency of NOS increases inflammatory injury. A number of mechanisms may mediate this protective effect of $\cdot$NO (Fig. 24.5). NO prevents platelet adherence and aggregation at sites of vascular injury, compensating for disruption of microvascular integrity. $\cdot$NO may play an anti-inflammatory role by suppression of bacterial infection and through its effect on leukocyte recruitment; $\cdot$NO from iNOS in neutrophils and macrophages directly inhibits leukocyte and monocyte adhesion to endothelial cells and transendothelial neutrophil migration. $\cdot$NO scavenges oxygen radicals, providing cytoprotection against oxidant-mediated injury at least in part by reducing available O_2^-, but also by modulating oxidant-mediated signal transduction events such as activation of NF-κB, leading to adhesion molecule expression.[56] In large vessels, $\cdot$NO retards smooth muscle proliferation and migration and stimulates endothelial cell proliferation and blocks stress-induced endothelial cell apoptosis. The protective versus injurious role of $\cdot$NO may be a function of a number of factors, including cell or tissue specificity, concentration of $\cdot$NO within the cell, the enzyme isoform source of $\cdot$NO, interaction with other reactive molecules such as O_2^-, and effects on signal transduction events.

$\cdot$NO expression and function has been linked to heat shock proteins (HSPs), a family of protective molecules. When cells are subjected to stress conditions, most undergo irreversible injury and die. However, mild heat treatment before lethal injury provides tolerance to subsequent injury, a phenomenon associated with increased expression of HSPs. Protection mediated by HSPs is poorly understood but is attributed in some cells to the molecular chaperone function resulting in, among other effects, increased protein expression due to enhanced folding of nascent proteins, altered actin cytoskeleton, activation of Toll-like receptors, suppression of NADPH oxidase, and decrease in proinflammatory cytokines. Vascular endothelial cells express the ubiquitous HSP-70 and HSP-90 as well as HSP-25. HSP-70 is induced in whole lungs, is increased in lungs of patients with ARDS and asthma, and protects during sepsis and metabolic stress.[57,58] $\cdot$NO upregulates HSP expression and protects against TNF-α-induced apoptosis, while HSP (HSP-60) reduces NO release by macrophages in the setting of acute lung injury. HSPs, perhaps in conjunction with NO, play a role in the host response to sepsis and lung injury.[59] The vascular endothelial cells have a central position in maintaining the intracellular and extracellular oxidant balance important for the maintenance of tissue homeostasis. During inflammation, this oxidant balance is tipped toward either tissue and cell injury or protection against oxidant-mediated injury.

ENDOTHELIAL REPAIR MECHANISMS

After injury, endothelial and vascular repair mechanisms are initiated to replace cells in denuded areas and to institute new vessels. In some cases, existing cells are capable of migrating and differentiating to form

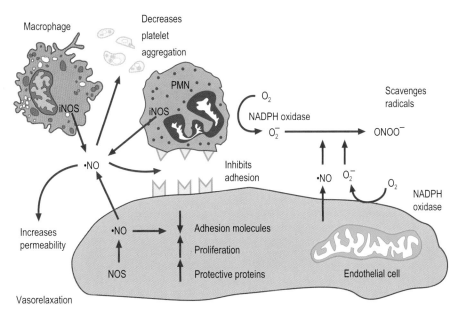

Fig. 24.5. Nitric oxide-mediated protective mechanisms in acute lung injury. Nitric oxide ($^\cdot$NO) from inducible nitric oxide synthase (iNOS) in macrophages and neutrophils and from NOS in endothelial cells stimulates protein leakage, and relaxation of smooth muscle but also decreases platelet aggregation, reduces neutrophil adhesion to endothelium, and scavenges toxic oxygen radicals. Within endothelial cells, $^\cdot$NO stimulates protective heat shock protein expression and endothelial cell proliferation.

new vessels, a process termed *angiogenesis*. When endothelial cells are replenished by incorporation of cells from the circulation, the process is termed *vasculogenesis*.[5] In the latter, endothelial progenitor cells (EPCs) originate in bone marrow, are released into the circulation, migrate into tissues and play an important role in endothelial cell maintenance and repair.[60] Increased numbers of EPCs in the circulation are associated with a variety of disease states in which vascular injury occurs.[61] EPCs are recruited from the bone marrow by several factors including growth factors such as GM-CSF, HGF, erythropoietin, and VEGF as well as inflammatory mediators such as IL-8 and SDF-1. Increased numbers of circulating EPCs have been found in patients with pneumonia[62] and are associated with increased survival in patients with acute lung injury.[63] EPCs develop endothelial cell phenotypes when incorporated into experimentally injured lungs in LPS-induced injury and elastase-induced emphysema.[64] As these cells differentiate into resident endothelial cells, they express eNOS, a variety of growth factors, cytokines, and antioxidants, thereby developing high resistance to oxidative stress. While their role in repair has not been fully delineated, EPCs appear to be able to provide a reservoir of repair cells to replace dysfunctional or lost endothelium and to release growth factors that may act on other resident cells to mediate lung injury repair.[65,66]

Endothelial cell migration and proliferation occur during angiogenesis. Vascular endothelial growth factor (VEGF) is expressed in the distal airway epithelial cells and the basement membrane subjacent to the airway epithelial cells. A potent stimulator of permeability as well as EPC recruitment, it is also critical for vessel growth during development and for endothelial cell survival. VEGF expression, signaling via the endothelial cell VEGF receptors Flt-1 and Flk-1, and endothelial cell proliferation are associated with the vascular lesions of pulmonary

hypertension.[67–69] Early in severe sepsis, circulating levels of VEGF, PIGF, and soluble VEGF receptor, sFlt-1 are increased, and VEGF signaling in the endothelium appears to contribute to the associated vascular leakage and inflammation.[70] In contrast, in ARDS patients compared to control patients, lung tissue contains less VEGF, lower vascular bed density, and increased endothelial cell apoptosis, suggesting a role for decreased VEGF concentration in the development of severe endothelial cell injury and subsequent decrease in lung capillary density.[71] Another molecule responsible for activation of endothelial cell migration and angiogenesis is sphingosine 1-phosphate (SIP) from activated platelets.[72] This sphingolipid is recognized by members of the endothelial differentiation gene receptor (Edg) family, also known to be involved in angiogenesis.[73]

Intriguing interactions between endothelial cells and pericytes suggest that a relationship between them may regulate vascular proliferation and repair, but an unambiguous role in pathophysiologic processes is not yet certain.[74] The complex balance of mediators regulates endothelial cell permeability, apoptosis, migration, and proliferation, triggering first endothelial injury and then repair.

■ ENDOTHELIAL CELLS IN ALLERGY AND ASTHMA ■

Accumulation of inflammatory cells, including lymphocytes, monocytes, basophils, neutrophils, and especially eosinophils, is the hallmark of pulmonary allergic inflammation and asthma. Lung eosinophil accumulation is central to the pathogenesis of disease and correlates with airway hyperresponsiveness. Trafficking of eosinophils to sites

Table 24.1 Cytokines/chemokines relevant to pulmonary vascular endothelial cell (EC) biology

Acting on ECs	Generated by ECs	Receptors on ECs
Growth factors		
GM-CSF	GM-CSF	GM-CSFRα (CD116)
G-CSF	G-CSF	G-CSFR (CD114)
VEGF	VEGF	VEGFR-$_2$ (Flt-1, Flk-1)
βFGF	βFGF	FGFR-1,-2,-3
	M-CSF	
Inflammatory cytokines		
Interleukin-1	Interleukin-1α	IL-1R (CD121
Interleukin-3		IL-3R (CDw123)
Interleukin-4		IL-4Rα (CD124)
Interleukin-5		IL-5Rα (CDw125)
Interleukin-6	Interleukin-6	IL-6Rβ (CDw130)
Interleukin-13		IL-13Rα (CD213a)
Interferon-γ		IFNγR (CD119)
TNF-α		TNFR-1 (CD120a,b)
CXC chemokines		CXC receptor
CXCL1, 2, 3	CXCL2	CXCR1
CXCL8	CXCL5	CXCR2
CXCL10	CXCL7	CXCR3
CXCL12		CXCR4
CC chemokines		CC receptor
CCL1	CCL2	CCR1
CCL2	CCL3	CCR2
CCL8	CCL4	CCR3
CCL11	CCL5	CCR4
CCL23	CCL7	CCR5
CCL27	CCL8	CCR8
	CCL13	
	CCL17	
	CCL26	
CX3C chemokines		
	CX3CL1	

GM-CSF, granulocyte-macrophage colony-stimulating factor; G-CSF, granulocyte colony-stimulating factor; M-CSF, macrophage colony-stimulating factor; βFGF, basic fibroblast growth factor; VEGF, vascular endothelial growth factor; CXCL1, 2, 3 (Gro-α, -β, -γ, growth-related oncogene); CXCL5, ENA-78, epithelial-neutrophil activating peptide 78; CXCL6, GCP-2, granulocyte chemotactic protein 2; CXCL7, NAP-2, neutrophil-activating protein-2; CXCL8, IL-8, interleukin 8; CXCL10, IP-10, interferon gamma-inducible protein-10; CXCL12, SDF-1α, stromal cell-derived factor; CCL1, I-309; CCL2, MCP-1, monocyte chemoattractant protein 1; CCL3, MIP-1α, macrophage inflammatory protein-1α; CCL4, MIP-1β, macrophage inflammatory protein-β; CCL5, RANTES, regulated on activation, normal T cells expressed and secreted; CCL7, MCP-3, monocyte chemoattractant protein 3; CCL8, MCP-2, monocyte chemoattractant protein 2; CCL13, MCP-4, monocyte chemoattractant protein 4; CCL17, TARC, thymus and activation regulated chemokine; CCL23, MIP-3, macrophage inflammatory protein 3; CCL26, eotaxin-3; CCL27, CTACK, cutaneous T cell attracting chemokine; CX3CL1, fractalkine.

of allergic reaction is regulated by (1) surface adhesion molecules on eosinophils and endothelial cells; (2) activating factors, including cytokines, products of leukocytes present at the inflammatory site, and complement activation products; and (3) chemoattractants, including PAF, leukotrienes, and chemokines. Endothelial cells play an active role in eosinophil recruitment by expression of surface adhesion molecules and by generation of, and response to, activating factors.[75] In a manner similar to neutrophil recruitment, eosinophil extravasation from the bloodstream into extravascular tissues is a regulated process involving a coordinated series of interactions between eosinophils and endothelial cells, including the sequential expression of adhesion molecules. Cytokines important in allergic responses, including IL-1β, TNF-α, IL-4, and IL-13, induce upregulation of adhesion molecules.[76,77] All three families of adhesion molecules that participate in acute inflammatory lung injury also play a role in allergic lung inflammation (see Chapter 9). In contrast to neutrophils, however, eosinophils constitutively express the β_1 integrin $\alpha_4\beta_1$ (very late antigen-4, VLA-4), which interacts with the endothelial cell molecule VCAM-1.[76,78] Induction of VCAM-1 expression by cytokines in allergic reactions may be one of the mechanisms allowing for the selective recruitment of eosinophils, and adhesion molecule engagement (particularly ICAM-1) also activates eosinophils.[78,79]

By necessity, the lungs are under constant exposure to aeroallergens, and the immunologic milieu in the lung permits or prohibits allergic sensitization. A distinct cytokine profile characterizes the inflammation associated with a specific immune response. Again, sepsis is the prototypical disease in which the role of cytokines in the coordination and persistence of the inflammatory response has been defined. Alterations in cytokine expression in the lung are associated with clinical outcome in ARDS; similarly, the cytokine response in asthma correlates with disease severity.[80,81] Less well characterized is the role of endothelial cell-derived cytokines and chemokines in the allergic response (Table 24.1). Endothelial cells secrete significant RANTES, IL-8, IL-6, and MCP-1 as well as growth factors and other cytokines. Since endothelial cells express many of the known cytokine receptors, it is likely that cytokines with important inflammatory effects influence these cells and the allergic response in ways yet to be elucidated.

Complement activation products are among the many mediators of eosinophil activation and recruitment into extravascular tissue during allergic inflammation.[82] Complex events occur, at least in part, by the direct and indirect effects of complement components on vascular endothelial cells, evoking activation of endothelial cells, release of soluble mediators, and increased adhesion of eosinophils to endothelial cells. The complement anaphylatoxins C3a and C5a and the distal terminal complement components, C5b-9 (the membrane attack complex, MAC) activate endothelial cells. C3a is chemotactic for eosinophils and induces rapid and stable adhesion and rolling of eosinophils on endothelial cells while C5a is chemotactic for neutrophils as well as eosinophils and induces not only the adhesion and rolling but also transmigration through endothelium and upregulation of endothelial cell adhesion molecules. MAC assembly stimulates expression of several soluble proinflammatory mediators including prostacyclin, TNFα, IL-1, βFGF, PDGF, IL-8, MCP-1, and RANTES. As well as being activated by complement products, the endothelium also mediates activation of the complement pathway. For example, human endothelial cells exposed to oxidative stress activate the lectin complement pathway (LCP) through binding of mannose-binding lectin.[83]

Inflammatory cell influx into bronchial tissue and increased permeability of the bronchial vasculature are present in asthma. Inadequate control of vascular permeability may be a critical component of the asthmatic response; histamine, bradykinin, lipoxygenase metabolites of arachidonic acid (leukotrienes C4, D_4, and E_4), cyclooxygenase (COX) products (thromboxane A_2), PAF, and certain neurogenic peptides, such as neurokinin A and neurokinin B contribute to increased vascular permeability in the asthmatic airway. These mediators are generated locally during an asthmatic attack, either from resident cells or from infiltrating leukocytes, and act directly on the endothelium to alter permeability.

■ CONCLUSIONS ■

The vascular endothelium has a number of important functions that are necessary for the maintenance of tissue homeostasis. Likewise, the endothelium has important roles to play in regulating the acute inflammatory response. When the endothelium is injured during the course of an inflammatory attack, mechanisms are activated to protect the cells and tissues. When these protective responses are overwhelmed, cell death and tissue damage is the result. When this occurs in the lung, the immediate consequence includes dysfunctional gas exchange, which can prove to be fatal. If death does not occur, the lung may heal with minimal structural damage and minimal long-term effect. Alternatively, the healing process may not occur normally and may result in the fibrotic state, in which case the consequence is permanent lung dysfunction.

The role of the endothelium in chronic allergic diseases such as asthma is not as well understood as in acute inflammation. Nevertheless, as mechanisms of diseases such as asthma become better delineated, a number of parallels with acute inflammatory injury are evident.

References

The endothelium and regulation of the inflammatory response

1. Aird W. Endothelial cell heterogeneity. Crit Care Med 2003; 31:S221–S230.
2. Stevens T. Molecular and cellular determinants of lung endothelial cell heterogeneity. Chest 2000; 128:538–584.
3. Thorin E, Stevens T, Patterson CE. Heterogeneity of lung endothelial cells. perspectives on lung endothelial barrier function. Adv Mol Cell Biol 2005; 35:277–310.
4. Price GC, Thompson SA, Kam PCA. Tissue factor and tissue factor pathway inhibitor. Anaesthesia 2004; 59:483–493.
5. Cines DB, Pollak ES, Buck CA, et al. Endothelial cells in physiology and in the pathophysiology of vascular disorders. Blood 1998; 91:3527–3561.
6. Okajima K. Regulation of inflammatory responses by activated protein C: the molecular mechanism(s) and therapeutic implications. Clin Chem Lab Med 2004; 42:132–141.
7. Miyauchi T, Masaki T. Pathophysiology of endothelin in the cardiovascular system. Annu Rev Physiol 1999; 61:391–415.
8. Zhou Y, Mitra S, Varadharaj S, et al. Increased expression of cyclooxygenase-2 mediates enhanced contraction to endothelin ETA receptor stimulation in endothelial nitric oxide synthase knockout mice. Circ Res 2006; 98:1439–1445.
9. Marletta MA. Nitric oxide synthase structure and mechanism. J Biol Chem 1993; 268:12231–11234.
10. Forstermann U, Munzel T. Endothelial nitric oxide synthase in vascular disease: from marvel to menace. Circulation 2006; 113:1708–1714.
11. Budhiraja R, Tuder RM, Hassoun P. Endothelial dysfunction in pulmonary hypertension. Circulation 2004; 109:159–165.
12. McVerry BJ, Garcia JGN. In vitro and in vivo modulation of vascular barrier integrity by sphingosine 1-phosphate: mechanistic insights. Cell Signal 2005; 17:131–139.
13. Patterson CE, Matthay MA. The cellular and molecular foundations of pulmonary edema. Perspectives on lung endothelial barrier function. Adv Mol Cell Biol 2005; 35:1–24.
14. Claesson-Welsh L. Signal transduction by vascular endothelial growth factor receptors. Biochem Soc Trans 2003; 31:20–24.

IMMUNOLOGY

15. Groeneveld ABJ. Vascular pharmacology of acute lung injury and acute respiratory distress syndrome. Vasc Pharmacol 2003; 39:247–256.
16. Lee YC. The involvement of VEGF in endothelial permeability: a target for anti-inflammatory therapy. Curr Opin Investig Drugs 2005; 6:1124–1130.
17. Itoh Y, Sendo T, Oishi R. Physiology and pathophysiology of proteinase-activated receptors (PARs): role of tryptase/PAR-2 in vascular endothelial barrier function. J Pharmacol Sci 2005; 97:14–19.
18. Kawabata A, Kawao N. Physiology and pathophysiology of proteinase-activated receptors (PARs): PARs in the respiratory system: cellular signaling and physiological/pathological roles. J Pharmacol Sci 97:20–24.
19. Lentsch AB, Ward PA. Regulation of inflammatory vascular damage. J Pathol 2000; 190(3):343–348.
20. Patterson CE. Perspectives on lung endothelial barrier function. Amsterdam: Elsevier, 2005.
21. Imhof BA, Dunon D. Leukocyte migration and adhesion. Adv Immunol 1995; 58:345.
22. Kubes P, Kerfoot SM. Leukocyte recruitment in the microcirculation: the rolling paradigm revisited. News Physiol Sci 2001; 16:76–80.
23. Tedder T, Steeber D, Chen A, et al. The selectins: vascular adhesion molecules. FASEB J 1995; 9:866–873.
24. Adams DH, Shaw S. Leucocyte-endothelial interactions and regulation of leucocyte migration. Lancet 1994; 343:831–836.

Endothelial cell injury during acute inflammation

25. Murphy HS, Varani J, Ward PA. Endothelial cell injury and defense in perspectives in lung endothelial cell barrier function. Adv Mol Cell Biol 2004; 35:335–364.
26. Zurawska J, Sze M, Lee J, et al. Dynamic microfilaments and microtubules regulate endothelial function. In: perspectives on lung endothelial barrier function. Adv Mol Cell Biol 2005; 35:205–236.
27. Dudek SM, Garcia JGN. Cytoskeletal regulation of pulmonary vascular permeability. J Appl Physiol 2001; 91:1487–1500.
28. Carden D, Xiao F, Moak C, et al. Neutrophil elastase promotes lung microvascular injury and proteolysis of endothelial cadherins. Am J Physiol Heart Circ Physiol 1998; 275:H385–H92.
29. Hermant B, Bibert S, Concord E, et al. Identification of proteases involved in the proteolysis of vascular endothelium cadherin during neutrophil transmigration. J Biol Chem 2003; 278:14002–14012.
30. Edens HA, Parkos CA. Neutrophil transendothelial migration and alteration in vascular permeability: focus on neutrophil-derived azurocidin. Curr Opin Hematol 2003; 10:25–30.
31. Alexander JS, Zhu Y, Elrod JW, et al. Reciprocal regulation of endothelial substrate adhesion and barrier function. Microcirculation 2002; 8:389–410.
32. Nilhand S, Cremer A, Fluck J, et al. Contraction-dependent apoptosis of normal dermal fibroblasts. J Invest Dermatol 2001; 116:686–692.
33. Tian B, Lessan K, Kahm J, et al. [beta]1 integrin regulates fibroblast viability during collagen matrix contraction through a phosphatidylinositol 3-kinase/Akt/protein kinase B signaling pathway. J Biol Chem 2004; 277:24667–24675.
34. Griendling K, Sorescu D, Ushio-Fukai M. NAD(P)H oxidase: role in cardiovascular biology and disease. Circ Res 2000; 86:494.
35. Zueleta J, Yu F, Hertig I, et al. Release of hydrogen peroxide in response to hypoxia-reoxygenation: role of and NAD(P)H oxidase-like enzyme in endothelial cell plasma membrane. Am J Respir Cell Mol Biol 1995; 12:41.
36. Al-Mehdi A, Zhao G, Dodia C, et al. Endothelial cell NADPH oxidase as source of oxidants in lungs exposed to ischemia. Circ Res 1998, 83.730–737.
37. Murphy HS, Yu C, Quddus J. Functional expression of NAD(P)H oxidase p47 in lung microvascular endothelial cells. Biochem Biophys Res Commun 2000; 278:584–589.
38. Channon KM, Guzik TJ. Mechanisms of superoxide production in human blood vessels: relationship to endothelial dysfunction, clinical and genetic risk factors. J Physiol Pharmacol 2002; 53:515–524.
39. Lubec G. The hydroxyl radical: from chemistry to human disease. J Invest Med 1996; 44:324.
40. Boehme MW, Galle P, Stremmel W. Kinetics of thrombomodulin release and endothelial cell injury by neutrophil-derived proteases and oxygen radicals. Immunol Today 2002; 107:340–349.
41. Hensley K, Robinson KA, Gabbita SP, et al. Reactive oxygen species, cell signaling, and cell injury. Free Radic Biol Med 2000; 28(10):1456–1462.
42. Gipson T, Bless N, Shanley T, et al. Regulatory effects of endogenous protease inhibitors in acute lung inflammatory injury. J Immunol 1999; 162:3653.
43. Nonas S, Miller I, Kawkitinarong K, et al. Oxidized phospholipids reduce vascular leak and inflammation in rat model of acute lung injury. Am J Respir Crit Care Med 2006; 173:1130–1138.
44. Bochkov VN, Kadl A, Huber J, et al. Protective role of phospholipid oxidation products in endotoxin-induced tissue damage. Nat Immunol 2002; 419:77–81.
45. Droge WK, Schulze-Osthoff S, Mihm D, et al. Functions of glutathione and glutathione disulfide in immunology and immunopathology. FASEB J 1994; 8:1131–1138.
46. Mehta S. The effects of nitric oxide in acute lung injury. Vasc Pharmacol 43:390–403.
47. Rahman I, Macnee W. Regulation of redox glutathione levels and gene transcription in lung inflammation: therapeutic approaches. Free Radic Biol Med 2000; 28:1405.
48. Guo F, Comhair S, Zheng S, et al. Molecular mechanisms of increased nitric oxide (NO) in asthma: evidence for transcriptional and post-translational regulation of NO synthesis. J Immunol 2000; 164:5970.
49. Berlyne G, N NB. No role for NO in asthma? Lancet 2000; 355:1029.
50. Murray P, Wylam M, Umans J. Nitric oxide and septic vascular dysfunction. Anesth Analg 2000; 90:89.
51. Stuehr DJ. Nitric oxide synthesis and breakdown. Biochim Biophys Acta 1999; 1411:217.
52. Bronte V, Zanovello P. Regulation of immune responses by L-arginine metabolism. Nat Rev Immunol 2005; 5:641–654.
53. Speyer C, Neff T, Warner R, et al. Regulatory effects of iNOS on acute lung inflammatory responses in mice. Am J Pathol 2003; 163:2319–2328.
54. Laroux FS, Lefer DJ, Kawachi S, et al. Role of nitric oxide in the regulation of acute and chronic inflammation. Antiox Redox Signal 2000; 2:391–396.
55. Mehta S. The effects of nitric oxide in acute lung injury. Vasc Pharmacol 2005; 43:390–403.
56. Gutierrez H, Nieves B, Chemley P, et al. Nitric oxide regulation of superoxide-dependent lung injury: oxidant-protective actions of endogenously produced and exogenously administered nitric oxide. Free Radic Biol Med 1996; 21:43.
57. Singleton KD, Wischmeyer PE. Effects of HSP70.1/3 gene knockout on acute respiratory distress syndrome and the inflammatory response following sepsis. Am J Physiol Lung Cell Mol Physiol 2006; 290:L956–L961.
58. Bromberg Z, Deutschman CS, Weiss YG. Heat shock protein 70 and the acute respiratory distress syndrome. J Anesth 2005; 19:236–242.
59. Sartori C, Scherrer U. Turning up the heat in the lungs. A key mechanism to preserve their function. Adv Exp Med Biol 2003; 543:263–275.
60. Asahara T, Murohara T, Sullivan A, et al. Isolation of putative progenitor endothelial cells for angiogenesis. Science 1997; 275:964–966.
61. Lemanske RF Jr. Inflammatory events in asthma: an expanding equation. J Allergy Clin Immunol 2000; 105(6 Pt 2):S633–S636.
62. Yamada M, Kubo H, Ishizawa K, et al. Increased circulating endothelial progenitor cells in patients with bacterial pneumonia: evidence that bone marrow derived cells contribute to lung repair. Thorax 2005; 60:410–413.
63. Burnham EL, Taylor WR, Quyyumi AA, et al. Increased circulating endothelial progenitor cells are associated with survival in acute lung injury. Am J Respir Crit Care Med 2005; 172:854–860.
64. Doerschuk CM. Circulating endothelial progenitor cells in pulmonary inflammation. Thorax 2005; 60:362–364.
65. Urbich C, Aicher A, Heeschen C, et al. Soluble factors released by endothelial progenitor cells promote migration of endothelial cells and cardiac resident progenitor cells. J Mol Cell Cardiol 2005; 39:733–742.
66. Körbling M, Estrov Z. Medical progress: adult stem cells for tissue repair - a new therapeutic concept? News Physiol Sci 2003; 349:570–582.
67. Healy AM, Morgenthau L, Zhu X, et al. VEGF is deposited in the subepithelial matrix at the leading edge of branching airways and stimulates neovascularization in the murine embryonic lung. Dev Dyn 2000; 219:341–352.
68. Thébaud B, Ladha F, Michelakis ED, et al. Vascular endothelial growth factor gene therapy increases survival, promotes lung angiogenesis, and prevents alveolar damage in hyperoxia-induced lung injury: evidence that angiogenesis participates in alveolarization. Circ Res 2005; 112:2477–2486.
69. Voelkel NF, Cool C, Taraceviene-Stewart L, et al. Janus face of vascular endothelial growth factor: the obligatory survival factor for lung vascular endothelium controls precapillary artery remodeling in severe pulmonary hypertension. Crit Care Med 2002; 30:S251–S6.
70. Yano K, Liaw PC, Mullington JM, et al. Vascular endothelial growth factor is an important determinant of sepsis morbidity and mortality. J Exp Med 2006; 203:1447–1458.
71. Abadie Y, Bregeon F, Papazian L, et al. Decreased VEGF concentration in lung tissue and vascular injury during ARDS. Eur Respir J 2005; 25:139–146.
72. Natarajan V, Jayaram H, Scribner W, et al. Activation of endothelial cell phospholipase D by sphingosine and sphingosine-1-phosphate. Am J Respir Cell Mol Biol 1994; 11:221–229.
73. Windh R, Lee M, Hla T, et al. Differential coupling of the sphingosine 1-phosphate receptors Edg-1, Edg-3, and H218/Edg-5 to the Gi, Gq, and G12 families of heterotrimeric G proteins. J Biol Chem 1999; 274:27351–27358.
74. Armulik A, Abramsson A, Betsholtz C. Endothelial/pericyte interactions. Circ Res 2005; 97:512–523.

Endothelial cells in allergy and asthma

75. Ward P. Recruitment of inflammatory cells into lung: roles of cytokines, adhesion molecules, and complement. J Lab Clin Med 1997; 129:400.
76. Ulfman LH, Kuijper PH, van der Linden JA, et al. Characterization of eosinophil adhesion to TNF-alpha-activated endothelium under flow conditions: alpha 4 integrins mediate initial attachment, and E-selectin mediates rolling. J Immunol 1999; 163:343–350.
77. Shahabuddin S, Ponath P, RP RS. Migration of eosinophils across endothelial cell monolayers: interactions among IL-5, endothelial-activating cytokines, and C-C chemokines. J Immunol 2000; 164:3847.
78. Chihara J, Yamamoto T, Kayaba H, et al. Degranulation of eosinophils mediated by intercellular adhesion molecule-1 and its ligands is involved in adhesion molecule expression on endothelial cells-selective induction of VCAM-1. J Allergy Clin Immunol 1999; 103:S452–S456.
79. Fernvik E, Hallden G, Lundahl J, et al. Allergen-induced accumulation of eosinophils and lymphocytes in skin chambers is associated with increased levels of interleukin-4 and sVCAM-1. Allergy 1999; 54:455–463.
80. Lukacs NW, Tekkanat KK. Role of chemokines in asthmatic airway inflammation. Immunol Rev 2000; 177:21–30.
81. Gonzalo JA, Lloyd CM, Kremer L, et al. Eosinophil recruitment to the lung in a murine model of allergic inflammation. The role of T cells, chemokines, and adhesion receptors. J Clin Invest 1996; 98:2332–245.
82. Ward PA. Recruitment of inflammatory cells into lung: roles of cytokines, adhesion molecules, and complement. J Lab Clin Med 1997; 129:400–404.
83. Collard CD, Montalto MC, Reenstra WR, et al. Endothelial oxidative stress activated the lectin-complement pathway. Am J Pathol 2001; 159:1045–1054.

Biology of Airway Smooth Muscle Cells

25

Yassine Amrani, Omar Tliba, and Reynold A Panettieri Jr

CONTENTS

SUMMARY OF IMPORTANT CONCEPTS

>> The traditional view of airway smooth muscle (ASM) in asthma, that of a purely contractile tissue, is rapidly changing. New evidence suggests that ASM cells play an important role not only in regulating bronchomotor tone but also in the perpetuation of airway inflammation and the remodeling of airways. ASM cells are capable of secreting immunomodulatory cytokines and chemokines and express cell surface receptors that are important for cell adhesion and leukocyte activation. Evidence also suggests that cytokine stimulation of ASM can render the myocyte insensitive to glucocorticoid stimulation. Although ASM has been a target tissue for pharmacologic agents that promote bronchodilatation, the newly described function of ASM as immunomodulatory will also offer the development of novel antiinflammatory agents

▓ INTRODUCTION ▓

The traditional view of airway smooth muscle (ASM) in asthma, that of a purely contractile tissue, is rapidly changing. New evidence suggests that ASM cells play an important role, not only in regulating bronchomotor tone but also in the perpetuation of airway inflammation and

in the remodeling of the airways. In this chapter, we will discuss three distinct functions of ASM cells. We will review the process of excitation-contraction coupling, with a particular focus on the role of cytokines in modulating calcium responses. We will next examine the processes of smooth muscle cell proliferation and migration. Finally, we will discuss the synthetic function of ASM cells, defined as the ability to secrete immune modulatory cytokines and chemokines and to express surface receptors that are important for cell adhesion and leukocyte activation. We will also examine pharmacologic approaches to modifying the synthetic function of ASM cells and discuss how altered synthetic function may contribute to airway remodeling.

AIRWAY SMOOTH MUSCLE PLAYS A ROLE IN THE DEVELOPMENTAL REGULATION OF LUNG GROWTH

ASM probably plays a key role in modulating lung development. Throughout embryogenesis, ASM expresses smooth muscle actin and is mechanically active as demonstrated by the spreading of spontaneous periodic calcium waves that propagate peristaltic waves.[1,2] The consequences of ASM peristalsis promote lung development.[3] Interestingly, normal epithelial growth and branching during embryogenesis requires fibroblast growth factor 10 (FGF-10) derived from ASM. In a rare disease, congenital diaphragmatic hernia syndrome,[4] lung growth is impaired as a result of the abnormal expression of serum response factor (SRF) isoforms and impaired SRF-mediated, ASM-specific gene expression.[5] This intrinsic ASM abnormality profoundly affects epithelial cell growth and branching in an SRF- and FGF-10-dependent manner. In in vivo animal models of pulmonary hyperplasia, using nitrofen administration to pregnant rats, a similar abnormality is manifested. Developmental regulation of ASM shortening, therefore, appears to be subject to epithelial–mesenchymal interactions that direct morphogenesis. Such epithelial–mesenchymal cell interaction has also been proposed to be critical in promoting airway remodeling secondary to airway inflammation in diseases of asthma and COPD. Collectively, ASM plays a role in providing airway peristalsis and in the development of the lung in morphogenesis. Whether such processes are important in airway remodeling remains to be explored.

ASM CONTRACTION AND AIRWAY HYPERRESPONSIVENESS

In normal airways, smooth muscle cell contraction regulates airway caliber and bronchomotor tone. Using isolated bronchial preparations, studies have compared the isotonic length and/or force generation of tissues derived from asthmatics and non-asthmatics. Interestingly, not all studies demonstrated an increased force generation in asthmatic tissues when compared to control tissues.[6] These conflicting data likely can be attributed to differences in the experimental and methodological approaches used.[7] Several parameters, such as the degree of tissue elastance, smooth muscle mass, and knowledge of the optimal length, were found to be important factors when evaluating the force-generating capacity of ASM preparations derived from asthmatics.[6,7]

Although there appear to be conflicting data in studies comparing smooth muscle responsiveness between normal and asthmatic patients, a number of studies report that passive sensitization of human ASM with asthmatic serum induces a non-specific increase in smooth muscle cell responsiveness,[8–11] demonstrating the existence of mediators in the serum of asthmatic patients that promote airway responsiveness. While the precise nature of these mediators has not been completely defined, evidence suggests that TNFα or IL-1β can induce bronchial hyperreactivity in both humans and animals. Cytokines also can 'prime' ASM to become hyperresponsive to contractile agonists in vitro, supporting the concept that cytokines modulate agonist-induced ASM contractile function. Other pro-inflammatory mediators, such as lysophosphatidic acid, a bioactive lipid released from activated platelets, phospholipase A_2, and leukotriene C4, also enhance ASM responsiveness in vitro to contractile agonists such as acetylcholine, methacholine, and serotonin. Together, these studies suggest that pro-inflammatory mediators induce airway hyperresponsiveness (AHR) by enhancing ASM contraction and/or altering ASM relaxation (Fig. 25.1). Understanding the mechanisms by which inflammatory mediators modulate ASM contractile reactivity may offer new insight into the molecular mechanisms that modulate AHR in asthma.[12]

MOLECULAR BASIS OF ASM CONTRACTION

In smooth muscle cells, the level of intracellular calcium regulates, in part, ASM shortening. Activation of an ASM cell by an agonist induces a rapid rise in $[Ca^{2+}]_i$, associated with the release of intracellular calcium stores, to a peak level roughly tenfold higher than the resting level (100 nM to >1 μM with maximum agonist stimulation). Following this peak, calcium levels fall but remain elevated provided that the excitatory stimulus remains present. The elevation in $[Ca^{2+}]_i$ activates the calcium/calmodulin-sensitive myosin light chain kinase (MLCK), leading to phosphorylation of the regulatory myosin light chain (MLC_{20}) at serine 19. Phosphorylation of this residue by myosin ATPase activity initiates crossbridge cycling between myosin and actin. ATP binding, hydrolysis, and ADP release continue as long as MLC_{20} is phosphorylated; dephosphorylation by the MLC phosphatase terminates crossbridge cycling and relaxes smooth muscle.[13]

MOLECULAR MECHANISMS REGULATING ASM SHORTENING

Enhanced function of contractile receptors

Considering the central role of Ca^{2+} in regulating ASM contractile function, investigators postulate that alterations in Ca^{2+}-regulatory mechanisms likely impair ASM contractility. Studies using cultured human tracheal or bronchial smooth muscle cells, as in vitro models of ASM responsiveness, convincingly demonstrated that G protein-coupled receptor (GPCR)-associated signaling in ASM can be modulated by a variety of inflammatory stimuli. Cytokines, such as TNF-α, augment agonist-induced ASM contractility by enhancing, in a non-specific manner, agonist-evoked Ca^{2+} transients (to bradykinin, carbachol).[12] The hypothesis that changes in GPCR-associated Ca^{2+} signaling represent an important mechanism underlying the development of AHR has also been supported by other studies. Tao and colleagues showed that ASM cells derived from hyperresponsive inbred rats have an augmented bradykinin-induced Ca^{2+} responses when compared to ASM cells derived from normoresponsive rats.[14] Deshpande and colleagues demonstrated that, in addition to TNF-α, other cytkines including IL-1β and, in to a lesser degree, IFN-γ augment Ca^{2+} responses induced by carbachol, bradykinin, and thrombin.[15] In a similar manner, IL-13, a Th2 type important

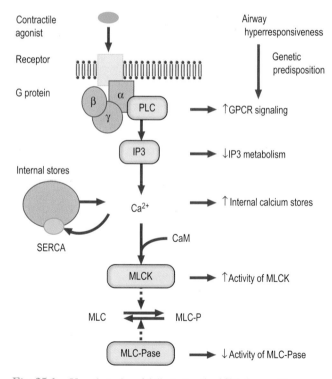

Fig. 25.1. Hypothetical model illustrating the ASM abnormalities that can cause airway hyperresponsiveness in asthma. Although the causal relationship between ASM dysfunction and airway hyperresponsiveness is still unknown, recent evidence suggests that at least two major pathways may promote an exaggerated contractility of ASM in asthma. This includes increased responsiveness to contractile agonists due to a potentiation of the calcium signaling associated with contractile agonists. Investigators also reported that cytokines can induce a hyporesponsiveness to β-adrenergic stimulation, an effect that involves an impairment of the β_2-adrenergic receptor function.

mediator in allergic asthma,[16] also non-specifically increased Ca^{2+} responses to agonists.[17-20] Microarray technology used to study the modulation of gene expression of ASM by IL-13 revealed a diversity of potential molecular mechanisms influencing ASM responsiveness, including changes in cytoskeletal proteins, receptors or calcium regulators.[21] Together, these data show that 'pro-asthmatic' cytokines, in a non-specific manner, enhance GPCR-associated Ca^{2+} responses in ASM, a mechanism likely to affect ASM contractility.

RhoA/Rho kinase expression and/or activity also modulates agonist responsiveness

Reports in C3H/HeJ, Balb/C and A/J mice revealed that differences in ASM contractility among species may not require changes in GPCR agonist-induced Ca^{2+} responses but rather involve changes in the Ca^{2+} sensitivity of the contractile apparatus.[22] A possible mechanism involves the small monomeric G protein Rho that can augment ASM contractility by increasing levels of MLC phosphorylation via the Rho-activated kinase (ROCK) dependent suppression of MLC phosphatase.[23,24] Both RhoA and ROCK are activated by a variety of stimuli associated with the development of AHR including cytokines,[25-28] sphingolipids,[29-31] mechanical stress,[32] and isoprostane.[33] The RhoA/Rho kinase pathway regulates the expression of serum response factor-dependent smooth muscle specific genes in canine ASM cells,[34] a mechanism that identifies the importance of the Rho-kinase pathway in maintaining a contractile phenotype recently described in bovine ASM tissues.[35] Rho pathways modulate diverse cellular responses in ASM cells including the regulation of Ca^{2+} influx[36] and cell proliferation.[37] Possibly, abnormal RhoA activity and/or expression will dramatically alter ASM contractility not only via the Ca^{2+} sensitization but also through the increased expression of Rho-dependent contractile proteins. A recent report using the Y-27632 inhibitor confirmed that the non-specific ASM hyperresponsiveness as well as the specific allergen responsiveness induced by passive sensitization require the activation of Rho-kinase.[38]

Changes in ASM contractile properties play an important role in the development of AHR associated with chronic airway diseases such as asthma. In vitro studies support the concept that a variety of 'pro-asthmatic' signals such as physical (repeated stretch) or chemical exposures (cytokines) drastically augment ASM contractile force by altering multiple key pathways: (1) via the aberrant activation of contractile and/or impaired function of relaxant receptors (desensitization), (2) the alteration of Ca^{2+} regulatory signaling molecules (CD38, SERCA, Ca^{2+} channels), and (3) the activity of elements of the contractile apparatus through Rho-dependent pathways. Defining the inflammatory signals (factors and associated mechanisms) involved in the regulation of ASM responsiveness may represent a potential new target for the treatment of AHR.

MODULATION OF RECEPTOR SIGNALING

Expression of contractile agonist receptors

Pro-inflammatory mediators can modulate the density of contractile agonist receptors on ASM cells. TNF-α induced a dramatic decrease in muscarinic receptor density. In contrast, expression of the bradykinin B_2 receptor was rapidly increased in ASM exposed to IL-1β or TNF-α

by a prostanoid-dependent regulation of gene transcription and by the activation of the Ras/Raf/MEK pathway. Surprisingly, the β_2-agonist fenoterol or the steroid methylprednisolone also increased expression of the histamine H_1 and bradykinin B_2 receptors, an effect that involved both increased gene expression and mRNA stability. This increase in H_1 receptor expression was associated with an increase in the contractile response to histamine. Whether β_2-agonists and steroids induce such effects in vivo remains unclear. These studies, however, suggest that current asthma therapy may also modulate airway hyperreactivity by altering contractile agonist receptor expression in ASM.[12]

Modulation of G-protein-coupled signal transduction

In human ASM cells, contractile agonists bind Gq-protein-coupled receptors, leading to the activation of phospholipase C. The subsequent hydrolysis of phosphatidylinositol 4,5-bisphosphate into inositol trisphosphate and diacylglycerol ultimately results in an increase in $[Ca^{2+}]_i$.[13] Since most of the inflammatory agents do not evoke either a calcium response or phosphoinositide hydrolysis in human ASM, modulation of agonist-induced increases in $[Ca^{2+}]_i$ by extracellular stimuli may be due to the modulation of downstream GPCR signaling. TNF-α increased the amount, as well as the activity, of G proteins in several cell types including ASM.[39-42] The finding that TNF-α potentiated calcium mobilization in response to NaF,[43] an agent that bypasses membrane receptors and directly activates G proteins,[44,45] supports the notion that TNF-α may act directly at the level of G proteins.

Recent studies showed that bradykinin-evoked phosphoinositide accumulation in human ASM is significantly enhanced by various cytokines such as TNF-α and IL-1β.[43,46-48] The effect of cytokines on agonist-evoked calcium responses seems to be stimulus-specific, however, since pretreatment of ASM cells with IL-1β diminished phosphoinositide metabolism induced by histamine.[49] In addition to their effect on calcium signaling, cytokines may also modulate β_2-adrenergic function. TNF-α as well as IL-1β also suppress isoproterenol-stimulated activation of adenylyl cyclase.[50-52] A recent report showed that IL-13 is also able to impair ASM responsiveness to β_2-adrenergic stimuli,[53] showing that cytokines may promote AHR by impairing β_2-adrenergic responsiveness in ASM cells.

Pro-inflammatory cytokines affect ASM contractility on many levels. Alterations in calcium homeostasis and sensitivity, as well as contractile agonist receptor expression and signal transduction pathways, have profound effects on airway hyperreactivity. The ability of antiinflammatory therapies, such as corticosteroids, to modulate these effects will be discussed later in this chapter.[12,54]

■ CELLULAR AND MOLECULAR MECHANISMS REGULATING AIRWAY SMOOTH MUSCLE CELL GROWTH ■

Early pathologic studies of patients with asthma described the increase in both size and number of ASM[55,56] and the correlation with airway hyperreactivity and increased airways resistance. Increased numbers of ASM cells (hyperplasia) also occur in subjects with mild asthma.[57] Over the past decade, significant advances have been made in identifying the many diverse mitogens and signal transduction pathways that modulate ASM growth.[58] As progression of ASM through the cell cycle is a fundamental event in regulating cell proliferation, recent studies have also examined the signal transduction pathways that regulate specific cell cycle protein expression in ASM cells. This section examines the signaling pathways that stimulate ASM cell proliferation and identifies the critical cell cycle events that regulate ASM growth.

AIRWAY SMOOTH MUSCLE PROLIFERATION

Many inflammatory mediators are increased in bronchoalveolar lavage (BAL) from asthmatic airways, and some have been shown to induce ASM mitogenesis in vitro. To date, mitogenic stimuli include: growth factors such as epidermal growth factor (EGF), insulin-like growth factors, platelet-derived growth factor (PDGF) isoforms BB and AB and basic fibroblast growth factor; plasma- or inflammatory cell-derived mediators, such as lysosomal hydrolases (β-hexoaminidases and β-glucuronidase), α-thrombin, tryptase, and sphingosine 1-phosphate (SPP); and contractile agonists, such as histamine, endothelin-1, substance P, phenylephrine, serotonin, thromboxane A_2, and leukotriene D4.[59,60]

Although the cytokines interleukin 1β (IL-1β), IL-6, and tumor necrosis factor α (TNF-α) are also increased in the BAL of asthmatics,[61] whether these cytokines stimulate ASM proliferation in vitro remains controversial. In 1995, De et al [62] reported that IL-1β and IL-6 cause hyperplasia and hypertrophy of cultured guinea pig ASM cells; however, other studies have shown that IL-1β [63] and IL-6 [64] are not mitogenic for human ASM cells. McKay et al [64] also reported that TNF-α (~ 30 pM) had no immediate mitogenic effect on human ASM cells. These results were in contrast to those of Stewart et al,[65] where the proliferative effect of TNF-α on human ASM cells appeared to be biphasic in which low concentrations of TNF-α (0.3–30 pM) were pro-mitogenic, while at

higher concentrations (300 pM), the mitogenic effect was abolished. Such conflicting reports may be due to cytokine-induced cyclo-oxygenase 2-dependent prostanoid production.[63] Cyclo-oxygenase products, such as prostaglandin E_2, inhibit DNA synthesis.[63] Therefore, cytokine-induced proliferative responses in ASM may be greater under conditions of cyclo-oxygenase inhibition, in which the expression of growth inhibitory prostanoids, such as prostaglandin E_2, is limited.[62,63,65]

Airway remodeling, a key feature of persistent asthma, is also characterized by the deposition of extracellular matrix (ECM) proteins in the airways.[66,67] ECM proteins (collagen I, III, V, fibronectin, tenascin, hyaluronan, versican, and laminin α_2/β_2) are increased in asthmatic airways.[66,68-70] Components of the ECM also modulate mitogen-induced ASM growth. Fibronectin and collagen I increase human ASM cell mitogenesis in response to PDGF-BB or α-thrombin, whereas laminin inhibits proliferation.[71] In this study, the increase in cell proliferation was accompanied by a decrease in expression of smooth muscle cell contractile proteins such as α-actin, calponin, and myosin heavy chain, suggesting that matrix may also modulate smooth muscle phenotype. Recently, human ASM cells were shown to secrete ECM proteins in response to asthmatic sera,[72] suggesting a cellular source for ECM deposition in airways, and implicating a novel mechanism in which ASM cells may modulate autocrine proliferative responses.

CELL CYCLE REGULATION

Extracellular stimuli transduce proliferative responses that move the cell through the cell cycle, which comprises distinct phases termed G_1, S (DNA synthesis), G_2, and M (mitosis) (Fig. 25.2). ASM growth appears to occur by activating cell cycle events similar to those described in other cell types. Hence, the following section provides an overview of the mammalian cell cycle[73,74] with particular emphasis on G_1–S transition, the most widely studied cell cycle phase in ASM biology shown

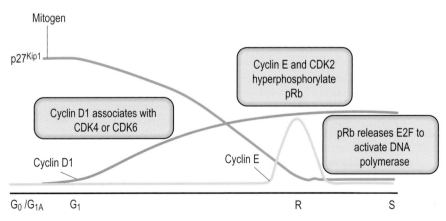

Fig. 25.2. Schematic representation of the G_1–S transition phase in the cell cycle. In response to mitogens, cells enter the cell cycle from the G_0/G_{1A} phase. D-type cyclins (D1 shown here) are expressed, while the levels of the CKI p27^{Kip1}, usually high in quiescent cells, fall in response to mitogenic stimulation. Progression through G_1 phase initially depends on holoenzymes composed of the D-type cyclins in association with cyclin-dependent kinases, CDK4 or CDK6. Most p27^{Kip1} becomes complexed with cyclin D-CDK, allowing activation of the cyclin E–CDK2 complex. Together, cyclin E and CDK2 act in a cascade to hyperphosphorylate pRb, which then releases the elongation factor E2F that activates DNA polymerase. Cell commitment to traverse completely through to mitosis is achieved on or near this point, termed the restriction point (R), in the cell cycle. Subsequently, cells initiate DNA synthesis (S phase). Reproduced from Ammit AJ, Panettieri Jr RP. Signal transduction in smooth muscle. J App Physiol 2001; 91:1431. Copyright, American Physiological Society, used with permission.

schematically in Figure 25.2. While many of the studies cited refer to ASM, the general phenomena are typical of other normal and malignant cell types.

To date, few studies have examined ASM cell growth in vivo. Proliferative responses in ASM cells are often studied using cell culture models. ASM cells are grown to confluence, and then growth-arrested in a low serum media or serum-free conditions for 24–48 h.[75,76] This experimental design synchronizes ASM cells in the G_0 or early G_1 phase (G_{1A}) of the cell cycle where ASM minimally incorporates [^{35}S]methionine and [^{3}H]thymidine.[75,76] As cells enter the cycle from G_0/G_{1A}, one or more D-type cyclins (D1, D2, and D3) are expressed as part of the delayed early response to mitogen stimulation as shown in Figure 25.2. Progression through G_1 phase initially depends on holoenzymes composed of one or more of the D-type cyclins (D1, D2, and/or D3) in association with cyclin-dependent kinases, CDK4 or CDK6. This is followed by activation of cyclin E–CDK2 complex as cells approach the G_1/S transition. Together, cyclin E and CDK2 act to hyperphosphorylate retinoblastoma protein (pRb), which then releases the elongation factor E2F that activates DNA polymerase. This step, termed the restriction point, represents the *point of no return*; cell commitment to undergo DNA synthesis (S phase) and mitosis is inevitable. In ASM cells, S phase is commonly detected by incorporation of radiolabeled thymidine,[75,76] or by immunofluorescent detection of the thymidine analogue 5-bromo-2'-deoxyuridine.[77] At each phase of G_1–S transition, CDK activities can also be constrained by CDK inhibitors (CKIs). CKIs are assigned to two families based on their structures and CDK targets: (1) the INK4 family (p16^{INK4a}, p15^{INK4b}, p18^{INK4c}, and p19^{INK4d}) specifically inhibits the catalytic subunits of CDK4 and CDK6; (2) the Cip/Kip family (p21^{Cip1}, p27^{Kip1}, and p57^{Kip2}) inhibits the activities of cyclin D-, E-, and A-dependent kinases.[78]

REGULATION OF CELL CYCLE IN AIRWAY SMOOTH MUSCLE CELL PROLIFERATION

ASM mitogens may act via different receptor-operated mechanisms,[58] as shown in Figure 25.3. While growth factors induce ASM cell mitogenesis by activating receptors with intrinsic protein tyrosine kinase (RTK) activity, contractile agonists released from inflammatory cells mediate their effects via activation of seven transmembrane GPCRs. Cytokines signal through cell surface glycoprotein receptors that function as oligomeric complexes consisting of typically two to four receptor chains,[79] coupled to Src family non-receptor tyrosine kinases, such as Lyn.[80]

Despite disparate receptor-operated mechanisms, recent evidence suggests that the small guanidine triphosphatase (GTPase), p21ras, acts as a point of convergence for diverse extracellular signal-stimulated pathways in ASM cells as shown in Figure 25.3.[77] Interestingly, synergy can occur between RTK and GPCRs that promotes human ASM mitogenesis and p21ras activation.[81] In their GTP-bound active state, p21ras proteins interact with downstream effectors, namely, Raf-1 and phosphatidylinositol 3-kinase (PI3K). By recruiting Raf-1, a 74-kDa cytoplasmic serine/threonine kinase, to the plasma membrane, GTP-bound p21ras activates the extracellular signal-regulated kinase (ERK) pathway, although Raf-1-independent signaling to ERK also has been shown.[82] P21ras also binds and activates PI3K by using specific regions termed switch I (Asp^{30}-Asp^{38}) and switch II (Gly^{60}-Glu^{76}).[83,84] Although alternative pathways do exist, e.g., protein kinase C-dependent

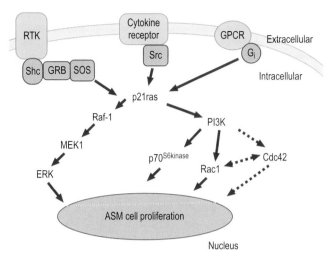

Fig. 25.3. Schematic representation of signal transduction mechanisms that regulate ASM cell proliferation. ASM mitogens act via RTKs, cytokine receptors or GPCRs to activate the small GTPase p21ras. p21ras proteins then interact with downstream effectors, Raf-1 and PI3K. Raf-1 activates MEK1, which then phosphorylates ERK. PI3K activates downstream effectors, p70^{S6k} or members of the Rho family GTPases, Rac1 and Cdc42 (although whether Cdc42 acts upstream of Rac1, or cross-talk exists is unknown at present, indicated by the dashed lines). ERK, PI3K and the downstream effectors of PI3K regulate cell cycle proteins, and thus the ERK and PI3K pathways are considered to be two major independent signaling pathways regulating ASM cell growth. Reproduced from Ammit AJ, Panettieri Jr RP. Signal transduction in smooth muscle. J App Physiol 2001; 91:1431. Copyright, American Physiological Society, used with permission.

pathways[58] or reactive oxygen-dependent pathways,[85] PI3K and ERK activation appears to be the dominant signal transduction pathway for RTK-, GPCR- or cytokine-stimulated growth of ASM cells.

Phosphatidylinositol 3-kinase pathway

PI3K isoforms are divided into three classes based on their structure and substrate specificity.[86] Class IA PI3Ks are cytoplasmic heterodimers composed of a 110 kDa (p110α, -β, or -δ) catalytic subunit and an 85 kDa (p85, p55, or p50) adaptor protein. Class IA isoforms can be activated by RTKs and non-receptor tyrosine kinases, whereas class IB p110γ is activated by Gβγ subunits of GPCRs. Class II isoforms are mainly associated with the phospholipid membranes and concentrated in the trans-Golgi network and present in clathrin-coated vesicles.[87] Class III isoforms are structurally related to the yeast vesicular sorting protein Vps34p.[88] Recent data[89] show that human ASM cells express class IA, II, and III PI3K but not the class IB p110γ isoform.

PI3K phosphorylates membrane phosphoinositides on the D3 hydroxyl of the inositol ring to form the phosphoinositides (PI) 3-phosphate, PI 3,4-diphosphate, and PI 3,4,5-triphosphate. These D3 phosphoinositides function as second messengers and activate downstream effector molecules, such as 70 kDa ribosomal S6 kinase (p70^{S6k}) [90,91] or members of the Rho family GTPases (Rac1[92] and Cdc42,[93] but not RhoA[93]) to regulate cell cycle protein expression and thus modulate cell cycle traversal in ASM cells.

The use of PI3K inhibitors has shown that activation of PI3K is critical for ASM cell cycle progression in human[90] and bovine ASM.[91,94]

Transfection or microinjection of cells with constitutively active class IA PI3K alone markedly increased DNA synthesis.[89] This is the first study to show that a constitutively active signaling molecule is capable of inducing DNA synthesis in human ASM cells. The extent of DNA synthesis stimulated in cells microinjected with constitutively active PI3K, however, was substantially less than that induced by receptor-mediated pathways. These data suggest that although active PI3K is sufficient to stimulate ASM DNA synthesis, other signaling events are also necessary to promote maximal ASM growth responses. Interestingly, PI3K inhibition does not alter ERK activation,[90] confirming that PI3K regulates DNA synthesis in an ERK-independent or possibly parallel manner.

In bovine[91] and human ASM,[90] rapamycin, an inhibitor of $p70^{S6k}$, attenuates growth factor-induced DNA synthesis, showing that $p70^{S6k}$ is an essential step in the pathway towards ASM cellular proliferation as shown in Figure 25.3. Through the phosphorylation of the 40S ribosomal protein, $p70^{S6k}$ upregulates the translation of mRNAs that contain an oligopyrimidine tract at their transcriptional start site. Such mRNA moieties encode proteins required for cell cycle progression in G_1 phase, such as the elongation factors E2F.[95]

Recent studies have also examined the involvement of the Rho GTPases, Rac1,[92] Cdc42,[93] and RhoA[93] in cyclin D1 upregulation and bovine ASM proliferation. Rac1 overexpression induced transcription of a cyclin D1 promoter construct, while a dominant-negative allele of Rac1 inhibited PDGF-induced cyclin D1 transcription.[92] Rac1-induced cyclin D1 promoter activation was also independent of ERK since inhibition of MEK1 had little effect.[92] In other studies, overexpression of the catalytically active subunit of PI3K ($p110^{PI3K}CAAX$) was sufficient to activate the cyclin D1 promoter, and cyclin D1 promoter activation could be attenuated by inhibitors of Rac1 signaling.[96] These results suggest that Rac1 may be downstream of PI3K; however, further study is necessary to confirm this observation. Other studies using overexpression constructs of Cdc42 and RhoA also showed that Cdc42 overexpression, but not RhoA, induced transcription from the cyclin D1 promoter in an ERK-independent manner.[93] In addition, $p110^{PI3K}CAAX$,[96] Rac1,[96] and Cdc42[93] were shown to activate the cyclin D1 promoter via the CREB/ATF-2 binding site. These results led the investigators to speculate that Cdc42 acts upstream of Rac1.[93] Whether this implicates PI3K in a linked signaling cascade remains unknown.

Extracellular signal-regulated kinase pathway

Raf-1 activation induces phosphorylation and activation of mitogen-activated protein (MAP) kinase/ERK kinase (MEK1). Activated MEK1 then directly phosphorylates (on both tyrosine and threonine residues) and activates the 42 kDa ERK2 and 44 kDa ERK1, also collectively referred to as p42/p44 MAP kinases as shown in Figure 25.3. In bovine ASM, inhibition of MEK1 and ERK activity attenuates PDGF-induced DNA synthesis, suggesting that activation of MEK1 and ERKs is required for proliferation.[97] In human ASM,[98] mitogens, including EGF, PDGF-BB, and thrombin, produced a robust and sustained activation of ERK1 and ERK2 that was correlated with ASM growth responses and was inhibited by MEK1 inhibition. Studies such as these suggest that the ERK pathway is a key signaling event mediating mitogen-induced ASM proliferation.

D-type cyclins (cyclins D1, D2, and D3) are key regulators of G_1 progression in mammalian cells, and consequently, cyclin D1 has been the most widely studied cyclin in ASM biology. In bovine ASM, mitogenic stimulation with PDGF induced cyclin D1 transcriptional activation and protein synthesis, with consequent hyperphosphorylation of pRb, while microinjection with a neutralizing antibody against cyclin D1 inhibited serum-induced S-phase traversal.[99] These studies suggested that cyclin D1 is a key downstream target of ERKs, and that downstream transcription factor targets of ERKs regulate cyclin D1 promoter transcriptional activity and cell cycle progression. This was also suggested in studies where MEK1 inhibitor and a dominant negative mutant of MEK1 or ERK abolished PDGF-induced cyclin D1 promoter activity or cyclin D1 expression.[100] Expression of a constitutively active p21ras induced ERK activation and transcriptional activation of the cyclin D1 promoter, postulating a role of p21ras in regulating the ERK pathway.[101]

Evidence now suggests that ERK activation induces expression of cyclin D1 in ASM cells. Hence, recent studies have focused on the transcriptional regulation of ERK-induced cyclin D1 accumulation. The promoter region of cyclin D1[102] contains multiple *cis*-elements potentially important for transcriptional activation, including binding sites for simian virus 40 protein 1 (Sp1), activator protein-1 (AP-1), signal transducers and activators of transcription (STAT), nuclear factor κB (NF-κB), and cAMP response element binding protein/activating transcription factor-2 (CREB/ATF-2).[103] Orsini et al showed that mitogen-induced ERK activation, thymidine incorporation, Elk-1, and AP-1 reporter activity were similarly abrogated by MEK1 inhibition.[98] Such studies suggest a linkage between ERK activation, transcription factor activation, cyclin D1 expression, and ASM proliferation. Similarly, MEK1 inhibition also attenuated expression of c-Fos,[104] suggesting that c-Fos may be one or both of the dimer pairs in the AP-1 transcription factor complex responsible for cyclin D1 expression in ASM cells. Whether ERK-dependent transcriptional regulation of cyclin D1 gene expression is via direct *cis*-activation with AP-1 dimers (composed of c-Fos), or via Elk-1-mediated *trans*-activation, still requires further investigation. In addition, cyclin D1 protein, but not mRNA levels, was affected by MEK1 inhibition,[105] suggesting that post-transcriptional control of cyclin D1 protein levels may also occur independently of the MEK1/ERK signaling pathways.

Another critical cell cycle protein is $p27^{Kip1}$, as shown in Figure 25.2.[74] In quiescent cells, the cytosolic protein levels of $p27^{Kip1}$ remain high. A coordinated increase of cyclin D1 expression promotes complexing of unbound $p27^{Kip1}$ molecules with cyclin D-dependent kinases, relieving cyclin E-CDK2 from CKI constraint, and thereby facilitating cyclin E-CDK2 activation later in G_1 phase.[74] In human ASM cells,[106] SPP, an agonist that activates multiple GPCRs, was shown to increase cyclin D1 levels and decrease $p27^{Kip1}$, possibly via an ERK-mediated pathway.[107] SPP also appeared to augment EGF- and thrombin-induced DNA proliferation by increasing G_1/S progression.[106] This was due to an enhancement of the stimulatory/inhibitory effect of EGF and thrombin on cyclin D1/$p27^{Kip1}$ expression by SPP.[106] A summary of the signal transduction pathways that modulate cell cycle events in ASM is described in Figure 25.3.

INHIBITION OF AIRWAY SMOOTH MUSCLE CELL PROLIFERATION BY ANTIASTHMA THERAPIES

The most widely used therapies for the control of asthma symptoms are the corticosteroids and the β_2-agonists. Inhaled corticosteroids inhibit inflammatory cell activation, while β_2-agonists are effective bronchodilators. In addition, these antiasthma therapies are potent inhibitors of ASM cell proliferation.

β_2-agonists activate the β_2-adrenergic receptor G_s-adenylyl cyclase pathway to elevate 3',5'-cyclic adenosine monophosphate (cAMP) in ASM cells. Because of their cAMP-elevating ability,[108] albuterol[109] and fenoterol[110] have been shown to inhibit mitogen-induced proliferation of human ASM cells. β_2-Adrenergic receptor agonists, and other cAMP-elevating agents, are thought to induce G_1 arrest by post-transcriptionally inhibiting cyclin D1 protein levels by action on a proteasome-dependent degradation pathway.[111] Musa et al[112] examined the effects of forskolin, an activator of adenylate cyclase, on DNA synthesis, cyclin D1 expression and cAMP response element-binding protein (CREB) phosphorylation and DNA binding in bovine ASM. By increasing cAMP in ASM cells, this study[112] showed that forskolin suppressed cyclin D_1 gene expression via phosphorylation and transactivation of CREB, suggesting that the effect of cAMP on cyclin D1 gene expression is via *cis*-repression of cyclin D1 promoter.

In human ASM,[113] corticosteroids dexamethasone and fluticasone propionate were shown to arrest ASM cells in the G_1 phase of the cell cycle. In this study, corticosteroids reduced thrombin-stimulated increases in cyclin D1 protein and mRNA levels, and attenuated pRb phosphorylation, via a pathway either downstream, or parallel, to the ERK cascade.[113] The difference between the relative inhibition of RTK- and GPCR-mediated ASM cell growth by dexamethasone suggests that steroid effects on ASM mitogenesis are complex. Further elucidation of the signaling and transcriptional targets for the inhibition of cell cycle progression by corticosteroids and β_2-agonists may indicate how these antiasthma therapies could be used optimally, and possibly in combination, to modulate airway wall remodeling in asthma.

■ SYNTHETIC FUNCTION OF ASM ■

CHEMOKINE AND CYTOKINE RELEASE BY AIRWAY SMOOTH MUSCLE CELLS

Following antigen exposure, eosinophils, macrophages, and lymphocytes that initiate and perpetuate airway inflammation are activated and/or recruited into the airways. The production of pro-inflammatory mediators by migratory inflammatory cells has a profound influence on ASM cells. Evidence suggests that exposure of ASM to cytokines or growth factors alters contractility and calcium homeostasis[13] and induces SMC hypertrophy and hyperplasia.[114] Recent data, however, convincingly demonstrate that ASM cells themselves can secrete a number of cytokines and chemoattractants. Studies of bronchial biopsies in mild asthmatics reveal constitutive staining for RANTES, a C-C chemokine, in ASM;[115] in vitro, RANTES secretion is induced by TNF-α and IFN-γ.[116–118] Similarly, the C-X-C chemokine IL-8 is also secreted by ASM in response to TNF-α, IL-1β, and bradykinin, a contractile agonist.[119–121] Other chemokines that are secreted by ASM cells include eotaxin, an eosinophil chemoattractant, and monocyte chemotactic protein (MCP)-1, MCP-2, MCP-3.[117,122,123]

IL-6, a pleiotropic cytokine, induces smooth muscle cell hyperplasia,[62] but also modulates B and T cell proliferation and immunoglobulin secretion. IL-6 secretion by ASM cells is inducible by multiple stimuli, including IL-1β, TNF-α, TGF-β, and sphingosine-1-phosphate, a recently described mediator in asthma.[64,106,118,121,124] Interestingly, transgenic expression of IL-6 in the murine lung evokes a peribronchiolar inflammatory infiltrate but promotes airway *hypo*responsiveness. This suggests an intriguing role for IL-6 in controlling local inflammation

and regulating airway reactivity[125,126] and is consistent with the known ability of IL-6 to inhibit TNF-α and IL-1β secretion. ASM cells may also play a role in promoting both the recruitment and survival of eosinophils by secretion of GM-CSF and IL-5.[127–129] Finally, additional cytokines that are secreted by human ASM cells include IL-1β, IFN-β, and other IL-6 family cytokines, such as leukemia inhibitory factor and IL-11, which are secreted following exposure of ASM cells to viral particles.[121,124,130–132]

RECEPTORS INVOLVED IN CELL ADHESION AND LYMPHOCYTE ACTIVATION

Cell adhesion molecules (CAMs) mediate leukocyte–endothelial cell interactions during the process of cell recruitment and homing.[133] The expression and activation of a cascade of CAMs that include selectins, integrins, and members of the immunoglobulin superfamily, as well as the local production of chemoattractants, leads to leukocyte adhesion and transmigration into lymph nodes and sites of inflammation involving non-lymphoid tissues. The mechanisms that regulate extravasation of leukocytes from the circulation during the establishment of a local inflammatory response are rapidly being delineated. Less defined are the subsequent interactions of the infiltrating leukocytes with other cell types in the bronchial submucosa or with the extracellular matrix, which may be important for sustaining the inflammatory response.

In addition to mediating leukocyte extravasation and transendothelial migration, CAMs promote submucosal or subendothelial contact with cellular and extracellular matrix components and serve as co-stimulatory molecules in the activation of leukocytes. New evidence suggests that CAMs mediate inflammatory cell–stromal cell interactions that may contribute to airway inflammation. ASM cells express ICAM-1 and VCAM-1, which are inducible by a wide range of inflammatory mediators.[134] In contrast, contractile agonists such as bradykinin and histamine have little effect on ASM CAM expression. ASM cells also constitutively express CD44, the primary receptor of the matrix protein hyaluronan.[134] Activated T lymphocytes adhere via LFA-1 and VLA-4 to cytokine-induced ICAM-1 and VCAM-1 on cultured human ASM cells. Moreover, an integrin-independent component of lymphocyte–smooth muscle cell adhesion appears to be mediated by CD44–hyaluronan interactions.[134]

CAMs can function as accessory molecules for leukocyte activation.[133,135,136] Whether CAMs expressed on smooth muscle serve this function, however, remains controversial. ASM cells do express MHC class II and CD40 following stimulation with interferon-γ (IFN-γ).[137,138] Studies also suggest that human ASM cells express low levels of CD80 (B7.1) and CD86 (B7.2).[139] The physiologic relevance of these findings remains unknown since ASM cells cannot present alloantigen to CD4 T cells, despite the expression of MHC class II and co-stimulatory molecules.[137]

Functionally, however, adhesion of stimulated CD4 T cells can induce smooth muscle cell DNA synthesis.[134] This appears to require direct cell–cell contact and is not mimicked by treatment of the cells with T cell conditioned medium. In addition, ligation of CD40, a co-stimulatory molecule upregulated by IFN-γ, increases intracellular calcium as well as IL-6 secretion; engagement of VCAM-1 on ASM cells activates phosphatidylinositol 3-kinase and augments growth factor-induced ASM cell proliferation.[138,140] Investigators have demonstrated that ASM cells express Fas in vivo. In vitro, expression of Fas is upregulated by

Table 25.1 Immunomodulatory proteins expressed by human ASM cells

Cytokines	Chemokines	CAMs	Other
IL-1β	IL-8	ICAM-1	CD40
IL-5	RANTES	VCAM-1	Fas
IL-6	MCP-1,-2,-3	CD44	HLA-DR
IL-8	Eotaxin	LFA-1	FcγRII
IL-11	GM-CSF	$\alpha_9\beta_1$	FcγRIII
LIF		$\alpha_5\beta_1$	NO
IFN-β		α_v, α_6 subunits	PGE$_2$
			CysLT receptors
			C3a/C5a receptors
			MMP/TIMP
			VEGF

TNF-α and, importantly, crosslinking of Fas induces smooth muscle cell apoptosis.[141] These studies highlight the finding that direct interactions between leukocytes and smooth muscle cells via immune receptors such as CD40 and Fas or adhesion receptors such as ICAM-1 and VCAM-1 contribute to the modulation of the local milieu resulting in smooth muscle cell activation and growth.

OTHER IMMUNOMODULATORY PROTEINS

Increased amounts of exhaled nitric oxide (NO) have been detected in patients with asthma.[142] NO appears to have a selective suppressive effect on the Th1 subset of helper T cells, suggesting that increased levels of NO may therefore lead to the predominantly Th2 type response associated with asthma. NO synthase has been demonstrated in cultured ASM cells where NO results in an inhibition of ASM cell proliferation.[143,144] In contrast, there is only indirect evidence that ASM cells produce NO in situ.[145] ASM cells also produce large amounts of PGE$_2$ and, to a lesser extent, other prostanoids, following stimulation with pro-inflammatory cytokines.[146] Although PGE$_2$ is a potent bronchodilator, it also has significant immunologic effects. For example, PGE$_2$ can decrease expression of CD23 (FcγRII), which has been shown to be expressed on human ASM cells[147] and may have a role as a negative regulator of airway inflammation and hyperresponsiveness.[148–150] PGE$_2$ inhibits cytokine-induced secretion of GM-CSF in vitro[151] and allergen-induced release of PGD$_2$ in patients with asthma.[152] In contrast, PGE$_2$ also primes dendritic cells towards a Th2-promoting capacity and synergizes with IL-4 to induce IgE synthesis.[153,154] Thus the roles of ASM-derived NO and PGE$_2$ need to be further defined, as they may have both beneficial and deleterious effects in the airway.

ASM cells express both receptors for the cysteinyl leukotrienes, LTC$_4$, LTD$_4$, and LTE$_4$.[155] Expression of the CysLT1 receptor is increased by exposure to IFN-γ and results in an increase in LTD$_4$-mediated force generation in cultured ASM cells.[156] The association between CysLT receptor expression and contractility may explain the increase in AHR following viral infection, a Th1-predominant environment. It also suggests that leukotriene receptor antagonists may have a therapeutic role in this clinical setting. Finally, receptors for the complement-derived anaphylatoxin peptides C3a and C5a have also been described on ASM cells. These peptides may play an important role in the pathogenesis of asthma by altering AHR, rather than airway inflammation.[157,158]

ASM cells provide a rich source of cytokines and chemokines, and under certain conditions, can express a wide variety of adhesion receptors, co-stimulatory molecules, and other immunomodulatory proteins (Table 25.1). Taken together, these data provide strong support for the potential role of ASM cells not only in perpetuating airway inflammation but also in leukocyte activation.

AIRWAY SMOOTH MUSCLE AS A TARGET FOR ANTIINFLAMMATORY THERAPY

To date, the most effective therapeutic approaches in asthma are corticosteroids and β-adrenergic receptor agonists, which abrogate airway inflammation and reverse bronchoconstriction, respectively. Given the new evidence that ASM cells secrete and express immunomodulatory proteins, investigators are now studying the cellular and molecular processes that regulate ASM synthetic function and examining the role of dexamethasone and β-agonists in modulating cytokine-induced synthetic responses.

Effects of [cAMP]$_i$ mobilizing agents on cytokine-induced synthetic responses

In asthma, β-agonists such as isoproterenol, albuterol, salmeterol, and formoterol are therapeutic agents that promote bronchodilation by stimulating receptors coupled to Gs, which in turn activates adenylyl cyclase, increases [cAMP]$_i$ and stimulates cAMP-dependent protein kinase (A-kinase) in ASM. In a similar manner, PGE$_2$, which is produced in large quantities at sites of inflammation, also increases [cAMP]$_i$ in human ASM cells and is a potent and effective bronchodilator.[159] New evidence suggests that $[cAMP]_i$-mobilizing agents in ASM cells also modulate cytokine-induced synthetic function. In TNF-α-stimulated ASM cells, both eotaxin and RANTES expression are effectively inhibited by isoproterenol, PGE_2, dibutyl-$[cAMP]_i$, or the phosphodiesterase inhibitors, rolipram and cilomast.[118,160,161] TNF-α-induced IL-8 secretion was also inhibited by the combination of $[cAMP]_i$ mobilizing agents and corticosteroids.[162] Similarly, sphingosine-1-phosphate, which activates a Gs protein-coupled receptor and increases $[cAMP]_i$, abrogated TNF-α-induced RANTES secretion in ASM cells.[106]

In contrast to the effects of $[cAMP]_i$ on chemokine secretion, pharmacological agents that increase $[cAMP]_i$ markedly stimulate secretion of IL-6 in human ASM cells.[118] This appears to be due to effects on basal IL-6 promoter activity.[163] Whether the secreted IL-6 modulates ASM cell function in an autocrine manner or alters leukocyte function in the submucosa remains unknown. However, since studies show that overexpression of IL-6 decreases acetylcholine responsiveness in transgenic mice,[125] the role of IL-6 in asthma may be that of an antiinflammatory signal. More recently, it has been shown that cAMP limits secretion of GM-CSF by ASM cells. Cyclo-oxygenase inhibitors reduce PGE_2 and enhance cytokine-induced secretion of GM-CSF,[151,164] while PDE type IV inhibitors reduce GM-CSF secretion in vitro and antigen-induced AHR in an animal model.[151,165] Taken together, current evidence suggests that some but not all pro-inflammatory functions in ASM cells are inhibited by $[cAMP]_i$-mobilizing agents.

Conflicting reports exist, however, concerning effects of increased $[cAMP]_i$ on lymphocyte adhesion and migration through cytokine-activated endothelial cells.[166,167] The controversy regarding the role of $[cAMP]_i$ in modulating cell adhesion likely reflects differences in the cytokines used to stimulate endothelial cells, or the temporal differences in the addition of the agonists used to increase $[cAMP]_i$. Far less is known concerning $[cAMP]_i$ effects on smooth muscle–leukocyte adhesion. In human ASM cells, activation of $[cAMP]_i$-dependent pathways inhibited, in part, both TNF-α-mediated induction of ICAM-1 and VCAM-1 expression and adhesion of activated T cells to ASM cells. Interestingly, the basal expression of ICAM-1 and VCAM-1, as well as the binding of activated T cells to unstimulated ASM, was resistant to increases in $[cAMP]_i$.[168] Together these studies show that cytokine-induced expression of cell adhesion molecules and T cell adhesion to ASM cells are modulated by changes in $[cAMP]_i$.

STEROID SIGNALING IN ASM CELLS

Molecular mechanisms of steroid actions

Most antiinflammatory effects of steroids are mediated via glucocorticoid (GC) receptor α-isoform (GRα) which suppresses expression of inflammatory genes through mechanisms known as transactivation or transrepression.[169] Transactivation occurs via direct binding of activated GRα to DNA sequences called GC responsive elements (GRE) present on the promoter of steroid-inducible genes such as IκB, Lipocortin-1, and IL-10. Transrepression defines a direct interaction of activated GRα with different transcription factors, such as NF-κB and AP-1, thus repressing their abilities to induce expression of pro-inflammatory genes. As a result of alternative splicing mechanisms, another glucocorticoid receptor isoform, namely GRβ, has been described.[170]

Differential effects of GC in ASM cells

Although steroid effects on human ASM cells have been investigated, the modulatory effects of steroids on gene expression remain complex and poorly characterized. First, the effects of steroids are gene-specific. Evidence suggests that dexamethasone effectively inhibits cytokine-induced IL-6, RANTES, eotaxin, or COX-2 expression, while steroids have little effect on cytokine-induced ICAM-1 expression.[160,163,171,172] Second, steroid suppressive effects are time-dependent, since dexamethasone partially abrogates cytokine-mediated ICAM-1 expression at early time points, but has no effect at later time points.[171] Third, steroid inhibitory action is also stimuli-specific. While dexamethasone significantly inhibits IL-1β-induced GM-GSF secretion, steroids have only partial effect on GM-GSF secretion induced by thrombin.[173] Finally, steroid suppressive effects are dramatically reduced in cells treated with multiple cytokines. We recently showed that the specific combination of TNF-α with IFNs, but not with IL-1β or IL-13, impairs the ability of fluticasone, dexamethasone, and budesonide to inhibit the expression of different pro-asthmatic genes such as CD38, RANTES, ICAM-1, and fractalkine.[174] The importance of IFNs in impairing steroid actions in ASM cells when acting in concert with TNF-α may explain, in part, the increased steroid requirements in severe asthma patients experiencing viral infections that produce high levels of IFNs in the airways.[175] These results support the concept that inflammation, through cytokine action, alters steroid function in airway structural cells.

Development of steroid resistance in ASM cells: role of GRβ

Although the role of GRβ isoform is not well understood, previous reports demonstrate a strong correlation between steroid resistance in asthmatics and the expression levels of GRβ. Indeed, GRβ may act as a dominant negative inhibitor of steroid action and has been associated with steroid resistance in different inflammatory diseases.[176] While most investigators studied GRβ function in either immune or transformed cells, its role in structural, non-transformed effector cells remains unexplored. We recently provided the first evidence that cytokine combination induced an upregulation of GRβ in mesenchymal cells. It is noteworthy to mention that transfection studies investigating the dominant negative activities of GRβ were carried out using exogenously expressed GRα and GRβ in cells that do not express endogenous GR (where the level of GR isoforms could be controlled) such as COS-1 and COS-7.[177] Interestingly, we demonstrated that GRβ overexpression in cells expressing endogenous GRα prevents the ability of steroids to (1) induce transactivation activity, and (2) inhibit cytokine-induced pro-inflammatory gene expression.[174] Collectively, upon pro-inflammatory cytokine stimulation, ASM cells become insensitive to GC action by a mechanism involving the upregulation of GRβ isoform, thus providing a novel in vitro cellular model to dissect GC resistance in primary cells. The implication of GRβ in asthma has been recently described by one study showing a high level of GRβ expression in asthmatic airways (epithelium).[178]

AIRWAY SMOOTH MUSCLE CELLS AND EXTRACELLULAR MATRIX

The importance of airway remodeling in chronic severe asthma has only recently been appreciated. ASM cells, by production of extracellular matrix (ECM) components, as well as matrix-modifying enzymes, may contribute to this process. ASM cell hypertrophy and hyperplasia is a hallmark of asthma. As has been discussed earlier in this chapter, ASM cells respond to exogenous growth factor stimulation by activating a complex array of signaling pathways that result in cell proliferation and growth. However, ASM cells may also produce endogenous growth factors that contribute to this process. Early reports demonstrated that IL-1β acts as a smooth muscle cell mitogen due to autocrine secretion of PDGF.[179] More recently, it has been shown that TGF-β is secreted from ASM cells and, in turn, induces smooth muscle cell synthesis of hyaluronan and collagen.[180–182]

ECM proteins are critical for maintaining the structure and function of the airways. The composition of the ECM is tightly controlled and involves a dynamic process of matrix deposition and degradation. In inflammatory processes such as asthma, this balance is disturbed, resulting not only in an abnormal amount of matrix deposition but also in an altered composition of matrix components. ASM cells secrete a wide variety of matrix proteins, including fibronectin, collagen, hyaluronan, laminin, and versican. In asthma, there is an increase in hyaluronan, fibronectin, tenascin, versican, laminin, and collagen types I, III, and V.[70,183] In vitro, serum from asthmatic patients increases smooth muscle cell release of fibronectin, laminin, perlecan, and chondroitin sulfate.[72] In addition, data suggest that fibronectin and collagen type I enhance smooth muscle cell proliferation in response to PDGF, whereas laminin reduced mitogen-induced proliferation.[71] However, treatment of cells with corticosteroids had no effect on the production of matrix proteins by ASM cells.[72] This has been borne out in human studies where inhaled corticosteroids had minimal effect on altering ECM composition in asthmatics.[66] These data support the finding that while corticosteroids are effective at inhibiting inflammation, newer therapies are needed to prevent and/or reverse airway fibrosis seen in asthma.

The derangement in matrix components seen in asthma likely is multifactorial. Not only is there increased matrix deposition but there is also an imbalance between matrix-degrading enzymes and inhibitors of these proteases. One class of proteins that has been intensively studied is the matrix metalloproteinase (MMP) family. MMP-1 expression is elevated in the smooth muscle cells of asthmatics, and studies have shown that LTD_4 increases expression of MMP-1, which acts to degrade insulin-like growth factor binding protein, a growth inhibitor.[184] TNF-α induces the release of MMP-9, which can degrade matrix but also plays a critical role in cleaving latent TGF-β to its active form.[185] Progelatinase A (MMP-2) is constitutively released by ASM cells, but remains inactive because of high levels of tissue inhibitor of metalloproteinases (TIMP)-2 on the cell membrane.[186] In contrast, TIMP-1 is secreted in large amounts into the conditioned media of ASM cells.[186] Membrane type 1 MMP is also found on ASM;[186] this proteinase can activate MMP-2 and has been shown to cleave CD44 from the cell surface and promote cell migration.[187] Clearly, ASM cells play an active role in modifying their environment. Further studies will be necessary to understand the interaction between ECM, MMPs, and TIMPs in the development of airway remodeling.

AIRWAY SMOOTH MUSCLE FUNCTION IN SUBJECTS WITH ASTHMA

Since ASM primarily modulates bronchomotor tone, investigators hypothesize there exists an intrinsic abnormality in ASM in asthma; however, this concept remains controversial. Evidence, using ASM derived from subjects with asthma in vitro, demonstrates that ASM cells derived from asthmatics proliferate at a faster rate than those of healthy subjects.[188] Physiologically, increases in ASM cell number may contribute to increases in ASM mass and thus irreversible airway obstruction in severe asthma.[57] In parallel, other in vitro studies suggest that ASM cells derived from patients with asthma respond differentially to TGF-β compared with those from healthy subjects. TGF-β induced increased levels of connective tissue growth factor and produced less PGE_2 due to lower COX2 expression in ASM.[189,190] The reduced levels of PGE_2 may promote a pro-inflammatory phenotype in the ASM as well as provide less autocrine airway bronchodilation in response to agonist-induced ASM shortening. Collectively, these in vitro studies suggest that ASM derived from asthmatic subjects appears different from that of healthy subjects. Whether such findings correlate with AHR and increased ASM mass in vivo needs to be addressed.

SUMMARY

The biology of ASM is complex and fascinating. The myriad pathways regulating cell growth and proliferation, combined with the emerging role of ASM as a modulator of inflammation, provide a rich area of investigation. Future studies will focus on mechanisms regulating both acute inflammation and the chronic repair processes leading to airway remodeling.

References

Introduction

1. Featherstone NC, Jesudason EC, Connell MG, et al. Spontaneous propagating calcium waves underpin airway peristalsis in embryonic rat lung. Am J Respir Cell Mol Biol 2005; 33:153.
2. Jesudason EC, Smith NP, Connell MG, et al. Developing rat lung has a sided pacemaker region for morphogenesis-related airway peristalsis. Am J Respir Cell Mol Biol 2005; 32:118.
3. Liu M, Tanswell AK, Post M. Mechanical force-induced signal transduction in lung cells. Am J Physiol (Lung Cell Mol Physiol) 1999; 277:L667.
4. Smith NP, Jesudason EC, Featherstone NC, et al. Recent advances in congenital diaphragmatic hernia. Arch Dis Child 2005; 90:426.
5. Yang Y, Beqaj S, Kemp P, et al. Stretch-induced alternative splicing of serum response factor promotes bronchial myogenesis and is defective in lung hypoplasia. J Clin Invest 2000; 106:1321.

ASM contraction and airway hyperresponsiveness

6. Seow CY, Schellenberg RR, Paré PD. Structural and functional changes in the airway smooth muscle of asthmatic subjects. Am J Respir Crit Care Med 1998; 158:S179.
7. James A, Carroll N. Airway smooth muscle in health and disease: methods of measurement and relation to function. Eur Respir J 2000; 15:782.
8. Schmidt D, Ruehlmann E, Branscheid D, et al. Passive sensitization of human airways increases responsiveness to leukotriene C4. Eur Respir J 1999; 14:315.
9. Black JL, Marthan R, Armour CL, et al. Sensitization alters contractile responses and calcium influx in human airway smooth muscle. J Allergy Clin Immunol 1989; 84:440.
10. Marthan R, Crevel H, Guenard H, et al. Responsiveness to histamine in human sensitized airway smooth muscle. Respir Physiol 1992; 90:239.
11. Roux E, Hyvelin JM, Savineau JP, et al. Calcium signaling in airway smooth muscle cells is altered by in vitro exposure to the aldehyde acrolein. Am J Respir Cell Mol Biol 1998; 19:437.
12. Amrani Y, Panettieri RA Jr. Modulation of calcium homeostasis as a mechanism for altering smooth muscle responsiveness in asthma. Curr Opin Allergy Clin Immunol 2002; 2:39.
13. Amrani Y, Panettieri RA Jr. Cytokines induce airway smooth muscle cell hyperresponsiveness to contractile agonists. Thorax 1998; 53:713.
14. Tao FC, Shah S, Pradhan AA, et al. Enhanced calcium signaling to bradykinin in airway smooth muscle from hyperresponsive inbred rats. Am J Physiol (Lung Cell Mol Physiol) 2003; 284:L90.
15. Deshpande DA, Walseth TF, Panettieri RA, et al. CD38/cyclic ADP-ribose-mediated Ca^{2+} signaling contributes to airway smooth muscle hyper-responsiveness. FASEB J 2003; 17:452.
16. Wills-Karp M. IL-12/IL-13 axis in allergic asthma. J Allergy Clin Immunol 2001; 107:9.
17. Deshpande DA, Dogan S, Walseth TF, et al. Modulation of calcium signaling by interleukin-13 in human airway smooth muscle: role of CD38/cyclic adenosine diphosphate ribose pathway. Am J Respir Cell Mol Biol 2004; 31:36.

18. Deshpande DA, White TA, Dogan S, et al. CD38/cyclic ADP-ribose signaling: role in the regulation of calcium homeostasis in airway smooth muscle. Am J Physiol (Lung Cell Mol Physiol) 2005; 288:L773.
19. Kellner J, Gamarra F, Welsch U, et al. IL-13Ralpha2 reverses the effects of IL-13 and IL-4 on bronchial reactivity and acetylcholine-induced Ca signaling. Int Arch Allergy Immunol 2006; 142:199.
20. Tliba O, Deshpande D, Chen H, et al. IL-13 enhances agonist-evoked calcium signals and contractile responses in airway smooth muscle. Br J Pharmacol 2003; 140:1159.
21. Syed F, Panettieri RA Jr, Tliba O, et al. The effect of IL-13 and IL-13R130Q, a naturally occurring IL-13 polymorphism, on the gene expression of human airway smooth muscle cells. Respir Res 2005; 6:9.
22. Bergner A, Sanderson MJ. Airway contractility and smooth muscle Ca(2+) signaling in lung slices from different mouse strains. J Appl Physiol 2003; 95:1325.
23. Amrani Y, Chen H, Panettieri RA Jr. Activation of tumor necrosis factor receptor 1 in airway smooth muscle: a potential pathway that modulates bronchial hyper-responsiveness in asthma? Respir Res 2000; 1:49.
24. Ito S, Kume H, Honjo H, et al. Possible involvement of Rho kinase in Ca^{2+} sensitization and mobilization by MCh in tracheal smooth muscle. Am J Physiol (Lung Cell Mol Physiol) 2001; 280:L1218.
25. Hunter I, Cobban HJ, Vandenabeele P, et al. Tumor necrosis factor-alpha-induced activation of RhoA in airway smooth muscle cells: role in the Ca^{2+} sensitization of myosin light chain20 phosphorylation. Mol Pharmacol 2003; 63:714.
26. Parris JR, Cobban HJ, Littlejohn AF, et al. Tumor necrosis factor-α activates a calcium sensitization pathway in guinea-pig bronchial smooth muscle. J Physiol 1999; 518:561.
27. Sakai H, Otogoto S, Chiba Y, et al. Involvement of p42/44 MAPK and RhoA protein in augmentation of ACh-induced bronchial smooth muscle contraction by TNF-alpha in rats. J Appl Physiol 2004; 2154:97.
28. Sakai H, Otogoto S, Chiba Y, et al. TNF-alpha augments the expression of RhoA in the rat bronchus. J Smooth Muscle Res 2004; 40:25.
29. Kume H, Takeda N, Oguma T, et al. Sphingosine 1-phosphate causes airway hyperreactivity by rho-mediated myosin phosphatase inactivation. J Pharmacol Exp Ther 2007; 320:763–773.
30. Rosenfeldt HM, Amrani Y, Watterson KR, et al. Sphingosine-1-phosphate stimulates contraction of human airway smooth muscle cells. FASEB J 1789; 2003:17.
31. Sakai J, Oike M, Hirakawa M, et al. Theophylline and cAMP inhibit lysophosphatidic acid-induced hyperresponsiveness of bovine tracheal smooth muscle cells. J Physiol 2003; 549:171.
32. Smith PG, Roy C, Zhang YN, et al. Mechanical stress increases RhoA activation in airway smooth muscle cells. Am J Respir Cell Mol Biol 2003; 28:436.
33. Liu C, Tazzeo T, Janssen LJ. Isoprostane-induced airway hyperresponsiveness is dependent on internal Ca^{2+} handling and Rho/ROCK signaling. Am J Physiol (Lung Cell Mol Physiol) 2006; 291:L1177.
34. Liu HW, Halayko AJ, Fernandes DJ, et al. The RhoA/Rho kinase pathway regulates nuclear localization of serum response factor. Am J Respir Cell Mol Biol 2003; 29:39.
35. Gosens R, Schaafsma D, Meurs H, et al. Role of Rho-kinase in maintaining airway smooth muscle contractile phenotype. Eur J Pharm 2004; 483:71.
36. Ito S, Kume H, Oguma T, et al. Roles of stretch-activated cation channel and Rho-kinase in the spontaneous contraction of airway smooth muscle. Eur J Pharm 2006; 552:135.
37. Takeda N, Kondo M, Ito S, et al. Role of RhoA inactivation in reduced cell proliferation of human airway smooth muscle by simvastatin. Am J Respir Cell Mol Biol 2006; 35:722.
38. Schaafsma D, Zuidhof AB, Nelemans SA, et al. Inhibition of rho-kinase normalizes nonspecific hyperresponsiveness in passively sensitized airway smooth muscle preparations. Eur J Pharm 2006; 531:145.
39. Reithmann C, Gierschik P, Werdan K, et al. Tumor necrosis factor-alpha up-regulates Gi alpha and G beta proteins and adenylyl cyclase responsive in rat cardiomyocytes. Eur J Pharmacol 1991; 206:53.
40. Klein JB, Scherzer JA, Harding G, et al. TNF-alpha stimulates increased plasma membrane guanine nucleotide binding protein activity in polymorphonuclear leukocytes. J Leuko Biol 1995; 57:500.
41. Scherzer JA, Lin Y, McLeish KR, et al. TNF translationally modulates the expression of G1 protein alpha(i2) subunits in human polymorphonuclear leukocytes. J Immunol 1997; 158:913.
42. Hakonarson H, Herrick DJ, Grunstein MM. Mechanism of impaired beta-adrenoceptor responsiveness in atopic sensitized airway smooth muscle. Am J Physiol (Lung Cell Mol Physiol) 1995; 269:L645.
43. Amrani Y, Krymskaya V, Maki C, et al. Mechanisms underlying TNFalpha effects on agonist-mediated calcium homeostasis in human airway smooth muscle cells. Am J Physiol (Lung Cell Mol Physiol) 1997; 273:L1020.
44. Hall IP, Donaldson J, Hill SJ. Modulation of fluoroaluminate-induced inositol phosphate formation by increases in tissue cyclic AMP content in bovine tracheal smooth muscle. Br J Pharmacol 1990; 100:646.
45. Hardy E, Farahani M, Hall IP. Regulation of histamine H1 receptor coupling by dexamethasone in human cultured airway smooth muscle. Br J Pharmacol 1996; 118:1079.
46. Hsu Y, Chiu C, Wang C, et al. Tumour necrosis factor-alpha enhances bradykinin-induced signal transduction via activation of Ras/Raf/MEK/MAPK in canine tracheal smooth muscle cells. Cell Signal 2001; 13:633.
47. Yang CM, Chien CS, Wang CC, et al. Interleukin-1beta enhances bradykinin-induced phosphoinositide hydrolysis and Ca^{2+} mobilization in canine tracheal smooth-muscle cells: involvement of the Ras/Raf/mitogen-activated protein kinase (MAPK) kinase (MEK)/MAPK pathway. Biochem J 2001; 354:439.
48. Schmidlin F, Scherrer D, Daeffler L, et al. Interleukin-1beta induces bradykinin B2 receptor gene expression through a prostanoid cyclic AMP-dependent pathway in human bronchial smooth muscle cells. Mol Pharmacol 1998; 53:1009.
49. Pype JL, Xu H, Schuermans M, et al. Mechanisms of interleukin 1beta-induced human airway smooth muscle hyporesponsiveness to histamine. Involvement of p38 MAPK NF-kB. Am J Respir Crit Care Med 2001; 163:1010.
50. Emala CW, Kuhl J, Hungerford CL, et al. TNFalpha inhibits isoproterenol-stimulated adenylyl cyclase activity in cultured airway smooth muscle cells. Am J Physiol (Lung Cell Mol Physiol) 1997; 272:L644.
51. Shore SA, Laporte J, Hall IP, et al. Effect of IL-1beta on responses of cultured human airway smooth muscle cells to bronchodilator agonists. Am J Respir Cell Mol Biol 1997; 16:702.
52. Moore PE, Lahiri T, Laporte JD, et al. Selected contribution: synergism between TNF-alpha and IL-1beta in airway smooth muscle cells: implications for beta-adrenergic responsiveness. J Appl Physiol 2001; 91:1467.
53. Laporte JD, Moore PE, Baraldo S, et al. Direct effects of interleukin-13 on signaling pathways for physiological responses in cultured human airway smooth muscle cells. Am J Respir Crit Care Med 2001; 164:141.
54. Amrani Y, Tliba O, Deshpande DA, et al. Bronchial hyperresponsiveness: insights into new signaling molecules. Curr Opin Pharmacol 2004; 4:230.

Cellular and molecular mechanisms regulating airway smooth muscle cell growth

55. Ebina M, Takahashi T, Chiba T, et al. Cellular hypertrophy and hyperplasia of airway smooth muscle underlying bronchial asthma. A 3-D morphometric study. Am Rev Resp Dis 1993; 148:720.
56. Jeffery PK. Morphology of the airway wall in asthma and in chronic obstructive pulmonary disease. Am Rev Respir Dis 1991; 143:1152.
57. Woodruff PG, Dolganov GM, Ferrando RE, et al. Hyperplasia of smooth muscle in mild to moderate asthma without changes in cell size or gene expression. Am J Respir Crit Care Med 2004; 169:1001.
58. Hirst SJ, Walker TR, Chilvers ER. Phenotypic diversity and molecular mechanisms of airway smooth muscle proliferation in asthma. Eur Respir J 2000; 16:159.
59. Panettieri RA Jr, Tan EML, Ciocca V, et al. Effects of LTD4 on human airways smooth muscle cell proliferation, matrix expression, and contraction in vitro: differential sensitivity to cysteinyl leukotriene receptor antagonists. Am J Respir Cell Mol Biol 1998; 19:453.
60. Ammit AJ, Panettieri RA Jr. Signal transduction in smooth muscle. Invited review: the circle of life – cell cycle regulation in airway smooth muscle. J Appl Physiol 2001; 91:1431.
61. Broide DH, Lotz M, Cuomo AJ, et al. Cytokines in symptomatic asthma airways. J Allergy Clin Immunol 1992; 89:958.
62. De S, Zelazny ET, Souhrada JF, et al. IL-1beta and IL-6 induce hyperplasia and hypertrophy of cultured guinea pig airway smooth muscle cells. J Appl Physiol 1995; 78:1555.
63. Belvisi MG, Saunders M, Yacoub M, et al. Expression of cyclo-oxygenase-2 in human airway smooth muscle is associated with profound reductions in cell growth. Br J Pharmacol 1998; 125:1102.
64. McKay S, Hirst SJ, Bertrand-de Haas M, et al. Tumor necrosis factor-α enhances mRNA expression and secretion of interleukin-6 in cultured human airway smooth muscle cells. Am J Respir Cell Mol Biol 2000; 23:103.
65. Stewart AG, Tomlinson PR, Fernandes DJ, et al. Tumor necrosis factor-α modulates mitogenic responses of human cultured airway smooth muscle. Am J Respir Cell Mol Biol 1995; 12:110.
66. Laitinen LA, Laitinen A. Inhaled corticosteroid treatment and extracellular matrix in the airways in asthma. Int Arch Allergy Immunol 1995; 107:215.
67. Roberts CR. Is asthma a fibrotic disease? Chest 1995; 107:111S.
68. Altraja A, Laitinen A, Virtanen I, et al. Expression of laminins in the airways in various types of asthmatic patients: a morphometric study. Am J Respir Cell Mol Biol 1996; 15:482.
69. Bousquet J, Vignola AM, Chanez P, et al. Airways remodelling in asthma: no doubt, no more? Int Arch Allergy Immunol 1995; 107:211.
70. Roberts CR, Burke A. Remodelling of the extracellular matrix in asthma: proteoglycan synthesis and degradation. Can Respir J 1998; 5:48.
71. Hirst SJ, Twort CHC, Lee TH. Differential effects of extracellular matrix proteins on human airway smooth muscle cell proliferation and phenotype. Am J Respir Cell Mol Biol 2000; 23:335.
72. Johnson PRA, Black JL, Cralin S, et al. The production of extracellular matrix proteins by human passively sensitized airway smooth-muscle cells in culture; the effect of beclomethasone. Am J Respir Crit Care Med 2000, 2145:162.
73. Sherr CJ. G1 phase progression: cycling on cue. Cell 1994; 79:551.
74. Sherr CJ, Roberts JM. CDK inhibitors: positive and negative regulators of G1-phase progression. Genes Develop 1999; 13:1501.
75. Panettieri RA Jr, Murray RK, DePalo LR, et al. A human airway smooth muscle cell line that retains physiological responsiveness. Am J Physiol: Cell Physiol 1989; 256:C329.
76. Panettieri RA Jr, Yadvish PA, Kelly AM, et al. Histamine stimulates proliferation of airway smooth muscle and induces c-fos expression. Am J Physiol (Lung Cell Mol Physiol) 1990; 259:L365.
77. Ammit AJ, Kane SA, Panettieri RA Jr. Activation of K-p21ras and N-p21ras, but not H-p21ras, is necessary for mitogen-induced human airway smooth muscle proliferation. Am J Respir Cell Mol Biol 1999; 21:719.
78. Sherr CJ, Roberts JM. Inhibitors of mammalian G1 cyclin-dependent kinases. Genes Dev 1995; 9:1149.
79. Bagley CJ, Woodcock JM, Stomski FC, et al. The structural and functional basis of cytokine receptor activation: lessons from the common beta subunit of the granulocyte-macrophage colony-stimulating factor, interleukin-3 (IL-3), and IL-5 receptors. Blood 1997; 89:1471.
80. Bolen JB, Brugge JS. Leukocyte protein tyrosine kinases: potential targets for drug discovery. Annu Rev Pharmacol Toxicol 1997; 15:371.
81. Krymskaya VP, Orsini MJ, Eszterhas AJ, et al. Mechanisms of proliferation synergy by receptor tyrosine kinase and G protein-coupled receptor activation in human airway smooth muscle. Am J Respir Cell Mol Biol 2000; 23:546.
82. Kartha S, Naureckas ET, Li J, et al. Partial characterization of a novel mitogen-activated protein kinase/extracellular signal-regulated kinase activator in airway smooth-muscle cells. Am J Respir Cell Mol Biol 1999; 20:1041.

83. Pacold ME, Suire S, Perisic O, et al. Crystal structure and functional analysis of Ras binding to its effector phosphoinositide 3-kinase gamma. Cell 2000; 103:931.
84. Rodriguez-Viciana P, Warne PH, Dhand R, et al. Phosphatidylinositol-3-OH kinase as a direct target of Ras. Nature 1994; 370:527.
85. Brar SS, Kennedy TP, Whorton AR, et al. Requirement for reactive oxygen species in serum-induced and platelet-derived growth factor-induced growth of airway smooth muscle. J Biol Chem 1999; 274:20017.
86. Rameh LE, Cantley LC. The role of phosphoinositide 3-kinase lipid products in cell function. J Biol Chem 1999; 274:8347.
87. Domin J, Gaidarov I, Smith MEK, et al. The class II phosphoinositide 3-kinase PI3K-C2apha is concentrated in the trans-Golgi network and present in clathrin-coated vesicles. J Biol Chem 2000; 275:11943.
88. Volinia S, Dhand R, Vanhaesebroeck B, et al. A human phosphatidylinositol 3-kinase complex related to the yeast Vps34p-Vps15p protein sorting system. EMBO J 1995; 14:3339.
89. Krymskaya VP, Ammit AJ, Hoffman RK, et al. Activation of class IA phosphatidylinositol 3-kinase stimulates DNA synthesis in human airway smooth muscle cells. Am J Physiol (Lung Cell Mol Physiol) 2001; 280:L1009.
90. Krymskaya VP, Penn RB, Orsini MJ, et al. Phosphatidylinositol 3-kinase mediates mitogen-induced human airways smooth muscle cell proliferation. Am J Physiol (Lung Cell Mol Physiol) 1999; 277:L65.
91. Scott PH, Belham CM, Al-Hafidh J, et al. A regulatory role for cAMP in phosphatidylinositol 3-kinase/p70 ribosomal S6 kinase-mediated DNA synthesis in platelet-derived-growth-factor-stimulated bovine airway smooth-muscle cells. Biochem J 1996; 318:965.
92. Page K, Li J, Hodge JA, et al. Characterization of a Rac1 signaling pathway to cyclin D(1) expression in airway smooth muscle cells. J Biol Chem 1999; 274:22065.
93. Bauerfeld CP, Hershenson MB, Page K. Cdc42, but not RhoA, regulates cyclin D1 expression in bovine tracheal myocytes. Am J Physiol (Lung Cell Mol Physiol) 2001; 280:L974.
94. Walker TR, Moore SM, Lawson MF, et al. Platelet-derived growth factor-BB and thrombin activate phosphoinositide 3 kinase and protein kinase B: role in mediating airway smooth muscle proliferation. Mol Pharmacol 1998; 54:1007.
95. Brennan P, Babbage JW, Thomas G, et al. p70(s6k) integrates phosphatidylinositol 3-kinase and rapamycin-regulated signals for E2F regulation in T lymphocytes. Mol Cell Biol 1999; 19:4729.
96. Page K, Li J, Wang Y, et al. Regulation of cyclin D(1) expression and DNA synthesis by phosphatidylinositol 3-kinase in airway smooth muscle cells. Am J Respir Cell Mol Biol 2000; 23:436.
97. Karpova AK, Abe MK, Li J, et al. MEK1 is required for PDGF-induced ERK activation and DNA synthesis in tracheal monocytes. Am J Physiol (Lung Cell Mol Physiol) 1997; 272:L558.
98. Orsini MJ, Krymskaya VP, Eszterhas AJ, et al. MAPK superfamily activation in human airway smooth muscle: mitogenesis requires prolonged p42/p44 activation. Am J Physiol (Lung Cell Mol Physiol) 1999; 277:L479.
99. Xiong W, Pestell RG, Watanabe G, et al. Cyclin D1 is required for S phase traversal in bovine tracheal myocytes. Annu Rev Physiol 1997; 272:L1205.
100. Ramakrishnan M, Musa NL, Li J, et al. Catalytic activation of extracellular signal-regulated kinases induces cyclin D1 expression in primary tracheal myocytes. Am J Respir Cell Mol Biol 1998; 18:736.
101. Page K, Li J, Hershenson MB. Platelet-derived growth factor stimulation of mitogen-activated protein kinases and cyclin D1 promoter activity in cultured airway smooth-muscle cells. Am J Respir Cell Mol Biol 1999; 20:1294.
102. Herber B, Truss M, Beato M, et al. Inducible regulatory elements in the human cyclin D1 promoter. Oncogene 1994; 2105:9.
103. Nagata D, Suzuki E, Nishimatsu H, et al. Transcriptional activation of the cyclin D1 gene is mediated by multiple cis-elements, including SP1 sites and a cAMP-responsive element in vascular endothelial cells. J Biol Chem 2000; 276:662.
104. Lee J-H, Johnson PRA, Roth M, et al. ERK activation and mitogenesis in human airway smooth muscle cells. Am J Physiol (Lung Cell Mol Physiol) 2001; 280:L1019.
105. Ravenhall C, Guida E, Harris T, et al. The importance of ERK activity in the regulation of cyclin D1 levels and DNA synthesis in human cultured airway smooth muscle. Br J Pharmacol 2000; 131:17.
106. Ammit AJ, Hastie AT, Edsall LC, et al. Sphingosine 1-phosphate modulates human airway smooth muscle cell functions that promote inflammation and airway remodeling in asthma. FASEB J 2001; 15:1212.
107. Pyne S, Pyne NJ. The differential regulation of cyclic AMP by sphingomyelin-derived lipids and the modulation of sphingolipid-stimulated extracellular signal regulated kinase-2 in airway smooth muscle. Biochem J 1996; 315:917.
108. Tomlinson PR, Wilson JW, Stewart AG. Salbutamol inhibits the proliferation of human airway smooth muscle cells grown in culture: relationship to elevated cAMP levels. Biochem Pharmacol 1995; 49:1809.
109. Tomlinson PR, Wilson JW, Stewart AG. Inhibition by salbutamol of the proliferation of human airway smooth muscle cells grown in culture. Br J Pharmacol 1994; 111:641.
110. Stewart AG, Tomlinson PR, Wilson JW. Beta 2-adrenoceptor agonist-mediated inhibition of human airway smooth muscle cell proliferation: importance of the duration of beta 2-adrenoceptor stimulation. Br J Pharmacol 1997; 121:361.
111. Stewart AG, Harris T, Fernandes DJ, et al. beta 2-adrenergic receptor agonists and cAMP arrest human cultured airway smooth muscle cells in the G1 phase of the cell cycle: role of proteasome degradation of cyclin D1. Mol Pharmacol 1999; 56:1079.
112. Musa NL, Ramakrishnan M, Li J, et al. Forskolin inhibits cyclin D1 expression in cultured airway smooth-muscle cells. Am J Respir Cell Mol Biol 1999; 20:352.
113. Fernandes D, Guida E, Koutsoubos V, et al. Glucocorticoids inhibit proliferation, cyclin D1 expression, and retinoblastoma protein phosphorylation, but not activity of the extracellular-regulated kinases in human cultured airway smooth muscle. Am J Respir Cell Mol Biol 1999; 21:77.

Synthetic function of ASM

114. Lazaar AL, Amrani Y, Panettieri RA Jr. The role of inflammation in the regulation of airway smooth muscle cell function and growth. In: Busse W, Holgate S, eds. Asthma and rhinitis. Oxford: Blackwell, 2000:1402.
115. Berkman N, Krishnan VL, Gilbey T, et al. Expression of RANTES mRNA and protein in airways of patients with mild asthma. Am J Respir Crit Care Med 1996; 154:1804.
116. John M, Hirst SJ, Jose PJ, et al. Human airway smooth muscle cells express and release RANTES in response to T helper 1 cytokines. Regulation by T helper 2 cytokines and corticosteroids. J Immunol 1997; 158:1841.
117. Pype JL, Dupont LJ, Menten P, et al. Expression of monocyte chemotactic protein (MCP)-1, MCP-2, and MCP-3 by human airway smooth-muscle cells. Modulation by corticosteroids and T-helper 2 cytokines. Am J Respir Cell Mol Biol 1999; 21:528.
118. Ammit AJ, Hoffman RK, Amrani Y, et al. TNFalpha-induced secretion of RANTES and IL-6 from human airway smooth muscle cells: modulation by cAMP. Am J Respir Cell Mol Biol 2000; 23:794.
119. John M, Au B-T, Jose PJ, et al. Expression and release of interleukin-8 by human airway smooth muscle cells: inhibition by Th-2 cytokines and corticosteroids. Am J Respir Cell Mol Biol 1998; 18:84.
120. Pang L, Knox AJ. Bradykinin stimulates IL-8 production in cultured human airway smooth muscle cells: role of cyclooxygenase products. J Immunol 1998; 161:2509.
121. Hedges JC, Singer CA, Gerthoffer WT. Mitogen-activated protein kinases regulate cytokine gene expression in human airway myocytes. Am J Respir Cell Mol Biol 2000; 23:86.
122. Ghaffar O, Hamid Q, Renzi PM, et al. Constitutive and cytokine-stimulated expression of eotaxin by human airway smooth muscle cells. Am J Respir Crit Care Med 1999; 159:1933.
123. Chung KF, Patel HJ, Fadlon EJ, et al. Induction of eotaxin expression and release from human airway smooth muscle cells by IL-1beta and TNFalpha: effects of IL-10 and corticosteroids. Br J Pharmacol 1999; 127:1145.
124. Elias JA, Wu Y, Zheng T, et al. Cytokine- and virus-stimulated airway smooth muscle cells produce IL-11 and other IL-6-type cytokines. Am J Physiol (Lung Cell Mol Physiol) 1997; 273:L648.
125. DiCosmo BF, Geba GP, Picarella D, et al. Airway epithelial cell expression of interleukin-6 in transgenic mice. Uncoupling of airway inflammation and bronchial hyperreactivity. J Clin Invest 1994; 94:2028.
126. Wang J, Homer RJ, Chen Q, et al. Endogenous and exogenous IL-6 inhibit aeroallergen-induced Th2 inflammation. J Immunol 2000; 165:4051.
127. Saunders MA, Mitchell JA, Seldon PM, et al. Release of granulocyte-macrophage colony stimulating factor by human cultured airway smooth muscle cells: suppression by dexamethasone. Br J Pharmacol 1997; 120:545.
128. Hallsworth MP, Soh CPC, Twort CHC, et al. Cultured human airway smooth muscle cells stimulated by interleukin-1β enhance eosinophil survival. Am J Respir Cell Mol Biol 1998; 19:910.
129. Hakonarson H, Maskeri N, Carter C, et al. Autocrine interaction between IL-5 and IL-1beta mediates altered responsiveness of atopic asthmatic sensitized airway smooth muscle. J Clin Invest 1999; 104:657.
130. Knight DA, Lydell CP, Zhou D, et al. Leukemia inhibitory factor (LIF) and LIF receptor in human lung: distribution and regulation of LIF release. Am J Respir Cell Mol Biol 1999; 20:834.
131. Hakonarson H, Carter C, Maskeri N, et al. Rhinovirus-mediated changes in airway smooth muscle responsiveness: induced autocrine role of interleukin-1beta. Am J Physiol (Lung Cell Mol Physiol) 1999; 277:L13.
132. Rodel J, Assefa S, Prochnau D, et al. Interferon-β induction by Chlamydia pneumoniae in human smooth muscle cells. FEMS Immunol Med Microbiol 2001; 32:9.
133. Springer TA. Adhesion receptors of the immune system. Nature 1990; 346:425.
134. Lazaar AL, Albelda SM, Pilewski JM, et al. T lymphocytes adhere to airway smooth muscle cells via integrins and CD44 and induce smooth muscle cell DNA synthesis. J Exp Med 1994; 180:807.
135. Dustin ML, Springer TA. Role of lymphocyte adhesion receptors in transient interactions and cell locomotion. Annu Rev Immunol 1991; 9:27.
136. van Seventer GA, Newman W, Shimuzu Y, et al. Analysis of T cell stimulation by superantigen plus major histocompatibility complex class II molecules or by CD3 monoclonal antibody: co-stimulation by purified adhesion ligands VCAM-1, ICAM-1, but not ELAM-1. J Exp Med 1991; 174:901.
137. Lazaar AL, Reitz HE, Panettieri RA Jr et al. Antigen receptor-stimulated peripheral blood and bronchoalveolar lavage-derived T cells induce MHC class II and ICAM-1 expression on human airway smooth muscle. Am J Respir Cell Mol Biol 1997; 16:38.
138. Lazaar AL, Amrani Y, Hsu J, et al. CD40-mediated signal transduction in human airway smooth muscle. J Immunol 1998; 161:3120.
139. Hakonarson H, Kim C, Whelan R, et al. Bi-directional activation between human airway smooth muscle cells and T lymphocytes: role in induction of altered airway responsiveness. J Immunol 2001; 166:293.
140. Lazaar AL, Krymskaya VP, Das SK. VCAM-1 activates phosphatidylinositol 3-kinase and induces p120(Cbl) phosphorylation in human airway smooth muscle cells. J Immunol 2001; 166:155.
141. Hamann KJ, Vieira JE, Halayko AJ, et al. Fas cross-linking induces apoptosis in human airway smooth muscle cells. Am J Physiol (Lung Cell Mol Physiol) 2000; 278:L618.
142. Gaston B, Drazen JM, Loscalzo J, et al. The biology of nitrogen oxides in the airways. Am J Respir Crit Care Med 1994; 149:538.
143. Hamad AM, Johnson SR, Knox AJ. Antiproliferative effects of NO and ANP in cultured human airway smooth muscle. Am J Physiol 1999; 277:L910.
144. Patel HJ, Belvisi MG, Donnelly LE, et al. Constitutive expressions of type I NOS in human airway smooth muscle cells: evidence for an antiproliferative role. FASEB J 1810; 1999:13.
145. Gow AJ, Chen Q, Hess DT, et al. Basal and stimulated protein S-nitrosylation in multiple cell types and tissues. J Biol Chem 2002; 277:9637.

146. Belvisi MG, Saunders MA, Haddad E-B, et al. Induction of cyclo-oxygenase-2 by cytokines in human cultured airway smooth muscle cells: novel inflammatory role of this cell type. Br J Pharmacol 1997; 120:910.

147. Hakonarson H, Grunstein MM. Autologously up-regulated Fc receptor expression and action in airway smooth muscle mediates its altered responsiveness in the atopic asthmatic sensitized state. Proc Natl Acad Sci USA 1998; 95:5257.

148. Cernadas M, De Sanctis GT, Krinzman SJ, et al. CD23 and allergic pulmonary inflammation: potential role as an inhibitor. Am J Respir Cell Mol Biol 1999; 20:1.

149. Dasic G, Juillard P, Graber P, et al. Critical role of CD23 in allergen-induced bronchoconstriction in a murine model of allergic asthma. Eur J Immunol 1999; 29:2957.

150. Haczku A, Takeda K, Hamelmann E, et al. CD23 exhibits negative regulatory effects on allergic sensitization and airway hyperresponsiveness. Am J Respir Crit Care Med 2000; 161:952.

151. Lazzeri N, Belvisi MG, Patel HJ, et al. Effects of prostaglandin E(2) and cAMP elevating drugs on GM-CSF release by cultured human airway smooth muscle cells. Relevance to asthma therapy. Am J Respir Cell Mol Biol 2001; 24:44.

152. Hartert TV, Dworski RT, Mellen BG, et al. Prostaglandin E2 decreases allergen-stimulated release of prostaglandin D2 in airways of subjects with asthma. Am J Respir Crit Care Med 2000; 162:637.

153. Kapsenberg ML, Hilkens CM, Wierenga EA, et al. The paradigm of type 1 and type 2 antigen-presenting cells. Implications for atopic allergy. Clin Exp Allergy 1999; 29(Suppl 2):33.

154. Roper RL, Conrad DH, Brown DM, et al. Prostaglandin E2 promotes IL-4-induced IgE and IgG1 synthesis. J Immunol 1990; 145:2644.

155. Lynch KR, O'Neill GP, Liu Q, et al. Characterization of the human cysteinyl leukotriene CysLT1 receptor. Nature 1999; 399:789.

156. Amrani Y, Moore PE, Hoffman R, et al. Interferon-gamma modulates cysteinyl leukotriene receptor-1 expression and function in human airway myocytes. Am J Respir Crit Care Med 2001; 2098:164.

157. Humbles AA, Lu B, Nilsson CA, et al. A role for the C3a anaphylatoxin receptor in the effector phase of asthma. Nature 2000; 406:998.

158. Karp CL, Grupe A, Schadt E, et al. Identification of complement factor 5 as a susceptibility locus for experimental allergic asthma. Nat Immunol 2000; 1:221.

159. Hall IP, Widdop S, Townsend P, et al. Control of cyclic AMP levels in primary cultures of human tracheal smooth muscle cells. Br J Pharmacol 1992; 107:422.

160. Pang L, Knox AJ. Regulation of TNF-alpha-induced eotaxin release from cultured human airway smooth muscle cells by beta2-agonists and corticosteroids. FASEB J 2001; 115:261.

161. Hallsworth MP, Twort CH, Lee TH, et al. beta2-adrenoceptor agonists inhibit release of eosinophil-activating cytokines from human airway smooth muscle cells. Br J Pharmacol 2001; 132:729.

162. Pang L, Knox AJ. Synergistic inhibition by beta2-agonists and corticosteroids on tumor necrosis factor-alpha-induced interleukin-8 release from cultured human airway smooth-muscle cells. Am J Respir Cell Mol Biol 2000; 23:79.

163. Ammit AJ, Lazaar AL, Irani C, et al. Tumor necrosis factor-alpha-induced secretion of RANTES and interleukin-6 from human airway smooth muscle cells: modulation by glucocorticoids and beta-agonists. Am J Respir Cell Mol Biol 2002; 26:465.

164. Bonazzi A, Bolla M, Buccellati C, et al. Effect of endogenous and exogenous prostaglandin E2 on interleukin-1beta-induced cyclooxygenase-2 expression in human airway smooth-muscle cells. Am J Respir Crit Care Med 2000; 162:2272.

165. Kanehiro A, Ikemura T, Makela MJ, et al. Inhibition of phosphodiesterase 4 attenuates airway hyperresponsiveness and airway inflammation in a model of secondary allergen challenge. Am J Respir Crit Care Med 2001; 163:173.

166. Oppenheimer-Marks N, Kavanaugh AF, Lipsky PE. Inhibition of the transendothelial migration of human T lymphocytes by prostaglandin E2. J Immunol 1994; 152:5703.

167. To SS, Schreiber L. Effect of leukotriene B4 and prostaglandin E2 on the adhesion of lymphocytes to endothelial cells. Clin Exp Immunol 1990; 81:160.

168. Panettieri RA Jr, Lazaar AL, Puré E, et al. Activation of cAMP-dependent pathways in human airway smooth muscle cells inhibits TNF-alpha-induced ICAM-1 and VCAM-1 expression and T lymphocyte adhesion. J Immunol 1995; 154:2358.

169. Leung DY, Bloom JW. Update on glucocorticoid action and resistance. J Allergy Clin Immunol 2003; 111:3.

170. Hollenberg SM, Weinberger C, Ong ES, et al. Primary structure and expression of a functional human glucocorticoid receptor cDNA. Nature 1985; 318:635.

171. Amrani Y, Lazaar AL, Panettieri RA Jr. Up-regulation of ICAM-1 by cytokines in human tracheal smooth muscle cells involves an NF-κB-dependent signaling pathway that is only partially sensitive to dexamethasone. J Immunol 1999; 163:2128.

172. Vlahos R, Stewart AG. Interleukin-1alpha and tumour necrosis factor-alpha modulate airway smooth muscle DNA synthesis by induction of cyclo-oxygenase-2: inhibition by dexamethasone and fluticasone propionate. Br J Pharmacol 1999; 126:1315.

173. Tran T, Fernandes DJ, Schuliga M, et al. Stimulus-dependent glucocorticoid-resistance of GM-CSF production in human cultured airway smooth muscle. Br J Pharmacol 2005; 145:123.

174. Tliba O, Cidlowski JA, Amrani Y. CD38 expression is insensitive to steroid action in cells treated with tumor necrosis factor-alpha and interferon-gamma by a mechanism involving the up-regulation of the glucocorticoid receptor beta isoform. Mol Pharmacol 2006; 69:588.

175. Yamada K, Elliott WM, Hayashi S, et al. Latent adenoviral infection modifies the steroid response in allergic lung inflammation. J Allergy Clin Immunol 2000; 106:844.

176. Pujols L, Mullol J, Torrego A, et al. Glucocorticoid receptors in human airways. Allergy 2004; 59:1042.

177. Bamberger CM, Bamberger AM, de Castro M, et al. Glucocorticoid receptor beta, a potential endogenous inhibitor of glucocorticoid action in humans. J Clin Invest 1995; 95:2435.

178. Bergeron C, Fukakusa M, Olivenstein R, et al. Increased glucocorticoid receptor-[beta] expression, but not decreased histone deacetylase 2, in severe asthma. J Allergy Clin Immunol 2006; 117:703.

179. De S, Zelazny ET, Souhrada JF, et al. Interleukin-1beta stimulates the proliferation of cultured airway smooth muscle cells via platelet-derived growth factor. Am J Respir Cell Mol Biol 1993; 9:645.

180. Black PN, Young PG, Skinner SJ. Response of airway smooth muscle cells to TGF-beta 1: effects on growth and synthesis of glycosaminoglycans. Am J Physiol (Lung Cell Mol Physiol) 1996; 271:L910.

181. McKay S, de Jongste JC, Saxena PR, et al. Angiotensin II induces hypertrophy of human airway smooth muscle cells: expression of transcription factors and transforming growth factor-beta1. Am J Respir Cell Mol Biol 1998; 18:823.

182. Coutts A, Chen G, Stephens N, et al. Release of biologically active TGF-β from airway smooth muscle cells induces autocrine synthesis of collagen. Am J Physiol (Lung Cell Mol Physiol) 2001; 280:L999.

183. Laitinen A, Altraja A, Kampe M, et al. Tenascin is increased in airway basement membrane of asthmatics and decreased by an inhaled steroid. Am J Respir Crit Care Med 1997; 156:951.

184. Rajah R, Nunn S, Herrick D, et al. LTD-4 induces matrix metalloproteinase-1 which functions as an IGFBP protease in airway smooth muscle cells. Am J Physiol (Lung Cell Mol Physiol) 1996; 271:L1014.

185. Yu Q, Stamenkovic I. Cell surface-localized matrix metalloproteinase-9 proteolytically activates TGF-β and promotes tumor invasion and angiogenesis. Genes Develop 2000; 14:163.

186. Foda HD, George S, Rollo E, et al. Regulation of gelatinases in human airway smooth muscle cells: mechanism of progelatinase A activation. Am J Physiol (Lung Cell Mol Physiol) 1999; 277:L174.

187. Kajita M, Itoh Y, Chiba T, et al. Membrane-type 1 matrix metalloproteinase cleaves CD44 and promotes cell migration. J Cell Biol 2001; 153:893.

188. Johnson PR, Roth M, Tamm M, et al. Airway smooth muscle cell proliferation is increased in asthma. Am J Respir Crit Care Med 2001; 164:474.

189. Burgess JK, Johnson PR, Ge Q, et al. Expression of connective tissue growth factor in asthmatic airway smooth muscle cells. Am J Respir Crit Care Med 2003; 167:71.

190. Chambers LS, Black JL, Ge Q, et al. PAR-2 activation, PGE2, and COX-2 in human asthmatic and nonasthmatic airway smooth muscle cells. Am J Physiol (Lung Cell Mol Physiol) 2003; 285:L619.

Regulation of Cell Survival

Hans-Uwe Simon

26

CONTENTS

- Introduction 413
- Key regulators of cell survival 413
- Mast cells 415
- Eosinophils 416
- T cells 417
- Dendritic cells 418
- Resolution of inflammation 418
- Conclusions 419

SUMMARY OF IMPORTANT CONCEPTS

>> The most common form of cell death is apoptosis

>> Although apoptosis is a physiologic process, it can be dysregulated and subsequently contributes to many pathologic processes

>> Apoptosis is a key mechanism by which leukocytes are regulated both under normal and inflammatory conditions

>> Leukocyte apoptosis is often inhibited during inflammation and accelerated in its resolution. These processes are mainly regulated by cytokines

>> Inflammation is often associated with tissue damage, which can occur via both apoptotic and necrotic death pathways

INTRODUCTION

Cell survival and cell death are essential physiologic processes required for normal development and maintenance of tissue homeostasis. However, the lifespan of cells may be dysregulated and this may cause, or at least contribute to, a wide range of pathologic conditions. Since injured tissues are in most cases associated with inflammation, identifying the cellular and molecular mechanisms regulating cell survival and cell death of leukocytes is crucial to understanding of the induction, propagation, and resolution of such inflammatory response. Moreover, it appears that such insights are required for the development of novel and highly effective antiinflammatory therapies.

This chapter discusses ligands, receptors, signaling pathways, and intracellular proteins regulating the lifespan of cells. Specifically, the focus will be on mast cells, eosinophils, T cells, and dendritic cells, since these cells are major players in allergic inflammatory responses.

KEY REGULATORS OF CELL SURVIVAL

Cells of the immune system require the stimulation with cytokines for cell survival. Increased survival factor expression prolongs survival and therefore contributes to the induction and maintenance of an inflammatory response. Lack of survival factors within the environment of leukocytes results in the induction of cell death, which is apoptosis in most cases. The process of apoptosis plays an important role in the resolution of inflammatory responses. Cell survival can also be regulated by triggering death receptors of the tumor necrosis factor (TNF)/nerve growth factor (NGF) family. The active cell death, as a consequence of death receptor activation, probably functions to minimize the immunopathology that results from the highly toxic effector molecules produced by leukocytes.

In general, survival cytokines produced during inflammatory responses induce the expression of anti-apoptotic proteins in leukocytes, which then prevent apoptosis (intrinsic apoptosis). However, it is important to note that survival cytokines do not usually block death receptor-induced apoptosis (extrinsic apoptosis), leaving the possibility for rapid cell death induction even under inflammatory conditions. Survival cytokines control the expression of members of both Bcl-2 and inhibitor of apoptosis protein (IAP) families. Members of the Bcl-2 family control the release of pro-apoptotic factors from mitochondria, whereas members of the IAP family act distal to mitochondria to block aspartic acid-specific cysteine proteases (caspases).

413

There are many excellent reviews on both intrinsic and extrinsic pro-apoptotic pathways.[1–4] Figure 26.1 represents a highly simplified view that is, however, sufficient for the general understanding of how apoptosis is regulated in leukocytes. In the following, the Bcl-2 and IAP families will be introduced, since their expression is largely regulated by survival cytokines.

THE FAMILY OF Bcl-2 PROTEINS

Three groups of Bcl-2 family members can be distinguished: (1) the anti-apoptotic proteins, most of which contain a C-terminal membrane anchor and the four Bcl-2 homology (BH) domains. Bcl-2 and

Bcl-xL are the best known anti-apoptotic members of the Bcl-2 family; (2) The pro-apoptotic members, which lack some of the four BH domains. Bax and Bak are the best known pro-apoptotic members of the Bcl-2 family; (3) The BH3-only proteins, which contain only the third BH domain. Well studied BH3-only proteins are Bid, Bim, Bad, and Bik. The relative levels of pro- and anti-apoptotic proteins determine a cell's susceptibility to apoptosis (rheostat hypothesis).[5] Figure 26.2 provides a diagrammatic representation of the Bcl-2 family. In general, members of the Bcl-2 family are believed to be involved in the regulation of the formation of pores in mitochondrial membranes.[6]

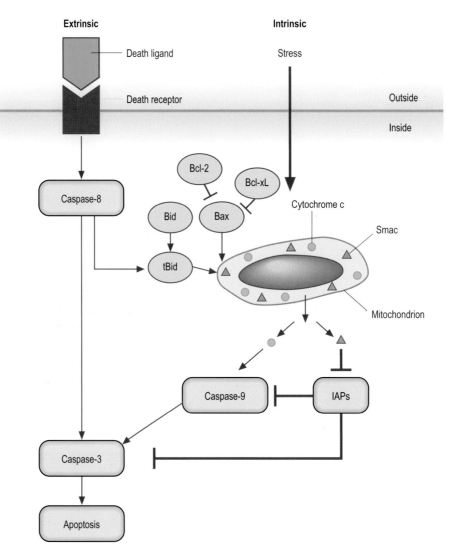

Fig. 26.1. Apoptotic pathways and their main regulators. Apoptosis can be initiated by the death receptor (extrinsic) pathway that acts through caspase-8. Intracellular stress signals result in the activation of the mitochondrial (intrinsic) pathway, which is regulated by members of the Bcl-2 family. There is a potential cross-talk between these two pathways via Bid. Both pathways converge to activate caspase-3 and other effector caspases, which mediate apoptosis. Bcl-2 proteins are thought to regulate the mitochondria permeability transition by inhibiting (Bcl-2, Bcl-xL) or promoting (Bax and Bid) the release of pro-apoptotic factors (cytochrome c, Smac), whereas IAPs act distal to inhibit caspases.

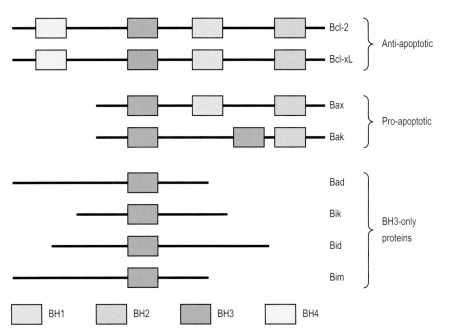

Fig. 26.2. Schematic representation of selected members of the human Bcl-2 family. Members have at least one Bcl-2 homology (BH) domain. The pro-apoptotic members of the Bcl-2 family can be subdivided into two groups: (1) Bax/Bak-like proteins, and (2) BH3-only proteins.

THE FAMILY OF IAPs

IAPs are characterized by the presence of at least one baculovirus IAP domain (BIR) that inhibit caspases.[7] In addition, many IAPs have additional functional domains, some of them (RING, UBC) are required to interact with the ubiquitin-proteasome degradation system (Figure. 26.3). The mammalian cIAP1, cIAP2, and XIAP contain three tandem copies of BIR domains, whereas survivin contains only one BIR domain.[8] In general, IAPs are believed to terminate the activity of caspases either by removing them from the cell through use of the ubiquitin-targeted proteasome degradation machinery or direct inhibition of their enzymatic activity.[9] Therefore, in contrast to anti-apoptotic Bcl-2 family members, IAPs may block both intrinsic and extrinsic death pathways.

▓ MAST CELLS ▓

Mast cells are resident in all normal tissues, where they are believed to play an important role in tissue homeostasis, wound healing, and host defense. Mast cell activation is a characteristic feature of allergic responses, and mast cells may also be involved in the mechanisms leading to bronchial hyperreactivity.[10] Mast cell numbers are increased in allergic inflammatory responses,[11] and preventing apoptosis might contribute to this phenomenon. Stem cell factor (SCF), interleukin (IL)-3, IL-4, IL-5, IL-6, and NGF have been described to promote mast cell survival.[12–14]

SCF is considered as being the most crucial survival factor for mast cells. The crucial role of SCF for regulating mast cell numbers is best reflected by experimental in vivo models. Mice with deficient expression of SCF, or its receptor kit, have almost complete lack of mast cells in

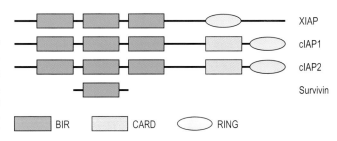

Fig. 26.3. Schematic representation of selected members of the human IAP family. Members have at least one baculoviral (IAP) repeat (BIR) domain. The really interesting new gene (RING) domain is an E3 ligase that directs targets to the ubiquitin-proteasome degradation system. The caspase-recruitment domain (CARD) in cIAP1 and cIAP2 serves to mediate homotypic protein–protein interactions, although the binding partners remain unclear.

their tissues.[15,16] SCF is secreted from several cell types, such as stromal cells, fibroblasts, endothelial cells, and mast cells themselves.[17,18] Injection of SCF to the skin increases mast cell numbers. Moreover, a gain of functional mutations of kit causes systemic mastocytosis.[19]

Following binding of SCF to kit, kit is dimerized and autophosphorylated on tyrosine residues. This initiates multiple intracellular signaling pathways, which involve phosphatidylinositol-3-kinase (PI3K), mitogen activated protein kinase (MAPK), phospholipase C (PLC)-γ, Src kinase, and Janus kinase/signal transducers and activators of transcription (Jak/STAT), resulting in gene activation.[20] It was found that Bim is both inactivated and reduced due to SCF stimulation of mast cells (Fig. 26.4).[21]

MAST CELLS

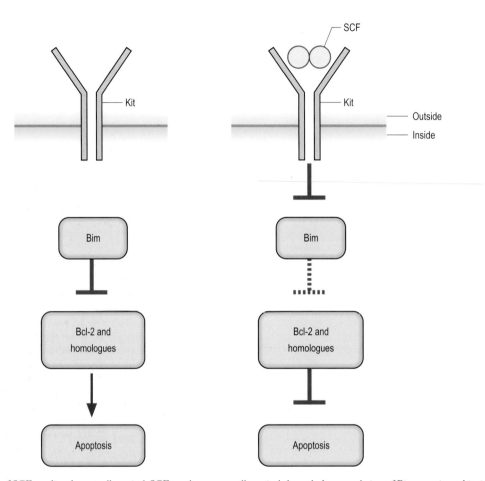

Fig. 26.4. A model of SCF-mediated mast cell survival. SCF regulates mast cell survival through downregulation of Bim protein and its inactivation by phosphorylation. Anti-apoptotic members of the Bcl-2 family are therefore active and prevent apoptosis.

Interestingly, cross-linking of the high-affinity IgE receptor also leads to apoptosis inhibition, which is mediated by increased Bcl-xL and A1 expression.[22] Increased survival following mast cell activation may also be the consequence of the release of survival factors, which then act in an autocrine manner.[23]

Besides the anti-apoptotic mechanisms, mast cells also carry functional death receptors. For instance, mast cell apoptosis can be induced following ligation of Fas and TNF-related apoptosis inducing ligand (TRAIL) receptors.[24,25] Interestingly, immunoglobulin E (IgE)-mediated activation of mast cells increased their sensitivity to undergo TRAIL-induced apoptosis, although the mechanism(s) responsible for these functional effects remain to be investigated.[25]

◼ EOSINOPHILS ◼

Eosinophils are prominent effector cells in many allergic and parasitic inflammatory responses.[26] They are constantly generated in the bone marrow and are short-lived.[27] Moreover, eosinophils are relatively rare

and their contribution to blood leukocyte numbers does not exceed 4% under physiologic conditions. IL-5 represents a crucial cytokine for eosinophil differentiation, activation, and survival.[28] Therefore, in diseases with elevated levels of IL-5, increased numbers of eosinophils are observed.[29] The importance of IL-5 for delayed eosinophil apoptosis in tissues has been directly demonstrated in nasal polyp explants.[30] Other eosinophil survival cytokines are IL-3 and granulocyte/macrophage colony-stimulating factor (GM-CSF). Interestingly, leptin[31] and CD40 ligand[32] are also able to prolong eosinophil survival.

The molecular mechanisms involved in cytokine-mediated enhanced eosinophil survival include increased expression of Bcl-xL,[33] inhibition of Bax translocation to mitochondria,[34] and delayed Bax cleavage,[31] resulting in delayed mitochondrial cytochrome c and second mitochondria-derived activator of caspase (Smac) release and caspase activation.[31,34] IL-5 has also been shown to induce cIAP2 and survivin, suggesting that delay of apoptosis can also be achieved by blocking caspases.[35] The signal transduction mechanisms leading to gene expression of anti-apoptotic proteins involve tyrosine kinases,[36,37] MAPK,[36]

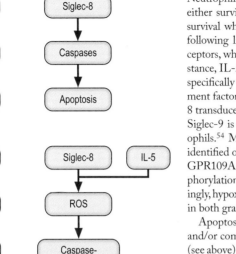

Fig. 26.5. Regulation of cell death in eosinophils. Both Fas and Siglec-8 ligation results in accelerated eosinophil apoptosis in the absence of IL-5 and other eosinophil hematopoietins (A). In the presence of IL-5, Siglec-8-mediated cell death is even more pronounced and partially caspase-independent, but dependent on reactive oxygen species (ROS). In contrast, Fas-mediated apoptosis is not influenced by concurrent IL-5 stimulation (B).

PI3K,[38] Jak/STAT,[39,40] and NF-κB pathways.[41] Currently, there are no data on the role of BH3-only proteins in eosinophils available.

Eosinophils also carry functional death receptors. For instance, eosinophils express Fas receptors that initiate apoptosis upon activation, even in the presence of survival cytokines.[42] In contrast, nitric oxide, that is increasingly generated during allergic inflammatory responses, counter-regulates Fas receptor-induced apoptosis.[43] TRAIL and TNF receptors are also expressed on eosinophils, and mediate eosinophil survival.[44,45] In contrast, eosinophil apoptosis can also be induced as a consequence of sialic acid binding immunoglobulin-like lectin (Siglec)-8 ligation.[46] Moreover, IL-5 increases Siglec-8 mediated death in a partially caspase-independent manner.[47] Recently, a natural ligand for Siglec 8 has been identified.[48] Interestingly, Siglec-8 can also be ligated by physiologic anti-Siglec-8 autoantibodies.[49] A summary of the described mechanisms regulating eosinophil survival is provided in Figure 26.5.

Glucocorticoids are often used as an antiinflammatory drug in allergic inflammatory responses to directly induce eosinophil apoptosis, although the molecular mechanism of this drug's action on cell survival remains unclear.[50] Nevertheless, this effect might be important as asthmatic patients exhibit an increased proportion of apoptotic eosinophils in their airway secretions following clinical improvement with successful glucocorticoid therapy.[51] Theophylline has also been reported to induce eosinophil apoptosis,[52] but the clinical significance of this finding is unclear. Agents that increase intracellular cAMP may also modify eosinophil apoptosis, depending on the inflammatory cytokine environment.[53]

Although neutrophils are usually not dominant in allergic inflammatory responses, it is interesting to compare the regulation of apoptosis between eosinophils and neutrophils, since both cell types are granulocytes.

Neutrophils and eosinophils express surface molecules, which initiate either survival or death signals. Both cell types respond with enhanced survival when stimulated with GM-CSF and with enhanced apoptosis following ligation of Fas receptors. However, there are also surface receptors, which are expressed on either eosinophils or neutrophils. For instance, IL-5 is a specific survival factor for eosinophils, whereas G-CSF specifically prolongs the lifespan of neutrophils. In addition, the complement factor C5a enhances neutrophil, but not eosinophil survival. Siglec-8 transduces death signals in eosinophils, but not neutrophils. In contrast, Siglec-9 is a death receptor on neutrophils, but not expressed in eosinophils.[54] Moreover, the nicotinic acid receptor GPR109A was recently identified on the surface of neutrophils, but not eosinophils. Activation of GPR109A results in a drop of intracellular cAMP, followed by dephosphorylation of Bad and accelerated apoptosis in neutrophils.[55] Interestingly, hypoxia, which induces apoptosis in most cell types, delays apoptosis in both granulocyte types.

Apoptosis in eosinophils and neutrophils is also regulated by drugs and/or compounds. Glucocorticoids, which induce eosinophil apoptosis (see above), delay the neutrophil apoptotic program.[50] On the other hand, nitric oxide donors promote neutrophil apoptosis, but somehow block eosinophil apoptosis.[43] Furthermore, the effect of phenylarsine oxide on apoptosis is different in neutrophils and eosinophils at a given concentration.[56] These data suggest that differences exist in the expression of intracellular components of cell death pathways between eosinophils and neutrophils. Indeed, caspases, although present, are somehow more difficult to activate in eosinophils compared with neutrophils. In contrast, the expression of Bcl-2 family members seems to be similar in eosinophils and neutrophils. Interestingly, Bcl-2, although present in immature precursors, is no longer present in both granulocyte types upon full maturation.[57] This observation may, at least partially, explain the short lifespan of these cells. Bim, a BH3-only protein, seems to play a major role in the regulation of neutrophil apoptosis.[58] The expression and function of Bim in eosinophils remains to be investigated. Taken together, the regulation of apoptosis in eosinophils and neutrophils is partially different, providing the opportunity to selectively target one granulocyte type without affecting the other by pharmacological means.

▪ T CELLS ▪

T cells, in particular T cells producing T helper (Th)2 cytokines, play an important role in allergic inflammatory responses. For instance, IL-4 and IL-13 enhance IgE production; IL-4, IL-9, and IL-10 enhance mast cell growth; and IL-5 promotes eosinophil accumulation.[59] This Th2 response is the result of clonal expansion of allergen-specific T cells and involves both increased proliferation and inhibition of apoptosis. Although some observations in allergic inflammatory responses suggest prolonged survival of Th2 cells,[60] most of our information on the role of T cell apoptosis in immune responses comes from experimental models. Bcl-2 expression is required for the survival of mature, resting T cells.[61] IL-4, IL-6, or IL-7 are required to maintain Bcl-2 and Bcl-xL levels in these cells.[62,63] Interaction of the T cell receptor (TCR) with major histocompatibility complex (MHC) class II molecules is required to keep memory T cells alive.[64]

The antigen-mediated stimulation of T cells results in a change in requirements for survival. Activated T cells produce IL-2 and are dependent on IL-2, and related cytokines, for their survival.[62,65] IL-2 and related cytokines maintain Bcl-2 and Bcl-xL levels,[62,63] and IL-2 withdrawal requires

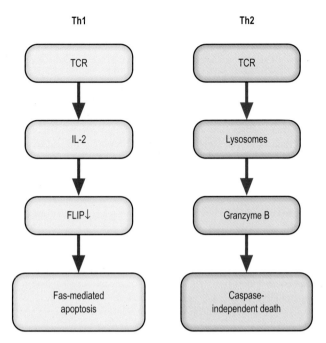

Fig. 26.6. Distinct T cell receptor (TCR)-mediated death pathways in Th1 and Th2 cells. Whereas Th1 cells gain Fas sensitivity due to IL-2-dependent downregulation of FLIP during an immune response, it seems that Th2 cells stay Fas resistant following TCR activation. Granzyme B is released from lysosomes and mediates death in Th2 cells, but not in Th1 cells.

activation of Bim to induce death.[66] Repeated TCR activation sensitizes T cells to apoptosis, a process known as activation-induced cell death. Upon activation, Th1 cells are initially resistant to Fas ligand-induced death, but they gain sensitivity after several days.[4] This increased susceptibility towards Fas receptor-mediated apoptosis has been attributed to lower levels of FLICE-like inhibitory protein (FLIP) and is IL-2-dependent.[67] In Th2 cells, however, FLIP levels may not decrease and are Fas resistant.[68]

In the resolution phase of inflammatory responses, most activated T cells are killed. T cell apoptosis may occur by two mechanisms: (1) by repeated stimulation of the TCR with antigen in conjunction with MHC class II molecules, and (2) by reduction in cytokine levels due to decreased inflammation. The first mechanism requires Fas in Th1 cells, and Fas-deficient patients develop a lymphoproliferative disease.[69,70] In Th2 cells, which are Fas resistant,[68] granzyme B is critical for activation-induced cell death (Fig. 26.6).[71] This second mechanism requires Bim[66] and can be blocked by high levels of Bcl-2.[72]

Almost nothing is known about the regulation of apoptosis of regulatory T cells. It is tempting to speculate, however, that dysregulated apoptosis in these cells contributes to the pathogenesis of allergic inflammatory responses.

■ DENDRITIC CELLS ■

The role of dendritic cells in driving Th2 allergic responses has received considerable attention in recent years. Dendritic cells have direct contact to incoming antigens. In the presence of a danger signal, dendritic cells mature to professional antigen-presenting cells, and interact with naive T cells in draining lymph nodes. Dendritic cells can influence polarization of T cells by the release of cytokines[73] and their expression of co-stimulatory molecules[74] that are both influenced by the local environment.[75] Dendritic cells have been shown to be essential in the pathogenesis of allergic diseases.[76,77]

The lifespan of mature dendritic cells is thought to be approximately 3 days.[78] This short time may limit the availability of antigen for T cells, and apoptosis induction in dendritic cells may serve to regulate immune responses. The lifespan of dendritic cells is determined by both antigen-mediated and T cell signals. For instance, ligands for Toll-like receptors (TLRs), CD40 ligand, or tumor necrosis factor-related activation-induced cytokine (TRANCE) promote dendritic cell survival via nuclear factor (NF)-κB pathways.[79–81] One of the NF-κB target genes is Bcl-xL, which is induced by both TLR ligands and T cell signals. In addition, TLR ligands, but not T cell signals, reduce Bcl-2 and induce Bim, thus limiting the lifespan of dendritic cells.[82] One might, therefore, speculate that immature dendritic cells receive first TLR ligands, which are likely to set the lifespan of dendritic cells, before they even enter the lymph node. A function of T cells might be to prolong the survival of dendritic cells, possibly leading to a temporary and local enrichment of dendritic cells. It is has been demonstrated that increasing the lifespan of mature dendritic cells is an important factor to strengthen the inflammatory response under in vivo conditions.[82] However, although likely, it is currently unclear whether increased dendritic cell survival plays a role in allergic inflammatory responses.

■ RESOLUTION OF INFLAMMATION ■

In addition to the processes involved in the induction and propagation of the inflammatory response, the mechanisms controlling its resolution are also critical in determining the ultimate outcome of the inflammatory response.[83,84]

In resolving beneficial inflammation, the majority of senescent cells at sites of inflammation are recognized by nearby phagocytes. It was shown that cells including inflammatory cells had to undergo apoptosis before they were rapidly and efficiently recognized and ingested by macrophages.[85] The macrophages can ingest several apoptotic cells at a time, and importantly, there is no detectable release of potentially injurious contents from the apoptotic target. Moreover, ingestion of apoptotic cells does not result in pro-inflammatory mediator release from macrophages.[86] In addition, increasing evidence suggests that macrophage phagocytosis of apoptotic cells triggers production and release of agents (TGF-β, IL-10) that have antiinflammatory capacity.[87,88] This non-inflammatory clearance mechanism is thought to be caused by the molecular mechanisms by which phagocytes recognize and ingest apoptotic cells. In contrast, when phagocytes ingest particles such as zymosan (yeast cell walls) in vitro, they liberate proinflammatory mediators (e.g., eicosanoids, granular enzymes, cytokines).

Although macrophages are believed to remove the majority of apoptotic cells, multiple other cells have been shown to uptake apoptotic cells. Several molecular interactions for recognition of apoptotic cells have been identified that are required for this process.[89] Apoptotic cells signal that they should be removed by the expression of specific surface structures,

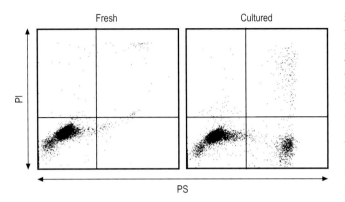

Fig. 26.7. Redistribution of phosphatidylserine (PS) within the plasma membrane of apoptotic cells. PS is normally confined to the inner plasma membrane leaflet. In contrast, PS appears on the external leaflet in apoptotic cells. Annexin V is a PS-binding protein and can be used to detect apoptotic cells. Apoptotic cells exclude DNA-staining dyes, such as propidium iodide (PI), since the plasma membrane stays intact. However, under in vitro conditions, the plasma membrane of apoptotic cells disintegrates over time and cells undergo secondary necrosis, characterized by PI uptake. The figure demonstrates flow cytometric results of freshly isolated and cultured eosinophils following staining with PI and FITC-labelled annexin V. A subgroup of cultured eosinophils binds annexin V, suggesting that these cells are apoptotic.

such as phosphatidylserine (PS). PS is used to detect apoptotic cells and can be identified by binding of fluorescence-labeled annexin V (Fig. 26.7) using flow cytometry. Macrophages engage apoptotic cells by using multiple surface molecules, such as thrombospondin-1, $\alpha_v\beta_3$ integrin, CD36, and phosphatidylserine-recognition structures.[89]

In chronic inflammatory diseases, persistent accumulation of inflammatory cells is usually associated with the release of toxic intracellular products, leading to tissue injury, scarring, and architectural disruption, which consequently results in loss of organ function. Such a scenario is best illustrated in patients suffering from the hypereosinophilic syndrome, in which eosinophil-mediated end-organ damage has often been described.[90] Since eosinophils have been shown to undergo disintegration (cytolysis) in allergic diseases,[91] it is indeed possible that at least some of the tissue damage is the consequence of the release of histotoxic content in the process of such non-apoptotic death. Whether eosinophil cytolysis is due to ineffective macrophage recognition and clearance mechanisms under such conditions remains to be investigated. On the other hand, caspase-independent non-apoptotic death of eosinophils has been observed following ligation of Siglec-8 in the presence of IL-5,[47] suggesting that eosinophil death associated with the liberation of toxic intracellular products might be triggered by more than one mechanism.

■ CONCLUSIONS ■

Apoptosis of inflammatory cells plays an important role in the pathogenesis of allergic diseases, and in this situation there is evidence that mechanisms exist to prevent timely apoptosis in eosinophils, mast cells, T cells, and dendritic cells. The increased lifespan of the

inflammatory cells leads to their accumulation and consequently contributes to the inflammatory response. Interestingly, the intracellular molecular mechanisms leading to prolonged survival in inflammatory cells and cancer cells are similar. For instance, anti-apoptotic molecules of the Bcl-2 and IAP families play an important role in cancer pathogenesis and chemoresistance.[92] In addition to the problem of the increased lifespan, it is possible that the long-living inflammatory cells die via non-apoptotic mechanisms associated with the release of intracellular content, resulting in additional tissue damage. However, we have currently only little information about the mechanisms that are responsible for such a scenario. Elucidation of the mechanisms that regulate the resolution of the inflammatory process should lead to the development of novel therapeutic targets. In particular, development of strategies to induce apoptosis selectively in specific inflammatory cells, together with augmentation of macrophage clearance mechanisms, will have implications for the control of inflammatory disorders, including allergic diseases. Although not discussed in this article, it should be noted that, in contrast to inflammatory cells, apoptosis of epithelial cells (e.g., bronchial epithelial cells in asthma, keratinocytes in atopic dermatis) is increased in association with allergic inflammation.[93,94]

Acknowledgment

Work in the author's laboratory is supported by the Swiss National Science Foundation (grant No. 310000-107526), the Stanley Thomas Johnson Foundation, Bern, and the OPO-Foundation, Zurich.

References

Key regulators of cell survival

1. Marsden VS, Strasser A. Control of apoptosis in the immune system: Bcl-2, BH3-only proteins and more. Annu Rev Immunol 2003; 21:71.
2. Strasser A. The role of the BH3-only proteins in the immune system. Nat Rev Immunol 2005; 5:189.
3. Green DR. Apoptosis pathways: ten minutes to dead. Cell 2005; 121:671.
4. Arnold R, Brenner D, Becker M, et al. How T lymphocytes switch between life and death. Eur J Immunol 2006; 36:1654.
5. Korsmeyer SJ. Regulators of cell death. Trends Genet 1995; 11:101.
6. Danial NN, Korsmeyer SJ. Cell death: critical control points. Cell 2004; 116:205.
7. Salvesen GS, Duckett CS. IAP proteins: blocking the road to death's door. Nat Rev Mol Cell Biol 2002; 3:401.
8. Altieri DC. Validating survivin as a cancer therapeutic target. Nature Rev 2003; 3:46.
9. Vaux DL, Silke J. IAPs, RINGs and ubiquitylation. Nat Rev Mol Cell Biol 2005; 6:287.

Mast cells

10. Bradding P, Walls AF, Holgate ST. The role of mast cells in the pathophysiology of asthma. J Allergy Clin Immunol 2006; 117:1277.
11. Gibson PG, Allen CJ, Yang JP, et al. Intraepithelial mast cells in allergic and nonallergic asthma. Assessment using bronchial brushings. Am Rev Respir Dis 1993; 148:80.
12. Mekori YA, Oh CK, Metcalfe DD. IL-3-dependent murine mast cells undergo apoptosis on removal of IL-3. Prevention of apoptosis by c-kit ligand. J Immunol 1993; 151:3775.
13. Iemura A, Tsai M, Ando A, et al. The c-kit ligand, stem cell factor, promotes mast cell survival by suppressing apoptosis. Am J Pathol 1994; 144:321.
14. Yanagida M, Fukamachi H, Ohgami K, et al. Effects of T-helper 2-type cytokines, interleukin-3 (IL-3), IL-4, IL-5, and IL-6 on the survival of cultured human mast cells. Blood 1995; 86:3705.
15. Kitamura Y, Go S, Hatanaka K. Decrease of mast cells in W/Wv mice and their increase by bone marrow transplantation. Blood 1978; 52:447.
16. Kitumara Y, Go S. Decreased production of mast cells in S1/S1d anemic mice. Blood 1979; 53:492.
17. Heinrich MC, Dooley DC, Freed AC, et al. Constitutive expression of steel factor gene by human stromal cells. Blood 1993; 82:771.

18. Zhang S, Anderson DF, Bradding P, et al. Human mast cells express stem cell factor. J Pathol 1998; 186:59.
19. Wershil BK, Tsai M, Geissler EN, et al. The rat c-kit ligand, stem cell factor, induces c-kit receptor-dependent mouse mast cell activation in vivo. Evidence that signaling through the c-kit receptor can induce expression of cellular function. J Exp Med 1992; 175:245.
20. Reber L, Da Silva CA, Frossard N. Stem cell factor and its receptor c-Kit as targets for inflammatory diseases. Eur J Pharmacol 2006; 533:327.
21. Möller C, Alfredsson J, Engström M, et al. Stem cell factor promotes mast cell survival via inactivation of FOXO3a-mediated transcriptional induction and MEK-regulated phosphorylation of the proapoptotic protein Bim. Blood 2005; 106:1330.
22. Alfredsson J, Puthalakath H, Martin H, et al. Proapoptotic Bcl-2 family member Bim is involved in the control of mast cell survival and is induced together with Bcl-xL upon IgE-receptor activation. Cell Death Differ 2004; 12:136.
23. Kalesnikoff J, Huber M, Lam V, et al. Monomeric IgE stimulates signaling pathways in mast cells that lead to cytokine production and cell survival. Immunity 2001; 14:801.
24. Hartmann K, Wagelie-Steffen AL, von Stebut E, et al. Fas (CD95, APO-1) antigen expression and function in murine mast cells. J Immunol 1997; 159:4006.
25. Berent-Maoz B, Piliponsky AM, Daigle I, et al. Human mast cells undergo TRAIL-induced apoptosis. J Immunol 2006; 176:2272.

Eosinophils

26. Simon D, Simon HU. Eosinophilic disorders. J Allergy Clin Immunol 2007; 119:1291.
27. Rothenberg ME, Hogan SP. The eosinophil. Annu Rev Immunol 2006; 24:147.
28. Sanderson CJ. Interleukin-5, eosinophils, and disease. Blood 1992; 79:3101.
29. Owen WF, Rothenberg ME, Petersen J, et al. Interleukin 5 and phenotypically altered eosinophils in the blood of patients with the idiopathic hypereosinophilic syndrome. J Exp Med 1989; 170:343.
30. Simon HU, Yousefi S, Schranz C, et al. Direct demonstration of delayed eosinophil apoptosis as a mechanism causing tissue eosinophilia. J Immunol 1997; 158:3902.
31. Conus S, Bruno A, Simon HU. Leptin is an eosinophil survival factor. J Allergy Clin Immunol 2005; 116:1228.
32. Bureau F, Seumois G, Jaspar F, et al. CD40 engagement enhances eosinophil survival through induction of cellular inhibitor of apoptosis protein 2 expression: possible involvement in allergic inflammation. J Allergy Clin Immunol 2002; 110:443.
33. Dibbert B, Daigle I, Braun D, et al. Role for Bcl-xL in delayed eosinophil apoptosis by granulocyte-macrophage colony-stimulating factor and interleukin-5. Blood 1998; 92:778.
34. Dewson G, Cohen GM, Wardlaw AJ. Interleukin-5 inhibits translocation of Bax to mitochondria, cytochrome c release, and activation of caspases in human eosinophils. Blood 2001; 98:2239.
35. Vassina EM, Yousefi S, Simon D, et al. cIAP-2 and survivin contribute to cytokine-mediated delayed eosinophil apoptosis. Eur J Immunol 2006; 36:1975.
36. Pazdrak K, Schreiber D, Forsythe P, et al. The signal transduction mechanism of IL-5 in eosinophils: the involvement of Lyn tyrosine kinase and the ras-raf 1-MEK-MAP kinase pathway. J Exp Med 1995; 181:1827.
37. Yousefi S, Hoessli DC, Blaser K, et al. Requirement of Lyn and Syk tyrosine kinases for the prevention of apoptosis by cytokines in human eosinophils. J Exp Med 1996; 183:1407.
38. Pinho V, Souza DG, Barsante MM, et al. Phosphoinositide-3 kinases critically regulate the recruitment and survival of eosinophils in vivo: importance for the resolution of allergic inflammation. J Leukoc Biol 2005; 77:800.
39. van der Bruggen T, Caldenhoven E, Kanters D, et al. Interleukin-5 signaling in human eosinophils involves JAK2 tyrosine kinase and STAT1α. Blood 1995; 85:1442.
40. Simon HU, Yousefi S, Dibbert B, et al. Anti-apoptotic signals of granulocyte-macrophage colony-stimulating factor are transduced via Jak2 tyrosine kinase in eosinophils. Eur J Immunol 1997; 27:3536.
41. Fujihara S, Jaffray E, Farrow SN, et al. Inhibition of NF-kappa B by a cell permeable form of I kappa B alpha induces apoptosis in eosinophils. Biochem Biophys Res Commun 2005; 326:632.
42. Matsumoto K, Schleimer RP, Saito H, et al. Induction of apoptosis in human eosinophils by anti-Fas antibody treatment in vitro. Blood 1995; 86:1437.
43. Hebestreit H, Dibbert B, Balatti I, et al. Disruption of Fas receptor signaling by nitric oxide in eosinophils. J Exp Med 1998; 187:415.
44. Daigle I, Simon HU. Alternative functions for TRAIL receptors in eosinophils and neutrophils. Swiss Med Wkly 2001; 131:231.
45. Temkin V, Levi-Schaffer F. Mechanisms of tumour necrosis factor alpha mediated eosinophil survival. Cytokine 2001; 15:20.
46. Nutku E, Aizawa H, Hudson SA, et al. Ligation of Siglec-8: a selective mechanism for induction of human eosinophil apoptosis. Blood 2003; 101:5014.
47. Nutku E, Hudson SA, Bochner BS. Mechanism of Siglec-8-induced human eosinophil apoptosis: role of caspases and mitochondrial injury. Biochem Biophys Res Commun 2005; 336:918.
48. Bochner BS, Alvarez RA, Mehta P, et al. Glycan array screening reveals a candidate ligand for Siglec-8. J Biol Chem 2005; 280:4307.
49. von Gunten S, Vogel M, Schaub A, et al. Intravenous immunoglobulin preparations contain anti-Siglec-8 autoantibodies. J Allergy Clin Immunol 2007; 119:1005.
50. Meagher LC, Cousin JM, Seckl JR, et al. Opposing effects of glucocorticoids on the rate of apoptosis in neutrophilic and eosinophilic granulocytes. J Immunol 1996; 156:4422.
51. Woolley KL, Gibson PG, Carty K, et al. Eosinophil apoptosis and the resolution of airway inflammation in asthma. Am J Respir Crit Care Med 1996; 154:237.
52. Yasui K, Hu B, Nakazawa T, et al. Theophylline accelerates human granulocyte apoptosis not via phosphodiesterase inhibition. J Clin Invest 1997; 100:1677.
53. Hallsworth MP, Giembycz MA, Barnes PJ. Cyclic AMP-elevating agents prolong or inhibit eosinophil survival depending on prior exposure to GM-CSF. Br J Pharmacol 1996; 117:79.

54. von Gunten S, Yousefi S, Seitz M, et al. Siglec-9 transduces apoptotic and nonapoptotic death signals into neutrophils depending on the proinflammatory cytokine environment. Blood 2005; 106:1423.
55. Kostylina G, Simon D, Fey MF, et al. Neutrophil apoptosis mediated by nicotinic acid receptors (GPR109A). Cell Death Differ 2008; 15:134.
56. Yousefi S, Green DR, Blaser K, et al. Protein-tyrosine phosphorylation regulates apoptosis in human eosinophils and neutrophils. Proc Natl Acad Sci USA 1994; 91:10868.
57. Altznauer F, Martinelli S, Yousefi S, et al. Inflammation-associated cell cycle-independent block of apoptosis by survivin in terminally differentiated neutrophils. J Exp Med 2004; 199:1343.
58. Villunger A, Scott C, Bouillet P, et al. Essential role for the BH3-only protein Bim, but redundant roles for Bax, Bcl-2 and Bcl-w in the control of granulocyte survival. Blood 2003; 101:2393.

T cells

59. Umetsu DT, DeKruyff RH. The regulation of allergy and asthma. Immunol Rev 2006; 212:238.
60. Akdis CA, Blaser K, Akdis M. Apoptosis in tissue inflammation and allergic disease. Curr Opin Immunol 2004; 16:717.
61. Veis DJ, Sorenson CM, Shutter JR, et al. Bcl-2-deficient mice demonstrate fulminant lymphoid apoptosis, polycystic kidneys, and hypopigmented hair. Cell 1993; 75:229.
62. Vella AT, Dow S, Potter TA, et al. Cytokine-induced survival of activated T cells in vitro and in vivo. Proc Natl Acad Sci USA 1998; 95:3810.
63. Li XC, Demirci G, Ferrari-Lacraz S, et al. IL-15 and IL-2: a matter of life and death for T cells in vivo. Nat Med 2001; 7:114.
64. Kirberg J, Berns A, von Boehmer H. Peripheral T cell survival requires continual ligation of the T cell receptor to major histocompatibility complex-encoded molecules. J Exp Med 1997; 186:1269.
65. Duke RC, Cohen JJ. IL-2 addiction: withdrawal of growth factor activates a suicide program in dependent T cells. Lymphokine Res 1986; 5:289.
66. Hildeman DA, Zhu Y, Mitchell TC, et al. Activated T cell death in vivo mediated by pro-apoptotic Bcl-2 family member. Bim. Immunity 2002; 16:759.
67. Refaeli Y, Von Parijs L, London CA, et al. Biochemical mechanisms of IL-2-regulated Fas-mediated T cell apoptosis. Immunity 1998; 8:615.
68. Zhang XR, Zhang LY, Devadas S, et al. Reciprocal expression of TRAIL and CD95L in Th1 and Th2 cells: role of apoptosis in T helper subset differentiation. Cell Death Differ 2003; 10:216.
69. Rieux-Laucat F, Le Deist F, Hivroz C, et al. Mutations in Fas associated with human lymphoproliferative syndrome and autoimmunity. Science 1995; 268:1347.
70. Fisher GH, Rosenberg FJ, Straus SE, et al. Dominant interfering Fas gene mutations impair apoptosis in a human autoimmune lymphoproliferative syndrome. Cell 1995; 81:935.
71. Devadas S, Das J, Liu C, et al. Granzyme B is critical for T cell receptor-induced cell death of type 2 helper T cells. Immunity 2006; 25:237.
72. Strasser A, Harris AW, Cory S. Bcl-2 transgene inhibits T cell death and perturbs thymic self-censorship. Cell 1991; 67:889.

Dendritic cells

73. Maldonado-Lopez R, Maliszewski C, Urbain J, et al. Cytokines regulate the capacity of CD8alpha(+) and CD8alpha(–) dendritic cells to prime Th1/Th2 cells in vivo. J Immunol 2001; 167:4345.
74. Harris NL, Ronchese F. The role of B7 costimulation in T-cell immunity. Immunol Cell Biol 1999; 77:304.
75. Vieira PL, de Jong EC, Wierenga EA, et al. Development of Th1-inducing capacity in myeloid dendritic cells requires environmental instructions. J Immunol 2000; 164:4507.
76. van Rijt LS, Jung S, Kleinjan A, et al. In vivo depletion of lung CD11c+ dendritic cells during allergen challenge abrogates the characteristic features of asthma. J Exp Med 2005; 201:981.
77. Kleinjan A, Willart M, van Rijt LS, et al. An essential role for dendritic cells in human and experimental allergic rhinitis. J Allergy Clin Immunol 2006; 118:1117.
78. Ingulli E, Mondino A, Khoruts A, et al. In vivo detection of dendritic cell antigen presentation to CD4+ T cells. J Exp Med 1997; 185:2133.
79. Park Y, Lee SW, Sung YC. Cutting edge: CpG DNA inhibits dendritic cell apoptosis by up-regulating cellular inhibitor of apoptosis proteins through the phosphatidylinositide-3′-OH kinase pathway. J Immunol 2002; 168:5.
80. Rescigno M, Martino M, Sutherland CL, et al. Dendritic cell survival and maturation are regulated by different signaling pathways. J Exp Med 1998; 188:2175.
81. Wong BR, Josien R, Lee SY, et al. TRANCE (tumor necrosis factor [TNF]-related activation-induced cytokine), a new TNF family member predominantly expressed in T cells, is a dendritic cell-specific survival factor. J Exp Med 1997; 186:2075.
82. Hou WS, Parijs LV. A Bcl-2-dependent molecular timer regulates the lifespan and immunogenicity of dendritic cells. Nat Immunol 2004; 5:583.

Resolution of inflammation

83. Haslett C. Granulocyte apoptosis and its role in the resolution and control of lung inflammation. Am J Respir Crit Care Med 1999; 160:S5.
84. Savill J, Dransfield I, Gregory C, et al. A blast from the past: clearance of apoptotic cells regulates immune responses. Nat Rev Immunol 2002; 2:965.

85. Savill JS, Wyllie AH, Henson JE, et al. Macrophage phagocytosis of aging neutrophils in inflammation: programmed cell death in the neutrophil leads to its recognition by macrophages. J Clin Invest 1989; 83:865.
86. Meagher LC, Savill JS, Baker A, et al. Phagocytosis of apoptotic neutrophils does not induce macrophage release of thromboxane B2. J Leukoc Biol 1992; 52:269.
87. Fadok VA, Bratton DL, Konowal A, et al. Macrophages that have ingested apoptotic cells in vitro inhibit proinflammatory cytokine production through autocrine/paracrine mechanisms involving TGF-β, PGE2, and PAF. J Clin Invest 1998; 101:890.
88. Voll RE, Herrmann M, Roth EA, et al. Immunosuppressive effects of apoptotic cells. Nature 1997; 390:350.
89. Serhan CN, Savill J. Resolution of inflammation: the beginning programs the end. Nat Immunol 2005; 6:1191.
90. Klion A, Bochner BS, Gleich GJ, et al. Approaches to the treatment of hypereosinophilic syndromes: a workshop summary report. J Allergy Clin Immunol 2006; 117:1292.
91. Erjefalt JS, Greiff L, Andersson M, et al. Allergen-induced eosinophil cytolysis is a primary mechanism for granule protein release in human upper airways. Am J Respir Crit Care Med 1999; 160:304.

Conclusions

92. Kaufmann SH, Vaux DL. Alterations in the apoptotic machinery and their potential role in anticancer drug resistance. Oncogene 2003; 22:7414.
93. Trautmann A, Akdis M, Kleemann D, et al. T cell-mediated Fas-induced keratinocyte apoptosis plays a key pathogenetic role in eczematous dermatitis. J Clin Invest 2000; 106:25.
94. Trautmann A, Schmid-Grendelmeier P, Kruger K, et al. T cells and eosinophils cooperate in the induction of bronchial epithelial cell apoptosis in asthma. J Allergy Clin Immunol 2002; 109:329.

REFERENCES

Protease-Activated Pathways of Inflammation

27

Hirohito Kita, Charles E Reed, and Catherine R Weiler

CONTENTS

SUMMARY OF IMPORTANT CONCEPTS

>> Protease-activated receptors (PARs) initiate the complex intracellular signal cascades of platelet activation after blood clotting, wound healing and scarring after injury, and the inflammation of allergic and immune diseases. They are present on virtually every cell

>> PARs function as an innate immune response. In this respect they are analogous to endotoxin activated toll-like receptor innate immunity to bacteria and viruses, but they are directed to multicellular organisms – parasites, and insects – by activating, attracting, and degranulating eosinophils. PAR effects resemble Th2 immunity; toll-like receptor effects resemble Th1 immunity

>> Mast cell tryptase stimulation of PAR-2 of respiratory epithelium disrupts tight junctions, and produces cytokines, chemokines, and adhesion molecules. Tryptase also contracts smooth muscle, and increases sensory neuron response. Chymase increases mucus secretion. Together these mast cell proteases generate airway remodeling

>> Proteases from environmental sources, especially mites and molds, can also activate PARs. However, some exogenous proteases seem to activate similar signaling pathways by incompletely characterized cleavage reactions

>> Proteases increase IgE production and can promote IgE antibody productions to accompanying antigens. It is significant that most airborne allergens have proteases as part of their molecular makeup

>> Continuing investigation of this field holds promise of explaining many things about allergic diseases that are still obscure

INTRODUCTION

Knowledge of the effect of proteases acting through specific cell membrane receptors has greatly increased our understanding of inflammation, especially allergic inflammation. Protease-activated receptors (PARs) were first identified as a mechanism for the interaction between blood clotting and platelet activation.[1] Later investigations expanded to the interaction of various coagulation factors with endothelial cells and fibroblasts in angiogenesis and scarring of wound healing after injury. More recent research has further demonstrated that PARs are important in many diseases, including innate immune response to parasitic invasion, proliferation and spread of cancer cells, autoimmune diseases, and allergic diseases. Four specific PARs have been identified and cloned. These receptors are expressed on almost all cells and are stimulated by serine proteases present in connective tissue fluid. Of particular interest for allergic diseases, mast cell tryptase activates PAR-2. PARs couple to G protein signaling cascades producing phospholipase C, which leads to increased intracellular Ca^{2+}, with secretion, degranulation, and smooth muscle contraction. PAR stimulation also generates transcriptional responses through protein kinases and $NF\kappa B$, producing integrins, chemokines and cytokines and cyclooxygenase-2. Important results of PAR stimulation are enhancement of IgE production, granulocyte infiltration, airway hyperresponsiveness, angiogenesis, fibrosis, smooth muscle hypertrophy, sensitization of sensory neurons with airway hyperresponsiveness and itching, and epidermal thickening. The different PARs may couple to different G proteins and specific coupling varies between different cells. Also, the specific cellular response doubtless depends upon interaction with other signal cascades stimulated by cytokines, chemokines or neurotransmitters. In addition to proteases in tissue fluids, environmental proteases also stimulate PARs.

Like stimulation of toll-like receptor 4 by Gram-negative lipopolysaccharide, stimulation of PARs can be considered a form of innate immunity.[2,3] But it is a very different form. Lipopolysaccharide stimulation resembles and enhances Th-1 immunity, while protease stimulation resembles and enhances Th-2-like responses. Synergistic co-stimulation of the two pathways enhances the severity of the inflammatory response.[4] Protease-driven innate immunity is effective against multicellular organisms like parasites that are too large to be phagocytosed. Instead, it attacks the invader with toxic granules from eosinophils, neutrophils, basophils, and mast cells.

Although investigation of the role of protease activation in the pathogenesis of allergic diseases is just beginning, it is apparent that this process is intimately involved in the production of IgE antibodies. In the airways it contributes to hyperresponsiveness, airway inflammation, and airway remodeling (including nasal polyp formation). They are similarly involved in allergic diseases of skin and other organs.

■ STRUCTURE AND INTRACELLULAR SIGNALING OF PROTEASE-ACTIVATED RECEPTORS ■

Apart from their ability to function as digestive enzymes or to generate active polypeptides from precursors, proteases are now known to play critical roles in coagulation, inflammation, and homeostasis of various organs. Certain proteases can signal directly to cells by cleaving protease-activated receptors, members of the G-protein-coupled receptor (GPCR) family.

Four PARs have been cloned and an emerging theme is that a single protease agonist can activate several distinct receptors, albeit with graded potency.[5] Thrombin is the earliest example of a protease with multiple actions. It is generated in the circulation during coagulation and it has direct receptor-mediated effects on platelets, endothelial cells, leukocytes,

fibroblasts, myocytes, epithelial cells, and neurons. Thrombin activates PAR-1, PAR-3, and PAR-4 (potency PAR-1>PAR-3>PAR-4). At low concentrations thrombin triggers platelet aggregation principally through PAR-1, and PAR-4 mediates responses to high thrombin concentrations. This dual system allows platelets to respond in a regulated manner to a range of thrombin concentrations. Coagulation factor Xa activates PAR-1 and coagulation factor VIIa activates PAR-2. Trypsin, which is found in the lumen of intestine and also expressed in respiratory epithelium and other tissues, activates PAR-2 and PAR-4 (potency PAR-2>PAR-4). Of particular interest for inflammation, enzymes released from the granules of mast cells and neutrophils trigger PAR activation. PARs are widely expressed on cells in blood vessels, connective tissue, leukocytes, platelets, and epithelium, and the expression pattern of PARs differs depending on the cell types. For example, human platelets express PAR-1 and PAR-4 and airway epithelial cells express PAR-1 and PAR-2 (Fig. 27.1). Thus, given that several different proteases can activate one or more receptors and that different cell types express different sets of PARs, the physiologically relevant proteases for PAR activation vary from tissue to tissue.

PARs use a unique mechanism for their activation. PARs can be viewed as a peptide receptor that carries its own ligand; the latter remains silent until activated by cleavage of the PAR N-terminus exodomain. PAR-protease interactions are accounted for by peptide sequences surrounding the cleavage site within the N-terminal exodomain of the receptor, and cleavage at this site is considered both necessary and sufficient for PAR activation. For example, thrombin binds to PAR-1 at two sites within the extracellular N-terminus of the receptor that straddle the cleavage sites. These binding sites can be considered analogous to CD14 binding of endotoxin before it stimulates toll-like receptor 4. Thrombin then cleaves PAR-1 between Arg41 and Ser42 to expose a new N-terminal tethered ligand domain with the sequence SFLLRN (mouse PAR-1). The tethered ligand interacts with domains in extracellular loop 2 of the receptor, which alters the conformation of the receptor to permit coupling and activation of G proteins. As shown in Fig. 27.1, trypsin cleaves PAR-2 between Arg36 and Ser37 to expose the tethered ligand SLIGKV. The SLIGKV peptide bends back to interact with extracellular loop2, activating G protein signal transduction. Cofactors can enhance the capacity of other proteases to activate PAR-2.

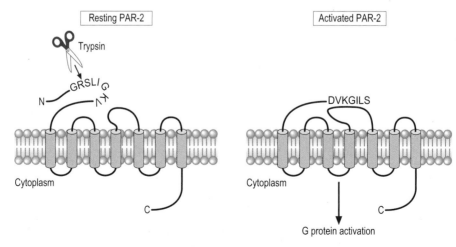

Fig. 27.1. Mechanism of PAR-2 activation.

The ability of FVIIa to activate depends on the presence of tissue factor (TF), an integrated membrane protein that localizes FVIIa to the cell surface and enhances its activity by more than 100-fold.[6]

Once activated, PARs couple to several heterotrimeric G proteins and thereby trigger a cascade of signaling events that result in a variety of cellular responses (Fig. 27.2). PAR-1 couples to $G_{12/13}$, G_q, and G_i families, whereas PAR-2 couples mainly to G_q. This coupling activates signaling pathways that alter cell motility, secretion, shape, growth, survival, and gene transcription. For example, the α-subunits of G_{12} and G_{13} ($G\alpha_{12}$ and $G\alpha_{13}$, respectively) binds RhoGEFs (guanine-nucleotide exchange factors, which activate small G proteins such as Rho), providing a pathway to Rho-dependent cytoskeletal responses that are likely to be involved in shape changes in platelets and migration in endothelial cells. $G\alpha_q$ activates phospholipase Cβ, triggering phosphoinositide hydrolysis, which results in Ca^{2+} mobilization and activation of protein kinase C (PKC). This response provides a pathway to calcium-regulated kinases and phosphatases, GEFs, mitogen-activated protein kinases (MAPK), and other proteins that mediate cellular responses ranging from granule secretion, integrin activation and platelet aggregation, to transcriptional regulation. $G\alpha_i$ inhibits adenylate cyclase, an action known to regulate cellular responses. The complex of the β- and γ-subunits of G proteins (G$\beta\gamma$ subunits) can activate phosphoinositide 3-kinases (PI3K) and other lipid-modifying enzymes, protein tyrosine kinases and ion channels. PI3K modifies the inner leaflet of the plasma membrane to provide attachment sites for a host of signaling proteins. PAR-1 activates the MAPK cascade by transactivation of the EGF receptor. Such pleiotropic effects of PAR activation are consistent with many actions of endogenous and exogenous proteases.[5]

The mechanism by which PAR is activated is striking in several ways compared to other GPCRs. First, one protease molecule might cleave and activate several molecules of PARs; therefore, one 'ligand' may activate several receptors. Second, cleavage of the receptor is irreversible, and the 'peptide agonist' unmasked by cleavage remains tethered to the receptor, which would result in continued signaling unless there are efficient mechanism of receptor uncoupling and desensitization. In common with many GPCRs, desensitization of PARs requires receptor phosphorylation and uncoupling from effector mechanisms. Activation of PAR-1 and PAR-2 induces receptor phosphorylation by GPCR kinases (GRKs) and PKC. Within minutes of activation of PAR-2, β-arrestins translocate from the cytosol to the plasma membrane to interact with phosphorylated PARs, mediating uncoupling with the G proteins. Thus after activation PAR rapidly internalize at sites of clathrin-coated pits into endosomes, where it is degraded. Renewal of cellular responses to proteases requires either recruitment from preformed pools of receptors or the synthesis of new receptors. The relative importance of these resensitization mechanisms depends on the

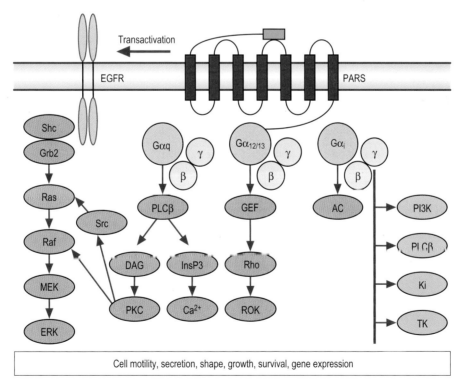

Fig. 27.2. Summary of PAR signal transduction. PARs couple to G_q, $G_{12/13}$, and G_i. $G\alpha_q$ activates phospholipase Cβ to generate inositol triphosphate (InsP3) and diacylglycerol (DAG), which mobilize Ca^{2+} and activate protein kinase C (PKC), respectively. $G\alpha_{12/13}$ couples to guanine nucleotide exchange factors (GEF), resulting in activation of Rho and Rho-kinase (ROK). $G\alpha_i$ inhibits adenylyl cyclase (AC) to reduce cyclic AMP. G$\beta\gamma$ subunits couple PARs to other pathways, such as phosphoinositide 3-kinase (PI3K), potassium channels (Ki), and non-receptor tyrosine kinases (TK). PAR can activate the mitogen-activated protein kinase cascade through transactivation of the EGF receptor (EGFR) and through activation of PKC. Modified from Ossovskaya and Bunnett. Physiol Rev. 2004; 84:579–621. Copyright, American Physiological Society.

STRUCTURE AND INTRACELLULAR SIGNALING OF PROTEASE-ACTIVATED RECEPTORS

Table 27.1 Endogenous enzymes that stimulate protease-activated receptors

PAR-1	PAR-2	PAR-3	PAR-4
Thrombin	Airway trypsin-like protease (Trypsin IV) from bronchial and other epithelial cells, and keratinocytes Pancreatic trypsin I	Thrombin	Thrombin Trypsin
Coagulation factor Xa	Coagulation factor Xa		
Plasmin			Plasmin
Neutrophil cathepsin G	Neutrophil proteases: elastase, proteinase-3 and cathepsin G.	Neutrophil cathepsin G	Neutrophil cathepsin G
Mast cell chymase	Mast cell tryptase and chymase Tryptase α_1 and β_1 have different effects		
Kallikrein	Kallikrein		

cell type. For example, resensitization of PAR-1 responses in fibroblasts and endothelial cells requires mobilization of intracellular pools, whereas recovery of PAR-1 responses in megakaryocytes requires synthesis of new receptors.

The rate of coupling and uncoupling of PARs and G proteins determines the overall cellular responses to a protease. In addition, the extent of PAR glycosylation has profound effects on the capacity of proteases to activate PARs.[7] The potency of tryptase varies greatly between cells; tryptase does not activate PAR-2 at all in some cells. PAR-2 contains glycosylation sequence in close proximity to the activation site in the N-terminal tail. The potency of tryptase (but not trypsin) to activate PAR-2 is dramatically increased if glycosylation is absent by mutation of this sequence, or by enzymatic deglycosylation, or by expression of PAR in glycosylation-defective cells. Thus, it would be of great interest to better understand the mechanisms that can regulate PAR glycosylation and to determine whether deglycosylation by exogenous glycolytic enzymes may alter the ability of other proteases to signal and to understand the mechanisms of PAR activation.

Finally, a polymorphic form of human PAR-2 has been identified with a point mutation in extracellular loop 2 (PAR-2-F204S). This variant displays diminished sensitivity to trypsin and a PAR-2 activating peptide, SLIGKV, but enhanced sensitivity to PAR-4 activating peptide, as determined by measurement of Ca^{2+} response and inhibition of cell growth.[7] It would be important to know whether there are polymorphic variants of other PARs in humans and if their expression is associated with human disease.

PROTEASES THAT ACTIVATE PARs

ENDOGENOUS PROTEASES

As described above, PARs are disposable 'one-shot' receptors. Given this irreversible and seemingly wasteful mechanism of activation, it is unlikely that PARs mediate routine intracellular signaling events under most circumstances. Rather, it is considered that proteases

and PARs play important roles in 'emergency situations' – when coagulation or tissue injury occurs, when mast cells degranulate, or when pathogens invade. A major endogenous stimulating protease, thrombin, is generated during injury when there is activation of the coagulation cascade. Thrombin cleaves PAR-1, PAR-3, and PAR-4. Most of the biological responses to thrombin are related to tissue response to injury and recovery.

The important proteases that cause inflammation are released from granules of neutrophils and mast cells, and secreted from epithelial cells (Table 27.1). Trypsins and mast cell tryptase are the primary endogenous stimuli for PAR-2, the most important PAR involved in allergic inflammation. Airway epithelium, like gastrointestinal mucosa, is an important source of trypsin. Mast cell chymase activates PAR-1. Subtle but possibly significant differences exist between tryptases and chymases from different mast cells. Tryptase is stabilized and its activity promoted by interaction with heparin. Also monomeric and tetrameric forms of β-tryptase have different activity (see Chapter 19). Tryptase is a member of a large family of serine proteases, granzymes, present in leukocytes including lymphocytes.[8] Proteases from neutrophils, elastase, and cathepsin G, are particularly important stimuli for mucus secretion.[9] The role of other granzymes in inflammation has not yet been studied.

Human tissue kallikreins represent a family of secreted serine proteases with potent trypsin-like activity.[10] As well as producing bradykinin, kallikreins can induce inflammation by cleaving and activating PAR-1, PAR-2, or PAR-4.[11]

EXOGENOUS PROTEASES

Exogenous proteases from environmental allergens and microbial organisms directly activate PARs, in particular PAR-2 (Table 27.2). For example, the mite cysteine proteases, Der p 1 and Der f 1, cleave and activate PAR-2, of airway epithelial cells, eosinophils, and fibroblasts.[12,13] Furthermore, aspartate protease from *Alternaria alternata* cleaves PAR-2 peptides one amino acid distal to the typical trypsin-cleavage site (i.e., Ser37 and Leu38), and induces activation and degranulation of human eosinophils. Thus, some non-serine

Table 27.2 Exogenous proteases with inflammatory activity on respiratory epithelium or skin

Pollens:	Mite:
Ambrosia artemisiifolia (short ragweed)	*Dermatophagoides farinae*:[a] Der f1, Der f3, Der f6, Der f9
Lolium perenne (ryegrass)	*Dermatophagoides pteronyssinus*:[a] Der p1, Der p3, Der p6, Der p9
Poa pratensis (Kentucky bluegrass)	*Blomia tropicalis*:[a] Blot 1, Blo t3, Blo t6, Blo t9
Phleum pretense (Timothy grass) Phl p1	*Dermatophagoides siboney*:[a] Der s1, Der s 3
Cynodon dactylon (Bermuda grass)	*Euroglyphus maynei*:[a] Eur m1, Eur m3
Betula spp (birch)	
Acacia longifolia (Sydney golden wattle)	**Cockroach:**
Casuarina distyla (she-oak)	*Blattella germanica* Bla g2
	Periplaneta Americana
Fungi:	
Alternaria alternata	**Hymenoptera:**
Aspergillus fumigatus	*Polistes dominulus* (wasp)
Aspergillus flavus	*Apis mellifera* (bee)
Aspergillus niger[a]	*Bombus pennsylvanicus* (bumble bee)
Aspergillus oryzae[a]	Cat dander Fel d3
Candida albicans[a]	
Cladosporium cladosporiodes[a]	**Other protease-containing organisms**
Cladosporium herbarum	*Pseudomonas aeruginosa*
Curvularia lunata[a]	*Staphylococcus aureus*
Epicoccum purpurascens	*Entamoeba histolytica*
Fusarium culmorum	Rhinovirus
Penicillium chrysogenum	Influenza virus
Penicillium notatum	*Bacillus subtilis*
Penicillium citrinum	Subtilisin
Rhodotorula mucilaginosa[a]	Papain and other proteases derived from foods
Trichophyton rubrum[a]	

[a]Listed in Allergome database.

environmental proteases also activate PARs of inflammatory cells. The mechanisms involved in regulating PAR activation are probably more complex than anticipated; they may involve cleavage of receptor peptides at atypical sites.

In a mouse model fungal protease allergens delivered to the airways elicit an IgE response, but non-protease antigens such as ovalbumin do not; they require priming with a remote adjuvant to overcome airway tolerance.[14] Addition of a protease prevented this tolerance and induced an allergic response in the airway to the non-protease allergen, ovalbumin. Thus, exogenous proteases may be required to overcome the innate resistance to development of Th2 activation and allergic inflammation. Intratracheal administration of the protease Der p 1 increases both specific and total IgE.[12] This may well account for the allergenic activity of complex airborne agents like mites, pollen, and fungi that all include proteases. Cysteine proteases from mites (Der p 1 and Der f 1) stimulate production of prostaglandin D_2 in airway epithelial cells, and activate eosinophils. The proteolytic activity of Der p 1 is inhibited by specific inhibitors of both serine and cysteine proteases. Their stimulation of epithelial cells to produce IL-6 and IL-8 is at least in part the result of activation of PAR-2.[13] Other investigators have reported that this activity in stimulating the production of IL-8 in epithelial cells is also through the ERK1/2 MAP

kinase and AP-1 signaling pathway. Group 3 mite allergens also are proteases that can activate cells, and an elastase from mites degranulates mast cells. Not surprisingly cockroach extracts, like mite extracts, have proteases that can activate PARs.

Fungi, especially *Aspergillus* and *Alternaria* secrete proteases that directly induce epithelial cell detachment and IL-8 production, and degranulation of eosinophils.[15,16] This effect is inhibited by cysteine protease inhibitors, but not by serine protease inhibitors including α_1-antitrypsin. Fungi require proteins in the culture medium to produce proteases. Thus, fungal extracts prepared on synthetic media do not have all the allergens, especially proteases, that fungi growing in their natural environment or on the respiratory mucosa produce.

In addition to mites and fungi, many other allergenic organisms produce proteases, but there are as yet no data about an effect on PARs or similar receptors. Freshly prepared grass and birch pollen extracts contain proteases that can disrupt epithelial cell integrity.[17] One of them, Phl p 1, is a cysteine protease.[18] *Ambrosia artemisiifolia* contains two serine proteases with trypsin-like activity. Some vespid extracts contain serine and cysteine proteases.[19] Protease allergens in some fruits may be involved in the oral allergy syndrome. Proteases in foods may be involved in the development of food allergy, as they are in mite and mold allergy. The Allergome database of allergenic molecules lists more than 50 proteases, but many of them have not been classified for substrate specificity or tested for possible activation of inflammation (www.allergome.org).

Bacterial proteases may also be involved in the pathogenesis of inflammation, but there are no data yet on the effect of bacterial proteases on PARs. *Pseudomonas aeruginosa* produces several serine proteases. One of them, elastase, inactivates important mucosal protease inhibitors, α_1-antitrypsin, and secretory leukocyte proteinase inhibitor. *Staphylococcus* produces several extracellular proteases, including a serine protease, a cysteine protease, a metalloprotease, and epidermolytic toxin. *Staphylococcus* protease V8 shares considerable substrate specificity with mast cell tryptase and chymase, and with neutrophil elastase. Respiratory viruses, too, produce proteases, but they have not yet been studied for ability to activate PARs.

◼ FUNCTIONS OF PARs AND PROTEASES IN INDIVIDUAL CELL TYPES ◼

Proteases stimulate most of the cells involved in inflammation: leukocytes, blood vessels, connective tissue, and organs (Table 27.3).[20] Of course the response depends on the cell's function. Some of these effects are enhanced by lipopolysaccharide.

PAR stimulation of airway epithelium produces metalloproteinase-9 (an enzyme that opens tight junctions between cells), the cytokines IL-6 and GM-CSF, the chemokines IL-8 and eotaxins, platelet-derived growth factor (PDGF) and ICAM-1. Intracellular Ca^{2+} is increased and cyclooxygenase activation generates prostaglandin D_2. Interestingly, stimulation of epithelial cell PARs causes bronchial relaxation, but PAR activation of smooth muscle itself causes contraction. Stimulation of PAR-1 and -2 of goblet cells produces mucus secretion, and PAR-2 peptide agonists stimulate mucus production by salivary and gastric glands. Mast cell chymase and neutrophil elastase stimulate secretion by tracheal mucus glands.[9] The hypertrophy of submucosal glands is not likely to be the direct effect of proteases on the glands, but rather an indirect effect of production of growth factors and growth factor receptors by cytokines released from other cells.

PAR-1 agonists increase endothelial cell expression of E- and P-selectins, and ICAM-1 and VCAM-1, as well as production of the chemokines IL-8 and MCP-1, thereby recruiting inflammatory cells. Agonists of PAR-2 of blood vessels cause nitric oxide dependent dilatation, induce extravasation of plasma proteins, promote leukocyte adhesion to endothelial cells and infiltration of inflammatory cells into the tissues, and stimulate secretion of pro-inflammatory cytokines.

PAR-2 stimulation of rat peritoneal mast cells induces heparin and hexosaminidase release. Thrombin stimulates murine mast cells to produce metalloprotease-9 and IL-6, and to adhere to fibronectin, and to enhance mast cell response to low level stimulation of FcεR1. Human mast cells express PAR-1 and PAR-2; stimulation of these receptors leads to mast cell degranulation and cytokine production. It is especially significant that tryptase itself degranulates other mast cells.[21] However, more information is needed about human mast cells: Does mucosal and connective tissue mast tryptase differ, and do human mast cells located in different sites respond differently?

Stimulation of eosinophil PAR-2 results in superoxide production and degranulation.[22,23] Eosinophils respond similarly to cysteine proteases, papain, and Der f 1. The response to cysteine proteases was enhanced by IL-5. Neutrophils are only weakly activated by PARs. Basophils lack protease receptors,[24] but they produce IL-4, IL-5, and IL-13 after stimulation with Der p1.[25]

Proteases contribute to airway remodeling in asthma and dermal thickening in eczema. They stimulate epithelial cells to produce GM-CSF, and growth factors, and promote maturation, proliferation, and collagen production of fibroblasts. PAR-1 stimulation also proliferates keratinocytes, although PAR-2 stimulation inhibits their growth.[26] Mast cell tryptase of asthmatic patients not only increases contractility of airway smooth muscle but also is a potent mitogen for airway smooth muscle, and increases the expression of epidermal growth factor receptor on fibroblasts.

As mentioned above, mite and fungal proteases deposited in the airways not only induce IgE antibody to themselves but also to other antigens that otherwise would not be allergenic. PAR-2 has a critical effect on ovalbumin challenge of immunized mice. Compared with wild-type animals, eosinophil infiltration was inhibited by 73% in mice lacking PAR-2 and increased by 88% in mice over-expressing PAR-2.[27]

Compared with wild-type animals, airway hyperreactivity to inhaled methacholine was diminished 38% in mice lacking PAR-2 and increased by 52% in mice overexpressing PAR-2. PAR-2 deletion also reduced IgE levels to ovalbumin sensitization 4-fold compared with those of wild-type animals. Proteases also increase IgE antibody response to other allergenic proteins. The intercellular pathways are complex. Stimulated basophils and mast cells produce IL-4 and IL-13.[28] Antigen-presenting cells express PAR-1 and PAR-2, which are increased by GM-CSF and decreased by IL-4. Stimulation of PAR-1 engenders proliferation of both T and B lymphocytes, and augments CD3 lymphocyte proliferation and expression of IL-2R. Ligation of PAR-1 co-stimulates lymphocyte proliferation in the presence of IL-2. Macrophages, epithelial, and endothelial cells produce IL-6, which increases the B lymphocyte response to IL-4 and IL-13.

The esophageal muscularis mucosa has PAR-1 and PAR-4; gastric smooth muscle, intestinal smooth muscle, and intestinal mucosa have PAR-1 and PAR-2.[29] Enterocytes, myenteric and submucosal neurons as well as mast cells, fibroblasts, and endothelium express PAR-1 and PAR-2. PAR-3 receptors are detected in the stomach and the small intestine but the cell type they are expressed on is yet to be identified. PAR-4 is expressed on enterocytes, submucosa, and enteric neurons. PARs-1, -2, and -3 are expressed on immune cells in the bowel wall. Activation of PARs modulates ion transport, bowel permeability, motility, inflammation, sensory function, and proliferation.

◼ PROTEASE INHIBITORS ◼

Protease inhibitors reduce inflammation (Table 27.4). The actions of different inhibitors are quite specific. The best known clinically is α_1-antitrypsin inhibition of neutrophil elastase and prevention of emphysema. Also a low level of α_1-antitrypsin is associated with asthma.[30] However, a more important inhibitor in asthma is secretory leukocyte protease inhibitor which blocks chymase and tryptase and reduces eosinophil and

Table 27.3 Effects of protease-activated receptor stimulation on individual cells

Cell	PAR-1	PAR-2	Exogenous proteases
Airway epithelium	Production of IL-6. IL-8, PGE_2, but less than PAR-2 Production of PDGF	Intracellular Ca^{2+} increase Increased ion transport Production of IL-6 and IL-8, GM-CSF and eotaxin, β-defensin, metalloproteinases-2 and -9 Production of COX-2 and PGE_2 with relaxation of bronchus Expression of ICAM-1	Disruption of tight junctions Desquamation Production of IL-6, IL-8, GM-CSF, and PGE_2
Intestinal epithelium	Ion transport Absorption	Ion transport Absorption	
Oral epithelial cells	Production of IL-6	Production of IL-2 and β-defensin, IL-8 and MCP-1	
Mucus glands	Mucus secretion		
Mast cells	Differentiation and activation Mediator release from rat subcutaneous and peritoneal mast cells Adhesion to fibronectin Metalloprotease-9 and IL-6 production in mouse Augments response to $Fc\varepsilon R1$	Mediator release from rat peritoneal cells PAR-2 activating peptide releases tryptase and chymase from rat peritoneal cells, but tryptase or trypsin does not Intracellular Ca^{2+} increase and mediator release from human subcutaneous mast cells TNF-α and other cytokine production	
Eosinophils	Increased migration and infiltration.	Activation, airway infiltration Degranulation, mediator release Superoxide production Leukotriene production	Activation and degranulation Superoxide production Increased response to IL-5
Basophils			IL-4, IL-5, and IL-13 production
Neutrophils	Chymase increases migration (which PAR not identified)	Expression of adhesion molecule CD11b Migration and excretion of IL-1β, IL-8, IL-6	
Lymphocytes	Ca^{2+} mobilization T and B cell proliferation Increased expression of IL-2R Augments IL-2 response	Ca^{2+} mobilization Increased production of IgE to ovalbumin	Increased total and specific IgE production, mechanism not defined
Alveolar macrophages	Action not defined	Action not defined	
Peritoneal macrophages	Thrombin stimulates IL-6 and MCP-1 production, possibly through a receptor other than PAR		
Monocytes and dendritic cells	MCP-1 and IL-10 production Inhibition of IL-12 production	Increased intracellular Ca^{2+}. IL-8 production	
Platelets	Aggregation Degranulation	Aggregation	

(Continued)

PROTEASE INHIBITORS

Table 27.3 Effects of protease-activated receptor stimulation on individual cells—cont'd

Cell	PAR-1	PAR-2	Exogenous proteases
Airway smooth muscle	Contraction DNA synthesis and proliferation	Increased Ca^{2+} Contraction in humans, with increased response to histamine and methacholine Contraction enhanced by indomethacin DNA synthesis and proliferation	
Vascular smooth muscle	Mitogenesis Contraction	Contraction	
Intestinal smooth muscle	Contraction	Contraction	
Salivary and bronchial glands	Secretion and proliferation	Secretion and proliferation	
Endothelial cells	Production of IL-6, IL-8, MCP-1, E-selectin, VCAM-1, and ICAM-1, PDGF, P-selectin, macrophage migration inhibitory factor, vascular endothelial growth factor, matrix metalloproteinase (MMP-1, MMP-2), and COX-2 Response varies at different sites. Production of IL-6 is enhanced by lipopolysaccharide and TNF-α	Proliferation Production of P-selectin, IL-6, IL-8, MCP-1, and NFκB Also COX-2 and NO	
Keratinocytes	Activation Production of metalloproteinase-2, IL-6, IL-8, and GM-CSF	Ca^{2+} mobilization	
Fibroblast precursors	Development and collagen production	Development and collagen production	
Fibroblasts	Mitogenesis Proliferation and collagen production Production of PDGF, VEGF, IL-6, RANTES, hepatic growth factor, COX-2, and PGE$_2$	Chemotaxis, proliferation, and collagen production Production of IL-8 and MCP-1	
Neurons	Reduced nociception Release substance P and VIP Excitation	May release substance P and VIP Excitation Activation of sensory neurons increases lung inflammation from PAR-2 AP stimulation of other cells	

IL-1β, -2, -5, -6, -8, -10, -12, interleukins 1β, 2, 5, 6, 8, 10, and 12; GM-CSF, granulocyte-macrophage colony stimulating factor; COX-2, cyclooxygenase 2; PGE$_2$, prostaglandin E$_2$; MCP-1, monocyte chemotactic protein 1; PAR-2 AP, protease-activated receptor 2 activating peptide; FcεR$_1$, high-affinity IgE receptor; IL-2R, interleukin 2 receptor; PDGF, platelet-derived growth factor; TGF-β, tumor growth factor beta; VEGF, vascular endothelial growth factor; TNF-α, tumor necrosis factor alpha; INF-γ, interferon gamma; VCAM-1, vascular cell adhesion molecule 1; ICAM-1, intercellular adhesion molecule 1; RANTES, regulated on activation, normal T cells expressed and secreted.

Table 27.4 Endogenous protease inhibitors

Inhibitor	Substrates	Action	Location
α_1-antitrypsin	Neutrophil elastase Capase-3, an intracellular cysteine protease involved in apoptosis Chymase	Inhibits neutrophil inflammation, and IgεR1 degranulation of mast cells	Plasma and secretions
Secretory leukocyte protease inhibitor	Chymase, tryptase Neutrophil elastase	Blocks eosinophil infiltration Blocks tryptase-induced bronchoconstriction	Respiratory and gastric epithelium, skin Macrophages
C1 esterase inhibitor	Complement 1 and complement cascade Plasmin Coagulation factors Kallikrein	Blocks formation of bradykinin	Plasma and interstitial fluid

lymphocyte infiltration and bronchoconstriction and hyperresponsiveness.[31] It also reduces scarring during wound healing. Epidermal growth factor stimulates its production, which is further enhanced by glucocorticoids. C1 esterase inhibitor blocks the formation of kallikrein. C1 esterase deficiency is the cause of hereditary angioedema.

■ DISEASE CORRELATIONS ■

RESPIRATORY DISEASES
Allergic rhinitis and asthma

Proteases play a critical role in the pathogenesis of respiratory tract allergy in several ways:
1. They amplify and even initiate the Th2 response with production of IgE antibodies.
2. They increase sneezing and bronchial hyperresponsiveness by activating sensory neurons.
3. They increase mast cell mediator release, degranulation, and cytokine production.
4. They attract and activate eosinophils, neutrophils, monocyte/macrophages, and lymphocytes.
5. They proliferate goblet cells and mucus glands and stimulate mucus production.
6. Mucosal mast cell tryptase stimulates epithelial cell ICAM-expression, thereby increasing susceptibility to rhinovirus infection.
7. Mast cell proteases contribute to airway remodeling by promoting smooth muscle proliferation and multiplying fibroblasts with stimulation of collagen production.

Virtually all of the cells in the airways have PARs (Table 27.3). Especially significant is that PAR-2 is overexpressed on respiratory epithelial cells of patients with asthma.[32] In rabbits, bacterial lipopolysaccharide increases PAR-2 expression, and in mice influenza virus infection increases both PAR-1 and PAR-2.[33]

A simplified scenario is: proteases from allergenic particles or tryptase released from allergen-activated mast cells in the airway lumen stimulate epithelial cells to release metalloproteases-9 and open up tight junctions promoting allergen penetration into the submucosa. The stimulated epithelial cells release trypsin, another stimulus of PAR-2. Then, activation of PARs on the epithelium and other cells in the airway by both endogenous and exogenous proteases increases production of IgE antibody, promotes infiltration of leukocytes and mucus production by both goblet cells and submucosal glands. Smooth muscle contraction is enhanced, nerves are made more reactive, and airway responsiveness is increased. Eosinophils and mast cells are degranulated, and stimulated to produce inflammatory molecules. Furthermore, tryptase and chymase acting on fibroblasts and smooth muscle cells produce submucosal fibrosis and smooth muscle hypertrophy.

Although these effects of PARs leave little doubt that they have a significant role in the pathophysiology of rhinitis and asthma, there are many issues that still require investigation: What are the details of the function of the different mast cell tryptases and chymase? Are there significant genotypic differences in PARs, especially PAR-2, and if so, do these differences help explain differences in the occurrence, type and severity of asthma and rhinitis in different individuals? Are there other factors that enhance the action of PARs through cross-talk between signal transduction pathways? Are there genetic differences in secretory protease inhibitor and other inhibitors like there are in α_1-antitrypsin?

Hyperplastic rhinosinusitis, nasal polyps, and intrinsic asthma

It has been almost 80 years since Francis Rackemann introduced the classification of asthma into 'allergic' and 'intrinsic' but the etiology and pathogenesis of intrinsic asthma, rhinitis, and nasal polyps are little better understood now than they were then. Although these patients do not have the familial clustering that allergic patients do, many have modestly increased serum IgE. The effect of stimulation of PARs in the cells of the airway by proteases from fungi growing there provides one explanation of the mechanisms of intrinsic asthma, if not its cause.

Ponikau and associates reported that 96% of nasal cultures of patients with chronic rhinosinusitis are positive for common fungi, particularly *Alternaria, Aspergillus,* and *Cladosporium.*[34] Normal control subjects had similar frequency of positive cultures, but the chronic hyperplastic rhinitis patients had hyphae in the mucus of 86% of surgical histologic specimens, indicating that the fungi were growing on the mucosa. Although the total serum IgE was elevated in a third of patients, serum IgE or skin tests specific to fungi were positive in less than half of the patients. Similar correlation of the growth of fungi with rhinosinusitis has been reported from Europe and Australia.[35,36] Subsequently, the Mayo group reported that extracts of mucus and nasal tissue from these patients attracted peripheral blood eosinophils in a tissue culture, and that the eosinophils from patients with chronic rhinosinusitis were more responsive than those from healthy controls.[37] Extracts of molds, especially *Alternaria*, increase expression of PAR-2 and PAR-3 on nasal epithelial cells and activate them to produce IL-8, and eotaxin with attraction of neutrophils and eosinophils.[38]

Thus, fungal proteases produced locally and activating PARs offer a plausible explanation for the pathogenesis of hyperplastic rhinitis and polyps with eosinophilia, edema, angiogenesis, and fibrosis, as well as the increased production of specific and non-specific IgE. Asthma may result from the inflammation in the upper airway or by fungal proteases deposited in the bronchi. Of course, these patients' response to the fungi is strikingly different from the normal population for reasons still to be determined.

Respiratory diseases related to damp, moldy buildings

There has as yet been little direct research of the role of PARs in other allergic diseases, but by extension of what is known about their cellular pathogenesis and PAR expression, a number of testable hypotheses are logical.

Rhinitis, asthma, and other respiratory diseases have been linked to exposure to mites and molds growing in damp or water-damaged buildings, but symptoms are not necessarily linked to specific IgE.[39] Most of the data supporting this link with molds have been based on fungal spore cultures. Assays for airborne proteases, notably papain, and bacterial subtilisin have been valuable in identifying and controlling asthma from these occupational allergens, so assay for fungal, mite, or bacterial proteases would be a much more effective means of correlating environmental exposure to disease.

Allergic bronchopulmonary aspergillosis

This complication of asthma and cystic fibrosis caused by *Aspergillus fumigatus* growing in the bronchi is characterized by exuberant production of antibodies. Levels of total serum IgE are extremely high and not all of it is specific antibody to *Aspergillus* antigens. The pathology includes central bronchiectasis and eosinophilic pneumonitis, and segmental pulmonary fibrosis. The segmental fibrosis is likely to be the result of connective tissue mast cell proteases. In this regard it is relevant that idiopathic pulmonary fibrosis is the lung disease with the greatest density of mast cells. Although *Aspergillus* proteases play a large role in the pathogenesis of bronchopulmonary aspergillosis, a major question remains: what is different about the few patients who develop this disease?

ANAPHYLAXIS

Ever since its discovery, anaphylaxis has been the epitome of the immediate allergic reaction. But allergen binding to IgE is neither necessary nor sufficient for anaphylaxis to occur. Idiopathic anaphylaxis occurs without an allergen, and many individuals with high titers of IgE to vespids have only large late local reactions at the site of the sting. Anaphylaxis affects organs distant from the site of the primary allergen contact and is typified by high levels of tryptase circulating in the plasma.

A hypothetical scenario of anaphylaxis is that there is a unique structural difference in mast cell PAR-2 (such as lack of glycosylation) which causes mast cells to over-respond to circulating tryptase released from distant mast cells. This hypothesis explains the apparent feedback amplification nature of anaphylaxis, and can explain idiopathic anaphylaxis. Two observations in mice encourage the testing of this hypothesis. Some inbred strains are more vulnerable to anaphylaxis than others. And pertussis toxin increases the severity of anaphylaxis by inhibiting the action of G_i signal transduction. Activation of the G_i pathway inhibits the effect of activation of the stimulatory G_q or $G_{12/13}$ pathway by tryptase.

GASTROINTESTINAL DISEASES

PAR-1 is detected in the lamina propria, submucosa, endothelial cells, and nerves of the gastrointestinal (GI) tract. Both the parotid and sublingual glands contain PAR-2, as does the pancreas. The GI tract expresses relatively high levels of PAR-1 mRNA compared with other tissues. PAR-1 is overexpressed in the colon of inflammatory bowel disease (IBD) patients.[40] PAR-2 is highly expressed by enterocytes. Moreover, myocytes as well as neuronal elements are also immunoreactive for PAR-2. Several studies suggest that a role for PAR-1 in regulating GI physiology, including motility, secretory pathways, and barrier functions. For example, intracolonic administration of PAR-1 agonists caused inflammation and disruption of intestinal barrier integrity.[41] Moreover, PAR-1 activation exacerbated and prolonged inflammation in a mouse model of inflammatory bowel disease; PAR-1 antagonism or PAR-1 deficiency attenuated the disease.[42] Trypsin may regulate enterocytes by cleaving and triggering PAR-2 to induce the generation of PGE_2 and PGF_{1a}. In addition, a role for PAR-2 in the protection against colon inflammation in mice induced by a hapten, 2,4,6-trinitrobenzene sulfonic acid (TNBS) was explored by the use of a synthetic PAR-2 tethered ligand, SLIGRL.[43] In contrast, soybean trypsin inhibitor or PAR-2 deficiency substantially reduced colonic inflammatory indices in mice infected with *Citrobacter rodentium* equivalent of *Escherichia coli* infection in humans.[44] Taken together, these results suggest a proinflammatory role of PARs and proteases in Crohn's disease and ulcerative colitis. In patients with Crohn's disease PAR-1 is upregulated and in patients with ulcerative colitis both PAR-1 and PAR-2 are unregulated.[45,46]

SKIN DISEASES

PAR-2 plays an important role in cutaneous inflammation. Keratinocytes, dermal endothelial cells, and dermal sensory nerves express functional PAR-2.[46] Potential endogenous activators of PAR-2 in human skin are mast cell tryptase, the trypsin-like enzyme granzyme A, and proteinases of the fibrinolytic cascade, such as FVIIa and FXa, which could be released during inflammation and wound healing. Exogenous activators of PAR-2 may be serine proteases generated by bacteria (especially *Staphylococcus aureus*), fungi, and house dust mite, although direct evidence on keratinocytes is still lacking. Indirect evidence for bacterial-induced activation of PAR-2 is the observation that bacterial gingipain activates buccal keratinocytes.[47] Furthermore, intradermal injection of tryptase into the skin results in vasodilatation and erythema, followed by leukocyte infiltration and local induration. In murine models of allergic contact dermatitis, a proinflammatory role of PAR-2 agonists was demonstrated.[48] Sensory neuron PAR-2s are involved in neurogenic inflammation and itching.[51,52]

Atopic dermatitis

There are two types of atopic dermatitis - like asthma: an extrinsic type characterized by high levels of IgE antibodies and an intrinsic type without this feature.[49] The histopathology of both types is similar and is characterized by infiltration of mast cells, eosinophils, Th2 cells, and Langerhans'-type cells.[50] PAR-2 expression on keratinocytes is increased in inflamed skin, especially in the granular layer.[56] The level of mast cell chymase is also higher in patients with atopic dermatitis than those without it.[51] Mast cell chymase increases eosinophil infiltration in the skin.[52] Furthermore, mice with spontaneous atopic dermatitis improve when treated with a chymase inhibitor, both clinically and upon pathologic evaluation of the skin. Thus, mast cell proteases are doubtless involved in the pathophysiology of atopic dermatitis causing cellular infiltration, dermal thickening by proliferation of keratinocytes, and pruritus by activating neurons.

Urticaria

The full pathophysiology of chronic urticaria, especially idiopathic urticaria, is yet to be understood, but mast cell numbers are increased and are activated with release of mast cell mediators. One-third of the patients with chronic urticaria have autoantibodies to the IgE receptors on the surface of mast cells causing mast cell activation and degranulation. Increased tryptase has been reported in a suction blister fluid in both lesional and non-lesional skin from a patient with chronic urticaria suggesting a role for tryptase in the pathogenesis in the disease.[53] Patients with urticaria and angioedema have reduced plasma levels of protease inhibitors.[54] Therefore, PAR-2 hypothetically plays a pathophysiologic role in chronic urticaria by activating mast cells, and by stimulating pruritus by increasing the neuronal response to histamine.

Hereditary angioedema

Hereditary angioedema (HAE) results from C1 esterase inhibitor (C1-INH) deficiency. C1-INH inhibits serine proteases. The edema results from increased levels of bradykinin.[55] C1-INH increases bradykinin production by inhibiting four biological cascades: the complement cascade, coagulation cascade, tissue kallikrein pathway, and the fibrinolytic cascade. Although the pathogenesis of HAE is due to increased protease activity, the proteases act by cleaving tissue fluid proteins to generate bradykinin, not by cleaving PARs. However, two of the proteases, plasmin and kallikrein, are known to activate PARs and as they are increased by the deficiency of C1-INH, they may contribute to the inflammation of the disease.

■ MODULATION OF PAR FUNCTIONS AS A POTENTIAL TREATMENT ■

Development of specific PAR antagonists has concentrated on antithrombolytic agents, and has focused on two sites: blocking the tethered ligand receptor, and modulating G protein signaling. In recent years,

there has been considerable progress in developing synthetic peptides that block cleavage of PARs. This tethered ligand approach developed a lead compound termed RWJ-56110, which inhibits platelet aggregation and smooth muscle and fibroblast proliferation.[56] The second strategy for inhibiting PARs is pepducins that modulate receptor-G protein signaling on the inside of receptor.[57] Cell-penetrating pepducins are lipidated peptides based on the intracellular loop sequences of the G-protein-coupled receptor of interest and designed to bind to the receptor-G protein on its interface on the inner leaflet of the plasma membrane. Pepducins have been studied extensively in the context of PAR-1 and PAR-4 signaling in platelets and in animal models' thrombosis, inflammation, and angiogenesis.

Several PAR-1 antagonists have shown in vivo efficacy in guinea pigs, monkeys, and baboons.[58] In addition, two pharmaceutical companies have announced that they have orally active PAR-1 antagonists in clinical trials for acute coronary syndrome. Coumarins that inhibit thrombin and elastase appear to be promising in reducing inflammation and mucus production. Therefore, novel compounds that can modulate PAR function may be potent candidate for the treatment of inflammatory or immune diseases.

Meanwhile, the current antiinflammatory treatments are effective. Agents that increase intracellular cAMP, including β-adrenergic agonists, prostaglandins, and theophylline, inhibit intracellular Ca^{2+} increase, and prevent PAR-stimulated eosinophil and mast cell degranulation, mediator release, and smooth muscle contraction. Theophylline also blocks of the adenosine receptor of mast cells, thereby inhibiting degranulation. Also, glucocorticoids prevent PAR-stimulated DNA transcription and production of cytokines and other inflammatory molecules.

■ CONCLUSION ■

Study of the effects of the PAR pathways of inflammation has explained many previously obscure things about allergic diseases, and future research promises to increase our understanding still more. Mast cell granule enzymes, tryptase and chymase, released by binding of FcεR1, contribute substantially to the inflammation of allergic diseases. Mast cell tryptase activates PAR-2. Chymase activates both PAR-1 and PAR-2. PAR-2 amplifies IgE production and the response of other mast cells to FcεR1 stimulation. Activation of PAR-2 stimulates respiratory epithelium to produce chemokines, cytokines, and metalloproteinases that disrupt the tight junctions that bind epithelial cells to each other and to the basement membrane. PARs stimulate expression of adhesion molecules on endothelium and promote fluid extravasation and edema. PARs recruit and activate inflammatory cells, and degranulate eosinophils. They stimulate mucus production. Mast cell tryptase increases the contractile response of airway smooth muscle; and, with chymase, remodels the airways with smooth muscle hypertrophy and fibroblast proliferation. Of course, these effects of mast cell proteases occur in parallel with other well-known effects of histamine and leukotrienes, and serve to amplify the reactions. Chymase probably plays a special role in fibrosis and dermal thickening.

Exogenous proteases from mites and molds (and possibly other organisms) are also important stimuli of inflammation. Some of the effects are due to activation of specific PARs, but other similar effects are due to activation of cells by a different route. In a mouse model, simultaneous exposure to proteases is required to overcome the airway tolerance for IgE antibody productions to non-protease antigens like ovalbumin. Extending this observation to humans helps to explain sensitization to common allergens; pollens, mites, molds, and cat dander all include proteases.

PAR-stimulated attack of invading multicellular organisms can be considered a type of innate immunity similar to the innate immunity stimulated by endotoxin. But it is different. Endotoxin innate immunity resembles a Th-1 response; PAR innate immunity resembles Th-2. Just as exposure to endotoxin at an early age protects against asthma, exposure to airborne proteases from mites and molds may predispose to asthma. Digestive proteases released into the surrounding environment by *Aspergillus* hyphae contribute to the exuberant IgE, IgG production and granulomatous response of allergic bronchopulmonary aspergillosis. Similar proteases from molds germinating on the respiratory mucosa have been recently been implicated in the pathogenesis of chronic hyperplastic rhinitis and polyps, and by extension of intrinsic asthma. And finally, proteases from mites and fungi growing in damp water-damaged buildings may be the basis for the increased prevalence in these buildings of rhinitis, asthma, and other respiratory diseases.

Protease activation of inflammation is involved in gastrointestinal allergy and other bowel diseases like ulcerative colitis and Crohn's disease. Proteases also contribute to the pathogenesis of allergic skin diseases: atopic dermatitis, urticaria, and angioedema.

Treatment of protease-activated inflammation is under considerable investigation, and new specific agents are on the distant horizon. Meanwhile, agents that increase intracellular cAMP, like β-adrenergic agonists and theophylline, are effective in reducing PAR-stimulated degranulation of mast cells and eosinophils and smooth muscle contraction. Glucocorticoids reduce cell proliferation and other responses due to gene transcription for production of cytokines, chemokines, and adhesion molecules.

This summary of the present state of knowledge about protease activation of the cells involved in allergic diseases has deliberately included hypotheses for further investigation, for without a hypothesis to guide the search, facts will not be found.

References

Introduction

1. Coughlin SR. Protease-activated receptors and platelet function. Thromb Haemost 1999; 82:353–356.
2. Cirino G, Vergnolle N. Proteinase-activated receptors (PARs): crossroads between innate immunity and coagulation. Curr Opin Pharmacol 2006; 6:428–434.
3. Donnelly S, Dalton JP, Loukas A, et al. Proteases in helminth- and allergen-induced inflammatory responses. Chem Immunol Allergy 2006; 90:45–64.
4. Chi L, Li Y, Stehno-Bittel L, et al. Interleukin-6 production by endothelial cells via stimulation of protease-activated receptors is amplified by endotoxin and tumor necrosis factor-alpha. J Interferon Cytokine Res 2001; 21:231–240.

Structure and intracellular signaling of protease-activated receptors

5. Ossovskaya VS, Bunnett NW. Protease-activated receptors: contribution to physiology and disease. Physiol Rev 2004; 84:579–621.
6. Camerer E, Huang W, Coughlin SR. Tissue factor- and factor X-dependent activation of protease-activated receptor 2 by factor VIIa. Proc Natl Acad Sci USA 2000; 97:5255–5260.
7. Compton SJ, Cairns JA, Palmer KJ, et al. A polymorphic protease-activated receptor 2 (PAR2) displaying reduced sensitivity to trypsin and differential responses to PAR agonists. J Biol Chem 2000; 275:39207–39212.

Proteases that activate PARs

8. Buzza MS, Bird PI. Extracellular granzymes: current perspectives. Biol Chem 2006; 387:827–837.
9. Nadel JA. Role of mast cell and neutrophil proteases in airway secretion. Am Rev Respir Dis 1991; 144:S48–S51.
10. Borgono CA, Diamandis EP. The emerging roles of human tissue kallikreins in cancer. Nat Rev Cancer 2004; 4:876–890.
11. Oikonomopoulou K, Hansen KK, Saifeddine M, et al. Proteinase-mediated cell signalling: targeting proteinase-activated receptors (PARs) by kallikreins and more. Biol Chem 2006; 387:677–685.
12. Gough L, Campbell E, Bayley D, et al. Proteolytic activity of the house dust mite allergen Der p 1 enhances allergenicity in a mouse inhalation model. Clin Exp Allergy 2003; 33:1159–1163.
13. Kauffman HF, Tamm M, Timmerman JA, et al. House dust mite major allergens Der p 1 and Der p 5 activate human airway-derived epithelial cells by protease-dependent and protease-independent mechanisms. Clin Mol Allergy 2006; 4:5.
14. Kheradmand F, Kiss A, Xu J, et al. A protease-activated pathway underlying Th cell type 2 activation and allergic lung disease. J Immunol 2002; 169:5904–5911.
15. Borger P, Koeter GH, Timmerman JA, et al. Proteases from Aspergillus fumigatus induce interleukin (IL)-6 and IL-8 production in airway epithelial cell lines by transcriptional mechanisms. J Infect Dis 1999; 180:1267–1274.
16. Kauffman HF, Tomee JF, van de Riet MA, et al. Protease-dependent activation of epithelial cells by fungal allergens leads to morphologic changes and cytokine production. J Allergy Clin Immunol 2000; 105:1185–1193.
17. Hassim Z, Maronese SE, Kumar RK. Injury to murine airway epithelial cells by pollen enzymes. Thorax 1998; 53:368–371.
18. Petersen A, Grobe K, Schramm G, et al. Implications of the grass group I allergens on the sensitization and provocation process. Int Arch Allergy Immunol 1999; 118:411–413.
19. Hoffman DR. Hymenoptera venom allergens. Clin Rev Allergy Immunol 2006; 30:109–128.

Functions of PARs and proteases in individual cell types

20. Vergnolle N, Wallace JL, Bunnett NW, et al. Protease-activated receptors in inflammation, neuronal signaling and pain. Trends Pharmacol Sci 2001; 22:146–152.
21. D'Andrea MR, Rogahn CJ, Andrade-Gordon P. Localization of protease-activated receptors-1 and -2 in human mast cells: indications for an amplified mast cell degranulation cascade. Biotech Histochem 2000; 75:85–90.
22. Miike S, McWilliam AS, Kita H. Trypsin induces activation and inflammatory mediator release from human eosinophils through protease-activated receptor-2. J Immunol 2001; 167:6615–6622.
23. Miike S, Kita H. Human eosinophils are activated by cysteine proteases and release inflammatory mediators. J Allergy Clin Immunol 2003; 111:704–713.
24. Falcone FH, Morroll S, Gibbs BF. Lack of protease activated receptor (PAR) expression in purified human basophils. Inflamm Res 2005; 54(Suppl 1):S13–S14.
25. Phillips C, Coward WR, Pritchard DI, et al. Basophils express a type 2 cytokine profile on exposure to proteases from helminths and house dust mites. J Leukoc Biol 2003; 73:165–171.
26. Derian CK, Eckardt AJ, Andrade-Gordon P. Differential regulation of human keratinocyte growth and differentiation by a novel family of protease-activated receptors. Cell Growth Differ 1997; 8:743–749.
27. Takizawa T, Tamiya M, Hara T, et al. Abrogation of bronchial eosinophilic inflammation and attenuated eotaxin content in protease-activated receptor 2-deficient mice. J Pharmacol Sci 2005; 98:99–102.
28. Gessner A, Mohrs K, Mohrs M. Mast cells, basophils, and eosinophils acquire constitutive IL-4 and IL-13 transcripts during lineage differentiation that are sufficient for rapid cytokine production. J Immunol 2005; 174:1063–1072.
29. Kawabata A. Gastrointestinal functions of proteinase-activated receptors. Life Sci 2003; 74:247–254.

Protease inhibitors

30. Eden E, Strange C, Holladay B, et al. Asthma and allergy in alpha-1 antitrypsin deficiency. Respir Med 2006; 100:1384–1391.
31. Forteza RM, Ahmed A, Lee T, et al. Secretory leukocyte protease inhibitor, but not alpha-1 protease inhibitor, blocks tryptase-induced bronchoconstriction. Pulm Pharmacol Ther 2001; 14:107–110.

Disease correlations

32. Knight DA, Lim S, Scaffidi AK, et al. Protease-activated receptors in human airways: upregulation of PAR-2 in respiratory epithelium from patients with asthma. J Allergy Clin Immunol 2001; 108:797–803.
33. Lan RS, Stewart GA, Goldie RG, et al. Altered expression and in vivo lung function of protease-activated receptors during influenza A virus infection in mice. Am J Physiol Lung Cell Mol Physiol 2004; 286:L388–L398.
34. Ponikau JU, Sherris DA, Kern EB, et al. The diagnosis and incidence of allergic fungal sinusitis. [comment]. Mayo Clinic Proc 1999; 74:877–884.
35. Braun H, Buzina W, Freudenschuss K, et al. 'Eosinophilic fungal rhinosinusitis': a common disorder in Europe? Laryngoscope 2003; 113:264–269.
36. Carney AS, Tan LW, Adams D, et al. Th2 immunological inflammation in allergic fungal sinusitis, nonallergic eosinophilic fungal sinusitis, and chronic rhinosinusitis. Am J Rhinol 2006; 20:145–149.

37. Inoue Y, Shin S-H, Ponikau JU, et al. The fungus, Alternaria, induces activation and degranulation of human eosinophils. J Allergy Clin Immunol 2002; 109:S165.
38. Shin SH, Lee YH, Jeon CH, et al. Protease-dependent activation of nasal polyp epithelial cells by airborne fungi leads to migration of eosinophils and neutrophils. Acta Otolaryngol 2006; 126:1286–1294.
39. Ruoppi PI, Husman TM, Reiman MH, et al. Nasal symptoms among residents in moldy housing 1. Scand J Work Environ Health 2003; 29:461–467.
40. Vergnolle N. Clinical relevance of proteinase activated receptors (pars) in the gut. Gut 2005; 54:867–874.
41. Chin AC, Vergnolle N, MacNaughton WK, et al. Proteinase-activated receptor 1 activation induces epithelial apoptosis and increases intestinal permeability. Proc Natl Acad Sci USA 2003; 100:11104–11109.
42. Vergnolle N, Cellars L, Mencarelli A, et al. A role for proteinase-activated receptor-1 in inflammatory bowel diseases. J Clin Invest 2004; 114:1444–1456.
43. Fiorucci S, Mencarelli A, Palazzetti B, et al. Proteinase-activated receptor 2 is an anti-inflammatory signal for colonic lamina propria lymphocytes in a mouse model of colitis. Proc Natl Acad Sci U S A 2001; 98:13936–13941.
44. Hansen KK, Sherman PM, Cellars L, et al. A major role for proteolytic activity and proteinase-activated receptor-2 in the pathogenesis of infectious colitis. Proc Natl Acad Sci USA 2005; 102:8363–8368.
45. Kim JA, Choi SC, Yun KJ, et al. Expression of protease-activated receptor 2 in ulcerative colitis. Inflamm Bowel Dis 2003; 9:224–229.
46. Santulli RJ, Derian CK, Darrow AL, et al. Evidence for the presence of a protease-activated receptor distinct from the thrombin receptor in human keratinocytes. Proc Natl Acad Sci USA 1995; 92:9151–9155.
47. Lourbakos A, Potempa J, Travis J, et al. Arginine-specific protease from Porphyromonas gingivalis activates protease-activated receptors on human oral epithelial cells and induces interleukin-6 secretion. Infect Immun 2001; 69:5121–5130.
48. Seeliger S, Derian CK, Vergnolle N, et al. Proinflammatory role of proteinase-activated receptor-2 in humans and mice during cutaneous inflammation in vivo. FASEB J 2003; 17:1871–1885.

49. Morar NW-OSMMCWO. The genetics of atopic dermatitis. J Allergy Clin Immunol 2006; 118:24–34.
50. Breuer K, Werfel T, Kapp A. Allergic manifestations of skin diseases – atopic dermatitis 6. Chem Immunol Allergy 2006; 91:76–86.
51. Badertscher K, Bronnimann M, Karlen S, et al. Mast cell chymase is increased in chronic atopic dermatitis but not in psoriasis. Arch Dermatol Res 2005; 296:503–506.
52. Tomimori Y, Muto T, Fukami H, et al. Chymase participates in chronic dermatitis by inducing eosinophil infiltration 13. Lab Invest 2002; 82:789–794.
53. Deleuran B, Kristensen M, Larsen CG, et al. Increased tryptase levels in suction-blister fluid from patients with urticaria 7. Br J Dermatol 1991; 125:14–17.
54. Eftekhari N, Ward AM, Allen R, et al. Protease inhibitor profiles in urticaria and angio-oedema. Br J Dermatol 1980; 103:33–39.
55. Kaplan AP, Joseph K, Silverberg M. Pathways for bradykinin formation and inflammatory disease. J Allergy Clin Immunol 2002; 109:195–209.
56. Andrade-Gordon P, Derian CK, Maryanoff BE, et al. Administration of a potent antagonist of protease-activated receptor-1 (PAR-1) attenuates vascular restenosis following balloon angioplasty in rats. J Pharmacol Exp Ther 2001; 298:34–42.

Modulation of PAR functions as a potential treatment

57. Covic L, Gresser AL, Talavera J, et al. Activation and inhibition of G protein-coupled receptors by cell-penetrating membrane-tethered peptides. Proc Natl Acad Sci USA 2002; 99:643–648.
58. Derian CK, Damiano BP, Addo MF, et al. Blockade of the thrombin receptor protease-activated receptor-1 with a small-molecule antagonist prevents thrombus formation and vascular occlusion in nonhuman primates. J Pharmacol Exp Ther 2003; 304:855–861.

REFERENCES

Animal Models of Allergen-Induced Asthma

28

Ian P Lewkowich and Marsha Wills-Karp

CONTENTS

SUMMARY OF IMPORTANT CONCEPTS

>> Allergen exposure of experimental animals, particularly mice, replicates many features of human asthma. The specific features manifest in each model are dependent upon several factors including the genetic background of the host, the nature of the allergen, and the timing and route of exposure to the inciting allergen

>> The use of gene targeting approaches and the availability of immunological reagents for the study of specific genes/pathways in mice provides a powerful approach for dissecting the underlying pathways involved in allergic lung inflammation

>> The ease of genetic manipulation of inbred murine strains has led to the identification of novel susceptibility genes including TIM-1 and C5, both of which were later shown to be associated with susceptibility to human asthma

>> Utilization of these models has led to the discovery of the importance of $CD4^+$ T-cell subsets in conveying either susceptibility (Th2, iNKT) or tolerance (Treg) to the development of allergic lung inflammation

>> The use of animal models has facilitated dissection of early innate immune events, specifically, those processes through which dendritic cells and epithelial cells recognize allergens and orchestrate T-cell differentiation/activation and disease development

INTRODUCTION

Asthma is a chronic debilitating disease that has been steadily increasing in prevalence and morbidity over the last few decades. Unfortunately, despite intense efforts to identify and target the underlying pathogenic mechanisms of disease, the development of effective therapeutic strategies has not kept pace with the explosion in asthma incidence. Although the etiology of asthma is not fully understood, there is a consensus that allergic asthma develops as a result of inappropriate immune responses to innocuous environmental triggers in genetically predisposed individuals. Exploration of the factors that predispose to, initiate, or perpetuate the inflammatory process in human asthma has been hampered by the complex etiology of disease, variability in expression of disease parameters, and ethical concerns related to procurement of relevant tissues for study, especially in early life. In this regard, the study of asthma pathogenesis in animal models has provided a wealth of information into the pathogenic mechanisms underlying disease development. Specifically, these models have played an important role in the discovery of the importance of T cells and Th2 cytokines in the development of allergic inflammation and associated changes in pulmonary function. In particular, the murine model has proven to be a valuable model of asthma for many reasons including: (1) the wide array of immunologic reagents available for study of immune pathways in this species; (2) the availability of over 200 well-characterized inbred strains for genetic studies; and (3) the ease of manipulation of specific genes through knockout and transgenic technologies. In this chapter, we will review important considerations for establishment of animal models of allergen-induced asthma, the salient characteristics of these models, the limitations and advantages of their use in exploring pathogenic mechanisms of disease, and the insights into disease pathogenesis resulting from their use to-date.

CHARACTERISTICS OF ANIMAL MODELS OF ALLERGIC ASTHMA

Experimental animal models of allergic asthma allow researchers to identify novel mechanisms of disease, and test the ability of therapeutic interventions to limit the severity or induction of allergic asthmatic inflammation. As in human disease, there are many determinants of the susceptibility of a given individual to the development of various features of allergic asthma. Among these are the host genetic background; the nature of the allergen; and the timing and route of exposure to the inciting allergen. Accordingly, it is important to select the appropriate model for the specific questions being addressed. Some important considerations for the development of and study of animal models of allergic asthma are discussed below.

CHOICE OF SPECIES AND STRAIN

Like humans, several other animal species including horses, felines, and canines spontaneously develop recurrent airway obstruction.[1,2] However, although rodents do not spontaneously develop asthma, they are typically used to study asthma due to their small size, and the relatively low costs associated with their purchase and housing.[3–7] Additionally, their short gestational periods and large litter size make rodents ideal for breeding experiments and genetic manipulations. Guinea pigs and rats had been traditionally used for physiological studies, as their larger size allows for greater ease of manipulations. However, development of methods for measurement of AHR in mice has extended this capability to mice (see section entitled 'Measuring airway function'). For immunological studies, mice are the most frequently used species due to the widespread availability of blocking reagents (e.g., monoclonal antibodies) and recombinant proteins (e.g., cytokines). Moreover, the fact that the mouse genome has been completely sequenced, makes dissection of specific immunological mechanisms possible. As such, this chapter focuses primarily on murine models of allergic asthma.

The ability to induce parameters of allergic asthma that are similar to those observed in human disease in mice varies greatly between strains, and thus selecting an appropriate strain is critical for the development of a relevant murine model of allergic asthma. Strains like A/J and AKR/J mice display high levels of allergen-induced airway hyperreactivity (AHR) after allergen sensitization and challenge (Fig. 28.1).[8] In contrast, C3H/HeJ and DBA/2 mice are comparatively resistant to the development of allergen-induced AHR.[8,9] However, the mouse strains most commonly used are BALB/c and C57Bl/6 mice. BALB/c and C57Bl/6 mice typically mount Th2- or Th1-dominated immune responses, respectively, and, as such, the induction of parameters of allergic asthma is robust in BALB/c mice, but comparatively limited in C57Bl/6 mice.[8,9] An additional convenience of using one or both of these strains to model human allergic asthma is that the majority of transgenic or knockout strains (see below) are initially generated on one or both of these genetic backgrounds. Thus, use of these strains ensures that appropriate wild-type controls for knockout or transgenic experiments are readily available without the need for extensive and time consuming back-crossing normally required to confirm that differences observed between control and knockout mice are not due to genetic differences between strains.

MODEL ALLERGENS

Chicken egg ovalbumin (OVA) is the most commonly used model allergen as it is inexpensive, can be obtained in high purity, and the immunodominant epitopes to which most immune responses are mounted have been identified. However, as inhalation of pure OVA induces the development of tolerance, rather than overt asthma-like airway responses,[10,11] there is a growing sentiment that OVA-based models bear little resemblance to human disease. The failure of OVA inhalation to induce asthma-like symptoms is perhaps not surprising, given that it is highly purified and functionally inert, bearing little resemblance to the complex mixture of proteins, many with enzymatic activity (e.g., pollens, dander, house-dust mite fecal pellets), that normally trigger the development of allergic asthma. Thus, while such complexity limits our ability to pinpoint specific allergenic epitopes to which the response is generated, investigators are increasingly making use of extracts or purified proteins derived from potent human allergens. Examples of such allergens include ragweed,[12–15] house-dust mite,[16–18] and *Aspergillus fumigatus*.[19–21]

METHODS OF ALLERGEN SENSITIZATION

To generate asthmatic responses to protein allergens (e.g. OVA), it is generally necessary to 'sensitize' mice through systemic, usually intraperitoneal (i.p.), administration of allergen. To further enhance the immunogenicity of the sensitizing allergen, it is frequently adsorbed to aluminum hydroxide (alum), a powerful Th2 skewing adjuvant. However, use of adjuvants is not absolutely required, particularly in mice normally susceptible to the development of allergic disease (e.g. BALB/c or A/J). Moreover, it has been demonstrated that allergen sensitization occurs through different mechanisms in the presence and absence of adjuvants like alum. Specifically, in the absence of alum, sensitization occurs through mast cell-dependent mechanisms, while in the presence of alum, sensitization does not require the presence of mast cells.[22] Thus, the use of powerfully Th2 skewing adjuvants to induce the development of allergic disease may ultimately impact the mechanisms through which the immune response develops, and therefore affect the results obtained.

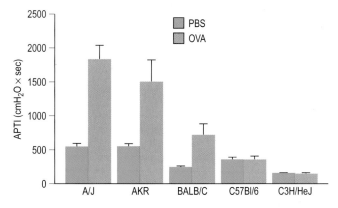

Fig. 28.1. Genetic variation in airway responses among murine strains. The indicated murine strains were sensitized by an intraperitoneal injection of OVA (200 μl), and challenged with PBS or OVA (50 μl of a 5% solution of OVA) intratracheally (i.t.) as indicated. Changes in airway pressure in response to acetylcholine were represented as integrated change in airway pressure time index (APTI). PBS, phosphate buffered saline; OVA, ovalbumin.

INDUCTION OF AIRWAY RESPONSES

The sensitization protocols described above trigger the production of readily detectable quantities of IgE and promote the production of type 2 cytokines (IL-4, IL-5, and IL-13). However, despite the induction of type 2 immunity, there is generally limited eosinophilic infiltration, mucus production or alteration in airway function following allergen sensitization. To induce these features of allergic asthma, allergen must be administered directly to the airways, either through aerosol inhalation, intratracheal injection or instillation (Fig. 28.2). Moreover, the development of eosinophilic inflammation, mucus hypersecretion, and decreased airway function is typically seen only after exposure of the airways to allergen for 3–7 consecutive days and is typically measured 24 h after the final OVA exposure.[23–25] Thus, the development of asthma-like alterations can occur in a relatively short period of time following airway allergen exposure in previously sensitized mice.

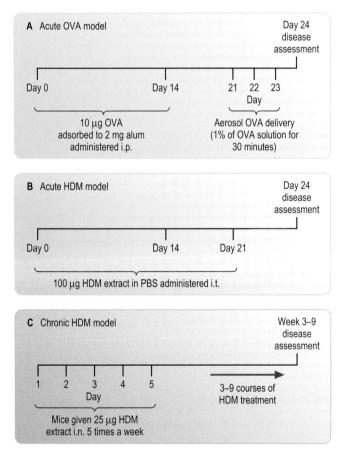

A Acute OVA model — Day 24 disease assessment

Day 0 — Day 14 — 21 22 23 Day

10 μg OVA adsorbed to 2 mg alum administered i.p.

Aerosol OVA delivery (1% of OVA solution for 30 minutes)

B Acute HDM model — Day 24 disease assessment

Day 0 — Day 14 — Day 21

100 μg HDM extract in PBS administered i.t.

C Chronic HDM model — Week 3–9 disease assessment

1 2 3 4 5 Day

3–9 courses of HDM treatment

Mice given 25 μg HDM extract i.n. 5 times a week

Fig. 28.2. Standard murine models of allergic asthma. Commonly used murine models of allergic asthma include acute OVA-driven models where sensitization occurs via the intraperitoneal route, following by airway inhalational exposure to induce airway responses (A). In HDM-based models, airway responses can be induced by exclusively airway allergen administration (B). To induce changes in airway structure more chronic allergen exposures are generally required (C). At sacrifice, various measures of disease severity such as airway function, eosinophilia, Th2 cytokine production, and IgE synthesis can be made.

AIRWAY ALLERGEN SENSITIZATION

The use of protocols involving systemic sensitization followed by airway exposure to induce airway responses in animal models is increasingly being regarded as unacceptable, particularly in light of the fact that in human disease, sensitization seems to occur following aeroallergen inhalation. However, attempts to sensitize mice exclusively through airway exposure to OVA have failed in the absence of adjuvants such as LPS, a low-level contaminant of most commercially available OVA preparations. Instillation of LPS-free OVA into the airways induces the development of tolerance rather than overt immunity, demonstrating the relatively poor immunogenicity of pure OVA.[10,11] In contrast, administration of extracts of house-dust mite (HDM), ragweed, or *Aspergillus fumigatus* is sufficient to induce robust changes in airway function after as little as two exposures (Fig. 28.2).[14,16,18,20] The observation that exposure to such allergen extracts induces similar disease in humans and animals following airway administration suggests that natural allergens possess unique properties that contribute to their ability to induce allergic disease. Identification of what makes an allergen uniquely allergenic remains the subject of ongoing speculation.[26]

ALTERNATIVE METHODS OF SENSITIZATION

Due to its widespread usage, the immunodominant epitopes of OVA responsible for triggering immune responses to OVA have been identified, and the T-cell receptor (TCR) chains that recognize these peptides in the context of different MHC class II molecules have been cloned. By engineering T cells that express OVA-specific TCRs, large numbers of T cells specific for OVA presented in the context of certain MHC molecules can be generated. Transfer of these OVA-specific T-cell clones to mice bearing the appropriate MHC molecules sensitizes mice to OVA without the need for immunization with native OVA.[27] Upon subsequent OVA inhalation, mice sensitized with OVA-specific T cells develop asthma-like symptoms,[27] demonstrating the importance of T cells in asthma pathogenesis. Such sensitization of mice circumvents the inherently low immunogenicity of OVA and the need for adjuvant and allows the study of the migration, proliferation, and cytokine production of those T cells involved in initiating the development of allergic disease if the sensitizing T cells are appropriately labeled (e.g., with fluorescent dye).

Alternatively, mice can be sensitized via administration of dendritic cells (DCs), which can be expanded from precursors in the bone marrow by culturing for 6–8 days in medium containing GM-CSF. Addition of allergen to cultures around day 6 allows the bone marrow DCs to take-up allergen and present it on their surface in the context of MHC class II molecules. If these allergen-presenting DCs are administered directly to the airways of mice, sensitization occurs, and subsequent exposure to allergen (either free allergen, or additional allergen-pulsed DCs) induces the development of an asthma-like phenotype.[28–31] Such experiments have highlighted the importance of dendritic cells in control of allergic asthma.[32]

MODELS OF AIRWAY REMODELING

Despite the fairly rapid induction of altered airway function and airway inflammation observed after airway challenge, structural changes usually associated with allergic asthma are generally not observed after such limited allergen exposures. To observe such features, usually termed airway remodeling, allergen exposures typically need to occur multiple times a week, over a span of several months.[16,33,34] Repetitive HDM administration to the airways of animals induces severe peribronchial and perivascular eosinophilic infiltration, increased mucus production, goblet cell metaplasia, extensive collagen deposition around the airways, and an increase in smooth muscle actin, all changes also seen in the lung of severely asthmatic individuals (Fig. 28.2).[16,33,34] Similar changes in airway structure can be observed in mice following instillation of cytokines directly into the airways, and in cytokine transgenic animals,[35–38] suggesting that cytokines play an important role in airway remodeling observed in allergic asthma.

CHARACTERISTICS AND ASSESSMENT OF THE ALLERGIC ASTHMA PHENOTYPE

The relevance of any animal model of disease relies on how closely it resembles disease in human patients. In this section, we will discuss the nature of the allergic phenotype elicited in murine models by allergen exposure, and how these parameters are typically assessed in animal models of allergen-induced asthma.

MEASURING AIRWAY FUNCTION

The primary physiological hallmark of allergic asthma is reversible airways obstruction, accompanied by airway hyperreactivity to cholinergic agonists. In humans, this is typically indicated by a decrease in FEV_1 or FVC observed following inhalation of cholinergic agonists or other substances. In humans, allergen exposure can induce early- and/or late-phase responses to allergen challenge. Although early responses have been assessed in mouse models, most investigators typically assess changes in airway responsiveness occurring between 24 and 72 h after allergen challenge. Allergen exposure of mice, as in humans, results in significant increases in responsiveness to cholinergic agonist stimulation when compared with their non-exposed controls (Fig. 28.3). However, several different methods are used to measure changes in airway responsiveness in mice. Invasive protocols, which represent the 'gold standard' of airway measurements, typically measure pulmonary resistance (RL) and dynamic compliance (Cdyn) in response to increasing doses of inhaled or intravenously administered cholinergic agonist (e.g., methacholine). However, these techniques generally require the animal to be anesthetized and artificially respirated, and are typically more technically challenging. However, the increasing availability of commercial systems for the invasive measurement of airway responses should facilitate more widespread, and consistent measurement of these parameters.[39]

The greatest shortcoming of such invasive techniques is that repeated airway measurements cannot be made in the same animal over time. Non-invasive techniques measure sensitivity to cholinergic agonists in unrestrained, fully conscious, spontaneously breathing mice. The greatest advantage of non-invasive techniques is that multiple measurements can be made in the same animal because extensive surgical preparation is not required, thus allowing the researcher to assess the kinetics of disease pathology or the impact of specific therapeutic interventions on

airway responses in the same animal. These studies typically use whole body plethysmography to measure enhanced pause (Penh), a dimensionless value that correlates with airway resistance, impedance, and intrapleural pressure.[40] However, while the ability to measure airway responses over time in the same animal proves to be a great convenience, there is a growing concern that changes in Penh do not represent changes in airway function as accurately as changes in RL or Cdyn. Thus, multiple factors should be considered when deciding which method to use to assess airway function.

SERUM IMMUNOGLOBULINS

As in humans, experimental asthma is usually associated with the production of allergen-specific immunoglobulins, including IgE and IgG1 and IgG2a (Fig. 28.3). ELISA can be used to measure the levels of total and allergen-specific immunoglobulins in serum samples collected many times over the course of the experiment. Thus, monitoring of immunoglobulin levels is a useful way of monitoring allergic sensitization. However, while ELISA reliably quantify total IgE levels, the low levels of allergen-specific IgE make detection by ELISA problematic. Alternatively, bioassays like passive cutaneous anaphylaxis (PCA) can be used to quantify antigen-specific IgE in the collected serum samples. Briefly, an unimmunized rat is given subcutaneous injections of mouse serum containing unknown quantities of allergen-specific IgE. Subsequent intravenous administration of allergen to the rat results in the development of a localized wheal and flare reaction. By administering serial dilutions of the mouse serum tested to the same animal, it is possible to determine the titer at which such responses are no longer detectable, and thus to compare the level of allergen-specific IgE in different serum samples. While PCA assays are laborious, expensive (as it requires housing additional animals), and subjective, they provide a method of directly assaying the levels of biologically active, allergen-specific IgE present in a serum sample.

Allergen sensitization is typically associated with a significant increase in the levels of circulating total and allergen-specific IgE. IgE titers typically peak around 10–14 days after initial sensitization, while the peak of IgE synthesis occurs around 7 days after each subsequent allergen exposure. However, while IgE levels are substantially increased following allergen sensitization, the requirement of IgE for the development of allergic asthma in mice remains controversial. For example, mice lacking B cells,[41,42] or IgE,[43,44] display levels of airway eosinophilia and AHR indistinguishable from control animals. Furthermore, following OVA inhalation, naive mice sensitized to OVA by adoptive transfer of OVA-specific Th2 cells, mount robust airway responses and display eosinophil-dominated airway inflammation 8 days post-transfer, a time period too short for de novo induction of substantial OVA-specific IgE responses.[45] However, transfer of IgE from OVA-sensitized into naive animals can induce the development of eosinophilia and AHR upon re-exposure to OVA, demonstrating that allergen-IgE is sufficient to induce an asthma-like phenotype.[46] Moreover, IgE enhances allergen uptake by antigen-presenting cells[47] and IgE binding to mast cell surface FcεR1 can directly activate mast cell function,[48,49] suggesting additional mechanisms by which IgE can contribute to the development of allergic asthma. The controversial role of IgE may, in part, be explained by differences in experimental protocols used. For example, mice lacking mast cells, an important mediator of many IgE-mediated activities, develop AHR normally if immunized

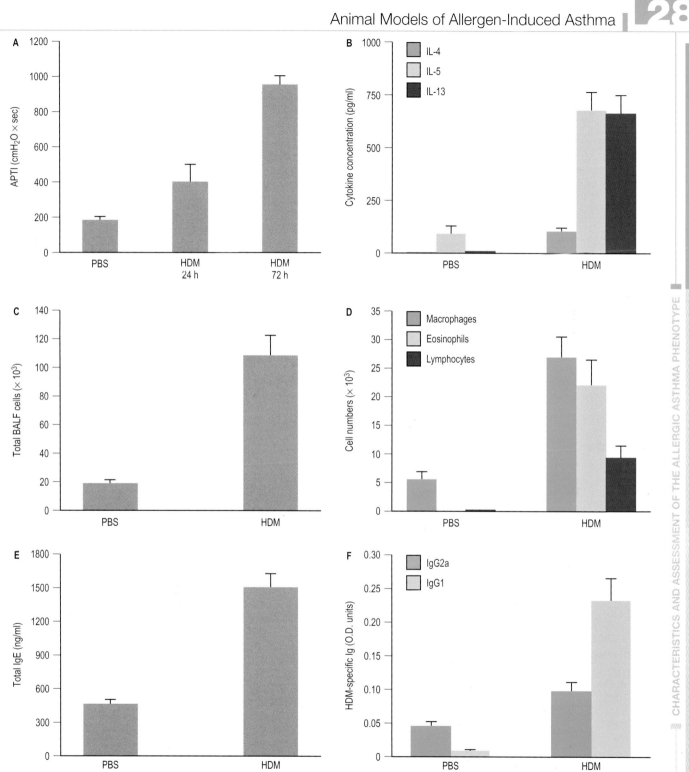

Fig. 28.3. House-dust mite induction of the asthma phenotype. Mice were given 100 µg of HDM extract, administered directly to the airways, three times over the span of 3 weeks. Such an exposure induces a progressive enhancement of AHR (measured by airway pressure time index (APTI)) compared with PBS-treated controls (A). Lung cells from HDM-treated mice, cultured in the presence of HDM, also produce substantial amounts of the Th2 cytokines IL-4, IL-5, and IL-13 while lung cells from PBS-treated animals produce low levels of cytokines (B). Airway allergen exposure also induces marked airway inflammation, markedly increasing the total cellular content of the BALF (C), with the largest increase seen in the eosinophil compartment (D). Allergen exposure significantly increases total IgE (E), and HDM-specific IgG1 levels in the serum, but has little impact on the production of IgG2a, an isotype associated with a Th1-dominated response (F). PBS, phosphate buffered saline; HDM, house-dust mite.

in the presence of alum, but fail to develop AHR if sensitized in the absence of alum[22] or using protocols that induce limited eosinophilia.[50] Moreover, while exposure to multiple rounds of inhaled OVA exposure induces progressively more robust, and rapid AHR responses in OVA-sensitized mice, in mice lacking FcεR1, airway responses always resemble those observed in animals receiving only one course of inhaled OVA.[51] Collectively, these results suggests that, as in human asthma, IgE may not be essential for development of asthma but may contribute to pathophysiology due to sensitivity to the specific allergen it is directed against.

EOSINOPHILIA

As in human disease, the development of asthma in murine models is frequently accompanied by the development of a predominantly eosinophilic inflammatory response in the airways. Eosinophil infiltration is typically determined by quantifying the number of eosinophils present in the bronchoalveolar lavage fluid (BALF) or by histological examination of pulmonary tissue after challenge. While there is a significant increase in the number of lymphocytes, monocytes, neutrophils, and epithelial cells following allergen treatment in experimental animal models, the largest increase observed is in the eosinophil lineage, which increase from nearly undetectable levels to as high as 50% of the cells in the BALF (Fig. 28.3). Similar increases are not observed in mice treated with PBS alone, demonstrating the allergen dependence of the eosinophil dominated airway inflammation observed in these models.

CYTOKINE PRODUCTION

Similar to human asthmatics, induction of an allergen-induced asthma-like phenotype in animal models is strongly associated with a polarized type 2 cytokine production in the lung. One convenient way of measuring cytokine production is to quantify cytokine mRNA in the whole lung of sensitized animals, a technique that allows the measurement of a large number of cytokines in the same sample and facilitates a direct indication of cytokine produced in situ. The principal drawback to this approach is that mRNA levels do not always correlate with protein levels in tissues and this approach does not allow determination of the cell type producing the cytokine. As an alternative approach, the cytokine protein-producing capacity of lung cells can be measured by assaying supernatants from in vitro cultured lung cells stimulated with allergen or polyclonal stimuli (e.g., concanavalin A) by ELISA, a relatively simple and inexpensive technique. While this approach directly measurescytokine synthesis (as opposed to message levels), the number of cytokines measured is generally limited. Recently, a technique designed to assay the amount of cytokine produced in vivo has also been developed.[52] This assay allows researchers to directly assay the amount of cytokine produced during the course of an ongoing immune response.

Using these techniques, it is routinely demonstrated that allergen sensitization and challenge results in robust increases in allergen-stimulated IL-4, IL-5, and IL-13 production by T cells found in the lung, or in secondary lymphoid organs (e.g., lung-draining lymph nodes)(Fig. 28.3). In contrast, the levels of IFNγ, a Th1-associated cytokine, are unaffected by allergen administration. These data demonstrate that in animal models, just as in human disease, increased airway hyperresponsiveness is associated with a bias towards increased production of Th2 cytokines.

MUCUS PRODUCTION

Mucus overproduction and mucus cell hyperplasia are also hallmarks of allergic asthma in humans. Specifically, assessment of autopsy samples from fatal asthma reveal that extensive mucus plugging occurs in the airways of individuals with severe asthma.[53] Despite the fact that mice possess no submucosal glands beyond the trachea,[54] mucus hypersecretion and goblet cell hyperplasia has also been observed in allergen-sensitized and challenged animals. By staining lung sections obtained from control and allergen-challenged mice with periodic acid Schiff reagent (PAS), it has been observed that the number of mucus-containing cells increases markedly after allergen exposure. Alternatively, it is also possible to specifically quantify the levels of mucus present in the airways or BALF by assaying the concentration of Muc5AC in BALF samples by ELISA.[55]

■ DISSECTING MECHANISMS IN ANIMAL MODELS OF ALLERGIC ASTHMA ■

The chief value in developing animal models of human disease is to develop a greater understanding of the mechanisms underlying the development of, or resistance to, disease, and to identify potentially novel therapeutic approaches by identifying proteins or pathways uniquely involved in disease progression or pathology. To this end, elucidating the individual contributions of specific effector molecules or cell types to disease pathology can be approached in a number of ways. A particular strength of animal models is the ability to examine the early or initiating events in allergen sensitization. Some of the more common approaches are discussed here.

KNOCKOUT MICE

A useful way of dissecting the contribution of a given molecule to overall disease development is through the use of knockout mice genetically engineered to produce a defective or non-functional version of a gene of interest. To develop a knockout mouse, the gene to be knocked out (the target gene) is first sequenced, and then a version of the gene engineered to encode a non-functional protein is created. Through homologous recombination techniques, the engineered gene is used to specifically replace the normal gene throughout the organism, resulting in an animal which is identical to other mice of the same strain, save for its inability to express functional versions of the target gene. Disease development in knockout and control mice is monitored to determine the role that the targeted gene normally plays in development of disease.

Certain caveats to the use and development of knockout mice must be acknowledged. Perhaps most dramatic is the fact that knocking out certain genes, those inextricably required for the normal development of a viable embryo, results in an embryonic lethal phenotype. Moreover, due to the highly pleiotropic nature of most mediators of the immune response, the function provided by the chronically absent gene can frequently be replaced by one or more factors. Such 'compensatory mechanisms' are frequently seen in knockout models of disease and must be considered when interpreting data.

TRANSGENIC MICE

The goal of studies involving transgenic mice is to examine the impact of constitutive overexpression of a gene of interest on the course of disease development. Transgenic mice differ from knockout mice in that rather than functionally inactivating a gene of interest, extra copies of the gene are added to the genome. Up to 200 extra copies of the transgene can be inserted into the genome, and the copy number generally correlates with protein expression level. Moreover, it is also possible to target the expression of the transgene to a specific cell or tissue type by placing the transgene under the control of tissue or cell-specific promoter. For example, by placing transgenes under the control of the promoter for Clara cell 10 kDa protein (CC10) or surfactant protein c (SPC) promoter, proteins normally expressed in lung epithelial cells, it possibly to achieve lung-specific expression.

However, since target genes randomly insert throughout the chromosome, by inserting into the middle of an exon or promoter region, it can disrupt the expression of other genes. Thus, it is again possible to develop embryonic lethal transgenics if the transgene inserts into a gene required for embryonic development. More critically however, it is possible to disrupt the expression of genes important in control of disease development. Therefore, once animals expressing the transgene have been made, it is important to confirm that insertion did not disrupt expression of any additional genes.

■ EXAMINING THE KINETICS OF THE ASTHMATIC RESPONSE ■

Since neither the frequency nor the intensity of aeroallergen exposure can easily be controlled in human patients, it is not possible to reliably determine the role of specific proteins or cells at specific phases of the immune response. In contrast, as allergen exposures can be strictly controlled in animal models, it is possible to determine at which phase of the immune response individual molecules contribute to the development of allergic lung responses. Examples of how the temporal importance of given proteins may be determined are outlined below.

MONOCLONAL ANTIBODIES

Monoclonal antibodies (mAbs) are antibodies, produced by a single B-cell clone, that are specific for a specific epitope. The process of developing mAbs is technically complicated; however, once developed, mAbs may be used for a variety of purposes in vivo. mAbs selected for their ability to block receptor:ligand interactions (e.g., cytokine:cytokine receptor interactions) can be used to gain a greater appreciation of the role of that cytokine in controlling disease development. Alternatively, mAbs raised against cell-surface molecules can be used to specifically deplete cellular targets in vivo, allowing researchers to assess the importance of certain cell types at specific periods of the asthmatic response.

One caveat to the use of mAbs in cytokine blockade or cellular depletion experiments is that it is difficult to verify complete target neutralization or depletion, particularly with cytokines produced locally at high levels, or long-lived, tissue residing cell populations. Moreover, it is also possible that animals treated with the mAbs over long periods of time may develop an immune response against the mAbs, thus increasing the rapidity of mAb clearance and decreasing the overall effectiveness of the mAb at blocking cytokine:receptor interactions or depleting cells. Also,

to ensure that any effect observed following mAb administration is not due to Fc receptor-mediated activation of cellular processes, it is critical to include groups of control animals treated with immunoglobulins of the same isotype, but of irrelevant specificity.

INDUCIBLE TRANSGENE EXPRESSION

Another powerful way to examine the role of target molecules at specific stages of the immune response is through the use of inducible transgenic mice. In these animals, the transgene is not constitutively expressed, but rather placed under the control of a specific promoter, *tetO*, part of a bacterial tetracycline responsiveness system. Transcription from this promoter requires the presence of doxycycline (usually administered in the animal's drinking water) plus a transcriptional activator (called *rtTA*), which animals must be engineered to produce. Thus, to get inducible control of a transgene in an animal, transgenic mice expressing the transgene under the control of the *tetO* promoter must be bred to mice expressing the *rtTA* in the desired tissue type. Once both transgenes are expressed in the appropriate cell types, expression of the target gene can be turned on in the presence of doxycycline.

Using such a system, mice overexpressing IL-13 in the airway epithelium following doxycycline exposure have been generated. Evaluation of these mice has revealed that chronic IL-13 exposure induces lung eosinophilia and structural changes including increased collagen deposition, subepithelial fibrosis, and smooth muscle hyperplasia. Moreover, these structural changes were shown to be the result of IL-13-induced increases in MMP-9 activation of TGF-β.[56] Using a similar system, a series of experiments examining the impact of VEGF overexpression on the allergic phenotype have shown that VEGF overexpression significantly increased airway inflammation (primarily mononuclear cells and B and T lymphocytes), airway mucus production, smooth muscle hypertrophy, collagen deposition, production of IL-13 (but not other Th2 cytokines), production of OVA-specific IgG$_1$, and enhanced AHR following intranasal sensitization.[57] Interestingly, while inflammation and mucus production returned to baseline after VEGF expression was turned off (by withdrawing doxycycline), increased smooth muscle hypertrophy and AHR were observed for as long as 1 month following doxycycline removal suggesting that enhanced VEGF production may contribute to the development of chronic changes in airway function and structure.[57] Finally, Köhl et al developed mice that expressed a C5aR antagonist in the lung following doxycycline administration to examine the role that C5a plays at distinct phases of the asthmatic response. This study demonstrated that during allergen sensitization, the expression of C5a was protective, yet exacerbated the asthmatic response during the effector phase.[58] Thus, the use of inducible transgenic mice is a powerful method of probing the importance of specific mediators at distinct phases of the asthmatic response.

■ USING ANIMAL MODELS TO IDENTIFY NOVEL ASTHMA SUSCEPTIBILITY GENES ■

The study of complex genetic disorders in humans has been hampered by a number of factors, such as genetic heterogeneity across populations, variability in disease expression, phenocopies, and uncontrolled environmental influences. Inbred mouse models of disease are ideal for gene identification due to: (1) the great degree of homology between the mouse and human genome (98%); (2) the ability to control the mouse genome through selective breeding strategies; (3) the reduced genetic heterogeneity seen in inbred mouse stains; and (4) the ability to control potentially confounding environmental factors. Indeed, searches for the genetic underpinnings of airway hyperresponsiveness in mice have been conducted by several groups. By performing selective matings between resistant (C3H/HeJ or C57Bl/6) and susceptible (A/J) mice, and their progeny, such genetic approaches were used to identify quantitative trait loci (QTL) on chromosomes 2, 6, 7, 15, 17 that contributed to the differences in baseline responsiveness observed in these strains.[59–61] Similar genetic approaches were used to identify QTL on chromosomes 2, 9, 10, 11, and 17 that regulated the development of airway hyperreactivity following allergen exposure.[8,62] However, while these screens identified broad regions implicated in regulating airway responsiveness, these regions were sufficiently large to contain numerous genes, making identification of individual genes involved in regulating the asthma phenotype difficult. More recently however, two studies identified individual genes within larger QTL that had significant impact on the development of allergen-induced airway responses.

COMPLEMENT FACTOR 5

To identify chromosomal regions associated with susceptibility to allergen-induced AHR, Ewart and colleagues performed linkage analysis studies on A/J mice (susceptible to allergen-induced AHR), C3H/HeJ mice (resistant to allergen-induced AHR), and [A/J × (C3H/HeJ × A/J)F1] A/J backcross mice exposed to ovalbumin. They identified a pair of QTL strongly associated with allergen-induced AHR on murine chromosome 2, which the investigators termed allergen-induced bronchial hyperresponsiveness 1 (*Abbr1*) and *Abbr2*.[8] After subsequent microarray analysis of genes differentially expressed in the lungs of C3H/HeJ and A/J animals, only one gene was found to be expressed at sufficiently differing levels between the two strains, *and* be located within the identified region of chromosome 2 – complement factor 5 (C5).[63] They also demonstrated that expression of C5 was consistently higher in resistant C3H/HeJ mice and F1 intercrosses with low AHR suggesting that C5 expression protects from the development of asthma.[63] Moreover, highly susceptible strains such as A/J and AKR/J actually possess a natural 2 bp mutation in *C5* making them unable to express functional C5 protein.[63] In exploring potential mechanisms through which C5 might limit the development of allergic asthma, it was found that C5 elicits production of IL-12, a key mediator of Th1-dominated responses, and critically involved in asthma resistance.[64]

Subsequently, a role of complement cascade proteins in human disease was inferred by the observations that increased levels of activated complement components can be found in the BAL samples from asthmatic individuals.[65] Moreover linkage analysis studies of the human genome have found associations between asthma risk and regions encoding both C5, and the C5a receptor,[66–69] and specific mutations in C3, C3a receptor, and C5 genes.[70] Collectively, these data suggest that complement components may significantly impact the development of allergic asthma.

TIM-1

In humans, chromosome 5q23–35 has been identified in a number of studies as containing genes linked to the development of allergic asthma. To identify novel asthma candidate genes in this region, McIntire et al

recently developed a mouse strain in which sections syntenic to human chromosome 5q23–35 (murine chromosome 11) in susceptible BALB/c mice were replaced with the sequences from DBA mice, a strain that develops weak IL-4 and AHR responses.[9] The authors were able to demonstrate that both high IL-4 production, and susceptibility to the development of allergen-induced AHR were associated with a region of chromosome 11 not homologous to the areas of human chromosome 5 previously assumed to be involved in control of allergic asthma, namely the cytokine gene cluster (containing the *IL4*, *IL5*, *IL13*, and *IL9* genes), IL-12p40, or the β-adrenergic receptor. Instead, positional cloning of the locus, named *Tapr* (for T cell and airway phenotype regulatory), identified a novel family of genes, the T-cell immunoglobulin and mucin-containing molecules (TIM). Further analysis revealed that the sequences of two TIM family members, *Tim1* and *Tim3*, contained significant amino acid deletions in mice resistant to the development of allergen-induced AHR (DBA and C57Bl/6), suggesting that these deletions protect from the development of allergen-induced asthma.

Subsequent studies have focused primarily on Tim-1, which has previously been identified as the hepatitis A virus cellular receptor (hHAVcr-1) on human cells. Numerous polymorphisms in the TIM-1 gene have since been identified, and specific deletions have been associated with an increased prevalence of atopy and eczema in a number of populations.[71–73] One specific mutation, a 6 amino acid insertion in a region of the protein critical for the HAV entry and uncoating, has been demonstrated to be protective against the development of asthma in HAV seropositive individuals.[74] This is particularly interesting in light of the observation that the dramatic decrease in HAV seropositivity in Westernized nations, which has occurred since the early 1970s, is concomitant with a doubling of the prevalence of asthma. This suggests that HAV infection may directly influence the development of asthma.

The identification of the complement and TIM family of molecules demonstrates the power of animal models to identify unique asthma susceptibility genes. By making use of powerful genetic tools and genetic manipulations possible only in laboratory animals, investigators were able to identify novel genes whose roles in asthma pathogenesis had not been previously appreciated. The success of these approaches suggests that further such studies should be undertaken. Indeed, genome scans for multiple asthmatic phenotypes (e.g., indices of airway remodeling, such as mucus hypersecretion or subepithelial fibrosis) conducted with crosses between the more than 200 inbred strains of mice would greatly enhance our knowledge of the genetic basis of experimental asthma.

GENE PROFILING APPROACHES TO IDENTIFYING NOVEL ASTHMA SUSCEPTIBILITY GENES

In addition to whole genome searches for asthma susceptibility genes, several groups have utilized a gene profiling approach to identify novel targets for asthma. Interestingly, examination of lung gene expression patterns in various mouse models of allergen and/or cytokine driven asthma[75–77] have identified a set of genes which are commonly expressed across different models, including Ca^{2+}-activating chloride channel 3 (CLCA3),[78] FIZZ2,[79] trefoil factor 2,[75,76,80] acid mammalian chitinase (AMCase),[75] YM-1,[75] SPRR2A,[75,81] intelectin,[76] and arginase I.[75,77] Although the exact role of each of these candidate genes has not been fully elucidated, there is support for a role for several of these in disease pathogenesis. For example, Elias and colleagues[56] demonstrated that neutralization of AMCase ameliorated Th2 inflammation and airway hyperresponsiveness, in part, by inhibiting IL-13 pathway activation and chemokine induction. Moreover, they showed exaggerated expression of AMCase in tissues from asthmatic individuals.[82]

Zimmermann and colleagues found that arginase I, an enzyme that hydrolyzes arginine to ornithine and urea, was elevated in response to allergen and IL-13 exposure in a STAT6-dependent manner.[83] A functional role for arginase in allergen-induced airway hyperresponsiveness has been suggested in experiments in which arginase was blocked in vivo either through pharmacological (NOR-NOHA)[84] or RNA interference approaches.[85] Although the mechanisms by which altered levels of arginase may impact AHR are not known, alterations in arginine catabolism may lead to airway hyperresponsiveness in several ways. First, as both arginase and iNOS synthase use arginine as a common substrate, elevated arginase levels may compromise the ability to synthesize NO and lead to AHR. Alternatively, elevated levels of arginase may contribute to increased production of ornithine, a precursor for the synthesis of proline, thus leading to enhanced collagen deposition and airway remodeling. In support of the first possibility, Maarsingh and colleagues have shown that arginase strongly impairs iNOS-mediated airway smooth muscle relaxation in allergen-exposed guinea pigs.[86] Extending these findings to humans, elevated levels of arginase have been found in both BAL cells[77] and plasma[87] from asthmatics as compared with normals. Although single nucleotide polymorphisms (SNPs) in arginase I have not been found to date to be associated with increased risk of asthma in humans, SNPs in a related molecule, arginase II, were strongly associated with childhood asthma and atopy.[88] Although much remains to be learned about the role of these novel pathways in asthma pathogenesis, the information gained through gene profiling in mouse models will undoubtedly fuel further exploration into these pathways.

T-CELL MEDIATORS OF ALLERGIC ASTHMA

As the primary orchestrator of specific immune responses to foreign antigens, the T lymphocyte has been implicated in the pathogenesis of allergic diseases. Indeed numerous studies have demonstrated increased numbers of activated T lymphocytes in BALF and bronchial biopsies from asthmatic individuals[89] suggesting an important role for these cells. Although considerable descriptive evidence suggests that CD4+ T lymphocytes are important in the pathogenesis of atopic disorders in humans, definitive proof is of course difficult to obtain. As a result, experimental animal models have been extremely useful in mechanistic delineation of the role of CD4+ T-cells and T-cell-derived cytokines in the pathogenesis of allergic disorders. Murine models of antigen-driven asthma have consistently revealed a causal role for CD4+ T cells in the development of the symptoms of allergic airway disease.[89–92] In depletion studies, administration of anti-CD4 mAbs completely abrogated airway and BAL eosinophilia and airway responses normally observed after OVA sensitization and airway challenge.[90] Moreover, while RAG-/- mice, which lack T and B cells, fail to develop allergen-induced AHR, reconstitution with CD4+ T cells restored airway responses.[89] Also, transfer of CD4+ T cells from antigen-primed mice or rats to naive hosts is sufficient to transfer both eosinophilic inflammation and AHR,[91,92] demonstrating that CD4+ T cells are both necessary and sufficient to induce the development of allergic asthma.

Of the multiple CD4+ T-cell subsets described to date (Th2, Th1, Tregs), allergic asthma appears to be associated with an expansion of CD4+ T cells producing Th2 cytokines (IL-4, IL-5, IL-13, IL-9). An immunopathogenic role for Th2 cytokine-producing cells in the development of murine models of allergic asthma was definitely demonstrated by adoptive transfer studies in mice. Specifically, transfer of OVA-specific CD4+ T cells skewed in vitro into IL-4 producing Th2 cells was sufficient to induce eosinophilic airway inflammation, mucus production, and increased AHR to subsequent inhalational challenge with OVA.[27,45,93] In contrast, it was demonstrated that transfer of OVA-specific CD4+ T cells skewed in vitro into IFNγ-secreting Th1 cells caused the development of a neutrophil-dominated inflammatory response, with no induction of airway reactivity.[27,45]

TH2 CYTOKINES IN ASTHMA

The involvement of each of the specific Th2 cytokines in atopic airway responses has been demonstrated in studies in which IL-4, IL-5, IL-13, and IL-9 have been manipulated through either antibody blockade, or gene targeting. Collectively, the Th2 cytokines orchestrate the elicitation of the allergic response via their ability to regulate IgE production and recruitment and activation of various effector cells (e.g., mast cells, eosinophils, fibroblasts, epithelial cells). In particular, IL-4, through its critical role in Th2 differentiation, has been shown to be essential in the initiation of allergic airway responses.[94] IL-5 clearly plays a role in eosinophil development, recruitment, and activation at the site of Th2-inflammatory responses,[95] while IL-9 appears to be an important regulator of mast cell activation.[96] IL-13 has been shown to have a singular role in the effector phase of the allergic response. Specifically, it is sufficient to induce many of the manifestations of allergic disease, including airway inflammation, airway hyperresponsiveness, and mucus cell hypersecretion in allergic airway diseases.[38]

IL-4 AND IL-13

The Th2 cytokines IL-4 and IL-13 are structurally very similar to one another, are located adjacent to one another on murine chromosome 11 (human chromosome 5), and can both signal through the type 2 IL-4 receptor composed of the IL-13Rα1 and IL-4Rα chains. Despite these similarities, the general consensus is that these two Th2 cytokines play distinct roles in promoting the subsequent development of allergic asthma. Initial studies conducted in IL-4 deficient mice demonstrated that this cytokine was essential for the development of allergic symptoms.[94] However, subsequent studies using IL-4 specific mAbs to block IL-4 activity at different phases of the immune response demonstrated that IL-4 neutralization prior to OVA sensitization did indeed limit the development of AHR, IL-5 production, and IgE synthesis. In contrast, neutralization of IL-4 during the effector phase (immediately prior to OVA challenge) had no impact on these parameters.[97,98] These data support the present understanding that the primary role of IL-4 in allergic asthma is to induce the expansion and survival of Th2 effector cells which, through the release of additional Th2 effector cytokines, trigger the inflammation, remodeling, and changes in airway function normally seen in asthmatic individuals.

In contrast to the importance of IL-4 in initiating the asthmatic response, the IL-4 look-alike, IL-13, is now felt to be a critical mediator of the effector phase of the asthmatic response. Studies in which IL-13 alone was blocked in vivo in OVA sensitized animals dramatically reduced AHR and mucus hypersecretion with little impact on IgE synthesis, or airway eosinophilia,[38,99] even in the presence of normal levels of IL-4 and IL-5 production.[100] Moreover, direct instillation of IL-13 into the airways, or transgenic overexpression of IL-13 in the lungs induced the development of airway eosinophilia, epithelial cell hypertrophy, goblet cell metaplasia, mucus secretion, subepithelial fibrosis, and AHR in the absence of allergen challenge.[35,38]

Much effort has been exerted to delineate the mechanisms by which IL-13 may regulate the asthmatic phenotype. Interestingly, although IL-13 can regulate IgE synthesis, and recruit and activate mast cells and eosinophils, IL-13 induction of the features of experimental asthma occurs independently of T cells,[99] mast cells,[101] and eosinophils.[102] These cells may instead contribute to the allergic response via their ability to produce IL-13. Interestingly, recent evidence suggests that IL-13 induction of AHR and mucus cell metaplasia are solely dependent upon IL-13 activation of STAT6 signaling in the airway epithelium.[103] Indeed, IL-13 likely regulates mucus hypersecretion through its combined effects on goblet cell differentiation, mucin gene expression, and regulation of ion channel expression and function (e.g., CLCA3, ENAC) (Fig. 28.4). The exact mechanisms by which IL-13 induces AHR are not fully understood, but it appears to induce the release of bronchoactive substances such as leukotrienes and complement factors from the airway epithelium rather than acting as a bronchoconstrictor agonist itself.[103]

Although IL-13-dependent induction of subepithelial fibrosis and eosinophilic inflammation were not dependent upon signaling in the epithelium, potential mechanisms for these actions have been described. For example, IL-13 stimulates the production of pro-fibrotic factors such as arginase-1 and TGF-β, and can therefore promote the development of subepithelial fibrosis and smooth muscle hyperplasia normally observed in asthmatic individuals (Fig. 28.4). Additionally, IL-13 promotes eosinophilic inflammation (Fig. 28.4) by upregulating the expression of VCAM-1 by vascular endothelial cells, and stimulating the production of chemokines such as eotaxin, MCP-1, and TARC. Intriguingly, IL-13 was also recently shown to upregulate the production of acidic mammalian chitinase (AMCase).[82] Expression of this molecule was shown to be critical for disease pathogenesis. While humans do not produce chitin, the presumed substrate for AMCase, many chitin-containing organisms (cockroach, house-dust mite, fungi) are strongly sensitizing aeroallergens, suggesting that these endogenous chitinases may play an important role in development or maintenance of allergic asthma.

The importance of IL-13 in human asthma is supported by several lines of evidence, including the observation that IL-13 is consistently overexpressed in the lungs of asthmatic patients, and that polymorphisms in the IL-13 gene are strongly associated with susceptibility to development of several asthma traits.[104–107] Moreover, SNPs in the IL-4Rα chain are strongly associated with various asthma phenotypes.[108–111] Proof of concept of the role of IL-13 should be forthcoming as clinical trials designed to assess the efficacy of several IL-13 inhibitors in the treatment of allergic asthma are currently underway, as are efforts using bispecific antibodies engineered to neutralize both IL-4 and IL-13.

IL-5

The Th2 cytokine IL-5 is the primary regulator of eosinophil differentiation, recruitment, maturation, activation, and survival in tissues. Several lines of evidence support its primary role in regulation of pulmonary eosinophilia in asthma. Mice expressing an IL-5 transgene specifically in the lung demonstrate increased eosinophilia, mucus production, and AHR.[37] In contrast, a genetic deficiency in IL-5 results in marked, but not complete absence, of bone marrow and circulating eosinophils, as well as a reduction in BAL eosinophilia and AHR in mice sensitized and challenged with OVA,[112,113] suggesting an important role for IL-5 in promoting both eosinophilia and allergen-induced AHR. However, while eosinophilia is consistently diminished in models where IL-5 is neutralized with mAbs or soluble IL-5R, the impact of IL-5 blockade on the development of AHR is variable. In mice[114] and guinea pigs,[115] IL-5 blockade prevents the development of AHR, while other studies in mice,[64,97,116] guinea pigs,[117] or monkeys[118] report that IL-5 neutralization has no impact on the development of AHR. This dissociation between eosinophils and the late-phase response has recently been confirmed in studies of human asthmatics that demonstrated that while anti-IL-5 treatment suppressed pulmonary eosinophils by about 50%,[119] it did not inhibit either early or late physiologic responses to inhaled allergens or improve lung function,[119,120] despite marked reductions in blood, sputum, and tissue eosinophilia.[119–121] While multiple explanations for a lack of effect in this study can be made, including the small study size, dosing schedule, and/or acute nature of treatment, these studies suggest that blockade of eosinophils and IL-5 alone are not sufficient to improve symptoms of asthma. Arguably, the study was underpowered and the dosing regime did not result in complete ablation of eosinophils in lung tissues, leaving the question open as to whether complete ablation is necessary to achieve therapeutic benefit. In a follow-up study using a multiple dosing regime, it was shown that anti-IL-5 attenuated several indices of airway remodeling, including enhanced matrix protein deposition (procollagen, tenascin, laminin), pro-fibrotic molecule expression (TGF-β), and airway smooth muscle hypertrophy, without effects on airway physiology.[122] The failure of anti-IL-5 treatment to ameliorate allergic symptoms in humans has brought into question the importance of eosinophils in human asthma. However, as long as existing therapies do not completely eliminate tissue eosinophils, the issue will not be resolved.

In order to address this issue, several groups have undertaken the task of developing eosinophil-deficient mice.[123,124] One group generated an eosinophil-deficient mouse via insertion of a cytocidal protein (diphtheria toxin A) in the promoter of the eosinophil peroxidase (EPO) gene. These mice were reported to be completely devoid of eosinophils in all tissues.[124] Moreover, all features of the allergic phenotype were absent (AHR, mucus, eosinophilia, Th2 cytokine production) in these mice following allergen challenge. The other eosinophil-deficient mouse line harbors a deletion of a high-affinity GATA-binding site in the GATA-1 promoter (dbl-GATA mice), leading to the specific ablation of the eosinophil lineage.[123] In this line, eosinophil depletion had no effect on AHR, mucus production, or Th2 cytokine production, but did reduce airway remodeling assessed by collagen deposition. Interestingly, the results of this study mirror those observed in the human anti-IL-5 trials. However, the exact reasons for the discrepancies in the mouse models are unknown. However, they may be due to the presence of residual eosinophils in the dbl-GATA mice, to unappreciated hematological abnormalities, or to toxic effects of diphtheria toxin on non-eosinophils in the EPO-diphtheria toxin A mice. Further studies with these eosinophil-deficient mice will hopefully further define the role of the eosinophils in asthma.

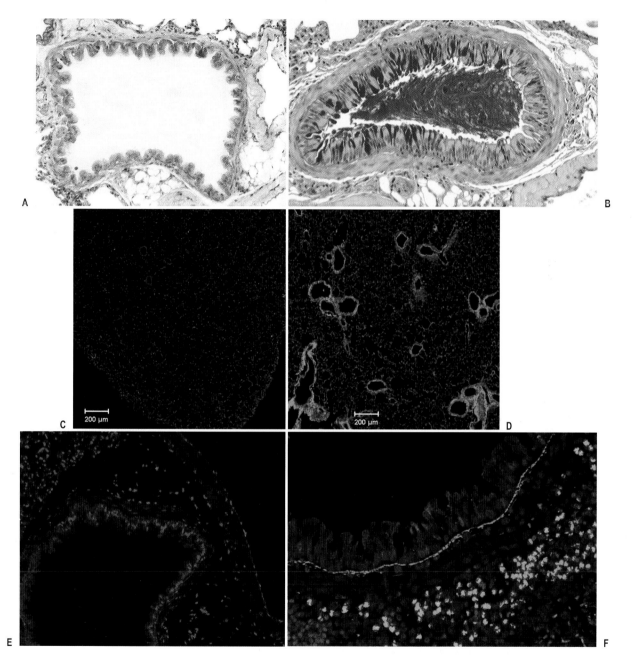

Fig. 28.4. IL-13 is sufficient to induce many parameters of allergic asthma. Mice were treated with 200 ng of IL-13 in 40 μl of PBS or PBS alone on days 0, 1, 2, 3, and sacrificed on day 4. Compared with control mice challenged with i.t. PBS (A), treatment with i.t. IL-13 administration induces substantial mucus production and the development of mucus plugs (B). To study the impact of IL-13 on smooth muscle proliferation, transgenic mice expressing GFP-labeled smooth muscle γ-actin were treated with PBS (C) or IL-13 (D). Histologic examination of GFP staining in these transgenic mice reveals that IL-13 enhances smooth muscle number. As compared with PBS-treated animals stained with a YFP-conjugated antibody to MBP (E), IL-13-treated mice demonstrated markedly enhanced MBP+ eosinophils (F).

iNKT CELLS

Although asthma has clearly been associated with polarized Th2 cytokine production in tissues, the source of these Th2 cytokines has been recently debated. Specifically, recent studies have implicated invariant TCR^+ CD1d-restricted $CD4^+$ natural killer T cells as one of the major sources of Th2 cytokines. iNKT cells are functionally distinguished by their capacity to produce extremely large amounts of IL-4, IL-13, and $IFN\gamma$ within hours after stimulation, and have thus been postulated to play important regulatory roles in regulating the development of allergic asthma.

Studies conducted in mice lacking iNKT cells ($CD1d^{-/-}$ mice or $J_\alpha 281^{-/-}$ mice) demonstrate that allergen-induced AHR, airway eosinophilia, production of OVA-specific IgE, and Th2 cytokine synthesis was completely abrogated in the absence of these cells.[25,125] Expression of both IL-4 and IL-13 by iNKT cells was shown to be crucial to their ability to induce the development of allergic asthma.[25] Moreover, intranasal administration of αGalCer, a glycolipid known to specifically activate iNKT cells, broke the tolerance normally observed during mucosal sensitization with OVA and induced the development of AHR, airway eosinophilia, and Th2 cytokine production.[126] However, a contrasting view of the role of iNKT cells comes from studies demonstrating that administration of αGalCer to previously sensitized animals protected mice from the development of asthma-like symptoms, decreasing AHR, mucus overproduction, IgE and Th2 cytokine production.[127,128] The protective effects of iNKT cells were dependent upon $IFN\gamma$ production, as blockade of $IFN\gamma$ reversed the protective effects of αGalCer administration.[127,128] Thus, iNKT cells clearly have a variable impact on the development of allergic asthma.

While the influences that determine whether iNKT potentiate or limit the development of allergic asthma remain undefined, a number of possibilities exist. The timing of iNKT activation may play an important role, as IL-4 production by these cells generally peaks at 2 h after activation, while $IFN\gamma$ peaks 24 h later[128] suggesting that induction of iNKT cells very early in the response might enhance allergen sensitization and thus promote the development of asthma. Alternatively, it has been demonstrated that repeated exposure to iNKT-stimulating ligands appears to powerfully tolerize these cells, preventing them from responding to further stimulation,[129] suggesting that repeated exposure to iNKT-activating ligands may limit their asthma-inducing capacity. Additionally, while ligands for iNKT cells have been identified from endogenous sources,[130] they have also been found in allergens and bacteria,[131,132] suggesting that iNKT cells may be activated by a number of different glycolipids. However, it is presently unclear whether activation of iNKT cells with different ligands results in qualitatively different signals that may influence the production of Th1 versus Th2-skewing cytokines.

In support of a role for NKT cells in human asthma, two independent groups have reported the presence of iNKT cells in the tissues of asthmatic individuals. In one study it was reported that as many as 60% of T cells found in the bronchial biopsies of human asthmatics were iNKT cells.[133] Similarly, Sen et al[134] found that a large number of $CCR9^+$ $V_\alpha24^+$ iNKT cells were present in both blood and bronchial biopsy samples from patients with asthma, but not from control subjects. They also showed that the numbers of $CCR9^+$ $V_\alpha24^+$ NKT cells from the peripheral blood of symptomatic patients with asthma decreased when asthma was clinically silent and after steroid treatment. Since subsequent reports have failed to confirm a role of iNKT cells in asthma,[135] further studies are needed to provide a better understanding of their role in allergic immune responses.

REGULATORY T CELLS

It has recently been hypothesized that under non-inflammatory conditions the outcome of immune responses to innocuous environmental allergens is the development of immunological tolerance. Moreover, it is thought that a loss of tolerance results in Th2-biased immune responses at mucosal surfaces. Although the specific immunological events that mediate tolerance in this setting are not well understood, recent studies have suggested that regulatory T cells (Tregs) protect against the development of allergic disease and that their function is impaired in genetically susceptible individuals. Regulatory T cells are a subset of $CD4^+$ T cells functionally distinguished by their low proliferative response, and capacity to limit the function and proliferation of other T cells, typically through IL-10 or TGF-β-dependent mechanisms.[136,137] As such, Tregs are generally considered to negatively regulate the development of immune responses. Indeed, Tregs are widely known to be important in controlling the development of autoimmune disease,[138] but have only just begun to be examined in the context of allergic asthma. Tregs generally fall within two broad categories: natural $CD4^+CD25^+$ Tregs (nTregs) and inducible Tregs (iTregs). nTregs are so-called because they develop in the thymus, following TCR:MHC interactions,[139] although thymic stromal lymphopoietin (TSLP)-activated dendritic cells have also been shown to play a role.[140] In contrast to nTregs, iTregs arise outside of the thymus, usually as a result of exposure to high levels of antigen, or in response to bacterial products. Identifying Tregs can be problematic as they are present in low levels (5–10% of circulating $CD4^+$ T cells), and although markers like CD25, CTLA-4, and glucocorticoid-induced TNF receptor (GITR) have been found to be constitutively expressed on nTregs, they are also expressed on activated effector T cells. As such, the most reliable way to identify Tregs is through expression of the forkhead transcription factor Foxp3, expression of which correlates with suppressor function.[139,141]

To examine the role of nTregs in control of allergic asthma, Jaffar et al transferred spleen cells from OVA transgenic TCR expressing mice to naive BALB/c mice and observed that depletion of nTregs resulted in enhanced airway eosinophilia compared with transfer of unfractionated spleen cells,[142] suggesting that nTregs may limit the development of allergic asthma. Similarly, transfer of purified OVA TCR transgenic nTregs cells to sensitized mice limited the development of AHR, Th2 cell recruitment, and cytokine production following airway allergen challenge by increasing host production of IL-10.[143] In a transgenic model where OVA was chronically expressed in the lungs of OVA TCR transgenic mice, recruitment of nTregs to the lungs prevented IL-4 production and the development of airway responses, despite dramatic, predominantly lymphocytic pulmonary inflammation.[144] Finally, nTreg depletion following administration of anti-CD25 mAbs was found to exacerbate asthmatic responses in mice resistant to the development of allergen-induced AHR, but not those normally susceptible to the development of asthma.[18] Collectively, these data suggest that while nTregs can limit the development of allergic asthma, such influences appear to be lacking in mice genetically predisposed to the development of experimental asthma.

Bacterial products typically regarded as strong inducers of Th1-dominated immunity have been demonstrated to promote resistance to the development of allergen-induced AHR through their ability to induce iTregs. For example, treatment of mice with heat-killed *Listeria monocytogenes* or killed *Mycobacterium vaccae* has been shown to induce the development of iTregs that significantly reduced airway inflammation, eosinophilia, and AHR through IL-10 and TGF-β-mediated mechanisms.[145,146] Interestingly, despite the Th2-dominated response elicited by helminthic parasitic infections, it has been demonstrated that infection with such parasites limits the development of allergic responses by promoting the development of iTregs. For example, infection with *Heligmosomoides polygyrus* or feeding *Schistosoma japonicum* eggs prior to allergen sensitization dramatically reduced airway inflammation, eosinophil number, and Th2 cytokine production in both BALB/c and C57Bl/6 mice following allergen challenge.[147,148] However, exposure to infectious agents or their products is not the only way to induce the development of protective iTregs. Feeding or inhalation of OVA prior to sensitization significantly reduced the development of airway inflammation, eosinophilia, and production of IgE and Th2 cytokines normally observed following aerosol challenges through a TGF-β-dependent mechanism.[149,150] Thus the development of mucosal tolerance in mice can be a result of populations of inducible Tregs. Interestingly, there is some evidence that the successful treatment of allergic diseases in humans following specific allergen immunotherapy or sublingual allergen immunotherapy is associated with the appearance of these antigen-specific inducible Tregs.[151] Taken together these studies suggest that impaired Treg function may lead to the loss of tolerance observed in human asthmatics and suggest that further elucidation of the factors regulating Treg development and function may inform the development of therapeutics to enhance Treg function in asthmatic individuals.

■ INNATE IMMUNE RESPONSES IN ASTHMA ■

While CD4+ Th2 cells are clearly important effectors of the asthmatic response, the factors that drive the aberrant expansion of pathogenic Th2 cells are not well understood. However, there is a growing appreciation that cells of the innate immune system, while not able to respond in an allergen-specific manner, can influence either the differentiation of naive T cells into Th1 or Th2 cytokine producing effectors, or control the activation status of previously differentiated, allergen-specific T cells. Two such cell types that have received a great deal of attention recently in this regard are dendritic cells and epithelial cells.

DENDRITIC CELLS

In the airways, dendritic cells (DCs) form an intricate cellular network just below the epithelial cell layer, a position from which they are well suited to sample inhaled antigens present in the airway lumen, and transport these allergens to lung-draining lymph nodes (LNs).[152–155] Once in the draining LNs, allergen-bearing DCs have the capacity to fully activate effector function in naive T cells due to their high level expression of MHC class II and co-stimulatory molecules like CD80/CD86 which interact with T-cell-expressed CD28. Indeed, transfer of allergen-bearing DCs to the airways of naive animals is sufficient to sensitize mice for subsequent development of allergic asthma,[156–158] suggesting that allergen-presenting DCs are sufficient to trigger T-cell activation and the development of allergic asthma. However, DCs also play an important role beyond sensitization by stimulating T-cell activation in the lung, as demonstrated by studies showing that administration of allergen-pulsed DCs to the airways of previously sensitized animals

is sufficient to trigger allergen-induced AHR,[30,31] and depletion of pulmonary DCs in sensitized hosts renders mice refractory to increases in AHR normally seen after allergen challenge.[153,159] Moreover, asthmatic humans have an increased number of intraepithelial DCs compared with healthy controls,[160,161] suggesting a similarly important role for pulmonary DCs in human disease. Collectively, these studies suggest a critical role for pulmonary DCs in both initial aeroallergen sensitization, and for inducing the development of asthma exacerbations.

One level of control through which DCs may influence the development or resistance to allergic asthma is via expression of different co-stimulatory molecules. For example, while CD80/CD86 and OX40L play important roles in promoting allergic disease,[162–164] ICOS-L expression promotes the development of IL-10-producing Tregs crucial for the development of inhalational tolerance.[165] Recently, B7-H1 (PD-L1) and B7-DC (PD-L2) were identified on the basis of homology to existing B7 family members. While there may be additional, unidentified T-cell ligands for these molecules,[166–168] both B7-DC and B7-H1 have been shown to bind to T-cell-expressed PD-1 and provide an inhibitory signal to limit T-cell activation.[169,170] Thus, the balance of inhibitory versus stimulatory molecules expressed on the surface of different DC subsets may in turn, contribute to the ability of these DC to stimulate asthmatic responses.

Recently, based on cell-surface marker expression, DCs have been divided into subsets that play differing roles in the development of allergen-induced asthma. Myeloid DCs (mDCs: CD11c+CD11b+Gr1-B220-) are effective stimulators of T-cell effector function and have been shown to be important mediators of allergic asthma, as transfer of these cells to the airways of naive animals is sufficient to induce the development of allergic asthma.[28] In contrast, plasmacytoid DCs (pDCs: CD11c+CD11b-Gr1+B220+) seem to induce the development of Tregs[11] and can markedly inhibit the ability of mDCs to fully activate T-cell effector functions, even in very low numbers.[58] Furthermore, transfer of allergen-pulsed pDCs prior to OVA (alum) sensitization was found to prevent the development of allergic inflammation in the lung, while depletion of pDCs using specific mAbs enhanced asthmatic responses.[11] Collectively, these studies in animal models demonstrate a tolerogenic role for pDCs in allergic asthma. Although no studies to date have examined the levels of various DC subsets in the lungs of asthmatics, an increase in pDCs in the nasal mucosa following allergen challenge has been noted in adult asthmatics,[171] while it has been noted that allergic children have a significantly decreased number of circulating pDCs.[172] However, the relationship between endogenous pulmonary DC subsets and asthma susceptibility or severity in humans remains to be determined.

AIRWAY EPITHELIAL CELLS

As the epithelial cells lining the airways are the first cells to encounter inhaled aeroallergens, they are uniquely poised to direct the subsequent immune responses to these substances. It is becoming increasingly evident that epithelial cells represent more than a simple physical barrier preventing exposure of the immune system to allergen. For example, airway epithelial cells express MHC class II molecules, CD80 and CD86, and can induce CD4+ T-cell proliferation and cytokine production, suggesting that epithelial cells may be able to directly induce T-cell activation.[173] It is clear, however, that epithelial cells also express, constitutively and in response to cytokine stimulation, B7-H1 and B7-DC, both of which limit T-cell activation by signaling through T-cell-expressed PD-1.[174] Indeed, blockade of B7-DC and B7-H1 significantly enhanced T-cell-derived cytokine production in co-cultures of epithelial cell lines and activated T-cells, suggesting that epithelial cells may be able to limit local T-cell activation by selective co-stimulatory molecule expression.[174]

More recently, epithelial cells were found to produce TSLP, a cytokine shown to directly increase the ability of DCs to stimulate Th2 effector function, and activate mast cells.[175] Arguing for an important role for epithelial cell production of TSLP in control or allergic asthma, mice rendered deficient in the TSLP receptor display reductions in both airway eosinophilia and goblet cell hyperplasia following systemic OVA sensitization and airway challenge.[176] Moreover, transgenic mice that overexpressed TSLP exclusively in the lungs (under the control of the human surfactant protein C (SPC) promoter) demonstrated a dramatic increase in the number of BAL eosinophils present, an increased frequency of IL-4, IL-5, and IL-13 expressing T cells, elevated serum IgE levels, and evidence of airway remodeling, all in the absence of allergen exposure.[176]

Another way epithelial cells have been demonstrated to contribute to disease pathology is through the production of pro-asthmatic factors in response to triggers of asthma. For example, epithelial cells are a source of TGF-β1 and can thus contribute to the airway remodeling seen in chronic asthmatics.[177] Epithelial cells are also a source of chemokines and cytokines and thus have the potential to recruit and activate both dendritic cells and inflammatory cells, thereby both initiating and perpetuating the development of the asthmatic response.[178] Indeed, epithelial cells from asthmatic individuals were found to express higher levels of the eosinophil-attracting chemokines CCL5, CCL11, and CCL15[179,180] and the DC-attracting chemokine CCL20 in response to allergen, cytokines or particulate matter.[181–183] Interestingly, there is also evidence that the epithelial cell plays a central role in the ability of IL-13 to induce both AHR and mucus hypersecretion as selective knockout of STAT6 in pulmonary epithelial cells results in a complete abrogation of these parameters in a murine model of asthma.[103] All of these studies suggest that the epithelium from asthmatic individuals may be fundamentally different from that found in healthy individuals. There is some evidence for this in humans as well, as asthmatic epithelium is more susceptible to apoptosis,[184,185] demonstrates greater fragility,[186] and has significantly increased expression of pro-inflammatory transcription factors.[187,188] Such changes can also be found in the epithelial cells of asthmatic children,[189,190] suggesting a potentially causative link between epithelial cell properties and development of asthma and suggesting that differences in epithelial cell response to injury or stimulation may play an important role in promoting tolerance or development of allergic asthma. Due to the important role that the epithelium plays in allergen recognition, initiation of inflammation, and in mediating responses to inflammatory mediators, delineation of the processes occurring at the epithelial interface with the environment is critical to the development of therapeutics aimed at modifying the course of disease.

CONCLUSION

In conclusion, because of the inherently greater experimental flexibility available in animal models, they offer uniquely attractive ways to identify basic pathogenic mechanisms and to validate novel therapeutic targets for the treatment of allergic asthma. Consequently, much of our current knowledge about the mechanisms involved in the development of

(Th2 cells/cytokines, iNTK cells, mDCs, airway epithelial cells) or the tolerance to (Tregs, pDCs) allergic inflammation has been generated in animal models. However, it is important to remember that while allergen exposure in mice replicates many features of human asthma, no animal model is a perfect representation of human disease. As such, it is important that those pathways identified as critical for the induction of allergic asthma in animal studies are demonstrated to be similarly associated with disease in human populations. Thus, just as the recent identification of TIM-1, C3, arginase I as asthma susceptible genes in diverse human populations was driven by initial genetic screening of phenotypically divergent murine strains, the insights gained from the genomic era will undoubtedly continue to be useful in the identification of novel mediators and pathways critical for the development of allergic asthma.[191,192]

References

Characteristics of animal models of allergic asthma

1. Moise NS, Wiedenkeller D, Yeager AE, et al. Clinical, radiographic, and bronchial cytologic features of cats with bronchial disease: 65 cases (1980–1986). J Am Vet Med Assoc 1989; 194:1467–1473.
2. Armstrong PJ, Derksen FJ, Slocombe RF, et al. Airway responses to aerosolized methacholine and citric acid in ponies with recurrent airway obstruction (heaves). Am Rev Respir Dis 1986; 133:357–361.
3. Levitt RC, Ewart SL. Genetic susceptibility to atracurium-induced bronchoconstriction. Am J Respir Crit Care Med 1995; 151:1537–1542.
4. Levitt RC, Mitzner W. Expression of airway hyperreactivity to acetylcholine as a simple autosomal recessive trait in mice. FASEB J 1988; 2:2605–2608.
5. Pauwels R, Van Der Straeten M, Weyne J, et al. Genetic factors in non-specific bronchial reactivity in rats. Eur J Respir Dis 1985; 66:98–104.
6. Eidelman DH, DiMaria GU, Bellofiore S, et al. Strain-related differences in airway smooth muscle and airway responsiveness in the rat. Am Rev Respir Dis 1991; 144:792–796.
7. Hirshman CA, Malley A, Downes H. Basenji–Greyhound dog model of asthma: reactivity to Ascaris suum, citric acid, and methacholine. J Appl Physiol 1980; 49:953–957.
8. Ewart SL, Kuperman D, Schadt E, et al. Quantitative trait loci controlling allergen-induced airway hyperresponsiveness in inbred mice. Am J Respir Cell Mol Biol 2000; 23:537–545.
9. McIntire JJ, Umetsu SE, Akbari O, et al. Identification of Tapr (an airway hyperreactivity regulatory locus) and the linked Tim gene family. Nat Immunol 2001; 2:1109–1116.
10. Eisenbarth SC, Piggott DA, Huleatt JW, et al. Lipopolysaccharide-enhanced, toll-like receptor 4-dependent T helper cell type 2 responses to inhaled antigen. J Exp Med 2002; 196:1645–1651.
11. de Heer HJ, Hammad H, Soullie T, et al. Essential role of lung plasmacytoid dendritic cells in preventing asthmatic reactions to harmless inhaled antigen. J Exp Med 2004; 200:89–98.
12. Barrett EG, Rudolph K, Bowen LF, et al. Effect of inhaled ultrafine carbon particles on the allergic airway response in ragweed-sensitized dogs. Inhal Toxicol 2003; 15:151–165.
13. Chapoval SP, Iijima K, Marietta EV, et al. Allergic inflammatory response to short ragweed allergenic extract in HLA-DQ transgenic mice lacking CD4 gene. J Immunol 2002; 168:890–899.
14. Kheradmand F, Kiss A, Xu J, et al. A protease-activated pathway underlying Th cell type 2 activation and allergic lung disease. J Immunol 2002; 169:5904–5911.
15. Santeliz JV, Van Nest G, Traquina P, et al. Amb a 1-linked CpG oligodeoxynucleotides reverse established airway hyperresponsiveness in a murine model of asthma. J Allergy Clin Immunol 2002; 109:455–462.
16. Johnson JR, Wiley RE, Fattouh R, et al. Continuous exposure to house dust mite elicits chronic airway inflammation and structural remodeling. Am J Respir Crit Care Med 2004; 169:378–385.
17. Obiefuna PC, Batra VK, Nadeem A, et al. A novel A1 adenosine receptor antagonist, L-97–1 [3-[2-(4-aminophenyl)-ethyl]-8-benzyl-7-{2-ethyl-(2-hydroxy-ethyl)-amino]- ethyl}-1-propyl-3,7-dihydro-purine-2,6-dione], reduces allergic responses to house dust mite in an allergic rabbit model of asthma. J Pharmacol Exp Ther 2005; 315:329–336.
18. Lewkowich IP, Herman NS, Schleifer KW, et al. CD4+CD25+ T cells protect against experimentally induced asthma and alter pulmonary dendritic cell phenotype and function. J Exp Med 2005; 202:1549–1561.
19. Baelder R, Fuchs B, Bautsch W, et al. Pharmacological targeting of anaphylatoxin receptors during the effector phase of allergic asthma suppresses airway hyperresponsiveness and airway inflammation. J Immunol 2005; 174:783–789.
20. Bryce PJ, Geha R, Oettgen HC. Desloratadine inhibits allergen-induced airway inflammation and bronchial hyperresponsiveness and alters T cell responses in murine models of asthma. J Allergy Clin Immunol 2003; 112:149–158.
21. Kurup VP, Choi H, Murali PS, et al. Role of particulate antigens of Aspergillus in murine eosinophilia. Int Arch Allergy Immunol 1997; 112:270–278.
22. Williams CM, Galli SJ. Mast cells can amplify airway reactivity and features of chronic inflammation in an asthma model in mice. J Exp Med 2000; 192:455–462.
23. Meyts I, Hellings PW, Hens G, et al. IL-12 contributes to allergen-induced airway inflammation in experimental asthma. J Immunol 2006; 177:6460–6470.

24. Jaradat M, Stapleton C, Tilley SL, et al. Modulatory role for retinoid-related orphan receptor α in allergen-induced lung inflammation. Am J Respir Crit Care Med 2006; 174:1299–1309.

25. Akbari O, Stock P, Meyer E, et al. Essential role of NKT cells producing IL-4 and IL-13 in the development of allergen-induced airway hyperreactivity. Nat Med 2003; 9:582–588.

26. Thomas WR, Hales BJ, Smith WA. Structural biology of allergens. Curr Allergy Asthma Rep 2005; 5:388–393.

27. Hansen G, Berry G, DeKruyff RH, et al. Allergen-specific Th1 cells fail to counterbalance Th2 cell-induced airway hyperreactivity but cause severe airway inflammation. J Clin Invest 1999; 103:175–183.

28. Lambrecht BN, De Veerman M, Coyle AJ, et al. Myeloid dendritic cells induce Th2 responses to inhaled antigen, leading to eosinophilic airway inflammation. J Clin Invest 2000; 106:551–559.

29. Hammad H, de Vries VC, Maldonado-Lopez R, et al. Differential capacity of CD8+ α or CD8– α dendritic cell subsets to prime for eosinophilic airway inflammation in the T-helper type 2-prone milieu of the lung. Clin Exp Allergy 2004; 34:1834–1840.

30. Gordon JR, Li F, Nayyar A, et al. CD8α+, but not CD8α–, dendritic cells tolerize Th2 responses via contact-dependent and -independent mechanisms, and reverse airway hyperresponsiveness, Th2, and eosinophil responses in a mouse model of asthma. J Immunol 2005; 175:1516–1522.

31. Kuipers H, Heirman C, Hijdra D, et al. Dendritic cells retrovirally overexpressing IL-12 induce strong Th1 responses to inhaled antigen in the lung but fail to revert established Th2 sensitization. J Leukoc Biol 2004; 76:1028–1038.

32. de Heer HJ, Hammad H, Kool M, et al. Dendritic cell subsets and immune regulation in the lung. Semin Immunol 2005; 17:295–303.

33. Cho JY, Miller M, McElwain K, et al. Remodeling associated expression of matrix metalloproteinase 9 but not tissue inhibitor of metalloproteinase 1 in airway epithelium: modulation by immunostimulatory DNA. J Allergy Clin Immunol 2006; 117:618–625.

34. Kim CH, Ahn JH, Kim SJ, et al. Co-administration of vaccination with DNA encoding T cell epitope on the Der p and BCG inhibited airway remodeling in a murine model of chronic asthma. J Asthma 2006; 43:345–353.

35. Zhu Z, Homer RJ, Wang Z, et al. Pulmonary expression of interleukin-13 causes inflammation, mucus hypersecretion, subepithelial fibrosis, physiologic abnormalities, and eotaxin production. J Clin Invest 1999; 103:779–788.

36. Rankin JA, Picarella DE, Geba GP, et al. Phenotypic and physiologic characterization of transgenic mice expressing interleukin 4 in the lung: lymphocytic and eosinophilic inflammation without airway remodeling. Proc Natl Acad Sci U S A 1996; 93:7821–7825.

37. Lee JJ, McGarry MP, Farmer SC, et al. Interleukin-5 expression in the lung epithelium of transgenic mice leads to pulmonary changes pathognomonic of asthma. J Exp Med 1997; 185:2143–2156.

38. Wills-Karp M, Luyimbazi J, Xu X, et al. Interleukin-13: central mediator of allergic asthma. Science 1998; 282:2258–2261.

Characteristics and assessment of the allergic asthma phenotype

39. Collins RA, Gualano RC, Zosky GR, et al. Hyperresponsiveness to inhaled but not intravenous methacholine during acute respiratory syncytial virus infection in mice. Respir Res 2005; 6:142.

40. Hamelmann E, Schwarze J, Takeda K, et al. Noninvasive measurement of airway responsiveness in allergic mice using barometric plethysmography. Am J Respir Crit Care Med 1997; 156: 766–775.

41. MacLean JA, Sauty A, Luster AD, et al. Antigen-induced airway hyperresponsiveness, pulmonary eosinophilia, and chemokine expression in B cell-deficient mice. Am J Respir Cell Mol Biol 1999; 20:379–387.

42. Korsgren M, Erjefalt JS, Korsgren O, et al. Allergic eosinophil-rich inflammation develops in lungs and airways of B cell-deficient mice. J Exp Med 1997; 185:885–892.

43. Oettgen HC, Martin TR, Wynshaw-Boris A, et al. Active anaphylaxis in IgE-deficient mice. Nature 1994; 370:367–370.

44. Mehlhop PD, van de Rijn M, Goldberg AB, et al. Allergen-induced bronchial hyperreactivity and eosinophilic inflammation occur in the absence of IgE in a mouse model of asthma. Proc Natl Acad Sci U S A 1997; 94:1344–1349.

45. Cohn L, Tepper JS, Bottomly K. IL-4-independent induction of airway hyperresponsiveness by Th2, but not Th1, cells. J Immunol 1998; 161:3813–3816.

46. Lack G, Oshiba A, Bradley KL, et al. Transfer of immediate hypersensitivity and airway hyperresponsiveness by IgE-positive B cells. Am J Respir Crit Care Med 1995; 152:1765–1773.

47. van der Heijden FL, Joost van Neerven RJ, van Katwijk M, et al. Serum-IgE-facilitated allergen presentation in atopic disease. J Immunol 1993; 150:3643–3650.

48. Matsuda K, Piliponsky AM, Iikura M, et al. Monomeric IgE enhances human mast cell chemokine production: IL-4 augments and dexamethasone suppresses the response. J Allergy Clin Immunol 2005; 116:1357–1363.

49. Kawakami T, Galli SJ. Regulation of mast cell and basophil function and survival by IgE. Nat Rev Immunol 2002; 2:773–786.

50. Kobayashi T, Miura T, Haba T, et al. An essential role of mast cells in the development of airway hyperresponsiveness in a murine asthma model. J Immunol 2000; 164:3855–3861.

51. Mayr SI, Zuberi RI, Zhang M, et al. IgE-dependent mast cell activation potentiates airway responses in murine asthma models. J Immunol 2002; 169:2061–2068.

52. Finkelman FD, Morris SC. Development of an assay to measure in vivo cytokine production in the mouse. Int Immunol 1999; 11:1811–1818.

53. Carroll NG, Mutavdzic S, James AL. Increased mast cells and neutrophils in submucosal mucous glands and mucus plugging in patients with asthma. Thorax 2002; 57:677–682.

54. Borthwick DW, West JD, Keighren MA, et al. Murine submucosal glands are clonally derived and show a cystic fibrosis gene-dependent distribution pattern. Am J Respir Cell Mol Biol 1999; 20:1181–1189.

55. Chorley BN, Crews AL, Li Y, et al. Differential Muc2 and Muc5ac secretion by stimulated guinea pig tracheal epithelial cells in vitro. Respir Res 2006; 7:35.

Examining the kinetics of the asthmatic response

56. Elias JA, Zheng T, Lee CG, et al. Transgenic modeling of interleukin-13 in the lung. Chest 2003; 123:339S–345S.

57. Lee CG, Link H, Baluk P, et al. Vascular endothelial growth factor (VEGF) induces remodeling and enhances TH2-mediated sensitization and inflammation in the lung. Nat Med 2004; 10:1095–1103.

58. Köhl J, Baelder R, Lewkowich IP, et al. A regulatory role for the C5a anaphylatoxin in type 2 immunity in asthma. J Clin Invest 2006; 116:783–796.

Using animal models to identify novel asthma susceptibility genes

59. De Sanctis GT, Merchant M, Beier DR, et al. Quantitative locus analysis of airway hyperresponsiveness in A/J and C57BL/6J mice. Nat Genet 1995; 11:150–154.

60. De Sanctis GT, Singer JB, Jiao A, et al. Quantitative trait locus mapping of airway responsiveness to chromosomes 6 and 7 in inbred mice. Am J Physiol 1999; 277:L1118–L1123.

61. Ewart SL, Mitzner W, DiSilvestre DA, et al. Airway hyperresponsiveness to acetylcholine: segregation analysis and evidence for linkage to murine chromosome 6. Am J Respir Cell Mol Biol 1996; 14:487–495.

62. Zhang Y, Lefort J, Kearsey V, et al. A genome-wide screen for asthma-associated quantitative trait loci in a mouse model of allergic asthma. Hum Mol Genet 1999; 8:601–605.

63. Karp CL, Grupe A, Schadt E, et al. Identification of complement factor 5 as a susceptibility locus for experimental allergic asthma. Nat Immunol 2000; 1:221–226.

64. Keane-Myers A, Wysocka M, Trinchieri G, et al. Resistance to antigen-induced airway hyperresponsiveness requires endogenous production of IL-12. J Immunol 1998; 161: 919–926.

65. Krug N, Tschernig T, Erpenbeck VJ, et al. Complement factors C3a and C5a are increased in bronchoalveolar lavage fluid after segmental allergen provocation in subjects with asthma. Am J Respir Crit Care Med 2001; 164:1841–1843.

66. Ober C, Cox NJ, Abney M, et al. Genome-wide search for asthma susceptibility loci in a founder population. The Collaborative Study on the Genetics of Asthma. Hum Mol Genet 1998; 7:1393–1398.

67. Wjst M, Fischer G, Immervoll T, et al. A genome-wide search for linkage to asthma. German Asthma Genetics Group. Genomics 1999; 58:1–8.

68. A genome-wide search for asthma susceptibility loci in ethnically diverse populations. The Collaborative Study on the Genetics of Asthma (CSGA). Nat Genet 1997; 15:389–392.

69. Bourgain C, Hoffjan S, Nicolae R, et al. Novel case-control test in a founder population identifies P-selectin as an atopy-susceptibility locus. Am J Hum Genet 2003; 73:612–626.

70. Hasegawa K, Tamari M, Shao C, et al. Variations in the C3, C3a receptor, and C5 genes affect susceptibility to bronchial asthma. Hum Genet 2004; 115:295–301.

71. Chae SC, Park YR, Lee YC, et al. The association of TIM-3 gene polymorphism with atopic disease in Korean population. Hum Immunol 2004; 65:1427–1431.

72. Gao PS, Mathias RA, Plunkett B, et al. Genetic variants of the T cell immunoglobulin mucin 1 but not the T cell immunoglobulin mucin 3 gene are associated with asthma in an African American population. J Allergy Clin Immunol 2005; 115:982–988.

73. Graves PE, Siroux V, Guerra S, et al. Association of atopy and eczema with polymorphisms in T cell immunoglobulin domain and mucin domain-IL-2-inducible T cell kinase gene cluster in chromosome 5 q 33. J Allergy Clin Immunol 2005; 116:650–656.

74. McIntire JJ, Umetsu SE, Macaubas C, et al. Immunology: hepatitis A virus link to atopic disease. Nature 2003; 425:576.

75. Follettie MT, Ellis DK, Donaldson DD, et al. Gene expression analysis in a murine model of allergic asthma reveals overlapping disease and therapy dependent pathways in the lung. Pharmacogen J 2006; 6:141–152.

76. Kuperman DA, Lewis CC, Woodruff PG, et al. Dissecting asthma using focused transgenic modeling and functional genomics. J Allergy Clin Immunol 2005; 116:305–311.

77. Zimmermann N, King NE, Laporte J, et al. Dissection of experimental asthma with DNA microarray analysis identifies arginase in asthma pathogenesis. J Clin Invest 2003; 111: 1863–1874.

78. Zhou Y, Dong Q, Louahed J, et al. Characterization of a calcium-activated chloride channel as a shared target of Th2 cytokine pathways and its potential involvement in asthma. Am J Respir Cell Mol Biol 2001; 25:486–491.

79. Stutz AM, Pickart LA, Trifilieff A, et al. The Th2 cell cytokines IL-4 and IL-13 regulate found in inflammatory zone 1/resistin-like molecule alpha gene expression by a STAT6 and CCAAT/enhancer-binding protein-dependent mechanism. J Immunol 2003; 170: 1789–1796.

80. Nikolaidis NM, Zimmermann N, King NE, et al. Trefoil factor-2 is an allergen-induced gene regulated by Th2 cytokines and STAT6 in the lung. Am J Respir Cell Mol Biol 2003; 29:458–464.

81. Zimmermann N, Doepker MP, Witte DP, et al. Expression and regulation of small proline-rich protein 2 in allergic inflammation. Am J Respir Cell Mol Biol 2005; 32:428–435.

82. Zhu Z, Zheng T, Homer RJ, et al. Acidic mammalian chitinase in asthmatic Th2 inflammation and IL-13 pathway activation. Science 2004; 304:1678–1682.

83. Zimmermann N, Mishra A, King NE, et al. Transcript signatures in experimental asthma: identification of STAT6-dependent and -independent pathways. J Immunol 2004; 172: 1815–1824.

84. Meurs H, McKay S, Maarsingh H, et al. Increased arginase activity underlies allergen-induced deficiency of cNOS-derived nitric oxide and airway hyperresponsiveness. Br J Pharmacol 2002; 136:391–398.

85. Yang M, Rangasamy D, Matthaei KI, et al. Inhibition of arginase I activity by RNA interference attenuates IL-13-induced airways hyperresponsiveness. J Immunol 2006; 177:5595–5603.

86. Maarsingh H, Leusink J, Bos IS, et al. Arginase strongly impairs neuronal nitric oxide-mediated airway smooth muscle relaxation in allergic asthma. Respir Res 2006; 7:6.

87. Morris CR, Poljakovic M, Lavrisha L, et al. Decreased arginine bioavailability and increased serum arginase activity in asthma. Am J Respir Crit Care Med 2004; 170:148–153.

88. Li H, Romieu I, Sienra-Monge JJ, et al. Genetic polymorphisms in arginase I and II and childhood asthma and atopy. J Allergy Clin Immunol 2006; 117:119–126.

T-cell mediators of allergic asthma

89. Corry DB, Grunig G, Hadeiba H, et al. Requirements for allergen-induced airway hyperreactivity in T and B cell-deficient mice. Mol Med 1998; 4:344–355.

90. Gavett SH, Chen X, Finkelman F, et al. Depletion of murine CD4+ T lymphocytes prevents antigen-induced airway hyperreactivity and pulmonary eosinophilia. Am J Respir Cell Mol Biol 1994; 10:587–593.

91. Watanabe A, Mishima H, Renzi PM, et al. Transfer of allergic airway responses with antigen-primed CD4+ but not CD8+ T cells in brown Norway rats. J Clin Invest 1995; 96:1303–1310.

92. Larsen GL, Renz H, Loader JE, et al. Airway response to electrical field stimulation in sensitized inbred mice. Passive transfer of increased responsiveness with peribronchial lymph nodes. J Clin Invest 1992; 89:747–752.

93. Cohn L, Homer RJ, Marinov A, et al. Induction of airway mucus production by T helper 2 (Th2) cells: a critical role for interleukin 4 in cell recruitment but not mucus production. J Exp Med 1997; 186:1737–1747.

94. Brusselle G, Kips J, Joos G, et al. Allergen-induced airway inflammation and bronchial responsiveness in wild-type and interleukin-4-deficient mice. Am J Respir Cell Mol Biol 1995; 12:254–259.

95. Rothenberg ME, Hogan SP. The eosinophil. Ann Rev Immunol 2006; 24:147–174.

96. Hultner L, Druez C, Moeller J, et al. Mast cell growth-enhancing activity (MEA) is structurally related and functionally identical to the novel mouse T cell growth factor P40/TCGFIII (interleukin 9). Eur J Immunol 1990; 20:1413–1416.

97. Corry DB, Folkesson HG, Warnock ML, et al. Interleukin 4, but not interleukin 5 or eosinophils, is required in a murine model of acute airway hyperreactivity. J Exp Med 1996; 183:109–117.

98. Coyle AJ, Le Gros G, Bertrand C, et al. Interleukin-4 is required for the induction of lung Th2 mucosal immunity. Am J Respir Cell Mol Biol 1995; 13:54–59.

99. Grunig G, Warnock M, Wakil AE, et al. Requirement for IL-13 independently of IL-4 in experimental asthma. Science 1998; 282:2261–2263.

100. Walter DM, McIntire JJ, Berry G, et al. Critical role for IL-13 in the development of allergen-induced airway hyperreactivity. J Immunol 2001; 167:4668–4675.

101. Venkayya R, Lam M, Willkom M, et al. The Th2 lymphocyte products IL-4 and IL-13 rapidly induce airway hyperresponsiveness through direct effects on resident airway cells. Am J Respir Cell Mol Biol 2002; 26:202–208.

102. Yang M, Hogan SP, Henry PJ, et al. Interleukin-13 mediates airways hyperreactivity through the IL-4 receptor-alpha chain and STAT-6 independently of IL-5 and eotaxin. Am J Respir Cell Mol Biol 2001; 25:522–530.

103. Kuperman DA, Huang X, Koth LL, et al. Direct effects of interleukin-13 on epithelial cells cause airway hyperreactivity and mucus overproduction in asthma. Nat Med 2002; 8:885–889.

104. Celedon JC, Soto-Quiros ME, Palmer LJ, et al. Lack of association between a polymorphism in the interleukin-13 gene and total serum immunoglobulin E level among nuclear families in Costa Rica. Clin Exp Allergy 2002; 32:387–390.

105. Graves PE, Kabesch M, Halonen M, et al. A cluster of seven tightly linked polymorphisms in the IL-13 gene is associated with total serum IgE levels in three populations of white children. J Allergy Clin Immunol 2000; 105:506–513.

106. Heinzmann A, Mao XQ, Akaiwa M, et al. Genetic variants of IL-13 signalling and human asthma and atopy. Hum Mol Genet 2000; 9:549–559.

107. van der Pouw Kraan TC, van Veen A, Boeije LC, et al. An IL-13 promoter polymorphism associated with increased risk of allergic asthma. Genes Immun 1999; 1:61–65.

108. Battle NC, Choudhry S, Tsai HJ, et al. Ethnicity-specific gene-gene interaction between IL-13 and IL-4Rα among African Americans with asthma. Am J Respir Crit Care Med 2007; 175:881–887.

109. Howard TD, Koppelman GH, Xu J, et al. Gene-gene interaction in asthma: IL4RA and IL13 in a Dutch population with asthma. Am J Hum Genet 2002; 70:230–236.

110. Howard TD, Whittaker PA, Zaiman AL, et al. Identification and association of polymorphisms in the interleukin-13 gene with asthma and atopy in a Dutch population. Am J Respir Cell Mol Biol 2001; 25:377–384.

111. Risma KA, Wang N, Andrews RP, et al. V75R576 IL-4 receptor alpha is associated with allergic asthma and enhanced IL-4 receptor function. J Immunol 2002; 169:1604–1610.

112. Foster PS, Hogan SP, Ramsay AJ, et al. Interleukin 5 deficiency abolishes eosinophilia, airways hyperreactivity, and lung damage in a mouse asthma model. J Exp Med 1996; 183:195–201.

113. Hamelmann E, Takeda K, Haczku A, et al. Interleukin (IL)-5 but not immunoglobulin E reconstitutes airway inflammation and airway hyperresponsiveness in IL-4-deficient mice. Am J Respir Cell Mol Biol 2000; 23:327–334.

114. Shardonofsky FR, Venzor J 3rd, Barrios R, et al. Therapeutic efficacy of an anti-IL-5 monoclonal antibody delivered into the respiratory tract in a murine model of asthma. J Allergy Clin Immunol 1999; 104:215–221.

115. Van Oosterhout AJ, Ladenius AR, Savelkoul HF, et al. Effect of anti-IL-5 and IL-5 on airway hyperreactivity and eosinophils in guinea pigs. Am Rev Respir Dis 1993; 147:548–552.

116. Yamaguchi S, Nagai H, Tanaka H, et al. Time course study for antigen-induced airway hyperreactivity and the effect of soluble IL-5 receptor. Life Sci 1994; 54:PL471–PL475.

117. Mauser PJ, Pitman A, Witt A, et al. Inhibitory effect of the TRFK-5 anti-IL-5 antibody in a guinea pig model of asthma. Am Rev Respir Dis 1993; 148:1623–1627.

118. Mauser PJ, Pitman AM, Fernandez X, et al. Effects of an antibody to interleukin-5 in a monkey model of asthma. Am J Respir Crit Care Med 1995; 152:467–472.

119. Flood-Page PT, Menzies-Gow AN, Kay AB, et al. Eosinophil's role remains uncertain as anti-interleukin-5 only partially depletes numbers in asthmatic airway. Am J Respir Crit Care Med 2003; 167:199–204.

120. Leckie MJ, ten Brinke A, Khan J, et al. Effects of an interleukin-5 blocking monoclonal antibody on eosinophils, airway hyper-responsiveness, and the late asthmatic response. Lancet 2000; 356:2144–2148.

121. Menzies-Gow A, Flood-Page P, Sehmi R, et al. Anti-IL-5 (mepolizumab) therapy induces bone marrow eosinophil maturational arrest and decreases eosinophil progenitors in the bronchial mucosa of atopic asthmatics. J Allergy Clin Immunol 2003; 111:714–719.

122. Flood-Page P, Menzies-Gow A, Phipps S, et al. Anti-IL-5 treatment reduces deposition of ECM proteins in the bronchial subepithelial basement membrane of mild atopic asthmatics. J Clin Invest 2003; 112:1029–1036.

123. Humbles AA, Lloyd CM, McMillan SJ, et al. A critical role for eosinophils in allergic airways remodeling. Science 2004; 305:1776–1779.

124. Lee JJ, Dimina D, Macias MP, et al. Defining a link with asthma in mice congenitally deficient in eosinophils. Science 2004; 305:1773–1776.

125. Bilenki L, Yang J, Fan Y, et al. Natural killer T cells contribute to airway eosinophilic inflammation induced by ragweed through enhanced IL-4 and eotaxin production. Eur J Immunol 2004; 34:345–354.

126. Kim JO, Kim DH, Chang WS, et al. Asthma is induced by intranasal coadministration of allergen and natural killer T cell ligand in a mouse model. J Allergy Clin Immunol 2004; 114:1332–1338.

127. Hachem P, Lisbonne M, Michel ML, et al. Alpha-galactosylceramide-induced iNKT cells suppress experimental allergic asthma in sensitized mice: role of IFN-gamma. Eur J Immunol 2005; 35:2793–2802.

128. Matsuda H, Suda T, Sato J, et al. Alpha-Galactosylceramide, a ligand of natural killer T cells, inhibits allergic airway inflammation. Am J Respir Cell Mol Biol 2005; 33:22–31.

129. Meyer EH, Goya S, Akbari O, et al. Glycolipid activation of invariant T cell receptor+ NK T cells is sufficient to induce airway hyperreactivity independent of conventional CD4+ T cells. Proc Natl Acad Sci U S A 2006; 103:2782–2787.

130. Zhou D, Mattner J, Cantu C 3rd, et al. Lysosomal glycosphingolipid recognition by NKT cells. Science 2004; 306:1786–1789.

131. Agea E, Russano A, Bistoni O, et al. Human CD1-restricted T cell recognition of lipids from pollens. J Exp Med 2005; 202:295–308.

132. Fischer K, Scotet E, Niemeyer M, et al. Mycobacterial phosphatidylinositol mannoside is a natural antigen for CD1d-restricted T cells. Proc Natl Acad Sci U S A 2004; 101:10685–10690.

133. Akbari O, Faul JL, Hoyte EG, et al. CD4+ invariant T cell-receptor+ natural killer T cells in bronchial asthma. N Engl J Med 2006; 354:1117–1129.

134. Sen Y, Yongyi B, Yuling H, et al. Vα24-invariant NKT cells from patients with allergic asthma express CCR9 at high frequency and induce Th2 bias of CD3+ T cells upon CD226 engagement. J Immunol 2005; 175:4914–4926.

135. Vijayanand P, Seumois G, Pickard C, et al. Invariant natural killer T cells in asthma and chronic obstructive pulmonary disease. N Engl J Med 2007; 356:1410–1422.

136. Piccirillo CA, Shevach EM. Naturally-occurring CD4+CD25+ immunoregulatory T cells: central players in the arena of peripheral tolerance. Semin Immunol 2004; 16:81–88.

137. Coombes JL, Robinson NJ, Maloy KJ, et al. Regulatory T cells and intestinal homeostasis. Immunol Rev 2005; 204:184–194.

138. Sakaguchi S. Naturally arising Foxp3-expressing CD25+CD4+ regulatory T cells in immunological tolerance to self and non-self. Nat Immunol 2005; 6:345–352.

139. Fontenot JD, Rasmussen JP, Williams LM, et al. Regulatory T cell lineage specification by the forkhead transcription factor foxp3. Immunity 2005; 22:329–341.

140. Watanabe N, Wang YH, Lee HK, et al. Hassall's corpuscles instruct dendritic cells to induce CD4+CD25+ regulatory T cells in human thymus. Nature 2005; 436:1181–1185.

141. Fontenot JD, Gavin MA, Rudensky AY. Foxp3 programs the development and function of CD4+CD25+ regulatory T cells. Nat Immunol 2003; 4:330–336.

142. Jaffar Z, Sivakuru T, Roberts K. CD4+CD25+ T cells regulate airway eosinophilic inflammation by modulating the Th2 cell phenotype. J Immunol 2004; 172:3842–3849.

143. Kearley J, Barker JE, Robinson DS, et al. Resolution of airway inflammation and hyperreactivity after in vivo transfer of CD4+CD25+ regulatory T cells is interleukin 10 dependent. J Exp Med 2005; 202:1539–1547.

144. Hadeiba H, Locksley RM. Lung CD25 CD4 regulatory T cells suppress type 2 immune responses but not bronchial hyperreactivity. J Immunol 2003; 170:5502–5510.

145. Hansen G, Yeung VP, Berry G, et al. Vaccination with heat-killed Listeria as adjuvant reverses established allergen-induced airway hyperreactivity and inflammation: role of CD8+ T cells and IL-18. J Immunol 2000; 164:223–230.

146. Zuany-Amorim C, Sawicka E, Manlius C, et al. Suppression of airway eosinophilia by killed Mycobacterium vaccae-induced allergen-specific regulatory T cells. Nat Med 2002; 8:625–629.

147. Wilson MS, Taylor MD, Balic A, et al. Suppression of allergic airway inflammation by helminth-induced regulatory T cells. J Exp Med 2005; 202:1199–1212.

148. Yang J, Zhao J, Yang Y, et al. Schistosoma japonicum egg antigens stimulate CD4 CD25 T cells and modulate airway inflammation in a murine model of asthma. Immunology 2007; 120:8–18.

149. Mucida D, Kutchukhidze N, Erazo A, et al. Oral tolerance in the absence of naturally occurring Tregs. J Clin Invest 2005; 115:1923–1933.

150. Ostroukhova M, Seguin-Devaux C, Oriss TB, et al. Tolerance induced by inhaled antigen involves CD4(+) T cells expressing membrane-bound TGF-beta and FOXP3. J Clin Invest 2004; 114:28–38.

151. Jutel M, Akdis M, Blaser K, et al. Mechanisms of allergen specific immunotherapy – T cell tolerance and more. Allergy 2006; 61:796–807.

Innate immune responses in asthma

152. Holt PG. Pulmonary dendritic cells in local immunity to inert and pathogenic antigens in the respiratory tract. Proc Am Thorac Soc 2005; 2:116–120.

153. Lambrecht BN, Salomon B, Klatzmann D, et al. Dendritic cells are required for the development of chronic eosinophilic airway inflammation in response to inhaled antigen in sensitized mice. J Immunol 1998; 160:4090–4097.

154. Huh JC, Strickland DH, Jahnsen FL, et al. Bidirectional interactions between antigen-bearing respiratory tract dendritic cells (DCs) and T cells precede the late phase reaction in experimental asthma: DC activation occurs in the airway mucosa but not in the lung parenchyma. J Exp Med 2003; 198:19–30.

155. Vermaelen KY, Carro-Muino I, Lambrecht BN, et al. Specific migratory dendritic cells rapidly transport antigen from the airways to the thoracic lymph nodes. J Exp Med 2001; 193:51–60.

156. Lambrecht BN, Pauwels RA, Fazekas De St Groth B. Induction of rapid T cell activation, division, and recirculation by intratracheal injection of dendritic cells in a TCR transgenic model. J Immunol 2000; 164:2937–2946.

157. Sung S, Rose CE, Fu SM. Intratracheal priming with ovalbumin- and ovalbumin 323–339 peptide-pulsed dendritic cells induces airway hyperresponsiveness, lung eosinophilia, goblet cell hyperplasia, and inflammation. J Immunol 2001; 166:1261–1271.

158. Graffi SJ, Dekan G, Stingl G, et al. Systemic administration of antigen-pulsed dendritic cells induces experimental allergic asthma in mice upon aerosol antigen rechallenge. Clin Immunol 2002; 103:176–184.

159. van Rijt LS, Jung S, Kleinjan A, et al. In vivo depletion of lung CD11c+ dendritic cells during allergen challenge abrogates the characteristic features of asthma. J Exp Med 2005; 201:981–991.

160. Bellini A, Vittori E, Marini M, et al. Intraepithelial dendritic cells and selective activation of Th2-like lymphocytes in patients with atopic asthma. Chest 1993; 103:997–1005.

161. Moller GM, Overbeek SE, Van Helden-Meeuwsen CG, et al. Increased numbers of dendritic cells in the bronchial mucosa of atopic asthmatic patients: downregulation by inhaled corticosteroids. Clin Exp Allergy 1996; 26:517–524.

162. Deurloo DT, van Berkel MA, van Esch BC, et al. CD28/CTLA4 double deficient mice demonstrate crucial role for B7 co-stimulation in the induction of allergic lower airways disease. Clin Exp Allergy 2003; 33:1297–1304.

163. Hoshino A, Tanaka Y, Akiba H, et al. Critical role for OX40 ligand in the development of pathogenic Th2 cells in a murine model of asthma. Eur J Immunol 2003; 33:861–869.

164. Keane-Myers AM, Gause WC, Finkelman FD, et al. Development of murine allergic asthma is dependent upon B7–2 costimulation. J Immunol 1998; 160:1036–1043.

165. Akbari O, Freeman GJ, Meyer EH, et al. Antigen-specific regulatory T cells develop via the ICOS-ICOS-ligand pathway and inhibit allergen-induced airway hyperreactivity. Nat Med 2002; 8:1024–1032.

166. Dong H, Zhu G, Tamada K, et al. B7-H1, a third member of the B7 family, co-stimulates T cell proliferation and interleukin-10 secretion. Nat Med 1999; 5:1365–1369.

167. Tseng SY, Otsuji M, Gorski K, et al. B7-DC, a new dendritic cell molecule with potent costimulatory properties for T cells. J Exp Med 2001; 193:839–846.

168. Wang S, Bajorath J, Flies DB, et al. Molecular modeling and functional mapping of B7-H1 and B7-DC uncouple costimulatory function from PD-1 interaction. J Exp Med 2003; 197:1083–1091.

169. Freeman GJ, Long AJ, Iwai Y, et al. Engagement of the PD-1 immunoinhibitory receptor by a novel B7 family member leads to negative regulation of lymphocyte activation. J Exp Med 2000; 192:1027–1034.

170. Latchman Y, Wood CR, Chernova T, et al. PD-L2 is a second ligand for PD-1 and inhibits T cell activation. Nat Immunol 2001; 2:261–268.

171. Jahnsen FL, Lund-Johansen F, Dunne JF, et al. Experimentally induced recruitment of plasmacytoid (CD123high) dendritic cells in human nasal allergy. J Immunol 2000; 165:4062–4068.

172. Hagendorens MM, Ebo DG, Schuerwegh AJ, et al. Differences in circulating dendritic cell subtypes in cord blood and peripheral blood of healthy and allergic children. Clin Exp Allergy 2003; 33:633–639.

173. Oei E, Kalb T, Beuria P, et al. Accessory cell function of airway epithelial cells. Am J Physiol Lung Cell Mol Physiol 2004; 287:L318–L331.

174. Kim J, Myers AC, Chen L, et al. Constitutive and inducible expression of b7 family of ligands by human airway epithelial cells. Am J Respir Cell Mol Biol 2005; 33:280–289.

175. Allakhverdi Z, Comeau MR, Jessup HK, et al. Thymic stromal lymphopoietin is released by human epithelial cells in response to microbes, trauma, or inflammation and potently activates mast cells. J Exp Med 2007; 204:253–258.

176. Zhou B, Comeau MR, De Smedt T, et al. Thymic stromal lymphopoietin as a key initiator of allergic airway inflammation in mice. Nat Immunol 2005; 6:1047–1053.

177. Duvernelle C, Freund V, Frossard N. Transforming growth factor-beta and its role in asthma. Pulm Pharmacol Ther 2003; 16:181–196.

178. Laberge S, El Bassam S. Cytokines, structural cells of the lungs and airway inflammation. Paediatr Respir Rev 2004; 5:S41–S45.

179. Sousa AR, Poston RN, Lane SJ, et al. Detection of GM-CSF in asthmatic bronchial epithelium and decrease by inhaled corticosteroids. Am Rev Respir Dis 1993; 147:1557–1561.

180. Taha RA, Minshall EM, Miotto D, et al. Eotaxin and monocyte chemotactic protein-4 mRNA expression in small airways of asthmatic and nonasthmatic individuals. J Allergy Clin Immunol 1999; 103:476–483.

181. Pichavant M, Taront S, Jeannin P, et al. Impact of bronchial epithelium on dendritic cell migration and function: modulation by the bacterial motif KpOmpA. J Immunol 2006; 177:5912–5919.

182. Reibman J, Hsu Y, Chen LC, et al. Airway epithelial cells release MIP-3α/CCL20 in response to cytokines and ambient particulate matter. Am J Respir Cell Mol Biol 2003; 28:648–654.

183. Reibman J, Hsu Y, Chen LC, et al. Size fractions of ambient particulate matter induce granulocyte macrophage colony-stimulating factor in human bronchial epithelial cells by mitogen-activated protein kinase pathways. Am J Respir Cell Mol Biol 2002; 27:455–462.

184. Bayram H, Rusznak C, Khair OA, et al. Effect of ozone and nitrogen dioxide on the permeability of bronchial epithelial cell cultures of non-asthmatic and asthmatic subjects. Clin Exp Allergy 2002; 32:1285–1292.

185. Bucchieri F, Puddicombe SM, Lordan JL, et al. Asthmatic bronchial epithelium is more susceptible to oxidant-induced apoptosis. Am J Respir Cell Mol Biol 2002; 27:179–185.

186. Shahana S, Jaunmuktane Z, Asplund MS, et al. Ultrastructural investigation of epithelial damage in asthmatic and non-asthmatic nasal polyps. Respir Med 2006; 100:2018–2028.

187. Mullings RE, Wilson SJ, Puddicombe SM, et al. Signal transducer and activator of transcription 6 (STAT-6) expression and function in asthmatic bronchial epithelium. J Allergy Clin Immunol 2001; 108:832–838.

188. Sampath D, Castro M, Look DC, et al. Constitutive activation of an epithelial signal transducer and activator of transcription (STAT) pathway in asthma. J Clin Invest 1999; 103:1353–1361.

189. Fedorov IA, Wilson SJ, Davies DE, et al. Epithelial stress and structural remodelling in childhood asthma. Thorax 2005; 60:389–394.

190. Kicic A, Sutanto EN, Stevens PT, et al. Intrinsic biochemical and functional differences in bronchial epithelial cells of children with asthma. Am J Respir Crit Care Med 2006; 174:1110–1118.

Conclusion

191. Shapiro SD. Animal models of asthma: Pro: Allergic avoidance of animal (model[s]) is not an option. Am J Respir Crit Care Med 2006; 174:1171–1173.

192. Wenzel S, Holgate ST. The mouse trap: it still yields few answers in asthma. Am J Respir Crit Care Med 2006; 174:1173–1178.

REFERENCES

Pathophysiology of Allergic Inflammation

Peter J Barnes

29

CONTENTS

- Introduction 455
- Inflammatory cells 456
- Inflammatory mediators 459
- Effects of inflammation 462
- Transcription factors 466
- Antiinflammatory mechanisms in allergy 467
- Future directions 468

SUMMARY OF IMPORTANT CONCEPTS

>> Asthma and other allergic diseases involve a complex inflammatory process with many infiltrating cells (mast cells, eosinophils, T lymphocytes, neutrophils) and resident cells (epithelial cells, dendritic cells, macrophages, airway smooth muscle, fibroblasts, endothelial cells, and nerves)

>> All of these cells produce multiple inflammatory mediators, including lipid mediators that have rapid effects, chemokines which attract inflammatory cells and cytokines, which orchestrate the complex inflammation. It follows that blocking a single mediator is unlikely to give much benefit in this complex network if in generating mediators

>> Structural cells in the airway, particularly epithelial cells and airway smooth muscle cells, are probably the major source of inflammatory mediators in chronic disease and are an important target for antiinflammatory therapy

>> In asthma, contraction of airway smooth muscle is a major mechanism of airway narrowing, but in all inflammatory diseases inflammation results in plasma exudation, edema, sensory nerve activation (coughing, sneezing, itching) and mucus secretion (asthma and rhinitis). Chronic inflammation may lead to structural changes, such as subepithelial fibrosis in asthma, angiogenesis, mucus hyperplasia, and increased mass of airway smooth muscle

>> The chronic inflammation of allergic disease involves the activation of several transcription factors, including nuclear factor-kappaB and activator-1 which switch on multiple inflammatory genes, and specific transcription factors such as GATA-3, which activates the Th2 genes IL-4, IL-5, and IL-13

INTRODUCTION

All allergic diseases are characterized by a specific pattern of inflammation that is largely driven via IgE-dependent mechanisms. Genetic factors play an important influence on whether atopy develops, and several genes have now been identified.[1,2] Indeed, most of the genetic linkages reported for asthma are common to all allergic diseases.[3] However, environmental factors appear to be more important in determining whether an atopic individual develops a particular allergic disease, although genetic factors may exert an influence on how severely the disease is expressed, and the extent of the allergic inflammatory response. It had been recognized for many years that patients who die of asthma attacks have grossly inflamed airways. The airway lumen is occluded by a tenacious mucus plug composed of plasma proteins exuded from airway vessels and mucus glycoproteins secreted from surface epithelial cells. The airway wall is edematous and infiltrated with inflammatory cells, which are predominantly eosinophils and lymphocytes. The airway epithelium is invariably shed in a patchy manner and clumps of epithelial cells are found in the airway lumen. Occasionally there have been opportunities to examine the airways of asthmatic patients who die accidentally and similar though less marked inflammatory changes have been observed. More recently, it has been possible to examine the airways of asthmatic patients by fiberoptic bronchoscopy, using bronchial biopsies and bronchoalveolar lavage (BAL). Direct bronchoscopy reveals that the airways of asthmatic patients are often reddened and swollen, indicating acute inflammation. Lavage has revealed an increase in the numbers of lymphocytes, mast cells, and eosinophils and evidence for activation of macrophages in comparison with non-asthmatic controls. Biopsies have revealed evidence for increased numbers and activation of mast cells, macrophages, eosinophils, and T lymphocytes.[4] These changes are found even in patients with mild asthma who have few symptoms, and this suggests that asthma is an inflammatory condition of the airways.

Similar inflammatory changes are described in rhinitis, with vasodilatation and infiltration of similar inflammatory cells,[5,6] although the components of inflammation differ between upper and lower respiratory tracts because of the preponderance of different structures (smooth muscle in lower airways, capacitance vessels in the upper airways). In atopic dermatitis, a very similar pathophysiological picture is evident, with the same spectrum of inflammatory cells and mediators.[7]

Inflammation is classically characterized by four cardinal signs: *calor* and *rubor* (due to vasodilatation), *tumor* (due to plasma exudation and edema), and *dolor* (due to sensitization and activation of sensory nerves). Inflammation is also characterized by an infiltration with inflammatory cells and that these will differ depending on the type of inflammatory process. It is important to recognize that inflammation is an important defense response that defends the body against invasion from microorganisms and against the effects of external toxins. Allergic inflammation is characterized by the fact that it is driven by exposure to allergens through IgE-dependent mechanisms, resulting in a characteristic pattern of inflammation. The inflammatory response seen in allergic diseases is characterized by an infiltration with eosinophils and resembles the inflammatory process mounted in response to parasite and worm infections.[8] The inflammatory response not only provides an acute defense against injury, but is also involved in healing and restoration of normal function after tissue damage as a result of infection of toxins. In allergic disease, the inflammatory response is activated inappropriately and is harmful rather than beneficial. For some reason, allergens such as house dust mite and pollen proteins activate an eosinophil inflammation. Normally such an inflammatory response would kill the invading parasite (or vice versa) and would therefore be self-limiting, but in allergic disease the inciting stimulus persists and the normally acute inflammatory response becomes converted into a chronic inflammation which may have structural consequences in the airways and skin.

The relationship between inflammation and clinical symptoms of allergy is not yet clear. There is evidence that the degree of inflammation is related to airway hyperresponsiveness (AHR), as measured by histamine or methacholine challenge. Increased airway responsiveness, is an exaggerated airway narrowing in response to many stimuli which is characteristic of asthma and the degree of AHR relates to asthma symptoms. Inflammation of the airways may increase airway responsiveness, which thereby allows triggers which would not narrow the airways to do so. But inflammation may also directly lead to an increase in asthma symptoms, such as cough and chest tightness, by activation of airway sensory nerve endings (Fig. 29.1). In rhinitis, nasal blockage is due to vasodilatation, and nasal discharge is due to plasma exudation and mucus secretion. The characteristic sneezing is a manifestation of hypersensitivity of sensory nerves and is the equivalent of cough in asthma. In the skin, itching is similarly due to sensory nerve sensitization.

Although most attention has focused on the acute inflammatory changes seen in allergic diseases, particularly asthma, these are chronic conditions with inflammation persisting over many years in most patients. The mechanisms involved in persistence of allergic inflammation are still poorly understood. Superimposed on this chronic inflammatory state are acute inflammatory episodes which correspond to exacerbations of asthma, rhinitis, or atopic dermatitis.

The purpose of this chapter is to provide an overview of allergic inflammatory mechanisms to integrate some of the preceding chapters,

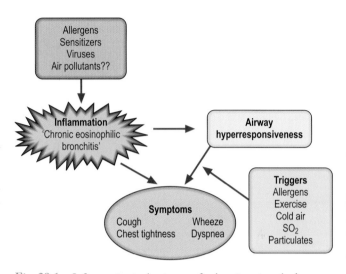

Fig. 29.1. Inflammation in the airways of asthmatic patients leads to airway hyperresponsiveness and symptoms. SO_2, sulfur dioxide.

where individual cells and mediators are discussed in detail. Allergic diseases often occur together; a large proportion of patients with asthma also have rhinitis, and many children with asthma also have atopic dermatitis.[9] No single cell or mediator can account for all the features of allergic disease and different cell and mediators may be more important in one manifestation of allergic disease than another. Thus, histamine clearly plays a key role in rhinitis, yet has a relatively minor role in asthma, as judged by the differences in efficacy of antihistamines in these conditions.

■ INFLAMMATORY CELLS ■

Many different inflammatory cells are involved in allergic inflammation, although the precise role of each cell type is not yet certain.[4,5,10] It is evident that no single inflammatory cell is able to account for the complex pathophysiology of allergic disease, but some cells predominate in allergic inflammation.

MAST CELLS

Mast cells play a key role in the symptomatology of asthma.[11] Mast cells are important in initiating the acute bronchoconstrictor responses to allergen and probably to many other indirect stimuli, such as exercise and hyperventilation (via osmolality or thermal changes), fog, and probably viral infection. Mast cells in airway smooth muscle appear to distinguish asthma from chromic eosinophilic bronchitis in which patients have chronic cough but not asthma.[12] They also play an important role in inducing symptoms of rhinitis after exposure to allergens, such as grass pollen. The number of mast cells in induced sputum in patients with seasonal allergic rhinitis is related to the degree of methacholine responsiveness. Treatment of asthmatic patients with prednisone results in a decrease in the number of tryptase-positive mast cells.[13] Furthermore, mast cell tryptase appears to play a role in airway remodeling, as this mast cell product stimulates human lung fibroblast proliferation.[14] Mast cells also secrete certain cytokines, such as interleukin (IL)-4 that may be involved in maintaining the allergic inflammatory response and tumor necrosis factor-α (TNF-α).[15] The cytokine stem cell factor (SCF) plays a critical role in the expression of mast cells at the airway mucosal surface and acts through the c-Kit receptor expressed on mast cells.[16]

The importance of mast cells in asthma has been highlighted by the clinical efficacy of anti-IgE therapy using omalizumab, which significantly reduces exacerbations of asthma and reduced maintenance doses of inhaled or oral corticosteroids.[17] This treatment is also effective in allergic rhinitis.

MACROPHAGES

Macrophages, which are derived from blood monocytes, may traffic into the airways in asthma and may be activated by allergen via low affinity IgE receptors (FcϵRII).[18] Leukotriene (LT)D$_4$ also stimulates macrophages to release inflammatory products, such as TNF-α and nitric oxide (NO).[19] The enormous immunological repertoire of macrophages allows these cells to produce many different products, including a large variety of cytokines that may orchestrate the inflammatory response. Macrophages have the capacity to initiate a particular type of inflammatory response via the release of a certain pattern of cytokines. Macrophages may both increase and decrease inflammation, depending on the stimulus. Alveolar macrophages normally have a *suppressive* effect on lymphocyte function, but this may be impaired in asthma after allergen exposure.[20] One antiinflammatory protein secreted by macrophages is IL-10 and its secretion is reduced in alveolar macrophages from patients with asthma.[21] Macrophages from normal subjects also inhibit the secretion of IL-5 from T lymphocytes, probably via the release of IL-12, but this is defective in patients with allergic asthma.[22] Macrophages may therefore play an important antiinflammatory role, by preventing the development of allergic inflammation.

Macrophages may also act as antigen-presenting cells which process allergen for presentation to T lymphocytes, although alveolar macrophages are far less effective in this respect than macrophages from other sites, such as the peritoneum. There may be subtypes of macrophages that perform different inflammatory, antiinflammatory or phagocytic roles in allergic disease. Immunological markers that can distinguish these subpopulations are beginning to emerge.[23] No differences in the macrophage population in induced sputum of allergic asthmatic compared to normal subjects have been detected, however.[24]

DENDRITIC CELLS

Dendritic cells are specialized macrophage-like cells that have a unique ability to induce a T lymphocyte-mediated immune response and therefore play a critical role in the development of allergic diseases. Dendritic cells in the respiratory tract form a network that is localized to the epithelium, and act as very effective antigen-presenting cells.[25] Dendritic cells in the skin, known as Langerhans' cells, play a critical role in sensitization responses. It is likely that they play a very important role in the initiation and maintenance of allergen-induced responses in allergic diseases.[26] Myeloid but not plasmacytoid dendritic cells have been shown to underlie AHR in experimental models of allergic asthma. Dendritic cells take up allergens, process them to peptides, and migrate to local lymph nodes, where they present the allergenic peptides to uncommitted T lymphocytes, and with the aid of co-stimulatory molecules, such as B7.1, B7.2, and CD40, they program the production of allergen-specific T cells. Animal studies have demonstrated that myeloid dendritic cells are critical to the development of Th2 cells and eosinophilia.[26] Immature dendritic cells in the respiratory tract promote Th2 cell differentiation and require cytokines such as IL-12 and TNF-α to promote the normally preponderant Th1 response. Dendritic cell-based immunotherapy may be developed in the future for the prevention and control of allergic diseases.[27]

EOSINOPHILS

Eosinophil infiltration is a characteristic feature of allergic inflammation. Asthma might more accurately be termed 'chronic eosinophilic bronchitis' (a term first used as early as 1916). Allergen inhalation results in a marked increase in eosinophils in bronchoalveolar lavage fluid at the time of the late reaction, and there is a correlation between eosinophil counts in peripheral blood or bronchial lavage and AHR. Eosinophils are linked to the development of AHR through the release of basic proteins and oxygen-derived free radicals.[28] Experimentally activated eosinophils have been shown to induce airway epithelial damage, which is a characteristic of patients with asthma.[29] However, similar shedding of nasal epithelial cells in patients with allergic rhinitis is not usually observed, indicating differential sensitivity of epithelial cells to the harmful effects of eosinophils.

Several mechanisms are involved in *recruitment* of eosinophils into the site of allergic inflammation. Eosinophils are derived from bone marrow precursors. After allergen challenge, eosinophils appear in BAL fluid during the late response, and this is associated with a decrease in peripheral eosinophil counts and with the appearance of eosinophil progenitors in the circulation.[30] The signal for increased eosinophil production is presumably derived from the inflamed airway. Eosinophil recruitment initially involves adhesion of eosinophils to vascular endothelial cells in the airway circulation, their migration into the submucosa, and their subsequent activation. The role of individual adhesion molecules, cytokines, and mediators in orchestrating these responses has been extensively investigated. Adhesion of eosinophils involves the expression of specific glycoprotein molecules on the surface of eosinophils (integrins) and the expression of such molecules as intercellular adhesion molecule-1 (ICAM-1) on vascular endothelial cells.[31] An antibody directed at ICAM-1 markedly inhibits eosinophil accumulation in the airways after allergen exposure and also blocks the accompanying hyperresponsiveness.[32] However, ICAM-1 is not selective for eosinophils and cannot account for the selective recruitment of eosinophils in allergic inflammation. The adhesion molecule very late antigen-4 (VLA4) expressed on eosinophils which interacts with VCAM-1 appears to be more selective for eosinophils[33] and IL-4 increases the expression of VCAM-1 on endothelial cells. Eosinophil migration may be due to the effects of lipid mediators, such as leukotrienes and possibly platelet-activating factor (PAF), and to the effects of cytokines, such as GM-CSF and IL-5, which may be very important for the survival of eosinophils in the airways and for 'priming' eosinophils to exhibit enhanced responsiveness.

Eosinophils from asthmatic patients show exaggerated responses to PAF and phorbol esters, compared to eosinophils from atopic nonasthmatic individuals[34] and this is further increased by allergen challenge,[35] suggesting that they may have been primed by exposure to cytokines in the circulation. There are several mediators involved in the migration of eosinophils from the circulation to the surface of the airway. The most potent and selective agents appear to be chemokines, such as RANTES, eotaxins 1–3, and MCP-4, that are expressed in epithelial cells. There appears to be a cooperative interaction between IL-5 and chemokines, so that both cytokines are necessary for the eosinophilic response in airways.[36] Once recruited to the airways, eosinophils require the presence of various growth factors, of which GM-CSF and IL-5 appear to be the most important.[37] In the absence of these growth factors eosinophils may undergo programmed cell death (apoptosis).

A humanized monoclonal antibody to IL-5 has been administered to asthmatic patients[38] and, as in animal studies, there is a profound and prolonged reduction in circulating eosinophils. Although the recruitment of eosinophils into the airway after inhaled allergen challenge is completely blocked, there is no effect on the response to inhaled allergen and no reduction in AHR. A clinical study with anti-IL-5 blocking antibody showed a similar profound reduction in circulating eosinophils, but no improvement in clinical parameters of asthma control.[39] However, eosinophils may not be completely depleted from the airways.[40] These data question the pivotal role of eosinophils in AHR and asthma, but it is possible that eosinophils may be playing an important role in the structural changes that occur in chronic asthma through the secretion of growth factors, such as transforming growth factor-β.[41]

NEUTROPHILS

While considerable attention has focused on eosinophils in allergic disease, there has been much less attention paid to neutrophils. Although neutrophils are not a predominant cell type observed in the airways of patients with mild to moderate chronic asthma, they appear to be a more prominent cell type in airways and induced sputum of patients with more severe asthma.[42–44] Also, large numbers of neutrophils are found in the airways of patients who die suddenly of asthma,[45] although this may reflect the rapid kinetics of neutrophil recruitment compared to eosinophil inflammation. The presence of neutrophils in severe asthma may reflect treatment with high doses of corticosteroids as steroids prolong neutrophil survival by inhibition of apoptosis.[46] However, it is possible that neutrophils are actively recruited in severe asthma. Neutrophils may be recruited to the airways in severe asthma and the concentrations of IL-8 are increased in induced sputum of these patients.[43] This in turn may be due to the increased levels of oxidative stress in severe asthma.[47] The role of neutrophils in asthma is also unknown and whether it pays a role in the pathophysiology of severe asthma needs to be determined, when selective inhibitors of IL-8 and its receptors become available. The fact that patients with even higher degrees of neutrophilic inflammation, such as in COPD and cystic fibrosis, do not have the pronounced AHR seen in asthma makes it unlikely that neutrophils are linked to increased airway responsiveness. However, it is possible that they may be associated with reduced responsiveness to corticosteroids that is seen in patients with severe asthma. Neutrophils may also play a role in acute exacerbations of asthma.

T LYMPHOCYTES

T lymphocytes play a very important role in coordinating the inflammatory response in asthma through the release of specific patterns of cytokines, resulting in the recruitment and survival of eosinophils and in the maintenance of mast cells in the airways. T lymphocytes are coded to express a distinctive pattern of cytokines, which are similar to that described in the murine T helper-2 (Th2) type of T lymphocytes, which characteristically express IL-4, IL-5, and IL-13.[48] This programming of T lymphocytes is presumably due to antigen-presenting cells, such as dendritic cells, which may migrate from the epithelium to regional lymph nodes or which interact with lymphocytes resident in the airway mucosa. The naive immune system is skewed to express the Th2 phenotype; data now indicate that children with atopy are more likely to retain this skewed phenotype than normal children.[49] There is some evidence that early infections or exposure to endotoxins might promote Th1-mediated responses to predominate and that a lack of infection or a clean environment in childhood may favor Th2 cell expression and thus atopic diseases.[50–52] Indeed, the balance between Th1 cells and Th2 cells is thought to be determined by locally released cytokines, such as IL-12, which tip the balance in favor of Th1 cells, or IL-4 or IL-13, which favor the emergence of Th2 cells (Fig. 29.2). There is some evidence that corticosteroid treatment may differentially affect the balance between IL-12 and IL-13 expression.[53] Data from murine models of asthma[54,55] have strongly suggested that IL-13 is both necessary and sufficient for induction of the asthmatic phenotype. Invariant natural killer T cells (iNKT), which express an invariant T cell receptor, are predominant in the airways of asthmatic patients and a major source of IL-4 and IL-13.[56] These cells are naturally activated by various glycolipids that are able to induce AHR in animal models independently of allergen exposure.[57] iNKT cells appear to be recruited into the asthmatic airways by the chemokines CCL25 acting on CCR9 that are selectively expressed by these cells.[58]

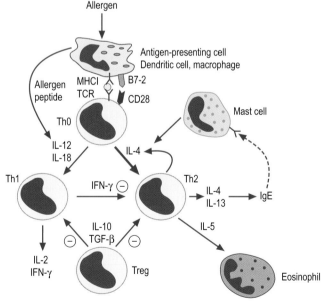

Fig. 29.2. Allergic inflammation is characterized by a preponderance of T helper 2 (Th2) lymphocytes over T helper 1 (Th1) cells. Regulatory T cells (Treg) have an inhibitory effect. MHCI, class I major histocompatibility complex; IL, interleukin; IFN-γ, interferon gamma; TGF-β, transforming growth factor beta; IgE, immunoglobulin E, Th0, uncommitted T cell.

Regulatory T (Treg) cells suppress the immune response through the secretion of inhibitory cytokines, such as IL-10 and TGF-β, and play an important role in immune regulation with suppression of Th1 and Th2 responses. CD4+CD25+ cells use the transcription factor FoxP3 to suppress the immune response.[59] There is evidence that these CD4+CD25+ regulatory T cells are defective in patients with allergic rhinitis.[60] Immunotherapy may target Tregs and induce their production of IL-10.[61]

CD8+ cells are not usually prominent in asthmatic airways but may become so in more severe asthma patients and have been linked to more rapid decline in lung function.[62] In experimental asthma LTB_4 is an important chemotactic factor for CD8+ cells which express BLT receptors.[63] CD8+ cells in asthma may express IL-4, IL-5, and IL-13 and are termed Tc2 cells.[64]

B LYMPHOCYTES

In allergic diseases, B lymphocytes secrete IgE and the factors regulating IgE secretion are now much better understood.[65] IL-4 is crucial in switching B cells to IgE production, and CD40 on T cells is an important accessory molecule that signals through interaction with CD40-ligand on B cells. There is increasing evidence for local production of IgE, even in patients with intrinsic asthma who have negative skin prick tests to allergens.[66]

BASOPHILS

The role of basophils in asthma is uncertain, as these cells have previously been difficult to detect by immunocytochemistry.[67] Using a basophil-specific marker, a small increase in basophils has been documented in the airways of asthmatic patients, with an increased number after allergen challenge.[68,69] However, these cells are far outnumbered by eosinophils (approximately 10:1 ratio) and their functional role is unknown.[68] There is also an increase in the numbers of basophils, as well as mast cells, in induced sputum after allergen challenge.[70] The role of basophils, as opposed to mast cells, is somewhat uncertain in asthma.[71] However, the role of basophils in allergic rhinitis appears to be more firmly established,[72] and in patients with atopic dermatitis basophils are present in similar numbers to eosinophils.[68]

PLATELETS

There is some evidence for the involvement of platelets in the pathophysiology of allergic diseases, since platelet activation may be observed and there is evidence for platelets in bronchial biopsies of asthmatic patients.[73] After allergen challenge there is a significant fall in circulating platelets,[74] and circulating platelets from patients with asthma show evidence of increased activation and release the chemokine RANTES.[75] Chemokines associated with Th2-mediated inflammation have recently been shown to activate and aggregate platelets.[76]

STRUCTURAL CELLS

Structural cells of the airways, including epithelial cells, endothelial cells, fibroblasts, and airway smooth muscle cells, may also be an important source of inflammatory mediators such as cytokines and lipid mediators in asthma.[77,78] Indeed, because structural cells far outnumber inflammatory cells, they may become the major source of mediators driving

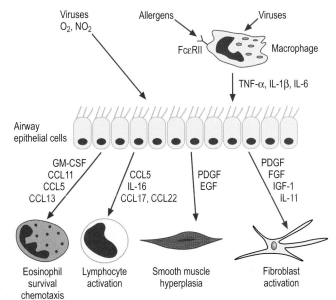

Fig. 29.3. Airway epithelial cells may play an active role in asthmatic inflammation through the release of many inflammatory mediators, cytokines, chemokines, and growth factors in response to several inhaled stimuli, including viruses, air pollutants (ozone and nitrogen dioxide), and allergens. TNF-α, tumor necrosis factor alpha; IL, interleukin, CCL, C-C chemokine, PDGF, platelet-derived growth factor; EGF, epidermal growth factor; FGF, fibroblast growth factor; IGF, insulin-like growth factor.

chronic inflammation in asthma and other allergic diseases. Epithelial cells may have a key role in translating inhaled environmental signals into an airway inflammatory response and are probably a major target cell for inhaled glucocorticoids (Fig. 29.3).

■ INFLAMMATORY MEDIATORS ■

Many different mediators have been implicated in asthma and they may have a variety of effects on the airways which could account for all of the pathological features of allergic diseases (Fig. 29.4).[7,79,80] Mediators such as histamine, prostaglandins, leukotrienes, and kinins contract airway smooth muscle, increase microvascular leakage, increase airway mucus secretion, and attract other inflammatory cells. Because each mediator has many effects, the role of individual mediators in the pathophysiology of asthma is not yet clear. The multiplicity and redundancy of effects of mediators makes it unlikely that preventing the synthesis or action of a *single* mediator will have a major impact in allergic diseases. However, some mediators may play a more important role if they are upstream in the inflammatory process. The effects of single mediators can only be evaluated through the use of specific receptor antagonists or mediator synthesis inhibitors. The role of mediators may differ between allergic diseases. Thus, antihistamines have a useful clinical effect in allergic rhinitis, whereas they are not useful in the treatment of asthma.[81] On the other hand, antileukotrienes have clinical effects in asthma but appear to be less useful in rhinitis.[82,83]

459

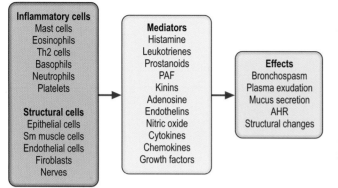

Fig. 29.4. Many cells and mediators are involved in asthma and lead to several effects on the airways. Th2, T helper 2 cells; Sm, smooth; PAF, platelet-activating factor; AHR, airway hyperresponsiveness.

LIPID MEDIATORS

Leukotrienes

The cysteinyl-leukotrienes (cys-LTs), LTC_4, LTD_4, and LTE_4, are potent constrictors of human airways and have been reported to increase AHR and may play an important role in asthma.[82] Cysteinyl-leukotriene receptors ($CysLT_1$) are increased in asthmatic airways due to infiltration with inflammatory cells, such as eosinophils, neutrophils, and macrophages, which express these receptors.[84] The introduction of potent specific leukotriene antagonists has recently made it possible to evaluate the role of these mediators in asthma. Potent LTD_4 antagonists protect (by about 50%) against exercise- and allergen-induced bronchoconstriction,[85–88] suggesting that leukotrienes contribute to bronchoconstrictor responses. Combining an antihistamine and an antileukotriene may be more effective in the treatment of asthma and rhinitis.[89,90] Chronic treatment with antileukotrienes improves lung function and symptoms in asthmatic patients, although the degree of lung function improvement is not as great as with inhaled corticosteroids, which have a much broader spectrum of effects.[91,92] In addition to their effects on airway smooth muscle and vessels, cys-LTs have weak inflammatory effects, with an increase in eosinophils in induced sputum,[93] but the antiinflammatory effects of antileukotrienes are small.[94]

LTB_4 has also been implicated in asthma. Not only is it a chemoattractant of neutrophils, which express BLT_1-receptors, but it is increasingly recognized as an important activator of T cells.[95]

Platelet-activating factor

Platelet-activating factor (PAF) is a potent inflammatory mediator that mimics many of the features of asthma, including eosinophil recruitment and activation and induction of AHR,[96] yet even potent PAF antagonists, such as modipafant, do not control asthma symptoms, at least in chronic asthma.[97–99] A genetic mutation that results in impaired function of the PAF metabolizing enzyme, PAF acetyl hydrolase, is associated with the presence of severe asthma in Japan,[100] suggesting that PAF may play a role in some forms of asthma.

Prostaglandins

Prostaglandins (PG) have potent effects on airway function and there is some evidence for increased expression of the inducible form of cyclo-oxygenase (COX-2) in asthmatic airways,[101] but inhibition of their synthesis with COX inhibitors, such as aspirin or ibuprofen, does not have any effect in most patients with asthma. Some patients have aspirin-sensitive asthma, which is more common in some ethnic groups, such as eastern Europeans and Japanese. It is associated with increased expression of LTC_4 synthase, resulting in increased formation of cys-LTs, possibly because of genetic polymorphisms.[102,103] Prostaglandin D_2 is a bronchoconstrictor prostaglandin produced predominantly by mast cells. Deletion of the PGD_2 receptors in mice significantly inhibits inflammatory responses to allergen and inhibits AHR, suggesting that this mediator may be important in asthma.[104] Recently, it has also been discovered that PGD_2 activates a novel chemoattractant receptor termed chemoattractant receptor of Th2 cells (CRTH2) or DP_2 receptor, which is expressed on Th2 cells, eosinophils, and basophils and mediates chemotaxis of these cell types and may provide a link between mast cell activation and allergic inflammation.[104] PGD_2 also activates classical DP_1 receptors on eosinophils and is therefore a potent eosinophil chemoattractant.[95,105]

5-oxo-ETE

5-oxo-eicosatetraenoic acid (5-oxo-ETE) is a product of 5-lipoxygenase and is a potent chemoattractant of eosinophils which express its distinct OXE receptors.[106]

Isoprostanes

Oxidation of arachidonic acid results in the formation of F2-isoprostanes from arachidonic acid and these are potent bronchoconstrictors and mediators of plasma exudation.[107]

CYTOKINES

Cytokines are increasingly recognized to be important in chronic inflammation and to play a critical role in orchestrating the type of inflammatory response (Fig. 29.5).[108] Many inflammatory cells (macrophages, mast cells, eosinophils, and lymphocytes) are capable of synthesizing and releasing these proteins, and structural cells such as epithelial cells, airway smooth muscle, and endothelial cells may also release a variety of cytokines and may therefore participate in the chronic inflammatory response.[109] While inflammatory mediators like histamine and leukotrienes may be important in the acute and subacute inflammatory responses and in exacerbations of asthma, it is likely that cytokines play a dominant role in maintaining chronic inflammation in allergic diseases. Almost every cell is capable of producing cytokines under certain conditions. Research in this area is hampered by a lack of specific antagonists, although important observations have been made using specific neutralizing antibodies that have been developed as novel therapies.[109]

Lymphokines

The cytokines which appear to be of particular importance in asthma include the lymphokines secreted by T lymphocytes: IL-4 which is critical in switching B lymphocytes to produce IgE and for expression of VCAM-1

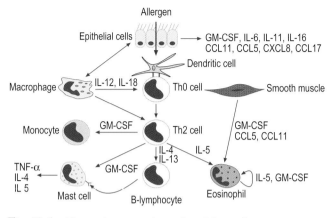
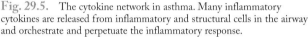

Fig. 29.5. The cytokine network in asthma. Many inflammatory cytokines are released from inflammatory and structural cells in the airway and orchestrate and perpetuate the inflammatory response.

on endothelial cells; IL-13, which acts similarly to IL-4 in IgE switching but also activates the release of growth factors to induce airway remodeling and mucus hypersecretion; and IL-5, which is of critical importance in the differentiation, survival, and priming of eosinophils. There is increased gene expression of IL-5 in lymphocytes in bronchial biopsies of patients with symptomatic asthma and allergic rhinitis.[110] The role of IL-5 in eosinophil recruitment in humans has been confirmed in a study in which administration of an anti-IL-5 antibody (mepolizumab) to asthmatic patients was associated with a profound decrease in eosinophil counts in the blood and induced sputum.[38] Interestingly in this study there was no effect on the physiology of the allergen-induced asthmatic response and this has been confirmed in a study in symptomatic asthmatic patients who showed no clinical improvement, despite a marked fall in circulating eosinophils. These studies question the critical role of eosinophils in asthma, although a more recent study showed that eosinophils were not completely reduced in the airways after this therapy.[40] IL-4 and IL-13 both play a key role in the allergic inflammatory response since they determine the isotype switching in B cells that results in IgE formation. IL-4, but not IL-13, is also involved in differentiation of Th2 cells and therefore may be critical in the initial development of atopy, whereas IL-13 is much more abundant in established disease and may therefore be more important in maintaining the inflammatory process.[111] Another Th2 cytokine, IL-9, may play a critical role is sensitizing responses the cytokines IL-4 and IL-5.[112]

Proinflammatory cytokines

Other cytokines, such as IL-1β, IL-6, TNF-α, and GM-CSF, are released from a variety of cells, including macrophages and epithelial cells, and may be important in amplifying the inflammatory response. TNF-α may be an amplifying mediator in asthma and is produced in increased amounts in asthmatic airways. Inhalation of TNF-α increased airway responsiveness in normal and asthmatic individuals.[113] TNF-α and IL-1β both activate the proinflammatory transcription factors, nuclear factor-κB (NF-κB) and activator protein-1 (AP-1) which then switch on many inflammatory genes in asthmatic airways, the nasal mucosa, and the skin. TNF-α appears to be more important in severe asthma where there is evidence for increased production.[114]

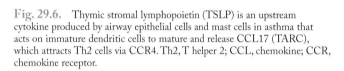

Fig. 29.6. Thymic stromal lymphopoietin (TSLP) is an upstream cytokine produced by airway epithelial cells and mast cells in asthma that acts on immature dendritic cells to mature and release CCL17 (TARC), which attracts Th2 cells via CCR4. Th2, T helper 2; CCL, chemokine; CCR, chemokine receptor.

IL-17

The IL-17 family of cytokines play a key role in the regulation of inflammation and result in a neutrophilic pattern of inflammation, and IL-17A is elevated in severe asthma.[115] IL-17A and IL-17F are released from a distinct subtype of CD4 cells termed Th17, which release IL-8, IL-6 and TNF-α. The production of Th17 cells is regulated by another cytokine IL-23, which is a member of the IL-12 family.[116]

Thymic stromal lymphopoietin

TSLP is an upstream IL-7-like cytokine that may initiate and propagate allergic immune responses.[117,118] TSLP is produced predominantly by epithelial cells and activated mast cells in the airways and by keratinocytes in the skin, and stimulates immature myeloid dendritic cells, which uniquely express the heterodimeric TSLP receptor to differentiate into mature dendritic cells. TSLP-activated dendritic cells promote naive CD4+ T cells to differentiate into a Th2 phenotype and promote the expansion of Th2 memory cells through the release of Th2 chemotactic cytokines, such as CCL17, and suppression of Th1 cytokines, such as interferon-γ (Fig. 29.6). TSLP may therefore play a pivotal role in the initiation of allergic asthma and atopic dermatitis and is highly expressed in the airways of asthmatic patients, and its expression is correlated with disease severity and the expression of CCL17.[119]

CHEMOKINES

Many chemokines are involved in the recruitment of inflammatory cells in asthma. Over 50 different chemokines are now recognized, and they activate more than 20 different surface receptors.[120] Chemokine

INFLAMMATORY MEDIATORS

receptors belong to the seven-transmembrane receptor superfamily of G-protein-coupled receptors, and this makes it possible to find small molecule inhibitors, which has not been possible for classical cytokine receptors.[121] Some chemokines appear to be selective for single chemokines, whereas others are promiscuous and mediate the effects of several related chemokines. Chemokines appear to act in sequence in determining the final inflammatory response and so inhibitors may be more or less effective depending on the kinetics of the response.[122]

Several chemokines, including CCL11 (eotaxin), CCL24 (eotaxin-2), CCL26 (eotaxin-3), CCL5 (RANTES), and CCL13 (macrophage chemoattractant protein-4, MCP-4), activate a common receptor on eosinophils termed CCR3.[123] There is increased expression of CCL11, CCL24, CCL13, and CCR3 in the airways of asthmatic patients and this is correlated with increased AHR.[124] Several small molecule inhibitors of CCR3, including UCB35625, SB-297006, and SB-328437, are effective in inhibiting eosinophil recruitment in allergen models of asthma, and drugs in this class are currently undergoing clinical trials in asthma.[125] Although it was thought that CCR3 were restricted to eosinophils, there is some evidence for their expression on Th2 cells and mast cells, so that these inhibitors may have a more widespread effect than on eosinophils alone, making them potentially more valuable in asthma treatment. CCL5, which shows increased expression in asthmatic airways,[126] also activates CCR3, but also has effects on CCR1 and CCR5, which may play a role in T cell recruitment.

CCL1 (MCP-1) activates CCR2 on monocytes and T lymphocytes. Blocking MCP-1 with neutralizing antibodies reduces recruitment of both T cells and eosinophils in a murine model of ovalbumin-induced airway inflammation, with a marked reduction in AHR.[127] MCP-1 also recruits and activates mast cells, an effect that is mediated via CCR2.[128] MCP-1 instilled into the airways induces marked and prolonged AHR in mice, associated with mast cell degranulation. A neutralizing antibody to MCP-1 blocks the development of AHR in response to allergen.[128] MCP-1 levels are increased in bronchoalveolar lavage fluid of patients with asthma.[129] Small molecule inhibitors of CCR2 are now in development.[121]

CCR4 are selectively expressed on Th2 cells and are activated by the chemokines CCL22 (monocyte-derived chemokine, MDC) and CCL17 (thymus and activation regulated chemokine, TARC).[130] Epithelial cells and myeloid dendritic of patients with asthma express CCL17, which may then recruit Th2 cells.[131] Increased concentrations of CCL17 are also found in BAL fluid of asthmatic patients, whereas CCL22 is only weakly expressed in the airways.[132] iNKT cells express CCR9, which is activated by CCL25 (thymus-expressed chemokine, TECK).[58]

CXC chemokines regulate neutrophilic inflammation, and there is evidence that CXCL8 (IL-8) is increased in the sputum of patients with severe asthma.[43]

OXIDATIVE STRESS

As in all inflammatory diseases, there is increased oxidative stress in allergic inflammation, as activated inflammatory cells, such as macrophages and eosinophils, produce reactive oxygen species. Evidence for increased oxidative stress in asthma is provided by the increased concentrations of 8-isoprostane (a product of oxidized arachidonic acid) in exhaled breath condensates[47] and increased ethane (a product of oxidative lipid peroxidation) in exhaled breath of asthmatic

patients.[133] There is also persuasive epidemiological evidence that a low dietary intake of antioxidants is linked to an increased prevalence of asthma.[134] Increased oxidative stress is related to disease severity and may amplify the inflammatory response and reduce responsiveness to corticosteroids, particularly in severe disease and during exacerbations.[134] One of the mechanisms whereby oxidative stress may be detrimental in asthma is through the reaction of superoxide anions with NO to form the reactive radical peroxynitrite, which may then modify several target proteins.

NITRIC OXIDE

Nitric oxide (NO) is produced by several cells in the airway by NO synthases.[135] Although the cellular source of NO within the lung is not known, inferences based on mathematical models suggest that it is the large airways which are the source of NO.[136] Current data indicate that the level of NO in the exhaled air of patients with asthma is higher than the level of NO in the exhaled air of normal subjects.[137] The elevated levels of NO in asthma are more likely reflective of an as yet to be identified inflammatory mechanism than of a direct pathogenetic role of this gas in asthma.[138,139] The combination of increased oxidative stress and NO may lead to the formation of the potent radical peroxynitrite, that may result in nitration of tyrosine residues in proteins in asthmatic airways.[140,141] NO production is also increased in allergic rhinitis.[142] Measurement of exhaled NO in asthma is increasingly used as a non-invasive way of monitoring the inflammatory process.[143]

■ EFFECTS OF INFLAMMATION ■

The acute and chronic allergic inflammatory responses have several effects on the target cells of the respiratory tract, resulting in the characteristic pathophysiologic changes associated with asthma or rhinitis (Fig. 29.7). Important advances have recently been made in understanding these changes, although their precise role in producing clinical symptoms is often not clear. There is considerable current interest in the structural changes that occur in the airways of patients with asthma that are loosely termed 'remodeling'. It is believed that these changes underlie the irreversible changes in airway function that occur in some patients with asthma.[144–146] However, many patients with asthma continue to have normal lung function throughout life, so it is likely that genetic factors may determine which patients develop these structural changes in the airways. Structural changes are much less pronounced in rhinitis, suggesting that there are particular cell types that drive the structural changes in the lower airways. It is possible that the distinct airway epithelial cells found in the lower airways orchestrate these structural changes in the airway, which are seen as an attempt to repair inflammation, whereas nasal epithelial cells are more robust and do not release the factors that induce such structural changes.

EPITHELIUM

Airway epithelial shedding is a characteristic feature of asthma and may be important in contributing to AHR, explaining how several different mechanisms, such as ozone exposure, virus infections, chemical sensitizers, and allergen exposure, can lead to its development, since all these

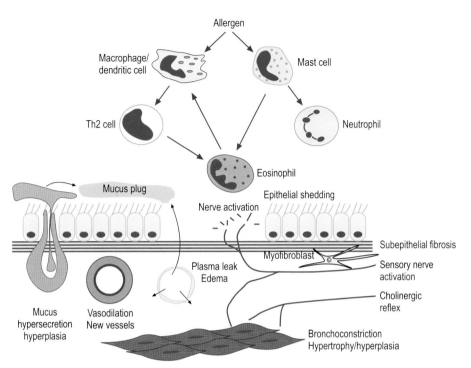

Fig. 29.7. The pathophysiology of asthma is complex, with participation of several interacting inflammatory cells resulting in acute and chronic inflammatory effects on the airway.

stimuli may lead to epithelial disruption. Epithelium may be shed as a consequence of inflammatory mediators such as eosinophil basic proteins and oxygen-derived free radicals, together with various proteases (particularly matrix metalloproteinase-9) released from inflammatory cells such as eosinophils. Epithelial cells are commonly found in clumps in the BAL or sputum (Creola bodies) of asthmatics, suggesting that there has been a loss of attachment to the basal layer or basement membrane. Epithelial damage may contribute to AHR in a number of ways, including loss of its barrier function to allow penetration of allergens, loss of enzymes (such as neutral endopeptidase) that normally degrade inflammatory mediators, loss of a relaxant factor (so-called epithelium-derived relaxant factor), and exposure of sensory nerves, which may lead to reflex neural effects on the airway. Epithelial shedding may be a feature of more severe asthma and the airway epithelium may be largely intact in patients with asthma, although it does appear to be more fragile. It is surprising that epithelial cells are not similarly friable in allergic rhinitis or in nasal polyps, despite the fact that a similar eosinophil inflammatory response is present.

As discussed above, epithelial cells appear to be an important source of mediators in allergic inflammation (Fig. 29.3). Release of mediators from epithelial cells may be stimulated by various inhaled substances, resulting in an increased inflammatory response. Epithelial cells may also release growth factors that stimulate structural changes in the airways, including fibrosis, angiogenesis, and proliferation of airway smooth muscle. These responses may be seen as an attempt to repair the damage caused by chronic inflammation.[147] Mechanical stimuli release growth factors from epithelial cells, which may be generated by the forces of bronchoconstriction.[148]

FIBROSIS

The basement membrane in asthma appears on light microscopy to be thickened, but on closer inspection by electron microscopy it has been demonstrated that this apparent thickening is due to subepithelial fibrosis with deposition of types III and V collagen below the true basement membrane.[149,150] The thickness of the deposited collagen is related to airway obstruction and AHR. The mechanism of the collagen deposition is not known, but appears to be related to activated eosinophils in the mucosa as it is also a feature of chronic eosinophilic bronchitis, which presents as cough without AHR or symptoms of asthma.[151] However, several profibrotic cytokines, including TGF-β and platelet-derived growth factor (PDGF), and mediators such as endothelin-1 can be produced by epithelial cells or macrophages in the inflamed airway.[152] The role of fibrosis in asthma is unclear; as subepithelial fibrosis has been observed even in mild asthmatics at the onset of disease, it is not certain whether the collagen deposition has any functional consequences. There is also evidence for fibrosis in airway smooth muscle and deeper in the airway and this is more likely to have functional consequences.[153] However, the fact that asthmatic patients are subject to chronic inflammation over many decades without gross fibrosis of the airways argues that there are likely to be powerful inhibitory mechanisms that prevent a fibrotic reaction to the multiple profibrotic mediators produced.

AIRWAY SMOOTH MUSCLE

There is still debate about the role of abnormalities in airway smooth muscle in asthmatic airways. Airway smooth muscle contraction plays a key role in the symptomatology of asthma and many inflammatory

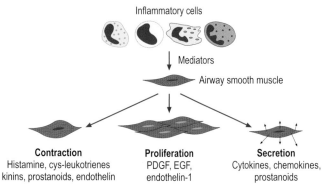

Fig. 29.8. Inflammation has several effects on airway smooth muscle cells, resulting in contraction, proliferation, and secretion of inflammatory mediators. Cys, cysteinyl; PDGF, platelet-derived growth factor; EGF, epidermal growth factor.

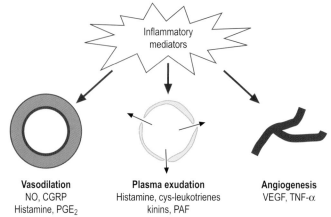

Fig. 29.9. Allergic inflammation has several vascular effects, including vasodilatation, plasma exudation from postcapillary venules, and new vessel formation (angiogenesis). NO, nitric oxide; CGRP, calcitonin gene-related peptide; PGE_2, prostaglandin E_2; PAF, platelet-activating factor; VEGF, vascular endothelial growth factor; TNF-α, tumor necrosis factor alpha.

mediators released in asthma have bronchoconstrictor effects. Recent studies using bronchial thermoplasty to eliminate airway smooth muscle cells have shown reduced airway responsiveness in patients with asthma.[154] It is now recognized that airway smooth muscle cells may also have other functions in asthmatic airways (Fig. 29.8).[155] In vitro airway smooth muscle from asthmatic patients usually shows no increased responsiveness to spasmogens. Reduced responsiveness to β-agonists has been reported in postmortem or surgically removed bronchi from asthmatics, although the number of β-receptors is not reduced, suggesting that β-receptors have been uncoupled.[156] These abnormalities of airway smooth muscle may be a reflection of the chronic inflammatory process. For example, chronic exposure to inflammatory cytokines, such as IL-1β, downregulates the response to β_2-adrenergic agonists in vitro and in vivo.[157,158] The reduced β-adrenergic responses in airway smooth muscle could be due to phosphorylation of the stimulatory G-protein-coupling β-receptors to adenylyl cyclase, resulting from the activation of protein kinase C by the stimulation of airway smooth muscle cells by inflammatory mediators and to increased activity of the inhibitory G protein (G_i) induced by proinflammatory cytokines.[157,159]

Inflammatory mediators may modulate the ion channels that serve to regulate the resting membrane potential of airway smooth muscle cells, thus altering the level of excitability of these cells. Furthermore, modulation of the activation kinetics of other ion channels by key inflammatory mediators can lead to altered contractile characteristics of smooth muscle.

In asthmatic airways there is also a characteristic *hypertrophy* and *hyperplasia* of airway smooth muscle, particularly in severe asthma,[160] which is presumably the result of stimulation of airway smooth muscle cells by various growth factors, such as platelet-derived growth factor (PDGF), or endothelin-1 released from inflammatory cells.[149,161] Cultured airway smooth muscle cells from asthmatic patients show a greater proliferative response to those from non-asthmatic airways, suggesting that either there is an intrinsic abnormality of airway smooth muscle cells or that their phenotypes have been changed by chronic inflammation. Airway smooth muscle also has a secretory role in asthma and has the capacity to release multiple cytokines, chemokines, and lipid mediators.[78,162]

VASCULAR RESPONSES

Allergic inflammation has several effects on blood vessels in the respiratory tract (Fig. 29.9). Vasodilatation occurs in inflammation, yet little is known about the role of the airway circulation in asthma, partly because of the difficulties involved in measuring airway blood flow. Recent studies using an inhaled absorbable gas have demonstrated an increased airway mucosal blood flow in asthma,[163] and this is correlated with an increased exhaled breath temperature.[164,165] The bronchial circulation may play an important role in regulating airway caliber, since an increase in the vascular volume may contribute to airway narrowing. Increased airway blood flow may be important in removing inflammatory mediators from the airway, and may play a role in the development of exercise-induced asthma. Increased shear stress due to high expiratory pressures may lead to gene transduction and enhanced production of NO by endothelial NO synthase.[166] Direct visualization shows a marked increase in vascularity of the airways of asthmatic patients, with a fine vascular network, representing new vessel formation.[167] The increase in the number of blood vessels in asthmatic airways[168] is a result of angiogenesis due to the release of growth factors such as vascular endothelial growth factor (VEGF) and TNF-α.[169] VEGF concentrations are increased in lavage fluid of asthmatic airways, and there is increased expression in the airway walls of VEGF and its receptor Ang-1 that is correlated with the increased numbers of blood vessels.[170]

Microvascular leakage is an essential component of the inflammatory response and many of the inflammatory mediators implicated in asthma produce this leakage.[171] There is good evidence for microvascular leakage in asthma, and it may have several consequences on airway function, including increased airway secretions, impaired mucociliary clearance, formation of new mediators from plasma precursors (such as kinins), and mucosal edema, which may contribute to airway narrowing and increased AHR.[172,173]

Vasodilatation is an important aspect of the inflammatory response in rhinitis and contributes to nasal blockage and increased nasal secretions.

Plasma leakage in rhinitis is also an important component of nasal secretions.[174]

MUCUS HYPERSECRETION

Mucus hypersecretion is a common inflammatory response in secretory tissues. Increased mucus secretion contributes to the viscid mucus plugs which occlude asthmatic airways, particularly in fatal asthma. There is evidence for hyperplasia of submucosal glands which are confined to large airways and of increased numbers of epithelial goblet cells in asthmatic airways and in the mucosa of patients with allergic rhinitis.[175,176] This increased secretory response may be due to inflammatory mediators acting on submucosal glands to increase the expression of the mucin genes MUC5AC and MUCB, and due to stimulation of neural elements. Th2 cytokines IL-4, IL-13, and IL-9 have all been shown to induce mucus hypersecretion in experimental models of asthma.[177] Epithelial growth factor (EGF) receptors, which may be activated by transforming growth factor-α, play an important role in mucus secretion of upper and lower airways and may be the final common pathway for many stimuli that stimulate mucus secretion, including IL-13 and oxidative stress (Fig. 29.10).[177] EGF stimulates the expression of MUC5AC, which shows increased expression in asthma.[178] The functional role of hypertrophy and hyperplasia of the mucus-secreting cells in asthma is not yet known as it is difficult to quantify mucus secretion in airways. AHR and mucus hypersecretion, together with MUC5AC expression, are associated with the expression of a specific calcium-activated chloride channel in goblet cells, designated gob-5, which has a human counterpart hCLCA1.[179] Overexpression of gob-5 induced marked AHR and mucus hypersecretion in mice, indicating that mucus hypersecretion may play a role in AHR;

however, gene knockout of gob-5 in mice or knockdown of hCLCA1 in human cells did not appear to reduce the mucus hypersecretion.[180]

NEURAL EFFECTS

Neural mechanisms play an important role in asthma and rhinitis, particularly in the context of symptomatology and AHR.[181] Autonomic nervous control of the respiratory tract is complex; in addition to classical cholinergic and adrenergic mechanisms, non-adrenergic non-cholinergic (NANC) nerves and several neuropeptides have been identified in the respiratory tract.[182,183] Abnormalities of autonomic function, such as enhanced cholinergic and α-adrenergic responses or reduced β-adrenergic responses, have been extensively investigated. However, these abnormalities are likely to be secondary to the disease, rather than primary defects.[181]

Nerve–inflammation interactions

There is a close interaction between nerves and inflammatory cells in allergic inflammation, as inflammatory mediators activate and modulate neurotransmission, whereas neurotransmitters may modulate the inflammatory response (Fig. 29.11). Inflammatory mediators may act on various prejunctional receptors on airway nerves to modulate the release of neurotransmitters.[184,185] Thus, thromboxane and PGD_2 facilitate the release of acetylcholine from cholinergic nerves in canine airways, whereas histamine inhibits cholinergic neurotransmission at both parasympathetic ganglia and postganglionic nerves via H_3 receptors. Inflammatory mediators may also activate sensory nerves, resulting in reflex cholinergic bronchoconstriction or release of inflammatory neuropeptides. Bradykinin is a potent activator of unmyelinated sensory nerves (C-fibers), but also sensitizes these nerves to other stimuli.[186]

Sensory nerves

Inflammatory products may also sensitize sensory nerve endings in the airway epithelium, so that the nerves become hyperalgesic. Hyperalgesia and pain (*dolor*) are cardinal signs of inflammation, and in the asthmatic airway may mediate cough and chest tightness, which are such characteristic symptoms of asthma. Sensory hyperalgesia also mediates sneezing in rhinitis and itching in atopic dermatitis. The precise mechanisms of

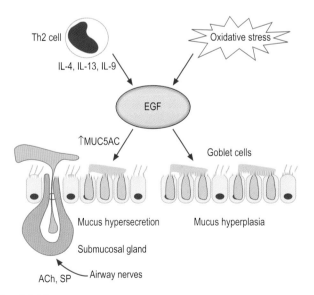

Fig. 29.10. Increased mucus secretion in allergic disease may be stimulated by T helper 2 (Th2) cytokines and oxidative stress. This may be mediated via epidermal growth factor (EGF), which may result in mucus hyperplasia and increased expression of the mucin gene MUC5AC. Mucus hypersecretion is also enhanced by neural mechanisms through the release of acetylcholine (ACh) and substance P (SP).

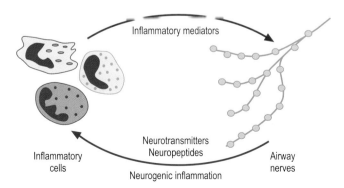

Fig. 29.11. There is a close interaction between allergic inflammation and neural mechanisms.

EFFECTS OF INFLAMMATION

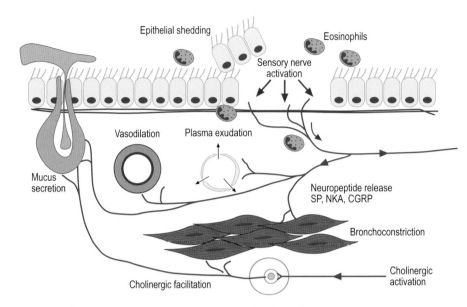

Fig. 29.12. Possible neurogenic inflammation in asthmatic airways via retrograde release of peptides from sensory nerves via an axon reflex. Substance P (SP) causes vasodilatation, plasma exudation, and mucus secretion, whereas neurokinin A (NKA) causes bronchoconstriction and enhanced cholinergic reflexes and calcitonin gene-related peptide (CGRP) vasodilatation.

hyperalgesia are not yet certain, but mediators such as prostaglandins, bradykinin, certain cytokines, and neurotrophins may be important. The activation of unmyelinated sensory nerves in the airways to several stimuli, including capsaicin, bradykinin, oxidative stress, and acid, is mediated via vanilloid-1 (TRP1) receptors.[187]

Neurotrophins

Neurotrophins, which may be released from various cell types in peripheral tissues, may cause proliferation and sensitization of airway sensory nerves.[188,189] Neurotrophins, such as nerve growth factor (NGF), may be released from inflammatory and structural cells in asthmatic airways and then stimulate the increased synthesis of neuropeptides, such as substance P, in airway sensory nerves, as well as sensitizing nerve endings in the airways. Thus, NGF is released from human airway epithelial cells after exposure to inflammatory stimuli.[190] Neurotrophins may play an important role in mediating AHR in asthma.

Bronchodilator nerves

Bronchodilator nerves, which are non-adrenergic, are prominent in human airways, and it has been suggested that these nerves may be defective in asthma.[191] In animal airways, vasoactive intestinal peptide (VIP) is a major neurotransmitter of these nerves and a striking absence of VIP-immunoreactive nerves has been reported in the lungs from patients with severe fatal asthma.[192] However, no difference in expression of VIP has been reported in bronchial biopsies from asthmatic patients.[193] It is likely that this loss of VIP immunoreactivity in severe asthma is explained by degradation by tryptase released from degranulating mast cells in the airways of asthmatics. In human airways, the single bronchodilator neurotransmitter appears to be NO.[194]

Neurogenic inflammation

Airway nerves may also release neurotransmitters which have inflammatory effects. Thus, neuropeptides such as substance P (SP), neurokinin A, and calcitonin-gene related peptide may be released from sensitized afferent nerves in the airways, which increase and extend the ongoing inflammatory response (Fig. 29.12).[195,196] There is evidence for an increase in SP-immunoreactive nerves in airways of patients with severe asthma,[197] which may be due to proliferation of sensory nerves and increased synthesis of sensory neuropeptides as a result of nerve growth factors released during chronic inflammation, although this has not been confirmed in milder asthmatic patients.[193] There may also be a reduction in the activity of enzymes, such as neutral endopeptidase, which degrade neuropeptides such as SP.[198] Chronic asthma may be associated with increased neurogenic inflammation, which may provide a mechanism for perpetuating the inflammatory response even in the absence of initiating inflammatory stimuli. At present, there is little direct evidence for neurogenic inflammation in asthma, but this is partly because it is difficult to make the appropriate measurements in the lower airways.[196] In rhinitis, there is more direct evidence for the existence of neurogenic inflammatory mechanisms.[199]

■ TRANSCRIPTION FACTORS ■

The chronic inflammation of asthma, allergic rhinitis, and atopic dermatitis is due to increased expression of multiple inflammatory proteins (cytokines, enzymes, receptors, adhesion molecules). In many cases, these inflammatory proteins are induced by transcription factors, DNA-binding factors that increase the transcription of selected target genes (Fig. 29.13).[200,201] One transcription factor that may play a critical

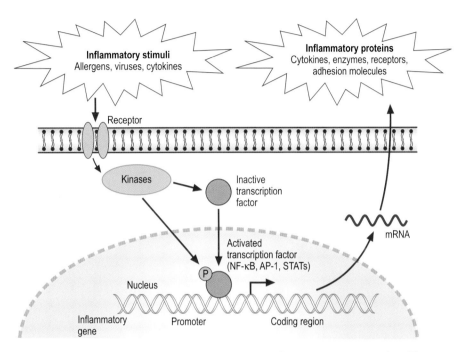

Fig. 29.13. Transcription factors play a key role in amplifying and perpetuating the inflammatory response in asthma. Transcription factors, including nuclear factor kappa-B (NF-κB), activator protein-1 (AP-1), and signal transduction-activated transcription factors (STATs), are activated by inflammatory stimuli and increase the expression of multiple inflammatory genes. mRNA, messenger ribonucleic acid.

role in asthma is NF-κB, which can be activated by multiple stimuli, including protein kinase C activators, oxidants, and proinflammatory cytokines (such as IL-1β and TNF-α).[202] There is evidence for increased activation of NF-κB in asthmatic airways, particularly in epithelial cells and macrophages.[203] NF-κB regulates the expression of several key genes that are overexpressed in asthmatic airways, including proinflammatory cytokines (IL-1β, IL-6, TNF-α, GM-CSF), chemokines (CCL1, CCL5, CCL11, CCL17), adhesion molecules (ICAM-1, VCAM-1), and inflammatory enzymes (COX-2 and iNOS). The c-Fos component of AP-1 is also activated in asthmatic airways and often cooperates with NF-κB in switching on inflammatory genes.[204] There is a common mechanism for inflammatory gene activation that involves activation of coactivator molecules by proinflammatory transcription factors, such as NF-κB, at the start site of transcription to induce acetylation of core histones, around which DNA is wound in the chromosome. This unwinds DNA, opening up the chromatin structure, and allows gene transcription to proceed.[205,206] These activated inflammatory genes are then switched off by the recruitment of histone deacetylase-2 (HDAC2), which is recruited by activated glucocorticoid receptors.[207]

Many other transcription factors are involved in the allergic inflammatory process in asthma and rhinitis. This includes transcription factors such as GATA-3, which regulates the expression of Th2 cytokine genes;[208,209] T-bet, which regulates Th1 cells;[210] and FOXP3, which regulates the activity of CD4+CD25+ Tregs.[211] The Th1/Th2 cell imbalance in allergic diseases may reflect an increase in GATA-3 and decrease in T-bet transcription factors, as demonstrated in experimental asthma.[212,213] There is increased expression of GATA-3 in T lymphocytes of asthmatic airways.[213]

■ ANTIINFLAMMATORY MECHANISMS IN ALLERGY ■

Although most emphasis has always been placed on inflammatory mechanisms, there are important antiinflammatory mechanisms that may be defective in asthma and other allergic diseases, resulting in increased inflammatory responses in the airways (Fig. 29.14).

Cortisol

Endogenous cortisol may be important as a regulator of the allergic inflammatory response, and nocturnal exacerbation of asthma may be related to the circadian fall in plasma cortisol. Blockade of endogenous cortisol secretion by metyrapone results in an increase in the late response to allergen in the skin.[214] Cortisol is converted to the inactive cortisone by the enzyme 11β-hydroxysteroid dehydrogenase II, which is expressed in the epithelium and endothelium of asthmatic airways and may be a determinant of corticosteroid sensitivity.[215] It is possible that this enzyme functions abnormally in asthma or may determine the severity of asthma.

Interleukin-1 receptor antagonist

Various cytokines have antiinflammatory actions.[216] IL-1 receptor antagonist (IL-1ra) inhibits the binding of IL-1 to its receptors and therefore has a potential antiinflammatory potential in asthma. It is reported to be effective in an animal model of asthma.[217] There is increased expression of IL-1ra in airway epithelial cells in asthma.[218]

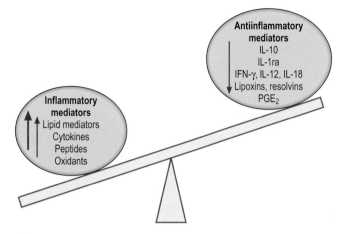

Fig. 29.14. There may be an imbalance between increased proinflammatory mediators and a deficiency in antiinflammatory mediators. IL, interleukin; IL-1ra, interleukin-1 receptor antagonist; IFN-γ, interferon gamma; PGE_2, prostaglandin E_2.

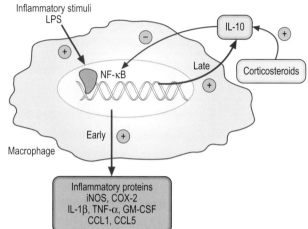

Fig. 29.15. Interleukin-10 (IL-10) is an antiinflammatory cytokine that may inhibit the expression of inflammatory mediators from macrophages. IL-10 secretion is deficient in macrophages from patients with asthma, resulting in increased release of inflammatory mediators. LPS, lipopolysaccharide; iNOS, inducible nitric oxide synthase; COX, cyclooxygenase; IL, interleukin; TNF-α, tumor necrosis factor alpha; GM-CSF, granulocyte-macrophage colony-stimulating factor; CCL; C-C chemokine.

Interleukin-12

IL-12 promotes the differentiation and, thus, the suppression of Th2 cells, resulting in a reduction in eosinophilic inflammation.[219] IL-12 infusions in patients with asthma indeed inhibit peripheral blood eosinophilia.[220] There is some evidence that IL-12 expression may be impaired in asthma.[53] IL-18 is similar to IL-12 and promotes Th1 cells. Its concentrations are reduced in sputum of asthmatic patients.[221]

Interleukin-10

IL-10 inhibits the expression of multiple inflammatory cytokines (TNF-α, IL-1β, GM-CSF) and chemokines, as well as inflammatory enzymes (iNOS, COX-2).[222] It may produce these widespread antiinflammatory action by inhibiting NF-κB activation, although this does not account for all of its antiinflammatory actions.[223] IL-10 secretion and gene transcription are defective in macrophages and monocytes from asthmatic patients;[21,224] this may lead to enhancement of inflammatory effects in asthma and may be a determinant of asthma severity (Fig. 29.15). IL-10 is also secreted by Tregs and may be an important regulator of the allergic immune response and mediate the effect of specific allergen immunotherapy.[225]

Lipid mediators

Other mediators may also have antiinflammatory and immunosuppressive effects. PGE_2 has inhibitory effects on macrophages, epithelial cells, and eosinophils. Exogenous PGE_2 inhibits allergen-induced airway responses and its endogenous generation may account for the refractory period after exercise challenge.[226] However, it is unlikely that endogenous PGE_2 is important in most asthmatics since non-selective COX inhibitors only worsen asthma in a minority of patients (aspirin-induced asthma). Other lipid mediators may also be antiinflammatory, including

15-HETE, which is produced in high concentration by airway epithelial cells. 15-HETE, which and lipoxins may inhibit cysteinyl-leukotriene effects on the airways and promote resolution of inflammation.[227] There is evidence that lipoxin production is reduced in severe asthma and aspirin-sensitive asthma. Resolvins are related antiinflammatory lipids molecules that are generated from omega-3-fatty acids in the diet that are involved in the resolution of acute inflammation, but their role in asthma is uncertain.[228]

The peptide adrenomcdullin, which is expressed in high concentrations in lung, has bronchodilator activity[229] and also appears to inhibit the secretion of cytokines from macrophages.[230] Its role in asthma is currently unknown.

■ FUTURE DIRECTIONS ■

Allergic inflammation is highly complex and involves multiple inflammatory proteins and cells with many effects. Although many of the individual components have now been characterized, there is still little understanding of the complex interactions between different cells and mediators. It is likely that genetic polymorphisms play an important role in determining the level of expression of many mediators involved in the allergic process and its resolution, and that the balance of these polymorphisms will determine the severity and possibly the site of allergic disease. Mechanisms of resolution are still not well understood and may be defective in chronic allergic disease, allowing the inflammation to persist even in the absence of driving allergens. The ready availability of gene microarrays and proteomics may make it easier to explore patterns of allergic inflammation and to identify logical therapeutic targets for future drug development.[231,232]

References

Introduction

1. Cookson W. The immunogenetics of asthma and eczema: a new focus on the epithelium. Nat Rev Immunol 2004; 4:978–988.
2. Cookson W, Moffatt M. Making sense of asthma genes. N Engl J Med 2004; 351:1794–1796.
3. Barnes KC. Evidence for common genetic elements in allergic disease. J Allergy Clin Immunol 2000; 106:S192–S200.
4. Busse WW, Lemanske RF. Asthma. N Engl J Med 2001; 344:350–362.
5. Howarth PH, Salagean M, Dokic D. Allergic rhinitis: not purely a histamine-related disease. Allergy 2000; 55(Suppl 64):7–16.
6. Wang DY, Clement P. Pathogenic mechanisms underlying the clinical symptoms of allergic rhinitis. Am J Rhinol 2000; 14:325–333.
7. Leung DY, Soter NA. Cellular and immunologic mechanisms in atopic dermatitis. J Am Acad Dermatol 2001; 44:S1–S12.
8. Leonardi-Bee J, Pritchard D, Britton J. Asthma and current intestinal parasite infection: systematic review and meta-analysis. Am J Respir Crit Care Med 2006; 174:514–523.
9. Bousquet J, Vignola AM, Demoly P. Links between rhinitis and asthma. Allergy 2003; 58:691–706.

Inflammatory cells

10. Boguniewicz M, Schmid-Grendelmeier P, Leung DY. Atopic dermatitis. J Allergy Clin Immunol 2006; 118:40–43.
11. Bradding P, Walls AF, Holgate ST. The role of the mast cell in the pathophysiology of asthma. J Allergy Clin Immunol 2006; 117:1277–1284.
12. Brightling CE, Bradding P, Symon FA, et al. Mast-cell infiltration of airway smooth muscle in asthma. N Engl J Med 2002; 346:1699–1705.
13. Bentley AM, Hamid Q, Robinson DS, et al. Prednisolone treatment in asthma. Reduction in the numbers of eosinophils, T cells, tryptase-only positive mast cells, and modulation of IL-4, IL-5, and interferon-gamma cytokine gene expression within the bronchial mucosa. Am J Respir Crit Care Med 1996; 153:551–556.
14. Reed CE, Kita H. The role of protease activation of inflammation in allergic respiratory diseases. J Allergy Clin Immunol 2004; 114:997–1008.
15. Galli SJ, Kalesnikoff J, Grimbaldeston MA, et al. Mast cells as 'tunable' effector and immunoregulatory cells: recent advances. Annu Rev Immunol 2005; 23:749–786.
16. Reber L, Da Silva CA, Frossard N. Stem cell factor and its receptor c-Kit as targets for inflammatory diseases. Eur J Pharmacol 2006; 533:327–340.
17. Fahy JV. Anti-IgE: lessons learned from effects on airway inflammation and asthma exacerbation. J Allergy Clin Immunol 2006; 117:1230–1232.
18. Peters-Golden M. The alveolar macrophage: the forgotten cell in asthma. Am J Respir Cell Mol Biol 2004; 31:3–7.
19. Menard G, Bissonnette EY. Priming of alveolar macrophages by leukotriene D(4): potentiation of inflammation. Am J Respir Cell Mol Biol 2000; 23:572–577.
20. Spiteri MA, Knight RA, Jeremy JY, et al. Alveolar macrophage-induced suppression of peripheral blood mononuclear cell responsiveness is reversed by in vitro allergen exposure in bronchial asthma. Eur Resp J 1994; 7:1431–1438.
21. John M, Lim S, Seybold J, et al. Inhaled corticosteroids increase IL-10 but reduce MIP-1α, GM-CSF and IFN-γ release from alveolar macrophages in asthma. Am J Respir Crit Care Med 1998; 157:256–262.
22. Tang C, Ward C, Reid D, et al. Normally suppressing CD40 coregulatory signals delivered by airway macrophages to TH2 lymphocytes are defective in patients with atopic asthma. J Allergy Clin Immunol 2001; 107:863–870.
23. Taylor PR, Martinez-Pomares L, Stacey M, et al. Macrophage receptors and immune recognition. Annu Rev Immunol 2005; 23:901–944.
24. Zeibecoglou K, Ying S, Meng Q, et al. Macrophage subpopulations and macrophage-derived cytokines in sputum of atopic and nonatopic asthmatic subjects and atopic and normal control subjects. J Allergy Clin Immunol 2000; 106:697–704.
25. Holt PG, Upham JW. The role of dendritic cells in asthma. Curr Opin Allergy Clin Immunol 2004; 4:39–44.
26. Hammad H, Lambrecht BN. Recent progress in the biology of airway dendritic cells and implications for understanding the regulation of asthmatic inflammation. J Allergy Clin Immunol 2006; 118:331–336.
27. Novak N. Targeting dendritic cells in allergen immunotherapy. Immunol Allergy Clin North Am 2006; 26:307–319. viii.
28. Rothenberg ME, Hogan SP. The eosinophil. Annu Rev Immunol 2006; 24:147–174.
29. Yukawa T, Read RC, Kroegel C, et al. The effects of activated eosinophils and neutrophils on guinea pig airway epithelium in vitro. Am J Respir Cell Mol Biol 1990; 2:341–354.
30. Woolley MJ, Denburg JA, Ellis R, et al. Allergen-induced changes in bone marrow progenitors and airway responsiveness in dogs and the effect of inhaled budesonide on these parameters. Am J Respir Cell Mol Biol 1994; 11:600–606.
31. Tachimoto H, Bochner BS. The surface phenotype of human eosinophils. Chem Immunol 2000; 76:45–62.
32. Wegner CD, Gundel L, Reilly P, et al. Intracellular adhesion molecule-1 (ICAM-1) in the pathogenesis of asthma. Science 1990; 247:456–459.
33. Wardlaw AJ. Molecular basis for selective eosinophil trafficking in asthma: a multistep paradigm. J Allergy Clin Immunol 1999; 104:917–926.
34. Chanez P, Dent G, Yukawa T, et al. Generation of oxygen free radicals from blood eosinophils from asthma patients after stimulation with PAF or phorbol ester. Eur Respir J 1990; 3:1002–1007.
35. Evans DJ, Lindsay MA, O'Connor BJ, et al. Priming of circulating human eosinophils following exposure to allergen challenge. Eur Respir J 1996; 9:703–708.

36. Collins PD, Marleau S, Griffiths-Johnson DA, et al. Cooperation between interleukin-5 and the chemokine eotaxin to induce eosinophil accumulation in vivo. J Exp Med 1995; 182:1169–1174.
37. Park CS, Choi YS, Ki SY, et al. Granulocyte macrophage colony-stimulating factor is the main cytokine enhancing the survival of eosinophils in asthmatic airways. Eur Respir J 1998; 12:872–878.
38. Leckie MJ, ten Brincke A, Khan J, et al. Effects of an interleukin-5 blocking monoclonal antibody on eosinophils, airway hyperresponsiveness and the late asthmatic response. Lancet 2000; 356:2144–2148.
39. Kips JC, O'Connor BJ, Langley SJ, et al. Effect of SCH55700, a humanized anti-human interleukin-5 antibody, in severe persistent asthma: a pilot study. Am J Respir Crit Care Med 2003; 167:1655–1659.
40. Flood-Page PT, Menzies-Gow AN, Kay AB, et al. Eosinophil's role remains uncertain as anti-interleukin-5 only partially depletes numbers in asthmatic airways. Am J Respir Crit Care Med 2003; 167:199–204.
41. Flood-Page P, Menzies-Gow A, Phipps S, et al. Anti-IL-5 treatment reduces deposition of ECM proteins in the bronchial subepithelial basement membrane of mild atopic asthmatics. J Clin Invest 2003; 112:1029–1036.
42. Wenzel SE, Szefler SJ, Leung DY, et al. Bronchoscopic evaluation of severe asthma. Persistent inflammation associated with high dose glucocorticoids. Am J Respir Crit Care Med 1997; 156:737–743.
43. Jatakanon A, Uasaf C, Maziak W, et al. Neutrophilic inflammation in severe persistent asthma. Am J Respir Crit Care Med 1999; 160:1532–1539.
44. Gibson PG, Simpson JL, Saltos N. Heterogeneity of airway inflammation in persistent asthma: evidence of neutrophilic inflammation and increased sputum interleukin-8. Chest 2001; 119:1329–1336.
45. Sur S, Crotty TB, Kephart GM, et al. Sudden onset fatal asthma: a distinct entity with few eosinophils and relatively more neutrophils in the airway submucosa. Am Rev Respir Dis 1993; 148:713–719.
46. Meagher LC, Cousin JM, Seckl JR, et al. Opposing effects of glucocorticoids on the rate of apoptosis in neutrophilic and eosinophilic granulocytes. J Immunol 1996; 156:4422–4428.
47. Montuschi P, Ciabattoni G, Corradi M, et al. Increased 8-isoprostane, a marker of oxidative stress, in exhaled condensates of asthmatic patients. Am J Respir Crit Care Med 1999; 160:216–220.
48. Kay AB. The role of T lymphocytes in asthma. Chem Immunol Allergy 2006; 91:59–75.
49. Prescott SL, Macaubas C, Smallacombe T, et al. Development of allergen-specific T-cell memory in atopic and normal children. Lancet 1999; 353:196–200.
50. Holt PG, Sly PD. Prevention of adult asthma by early intervention during childhood: potential value of new generation immunomodulatory drugs. Thorax 2000; 55:700–703.
51. Ball TM, Castro-Rodriguez JA, Griffith KA, et al. Siblings, day-care attendance, and the risk of asthma and wheezing during childhood. N Engl J Med 2000; 343:538–543.
52. Christiansen SC. Day care, siblings, and asthma – please, sneeze on my child. N Engl J Med 2000; 343:574–575.
53. Naseer T, Minshall EM, Leung DY, et al. Expression of IL-12 and IL-13 mRNA in asthma and their modulation in response to steroids. Am J Respir Crit Care Med 1997; 155:845–851.
54. Wills-Karp M, Luyimbazi J, Xu X, et al. Interleukin-13: central mediator of allergic asthma. Science 1998; 282:2258–2261.
55. Zhu Z, Homer RJ, Wang Z, et al. Pulmonary expression of interleukin-13 causes inflammation, mucus hypersecretion, subepithelial fibrosis, physiologic abnormalities, and eotaxin production. J Clin Invest 1999; 103:779–788.
56. Akbari O, Faul JL, Hoyte EG, et al. CD4+ invariant T-cell-receptor+ natural killer T cells in bronchial asthma. N Engl J Med 2006; 354:1117–1129.
57. Meyer EH, Goya S, Akbari O, et al. Glycolipid activation of invariant T cell receptor+ NK T cells is sufficient to induce airway hyperreactivity independent of conventional CD4+ T cells. Proc Natl Acad Sci U S A 2006; 103:2782–2787.
58. Sen Y, Yongyi B, Yuling H, et al. V alpha 24-invariant NKT cells from patients with allergic asthma express CCR9 at high frequency and induce Th2 bias of CD3+ T cells upon CD226 engagement. J Immunol 2005; 175:4914–4926.
59. Umetsu DT, Akbari O, DeKruyff RH. Regulatory T cells control the development of allergic disease and asthma. J Allergy Clin Immunol 2003; 112:480–487.
60. Ling EM, Smith T, Nguyen XD, et al. Relation of CD4+CD25+ regulatory T-cell suppression of allergen-driven T-cell activation to atopic status and expression of allergic disease. Lancet 2004; 363:608–615.
61. Akdis M, Blaser K, Akdis CA. T regulatory cells in allergy: novel concepts in the pathogenesis, prevention, and treatment of allergic diseases. J Allergy Clin Immunol 2005; 116:961–968.
62. van Rensen EL, Sont JK, Evertse CE, et al. Bronchial CD8 cell infiltrate and lung function decline in asthma. Am J Respir Crit Care Med 2005; 172:837–841.
63. Gelfand EW, Dakhama A. CD8+ T lymphocytes and leukotriene B4: novel interactions in the persistence and progression of asthma. J Allergy Clin Immunol 2006; 117:577–582.
64. Cho SH, Stanciu LA, Holgate ST, et al. Increased interleukin-4, interleukin-5, and interferon-gamma in airway CD4+ and CD8+ T cells in atopic asthma. Am J Respir Crit Care Med 2005; 171:224–230.
65. Gould HJ, Beavil RL, Vercelli D. IgE isotype determination: epsilon-germline gene transcription, DNA recombination and B-cell differentiation. Br Med Bull 2000; 56:908–924.
66. Humbert M, Menz G, Ying S, et al. The immunopathology of extrinsic (atopic) and intrinsic (non-atopic) asthma: more similarities than differences. Immunol Today 1999; 20:528–533.
67. Marone G, Triggiani M, de Paulis A. Mast cells and basophils: friends as well as foes in bronchial asthma? Trends Immunol 2005; 26:25–31.
68. Macfarlane AJ, Kon OM, Smith SJ, et al. Basophils, eosinophils, and mast cells in atopic and nonatopic asthma and in late-phase allergic reactions in the lung and skin. J Allergy Clin Immunol 2000; 105:99–107.
69. Braunstahl GJ, Overbeek SE, Fokkens WJ, et al. Segmental bronchoprovocation in allergic rhinitis patients affects mast cell and basophil numbers in nasal and bronchial mucosa. Am J Respir Crit Care Med 2001; 164:858–865.

REFERENCES

70. Gauvreau GM, Lee JM, Watson RM, et al. Increased numbers of both airway basophils and mast cells in sputum after allergen inhalation challenge of atopic asthmatics. Am J Respir Crit Care Med 2000; 161:1473–1478.

71. Holgate ST. The role of mast cells and basophils in inflammation. Clin Exp Allergy 2000; 30 (Suppl 1):28–32.

72. Knol EF, Mul FP, Lie WJ, et al. The role of basophils in allergic disease. Eur Respir J Suppl 1996; 22:126s–131s.

73. Herd CM, Page CP. Pulmonary immune cells in health and disease: platelets. Eur Respir J 1994; 7:1145–1160.

74. Sullivan PJ, Jafar ZH, Harbinson PL, et al. Platelet dynamics following allergen challenge in allergic asthmatics. Respiration 2000; 67:514–517.

75. Moritani C, Ishioka S, Haruta Y, et al. Activation of platelets in bronchial asthma. Chest 1998; 113:452–458.

76. Abi-Younes S, Si-Tahar M, Luster AD. The CC chemokines MDC and TARC induce platelet activation via CCR4. Thromb Res 2001; 101:279–289.

77. Johnson SR, Knox AJ. Synthetic functions of airway smooth muscle in asthma. Trends Pharmacol Sci 1997; 18:288–292.

78. Chung KF. Airway smooth muscle cells: contributing to and regulating airway mucosal inflammation? Eur Respir J 2000; 15:961–968.

Inflammatory mediators

79. Barnes PJ, Chung KF, Page CP. Inflammatory mediators of asthma: an update. Pharmacol Rev 1998; 50:515–596.

80. Wilson SJ, Lau L, Howarth PH. Inflammatory mediators in naturally occurring rhinitis. Clin Exp Allergy 1998; 28:220–227.

81. van Ganse E, Kaufman L, Derde MP, et al. Effcts of antihistamines in adult asthma: a meta-analysis of clinical trials. Eur Respir J 1997; 10:2216–2224.

82. Drazen JM, Israel E, O'Byrne PM. Treatment of asthma with drugs modifying the leukotriene pathway. N Engl J Med 1999; 340:197–206.

83. Pullerits T, Praks L, Skoogh BE, et al. Randomized placebo-controlled study comparing a leukotriene receptor antagonist and a nasal glucocorticoid in seasonal allergic rhinitis. Am J Respir Crit Care Med 1999; 159:1814–1818.

84. Zhu J, Qiu YS, Figueroa DJ, et al. Localization and upregulation of cysteinyl leukotriene-1 receptor in asthmatic bronchial mucosa. Am J Respir Cell Mol Biol 2005; 33:531–540.

85. Leff JA, Busse WW, Pearlman D, et al. Montelukast, a leukotriene-receptor antagonist, for the treatment of mild asthma and exercise-induced bronchoconstriction [see comments]. N Engl J Med 1998; 339:147–152.

86. Adelroth E, Inman MD, Summers E, et al. Prolonged protection against exercise-induced bronchoconstriction by the leukotriene D4-receptor antagonist cinalukast. J Allergy Clin Immunol 1997; 99:210–215.

87. Taylor IK, O'Shaughnessy KM, Fuller RW, et al. Effect of cysteinyl-leukotriene receptor antagonist ICI 204,219 on allergen-induced bronchoconstriction and airway hyperreactivity in atopic subjects. Lancet 1991; 337:690–694.

88. Hamilton A, Faiferman I, Stober P, et al. Pranlukast, a cysteinyl leukotriene receptor antagonist, attenuates allergen-induced early- and late-phase bronchoconstriction and airway hyperresponsiveness in asthmatic subjects. J Allergy Clin Immunol 1998; 102:177–183.

89. Roquet A, Dahlen B, Kumlin M, et al. Combined antagonism of leukotrienes and histamine produces predominant inhibition of allergen-induced early and late phase airway obstruction in asthmatics. Am J Respir Crit Care Med 1997; 155:1856–1863.

90. Meltzer EO, Malmstrom K, Lu S, et al. Concomitant montelukast and loratadine as treatment for seasonal allergic rhinitis: a randomized, placebo-controlled clinical trial. J Allergy Clin Immunol 2000; 105:917–922.

91. Borish LC, Nelson HS, Corren J, et al. Efficacy of soluble IL-4 receptor for the treatment of adults with asthma. J Allergy Clin Immunol 2001; 107:963–970.

92. Kim KT, Ginchansky EJ, Friedman BF, et al. Fluticasone propionate versus zafirlukast: effect in patients previously receiving inhaled corticosteroid therapy. Ann Allergy Asthma Immunol 2000; 85:398–406.

93. Diamant Z, Hiltermann JT, van Rensen EL, et al. The effect of inhaled leukotriene D4 and methacholine on sputum cell differentials in asthma. Am J Respir Crit Care Med 1997; 155:1247–1253.

94. Barnes PJ. Anti-leukotrienes: here to stay? Curr Opin Pharmacol 2003; 3:257–263.

95. Luster AD, Tager AM. T-cell trafficking in asthma: lipid mediators grease the way. Nat Rev Immunol 2004; 4:711–724.

96. Chung KF. Platelet-activating factor in inflammation and pulmonary disorders. Clin Sci (Lond) 1992; 83:127–138.

97. Freitag A, Watson RM, Mabos G, et al. Effect of a platelet activating factor antagonist, WEB 2086, on allergen induced asthmatic responses. Thorax 1993; 48:594–598.

98. Spence DPS, Johnston SL, Calverley PMA, et al. The effect of the orally active platelet-activating factor antagonist WEB 2086 in the treatment of asthma. Am J Respir Crit Care Med 1994; 149:1142–1148.

99. Kuitert LM, Angus RM, Barnes NC, et al. The effect of a novel potent PAF antagonist, modipafant, in chronic asthma. Am J Respir Crit Care Med 1995; 151:1331–1335.

100. Stafforini DM, Numao T, Tsodikov A, et al. Deficiency of platelet-activating factor acetylhydrolase is a severity factor for asthma. J Clin Invest 1999; 103:989–997.

101. Taha R, Olivenstein R, Utsumi T, et al. Prostaglandin H synthase 2 expression in airway cells from patients with asthma and chronic obstructive pulmonary disease. Am J Respir Crit Care Med 2000; 161:636–640.

102. Cowburn AS, Sladek K, Soja J, et al. Overexpression of leukotriene C4 synthase in bronchial biopsies from patients with aspirin-intolerant asthma. J Clin Invest 1998; 101:834–846.

103. Hirai H, Tanaka K, Yoshie O, et al. Prostaglandin D2 selectively induces chemotaxis in T helper type 2 cells, eosinophils, and basophils via seven-transmembrane receptor CRTH2. J Exp Med 2001; 193:255–261.

104. Kostenis E, Ulven T. Emerging roles of DP and CRTH2 in allergic inflammation. Trends Mol Med 2006; 12:148–158.

105. Ulven T, Kostenis E. Targeting the prostaglandin D2 receptors DP and CRTH2 for treatment of inflammation. Curr Top Med Chem 2006; 6:1427–1444.

106. Powell WS, Rokach J. Biochemistry, biology and chemistry of the 5-lipoxygenase product 5-oxo-ETE. Prog Lipid Res 2005; 44:154–183.

107. Montuschi P, Barnes PJ, Roberts LJ. Isoprostanes: markers and mediators of oxidative stress. FASEB J 2004; 18:1791–1800.

108. Chung KF, Barnes PJ. Cytokines in asthma. Thorax 1999; 54:825–857.

109. Barnes PJ. Cytokine-directed therapies for the treatment of chronic airway diseases. Cytokine Growth Factor Rev 2003; 14:511–522.

110. Greenfeder S, Umland SP, Cuss FM, et al. The role of interleukin-5 in allergic eosinophilic disease. Respir Res 2001; 2:71–79.

111. Wills-Karp M. Interleukin-13 in asthma pathogenesis. Immunol Rev 2004; 202:175–190. 175–190.

112. Zhou Y, McLane M, Levitt RC. Interleukin-9 as a therapeutic target for asthma. Respir Res 2001; 2:80–84.

113. Thomas PS. Tumour necrosis factor-alpha: the role of this multifunctional cytokine in asthma. Immunol Cell Biol 2001; 79:132–140.

114. Berry MA, Hargadon B, Shelley M, et al. Evidence of a role of tumor necrosis factor alpha in refractory asthma. N Engl J Med 2006; 354:697–708.

115. Kawaguchi M, Adachi M, Oda N, et al. IL-17 cytokine family. J Allergy Clin Immunol 2004; 114:1265–1273.

116. Iwakura Y, Ishigame H. The IL-23/IL-17 axis in inflammation. J Clin Invest 2006; 116:1218–1222.

117. Liu YJ. Thymic stromal lymphopoietin: master switch for allergic inflammation. J Exp Med 2006; 203:269–273.

118. Huston DP, Liu YJ. Thymic stromal lymphopoietin: a potential therapeutic target for allergy and asthma. Curr Allergy Asthma Rep 2006; 6:372–376.

119. Ying S, O'Connor B, Ratoff J, et al. Thymic stromal lymphopoietin expression is increased in asthmatic airways and correlates with expression of Th2-attracting chemokines and disease severity. J Immunol 2005; 174:8183–8190.

120. Rossi D, Zlotnik A. The biology of chemokines and their receptors. Annu Rev Immunol 2000; 18:217–242.

121. Wells TN, Power CA, Shaw JP, et al. Chemokine blockers – therapeutics in the making? Trends Pharmacol Sci 2006; 27:41–47.

122. Gutierrez-Ramos JC, Lloyd C, Kapsenberg ML, et al. Non-redundant functional groups of chemokines operate in a coordinate manner during the inflammatory response in the lung. Immunol Rev 2000; 177:31–42.

123. Gutierrez-Ramos JC, Lloyd C, Gonzalo JA. Eotaxin: from an eosinophilic chemokine to a major regulator of allergic reactions. Immunol Today 1999; 20:500–504.

124. Ying S, Meng Q, Zeibecoglou K, et al. Eosinophil chemotactic chemokines (eotaxin, eotaxin-2, RANTES, monocyte chemoattractant protein-3 (MCP-3), and MCP-4), and C-C chemokine receptor 3 expression in bronchial biopsies from atopic and nonatopic (Intrinsic) asthmatics. J Immunol 1999; 163:6321–6329.

125. Erin EM, Williams TJ, Barnes PJ, et al. Eotaxin receptor (CCR3) antagonism in asthma and allergic disease. Curr Drug Targets Inflamm Allergy 2002; 1:201–214.

126. Berkman N, Krishnan VL, Gilbey T, et al. Expression of RANTES mRNA and protein in airways of patients with mild asthma. Am J Respir Crit Care Med 1996; 15:382–389.

127. Gonzalo JA, Lloyd CM, Kremer L, et al. Eosinophil recruitment to the lung in a murine model of allergic inflammation. The role of T cells, chemokines, and adhesion receptors. J Clin Invest 1996; 98:2332–2345.

128. Campbell EM, Charo IF, Kunkel SL, et al. Monocyte chemoattractant protein-1 mediates cockroach allergen-induced bronchial hyperreactivity in normal but not CCR2-/- mice: the role of mast cells. J Immunol 1999; 163:2160–2167.

129. Holgate ST, Bodey KS, Janezic A, et al. Release of RANTES, MIP-1 alpha, and MCP-1 into asthmatic airways following endobronchial allergen challenge. Am J Respir Crit Care Med 1997; 156:1377–1383.

130. Lloyd CM, Delaney T, Nguyen T, et al. CC chemokine receptor (CCR)3/eotaxin is followed by CCR4/monocyte-derived chemokine in mediating pulmonary T helper lymphocyte type 2 recruitment after serial antigen challenge in vivo. J Exp Med 2000; 191:265–274.

131. Berin MC, Eckmann L, Broide DH, et al. Regulated production of the T helper 2-type T-cell chemoattractant TARC by human bronchial epithelial cells in vitro and in human lung xenografts. Am J Respir Cell Mol Biol 2001; 24:382–389.

132. Sekiya T, Miyamasu M, Imanishi M, et al. Inducible expression of a Th2-type CC chemokine thymus- and activation-regulated chemokine by human bronchial epithelial cells. J Immunol 2000; 165:2205–2213.

133. Paredi P, Kharitonov SA, Barnes PJ. Elevation of exhaled ethane concentration in asthma. Am J Respir Crit Care Med 2000; 162:1450–1454.

134. Barnes PJ. Reactive oxygen species in asthma. Eur Respir Rev 2000; 10:240–243.

135. Ricciardolo FL, Sterk PJ, Gaston B, et al. Nitric oxide in health and disease of the respiratory system. Physiol Rev 2004; 84:731–765.

136. Silkoff PE, Sylvester JT, Zamel N, et al. Airway nitric oxide diffusion in asthma: role in pulmonary function and bronchial responsiveness. Am J Respir Crit Care Med 2000; 161:1218–1228.

137. Kharitonov SA, Barnes PJ. Clinical aspects of exhaled nitric oxide. Eur Respir J 2000; 16:781–792.

138. Jatakanon A, Lim S, Kharitonov SA, et al. Correlation between exhaled nitric oxide, sputum eosinophils and methacholine responsiveness. Thorax 1998; 53:91–95.

139. Lim S, Jatakanon A, Meah S, et al. Relationship between exhaled nitric oxide and mucosal eosinophilic inflammation in mild to moderately severe asthma. Thorax 2000; 55:184–188.

140. Saleh D, Ernst P, Lim S, et al. Increased formation of the potent oxidant peroxynitrite in the airways of asthmatic patients is associated with induction of nitric oxide synthase: effect of inhaled glucocorticoid. FASEB J 1998; 12:929–937.

141. Sugiura H, Ichinose M, Tomaki M, et al. Quantitative assessment of protein-bound tyrosine nitration in airway secretions from patients with inflammatory airway disease. Free Radic Res 2004; 38:49–57.

142. Kharitonov SA, Rajakulasingam K, O'Connor BJ, et al. Nasal nitric oxide is increased in patients with asthma and allergic rhinitis and may be modulated by nasal glucocorticoids. J Allergy Clin Immunol 1997; 99:58–64.
143. Kharitonov SA, Barnes PJ. Exhaled markers of pulmonary disease. Am J Respir Crit Care Med 2001; 163:1693–1772.

Effects of inflammation

144. Lange P, Parner J, Vestbo J, et al. A 15-year follow-up study of ventilatory function in adults with asthma. N Engl J Med 1998; 339:1194–1200.
145. Ulrik CS, Lange P. Decline of lung function in adults with bronchial asthma. Am J Respir Crit Care Med 1994; 150:629–634.
146. James AL, Palmer LJ, Kicic E, et al. Decline in lung function in the Busselton Health Study: the effects of asthma and cigarette smoking. Am J Respir Crit Care Med 2005; 171:109–114.
147. Holgate ST, Davies DE, Lackie PM, et al. Epithelial-mesenchymal interactions in the pathogenesis of asthma. J Allergy Clin Immunol 2000; 105:193–204.
148. Tschumperlin DJ, Drazen JM. Chronic effects of mechanical force on airways. Annu Rev Physiol 2006; 68:563–583. 563–583.
149. Redington AE. Fibrosis and airway remodelling. Clin Exp Allergy 2000; 30(Suppl 1):42–45.
150. James A. Airway remodeling in asthma. Curr Opin Pulm Med 2005; 11:1–6.
151. Birring SS, Brightling CE, Bradding P, et al. Clinical, radiologic, and induced sputum features of chronic obstructive pulmonary disease in nonsmokers: a descriptive study. Am J Respir Crit Care Med 2002; 166:1078–1083.
152. Redington AE, Howarth PH. Airway wall remodelling in asthma [editorial]. Thorax 1997; 52:310–312.
153. Wilson JW, Li X. The measurement of reticular basement membrane and submucosal collagen in the asthmatic airway [see comments]. Clin Exp Allergy 1997; 27:363–371.
154. Cox G, Miller JD, McWilliams A, et al. Bronchial thermoplasty for asthma. Am J Respir Crit Care Med 2006; 173:965–969.
155. Barnes PJ. Pharmacology of airway smooth muscle. Am J Respir Crit Care Med 1998; 158:S123–S132.
156. Bai TR, Mak JCW, Barnes PJ. A comparison of beta-adrenergic receptors and in vitro relaxant responses to isoproterenol in asthmatic airway smooth muscle. Am J Respir Cell Mol Biol 1992; 6:647–651.
157. Koto H, Mak JCW, Haddad E-B, et al. Mechanisms of impaired β-adrenergic receptor relaxation by interleukin-1β in vivo in rat. J Clin Invest 1996; 98:1780–1787.
158. Laporte JD, Moore PE, Panettieri RA, et al. Prostanoids mediate IL-1beta-induced beta-adrenergic hyporesponsiveness in human airway smooth muscle cells. Am J Physiol 1998; 275:L491–L501.
159. Grandordy BM, Mak JCW, Barnes PJ. Modulation of airway smooth muscle β-receptor function by a muscarinic agonist. Life Sci 1994; 54:185–191.
160. Benayoun L, Druilhe A, Dombret MC, et al. Airway structural alterations selectively associated with severe asthma. Am J Respir Crit Care Med 2003; 167:1360–1368.
161. Hirst SJ, Walker TR, Chilvers ER. Phenotypic diversity and molecular mechanisms of airway smooth muscle proliferation in asthma. Eur Respir J 2000; 16:159–177.
162. Lazaar AL, Panettieri RA Jr. Airway smooth muscle as a regulator of immune responses and bronchomotor tone. Clin Chest Med 2006; 27:53–69, vi.
163. Kumar SD, Emery MJ, Atkins ND, et al. Airway mucosal blood flow in bronchial asthma. Am J Respir Crit Care Med 1998; 158:153–156.
164. Paredi P, Kharitonov SA, Barnes PJ. Faster rise of exhaled breath temperature in asthma. A novel marker of airway inflammation? Am J Respir Crit Care Med 2002; 165:181–184.
165. Paredi P, Kharitonov SA, Barnes PJ. Correlation of exhaled breath temperature with bronchial blood flow in asthma. Respir Res 2005; 6:15.
166. Malek AM, Jiang L, Lee I, et al. Induction of nitric oxide synthase mRNA by shear stress requires intracellular calcium and G-protein signals and is modulated by PI 3 kinase. Biochem Biophys Res Commun 1999; 254:231–242.
167. Tanaka H, Yamada G, Saikai T, et al. Increased airway vascularity in newly diagnosed asthma using a high-magnification bronchovideoscope. Am J Respir Crit Care Med 2003; 168:1495–1499.
168. Hashimoto M, Tanaka H, Abe S. Quantitative analysis of bronchial wall vascularity in the medium and small airways of patients with asthma and COPD. Chest 2005; 127:965–972.
169. Wilson JW. The bronchial microcirculation in asthma. Clin Exp Allergy 2000; 30(Suppl 1):51–53. 51–53.
170. Feltis BN, Wignarajah D, Zheng L, et al. Increased vascular endothelial growth factor and receptors: relationship to angiogenesis in asthma. Am J Respir Crit Care Med 2006; 173:1201–1207.
171. Chung KF, Rogers DF, Barnes PJ, et al. The role of increased airway microvascular permeability and plasma exudation in asthma. Eur Respir J 1990; 3:329–337.
172. Persson CG, Andersson M, Greiff L, et al. Airway permeability. Clin Exp Allergy 1995; 25:807–814.
173. Yager D, Martins MA, Feldman H, et al. Acute histamine-induced flux of airway liquid: role of neuropeptides. J Appl Physiol 1996; 80:1285–1295.
174. Raphael GD, Meredith SC, Baraniuk JN, et al. The pathophysiology of rhinitis. II Assessment of the sources of protein in histamine-induced nasal secretions. Am Rev Respir Dis 1989; 139:791–800.
175. Morcillo EJ, Cortijo J. Mucus and MUC in asthma. Curr Opin Pulm Med 2006; 12:1–6.
176. Martinez-Anton A, Roca-Ferrer J, Mullol J. Mucin gene expression in rhinitis syndromes. Curr Allergy Asthma Rep 2006; 6:189–197.
177. Burgel PR, Nadel JA. Roles of epidermal growth factor receptor activation in epithelial cell repair and mucin production in airway epithelium. Thorax 2004; 59:992–996.
178. Ordonez CL, Khashayar R, Wong HH, et al. Mild and moderate asthma is associated with airway goblet cell hyperplasia and abnormalities in mucin gene expression. Am J Respir Crit Care Med 2001; 163:517–523.
179. Nakanishi A, Morita S, Iwashita H, et al. Role of gob-5 in mucus overproduction and airway hyperresponsiveness in asthma. Proc Natl Acad Sci U S A 2001; 98:5175–5180.
180. Robichaud A, Tuck SA, Kargman S, et al. Gob-5 is not essential for mucus overproduction in preclinical murine models of allergic asthma. Am J Respir Cell Mol Biol 2005; 33:303–314.
181. Barnes PJ. Is asthma a nervous disease? Chest 1995; 107:119S–124S.
182. Barnes PJ, Baraniuk J, Belvisi MG. Neuropeptides in the respiratory tract. Am Rev Respir Dis 1991; 144:1187–1198. 1391–1399.
183. Joos GF, Germonpre PR, Pauwels RA. Role of tachykinins in asthma. Allergy 2000; 55:321–337.
184. Barnes PJ. Modulation of neurotransmission in airways. Physiol Rev 1992; 72:699–729.
185. Undem BJ, Kollarik M. The role of vagal afferent nerves in chronic obstructive pulmonary disease. Proc Am Thorac Soc 2005; 2:355–360.
186. Fox AJ, Lalloo UG, Belvisi MG, et al. Bradykinin-evoked sensitization of airway sensory nerves: a mechanism for ACE-inhibitor cough. Nature Med 1996; 2:814–817.
187. Geppetti P, Materazzi S, Nicoletti P. The transient receptor potential vanilloid 1: role in airway inflammation and disease. Eur J Pharmacol 2006; 533:207–214.
188. Nockher WA, Renz H. Neurotrophins and asthma: novel insight into neuroimmune interaction. J Allergy Clin Immunol 2006; 117:67–71.
189. Nassenstein C, Schulte-Herbruggen O, Renz H, et al. Nerve growth factor: the central hub in the development of allergic asthma? Eur J Pharmacol 2006; 533:195–206.
190. Fox AJ, Patel HJ, Barnes PJ, et al. Release of nerve growth factor by human pulmonary epithelial cells: role in airway inflammatory diseases. Eur J Pharmacol 2001; 424:159–162.
191. Lammers JWJ, Barnes PJ, Chung KF. Non-adrenergic, non-cholinergic airway inhibitory nerves. Eur Respir J 1992; 5:239–246.
192. Ollerenshaw S, Jarvis D, Woolcock A, et al. Absence of immunoreactive vasoactive intestinal polypeptide in tissue from the lungs of patients with asthma. N Engl J Med 1989; 320:1244–1248.
193. Howarth PH, Springall DR, Redington AE, et al. Neuropeptide-containing nerves in bronchial biopsies from asthmatic and non-asthmatic subjects. Am J Respir Cell Mol Biol 1995; 13:288–296.
194. Belvisi MG, Stretton CD, Barnes PJ. Nitric oxide is the endogenous neurotransmitter of bronchodilator nerves in human airways. Eur J Pharmacol 1992; 210:221–222.
195. Barnes PJ. Sensory nerves, neuropeptides and asthma. Ann NY Acad Sci 1991; 629:359–370.
196. Barnes PJ. Neurogenic inflammation in the airways. Respir Physiol 2001; 125:145–154.
197. Ollerenshaw SL, Jarvis D, Sullivan CE, et al. Substance P immunoreactive nerves in airways from asthmatics and non-asthmatics. Eur Resp J 1991; 4:673–682.
198. Nadel JA. Neutral endopeptidase modulates neurogenic inflammation. Eur Resp J 1991; 4:745–754.
199. Sanico AM, Atsuta S, Proud D, et al. Dose-dependent effects of capsaicin nasal challenge: in vivo evidence of human airway neurogenic inflammation. J Allergy Clin Immunol 1997; 100:632–641.

Transcription factors

200. Barnes PJ, Adcock IM. Transcription factors and asthma. Eur Respir J 1998; 12:221–234.
201. Barnes PJ. Transcription factors in airway diseases. Lab Invest 2006; 86:867–872.
202. Barnes PJ, Karin M. Nuclear factor-κB: a pivotal transcription factor in chronic inflammatory diseases. N Engl J Med 1997; 336:1066–1071.
203. Hart LA, Krishnan VL, Adcock IM, et al. Activation and localization of transcription factor, nuclear factor-kB, in asthma. Am J Respir Crit Care Med 1998; 158:1585–1592.
204. Demoly P, Basset-Seguin N, Chanez P, et al. c-Fos proto-oncogene expression in bronchial biopsies of asthmatics. Am J Respir Cell Mol Biol 1992; 7:128–133.
205. Barnes PJ, Adcock IM, Ito K. Histone acetylation and deacetylation: importance in inflammatory lung diseases. Eur Respir J 2005; 25:552–563.
206. Adcock IM, Ford P, Barnes PJ, et al. Epigenetics and airways disease. Respir Res 2006; 7:21.
207. Barnes PJ. How corticosteroids control inflammation. Br J Pharmacol 2006; 148:245–254.
208. Zhu J, Yamane H, Cote-Sierra J, et al. GATA-3 promotes Th2 responses through three different mechanisms: induction of Th2 cytokine production, selective growth of Th2 cells and inhibition of Th1 cell-specific factors. Cell Res 2006; 16:3–10.
209. Maneechotesuwan K, Xin Y, Ito K, et al. Regulation of Th2 cytokine genes by p38 MAPK-mediated phosphorylation of GATA-3. J Immunol 2007; 178:2491–2498.
210. Peng SL. The T-box transcription factor T-bet in immunity and autoimmunity. Cell Mol Immunol 2006; 3:87–95.
211. Li B, Samanta A, Song X, et al. FOXP3 ensembles in T-cell regulation. Immunol Rev 2006; 212:99–113.
212. Kiwamoto T, Ishii Y, Morishima Y, et al. Transcription factors T-bet and GATA-3 regulate development of airway remodeling. Am J Respir Crit Care Med 2006; 174:142–151.
213. Caramori G, Lim S, Ito K, et al. Expression of GATA family of transcription factors in T-cells, monocytes and bronchial biopsies. Eur Respir J 2001; 18:466–473.

Antiinflammatory mechanisms in allergy

214. Herrscher RF, Kasper C, Sullivan TJ. Endogenous cortisol regulates immunoglobulin E-dependent late phase reactions. J Clin Invest 1992; 90:593–603.
215. Orsida BE, Krozowski ZS, Walters EH. Clinical relevance of airway 11beta-hydroxysteroid dehydrogenase type II enzyme in asthma. Am J Respir Crit Care Med 2002; 165:1010–1014.
216. Barnes PJ, Lim S. Inhibitory cytokines in asthma. Mol Med Today 1998; 4:452–458.
217. Selig W, Tocker J. Effect of interleukin-1 receptor antagonist on antigen-induced pulmonary responses in guinea-pigs. Eur J Pharmacol 1992; 213:331–336.
218. Sousa AR, Lane SJ, Nakhosteen JA, et al. Expression of interleukin-1 beta (IL-1β) and interleukin-1 receptor antagonist (IL-1ra) on asthmatic bronchial epithelium. Am J Respir Crit Care Med 1996; 154:1061–1066.

219. Wills-Karp M. IL-12/IL-13 axis in allergic asthma. J Allergy Clin Immunol 2001; 107:9–18.
220. Bryan S, O'Connor BJ, Matti S, et al. Effects of recombinant human interleukin-12 on eosinophils, airway hyperreactivity and the late asthmatic response. Lancet 2000; 356:2149–2153.
221. McKay A, Komai-Koma M, Macleod KJ, et al. Interleukin-18 levels in induced sputum are reduced in asthmatic and normal smokers. Clin Exp Allergy 2004; 34:904–910.
222. Barnes PJ. Cytokine modulators for allergic diseases. Curr Opin Allergy Clin Immunol 2001; 1:555–560.
223. Wang P, Wu P, Siegel MI, et al. Interleukin (IL)-10 inhibits nuclear factor kappa B activation in human monocytes. IL-10 and IL-4 suppress cytokine synthesis by different mechanisms. J Biol Chem 1995; 270:9558–9563.
224. Borish L, Aarons A, Rumbyrt J, et al. Interleukin-10 regulation in normal subjects and patients with asthma. J Allergy Clin Immunol 1996; 97:1288–1296.
225. Jutel M, Akdis M, Budak F, et al. IL-10 and TGF-β cooperate in the regulatory T cell response to mucosal allergens in normal immunity and specific immunotherapy. Eur J Immunol 2003; 33:1205–1214.
226. Pavord ID, Tattersfield AE. Bronchoprotective role for endogenous prostaglandin E2. Lancet 1995; 344:436–438.
227. Serhan CN. Lipoxins and aspirin-triggered 15-epi-lipoxins are the first lipid mediators of endogenous antiinflammation and resolution. Prostaglandins Leukot Essent Fatty Acids 2005; 73:141–162.
228. Bannenberg GL, Chiang N, Ariel A, et al. Molecular circuits of resolution: formation and actions of resolvins and protectins. J Immunol 2005; 174:4345–4355.
229. Kanazawa H, Kurihara N, Hirata K, et al. Adrenomedullin, a newly discovered hypotensive peptide, is a potent bronchodilator. Biochem Biophys Res Commun 1994; 205:251–254.
230. Kamoi H, Kanazawa H, Hirata K, et al. Adrenomedullin inhibits the secretion of cytokine-induced neutrophil chemoattractant, a member of the interleukin-8 family, from rat alveolar macrophages. Biochem Biophys Res Commun 1995; 211:1031–1035.

Future directions

231. Barnes PJ. New drugs for asthma. Nat Rev Drug Discov 2004; 3:831–844.
232. Barnes PJ. New therapies for asthma. Trends Mol Med 2006; 12:512–520.

Immunopathology of Allergic Airway Inflammation

30

Susan Foley and Qutayba Hamid

CONTENTS

- Introduction 473
- Immunoglobulin E and receptors 473
- Key inflammatory cells in human allergic airways disease 475
- Th2 cytokine expression in human allergic airways disease 480
- Chemokines in allergic airways inflammation 485
- Transcription factors 488
- Summary 490

SUMMARY OF IMPORTANT CONCEPTS

>> Allergic disease is considered to result from an inappropriate balance between allergen activation of regulatory T cells and effector Th2 cells in susceptible individuals, a process in which dendritic cells are key players

>> Eosinophils are the predominant cell in the chronic inflammatory process characteristic of late-phase allergic responses and are the hallmark of allergic inflammation of the airways

>> Within allergic airways, IL-4 is presumed to be critical for the development of Th2 cells. IL-5 is critical for eosinophil survival and can regulate most aspects of eosinophils behavior

>> The immunosuppressive cytokine, IL-10, produced by regulatory T cells can inhibit Th1 and Th2 cytokine production and proliferation of other $CD4^+$ T cells

>> Recently, some biological therapies that specifically control inflammatory pathways in allergy have been shown to be effective in models of asthma but their therapeutic efficacy remains under study

INTRODUCTION

Allergic diseases are characterized by the IgE-dependent release of mast cell-derived mediators and cellular infiltration particularly of activated eosinophils and T lymphocytes that exhibit predominantly a Th2-type cytokine profile. It is evident that Th2 cytokines such as IL-4, IL-5, and IL-13 perform important regulatory roles in allergic inflammation since their gene expression has been localized in vivo at the involved tissue sites. These cytokines have been shown to be the driving force behind IgE production, eosinophil activation, and stimulation of the endothelium, epithelium, and other tissue-resident cells to produce mediators important in the inflammatory response.

Currently, both upper and lower allergic airway diseases are considered to be parts of the same syndrome, but in different locations. This has led to the concept of united airways disease and there is evidence that therapeutic control of rhinitis is beneficial for asthma. Prospective studies have identified allergic rhinitis as a risk for asthma and the risk factor increases with the severity of the symptoms; patients with allergic rhinitis have a two/three fold increased risk of developing asthma.

Most recent evidence suggests that other alterations in the immune response might contribute to the emergence of allergic disease. It has been proposed that allergy is the result of an improper balance between tolerance and immunity to harmless antigens. The recent identification of T regulatory (Treg) cells as key regulators in peripheral tolerance to allergens,[1] and the role that dendritic cells have on their generation,[2] open up new perspectives for the understanding of allergy pathogenesis and for the development of more efficient therapies. At the molecular and cellular levels, multiple mediators, cell types, and pathways are involved in the allergic inflammatory cascade that ensues after allergen exposure, and are subsequently reviewed.

IMMUNOGLOBULIN E AND RECEPTORS

The immunoglobulin E (IgE) molecule plays a central role in the pathogenesis of immediate hypersensitivity reactions because of its capacity to bind specifically to high-affinity IgE receptors on mast cells or basophils

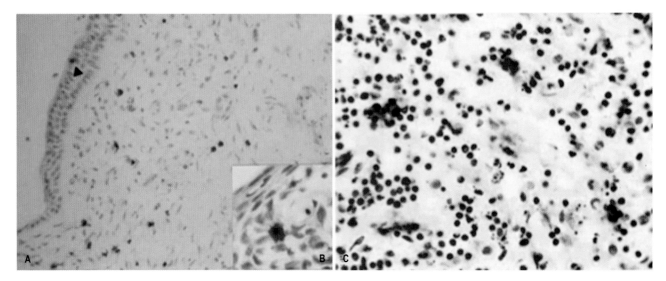

Fig. 30.1. B lymphocytes identified on the basis of CD20 immunoreactivity within allergic nasal mucosa cultured for 24 h in the presence of specific allergen (500 PNU/ml). B cells are present directly beneath the basement membrane (A), infiltrating the epithelial layer (inset B), and clustering within the submucosa in groups of three or four cells (C).

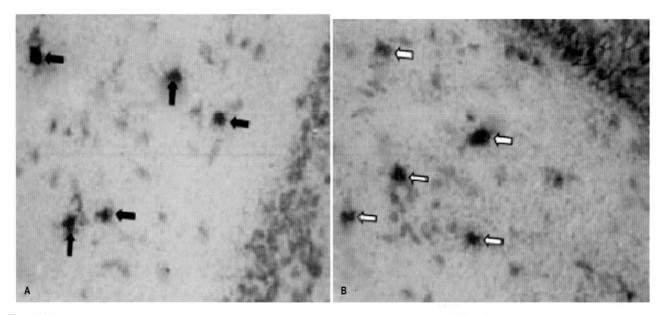

Fig. 30.2. (A) In situ hybridization for IgE mRNA (Cε RNA) in the nasal mucosa of an allergic patient. Black arrows point to positive cells. (B) Co-localization of IgE mRNA with resident CD20-positive B cells. In situ hybridization was performed with the same probe, whereas CD20-positive cells were determined with horseradish peroxidase immunocytochemistry. White arrows point to double-positive cells.

via the α-chain of Fc epsilon receptor type 1(FcεRI-α).[3] The cross-linking of bound IgE by allergen triggers degranulation, resulting in the release of a wide variety of both preformed and newly generated mediators. FcεRI has also been found on dendritic cells where it can facilitate the IgE-dependent trapping and presentation of allergen to T cells.

In addition to its ability to activate mast cells and basophils via FcεRI, IgE can bind to the low-affinity IgE receptor (CD23 or FcεRII) on B cells to augment cellular and humoral immune responses in allergic disease. Although IgE production has long been ascribed to B cells in secondary lymphoid tissue, bone marrow, and blood, recent studies have demonstrated that this phenomenon may also occur locally in allergic tissue. A resident population of B cells is present in the nasal mucosa (Fig. 30.1) and the factors required for induction of isotype switching to IgE are expressed within this tissue in individuals with allergic rhinitis.[4] IgE mRNA-positive B cells have been identified in nasal mucosa of patients with symptoms of allergy (Fig. 30.2). Increased numbers of

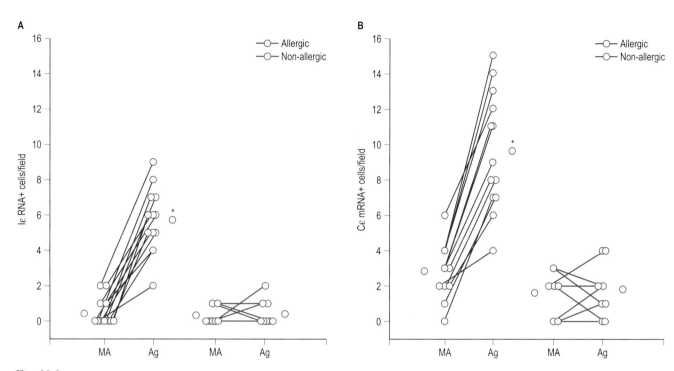

Fig. 30.3. Expression of ε RNA transcripts within explanted nasal mucosal tissue. Significantly higher numbers of Iε (A) and Cε (B) RNA-positive cells were observed in allergen-stimulated (Ag) compared with unstimulated (medium alone, MA) allergic tissue but not within tissue obtained from non-allergic patients.

ε-heavy chain germline (Iε) and ε-heavy chain constant region (Cε) ribonucleic acid-positive (RNA+) cells, in the absence of a change in B-cell number, have been observed in allergic nasal mucosa after allergen challenge and natural allergen exposure. To confirm that these increases were not merely the result of B-cell infiltration, Cameron et al[5] cultured nasal mucosal explants with allergen and demonstrated an increased number of Iε and Cε RNA+ cells (Fig. 30.3). These results confirm that ε-germline transcription occurs locally in the nasal mucosa and may be regulated by the local T cell and mast cell production of interleukin-4 (IL-4) and interleukin-13 (IL-13).

■ KEY INFLAMMATORY CELLS IN HUMAN ALLERGIC AIRWAYS DISEASE ■

Inflammation has always been a critical component of the allergic airways diathesis. It appears to involve a cascade of cells that become activated, including eosinophils, basophils, mast cells, T cells, epithelial and endothelial cells, neutrophils, and even smooth muscle cells. Although each cell has its proponents, and their interaction adds further complexity to the pathogenesis of allergic airway disease, substantial attention has been directed toward eosinophils and T cells. Sophisticated molecular biology tools now allow researchers to investigate the phenotype and profile of cytokine production of particular cell types.

EOSINOPHILS

Eosinophils are the predominant cell in the chronic inflammatory process characteristic of late-phase allergic responses and are the hallmark of allergic inflammation of the airways (Fig. 30.4). They can be detected in the mucosa of the upper and lower airways, and their number has been shown to correlate with disease severity and response to treatment. They have been associated with the characteristic pathologic features of allergic mucosa: namely, epithelial injury and desquamation, subepithelial fibrosis, and hyperresponsiveness.[6]

Eosinophils release an array of pro-inflammatory mediators, eosinophil cationic protein (ECP), eosinophil peroxidase (EPO), and major basic protein (MBP), and serve as a major source of granulocyte macrophage colony-stimulating factor (GM-CSF) and other cytokines. They are also a potent source of LTC_4, a mediator that is elevated in nasal lavage fluid of seasonal allergic rhinitis (SAR) patients after allergen challenge and that contributes to nasal blockage. Increased levels of MBP and ECP are also present within nasal mucosa and secretions in AR and have been shown to cause degranulation of other inflammatory cells as well as epithelial cell damage.

The presence of eosinophils within mucosal tissue of allergic airways disease is believed to be due to de novo infiltration of mature cells from the circulation. Using an explant system of human allergic nasal mucosa, Cameron et al[7] provided strong evidence that a subpopulation of immature eosinophils may also undergo local differentiation within the mucosa itself. Following ex-vivo stimulation with specific allergen

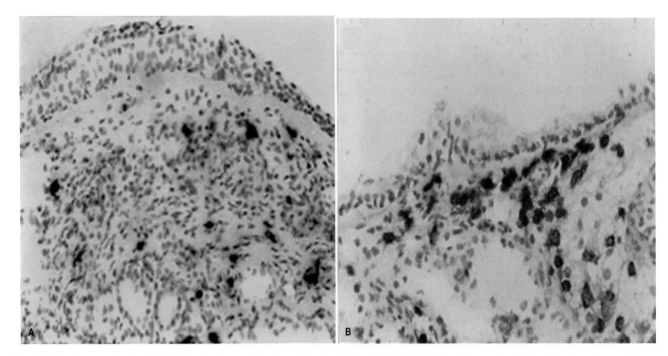

Fig. 30.4. Immunostaining for MBP showing increased numbers of eosinophils in allergic rhinitis (A) and the asthmatic lung (B) after antigen challenge.

or recombinant human (rh) IL-5, more MBP-immunoreactive and IL-5 mRNA$^+$ cells, along with fewer CD34$^+$/IL-5Rα cells, were found in nasal mucosal tissues (Fig. 30.5).[7] The process was found to be highly IL-5 dependent, implying that it might be regulated in vivo by endogenous production of sIL-5Rα. Since the alpha subunit of the IL-5 receptor (IL-5Rα) is expressed almost exclusively by eosinophils, the co-localization of CD34 immunoreactivity with IL-5Rα is considered to be a marker for precursor eosinophils (CD34$^+$/IL-5Rα^+).[8] Eosinophil precursors and IL-5 mRNA have been identified by Robinson et al[9] in the lungs of atopic asthmatic patients, and correlate with the number of MBP$^+$ cells, indicating that a similar process of local differentiation of eosinophils may occur within the asthmatic lung.

In most asthma phenotypes, there are increases in eosinophils in the tissues, blood, and bone marrow and in general, raised numbers correlate with disease severity (Fig. 30.6). It is thought, therefore that the eosinophil is the central effector cell responsible for ongoing airway inflammation. The cell has the potential to damage the airway mucosa and associated nerves through the release of granule-associated proteins, lipid mediators, and reactive oxygen species.

Animal and human studies point to an important role for eosinophils in the repair and remodeling process in asthma but the exact nature of this role is as yet unclear. The eosinophil is the source of several fibrogenic and growth factors, including transforming growth factor (TGF)-α, TGF-β, fibroblast growth factor (FGF)-2, vascular endothelial growth factor (VEGF), matrix metalloproteinase (MMP)-9, IL-13, and IL-17.

T LYMPHOCYTES

T lymphocytes are highly involved in allergic airway inflammation and both coordinate and mediate the adaptive immune response that the body elicits on exposure to a foreign antigen. An increased number of T lymphocytes is a frequent finding within the bronchial mucosa of patients with all forms of asthma, from newly diagnosed to severe disease.[10]

T lymphocytes are broadly subdivided into two distinct subsets according to their cell-surface markers and distinct effector functions: T cells expressing the CD4 antigen are involved in humoral immunity and are termed T-helper cells (Th cells), whereas those expressing the CD8 antigen are referred to as T-cytotoxic/suppressor cells (Tc cells). CD8$^+$ cytotoxic T cells orchestrate the cell-mediated response and interact with endogenously processed antigen presented in conjunction with major histocompatibility class (MHC) 1. In contrast, CD4$^+$ lymphocytes recognize foreign antigens processed in association with MHC II on the surface of professional antigen-presenting cells. As such, CD4$^+$ cells have attracted considerable attention in the pathogenesis of asthma and allergic rhinitis because of their ability to drive antigen-specific inflammatory responses and regulate immunoglobulin production.

CD4$^+$ T-helper cells are further divided into T-helper-1 (Th1) and T-helper-2 (Th2) based on the cytokines they produce. Naive Th cells (CD4$^+$ T cells never exposed to antigen), when activated by antigen-presenting cells, produce cytokines from both subsets and are known as Th0 cells.[11] If given the proper stimulus, naive Th cells can differentiate into the biased Th1 or Th2 subsets. Th1 cells produce interleukin (IL-2),

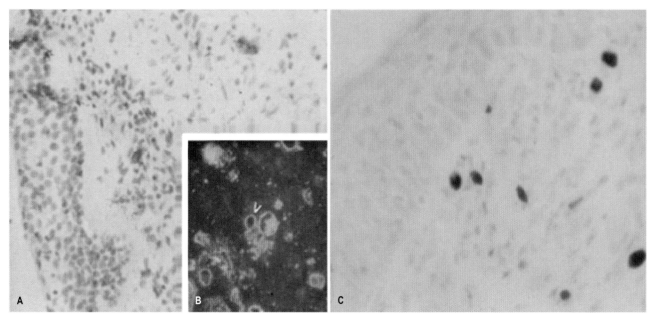

Fig. 30.5. Representative photos of nasal mucosal explant tissue 24h following culture. (A) The presence of CD34+ progenitor cells within tissue cultured in medium alone. Under dark field illumination, cells co-expressing both CD34 immunoreactivity and IL-5Rα mRNA are also seen within unstimulated tissue; these cells appear both orange and illuminated (B, note the arrow). (C) The considerable number of MBP+ cells within tissue cultured with ragweed allergen.

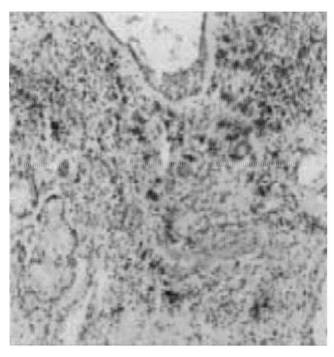

Fig. 30.6. Immunostaining for major basic protein (MBP) in a bronchial biopsy of a subject with severe asthma. Note the large number of positively stained cells. Reaction developed with fast red. (×200).

interferon-gamma (IFN-γ), and tumor necrosis factor-alpha (TNF-α). They are inducers of cell-mediated immunity or delayed-type hypersensitivity reactions. The major Th2 cytokines are IL-4, IL-5, and IL-13. They are helpers for B-cell antibody secretion, particularly IgE. During the last 15 years, it has largely been shown that allergic inflammation was caused by activated Th2 lymphocytes, leading to IgE production and eosinophil activation.

Another subset of T-helper cells, known as Th3 cells, secrete high levels of TGF-β but low levels, if any, of Th1 and Th2 cytokines.[12] Th3 cells suppress both Th1 and Th2 cytokine production and are thought to have a role in mucosal tolerance to antigen but their role in atopy is unclear.

Th1 and Th2 responses are capable of cross-regulating each other, thereby biasing the immune response in one direction or the other. IL-4 inhibits the production of IL-12 (a potent stimulator of IFN-γ production by T cells) by dendritic cells and macrophages. IL-4 also downregulates the IL-12Rβ2 chain decreasing the responsiveness of Th2 cells to IL-12,[13] while IFN-γ enhances its production.[14] Furthermore, IL-4 may inhibit T-helper cell production by IFN-γ and vice versa.[15]

CD4+ T lymphocytes are the predominant cells in allergic mucosal inflammation and help perpetuate the allergic response by providing a source of cytokines and amplifying and regulating local immune responses. There is a marked increase in the number of CD4+ T lymphocytes seen in nasal biopsy tissue obtained from individuals with allergic rhinitis 24h after allergen challenge outside the pollen season.[16] Furthermore, in situ hybridization with antisense complementary riboprobes has enabled detection of increased amounts of the Th2-type cytokines IL-3, IL-4, IL-5, IL-13, as well as GM-CSF mRNA+ cells within allergic nasal mucosa after local allergen provocation (Fig. 30.7).[17] These lymphocytes, both in bronchial and nasal mucosa, appear to be 'activated' as determined by their expression of the interleukin-2 (IL-2) receptor (CD25), suggesting that these cells are a cardinal feature of allergic airways inflammation.[18]

Whatever their actions, CD8+ T cells constitute a minority of CD3+ lymphocytes found in the bronchial mucosa and thus it is likely that they provide only a modulatory influence over CD4+-driven inflammation. Although both CD4+ and CD8+ T lymphocytes in bronchoalveolar lavage (BAL) fluid from asthmatic subjects expressed CD25, only the numbers of activated CD4+ cells correlated with numbers of BAL eosinophils and disease severity.[19] Some studies have shown that CD8+ T cells can produce IL-4 and stimulate B cells to produce IgE and IL-5 and are able to induce tissue eosinophilia.[20] CD8+ T cells may not play as great a role in orchestrating allergic inflammation as Th2 cells but they may help promote and maintain it.

REGULATORY T CELLS AND ALLERGIC AIRWAYS INFLAMMATION

CD4+CD25+ regulatory T cells (Tregs) are key regulators in peripheral tolerance to allergens. They account for 5–10% of peripheral CD4+ T cells. The expression of CD25 antigen, the IL-2 receptor α-unit, is induced in T cells upon antigen stimulation, but T-regulatory cells express high levels constitutively.[21] Unlike activated Th2 cells, they produce high levels of IL-10 and are involved in the maintenance of self-tolerance and in the suppression of the immune responses. Production of IL-10 by these cells can inhibit Th1 and Th2 cytokine production and proliferation of other CD4+ T cells.[22] A recently described transcription factor forkhead box P3 (Foxp3) is associated with regulatory T cells.[23] In humans, mutations in Foxp3 lead to an immunodysregulation, polyendocrinopathy, and enteropathy (IPEX) syndrome as a consequence of deficiency of regulatory T cells. Tregs are present in both atopic and non-atopic individuals, but those from atopic patients have a significantly lowered activity in inhibiting proliferation and Th2 cytokine production of other cells, especially during allergen exposure.[24]

MAST CELLS

Mast cells are key participants in allergic inflammation, containing a potent array of inflammatory mediators. They develop from bone marrow progenitor cells and are found in increased numbers in the airways of subjects with allergic rhinitis and asthma. These cells have unique characteristics and possess high-affinity IgE receptors. Circulating IgE binds to high-affinity Fc receptors (Fc-RI) on the surfaces of mast cells and basophils. Activation of the mast cells by specific antigen through cell-bound IgE leads to their explosive degranulation, resulting in the release of a complex cascade of both preformed and newly synthesized mediators that have synergistic effects on resident cells in tissues.[25]

Mast-cell degranulation is the critical initiating event of acute allergic symptoms. In the early phase following antigen challenge, mast cells secrete the autacoid mediators histamine, prostaglandin (PG)D$_2$, and leukotriene (LT) C$_4$. These mediators are capable of inducing bronchoconstriction, mucus secretion, and mucosal edema, features of allergic disease. Histamine appears to be a crucial mediator of the immediate allergic response because most of the symptoms can be initiated by histamine challenge. The cys-LTs and PGD$_2$ are considered to increase

vascular permeability and glandular secretion induced by the action of the cys-LTs and PGD$_2$ on sensory nerve fibers.

The serine proteases, tryptase, chymase, and carboxy-peptidase, are major secretory products of human mast cells that are believed to have proinflammatory proteolytic effects and can interact with various cell types via protease activated receptors (PARs) and by other processes to alter their behavior profoundly. Chymase may contribute to glandular hypersecretion.

Mast cells also synthesize a large number of proinflammatory cytokines (including IL-4, IL-5, and IL-13), which regulate both IgE synthesis and the development of eosinophilic inflammation and several profibrotic cytokines including TGF-β and FGF-2.[26]

In asthma, there is evidence that mast cells localize to the airway smooth muscle (ASM) as well as airway mucous glands and the bronchial epithelium. The mechanism of mast cell recruitment by asthmatic ASM involves the CCR3, CRTh2, CXCR3 axis and several mast cell mediators have profound effects on ASM function. The localization of mast cells within ASM in asthma facilitates specific interactions between these cells and ASM in terms of both localized mediator release and direct cell-to-cell contact. It is probable that these mast cells contribute to the development of hypertrophy and hyperplasia, smooth muscle dysfunction expressed as BHR, and variable airflow obstruction. Mast cells are also a potential source of products stimulating migration and proliferation of fibroblasts.

BASOPHILS

Although basophils are granulocytes that express FcεRI, Th2 cytokines, and histamine, they are believed to be a separate lineage from mast cells. They develop in the bone marrow and represent <1% of peripheral blood leukocytes. Due to their low levels in blood, it has been difficult to ascribe a physiologic function to the basophil but they may promote late-phase inflammation by Th2 cytokine production and may also promote IgE class switching as they also express CD40L.[27] They produce many mediators, including LTC$_4$, IL-4, and IL-13.[28] Unlike mast cells, PDG$_2$, TNF, and IL-5 are not produced by basophils.

Several studies have demonstrated infiltration of tissue basophils in human allergen-induced late responses occurring in the nose and bronchi. A proportion of these basophils express IL-4 mRNA and protein in the bronchial mucosa at 24h after challenge.[29] Basophil numbers are also increased in nasal lavage fluid obtained 24h after allergen challenge.[30] Similar to mast cells, basophils bind allergen by IgE/FcεRI and release histamine on activation. Because the level of histamine but not of tryptase and PGD$_2$ is increased during the late-phase response, it is attributed to basophil activation rather than to secondary mast cell degranulation. However, to date, none of the products released by basophils is unique to this cell type.

EPITHELIAL CELLS

The epithelium has long been considered to act mainly as a barrier participating in mucociliary clearance and removal of noxious agents. Loss of integrity of the epithelial layer, a feature of both allergic rhinitis and asthma, may promote exposure of the mucosa by allergen and promote further inflammation (Fig. 30.8). Apart from its barrier functions, however, the epithelium has been shown more recently to participate in inflammation by producing a wide array of mediators, including

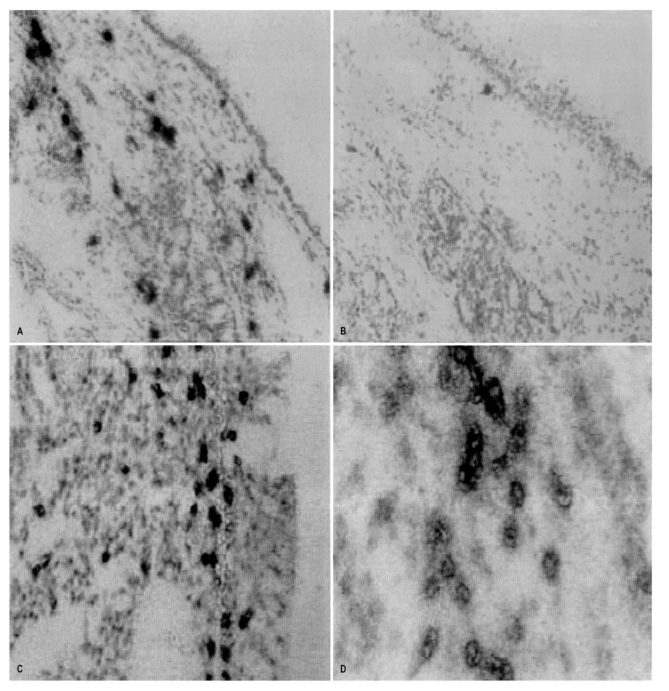

Fig. 30.7. Representative examples of in situ hybridization of nasal biopsy specimens in allergic rhinitis. Expression of IL-4 mRNA after antigen challenge (A) and diluent challenge (B). Expression of IL-13 mRNA after allergen challenge (C) and co-localization of IL-4 and IL-13 mRNA after allergen challenge (D).

cytokines, chemokines, eicosanoids, peptidases, and matrix proteins. Cytokines produced by epithelial cells include IL-1β, IL-6, IL-11, IL-13, IL-16, GM-CSF, and TGF-β. The chemokine eotaxin-1 (CCL-1), produced by the epithelium, recruits eosinophils and other cells from the blood for inflammatory reactions in the tissues.

Inducible nitric oxide synthase (iNOS) is synthesized in epithelial cells. NOS has vasodilating and bronchodilating effects and plays an important role in neurotransmission, immune defense, cytotoxicity, ciliary beat frequency, and mucus secretion.

Epithelial cells also perform an immune function through their capacity to express human leukocyte-associated antigen-DR (HLA-DR) and present antigen. In asthma, epithelial cells are likely to be important in repair processes. They release extracellular matrix proteins, including fibronectin, which appears important in cell regeneration.

NEUTROPHILS

Neutrophils are one of the first inflammatory cells to be recruited into the airways after either allergen exposure or injury. However, their precise role in allergic airways disease remains unclear. They are readily found in the sputum of asthmatic subjects but are reported in low numbers in BAL and bronchial biopsies. Increased numbers are found in the airways during the late-phase reaction after an allergen challenge (Fig. 30.9), in patients who died within hours of an asthma exacerbation, in nocturnal asthma, in long-standing asthma or in corticosteroid-dependent asthma.

Neutrophils are recruited to the site of lung inflammation by a number of chemokines, particularly CXCL8 (IL-8) (Fig. 30.10) produced predominantly by the lung epithelium. IL-8 is also the most potent activator of neutrophils and triggers the secretion of granular enzymes such as myeloperoxidase (MPO), β-glucuronidase, elastase, and gelatinase. In addition, IL-8 induces the production of LTB_4 and oxygen radicals by neutrophils and stimulates phagocytosis.

Evidence has been accumulating for the presence and involvement of neutrophils in severe asthma. Since neutrophils have been shown to be relatively steroid resistant, this increased neutrophilic inflammation may explain the poor response to steroids in these patients.

Neutrophils synthesize and release various proinflammatory mediators, proteases, and cytotoxic compounds as well as cytokines, particularly IL-9, TNF-α, and TGF-α, factors that may be involved in bronchoconstriction, tissue damage, and chronic airways inflammation.

Neutrophils also express receptors for a number of mediators including IL-8, IL-9, and, at least in asthmatics, the high-affinity IgE receptor (Fig. 30.11). This suggests that neutrophils may play a role in allergic inflammation through IgE-dependent mechanisms.

To date, little is known about neutrophils and their role in upper allergic airways diseases but their presence has been detected in nasal lavage from patients with allergic rhinitis obtained 6–24h after allergen challenge which correlated with the levels of LTB_4.[31]

■ Th2 CYTOKINE EXPRESSION IN HUMAN ALLERGIC AIRWAYS DISEASE ■

INTERLEUKIN-4

The IL-4 gene is present on chromosome 5 (5q31.1) alongside IL-3, IL-5, IL-9, IL-13, and GM-CSF, the so-called Th2 cytokine gene cluster. The major cellular sources of IL-4 mRNA within the airways

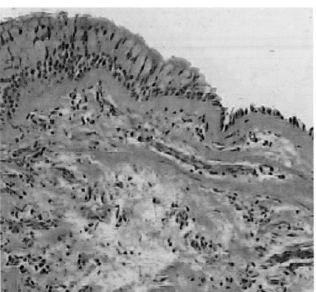

Fig. 30.8. Hematoxylin and eosin staining of a bronchial biopsy from a subject with severe asthma showing detachment of the epithelium.

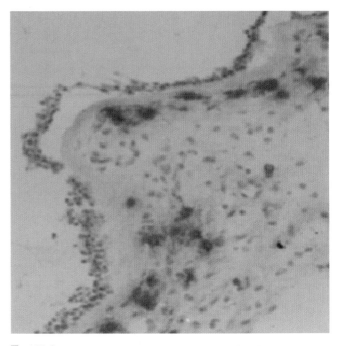

Fig. 30.9. Immunostaining for neutrophil elastase (pink) in a bronchial biopsy from an asthmatic subject after allergen challenge showing increased numbers of neutrophils in the submucosa. (×200).

of allergic subjects are $CD4^+$ T cells and to a lesser extent $CD8^+$ T cells, eosinophils, and mast cells (Fig. 30.7).[32,33] It mediates its actions through the IL-4 receptor composed of two subunits, IL-4 receptor α subunit (IL-4Rα) and the IL-2 receptor common γ subunit (γc).

Within allergic airways, IL-4 is presumed to be critical for the development of Th2 cells. It also inhibits the expression of the β2 subunit of the interleukin-12 receptor (IL-12Rβ2) in T cells. IL-4 has been shown to induce naive T cells to commence the production of Th2 cytokines, the production of NO, and the secretion of other proallergic cytokines. The predisposition of inflammatory cells for IL-4 production has been suggested because peripheral blood mononuclear cells (PBMCs) from patients with seasonal allergic rhinitis produce IL-4 in response to non-specific activation. IL-4 is critical in the switching of B cells to IgE production, although this effect can be enhanced by other cytokines, including IL-5, IL-10, and TNF-α.[34] After switching occurs, IL-4 potentiates IgE production. Furthermore, IL-4 enhances the IgE-mediated response by upregulating IgE receptors on inflammatory cells within the airway such as mast cells. IL-4 has also been shown to promote goblet cell metaplasia, mucus hypersecretion, and vascular cell adhesion molecule (VCAM)-1 expression in endothelial cells resulting in the recruitment of eosinophils. Also, inhalation of IL-4 causes the development of sputum eosinophilia and increased airway hyperreactivity (AHR).[35]

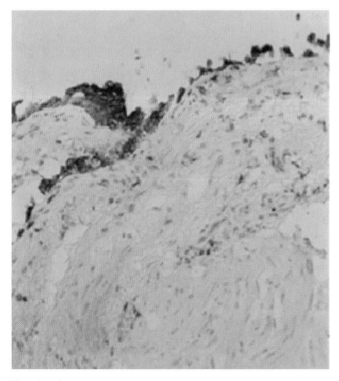

Fig. 30.10. Increased expression of IL-8 in the epithelium and submucosa in a bronchial biopsy from a patient with asthma. Positive staining is brown. (×200).

INTERLEUKIN-5

IL-5 is expressed by Th2 cells and to a lesser extent by eosinophils and activated mast cells. This cytokine is critical in the development of eosinophils in the bone marrow, influencing mainly terminal differentiation of CD34/CD33$^+$ progenitor cells. IL-5 releases both mature and immature eosinophils from the bone marrow, regulates the expression of the transmembrane isoform of its own receptor, and is essential for the terminal differentiation of committed eosinophil precursors. In addition to hematopoietic properties, IL-5, though a weak eosinophil chemoattractant, primes these cells for recruitment by other chemotactic agents such as eotaxin. IL-5 also stimulates the production of IgA from plasma cells which are extremely efficient at degranulating eosinophils when bound to antigen.

IL-5 mRNA expression has been identified by Robinson et al[9] in the lungs of asthmatic patients and has been shown to be closely related to lung function in asthmatic subjects.[36] Studies with explanted airways have shown that allergen challenge results in an increased number of IL-5 mRNA positive cells, suggesting that at least part of the cytokine production is from resident inflammatory cells.

IL-5 is the most important Th2 cytokine associated with eosinophils and it can regulate most aspects of eosinophil behavior. In addition, intravenous injections of antibodies that block IL-5 lead to a decrease in circulating eosinophils and allergen-induced asthmatic sputum eosinophilia. IL-5 promotes eosinophil survival by blocking apoptosis. It is also capable of activating eosinophil secretion, cytotoxicity, and chemotaxis. IL-5 activates eosinophils to upregulate integrin receptor expression which promotes adhesion to VCAM-expressing endothelial cells and eosinophil accumulation in the tissues.

INTERLEUKIN-9

IL-9 is a Th2 cytokine that is expressed and released by a variety of cells such as lymphocytes, eosinophils, mast cells, and neutrophils. IL-9 has pleiotropic activities on Th2 lymphocytes, mast cells, B cells, eosinophils, and airway epithelial cells. It promotes the proliferation and differentiation of mast cells and hematopoietic progenitors and it enhances the production of IgE by B cells. The production of IL-9 by human CD4$^+$ T cells is dependent on T-cell activation and may occur in vivo through stimulation by IL-2 or a combination of cytokines. Human peripheral eosinophils are capable of IL-9 production. Eosinophils from asthmatic subjects express high levels of biologically active IL-9 that is enhanced by TNF-α and IL-1β (Fig. 30.12).[37]

Like other Th2 cytokines, IL-9 has been linked to bronchial asthma. The locus of the IL-9 gene is associated with AHR and elevated levels of serum IgE. Bronchial biopsies of asthmatic patients show higher numbers of IL-9 mRNA$^+$ cells (Fig. 30.13).[38,39] Those cells were identified as CD3$^+$ lymphocytes (68%), eosinophils (16%), and neutrophils (8%).[38] Total numbers of IL-9 mRNA$^+$ cells correlated with FEV_1 and PC20 in those asthmatic patients.[38] In atopic asthmatics, segmental allergen challenge led to increased production of IL-9.[40] BAL lymphocytes were identified as the major source of IL-9 in that study. Selective overexpression of the IL-9 gene within the lungs of transgenic mice results in massive airway inflammation with eosinophils and lymphocytes as well as in the release of CC chemokines from airway epithelial cells. This reaction may be caused by the increase in other Th2 cytokines (IL-4, IL-5, IL-13) in response to IL-9 as other features seen in this

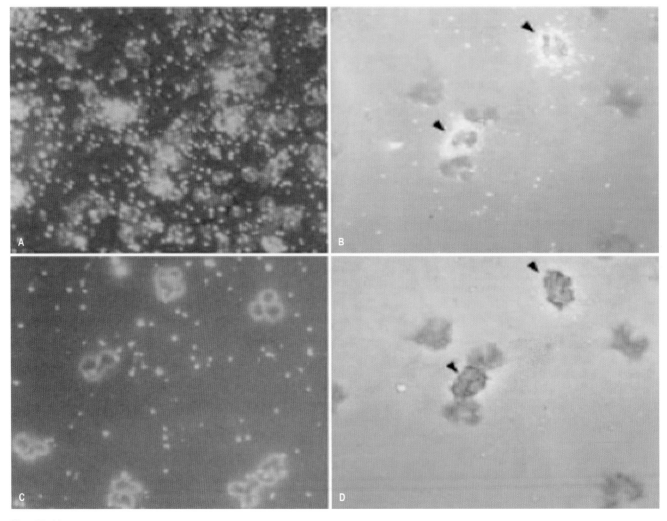

Fig. 30.11. Detection of FcεRIα chain mRNA in human PMNs by in situ hybridization. Positive signal was detected using antisense FcεRIα chain riboprobe in neutrophils from a subject with asthma (A). The FcεRIα chain positive cells (dark field, arrows in B) show neutrophil morphology with phase-contrast microscopy (arrows in D). No specific signal was detected with sense probe (C). (A ×200; B–D ×400).

model were mast cell hyperplasia, epithelial cell hypertrophy with mucus accumulation, subepithelial collagen deposition, and AHR. Intratracheal instillation of IL-9 in mice led to lung eosinophilia and increased serum IgE levels.

The receptor for IL-9 (IL-9R) is expressed by ASM in asthmatic subjects but not normal controls and IL-9 may play a direct role in the production of eosinophilia through induction of eotaxin 1/CCL11 in human ASM although the reports are conflicting.

There are conflicting results in relation to the exact role of IL-9 in allergic airways inflammation. In one mouse model of experimental asthma, blockade of IL-9 with an anti-IL-9 antibody inhibited the development of allergic inflammation and AHR. However, another group reported a persistence of the Th2 response to allergen after sensitization in IL-9 knockout mice. Clearly further studies are required in order to establish the potential role of blocking IL-9 as a therapeutic strategy for asthma, and such studies in humans should soon be underway.

INTERLEUKIN-13

There is mounting evidence that IL-13 is a key mediator of allergic airways disorders in humans, including asthma, atopic rhinitis, and chronic sinusitis. This cytokine has 70% sequence homology with IL-4 and has many similar actions because it shares the IL-4Rα subunit for its high-affinity receptor formation. It induces IgE production and the expression of VCAM-1 on endothelial cells and activates eosinophils by inducing the expression of CD69. IL-13 has been shown to downregulate the transcription of IFN-γ and IL-12 and thus may modulate the cytokine environment at the time of antigen presentation.

Due to redundancy in IL-4Rα binding, both IL-4 and IL-13 exhibit some degree of functional overlap. As in the case of IL-4, overexpression of IL-13 within the lungs results in the production of IgE, eotaxin, inflammation, mucus hypersecretion, eosinophilia, and upregulation of VCAM-1.

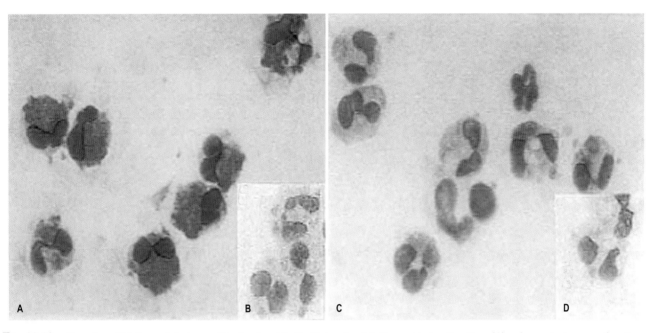

Fig. 30.12. Detection of IL-9 protein in human blood eosinophils. Purified eosinophils from subjects with asthma (A) and non-atopic, non-asthmatic, control subjects (C) were stained with goat polyclonal anti-IL-9 antibody. Goat IgG was used as a negative control (B and D). The staining was performed using goat anti-IL-9 followed by biotin-labeled, rabbit anti-goat streptavidin alkaline phosphatase, and counterstaining was with hematoxylin.

Although IL-13 does not appear to have direct effects on T-cell differentiation, it may perpetuate the effector arm of the Th2 immune response via several pathways. First, it induces the expression of several chemokines that are thought to selectively recruit Th2 cells, namely TARC and MDC. Second, it can recruit additional dendritic cells to the site of allergen exposure via the induction of MMP9 and TARC. Third, it appears to promote its own production via regulation of several mediators, such as adenosine and histamine, which in turn stimulate cells such as eosinophils, mast cells, basophils, and SMC to produce more IL-13. Through stimulation of these pathways, IL-13 may be an important contributor to the chronicity of allergic disease.

IL-13 is thought to be closely associated with the pathophysiology of allergic airways disease; the increased expression of IL-13 mRNA has been demonstrated in both asthma and allergic rhinitis (Fig. 30.7).[41] Numerous studies have shown that both message and protein levels of IL-13 are elevated in bronchial biopsy specimens and BAL cells from subjects with allergic asthma compared with those of control subjects.[42,43]

IL-13 is also a critical factor for mucin synthesis, a characteristic feature of asthma. Studies in murine models of allergen-induced airway inflammation have shown that blocking IL-13 results in the complete abrogation of mucin synthesis in airway epithelial cells. In another murine study, administration of IL-13 was sufficient to induce AHR and administration of soluble IL-13Rα_2 completely reversed IL-13-mediated AHR in albino Jackson (A/J) mice. There is thus a strong rationale for pursuing IL-13 or IL-13 signaling pathway inhibition as a therapy for asthma.

INTERLEUKIN-25

Interleukin-25 (IL-25) is a novel Th2 cytokine of the IL-17 family that plays a key role in allergic inflammation. It appears to have biological activities that are different from the other family members. Although it was originally thought to be exclusively expressed in polarized Th2 cells, IL-25 mRNA has since been detected in multiple other tissues such as colon, stomach, small intestine, kidney, uterus, and lung.

Systemic administration of IL-25 in mice results in eosinophilia through the production of IL-5,[44] while other IL-17 family cytokines induce predominantly neutrophilia. The viability of IL-25-treated eosinophils was greatly enhanced when compared with untreated ones, indicating that IL-25 may promote eosinophilia in allergic inflammation by delaying eosinophil apoptosis. IL-25 also induces increased gene expression of IL-4 and IL-13 in tissues, leading to elevated IgE levels and typical Th2-associated pathological changes in the tissues.[44] Animal studies have demonstrated IL-25-induced Th2 cytokine production occurs even in mice lacking T cells.[44] This suggests that IL-25 is capable of promoting an allergic inflammatory response even in the absence of Th2 cells. Mast cells have been shown to be potent IL-25 producers and may play a role in prolonging the Th2-type immune response.

While the physiological effects of IL-25 have been well illustrated in animal models, the cell populations that express the IL-25 receptor are still poorly recognized in humans. The receptor for IL-25 was first identified as IL-17B receptor (IL-17BR), also called IL-17 receptor homolog 1 (IL-17Rh1) and Evi27. Wong et al[45] showed that human

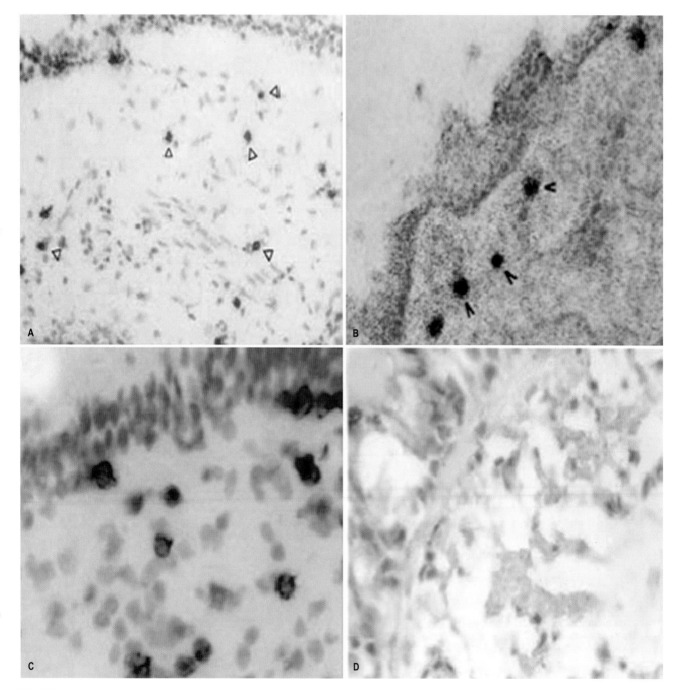

Fig. 30.13. Representative examples of in situ hybridization of IL-9 mRNA by use of S-labeled cRNA probes and ICC for IL-9 in bronchial biopsy specimens. In situ hybridization of IL-9 mRNA from asthmatic subject (×200) (positive cells indicated by arrows) (A) and high power of A (×400) (B). IL-9 immunoreactivity in bronchial biopsy specimen from atopic asthmatic subject (C) and from non-atopic healthy control subject (D).

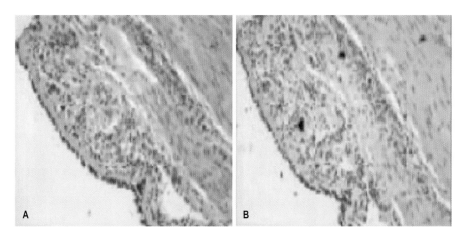

Fig. 30.14. Expression of IL-17BR in ASMC in asthma. Immunostaining showing expression of IL17BR in the smooth muscle layers of bronchial biopsy from a subject with asthma (A). (B), biopsy treated with isotype control. The APAAP method of immunostaining was used and the reaction was developed with fast red. (×200).

eosinophils constitutively express IL-17BR protein. They also found that the median plasma concentration of IL-25 in allergic asthmatic patients was significantly higher than that of normal control subjects. We have shown the receptor to be highly expressed by ASMC in asthma (Fig. 30.14).

Evidence is therefore accumulating for a role for IL-25 in allergic diseases, particularly in the enhancement and/or prolongation of Th2 cell-mediated allergic diseases such as asthma and allergic rhinitis.

■ CHEMOKINES IN ALLERGIC AIRWAYS INFLAMMATION ■

Chemokines and their receptors are involved at many levels in the allergic process and play an important role in the establishment and persistence of allergic disease. Their spectrum of activities is broad and encompasses effects on morphogenesis, proliferation, and recruitment/activation of inflammatory cell populations involved in allergic diseases, such as Th1 and Th2 cells.

Chemokines are a group of structurally related peptides and are subdivided into four families (C, CXC, CC, CX_3) on the basis of their cysteine residues. Members of the CC family include the majority of the chemokines that stimulate movement of cells associated with allergic responses, including monocytes, lymphocytes, basophils, and eosinophils. Thus, these cells are the most responsive to RANTES (regulated upon activation, normal T cell expressed and secreted), eotaxin types 1, 2, and 3, monocyte chemotactic protein (MCP) types 2, 3, and 4, and macrophage inflammatory protein (MIP) types 1α, 1β, 3α, and 3β.

Within the nasal mucosa in allergic rhinitis, there is a tendency for inflammatory cell accumulation within the epithelial layer, particularly of mast cells and eosinophils. This has been attributed to the ability of the epithelial cells to generate chemokines, particularly the CC chemokines, with chemotactic activity for eosinophils, mast cells, and T lymphocytes. After antigen challenge, the nasal mucosa of subjects with seasonal allergic rhinitis exhibit increased numbers of RANTES, eotaxin, and the MCPs. Co-localization studies have demonstrated

that within the submucosa mRNA coding for RANTES, MCP-3, MCP-4, and eotaxin is expressed mainly by macrophages, T cells, and eosinophils.[17]

Furthermore, these chemokines are induced by the cytokines IL-4, IL-13, and TNF-α. IL-8 is also expressed within the nasal mucosa by leukocytes as well as the epithelium after allergen exposure. This is a CXC chemokine and its expression by the epithelial layer has been suggested to mediate the recruitment of mast cells and eosinophils toward this layer, as observed in seasonal and perennial rhinitis. IL-8 is also the main chemokine involved in the recruitment of neutrophils to the site of lung inflammation in the asthmatic airway and is the most potent activator of neutrophils (Fig. 30.10).

Of the CC chemokines, eotaxin has attracted the most attention by far because of the potency and specificity of its actions on eosinophils. Originally described in the BAL fluid of allergen-challenged guinea-pigs, eotaxin is an eosinophil, basophil, and mast cell chemoattractant. Both eotaxin mRNA and protein have been detected at increased levels in nasal as well as bronchial epithelium and in submucosal inflammatory cells in patients with allergic rhinitis and asthma, respectively (Fig. 30.15).[46]

Structural cells, such as epithelial cells, endothelial cells, smooth muscle, and fibroblasts are also sources of chemokines within the airways. CCL5 (RANTES), CCL11 (eotaxin 1), and CCL13 (MCP-4), important chemoattractants for eosinophils, were strongly upregulated in epithelial cells of asthmatics compared to healthy controls.[47] TNF-α and IFN-γ have been shown to induce the production of eotaxin 1 from endothelial cells isolated from nasal mucosa of subjects with allergic rhinitis. This cytokine-induced production of eotaxin was higher in nasal mucosal endothelial cells of atopic subjects than atopic controls. MCP-4 has been described in the airways of asthmatic individuals. Moreover, using the nasal allergen challenge model, MCP-4 expression was shown to increase after allergen provocation (Fig. 30.16).[48]

Joubert et al[49] reported that the expression of CCR3 by ASMC is increased in asthmatics (Fig. 30.17) and that a CCR3 ligand, such as eotaxin, induces migration of ASMC in vitro. These results suggest that eotaxin could be involved in the increased smooth muscle mass observed

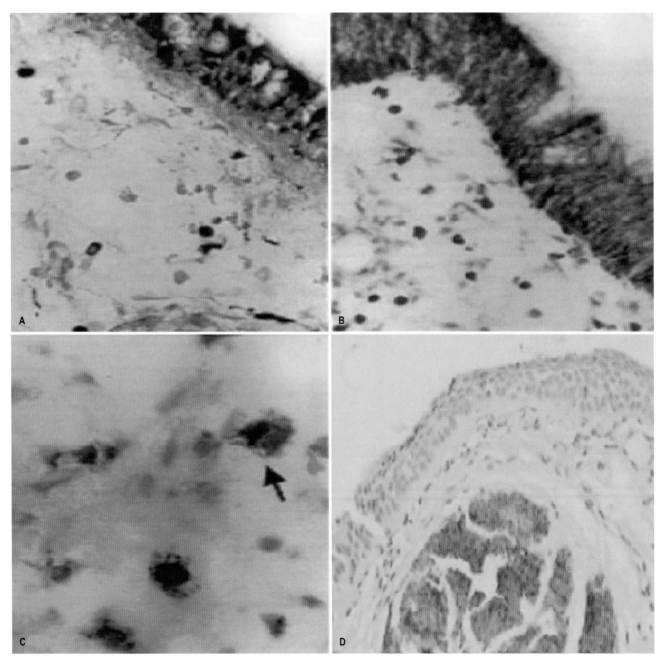

Fig. 30.15. Representative examples of in situ hybridization of nasal biopsies in (A) allergic rhinitis following allergen challenge using digoxigenin-labeled antisense cRNA probes coding for eotaxin mRNA. Positive eotaxin mRNA cells exhibited a dark purple staining. Also shown are the results of double immunocytochemistry for (B) eotaxin immunoreactivity (developed by fast red) and antikeratin (epithelial cells; developed by DAB), and (C) eotaxin immunoreactivity and CD68-positive macrophages in sections of nasal biopsies in allergic rhinitis following allergen challenge. Macrophages (brown staining) were a major cellular source of eotaxin immunoreactivity (red staining; arrow). (D) immunostaining for eotaxin in the airway smooth muscle of a severe asthmatic patient.

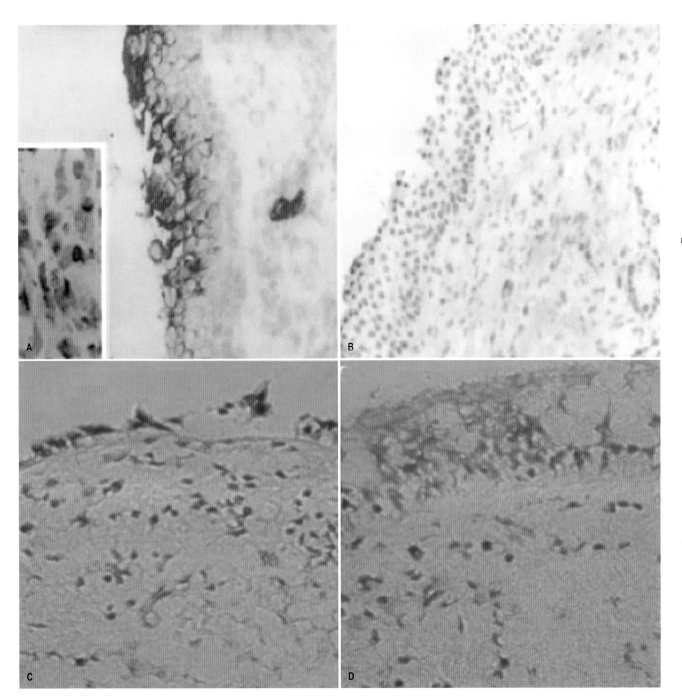

Fig. 30.16. Immunostaining for monocyte chemotactic protein (MCP)-4 in allergic rhinitis and asthma. (A) Positive staining in the nasal mucosa of a subject with allergic rhinitis after allergen challenge. The inset shows co-localization of MCP-4 immunoreactivity to CD3$^+$ T cells. (B) Nasal biopsy stained with non-specific mouse Ig (negative control) after antigen challenge showing no cellular staining. (C) Increased staining for MCP-4 protein both in the epithelium and submucosa of a bronchial biopsy from a subject with asthma compared with normal control subject (D). MCP-4 immunoreactivity was visualized with fast red chromagen. (×200).

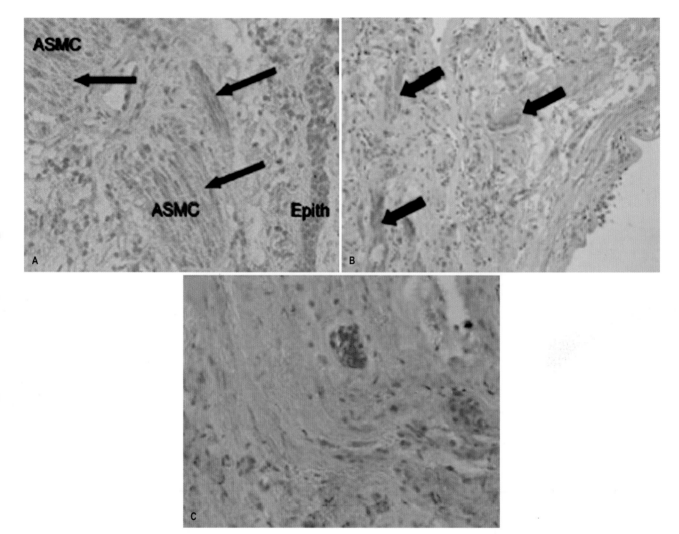

Fig. 30.17. Increased CCR3 immunostaining in airway smooth muscle bundles (ASMC) in a biopsy specimen from a subject with asthma (A) compared with control subject (B). (C) An example of staining with the isotype control. The reaction was developed with diaminobenzidine tetrahydrochloride (DAB) and positive staining is brown.

in asthmatics through the activation of CCR3. Airway epithelial cells in asthmatics also express CCR3 and react to CCR3 ligands.

■ TRANSCRIPTION FACTORS ■

Transcription factors are proteins that act to facilitate or inhibit RNA production. They operate by binding to specific recognition sites, usually located in the upstream promoter region of the gene, and they are central to the control of gene transcription. Both Th1 and Th2 cytokine responses in allergic disease are associated with transcription factors which control gene expression and lineage commitment by promoting transcription and chromatin remodeling.

The transcription factors activator protein-1 (AP-1) and nuclear factor kappa B (NF-κB) are particularly important in allergic diseases. They are responsible for the gene transcription of a wide range of cytokines implicated in allergic disease, including IL-1β, TNF-α, IL-2, IL-6, GM-CSF, MCP-1, and RANTES. In addition, one of the mechanisms by which corticosteroids are thought to act is by sequestration of AP-1.

c-Maf, a basic region/leucine zipper transcription factor, has also been implicated in Th2-specific gene transcription. It is expressed in Th2 but not Th1 clones and has been reported to activate the IL-4 promoter. Expression of c-Maf was first demonstrated in human asthmatic airways, suggesting a role in allergic inflammation.

GATA-3 is a master regulator of Th2 cell generation. It plays an important role in the development of Th2 reactions and is highly expressed by naive, freshly activated T cells and Th2 cells (but not Th1 cells, macrophages or B cells). GATA-3 is critical for the production of IL-5 and IL-13 but not for IL-4 and controls the expression of

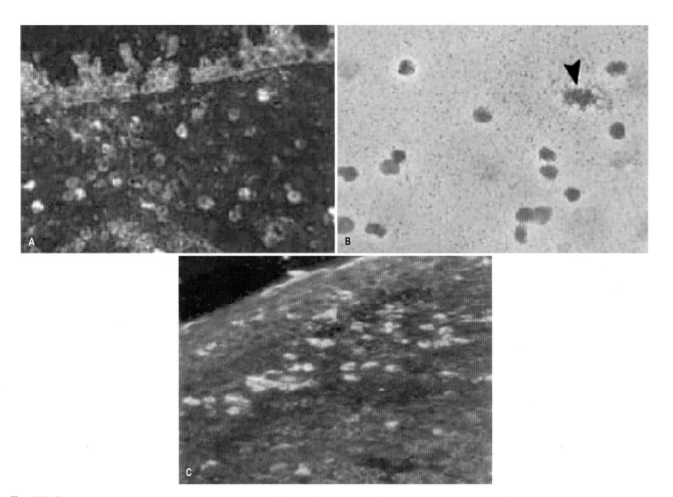

Fig. 30.18. (A) In situ hybridization was performed for GATA-3 mRNA by using 35S-labeled riboprobes in bronchial biopsy specimens from a subject with atopic asthma. Dark-field illumination was used to visualize the brightly staining positive cells. (B) Bronchoalveolar lavage fluid from atopic asthmatic subjects was probed with GATA-3 35S-labeled riboprobes (silver granule deposition from autoradiography) combined with IL-5 biotin-labeled riboprobes (brown staining from diaminobenzidine) to co-localize the two markers. The arrowhead points to an example of a GATA-3/IL-5 mRNA-positive cell. (C) In situ hybridization for GATA-3 mRNA with 35S-labeled riboprobes in the nasal tissue explant. The biopsy specimens were obtained from an allergic subject and were cultured for 24 h with ragweed allergen before processing.

IL-4, IL-5, and IL-13, and other factors. GATA-3 mRNA is elevated in bronchial biopsies of atopic asthmatic subjects and in the nasal mucosa of subjects with allergic rhinitis compared to controls (Fig. 30.18).[50,51] It is also increased in allergen sensitization models in mice. This suggests a significant role for GATA-3 in allergic disorders by biasing T cells in favor of Th2-type cytokine production.

Signal transducer and activator of transcription 6 (STAT-6) is also implicated in the pathogenesis of allergic diseases. Expression of STAT-6 is increased in the nasal mucosa of patients with allergic rhinitis and in bronchial biopsies of asthmatic subjects (Fig. 30.19).[52,53] STAT-6 knockout mice are protected from developing airway hyperresponsiveness and from producing excess mucus in response to allergen challenge. These mice also fail to mount allergen-specific IgE responses. Th2 commitment is associated with the transcription factors STAT-6 and

GATA-3. STAT-6 is activated by IL-4 and IL-13 and it controls transcription of GATA-3.

T-box expressed in T cells (T-bet), one of the main transcription factors associated with Th1 cells, transactivates and controls IFN-γ production in Th1 cells. It has the unique ability to redirect fully polarized Th2 cells into Th1 cells as demonstrated by simultaneous induction of IFN-γ and repression of IL-4 and IL-5. Expression of T-bet is decreased in airways of patients with asthma[54] compared with T cells from airways of non-asthmatic subjects, concordant with decreased Th1 cytokine production in asthma. This suggests that loss of T-bet might be associated with asthma.[54]

GATA-3 and STAT-6 are increased in the upper and lower airways in asthma and allergies. Th1 and Th2 associated transcription factors can further bias cytokine responses by inhibiting gene expression. T-bet

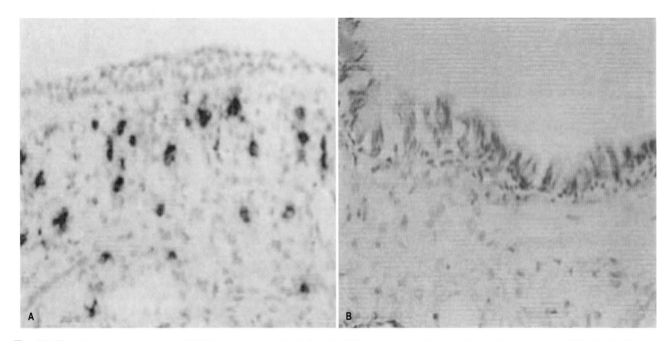

Fig. 30.19. Representative example of STAT-6 immunoreactivity in bronchial biopsy specimens from a subject with atopic asthma (A) and a healthy control subject (B).

represses Th2 lineage commitment by interfering with GATA-3 activity. STAT-6 and GATA-3 also inhibit IFN-γ production in Th1 cells and functions.

◼ SUMMARY ◼

Currently, allergic disease is considered to result from an inappropriate balance between allergen activation of regulatory T cells and effector Th2 cells in susceptible individuals, a process in which dendritic cells are key players. This lack of regulation in the immune response leads to an ongoing inflammatory process, in which different immune processes follow one another and accumulate over time. The presence of the allergen not only induces the activation of an effector response that is responsible for the clinical manifestations but also promotes an immunomodulatory process which may determine the evolution of the disease. In addition, the genetic and environmental susceptibility of each patient plays a role in the activation of the inflammatory response, leading to a highly variable inflammatory process and ultimately a wide range of clinical manifestations.

Recently, some biological therapies that specifically control inflammatory pathways in allergy have been shown to be effective in models of asthma but their therapeutic efficacy is still under study. Current research strategies seek to exploit recent knowledge in relation to Treg and dendritic cells in order to induce specific tolerance against allergens that would allow longer-lasting control of allergic diseases.

References

Introduction

1. Akdis M, Blaser K, Akdis CA. T regulatory cells in allergy: novel concepts in the pathogenesis, prevention, and treatment of allergic diseases. J Allergy Clin Immunol 2005; 116:961–968.
2. Grunig G, Banz A, de Waal Malefyt R. Molecular regulation of Th2 immunity by dendritic cells. Pharmacol Ther 2005; 106:75–96.

Immunoglobulin E and receptors

3. Turner H, Kinet JP. Signalling through the high-affinity IgE receptor FcepsilonRI. Nature 1999; 402:B24–B30.
4. Davidsson A, Karlsson MG, Hellquist HB. Allergen-induced changes of B-cell phenotypes in patients with allergic rhinitis. Rhinology 1994; 32:184–190.
5. Cameron L, Hamid Q, Wright E, et al. Local synthesis of e germline gene transcripts, IL-4, and IL-13 in allergic nasal mucosa after ex vivo allergen exposure. J Allergy Clin Immunol 2000; 106:46–52.

Key inflammatory cells in human allergic airways disease

6. Bousquet J, Chanez P, Lacoste JY, et al. Eosinophilic inflammation in asthma. N Engl J Med 1990; 323:1033–1039.
7. Cameron L, Christodoulopoulos P, Lavigne F, et al. Evidence for local eosinophil differentiation within allergic nasal mucosa: inhibition with soluble IL-5 receptor. J Immunol 2000; 164: 1538–1545.
8. Sehmi R, Wood LJ, Watson R, et al. Allergen-induced increases in IL-5 receptor alpha-subunit expression on bone marrow-derived CD34+ cells from asthmatic subjects. A novel marker of progenitor cell commitment towards eosinophilic differentiation. J Clin Invest 1997; 100:2466–2475.
9. Robinson DS, Damia R, Zeibecoglou K, et al. CD34(+)/interleukin-5Ralpha messenger RNA+ cells in the bronchial mucosa in asthma: potential airway eosinophil progenitors. Am J Respir Cell Mol Biol 1999; 20:9–13.
10. Jeffery PK, Wardlaw AJ, Nelson FC, et al. Bronchial biopsies in asthma. An ultrastructural, quantitative study and correlation with hyperreactivity. Am Rev Respir Dis 1989; 140: 1745–1753.

11. Kelso A. Th1 and Th2 subsets: paradigms lost? Immunol Today 1995; 16:374–379.
12. Weiner HL. Induction and mechanism of action of transforming growth factor-beta-secreting Th3 regulatory cells. Immunol Rev 2001; 182:207–214.
13. Szabo SJ, Jacobson NG, Dighe AS, et al. Developmental commitment to the Th2 lineage by extinction of IL-12 signaling. Immunity 1995; 2:665–675.
14. Szabo SJ, Dighe AS, Gubler U, et al. Regulation of the interleukin (IL)-12R beta 2 subunit expression in developing T helper 1 (Th1) and Th2 cells. J Exp Med 1997; 185:817–824.
15. Rousset F, Robert J, Andary M, et al. Shifts in interleukin-4 and interferon-gamma production by T cells of patients with elevated serum IgE levels and the modulatory effects of these lymphokines on spontaneous IgE synthesis. J Allergy Clin Immunol 1991; 87:58–69.
16. Varney VA, Jacobson MR, Sudderick RM, et al. Immunohistology of the nasal mucosa following allergen-induced rhinitis. Identification of activated T lymphocytes, eosinophils, and neutrophils. Am Rev Respir Dis 1992; 146:170–176.
17. Christodoulopoulos P, Cameron L, Durham S, et al. Molecular pathology of allergic disease. II: Upper airway disease. J Allergy Clin Immunol 2000; 105:211–222.
18. Bradley BL, Azzawi M, Jacobson M, et al. Eosinophils, T-lymphocytes, mast cells, neutrophils, and macrophages in bronchial biopsy specimens from atopic subjects with asthma: comparison with biopsy specimens from atopic subjects without asthma and normal control subjects and relationship to bronchial hyperresponsiveness. J Allergy Clin Immunol 1991; 88:661–674.
19. Walker C, Kaegi MK, Braun P, et al. Activated T cells and eosinophilia in bronchoalveolar lavages from subjects with asthma correlated with disease severity. J Allergy Clin Immunol 1991; 88:935–942.
20. Meissner N, Kussebi F, Jung T, et al. A subset of CD8+ T cells from allergic patients produce IL-4 and stimulate IgE production in vitro. Clin Exp Allergy 1997; 27:1402–1411.
21. Baecher-Allan C, Brown JA, Freeman GJ, et al. CD4+CD25high regulatory cells in human peripheral blood. J Immunol 2001; 167:1245–1253.
22. Annacker O, Pimenta-Araujo R, Burlen-Defranoux O, et al. CD25+ CD4+ T cells regulate the expansion of peripheral CD4 T cells through the production of IL-10. J Immunol 2001; 166:3008–3018.
23. Brunkow ME, Jeffery EW, Hjerrild KA, et al. Disruption of a new forkhead/winged-helix protein, scurfin, results in the fatal lymphoproliferative disorder of the scurfy mouse. Nat Genet 2001; 27:68–73.
24. Grindebacke H, Wing K, Andersson AC, et al. Defective suppression of Th2 cytokines by CD4CD25 regulatory T cells in birch allergics during birch pollen season. Clin Exp Allergy 2004; 34:1364–1372.
25. Gelfand EW. Inflammatory mediators in allergic rhinitis. J Allergy Clin Immunol 2004; 114 (5 Suppl):S135–S138.
26. Bradding P, Holgate ST. Immunopathology and human mast cell cytokines. Crit Rev Oncol Hematol 1999; 31:119–133.
27. Gauchat JF, Henchoz S, Mazzei G, et al. Induction of human IgE synthesis in B cells by mast cells and basophils. Nature 1993; 365:340–343.
28. Schroeder JT, MacGlashan DW Jr, Lichtenstein LM. Human basophils: mediator release and cytokine production. Adv Immunol 2001; 77:93–122.
29. Nouri-Aria KT, Irani AM, Jacobson MR, et al. Basophil recruitment and IL-4 production during human allergen-induced late response. J Allergy Clin Immunol 2001; 108:205–211.
30. Pawankar R, Okuda M, Yssel H, et al. Nasal mast cells in perennial allergic rhinitis exhibit increased expression of the FcepsilonRI, CD40L, IL-4, and IL-13, and can induce IgE synthesis in B cells. J Clin Invest 1997; 99:1492–1499.
31. Miadonna A, Milazzo N, Gibelli S, et al. Nasal response to a single antigen challenge in patients with allergic rhinitis – inflammatory cell recruitment persists up to 48 hours. Clin Exp Allergy 1999; 29:941–949.

Th2 cytokine expression in human allergic airways disease

32. Robinson DS, Hamid Q, Ying S, et al. Predominant TH2-like bronchoalveolar T-lymphocyte population in atopic asthma. N Engl J Med 1992; 326:298–304.
33. Ying S, Durham SR, Corrigan CJ, et al. Phenotype of cells expressing mRNA for TH2-type (interleukin 4 and interleukin 5) and TH1-type (interleukin 2 and interferon gamma) cytokines in bronchoalveolar lavage and bronchial biopsies from atopic asthmatic and normal control subjects. Am J Respir Cell Mol Biol 1995; 12:477–487.
34. Pene J, Rousset F, Briere F, et al. IgE production by normal human lymphocytes is induced by interleukin 4 and suppressed by interferons gamma and alpha and prostaglandin E2. Proc Natl Acad Sci U S A 1988; 85:6880–6884.
35. Shi HZ, Deng JM, Xu H, et al. Effect of inhaled interleukin-4 on airway hyperreactivity in asthmatics. Am J Respir Crit Care Med 1998; 157:1818–1821.
36. Lamkhioued B, Renzi PM, Abi-Younes S, et al. Increased expression of eotaxin in bronchoalveolar lavage and airways of asthmatics contributes to the chemotaxis of eosinophils to the site of inflammation. J Immunol 1997; 159:4593–4601.
37. Gounni AS, Nutku E, Koussih L, et al. IL-9 expression by human eosinophils: regulation by IL-1beta and TNF-alpha. J Allergy Clin Immunol 2000; 106:460–466.
38. Shimbara A, Christodoulopoulos P, Soussi-Gounni A, et al. IL-9 and its receptor in allergic and nonallergic lung disease: increased expression in asthma. J Allergy Clin Immunol 2000; 105:108–115.
39. Ying S, Meng Q, Kay AB, et al. Elevated expression of interleukin-9 mRNA in the bronchial mucosa of atopic asthmatics and allergen-induced cutaneous late-phase reaction: relationships to eosinophils, mast cells and T lymphocytes. Clin Exp Allergy 2002; 32:866–871.
40. Erpenbeck VJ, Hohlfeld JM, Volkmann B, et al. Segmental allergen challenge in patients with atopic asthma leads to increased IL-9 expression in bronchoalveolar lavage fluid lymphocytes. J Allergy Clin Immunol 2003; 111:1319–1327.
41. Ghaffar O, Laberge S, Jacobson MR, et al. IL-13 mRNA and immunoreactivity in allergen-induced rhinitis: comparison with IL-4 expression and modulation by topical glucocorticoid therapy. Am J Respir Cell Mol Biol 1997; 17:17–24.
42. Huang SK, Xiao HQ, Kleine-Tebbe J, et al. IL-13 expression at the sites of allergen challenge in patients with asthma. J Immunol 1995; 155:2688–2694.
43. Humbert M, Durham SR, Kimmitt P, et al. Elevated expression of messenger ribonucleic acid encoding IL-13 in the bronchial mucosa of atopic and nonatopic subjects with asthma. J Allergy Clin Immunol 1997; 99:657–665.
44. Cheung PF, Wong CK, Ip WK, Lam CW. IL-25 regulates the expression of adhesion molecules on eosinophils: mechanism of eosinophilia in allergic inflammation. Allergy 2006; 61:878–885.
45. Wong CK, Cheung PF, Ip WK, Lam CW. Interleukin-25-induced chemokines and interleukin-6 release from eosinophils is mediated by p38 mitogen-activated protein kinase, c-Jun N-terminal kinase, and nuclear factor-kappaB. Am J Respir Cell Mol Biol 2005; 33:186–194.

Chemokines in allergic airways inflammation

46. Minshall EM, Cameron L, Lavigne F, et al. Eotaxin mRNA and protein expression in chronic sinusitis and allergen-induced nasal responses in seasonal allergic rhinitis. Am J Respir Cell Mol Biol 1997; 17:683–690.
47. Devalia JL, Bayram H, Abdelaziz MM, et al. Differences between cytokine release from bronchial epithelial cells of asthmatic patients and non-asthmatic subjects: effect of exposure to diesel exhaust particles. Int Arch Allergy Immunol 1999; 118:437–439.
48. Christodoulopoulos P, Wright E, Frenkiel S, et al. Monocyte chemotactic proteins in allergen-induced inflammation in the nasal mucosa: effect of topical corticosteroids. J Allergy Clin Immunol 1999; 103:1036–1044.
49. Joubert P, Lajoie-Kadoch S, Labonte I, et al. CCR3 expression and function in asthmatic airway smooth muscle cells. J Immunol 2005; 175:2702–2708.

Transcription factors

50. Nakamura Y, Christodoulopoulos P, Cameron L, et al. Upregulation of the transcription factor GATA-3 in upper airway mucosa after in vivo and in vitro allergen challenge. J Allergy Clin Immunol 2000; 105:1146–1152.
51. Erpenbeck VJ, Hagenberg A, Krentel H, et al. Regulation of GATA-3, c-maf and T-bet mRNA expression in bronchoalveolar lavage cells and bronchial biopsies after segmental allergen challenge. Int Arch Allergy Immunol 2006; 139:306–316.
52. Ghaffar O, Christodoulopoulos P, Lamkhioued B, et al. In vivo expression of signal transducer and activator of transcription factor 6 (STAT-6) in nasal mucosa from atopic allergic rhinitis: effect of topical corticosteroids. Clin Exp Allergy 2000; 30:86.
53. Christodoulopoulos P, Cameron L, Nakamura Y, et al. Th2 cytokine-associated transcription factors in atopic and nonatopic asthma: evidence for differential signal transducer and activator of transcription 6 expression. J Allergy Clin Immunol 2001; 107:586.
54. Finotto S, Neurath MF, Glickman JN, et al. Development of spontaneous airway changes consistent with human asthma in mice lacking T-bet. Science 2002; 295:336–338.

section B

AEROBIOLOGY AND ALLERGENS

Air Pollution: Indoor and Outdoor

David B Peden

31

SUMMARY OF IMPORTANT CONCEPTS

>> Air pollutants are a clear cause of asthma exacerbation, and some studies suggest pollution may contribute to development of asthma

>> Increase in airway inflammation is a frequent mode of action of air pollutants in asthma

>> Exposure to air pollutants enhances response to allergens

>> Oxidant stress is an important element of response to pollutants, and genetic variability in antioxidant responses to pollutants likely account for increased susceptibility to pollutants

>> Antiinflammatory treatments are promising interventions for decreasing the response to pollutants

>> Community-wide approaches to decrease pollutant exposure have been shown to decrease exacerbations of disease due to pollution

INTRODUCTION

Air pollution and poor air quality is a worldwide problem. Though pollutants affect the entire population, specific subsets of the population are disproportionately affected, including the very young, the elderly, and people with pre-existing disease. Genetic risk factors also increase response to pollutants, and people of lower socioeconomic status may also have increased risk due to increased exposure to polluted environments associated with location and quality of housing stock.

Respiratory disease associated with poor air quality includes a number of occupational lung diseases (linked with occupation-specific air contaminants) and respiratory tract cancer (associated with radon exposure, outdoor pollutants, and second-hand tobacco smoke).[1] However, the most common adverse health effects associated with exposure to air pollutants are acute respiratory tract illnesses, including exacerbations of asthma or hospital admission for chronic obstructive pulmonary disease. Persons with allergic disorders of the airway are especially sensitive to the impact of air contaminants. Environmental pollutants may cause non-specific inflammatory or mechanical responses in the airway or modify Th2 response to allergen, either by promoting primary Th2 responses or enhancing recall response to environmental allergens in persons already sensitized, as summarized in Table 31.1.[2–7] The primary focus of this chapter is the impact of air pollutants on asthma and allergic inflammation.

NATURE OF AIRBORNE CONTAMINANTS

A variety of airborne contaminants are encountered in both indoor and outdoor environments, including carbon monoxide, lead, sulfur dioxide, oxides of nitrogen, ozone, particulate matter (PM), and biological agents, and are outlined in Table 31.2.[8] Except for carbon monoxide and lead, each of these pollutants has a reported impact on asthma. Some pollutants, such as sulfur dioxide, have primarily a bronchospastic effect. However, the majority of airborne pollutants have an inflammatory effect, despite the fact that these are a diverse group of molecules, including gases, metals, organic molecules, and biological compounds.

Table 31.1 Interactions between pollutant and allergen exposure: effects of in vivo airway challenge to ozone, diesel exhaust particles, and LPS on response to allergen in allergic volunteers

Observed effect of pollutant in humans	Ozone	DEP	LPS
Response to recall eosinophilic response to nasal allergen challenge	Increased	Increased	Increased
Immediate phase response to inhaled allergen (PD20)	Increased	Unknown	Increased
Effect on development of IgE response to a neoantigen	Unknown	Increased	Unknown
Effect on local (airway) IgE levels	Unknown	Increased	Unknown

DEP, diesel exhaust particles; LPS, lipopolysaccharide. (From: Peden.[6])

Table 31.2 Classification of air pollutants

A Primary/secondary pollutants

  i Primary: pollutants emitted directly into the atmosphere (e.g., SO_2, some NO_x species, CO, PM)
  ii Secondary: pollutants that form in the air as a result of chemical reactions with other pollutants and gases (e.g., ozone, NO_x, and some particulates)

B Indoor/outdoor pollutants

  i Indoor pollutants
    a Sources: cooking and combustion, particle resuspension, building materials, air conditioning, consumer products, smoking, heating, biologic agents
    b Products: combustion products (e.g., tobacco and wood smoke), CO, CO_2, SVOC (e.g. aldehydes, alcohol, alkanes, and ketones), microbial agents and organic dusts, radon, manmade vitreous fibers
  ii Outdoor pollutants
    a Sources: industrial, commercial, mobile, urban, regional, agricultural, natural
    b Products: SO_2, ozone, NO_x, CO, PM, SVOC

C Gaseous/particulate pollutants

  i Gaseous: SO_2, NO_x, ozone, CO, SVOC (e.g., PAH, dioxins, benzene, aldehydes, 1,3-butadiene)
  ii Particulate: coarse PM (2.5–10 μm; regulatory standard = PM_{10}), fine PM (0.1–2.5 μm; regulatory standard = $PM_{2.5}$); ultrafine PM (<0.1 μm; not regulated)

NO_x, nitrogen oxides; SVOC, specific volatile organic compounds. (From: Bernstein et al.[2])

The inflammatory actions of these pollutants account for the effect of pollutants in asthma.[2]

THE NATIONAL AMBIENT AIR QUALITY STANDARD (NAAQS)

The United States Environmental Protection Agency (EPA) oversees monitoring of specified air pollutants as outlined in the Clean Air Act of 1970, which has been most recently amended in 1990 with updated standards established in 1997.[9] The monitored (or criteria) pollutants include carbon monoxide, lead, sulfur dioxide (SO_2), nitrogen dioxide (NO_2), ozone (O_3), particulate matter (PM) <10 μm (PM_{10}, coarse mode) and 2.5 μm ($PM_{2.5}$, fine mode) in diameter. The NAAQS are outlined in Table 31.3.

To report air quality data to the general public, the air quality index (or AQI) was developed. AQI values have been developed for ozone, $PM_{2.5}$, CO, and SO_2, though at the time of this writing, only the AQI for ozone and $PM_{2.5}$ are routinely reported. For ozone, the AQI value of 100 is based on the 8-hour NAAQS for that pollutant (0.085 ppm ozone averaged over 8h). An AQI of 51–100 is considered 'moderate'

Table 31.3 National Ambient Air Quality Standards

Pollutant	Primary standards	Averaging times
Carbon monoxide	9 ppm (10 mg/m^3)	8 h
	35 ppm (40 mg/m^3)	1 h
Lead	1.5 μg/m^3	Quarterly average
Nitrogen dioxide	0.053 ppm (100 μg/m^3)	Annual (arithmetic mean)
Particulate matter (PM$_{10}$)	150 μg/m^3	24 h
Particulate matter (PM$_{2.5}$)	15.0 μg/m^3	Annual (arithmetic mean)
	35 μg/m^3	24 h
Ozone	0.08 ppm	8 h
	0.12 ppm	1 h (applies only in limited areas)
Sulfur oxides	0.03 ppm	Annual (arithmetic mean)
	0.14 ppm	24 h

Table 31.4 Air quality index (AQI)

Categories	AQI value and color	O$_3$ (ppm), 8 h	CO (ppm), 8 h	SO$_2$ (ppm), 24 h	PM$_{2.5}$ (μg/m^3), 24 h
Good	0–50 Green	0.000–0.064	0.0–4.4	0.000–0.034	0.0–15.4
Moderate	51–100 Yellow	0.065–0.084	4.5–9.4	0.035–0.144	15.5–40.4
Unhealthy for sensitive groups	101–150 Orange	0.085–0.104	9.5–12.4	0.145–0.224	40.5–65.4
Unhealthy	151–200 Red	0.105–0.124	12.5–15.4	0.225–0.304	65.5–150.4
Very unhealthy	201–300 Purple	0.125–0.374	15.5–30.4	0.305–0.604	150.5–250.4

and usually reported as a 'code yellow' level. AQIs of 101–150 are listed as unhealthy for 'sensitive groups' and reported as a 'code orange' day. A 'code red' condition exists when the AQIs is 151–200 and is considered unhealthy. An AQI over 200 is considered very unhealthy. A comparison of the NAAQS for the criteria pollutants and AQI scales for each pollutant are shown in Table 31.4.

In setting the NAAQS for a given pollutant, several types of data are reviewed, including those from epidemiological and human exposure studies. Epidemiological data are those that demonstrate increased occurrence of a disease outcome in correlation with increased exposure to an outdoor pollutant. Human exposure data are derived from studies in which human volunteers undergo experimental exposure to a given pollutant and undergo various types of measurements, including lung function, non-specific airway hyperresponsiveness, responsiveness to a specific allergen, and changes in airway inflammation.[10,11]

There are several problems associated with the establishment and enforcement of air pollution standards. First, it is difficult to establish a 'no-effect' level of response to air pollutants. Human variability is such that even very small levels of a pollutant can be found that have a deleterious effect on human health. Also, it is difficult to establish how large a susceptible population must be to invoke special protection under the Clean Air Act. Additionally, some areas may be out of compliance due to pollutants that are produced elsewhere, often hundreds of miles distant to where increased pollutant levels were observed.[10,11] While the EPA is charged with setting the NAAQS, state agencies are responsible for implementing the standards and carry out actual monitoring of air quality.

SOURCES OF OUTDOOR AIR POLLUTANTS

Outdoor air pollutants derive from a number of sources.[12] These are generally considered as *point sources* or *mobile sources*. Point sources include facilities that operate from a fixed location that routinely emit gaseous and particulate pollutants into the air and can include power plants, chemical plants, steel and other metallurgical processing facilities. Mobile sources include automobiles, trucks, and aircraft. Other sources that can be considered as mobile sources include lawn mowers, marine motors, farm vehicles, and snowmobiles.[9]

In the USA, it is estimated that point sources account for approximately 93% of SO_2 emissions, 51% of the emissions of nitrogen oxides (NO_x), 9% of CO emissions, and 52% of volatile organic compound (VOC) emissions. While it can be argued that a large fraction of PM_{10} derive from non-man-made sources, point sources contribute to these as well. Mobile sources account for 2% of SO_2 emissions, 45% of NO_x emissions, 81% of CO emissions, and 37% of VOCs. Mobile sources also contribute to PM production.

Nitrogen dioxide (NO_2), a precursor to photochemical smog, is found in ambient outdoor air in urban and industrial regions and results primarily in combustion of fossil fuels or natural gas. Ozone is a by-product of atmospheric reactions that require NO_x, VOCs, and ultraviolet light. Thus, ozone will be highest in areas with substantial amounts of sunlight, NO_x (which includes NO_2), and VOCs as well as weather conditions that allow for production of ozone. In most regions of the USA, ozone levels are increased from May through September, and on a daily basis,

peak in the afternoon. Figures 31.1 and 31.2 depict areas in the USA that exceed the NAAQS for ozone and PM_{10} >2 times/year. Figure 31.3 depicts the counties in the USA which were out of attainment for 1–3 of the monitored NAAQS pollutants in 2006.

DETERMINANTS OF INDOOR AIR QUALITY

Biomass burning represents a significant source of indoor air pollution, and includes burning of tobacco, wood, and other biologically derived plant fuels.[13–16] In general, biomass burning results in production of particulates which are rich in polyaromatic hydrocarbons and other organic molecules which can be metabolized to quinones and other oxidant species.[4] Environmental tobacco smoke (ETS) (sidestream smoke from the burning end of the cigarette and exhaled mainstream smoke from the smoker) is a major source of gases and respirable particles in indoor environments and is perhaps the most significant

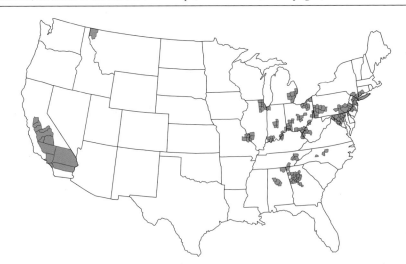

Non-attainnment areas (329 entire counties)
Non-attainment areas (37 partial counties)
Maintenance areas (108 entire or partial counties)
Partial counties, those with part of the county designated non-attainment and part attainment, are shown as full counties on the map

Fig. 31.1. Non-attainment and maintenance areas in the US 8-h ozone standard. Partial counties, those with part of the county designated non-attainment and part-attainment, are shown as full counties on the map. (*Source* US EPA; www.epa.gov.)

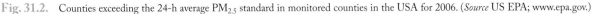

Fig. 31.2. Counties exceeding the 24-h average $PM_{2.5}$ standard in monitored counties in the USA for 2006. (*Source* US EPA; www.epa.gov.)

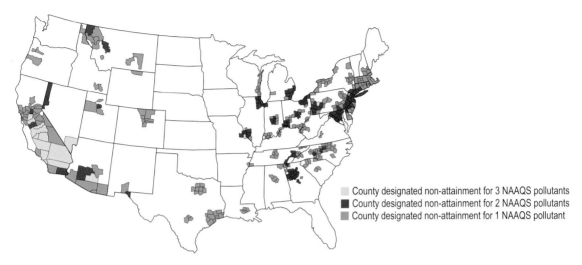

County designated non-attainment for 3 NAAQS pollutants
County designated non-attainment for 2 NAAQS pollutants
County designated non-attainment for 1 NAAQS pollutant

Fig. 31.3. Counties in the USA which were out of attainment for 1–3 monitored air pollutants in 2006. (*Source* US EPA; www.epa.gov.)

and remediable indoor air contaminant in the USA. An example of the impact of ETS on indoor particulates is shown in a study of 11 hospitality locations in Paducah, Kentucky. In these locations (primarily restaurants), the mean $PM_{2.5}$ concentration in smoking areas was $177\,\mu g/m^3$ and $87\,\mu g/m^3$ in the non-smoking section. The $PM_{2.5}$ concentration of the non-smoking section was 29 times higher than that in smoke-free air and six times higher than local outdoor air in Paducah.[17] Endotoxin levels of indoor particulates are also increased in locations where smoking occurs.[18] Burning of wood in indoor stoves and fireplaces also generates indoor particulates and gases, and is associated with increased respiratory tract illness. Thus, one significant determinant of indoor air quality is use of tobacco or wood fuel inside domestic settings.

Another significant indoor pollutant is nitrogen dioxide. While NO_2 is known to be a precursor for ozone, in indoor settings it likely exerts a direct effect in asthma. A primary source of indoor NO_2 is use of natural gas appliances, especially if they are poorly maintained or poorly vented. A number of studies have found that increased levels of NO_2 inside dwellings correlate with increased respiratory symptoms in children.[19] These studies also link increased reports of cough, wheeze, phlegm, and bronchitis with the annual average household NO_2 concentration as well as an enhancement of the effect of viral infection in asthma.[19–23]

Biological contaminants certainly contribute to poor air quality, including indoor endotoxin, products from Gram-positive bacteria, and 1,3 β-glucans from molds and may also impact airway inflammation in both atopic and non-atopic subjects. Many studies have shown that indoor levels of endotoxin are associated with increased respiratory tract illness in both allergic and non-allergic persons in domestic settings,[24] as well as occupational settings.[25,26] In domestic settings, the number of animals (dogs, cats, and evidence of rodents) and people living in the home correlates with the amount of endotoxin present. Older homes tend to have more environmental endotoxin. Some studies suggest that frequency of indoor cleaning is also linked with endotoxin levels.[27–29]

There are conflicting observations regarding the relationship between increased humidity and endotoxin levels. However, when humidity and dampness are examined independently of an association with endotoxin, there is a growing body of evidence that decreased levels of humidity are associated with decreased severity of asthma.[30,31] It is well known that humidity plays a role in allowing for increases in house dust mite allergen as well as mold growth. However, effects on mite allergen alone do not account for the entire effect of humidity in asthma. Nicolai et al[32] identified, in a large cross-sectional study of 4th grade school children in Munich, Germany, 234 children with active asthma (5% of the total cohort). Three years later, 155 of these children underwent measurement of lung function and non-specific airway reactivity. Dampness was associated with increased nighttime wheeze and shortness of breath but not with persisting asthma. Risk factors for bronchial hyperreactivity in adolescence included allergen exposure and damp housing conditions. Mite antigen levels were examined from homes of 70% of the asthma cohort and found to significantly correlate with dampness and bronchial hyperreactivity. However, the effect of dampness was not due to mite allergen alone, as bronchial hyperreactivity remained significantly correlated with humidity even when adjusting for mite allergen levels.

In summary, there are a number of features which contribute to indoor air quality. Biomass burning, including use of tobacco, is a primary cause of air pollution indoors. Other items which impact air quality include presence of household chemicals, mode of heating and cooking, maintenance of appropriate ventilation systems, presence of animals (either pets or vermin), and the number of persons present in the home or office. Humidity within buildings and water damage also contribute to indoor air quality, likely by allowing for increased allergen and microbial molecules in the indoor air shed.

BIOLOGICAL EFFECTS OF SPECIFIC AIR POLLUTANTS

PARTICULATE MATTER

Numerous studies have repeatedly demonstrated that increased exposure to respirable particulate matter (PM) (<10 μm size) is associated with exacerbation of asthma and other respiratory diseases in locations as varied as China, Brazil, Australia, New Zealand, and various locations in Europe and the USA. Studies performed in the Utah Valley offer a unique opportunity to link the effect of particulates to a particular point source, focusing on the relationship between airborne particulates and occurrence of respiratory disease associated with the activity of a steel mill which was inactive for 1 year due to a labor dispute.[33,34] Both respiratory disease and the level of particulates were markedly decreased during the strike year compared with those seen in the years preceding and following the strike, demonstrating a link between pollutant generation by the mill, levels of ambient air particulates, and occurrence of disease exacerbation in asthma and bronchitis.

Particulates from vehicles also impact on respiratory disease. One example of this is seen in a study of 1759 children who were enrolled at age 10 and followed through to age 18, from 12 Southern Californian cities. It was observed that exposure to a number of products of vehicular fuel use (NO_2, acid vapor, $PM_{2.5}$ and elemental carbon, but not O_3, PM_{10}, or elemental carbon) was significantly correlated to decreased lung function in the cohort. When examining the role of $PM_{2.5}$ on lung function, it was found that 1.6% of children had a FEV_1 of <80% of predicted with chronic exposure to 5μg/m^3 vs 7.9% of children exposed to 20 μg/m^3.[35]

Further evidence of the impact of vehicular traffic in asthma is found in studies of the relationship of proximity to a roadway on health measures. A survey of traffic exposure (estimated by traffic counts and an emission model which predicted soot, benzene, and nitrogen dioxide (NO_2) exposure) and its effect on allergen skin test response, presence of serum IgE, and lung function testing was conducted in approximately 6200 German children.[32] Traffic counts correlated with active asthma, cough and wheeze, and in children exposed to ETS, a positive skin test. Pollutant exposure was also linked to cough, wheeze, and asthma. In a study in Birmingham UK,[36] children aged <5 years who lived in a high traffic exposure area (>24000 vehicles/24h at the nearest segment of main road) were more likely to be admitted to hospital for asthma with traffic exposure (vehicles/24h) correlating well with admission in those living <500m from a road (p <0.006). Compared with well children, those admitted for respiratory reasons were more likely to live within 200m of a main road (p <0.02), consistent with results from a case (n = 417) /control (n = 461) study in Erie County, NY, of children aged 0–14 years, which indicated that exposure to high truck volume within a 200m distance was associated with increased risk for hospitalization due to asthma.[37] Likewise, in a study of adult veterans, there is a reported 1.7 relative risk of wheeze associated with living within 50m of a heavily traveled road compared with those living more than 400m from a road.[38] Other health outcomes, most notably myocardial infarction, have been associated with proximity to vehicular traffic.[39]

CHALLENGE STUDIES WITH CONCENTRATED AIR PARTICULATES

Another approach used in assessing the effect of PM in humans is to use particle concentrators, which allow ambient air particulates to be concentrated into a given volume of air, as reviewed by Ghio and Huang.[40] Air containing the concentrated air particulates (CAPs) is then vented into an exposure chamber and volunteers are exposed to air containing such samples, followed by sampling of the airway, typically via bronchoscopy. Studies of the effect of CAPs exposures have generally revealed that ambient air particulates (usually $PM_{2.5}$) can result in mild

airway inflammation. It has also been shown that changes in heart rate variability and other systemic effects can be observed following CAPs exposures.

CHALLENGE STUDIES WITH METAL-RICH PREPARATIONS

The ability of metals to induce airway inflammation in humans has been investigated in studies in which preparations made from particulates with high and low metal content were instilled into airway bronchial segments and recovered bronchoalveolar lavage fluid was assessed for evidence of inflammation. Particles recovered from ambient air from the Utah Valley studies outlined above were studied. Extracts of particles in equal mass amounts from the year of the labor stoppage as well as the years preceding and following the strike were instilled into the airways of normal volunteers using segmental bronchoscopic techniques. While each of these extracts induced some influx of neutrophils relative to a control challenge (saline), there was a marked decrease in inflammation associated with extracts from the strike year from those produced from particles collected during the years that the mill was active. Furthermore, in vitro oxidant activity was decreased in particles collected during the strike year. Both antioxidants and metal chelators blunted oxidant activity from the particulate samples.[41]

A similar study was conducted in which preparations from $PM_{2.5}$ samples were collected from the German cities of Hettstedt and Zerbst. Hettstedt is the location of a smelter and Zerbst is a non-industrial town, and epidemiological studies have shown that asthma exacerbations are more common in children from the Hettstedt region. $PM_{2.5}$ samples from the Hettstedt regions had markedly increased levels of copper, nickel, and, zinc than did those from Zerbst, and normal volunteers challenged with extracts from the Hettstedt samples had increased airway monocytes which had an enhanced oxidative burst relative to results following challenge with Zerbst sample preparations.[42] These results demonstrate that metals in particulates induce airway inflammation, likely due to oxidant activity associated with transition metal content of the particles, and contribute to the inflammatory response to PM.

CHALLENGE STUDIES WITH ENDOTOXIN

Biological agents such as endotoxin have also been identified on both $PM_{2.5}$ and PM_{10} particles[43–45] and have been associated with increased airway inflammation in human challenge studies.[25] Environmental endotoxin is perhaps been known in the context of the hygiene hypothesis, in which exposures to endotoxin in early life have been linked to decreased development of allergic disease and asthma. However, environmental endotoxin is also clearly linked to respiratory tract morbidity as well. Endotoxin-rich PM found in agricultural settings has been linked to occupational lung disease and ambient air endotoxin is associated with increased respiratory tract disease in allergic and non-allergic persons. Human challenge studies with endotoxin reveal increased airway neutrophilia at higher doses. Additionally, both higher and lower doses of endotoxin reveal changes in airway macrophages and monocytes in which cell-surface markers for both innate immune and antigen-presenting function are increased, suggesting that endotoxin may not only directly induce inflammation but also enhance response to antigens, including those associated with Th2 responses.[25,26,46]

A recent study examining the airway responses to inhaled bolus doses of coarse PM from ambient air reveal that both increased PMN numbers as well as increased expression of MHC class II molecules on macrophages can be induced by ambient air PM, but that heat treatment which denatures endotoxin blunts the effect of PM on macrophage surface marker expression.[47] Thus, it is possible that a major effect of low-level environmental endotoxin in asthma is enhancement of response to allergen via actions on antigen-presenting cells. Indeed, low-level endotoxin challenge has been shown to enhance immediate phase response to inhaled allergen as well as late phase to nasally applied allergen.[48,49] Finally, it should also be pointed out that allergen-induced inflammation enhances expression of molecules involved in response to endotoxin (most notably CD14 expression on airway monocytes), indicating that allergic individuals may have enhanced response to environmental endotoxin.[50,51]

RESPONSES TO DIESEL EXHAUST

The effect of diesel exhaust (DE) and diesel exhaust particles (DEPs) on airway inflammation and Th2 immune function has been very avidly studied. In general, many studies have shown that these agents induce airway inflammation and exert significant oxidant stress on airway cells and tissues. Diesel exhaust particles have been shown in numerous animal, in vitro, and human challenge studies to skew immune responses towards a Th2 response.[52–55] Numerous human challenge studies have examined the effect of DE and DEP on airway inflammation and lung function. In general, two approaches have been employed to examine the role of diesel on airway inflammation: one in which exposure to diluted DE (which will contain both particulates and gases such as NO_2) in real time has been employed, and another in which DEP are examined in nasal challenge or bronchial instillation studies.

Much of the action of DEP is due to oxidative stress induced by the metabolism of polyaromatic hydrocarbons (PAHs) to quinones and other oxidant species by enzymes such as cytochrome P450, and will be discussed in further detail below. The potency of specific forms of DE appears to be due, in part, to the amount of PAHs present on a given particle. This has been shown in animal studies comparing two types of DE (which vary on the basis of organic molecule content) in which the low-PAH-containing particles had much less effect on inflammation than did the PAH-rich preparations.[56] Likewise, in humans, airway challenge studies employing PAH-rich DEP particles yield much more pro-inflammatory and allergic responses compared with studies using DEPs with low organic molecule content.[57,58]

A series of studies conducted by a joint Swedish and British research team has focused on the effect of diluted DE on inflammatory, cytokine, and antioxidant responses of the airway of normal and allergic volunteers exposed in real time to a diluted DE at particle levels ranging from 100 to 300 µg diesel particles/m^3 air.[59–65] These investigators have reported that DE enhances non-specific airway reactivity, induces increased numbers of neutrophils, B-lymphocytes, and IL-6 in BAL fluid, and increases mast cell and neutrophil numbers in biopsy specimens. Analysis of biopsy specimens recovered after exposure to 300 µg/m^3 diesel particles also reveals that ICAM-1, VCAM-1, and IL-13 expression is increased in airway epithelium as is the presence of phosphorylated p38, NF-B (p65), and phosphorylated JNK as examined by immunostaining of the specimens.[61,62] It is intriguing that low-level diesel causes increase inflammation (PMNs, IL-6) in the airways of normal volunteers but not

mild asthmatics. However, there is an increase in IL-10 in the airways of asthmatics, though it is not clear if IL-10 minimizes inflammatory response due to DE.[65]

A study of 15 normal volunteers challenged with lower doses of DE (100 mg/m^3 diesel particles) and clean air reveals that there is an increase in neutrophil and mast cell numbers in the bronchial mucosa and neutrophils, IL-8, and myeloperoxidase concentrations in lavage of the bronchial region recovered 18 h after challenge, whereas no inflammatory response was noted in lavage fluid from the alveolar spaces. It is intriguing that there was an increase in the antioxidants glutathione (GSH) and urate in the alveolar lavage but not the bronchial lavage (the compartment in which inflammation was noted). An examination of airway antioxidant levels 6 h after exposure to this same level of diesel found no evidence of inflammation in lavage fluid from either the bronchial or alveolar compartments with an associated increase in glutathione present in nasal and bronchial samples. These results suggest that there is a compartmentalization of responses to inhaled DE, as well as temporally specific differences in response to DE in these compartments.[59,60]

Another approach to examining the effect of DE on airway inflammation and allergy is to conduct studies of DEPs. Numerous animal and in vitro studies have demonstrated that DEPs shift primary immune responses to antigens towards a Th2 phenotype, characterized by production of antigen-specific IgE, and enhances allergen-induced immune responses, including increasing IgE production and enhancing cytokines involved in eosinophilic or allergic inflammation, especially IL-4, IL-5, and GM-CSF, as well as airway hyperresponsiveness.[54] DEPs have been reported to induce B-lymphocyte immunoglobulin isotype switching to IgE.

Nasal challenge studies in humans employed by Diaz-Sanchez et al demonstrate that challenge of volunteers (four atopic and seven nonatopic) to DEP increased nasal IgE production 4 days after DEP challenge without any effect on IgG, IgA or IgM. There were also shifts in the ratio of the five isoforms of IgE noted with the challenge as well. This effect was very dose specific as only a dose of 0.3 mg DEP caused this result. In a series of studies (which are extensively reviewed elsewhere),[4,52,54,66] this group reported that DEP challenge of the nasal mucosa causes increased cytokine production by cells recovered in lavage fluid. When comparing nasal lavage fluid components recovered pre- and post-challenge with 0.3 mg of DEP, pre-challenge lavage cells had detectable mRNA levels for γ-interferon, IL-2, and IL-13, whereas cells recovered post-challenge had detectable levels of mRNA for IL-4, IL-5, IL-6, IL-10 (in addition to mRNA for IL-2, IL-13, and γ-interferon). When coupled with challenge with ragweed allergen in ragweed sensitized atopic subjects, DEP was found to yield an enhanced ragweed-specific IgE and IgG response to ragweed allergen when compared to ragweed alone. This effect included increased expression of IL-4, IL-5, IL-6, IL-10, IL-13 and decreased expression of γ-interferon and IL-2 and had no effect on total IgE and IgG.

DEP challenge can also shift primary immune responses of the nasal mucosa in humans to keyhole limpet hemocyanin (KLH, a neoantigen rarely encountered by humans) towards a Th2 phenotype, yielding KLH-specific IgE. Without DEPs, immune response to KLH is of the Th1 type characterized by KLH-specific IgE.[67] A recent report demonstrated that DEP treatment of murine dendritic cells prevented TLR4-induced activation of MHC class II and other accessory molecule which would promote Th1 responses, suggesting a cellular mechanism by which DEP modulates immune response.[68]

ENVIRONMENTAL TOBACCO SMOKE

Environmental tobacco smoke (ETS) exposure has been associated with increased occurrence of otitis media, upper and lower respiratory tract infections, wheezing, and even increased occurrence of cancer in persons living with active smokers. ETS is clearly a significant factor in exacerbating airway illnesses affecting airway mucosa. The evidence is overwhelming that ETS is a cause of airway disease, with numerous reviews detailing the role of ETS in asthma exacerbation and development of allergy.[4,69–71]

Supporting the epidemiological observations that indicate that ETS exposure, especially during early life, increases the occurrence of allergy and asthma, are murine studies that examine the impact of ETS or components of ETS on airway immune function. Studies by Seymour and colleagues have shown that mice exposed to ETS have increased levels of the Th2 cytokines IL-4 and IL-10 and eosinophils following allergen challenge.[72] Other studies by Diaz-Sanchez and colleagues also demonstrate that mice exposed to ETS during sensitization with ovalbumin (OVA) have marked increases in Th2-type recall responses to subsequent challenge with OVA not seen in animals exposed to ETS alone or following OVA sensitization without exposure to ETS.[73] Following up on this observation, these investigators examined the effect of experimental exposure to ETS on nasal responses to allergen in humans, and found a marked enhancement of allergen-induced specific IgE and IgG4, increased IL-4, IL-5, and IL-13, with decreased levels of γ-interferon, and increased amounts of post-allergen histamine in nasal lavage fluid.[74] It is notable that polyaromatic hydrocarbons, the same species of molecules that likely mediate the Th2-promoting actions of DEP as previously discussed, are also found in ETS. Taken together, these studies provide initial mechanistic support to the epidemiological reports suggesting that ETS exposure enhances development of atopy and asthma.[2,4,66]

■ GAS PHASE AIR POLLUTANTS ■

SULFUR DIOXIDE

The effects of SO_2 have been extensively reviewed.[8,75] Total emergency room visits for respiratory problems and increased hospital admission rates have been linked with increased ambient exposure to SO_2. In children, decreased lung function has been linked to increases in ambient sulfur dioxide levels and the likelihood of chronic asthma or obstructive lung disease likewise is associated with lifetime exposure to SO_2. However, in many of these studies, it is difficult to separate effects of sulfur dioxide from that of particulate air pollutants. Additionally, ambient SO_2 may contribute to acid aerosol (H_2SO_4) formation and may exert effects either as a gas or by contributing to H_2SO_4 particle formation.

Challenge studies with sulfur dioxide do not demonstrate substantial inflammatory effects at concentrations encountered in ambient air. However, this gas has potent bronchospastic effects, with most asthmatics reacting at 0.50 ppm. In contrast, normal volunteers are unaffected, with concentrations as high as 0.6 ppm while sensitive asthmatics FEV_1 can drop by as much as 60% at concentrations as low as 0.25 ppm. SO_2-related symptoms in asthmatics include wheezing, chest discomfort, and dyspnea. SO_2 has a rapid onset of action, with responses observed within 2 min into exposure, becoming maximal within 5–10 min. Spontaneous recovery occurs within 30 min and exposed asthmatics are refractory to

the effects of SO_2 for up to 4 h after initial exposure. Repeated exposures to SO_2 induce tachyphylaxis as well.

Nasal breathing has been shown to largely mitigate the effect of SO_2 in asthmatics, likely due to absorption of this water-soluble gas by the nasal mucosa. Exercise results in a shift from strictly nasal breathing to combined oral and nasal respiration, thus increasing the amount of SO_2 that will reach the lower airway, and possibly accounting for the effect of exercise on sensitivity to SO_2. Additionally, asthmatics have a high occurrence of nasal co-morbidities (such as allergic rhinitis or sinusitis), which may further decrease nasal airflow, possibly contributing to sensitivity to the effect of SO_2 by increasing effect dose to the lower airway.

NITROGEN DIOXIDE

Epidemiological studies have shown a strong association between ambient air NO_2 and both chronic and acute changes in lung function. In human challenge studies, NO_2 has been shown to enhance airway inflammation, a prominent feature of asthma. In non-asthmatics, NO_2 exposure is associated with an influx of airway PMNs. NO_2 has been shown to induce pro-inflammatory cytokine production in epithelial cells following in vitro pollutant exposure. Overall, these data suggest that NO_2 could influence airway function of asthmatics by increasing airway inflammation. However, most studies fail to show an effect of low levels of NO_2 on non-specific airway reactivity. Higher levels of NO_2 (4.0 ppm) may impact airway function of asthmatics.[8,75–77]

However, a number of studies have demonstrated that NO_2 has a more impressive effect on response to airway allergen challenge in allergic asthmatics.[78–81] Exposure to 0.4 ppm NO_2 for 4 h has been reported to enhance response to inhaled allergen. Additionally, a combination of 0.2 ppm SO_2 and 0.4 ppm NO_2 for 6 h enhances immediate bronchial responses of mild asthmatics to inhaled allergen. Exposure to NO_2 also enhances late-phase responses of asthmatics to inhaled allergen. Likewise, exposure to 0.4 ppm NO_2 for 6 h increases allergen-induced ECP in the nasal airways of allergic asthmatics. Taken together, these studies demonstrate that NO_2 can augment acute response to allergen in atopic subjects.

OZONE

An overwhelming number of studies demonstrate that there is an association between increased levels of ambient air ozone and exacerbations of asthma, as measured by hospitalizations, rescue medication use, and symptoms.[2,5,8,82] Of note is a 24–48 h time lag between the ozone exposure and occurrence of hospital admission. Gent et al reported that even ozone levels significantly less that the current NAASQ for ozone are also associated with increased exacerbations of asthma.[83] Overall, ozone exposure is strongly associated with increased asthma morbidity, and is a major trigger for asthma exacerbation in summer months.

While ozone is thought of as a major cause of asthma exacerbation, there is mounting evidence that chronic exposure to ozone is linked to increased occurrence of lung disease. A cohort of 3535 children with no history of asthma from 12 schools in southern California was studied for up to 5 years,[84] with 265 children developing a new diagnosis of asthma during this observation period. It was observed that participation in outdoor sports (presumably associated with increased minute ventilation) in areas of increased ozone concentration was a risk factor for asthma development relative to similar exercise in areas where ozone exposures were low. McDonnell and colleagues prospectively studied a cohort of 3091 adult non-smokers. Over a 15-year interval, new diagnoses of asthma by a physician occurred in 3.2% of men and 4.3% of women. In the men (but not the women) with newly diagnosed asthma, the 20-year mean 8-h average for ambient ozone levels was a significant risk factor associated with new asthma (relative risk (RR) of 2.09 for a 27 ppb increase in ambient air ozone).[85] As with NO_2, chronic exposure to O_3 is also associated with decreased lung function, as noted in a study of 255 college students from regions with high and low pollution levels. In this study, chronic ambient O_3 levels were linked to decreased measures of small airways function (as assessed by FEF75 and FEF25–75), which is not altered after accounting for a history of chronic respiratory disease, allergy, second-hand exposure to environmental tobacco smoke, exposure to PM_{10}, and NO_2.[86] Taken together, these and other reports indicate that chronic ozone exposure contributes to disease causation.

Controlled exposure studies have revealed two primary effects of ozone in humans. One of these effects is a relatively rapid decrease in FVC and FEV_1, accompanied by a sensation of chest discomfort when taking a deep breath and an increase in non-specific bronchial responsiveness. The second effect is development of neutrophilic inflammation which can be seen as early as 1 hour after exposure, but persists for as long as 24 h after exposure.[87,88] Despite the temporal relationship between these two general effects to acute ozone exposure, inflammatory and lung function changes do not correlate with each other, suggesting that they are mediated separately.

The effective dose of ozone is dependent on the concentration of ozone, duration of exposure, and the level of exercise (with corresponding increases in minute ventilation). Exposure to ozone without exercise usually exerts no effect on lung function at levels below 0.50 ppm. However, with exercise, ozone induces increases in respiratory frequency and the concentration of ozone required to cause decreases in FEV_1, FVC, airway resistance, and symptoms can be much less.[89,90] These observations have led to recommendations that exercise be minimized in persons who may be susceptible to the effect of ozone.

Human and animal studies confirm that ozone induces neutrophilic influx into the airway. In humans, this has been shown in both BAL fluid and in bronchial mucosal biopsies recovered from subjects following exposures ranging from 0.10 to 0.4 ppm. Neutrophil influx occurs early (1–6 h after exposure) and persists until at least the next day. Inflammatory mediators such as IL-6, IL-8, PGE_2, LTB_4, TXB_2, fibronectin, plasminogen activator, and elastase are also increased by ozone. Direct comparison of the kinetics of mediator response to ozone shows that changes in IL-6 and PGE_2 peak 1 hour after exposure, whereas fibronectin and plasminogen activator are higher 18 h after exposure.[8,91,92]

Tachyphylaxis to the effect of ozone has been reported in volunteers undergoing repeated exposure to ozone, with an initial augmentation of the effect on lung function, followed by an attenuation of the effect on spirometry.[93] There is also evidence that the inflammatory response to ozone is attenuated after repeated exposure to ozone.[94] A more recent study did not reveal a change in neutrophils but an influx in macrophages to the airway, suggesting that these cells may be important in regulating airway responses to ozone.[95] Other studies have reported that ozone induces influx of monocytes and macrophages with increased expression of CD11b and CD14, suggesting that ozone exposure may enhance response to other biological agents.[96] Overall, it seems likely that monocytes and macrophages may play a role in mediating the effects of this pollutant, and may be much more important with repeated exposures.

Asthmatic individuals may have increased response to the immediate effects of ozone on lung function, though results from different studies are mixed on this point.[97] There are also reports that asthmatics have different inflammatory response to ozone than non-asthmatics, with some studies revealing increased neutrophilic inflammation in the bronchial airways of asthmatics[98,99] and other studies demonstrating an eosinophilic response in the nasal and bronchial airways after ozone challenge.[100,101]

Ozone also has an effect on response to allergen challenge. Following an ozone exposure to 0.12 ppm for 1 h, some investigators have observed increased immediate response to inhaled allergen,[102] whereas others have either not shown a response of low-level ozone to allergen, or trends in responses to subsets of volunteers.[103] However, levels of 0.16 and 0.25 ppm ozone have clearly demonstrated increased response to inhaled allergen.[104,105] Repeated challenge with ozone (even at 0.125 ppm levels) also enhances response to inhaled allergen.[106] Nasal studies of allergic asthmatics demonstrate that the late-phase response to allergen is increased following exposure to 0.4 ppm ozone.[107] Experimental exposure to 0.27 ppm ozone after inhaled allergen challenge has also been shown to enhance the late-phase response to allergen as shown by enhanced eosinophil, but not neutrophil response to allergen.[108]

■ OXIDANT BIOLOGY AND EVIDENCE FOR GENETIC INFLUENCES ON THE RESPONSE TO POLLUTANTS ■

REACTIVE OXYGEN SPECIES AND INFLAMMATION

There is a growing body of evidence that oxidant/antioxidant biology is key to modulation of response to a variety of types of inflammatory stimuli.[109,110] As reviewed by Cross et al, a number of oxidant stressors on the airway are possible, including those by endogenous sources (inflammatory cells), pollutants, and cells activated by primary innate immune processes (viruses and LPS).[111] Asthmatics have been reported to have decreased antioxidant capabilities, and nutritional deficiencies in antioxidants like vitamin E, ascorbate, and selenium have been linked to asthma exacerbation and severity.[112–115] A number of pollutants, including O_3 and a number of components of PM, exert oxidant stress on airway tissues and cells. Particulates such as DEP and tobacco smoke particulates generate a large amount of polyaromatic hydrocarbons (PAHs) that are metabolized to quinone species, which act as intracellular oxidants. Given the role that oxidant stress has in inflammation, the decreased antioxidant defenses noted in asthma, and the oxidant nature of a number of pollutants, it is likely that genetic variation in antioxidant defenses would also account for increased susceptibility of asthmatics to pollutants.

Reactive oxygen species (ROS) have a multitude of actions, including activation of NF-κB, AP-1, and other signaling pathways, as well as participating in production of a number of inflammatory mediators, most notably eicosanoids.[116] Figure 31.4 depicts a hierarchical oxidative stress model for cellular response to DEP, which can be applied to a number of particulate air pollutants as well. ROS has even been reported to play a role in responses to innate immune stimuli, including LPS and viruses, as well as to acquired immune responses such as antigen interactions with IgE or IgG antibodies. ROS can derive from

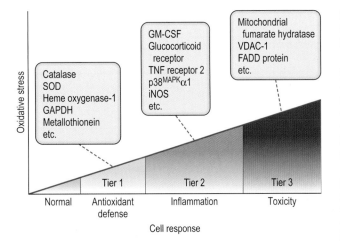

Fig. 31.4. Hierarchical oxidative stress model in response to DEP exposure: proteome analysis of oxidative stress proteins shows a hierarchical response. Incremental doses of organic DEP extracts induce a series of incremental cellular responses that include increased antioxidant offense, inflammation, and cytotoxicity. At a lower level of oxidative stress (tier 1), antioxidant enzymes are induced to restore cellular redox homeostasis. At an intermediate level of oxidative stress (tier 2), newly expressed proteins often exhibit proinflammatory activity. At a high level of oxidative stress (tier 3), perturbation of the mitochondrial permeability transition pore and disruption of electron transfer result in cellular apoptosis or necrosis. FADD, Fas-associating protein with death domain; GM-CSF, granulocyte-macrophage colony-stimulating factor; iNOS, inducible nitric oxide synthase; SOD, superoxide dismutase; TNF, tumor necrosis factor; VDAC-1, voltage-dependent anion channel 1. (From: Gilmour et al.[4] Published online 26 January 2006. DOI: 10.1289/ehp.8380. © This is an Open Access article: verbatim copying and redistribution of this article are permitted in all media for any purpose, provided this notice is preserved along with the article's original DOI.)

a number of endogenous or exogenous sources, including quinone species generated by the metabolism of PAHs from DE, tobacco, and wood smoke, Fenton chemistry involving metals, cellular oxidant processes which play a role in host defense (e.g. NADPH oxidase mediation of the oxidative burst), and a variety of oxidants which participate in signal transduction.[116–119]

EVIDENCE FOR GENETIC SUSCEPTIBILITY TO OXIDIZING POLLUTANTS

Regulation of oxidant stress is also achieved to a great extent by activation of the antioxidant response element (ARE) genes with subsequent production of phase II enzymes which interact in a variety of ways to handle ROS. These enzymes include NQO1, GSTM1, GSTP1, HO-1, and a variety of others.[120] A common feature of these ARE genes is that they are activated at a nuclear level by translocation of Nrf2 to the nucleus (after oxidative attack of critical-SG residues of KEAP1).[109,121,122] The importance of Nrf2 is highlighted by a series of studies in which lung injury due to exposure to allergen (IgE mediated), virus infection, LPS (CD14/TLR4), bleomycin, hyperoxia, and ozone are all markedly enhanced in Nrf2 knockout animals.[109,110,123–126] Furthermore, epidemiological, animal, and human challenge studies demonstrate that defects

in Nrf2-derived enzymes (GSTM1, NQO1, selenoproteins, such as GPX1–3) are associated with environmental asthma, viral injury of the lung, and response to PAHs[120] and O_3.[120,127,128]

Of the individual genes activated by Nrf2, perhaps the best studied are those which influence cellular glutathione. Glutathione S-transferase M1 (*GSTM1*), is a member of the μ family of GSTs. GSTM1 has a null allele (GSTM1*0) which results in no protein expression with resultant decreases in antioxidant capability. Approximately 40% of the population is affected by this allele. Another GST of interest is the GSTP1, in which the single nucleotide polymorphisms at the 105 position are important.

Glutathione S-transferase genes play a role in lung growth, as shown in a study of a large cohort of 1954 schoolchildren in Southern California, in which children with the *GSTM1* null allele or a *GSTP1* val105/val105 genotype had decreased lung function growth over a 4-year period.[129] Studies of children in Mexico City have examined the risk for asthma relative to lifetime ozone exposure. These studies indicate that expression of GST proteins is an important determinant of asthma severity. GSTM1 null children with asthma have decreased lung function associated with ozone exposure compared with those who are GSTM1 sufficient. Interestingly, within this group, if one also screens for a second antioxidant SNP, the Pro187Ser single nucleotide polymorphism for nicotinamide adenine dinucleotide (phosphate) reduced:quinone oxidoreductase (NQO1), those with the Pro/Pro allele genotype for NQO1 have significantly increased asthma risk ascribed to ozone exposure, compared with GSTM1 null children with other NQO1 genotypes.[127] Thus, while GSMT1 null state is associated with risk for ozone-induced asthma exacerbation, this risk may be mitigated by other protective genes. These investigators also studied the ability of dietary supplementation of vitamin C and E to protect asthmatics from ozone-induced exacerbation of disease. Overall, there was a significant protective effect observed in the entire group of asthmatics, but this effect was much more apparent in those children with the GSTM1 null genotype.[128]

In a Southern Californian study, children with the GSTM1 null genotype and born to mothers who smoked during pregnancy also have increased occurrence of early-onset asthma, persistent asthma, exercise-induced wheeze, need for rescue medication use, and emergency room visits for asthma compared with children with protective GST alleles or born to non-smoking mothers.[130] A German study from a cohort of 3504 children revealed that exposure to ETS was associated with a markedly increased risk of asthma and asthma symptoms in GSTM1 null individuals.[131] GSTM1 and GSTT1 insufficient children exposed to in utero ETS were also found to be decreased lung function. Taken together, these studies suggest that specific SNPs of GST genes modulate the response of asthmatics to a variety of oxidizing air pollutants.

Diesel exhaust challenge and environmental tobacco smoke have been shown to induce production of IgE and, like O_3, act as adjuvants for increased response to allergen. It has recently been reported that the adjuvant effect of DE on response to ragweed challenge of the nasal airway is greater in subjects having either the GSTM1 null or GSTP1 105 wild-type genotypes.[132,133] A similar genetic influence on the effect of environmental tobacco smoke has also been observed. Nrf2, a regulatory nuclear factor which activates phase II antioxidant pathways (including GSTM1 expression), has also been found to protect macrophages and epithelial cells from the adverse effects of diesel exhaust particles, demonstrating the role of GSTM1-related antioxidants in protection from the effects of DE.

INTERVENTIONS FOR THE EFFECTS OF POLLUTANTS ON AIRWAY PHYSIOLOGY

Air pollutants likely exert effects on asthmatics by a number of mechanisms, including impacting airway reflexes, activating eicosanoid metabolism, and through antiinflammatory mechanisms. Many pollutants may also exert a pro-oxidant effect on airway tissues, either because they have intrinsic oxidant activity, or because they induce production of endogenous oxidants. These actions suggest a number of potential pharmacological approaches to mitigating the effect of pollutants. Although it would be premature to suggest treatment guidelines for prophylaxis of pollutant-induced asthma exacerbation, a review of studies which examine the effect of pharmacotherapy on responses to pollutants is of interest and may provide clues as to important mechanisms by which such agents impact airway disease.

BRONCHODILATORS

Bronchodilators have a clear effect on SO_2-induced bronchospasm. Beta-agonists are the most effective at reversing SO_2-induced bronchospasm, with methyl xanthines and ipratropium bromide reported to have a modest effect on the effect of sulfur dioxide on lung function as well.[134] Unlike their effect in SO_2-induced bronchospasm, bronchodilators have little apparent effect on ozone-induced changes in lung function. While there is a report that β-agonists may block some ozone-induced decreases in lung function in normal subjects, most studies indicate that β-agonists have little effect on the impact of ozone on lung function.[135] Anticholinergic agents have not been found to reverse ozone-related decreases in spirometry, although they do have some effect on airway resistance.[136] Thus, vagal mechanisms may play a small role in the effect of ozone on lung mechanics whereas it is unlikely that β-adrenergic tone plays a substantial role in blocking the immediate effects of ozone on lung function.

ANALGESICS

The degree to which lung function is decreased correlates with levels of PGE_2 in BAL recovered after O_3 exposure and correlates with observed lung function decrements.[87] Additionally, multiple laboratories have shown in animals and humans that cyclooxygenase inhibitors, such as ibuprofen and indomethacin, inhibit ozone-induced decreases in spirometry, although they have little effect on inflammatory responses to ozone or changes in airway hyperreactivity.[137–141] The effect of narcotic analgesics on immediate responses to ozone in human volunteers has been examined as well. Volunteers treated with sufentanil (a short-acting narcotic) shortly after ozone exposure have a significant reversal in ozone-induced decrease in lung function.[142] Taken together, these studies suggest that the immediate decrease in lung function caused by ozone exposure is a pain response.

ANTIINFLAMMATORY AGENTS

Given the proinflammatory actions of a number of pollutants, including NO_2, O_3, particulates, and endotoxin, it is not surprising that agents with antiinflammatory actions decrease the response to pollutants. Cromolyn sodium or nedocromil have both been shown to blunt immediate spirometric responses to sulfur dioxide, environmental tobacco smoke, and endotoxin[77,134,143] in asthmatic volunteers. Corticosteroids have also been shown to blunt the effect of pollutants on airway inflammation. The effect of SO_2 and NO_2 on allergen-induced inflammation is blunted following treatment with fluticasone as is the effect of NO_2-induced eosinophilic inflammation in the nasal airway.[144] In non-asthmatic subjects, there are conflicting findings of the effect of corticosteroids on ozone-induced neutrophilic inflammation.[145,146] Corticosteroids have been shown to decrease ozone-induced inflammation in allergic asthmatics.[147]

Corticosteroids have also been examined for their impact on elements of particulate pollution, specifically DEPs and endotoxin. Topical fluticasone has little impact on DEP-induced production of IgE or Th2 cytokines, although equivalent doses did inhibit antigen-specific IgE and Th2 inflammatory responses following ragweed allergen challenge in allergic subjects.[148] Corticosteroid treatment prior to inhalation challenge with grain-dust extract, an endotoxin-rich preparation, has a mild protective effect against both inflammatory and bronchoconstrictive responses to such challenge in healthy subjects.[149] Studies done by our group in mild allergic asthmatics demonstrate that pre-treatment with inhaled fluticasone prior to challenge with 5 µg of nebulized endotoxin decreases both the expression of CD14 on airway monocytes and macrophages and the neutrophilic response to endotoxin in allergic asthmatics.[150]

ANTIOXIDANTS

It has been hypothesized that antioxidants in the airway epithelial lining fluid may be important in blunting the effect of oxidizing pollutants such as ozone and particulates. Examples of antioxidants found in airway fluids include uric acid, ascorbic acid, and glutathione.[111,151] In humans, there are reports that exposure to pollutants such as ozone cause decreases in airway urate levels or increases in glutathione or ascorbate, though these changes do not always predict protection from the effect of ozone.[151–155] Nonetheless, recent studies by Samet and colleagues examining the effect of an ascorbate-rich diet vs an ascorbate-depleting diet in humans suggest that antioxidants may be an important defense against the impact of ozone on lung function in healthy volunteers.[156] Trenga and colleagues[157] also examined the effect of vitamin E and C pre-treatment on ozone-induced airway responsiveness, using an SO_2 challenge to induce bronchospasm after ozone exposure. Antioxidant therapy was found to have a protective effect on airway function in challenged asthmatics. These studies suggest that antioxidants may play a role in protection from the impact of pollutants with oxidant activity.

ENVIRONMENTAL INTERVENTIONS

One approach that individuals can take to decrease exposure to pollutants is to avoid or minimize outdoor activities during times when ambient air pollutant levels will be increased. The AQI for criteria pollutants can be found on a number of publicly available media sources, including the website for the US EPA (www.epa.gov), as well as on websites maintained by many state governmental agencies generally updated on a daily basis. For ozone, the AQI is generally included as a routine part of television and print weather forecasts during the summer months, when ozone levels are increased.

In addition to personal avoidance strategies, public health approaches to decrease air pollutants have been shown to have a measurable effect on health outcomes. One example of this occurred in concert with the 1996 Olympic Games held in Atlanta. Coincident with attempts by the local government to decrease ozone generation by vehicle exhaust, there was not only a decrease in summer ozone levels but also there was a significant decrease in asthma morbidity noted during this time.[158] Likewise, in Dublin, Ireland, a ban on bituminous coal sales was implemented on September 1, 1990 to improve air quality.[159] In the 72 months following the ban, there was a 70% decrease in black smoke concentrations, a 5.7% decrease in non-trauma death rates, a 15.5% decrease in respiratory death rates, and a 10.3% decrease in cardiovascular death rates when compared with the 72 months preceding the ban.

Environmental interventions designed to decrease indoor air contamination are also a key approach to decreasing asthma onset and exacerbation. Allergen exposure (house-dust mite, cockroach, mold, mammalian pet, and vermin allergens, see Chapter 34), exposure to combustion products (gas stoves, tobacco smoke, wood smoke), exposure to non-allergenic bioaerosols (endotoxins), and humidity are all important elements which influence indoor air quality.[24,31,160–164] A number of approaches to decreasing exposures to these agents have been developed, including mattress and pillow encasings and washing bedding in hot water for mite allergen control, extermination and pest control for decreasing cockroach exposure, washing pets or removing them from the home to decrease animal allergen exposures, appropriate maintenance of gas-burning appliances, fireplaces, and decreasing (or eliminating) use of tobacco to decrease particulate exposures, use of dehumidifiers to decrease humidity inside houses, and use of high-efficiency particulate air cleaners to remove PM from indoor air.

The data are mixed concerning the effectiveness of environmental control maneuvers inside homes, especially when studies are focused on a specific intervention. However, there is a growing body of evidence that comprehensive and customized approaches to improving indoor air quality result in significant decreases in asthma symptoms and severity or even primary prevention of allergic disease.[165–167] Effective strategies have generally included assessment of a specific home environment, simultaneous use of multiple interventions relevant to the specific environment, and education approaches for family members focused on the need for intervention and how to employ the specific environmental control techniques. However, a uniform recommendation in each of these approaches is eliminating exposure to environmental tobacco smoke.

▪ SUMMARY ▪

Epidemiological studies demonstrate that exposure to both indoor and outdoor air pollution causes exacerbations of human airway disease. Many of these pollutants have a pro-oxidant effect, which contributes to airway inflammation. Furthermore, many pollutants modify response to allergens, resulting in increased sensitivity of allergic individuals to environmental allergens, even at pollutant doses that do not appear to independently impact lung function. Antiinflammatory agents may be helpful in mitigating pollutant-induced asthma exacerbation. Early studies also suggest that antioxidant approaches may be useful. Societal and home-based control of pollutants has also been shown to be effective in decreasing asthma exacerbation, and research aimed at developing better environmental control strategies will certainly provide more strategies to decrease environmentally induced exacerbations or airway disease.

References

Introduction

1. Alberg AJ, Brock MV, Samet JM. Epidemiology of lung cancer: looking to the future. J Clin Oncol 2005; 23:3175–3185.
2. Bernstein JA, Alexis N, Barnes C, et al. Health effects of air pollution. J Allergy Clin Immunol 2004; 114:1116–1123.
3. Delfino RJ. Epidemiologic evidence for asthma and exposure to air toxics: linkages between occupational, indoor, and community air pollution research. Environ Health Perspect 2002; 110:573–589.
4. Gilmour MI, Jaakkola MS, London SJ, et al. How exposure to environmental tobacco smoke, outdoor air pollutants, and increased pollen burdens influences the incidence of asthma. Environ Health Perspect 2006; 114:627–633.
5. Peden DB. Air pollution in asthma: effect of pollutants on airway inflammation. Ann Allergy Asthma Immunol 2001; 87:12–17.
6. Peden DB. The epidemiology and genetics of asthma risk associated with air pollution. J Allergy Clin Immunol 2005; 115:213–219.
7. Singh N, Davis GS. Review: occupational and environmental lung disease. Curr Opin Pulm Med 2002; 8:117–125.

Nature of airborne contaminants

8. Health effects of outdoor air pollution. Committee of the Environmental and Occupational Health Assembly of the American Thoracic Society. Am J Respir Crit Care Med 1996; 153:3–50.
9. US Clean Air Act. 2007. Online. Available: www.epa.gov/air/caa
10. Grant LD, Shoaf CR, Davis JM. United States and international approaches to establishing air standards and guidelines. In: Holgate ST, Samet JM, Koren HS, Maynard RL, eds. Air pollution and health. San Diego: Academic Press; 1999:947–982.
11. Lippmann M, Maynard RL. Air Quality Guidelines and Standards. In: Holgate ST, Samet JM, Koren HS, Maynard RL, eds. Air pollution and health. San Diego: Academic Press; 1999: 983–1018.
12. Holman C. Sources of air pollution. In: Holgate ST, Samet JM, Koren HS, Maynard RL, editors. Air pollution and health. San Diego: Academic Press; 1999:115–148.
13. Brims F, Chauhan AJ. Air quality, tobacco smoke, urban crowding and day care: modern menaces and their effects on health. Pediatr Infect Dis J 2005; 24:S152–S156, discussion.
14. Gupta D, Aggarwal AN, Chaudhry K, et al. Household environmental tobacco smoke exposure, respiratory symptoms and asthma in non-smoker adults: a multicentric population study from India. Indian J Chest Dis Allied Sci 2006; 48:31–36.
15. Mishra V. Effect of indoor air pollution from biomass combustion on prevalence of asthma in the elderly. Environ Health Perspect 2003; 111:71–78.
16. Schei MA, Hessen JO, Smith KR, et al. Childhood asthma and indoor woodsmoke from cooking in Guatemala. J Expo Anal Environ Epidemiol 2004; 14:S110–S117.
17. Jones SC, Travers MJ, Hahn EJ, et al. Secondhand smoke and indoor public spaces in Paducah, Kentucky. J Ky Med Assoc 2006; 104:281–288.
18. Larsson L, Szponar B, Pehrson C. Tobacco smoking increases dramatically air concentrations of endotoxin. Indoor Air 2004; 14:421–424.
19. Brunekreef B, Houthuijs D, Dijkstra L, et al. Indoor nitrogen dioxide exposure and children's pulmonary function. J Air Waste Manage Assoc 1990; 40:1252–1256.
20. Neas LM, Dockery DW, Ware JH, et al. Association of indoor nitrogen dioxide with respiratory symptoms and pulmonary function in children. Am J Epidemiol 1991; 134:204–219.
21. Chauhan AJ, Johnston SL. Air pollution and infection in respiratory illness. Br Med Bull 2003; 68:95–112.
22. Chauhan AJ, Inskip HM, Linaker CH, et al. Personal exposure to nitrogen dioxide (NO₂) and the severity of virus-induced asthma in children. Lancet 2003; 361:1939–1944.
23. van Strien RT, Gent JF, Belanger K, et al. Exposure to NO₂ and nitrous acid and respiratory symptoms in the first year of life. Epidemiology 2004; 15:471–478.
24. Thorne PS, Kulhankova K, Yin M, et al. Endotoxin exposure is a risk factor for asthma – The National Survey of Endotoxin in United States Housing. Am J Respir Crit Care Med 2005; 172:1371–1377.
25. Liu AH. Endotoxin exposure in allergy and asthma: reconciling a paradox. J Allergy Clin Immunol 2002; 109:379–392.
26. Reed CE, Milton DK. Endotoxin-stimulated innate immunity: a contributing factor for asthma. J Allergy Clin Immunol 2001; 108:157–166.
27. Bischof W, Koch A, Gehring U, et al. Predictors of high endotoxin concentrations in the settled dust of German homes. Indoor Air 2002; 12:2–9.
28. Park JH, Spiegelman DL, Burge HA, et al. Longitudinal study of dust and airborne endotoxin in the home. Environ Health Perspect 2000; 108:1023–1028.
29. Wickens K, Douwes J, Siebers R, et al. Determinants of endotoxin levels in carpets in New Zealand homes. Indoor Air 2003; 13:128–135.
30. van Strien RT, Gehring U, Belanger K, et al. The influence of air conditioning, humidity, temperature and other household characteristics on mite allergen concentrations in the northeastern United States. Allergy 2004; 59:645–652.
31. Tavernier G, Fletcher G, Gee I, et al. IPEADAM study: indoor endotoxin exposure, family status, and some housing characteristics in English children. J Allergy Clin Immunol 2006; 117:656–662.
32. Nicolai T, Carr D, Weiland SK, et al. Urban traffic and pollutant exposure related to respiratory outcomes and atopy in a large sample of children. Eur Respir J 2003; 21:956–963.

Biological effects of specific air pollutants

33. Pope CA, III. Respiratory hospital admissions associated with PM_{10} pollution in Utah, Salt Lake, and Cache Valleys. Arch Environ Health 1991; 46:90–97.

34. Pope CA, III. Respiratory disease associated with community air pollution and a steel mill, Utah Valley. Am J Public Health 1989; 79:623–628.

35. Gauderman WJ, Avol E, Gilliland F, et al. The effect of air pollution on lung development from 10 to 18 years of age. N Engl J Med 2004; 351:1057–1067.

36. Edwards J, Walters S, Griffiths RK. Hospital admissions for asthma in preschool children: relationship to major roads in Birmingham, United Kingdom. Arch Environ Health 1994; 49:223–227.

37. Lin S, Munsie JP, Hwang SA, et al. Childhood asthma hospitalization and residential exposure to state route traffic. Environ Res 2002; 88:73–81.

38. Garshick E, Laden F, Hart JE, et al. Residence near a major road and respiratory symptoms in U.S. Veterans. Epidemiology 2003; 14:728–736.

39. Peters A, von Klot S, Heier M, et al. Exposure to traffic and the onset of myocardial infarction. N Engl J Med 2004; 351:1721–1730.

40. Ghio AJ, Huang YC. Exposure to concentrated ambient particles (CAPs): a review. Inhal Toxicol 2004; 16:53–59.

41. Ghio AJ. Biological effects of Utah Valley ambient air particles in humans: a review. J Aerosol Med 2004; 17:157–164.

42. Schaumann F, Borm PJ, Herbrich A, et al. Metal-rich ambient particles (PM 2.5) cause airway inflammation in healthy subjects. Am J Respir Crit Care Med 2004; 170:898–903.

43. Carty CL, Gehring U, Cyrys J, et al. Seasonal variability of endotoxin in ambient fine particulate matter. J Environ Monit 2003; 5:953–958.

44. Mueller-Anneling L, Avol E, Peters JM, et al. Ambient endotoxin concentrations in PM_{10} from Southern California. Environ Health Perspect 2004; 112:583–588.

45. Osornio-Vargas AR, Bonner JC, Alfaro-Moreno E, et al. Proinflammatory and cytotoxic effects of Mexico City air pollution particulate matter in vitro are dependent on particle size and composition. Environ Health Perspect 2003; 111:1289–1293.

46. Singh J, Schwartz DA. Endotoxin and the lung: insight into the host-environment interaction. J Allergy Clin Immunol 2005; 115:330–333.

47. Alexis NE, Lay JC, Zeman K, et al. Biological material on inhaled coarse fraction particulate matter activates airway phagocytes in vivo in healthy volunteers. J Allergy Clin Immunol 2006; 117:1396–1403.

48. Boehlecke B, Hazucha M, Alexis NE, et al. Low-dose airborne endotoxin exposure enhances bronchial responsiveness to inhaled allergen in atopic asthmatics. J Allergy Clin Immunol 2003; 112:1241–1243.

49. Eldridge MW, Peden DB. Allergen provocation augments endotoxin-induced nasal inflammation in subjects with atopic asthma. J Allergy Clin Immunol 2000; 105:475–481.

50. Lensmar C, Prieto J, Dahlen B, et al. Airway inflammation and altered alveolar macrophage phenotype pattern after repeated low-dose allergen exposure of atopic asthmatic subjects. Clin Exp Allergy 1999; 29:1632–1640.

51. Virchow JC, Julius P, Matthys H, et al. CD14 expression and soluble CD14 after segmental allergen provocation in atopic asthma. Eur Respir J 1998; 11:317–323.

52. Diaz-Sanchez D, Proietti L, Polosa R. Diesel fumes and the rising prevalence of atopy: an urban legend? Curr Allergy Asthma Rep 2003; 3:146–152.

53. Peden DB. Pollutants and asthma: role of air toxics. Environ Health Perspect 2002; 110: 565–568.

54. Riedl M, Diaz-Sanchez D. Biology of diesel exhaust effects on respiratory function. J Allergy Clin Immunol 2005; 115:221–228.

55. Pandya RJ, Solomon G, Kinner A, et al. Diesel exhaust and asthma: hypotheses and molecular mechanisms of action. Environ Health Perspect 2002; 110:103–112.

56. Singh P, DeMarini DM, Dick CA, et al. Sample characterization of automobile and forklift diesel exhaust particles and comparative pulmonary toxicity in mice. Environ Health Perspect 2004; 112:820–825.

57. Diaz-Sanchez D, Dotson AR, Takenaka H, et al. Diesel exhaust particles induce local IgE production in vivo and alter the pattern of IgE messenger RNA isoforms. J Clin Invest 1994; 94:1417–1425.

58. Kongerud J, Madden MC, Hazucha M, et al. Nasal responses in asthmatic and nonasthmatic subjects following exposure to diesel exhaust particles. Inhal Toxicol 2006; 18:589–594.

59. Behndig AF, Mudway IS, Brown JL, et al. Airway antioxidant and inflammatory responses to diesel exhaust exposure in healthy humans. Eur Respir J 2006; 27:359–365.

60. Mudway IS, Stenfors N, Duggan ST, et al. An in vitro and in vivo investigation of the effects of diesel exhaust on human airway lining fluid antioxidants. Arch Biochem Biophys 2004; 423:200–212.

61. Pourazar J, Mudway IS, Samet JM, et al. Diesel exhaust activates redox-sensitive transcription factors and kinases in human airways. Am J Physiol Lung Cell Mol Physiol 2005; 289: L724–L730.

62. Pourazar J, Frew AJ, Blomberg A, et al. Diesel exhaust exposure enhances the expression of IL-13 in the bronchial epithelium of healthy subjects. Respir Med 2004; 98:821–825.

63. Rudell B, Ledin MC, Hammarstrom U, et al. Effects on symptoms and lung function in humans experimentally exposed to diesel exhaust. Occup Environ Med 1996; 53:658–662.

64. Salvi SS, Nordenhall C, Blomberg A, et al. Acute exposure to diesel exhaust increases IL-8 and GRO-alpha production in healthy human airways. Am J Respir Crit Care Med 2000; 161:550–557.

65. Stenfors N, Nordenhall C, Salvi SS, et al. Different airway inflammatory responses in asthmatic and healthy humans exposed to diesel. Eur Respir J 2004; 23:82–86.

66. Nel AE, Diaz-Sanchez D, Li N. The role of particulate pollutants in pulmonary inflammation and asthma: evidence for the involvement of organic chemicals and oxidative stress. Curr Opin Pulm Med 2001; 7:20–26.

67. Diaz-Sanchez D, Garcia MP, Wang M, et al. Nasal challenge with diesel exhaust particles can induce sensitization to a neoallergen in the human mucosa. J Allergy Clin Immunol 1999; 104:1183–1188.

68. Chan RC, Wang M, Li N, et al. Pro-oxidative diesel exhaust particle chemicals inhibit LPS-induced dendritic cell responses involved in T-helper differentiation. J Allergy Clin Immunol 2006; 118:455–465.

69. Etzel RA. How environmental exposures influence the development and exacerbation of asthma. Pediatrics 2003; 112:233–239.

70. Gergen PJ. Environmental tobacco smoke as a risk factor for respiratory disease in children. Respir Physiol 2001; 128:39–46.

71. Gold DR. Environmental tobacco smoke, indoor allergens, and childhood asthma. Environ Health Perspect 2000; 108:643–651.

72. Seymour BW, Schelegle ES, Pinkerton KE, et al. Second-hand smoke increases bronchial hyperreactivity and eosinophilia in a murine model of allergic aspergillosis. Clin Dev Immunol 2003; 10:35–42.

73. Rumold R, Jyrala M, Diaz-Sanchez D. Secondhand smoke induces allergic sensitization in mice. J Immunol 2001; 167:4765–4770.

74. Diaz-Sanchez D, Rumold R, Gong H Jr. Challenge with environmental tobacco smoke exacerbates allergic airway disease in human beings. J Allergy Clin Immunol 2006; 118: 441–446.

Gas phase air pollutants

75. Peden DB. Mechanisms of pollution-induced airway disease: in vivo studies. Allergy 1997; 52: 37–44.

76. Barnes PJ. Air pollution and asthma. Postgrad Med J 1994; 70:319–325.

77. Koenig JQ. Air pollution and asthma. J Allergy Clin Immunol 1999; 104:717–722.

78. Jenkins HS, Devalia JL, Mister RL, et al. The effect of exposure to ozone and nitrogen dioxide on the airway response of atopic asthmatics to inhaled allergen: dose- and time-dependent effects. Am J Respir Crit Care Med 1999; 160:33–39.

79. Tunnicliffe WS, Burge PS, Ayres JG. Effect of domestic concentrations of nitrogen dioxide on airway responses to inhaled allergen in asthmatic patients. Lancet 1994; 344:1733–1736.

80. Wang JH, Devalia JL, Duddle JM, et al. Effect of six-hour exposure to nitrogen dioxide on early-phase nasal response to allergen challenge in patients with a history of seasonal allergic rhinitis. J Allergy Clin Immunol 1995; 96:669–676.

81. Wang JH, Duddle J, Devalia JL, et al. Nitrogen dioxide increases eosinophil activation in the early-phase response to nasal allergen provocation. Int Arch Allergy Immunol 1995; 107: 103–105.

82. Balmes JR. The role of ozone exposure in the epidemiology of asthma. Environ Health Perspect 1993; 101:219–224.

83. Gent JF, Triche EW, Holford TR, et al. Association of low-level ozone and fine particles with respiratory symptoms in children with asthma. JAMA 2003; 290:1859–1867.

84. McConnell R, Berhane K, Gilliland F, et al. Asthma in exercising children exposed to ozone: a cohort study. Lancet 2002; 359:386–391.

85. McDonnell WF, Abbey DE, Nishino N, et al. Long-term ambient ozone concentration and the incidence of asthma in nonsmoking adults: the AHSMOG Study. Environ Res 1999; 80:110–121.

86. Tager IB, Balmes J, Lurmann F, et al. Chronic exposure to ambient ozone and lung function in young adults. Epidemiology 2005; 16:751–759.

87. Peden DB. Controlled exposures of asthmatics to air pollutants. In: Holgate S, Samet J, Koren HS, Maynard RL, eds. Air pollution and health, San Diego. Academic Press; 1999: 865–880.

88. Peden DB. Air pollution in asthma: effect of pollutants on airway inflammation. Ann Allergy Asthma Immunol 2001; 87:12–17.

89. McDonnell WF, Muller KE, Bromberg PA, et al. Predictors of individual differences in acute response to ozone exposure. Am Rev Respir Dis 1993; 147:818–825.

90. McDonnell WF, Horstman DH, Hazucha MJ, et al. Pulmonary effects of ozone exposure during exercise: dose-response characteristics. J Appl Physiol 1983; 54:1345–1352.

91. Bromberg PA, Koren HS. Ozone-induced human respiratory dysfunction and disease. Toxicol Lett 1995; 82–83:307–316.

92. Brunekreef B, Holgate ST. Air pollution and health. Lancet 2002; 360:1233–1242.

93. Folinsbee LJ, Horstman DH, Kehrl HR, et al. Respiratory responses to repeated prolonged exposure to 0.12 ppm ozone. Am J Respir Crit Care Med 1994; 149:98–105.

94. Christian DL, Chen LL, Scannell CH, et al. Ozone-induced inflammation is attenuated with multiday exposure. Am J Respir Crit Care Med 1998; 158:532–537.

95. Arjomandi M, Witten A, Abbritti E, et al. Repeated exposure to ozone increases alveolar macrophage recruitment into asthmatic airways. Am J Respir Crit Care Med 2005; 172: 427–432.

96. Alexis NE, Becker S, Bromberg P, et al. Circulating CD11b expression correlates with the neutrophil response and airway mCD14 expression is enhanced following ozone exposure in humans. Clin Immunol 2004; 111:126–131.

97. Koren HS, Bromberg PA. Respiratory responses of asthmatics to ozone. Int Arch Allergy Immunol 1995; 107:236–238.

98. Scannell C, Chen L, Aris RM, et al. Greater ozone-induced inflammatory responses in subjects with asthma. Am J Respir Crit Care Med 1996; 154:24–29.

99. Basha MA, Gross KB, Gwizdala CJ, et al. Bronchoalveolar lavage neutrophilia in asthmatic and healthy volunteers after controlled exposure to ozone and filtered purified air. Chest 1994; 106:1757–1765.

100. Bascom R, Naclerio RM, Fitzgerald TK, et al. Effect of ozone inhalation on the response to nasal challenge with antigen of allergic subjects. Am Rev Respir Dis 1990; 142:594–601.

101. Peden DB, Boehlecke B, Horstman D, et al. Prolonged acute exposure to 0.16 ppm ozone induces eosinophilic airway inflammation in asthmatic subjects with allergies. J Allergy Clin Immunol 1997; 100:802–808.

102. Molfino NA, Wright SC, Katz I, et al. Effect of low concentrations of ozone on inhaled allergen responses in asthmatic subjects. Lancet 1991; 338:199–203.

REFERENCES

103. Ball BA, Folinsbee LJ, Peden DB, et al. Allergen bronchoprovocation of patients with mild allergic asthma after ozone exposure. J Allergy Clin Immunol 1996; 98:563–572.
104. Kehrl HR, Peden DB, Ball B, et al. Increased specific airway reactivity of persons with mild allergic asthma after 7.6 hours of exposure to 0.16 ppm ozone. J Allergy Clin Immunol 1999; 104:1198–1204.
105. Jorres R, Nowak D, Magnussen H. The effect of ozone exposure on allergen responsiveness in subjects with asthma or rhinitis. Am J Respir Crit Care Med 1996; 153:56–64.
106. Holz O, Mucke M, Paasch K, et al. Repeated ozone exposures enhance bronchial allergen responses in subjects with rhinitis or asthma. Clin Exp Allergy 2002; 32:681–689.
107. Peden DB, Setzer RW Jr, Devlin RB. Ozone exposure has both a priming effect on allergen-induced responses and an intrinsic inflammatory action in the nasal airways of perennially allergic asthmatics. Am J Respir Crit Care Med 1995; 151:1336–1345.
108. Vagaggini B, Taccola M, Cianchetti S, et al. Ozone exposure increases eosinophilic airway response induced by previous allergen challenge. Am J Respir Crit Care Med 2002; 166: 1073–1077.

Oxidant biology and evidence for genetic influences on the response to pollutants

109. Kensler TW, Wakabayashi N, Biswal S. Cell survival responses to environmental stresses via the Keap1-Nrf2-ARE pathway. Annu Rev Pharmacol Toxicol 2007; 47:89–116.
110. Osburn WO, Wakabayashi N, Misra V, et al. Nrf2 regulates an adaptive response protecting against oxidative damage following diquat-mediated formation of superoxide anion. Arch Biochem Biophys 2006; 454:7–15.
111. Cross CE, Valacchi G, Schock B, et al. Environmental oxidant pollutant effects on biologic systems: a focus on micronutrient antioxidant-oxidant interactions. Am J Respir Crit Care Med 2002; 166:44S–50.
112. Fogarty A, Lewis S, Weiss S, et al. Dietary vitamin E, IgE concentrations, and atopy. Lancet 2000; 356:1573–1574.
113. Gilliland FD, Berhane KT, Li YF, et al. Children's lung function and antioxidant vitamin, fruit, juice, and vegetable intake. Am J Epidemiol 2003; 158:576–584.
114. Romieu I, Sienra-Monge JJ, Ramirez-Aguilar M, et al. Antioxidant supplementation and lung functions among children with asthma exposed to high levels of air pollutants. Am J Respir Crit Diaz-Sanchez D 2002; 166:703–709.
115. Seaton A, Devereux G. Diet, infection and wheezy illness: lessons from adults. Pediatr Allergy Immunol 2000; 11:37–40.
116. Balboa MA, Balsinde J. Oxidative stress and arachidonic acid mobilization. Biochim Biophys Acta 2006; 1761:385–391.
117. Bowler RP, Crapo JD. Oxidative stress in allergic respiratory diseases. J Allergy Clin Immunol 2002; 110:349–356.
118. Henricks PA, Nijkamp FP. Reactive oxygen species as mediators in asthma. Pulm Pharmacol Ther 2001; 14:409–420.
119. Kinnula VL, Crapo JD. Superoxide dismutases in the lung and human lung diseases. Am J Respir Crit Care Med 2003; 167:1600–1619.
120. Gilliland FD, Li YF, Saxon A, et al. Effect of glutathione-S-transferase M1 and P1 genotypes on xenobiotic enhancement of allergic responses: randomised, placebo-controlled crossover study. Lancet 2004; 363:119–125.
121. Kong AN, Owuor E, Yu R, et al. Induction of xenobiotic enzymes by the MAP kinase pathway and the antioxidant or electrophile response element (ARE/EpRE). Drug Metab Rev 2001; 33:255–271.
122. Lee JS, Surh YJ. Nrf2 as a novel molecular target for chemoprevention. Cancer Lett 2005; 224:171–184.
123. Biswal S, Rangasamy T, Tuder RM. Modifier role of Nrf2 in cigarette smoke-induced emphysema. Proc Am Thorac Soc 2006; 3:543a.
124. Rangasamy T, Guo J, Mitzner WA, et al. Disruption of Nrf2 enhances susceptibility to severe airway inflammation and asthma in mice. J Exp Med 2005; 202:47–59.
125. Rangasamy T, Cho CY, Thimmulappa RK, et al. Genetic ablation of Nrf2 enhances susceptibility to cigarette smoke-induced emphysema in mice. J Clin Invest 2004; 114: 1248–1259.
126. Thimmulappa RK, Lee H, Rangasamy T, et al. Nrf2 is a critical regulator of the innate immune response and survival during experimental sepsis. J Clin Invest 2006; 116:984–995.
127. David GL, Romieu I, Sienra-Monge JJ, et al. Nicotinamide adenine dinucleotide (phosphate) reduced:quinone oxidoreductase and glutathione S-transferase M1 polymorphisms and childhood asthma. Am J Respir Crit Care Med 2003; 168:1199–1204.
128. Romieu I, Sienra-Monge JJ, Ramirez-Aguilar M, et al. Genetic polymorphism of GSTM1 and antioxidant supplementation influence lung function in relation to ozone exposure in asthmatic children in Mexico City. Thorax 2004; 59:8–10.
129. Gilliland FD, Gauderman WJ, Vora H, et al. Effects of glutathione-S-transferase M1, T1, and P1 on childhood lung function growth. Am J Respir Crit Care Med 2002; 166:710–716.
130. Gilliland FD, Li YF, Dubeau L, et al. Effects of glutathione S-transferase M1, maternal smoking during pregnancy, and environmental tobacco smoke on asthma and wheezing in children. Am J Respir Crit Care Med 2002; 166:457–463.
131. Kabesch M, Hoefler C, Carr D, et al. Glutathione S transferase deficiency and passive smoking increase childhood asthma. Thorax 2004; 59:569–573.
132. Bastain TM, Gilliland FD, Li YF, et al. Intraindividual reproducibility of nasal allergic responses to diesel exhaust particles indicates a susceptible phenotype. Clin Immunol 2003; 109:130–136.
133. Gilliland FD, Li YF, Saxon A, et al. Effect of glutathione-S-transferase M1 and P1 genotypes on xenobiotic enhancement of allergic responses: randomised, placebo-controlled crossover study. Lancet 2004; 363:119–125.

Interventions for the effects of pollutants on airway physiology

134. Koenig JQ, Pierson WE. Air pollutants and the respiratory system: toxicity and pharmacologic interventions. J Toxicol Clin Toxicol 1991; 29:401–411.
135. Gong H Jr, Bedi JF, Horvath SM. Inhaled albuterol does not protect against ozone toxicity in nonasthmatic athletes. Arch Environ Health 1988; 43:46–53.
136. Beckett WS, McDonnell WF, Horstman DH, et al. Role of the parasympathetic nervous system in acute lung response to ozone. J Appl Physiol 1985; 59:1879–1885.
137. Alexis N, Urch B, Tarlo S, et al. Cyclooxygenase metabolites play a different role in ozone-induced pulmonary function decline in asthmatics compared to normals. Inhal Toxicol 2000; 12:1205–1224.
138. Hazucha MJ, Madden M, Pape G, et al. Effects of cyclo-oxygenase inhibition on ozone-induced respiratory inflammation and lung function changes. Eur J Appl Physiol Occup Physiol 1996; 73:17–27.
139. O'Byrne PM, Walters EH, Aizawa H, et al. Indomethacin inhibits the airway hyper-responsiveness but not the neutrophil influx induced by ozone in dogs. Am Rev Respir Dis 1984; 130:220–224.
140. Schelegle ES, Adams WC, Siefkin AD. Indomethacin pre-treatment reduces ozone-induced pulmonary function decrements in human subjects. Am Rev Respir Dis 1987; 136:1350–1354.
141. Ying RL, Gross KB, Terzo TS, et al. Indomethacin does not inhibit the ozone-induced increase in bronchial responsiveness in human subjects. Am Rev Respir Dis 1990; 142:817–821.
142. Passannante AN, Hazucha MJ, Bromberg PA, et al. Nociceptive mechanisms modulate ozone-induced human lung function decrements. J Appl Physiol 1998; 85:1863–1870.
143. Michel O, Ginanni R, Sergysels R. Protective effect of sodium cromoglycate on lipopoly-saccharide-induced bronchial obstruction in asthmatics. Int Arch Allergy Immunol 1995; 108:298–302.
144. Davies RJ, Rusznak C, Calderon MA, et al. Allergen-irritant interaction and the role of corticosteroids. Allergy 1997; 52:59–65.
145. Nightingale JA, Rogers DF, Fan CK, et al. No effect of inhaled budesonide on the response to inhaled ozone in normal subjects. Am J Respir Crit Care Med 2000; 161:479–486.
146. Holz O, Tal-Singer R, Kanniess F, et al. Validation of the human ozone challenge model as a tool for assessing anti-inflammatory drugs in early development. J Clin Pharmacol 2005; 45:498–503.
147. Vagaggini B, Taccola M, Conti I, et al. Budesonide reduces neutrophilic but not functional airway response to ozone in mild asthmatics. Am J Respir Crit Care Med 2001; 164:2172–2176.
148. Diaz-Sanchez D, Tsien A, Fleming J, et al. Effect of topical fluticasone propionate on the mucosal allergic response induced by ragweed allergen and diesel exhaust particle challenge. Clin Immunol 1999; 90:313–322.
149. Trapp JF, Watt JL, Frees KL, et al. The effect of glucocorticoids on grain dust-induced airway disease. Chest 1998; 113:505–513.
150. Alexis NE, Peden DB. Blunting airway eosinophilic inflammation results in a decreased airway neutrophil response to inhaled LPS in patients with atopic asthma: a role for CD14. J Allergy Clin Immunol 2001; 108:577–580.
151. Kelly FJ, Cotgrove M, Mudway IS. Respiratory tract lining fluid antioxidants: the first line of defence against gaseous pollutants. Cent Eur J Public Health 1996; 4:11–14.
152. Blomberg A, Mudway IS, Nordenhall C, et al. Ozone-induced lung function decrements do not correlate with early airway inflammatory or antioxidant responses. Eur Respir J 1999; 13:1418–1428.
153. Mudway IS, Blomberg A, Frew AJ, et al. Antioxidant consumption and repletion kinetics in nasal lavage fluid following exposure of healthy human volunteers to ozone. Eur Respir J 1999; 13:1429–1438.
154. Mudway IS, Krishna MT, Frew AJ, et al. Compromised concentrations of ascorbate in fluid lining the respiratory tract in human subjects after exposure to ozone. Occup Environ Med 1999; 56:473–481.
155. Mudway IS, Stenfors N, Blomberg A, et al. Differences in basal airway antioxidant concentrations are not predictive of individual responsiveness to ozone: a comparison of healthy and mild asthmatic subjects. Free Radic Biol Med 2001; 31:962–974.
156. Samet JM, Hatch GE, Horstman D, et al. Effect of antioxidant supplementation on ozone-induced lung injury in human subjects. Am J Respir Crit Care Med 2001; 164:819–825.
157. Trenga CA, Koenig JQ, Williams PV. Dietary antioxidants and ozone-induced bronchial hyperresponsiveness in adults with asthma. Arch Environ Health 2001; 56:242–249.
158. Friedman MS, Powell KE, Hutwagner L, et al. Impact of changes in transportation and commuting behaviors during the 1996 Summer Olympic Games in Atlanta on air quality and childhood asthma. JAMA 2001; 285:897–905.
159. Clancy L, Goodman P, Sinclair H, et al. Effect of air-pollution control on death rates in Dublin, Ireland: an intervention study. Lancet 2002; 360:1210–1214.
160. Eggleston PA, Bush RK. Environmental allergen avoidance: an overview. J Allergy Clin Immunol 2001; 107:S403–S405.
161. Eggleston PA. Environmental causes of asthma in inner city children. The National Cooperative Inner City Asthma Study. Clin Rev Allergy Immunol 2000; 18:311–324.
162. Eggleston PA, Rosenstreich D, Lynn H, et al. Relationship of indoor allergen exposure to skin test sensitivity in inner-city children with asthma. J Allergy Clin Immunol 1998; 102:563–570.
163. Matsui EC, Simons E, Rand C, et al. Airborne mouse allergen in the homes of inner-city children with asthma. J Allergy Clin Immunol 2005; 115:358–363.
164. Matsui EC, Eggleston PA, Buckley TJ, et al. Household mouse allergen exposure and asthma morbidity in inner-city preschool children. Ann Allergy Asthma Immunol 2006; 97:514–520.
165. Chan-Yeung M, Ferguson A, Watson W, et al. The Canadian Childhood Asthma Primary Prevention Study: outcomes at 7 years of age. J Allergy Clin Immunol 2005; 116:49–55.
166. Eggleston PA, Butz A, Rand C, et al. Home environmental intervention in inner-city asthma: a randomized controlled clinical trial. Ann Allergy Asthma Immunol 2005; 95:518–524.
167. Morgan WJ, Crain EF, Gruchalla RS, et al. Results of a home-based environmental intervention among urban children with asthma. N Engl J Med 2004; 351:1068–1080.

Aerobiology of Outdoor Allergens

Robert E Esch and Robert K Bush

32

SUMMARY OF IMPORTANT CONCEPTS

>> Exposure to outdoor aeroallergens may vary based on geographic region, season, weather, and time of day

>> The pollination of allergenic plants has distinct seasons, such that 'pollen seasons' can be predictable for a given species

>> Different methods for the detection and quantitation of aeroallergens have advantages and disadvantages and they need to be considered when devising a monitoring strategy

>> Fungal life cycles and taxonomy can be extremely complex, which limits our ability to assess the level of fungal allergen exposure using conventional methods

AEROALLERGENS AND SOURCES

Aeroallergens are air-borne particles that induce allergic reactions in sensitized subjects and can cause respiratory, cutaneous, or conjunctival allergy. Aeroallergens are a subset of diverse forms of aerosols ranging from submicronic particles to relatively larger pollen grains, fungal spores, animal emanations, and biogenic debris.[1] Pollens and fungal spores have been studied most extensively in the outdoor environment because they are relatively easy to sample and identify. Residential environments may present significantly more risk for allergic disease; most Americans spend most of their time indoors, and modern energy-efficient buildings result in higher aeroallergen concentrations, especially animal dander, house-dust mites, and fungi. Aeroallergen exposure in the workplace may also result in allergic sensitization and disease. Many of the biogenic or proteinaceous aeroallergens have long been recognized, with a growing list of industrial chemicals that become air-borne and cause allergic contact dermatitis or hypersensitivity pneumonitis (HP).

FACTORS INFLUENCING CLINICAL SIGNIFICANCE OF AEROALLERGENS

To be clinically significant, aeroallergens first must be buoyant, present in significant concentration, and allergenic. Grass pollens and *Alternaria* spores are typical examples of frequently encountered aeroallergens. In general, entomophilous (insect-pollinated) plants produce scant, heavy, or sticky pollens that do not become air-borne. *Anemophilous* (wind-pollinated) plants represent only about one-tenth of the more than 250000 pollen-producing species. Depending on their season, anemophilous spores can reach concentrations >100 grains/m^3, can remain air-borne for days, and can be carried hundreds of miles from their point of origin. In contrast to entomophilous plants, *anemophilous* plants possess large stamens borne on long, well-exposed filaments, often organized as catkins. Their flowers usually lack color, scent, and nectar and release large quantities of pollen in warm, dry weather.[2]

Particle size is a critical physical attribute of aeroallergens and an important consideration in the pathogenesis of allergic rhinitis, bronchial asthma, and HP. Protective mechanisms in the nasal mucosa and upper tracheobronchial passages remove larger particles, so only those of 5 micrometers (µm) or less reach the alveoli of the lungs. Intact pollen grains range in size from about 15 to 75 µm, and most fungal spores vary from about 5 to 30 µm. Thus, the conjunctivae and upper respiratory tract are exposed to the highest dose of aeroallergens. Until recently, pollen-induced asthma remained enigmatic because the available evidence suggested that inhalation of pollen grains encountered naturally could not reach the bronchial tree. Current evidence supports the importance of pollen allergens associated with submicronic aerosol fractions in asthma.[3–6]

Another important factor is the rapidity with which allergen molecules diffuse or leach out the particles.[7,8] Rapidly released allergens may induce immediate allergic reactions and may be adsorbed through the respiratory mucosa before the pollen grains or fungal spores are swallowed.

DETECTION OF AEROALLERGENS

The choice of sampling method requires an understanding of the environmental conditions that influence aeroallergens and the sampling equipment.[9] The selection of sampling device for a given study depends on the aeroallergen of interest (aerodynamic size, concentration, viability), the detection method used, and the technical skills of and facilities available to the investigator.

Site selection for sampling should be carefully determined. In urban environments, samples are taken mostly from unobstructed rooftops of buildings. Airflow patterns between tall buildings may significantly affect pollen concentrations at locations only a few hundred feet apart. If practical, samplers at multiple sites should be used. In rural areas, local agricultural activities and prevailing wind directions are important considerations. Studies requiring the sampling of indoor air or sampling in occupational settings require knowledge of the building's architecture, air-handling system, and use. Several options are available for indoor environments, including surface sampling and bulk material sampling as well as air sampling.

The anticipated aeroallergen concentration, aerodynamic properties of the particles of interest, and potential reservoirs should be considered before selecting the sampling device. Common samplers used for indoor environments include small-volume suction impactors, impingers, cyclones, and filtration samplers. For most pollens and larger fungal spores, a cost-effective choice has been to use the Rotorod and microscopic examination. However, the low trapping efficiency for fungal spores less than $10\,\mu m$ by rotating-arm samplers has led to the adoption of Hirst-type suction samplers in standardized sampling protocols.

A variety of sample analysis methods are available to identify and quantitate aeroallergens. The most common is direct examination for pollens, fungi, insects, and mites by microscopy.[10–12] Immunoassays for specific allergens and propagation of viable microorganisms on culture media can be used depending on the material under study and the type of information required.[3,4,13–15] Thus a comprehensive sampling strategy may require the use of multiple samplers, sampling sites, and detection methods.

SAMPLING DEVICES

The earliest studies, including those of Blackley with grass pollen, used sedimentation samplers for the microscopic assessment of pollens (Table 32.1). The standard device is the Durham Sampler, consisting of a microscope slide coated with petroleum jelly or silicone grease placed adhesive side up, between a pair of parallel circular plates 3 inches (7.5 cm) apart.[16] The slides are exposed for varying times to the ambient air, then stained with Calberla's solution, and the catches are identified and counted microscopically. The results are reported in terms of the number of pollen grains deposited per square centimeter (cm^2), and extrapolation to air-borne concentration is not possible. Exposed agar plates containing culture media can be substituted for the microscope slides to provide counts of viable fungi or algae. Results obtained with sedimentation samplers are purely qualitative and are biased toward

Table 32.1 Common aeroallergen sampling methods

Method	Device	Application
Sedimentation/gravity sampling	Durham Sampler Settle plates	Not quantitative; useful for describing common pollen and molds and their patterns of abundance
Rotating-arm impactor sampling	Rotorod	Simple to operate; intermittent, overlaid samples; less efficient for small ($<10\,\mu m$) particles or spores
Suction/cascade impactor sampling	Andersen Sampler	Separation of up to six size fractions; used with culture plates
	Allergenco MK-3 Burkard Personal Sampler	Non-wind-oriented, intermittent, discrete sampling; efficient with small particles
	Hirst-type samplers	Wind-oriented, continuous sampling; efficient with small particles
Impinger sampling	AGI-30 SKC Biosampler	Aerosols collected by suspension in liquid; no strict limit to sampling duration
Cyclone/centrifugal sampling	SKC Aluminum Cyclone	Sharp particle-size cutoff point ($4\,\mu m$); reduces particle impaction
Filtration sampling	Air-Sentinel	Continuous high-volume sampling; detection by immunoassay
	IOM Sampler	Lightweight sampler for inhalable particles up to $100\,\mu m$

large particles. Volumetric air sampling is preferred over sedimentation samplers for estimating aeroallergen concentration in ambient air, using impactors, suction traps, impingers, and filtration samplers.

Rotorod samplers, popular among allergists, employ plastic rods that are mechanically rotated to increase the trapping efficiency of the narrow collection surface.[17,18] This portable, inexpensive device is readily adaptable to a variety of environmental conditions. The adhesive rod assembly is rotated at about 2000 rpm to simulate increased wind velocity, and when used, transparent Lucite rods may be stained directly for microscopic examination. The volume sampled is calculated using the formula $V = 2wld\pi r \times 10^{-3}$, where V is volume sampled (L/min); w is width and l is length of sampling surface; d is diameter of circle swept; and r is speed of rotation (rpm). Commercially available devices can sample at rates equivalent to 100 L/min and can be operated intermittently to reduce overloading the sampling surface during extended collection times. Trapping efficiency is about 90% for particles 20 μm in diameter, and Rotorod samplers therefore are ideal for trapping pollen grains. The efficiency falls to below 20% for particles <5 μm in diameter, and Rotorod samplers thus are not suitable for most fungal spores.

Cascade impactors are suction devices that aspirate air through sequential stages, each with a trap for successively smaller particles. The stages at which the particles are collected can be used to estimate their aerodynamic diameters. The 'automatic volumetric spore trap' of Hirst[19] and later modifications allow for continuous monitoring of spore concentrations. The Hirst-type trap utilizes the second intake orifice (14×2 mm) of a four-stage cascade impactor, with air drawn into the device at a rate of 10 L/min. The original version trapped incoming particles on a microscope slide moving past the orifice. Current versions use transparent Milinex tape around a drum rotating at 2 mm/h. Scans across a 7-day collection period allow for the estimation of the number and type of particles during a particular interval. The particle concentration per cubic meter (particles/m³) is estimated for a standard device equipped with a 14 mm intake-slit width operating at a flow rate of 10 L/min and an exposure time of 24 h, using the following formula: $p/(X/14000) \times 14.4\,m^3$, where p is the number of particles counted in a microscope field and X is the field diameter of the objective. The Burkard trap, equipped with a wind vane to maintain proper orientation, recovers particles >5 μm with trapping efficiencies exceeding 50% under most environmental conditions. Thus the device allows for efficient sampling of pollen grains and most fungal spores. Hirst-type samplers have revolutionized aeroallergen sampling and become the sampler of choice in documenting the prevalence of outdoor aeroallergens.

The Andersen sampler collects particles directly on culture media positioned at one, two, or six stages, with each plate representing viable particles of a different size fraction.[15] Operating at 28.3 L/min, Andersen samplers have been employed to study fungal spores, bacteria, and algae with diameters of ≤1 μm. The sampler must be manually positioned toward the airflow in moving air and thus is usually restricted to indoor applications.

Other suction impactors suitable for indoor environments and specifically designed for estimating aeroallergen concentrations include the Burkard personal volumetric air sampler and the Allergenco MK-3. The Burkard sampler is a lightweight cylindrical device operating at 10 L/min with a 14×2 mm slit in the top. The particles impact onto an adhesive-coated microscope slide inserted through the side of the unit. The Allergenco MK-3 is a similar portable 'grab' sampling device that operates at 15 L/min through a 14×1 mm slot.[20] The user may set the collection time and intervals at will, from minutes to days, and samples are deposited on vertical traces spaced 2 mm apart on an adhesive-coated microscope slide. Both devices have optional rechargeable batteries that can operate the pump for 8 h continuously.

Liquid impingers are available in various sizes that operate at 0.3–55 L/min, and the collection efficiency is almost 100% over a wide range of particle sizes. The multistage all-glass liquid impinger is operated with a vacuum pump at 10–55 L/min and collects air-borne particles into three size fractions (1-, 3-, and 6-μm cutoffs).[21] The less complicated AGI-30 or SKC Biosampler operates at 2–13 L/min and is small enough for personal monitoring. The evaporation of water-based collection liquids during sampling may limit the sampling times, however, and fragile microorganisms may be damaged by shear forces through the jet or by impacting into the collection liquid. Also, air-borne fungal spores are highly water repellent and, when in contact with aqueous media, tend to adhere to surface films and clump together in minute air pockets.[22]

Filtration samplers are also available in various sizes and allow for a wide range of sampling rates.[23,24] Filters with defined porosity can be used to trap particles in various size ranges, and air-borne particles can be characterized microscopically. Alternatively, aeroallergens can be eluted directly from the filters using buffer solutions and measured using specific immunoassays. Filtration can be used in high-volume air sampling, operating up to 600 L/min to collect ragweed, *Alternaria*, and latex allergens, which in turn can be eluted from glass-fiber or Gortex-membrane filters and detected by immunoassay.[25,26] Gelatin-membrane filters are available for direct application onto culture media for counts of viable bacterial and fungi. Dehydration and reduction of viability during sampling can lead to an underestimation of microorganisms, and sampling times are therefore limited in these applications.

Cyclone samplers and centrifugal samplers are based on the creation of a vortex in which particles with sufficient inertia are deposited on the sampler's wall. Small personal cyclone samplers operating at about 2.5 L/min can be used to separate respirable from non-respirable particles.[27] Larger units operating at more than 500 L/min have been used for the collection of pollen source materials. Pressure decrease is minor across this type of sampler, so powerful vacuum sources are not required. The main disadvantage is that calculating aeroallergen concentration in air samples is difficult, because the theory of centrifugal sampling is complex and not well described.

ANALYTIC METHODS

Visual inspection is the most economical method of analysis and requires no specialized sampling devices (Table 32.2). The identification and survey of local flora provides valuable information regarding potential aeroallergen sources.[28–30] In indoor environments the presence of furry pets, water damage, and insect pests can yield clues that lead to more specific analytic approaches based on the identification of potential reservoirs.[31] The lack of visible evidence for potential aeroallergen sources, however, does not preclude their existence.

Direct microscopic examination is the most widely employed method for detecting and counting pollen and fungal spores.[32,33] Usually, pollen grains and fungal spores are identified and counted after mounting and staining using a compound light microscope fitted with a stage Vernier scale. A magnification of ×400 is used for pollen grains and ×1000 under oil for fungal spores. A calibrated eyepiece micrometer and a stage micrometer are required to determine the field of view and particle sizes.

Table 32.2 Aeroallergen detection and measurement methods

Method	Application
Visual inspection	Identification of potential aeroallergen reservoirs
Microscopic analysis	Identification and enumeration of pollen and fungal spora
Cultivation	Identification and enumeration of viable microorganisms (fungi, bacteria, protozoa)
Immunoassay	Specific allergen detection and measurement

Sampling tapes from Hirst-type samplers are secured to a microscope slide using 10% Gelvatol in water. Mounting medium with basic fuchsin stain or Calberla's solution is added to the exposed tape. A coverslip is gently placed on the slide to spread the mounting medium evenly before examination. Identification of pollens and spores can be achieved by consulting manuals or validated reference slide collections. Microscopic examination is limited to recognizable particles, and identification of pollens and fungi to the species level is not possible.

A variety of culture media are used in sampling and propagating fungal air and dust spora.[34–37] Enriched media (e.g., nutrient agar, V-8 agar, malt extract agar) permit the growth and identification of a wide range of fungi. Restrictive media contain components that limit colony overgrowth and allow in situ identification of some fungi (e.g., Bengal agar, Littman oxgall agar). Selective media contain components for isolation of particular groups of fungi. Positive identification of fungal isolates may require subculturing on media that promote sporulation because fungal taxonomy depends greatly on spore morphology. When liquid samplers are used (e.g., impingers), collecting fluids should be non-toxic and presterilized and should not allow trapped microorganisms to multiply before plating. Gelatin-phosphate solution or peptone water containing Tween-20 are common collection fluids used. Filter sampling may incorporate gelatin filters that reduce desiccation during sampling and allow for direct application of the sampling surface to culture media.

The total allergen concentration in the air often provides more useful information than air-borne particle counts alone. Pollen counts do not necessarily correlate with total allergen concentration; pollen grains may be void of allergens at times, whereas allergens often are found in high concentrations in small particle fractions when there are no air-borne pollen grains.[3,38,39] Fungal spores have distinctive morphologic features facilitating their identification. In contrast, fungal hyphae and hyphal fragments, which become air-borne in large numbers, are extremely difficult to classify taxonomically. The detection of such submicronic or amorphous aeroallergens usually requires sensitive immunoassays. A semiquantitative fluorescent immunostaining method was used to detect Bermuda grass pollen allergens directly on Burkard tapes, and antigenic material was found outside of the pollen grains associated with small size fractions.[3] Allergens can be eluted or extracted from bulk dust samples, sampling filters, or cascade impactor samples and analyzed by enzyme-linked immunosorbent assay (ELISA) or radioallergosorbent test (RAST) using allergen-specific antibodies.[40,41] Liquid samples from impinger samples can be assayed directly. Although highly specific,

immunoassays may be susceptible to interference by contaminants in dust and air samples.

Although a variety of methods are available for the detection and measurement of aeroallergens in air samples, no single method satisfies the wide range of performance criteria that need to be considered in a particular study. Current technology allows for the detection of very small samples and even of single submicronic particles, and various techniques can be employed to maximize recovery or detection of aeroallergens from an air sample. However, compromises among the technical effort needed to establish a method, assay sensitivity or specificity, time to obtain results, and cost may have to be reached. Ultimately, a method should be widely accepted by fellow investigators in order for the results to be comparable and generally applicable.

POLLEN AEROALLERGENS

POLLEN MORPHOLOGY

Only a cursory knowledge of pollen morphology is required for basic identification. Most comprehensive keys for pollen identifications rely on size, shape, germinal apertures, sculpture, and cell contents. The size of pollen of a particular species is predictable when mounts are prepared fresh with a consistent medium. Heating the glycerin mounting medium or slide for prolonged periods, or pressing the coverslip with force during slide preparations, can increase pollen size. Size may be the most important characteristic for identifying pollen grains from nettle (*Urtica*), which are among the smallest (10–12 µm) grains often trapped in air samplers.

Most pollen grains are described as spheroidal or ellipsoidal. Normal expansion and orientation of the pollen grain may be affected by the mounting medium or the adhesive used to trap the pollen. Thus, the native shape of a pollen grain may change during collection or mounting. Thin-walled pollens may even rupture on wetting. Despite these limitations and potential for artifacts, pollen shape observed in both equatorial and polar views has proved useful. The compound grains of *Acacia* and the 'wings' of the pines are examples in which shape is the primary characteristic used for identification.

The number and position of germinal apertures (pores and furrows) represent the most widely used characteristic in keys for pollen identification. *Porate* grains possess only pores, *colpate* grains possess only furrows, and colporate grains possess both pores and furrows. The positions of germinal apertures may be polar, equatorial, or meridional. *Inaperturate* grains are uncommon and represent a distinguishing feature for cottonwood *(Populus)* and cedar *(Juniperus)* pollen. In most dicotyledonous plants the number of apertures is three (triporate, tricolpate) or four (tetraporate, tetracolpate), and when radially symmetric, the centers of the apertures are *equatorial*. When pollens have more than five apertures, they are usually porate. *Periporate* pollens include the members of the Chenopodiaceae and Amaranthaceae families, which may have more than 50 pores on their surface; sweet gum *(Liquidambar)* and walnut *(Juglans)*, which may have up to 20; and plantain *(Plantago)*, up to 10 surface pores.

Pores and furrows may be surrounded by distinctive margins or thickenings, the pollen's sculpture. The shield-shaped thickenings, termed *aspides*, surrounding the three pores of birch *(Betula)* pollen is an example. An *operculum*, or covering of the apertural membrane, may be found in pollens stained with Calberla's solution. The operculi of the periporate plantain *(Plantago)* pollen give the apertures a characteristic 'doughnut' appearance. The outer wall of pollen grains *(exine)* may possess ornate striations, reticulated patterns, spines, and appendages. In pollen grains stained with basic fuchsin, the outer layers of the exine stain deep red, and the inner exine layers stain pink. The internal layer *(intine)*, which does not contain sporopollenin, does not stain.

Proper staining is required for precise observation of these features because the cell contents have a tendency to obscure details of the exine. The appearance of the intine or cell contents can be useful in pollen identification. Dock pollen *(Rumex)* bears prominent spherical inclusion bodies (starch granules), and members of the family Cupressaceae possess thin, featureless exines and unusually thick intines that aid in their identification.

THE GRASSES

There are more than 600 genera and 10000 species of grasses (Poaceae) in the world. More than 95% of the allergenically important grass species belong to the three subfamilies: Pooideae, Chloridoideae, and Panicoideae (Table 32.3).

The temperate zones are dominated by grasses belonging to the subfamily Pooideae. The genera account for approximately 70–85% of the grasses in Canada and north-western USA, 40–50% in middle-latitude states, and <15–25% in southern states. The cool-season turf grasses, bluegrass *(Poa)*, bent grass *(Agrostis)*, fescues *(Festuca)*, and ryegrass *(Lolium)* represent the major allergenic genera, along with orchard grass *(Dactylis glomerata)*, timothy grass *(Phleum pratense)*, and vernal grass *(Anthoxanthum odoratum)*, which are common in meadows, pastures, and waste places.

Bermuda grass *(Cynodon dactylon)*, the popular southern turf grass belonging to the subfamily Chloridoideae, is a major allergenic species throughout the warmer regions of the world. The Panicoideae are common in humid, tropical to subtropical environments. Allergenically

important species include Bahia grass *(Paspalum notatum)*, an important forage and erosion control grass in the Gulf Coast states, and Johnson grass *(Sorghum halepense)*, a forage grass and frequently a troublesome weed in the warmer and tropical regions of both hemispheres.

It is difficult, if not impossible, to distinguish morphologically the pollen from different grasses. The pollen grains are spheroidal to ovoidal, monoporate, and often with a visible annulus (Fig. 32.1). The size range is great, 20–110 µm, and the larger pollens (>50 µm) are produced by less allergenic, cultivated grasses such as *Secale cereale* and *Zea mays*. The pollens are also highly cross-reactive within subfamilies, which makes immunochemical differentiation difficult. Therefore, the relative importance of the various species in a given geographic area is usually determined by their regional presence.

THE TREES (TABLE 32.4)

The conifers

The conifers, which include the pine and cypress families, are found from the Arctic to the Southern Hemisphere. The Cupressaceae (including Taxodiaceae) is a diverse family representing about 30 genera and comprising both large and small trees and shrubs. They are mainly diecious and produce large quantities of pollen grains 25–35 µm in diameter with a thick intine and stellate cytoplasmic contents (Fig. 32.2). Pollens from two genera, *Cupressus (cypress)* and *Juniperus*, are allergenically important in the USA. *Juniperus ashei (sabinoides)*, or mountain cedar, has been identified as an important cause of allergic rhinitis in certain regions of Texas. Its unique pollination season in these regions makes mountain cedar allergy an ideal model for investigating seasonal allergic rhinitis. *J. virginiana*, commonly called the eastern red cedar or Virginia juniper, occurs throughout eastern states. The bald cypress *(Taxodium distichum)* is an important timber tree of the coastal swamps in southeastern states. In Japan, *Cryptomeria japonica* is considered an important cause of allergic rhinitis.

Table 32.3 Common allergenic grasses (family Poaceae)

Subfamily	Genus/species	Common name
Chloridoideae	Cynodon dactylon	Bermuda grass
Panicoideae	Paspalum notatum	Bahia grass
	Sorghum halepense	Johnson grass
Pooideae	Dactylis glomerata	Orchard grass
	Festuca pratensis (elatior)	Meadow fescue
	Lolium perenne	Perennial ryegrass
	Poa pratensis	Kentucky bluegrass
	Agrostis gigantea (alba)	Redtop, bent grass
	Anthoxanthum odoratum	Sweet vernal grass
	Phleum pratense	Timothy grass

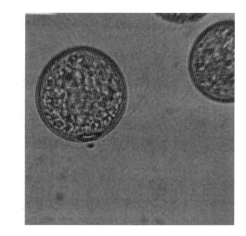

Fig. 32.1. Typical monoporate grass *(Phleum)* pollen (32 µm) with visible annulus, or thickened, slightly raised exine surrounding the pore.

513

Table 32.4 Common allergenic trees

Family	Genus/species	Common name
Aceraceae	*Acer negundo*	Box elder
	Acer saccharum	Sugar maple
Betulaceae	*Alnus incana*	Tag alder
	Corylus americana	American hazelnut
	Betula nigra	Red birch
	Betula populifolia	White birch
Casuarinaceae	*Casuarina equisetifolia*	Australian pine
Cupressaceae	*Cupressus arizonica*	Arizona cypress
	Juniperus ashei	Mountain cedar
	Juniperus virginiana	Red cedar
	Taxodium distichum	Bald-cypress
Fabaceae	*Acacia* spp	Acacia
	Prosopis glandulosa	Mesquite
Fagaceae	*Fagus grandifolia*	American beech
	Quercus velutina	Black oak
	Quercus rubra	Red oak
	Quercus alba	White oak
	Quercus agrifolia	California live oak
Hamamelidaceae	*Liquidambar styraciflua*	Sweet gum
Juglandaceae	*Carya alba*	White hickory
	Carya illinoensis	Pecan
	Juglans nigra	Black walnut
	Juglans regia	English walnut
Moraceae	*Broussonetia papyrifera*	Paper mulberry
	Morus rubra	Red mulberry
Myricaceae	*Myrica cerifera*	Bayberry/wax myrtle
Oleaceae	*Olea europaea*	Olive
	Fraxinus pennsylvanica	Red/green ash
	Ligustrum vulgare	Privet
Platanaceae	*Platanus occidentalis*	American sycamore
	P. racemosa	California sycamore
	Platanus x acerifolia	London plane
Salicaceae	*Populus monilifera*	Western cottonwood
	Populus deltoides	Eastern cottonwood
	Populus alba	White poplar
	Salix nigra	Black willow
Ulmaceae	*Ulmus americana*	American elm
	Celtis occidentalis	Hackberry

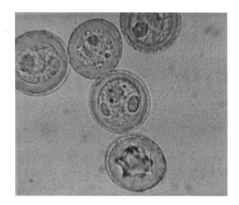

Fig. 32.2. Cedar *(Juniperus)* pollen (25–30 µm) with thin exine and distinctly stellate intine.

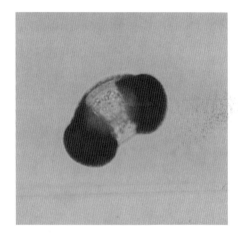

Fig. 32.3. 'Winged' pine *(Pinus)* pollen grain, approximately 75 µm across.

Pines are monoecious and have pollen grains 50–100 µm in diameter with two bladders or 'wings' (Fig. 32.3). Because of pollen size and weight, the pines are only occasionally implicated in allergy.

Sweet gum

The Hamamelidaceae comprises 24 genera of trees and shrubs in the subtropical and warm-temperate regions of the world. Most species are in Asia, and only the sweet gum *(Liquidambar styraciflua)* is common and of allergenic importance in North America. Sweet gum grows from Connecticut southward throughout eastern states to central Florida and eastern Texas. It can be found in Oklahoma, Arkansas, and Missouri into southern Illinois. *L. styraciflua* also grows in scattered locations in northwestern and central Mexico, Guatemala, Belize, Salvador, Honduras, and Nicaragua. The pollen grains, 34–45 µm in size, are spheroidal and periporate (Fig. 32.4).

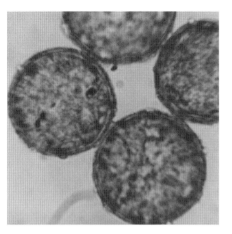

Fig. 32.4. Sweet gum *(Liquidambar)* pollen (35 μm) with coarse, netlike sculpturing on surface and periporate apertures distributed globally.

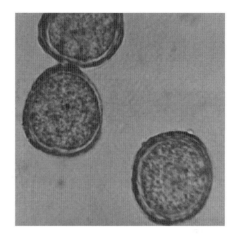

Fig. 32.6. Thick, rippled exine of typical elm *(Ulmus)* pollen grains (35–40 μm).

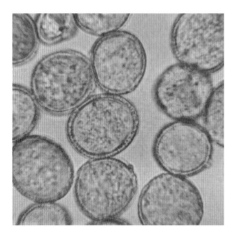

Fig. 32.5. Sycamore *(Platanus)* pollen grains (20–23 μm) with fine reticulate pits viewed on cross section.

Sycamores

Two major species of sycamore or plane (Platanaceae) occur in North America: the eastern sycamore *(Platanus occidentalis)* and western or California sycamore *(P. racemosa)*. The eastern sycamore occurs in mixture with sweet gum, box elder, maple, cottonwood, and willows, especially on frequently disturbed river bottoms. The sycamore flowers appear in May in the northern parts of its range, and as early as late March in southern states. The pollen grains are suboblate, 17–20 μm in size, and tricolpate, and the exine is thin with fine reticulate pits (Fig. 32.5).

Elms and Hackberries

The elms (Ulmaceae) in North America occurring east of the Rocky Mountains are represented by the American elm *(Ulmus americana)* and hackberry *(Celtis occidentalis)*. There are no native elms west of the Rockies, although the Siberian *(Ulmus pumila)* and Chinese elm

(U. parvifolia) have been introduced. Elm pollen is 35–40 μm in diameter and typically has five pores and a thick, rippled exine (Fig. 32.6). The American elm produces large quantities of pollen and is a major cause of allergy despite its destruction by Dutch elm disease. *U. americana* is still abundant in the Mississippi and the Ohio River Valley and their tributaries.

Birches, alders, and hazels

The birches, alders, hornbeams, and hazels (Betulaceae) can be found throughout the temperate, boreal, and arctic zones of the Northern Hemisphere. The birches are important causes of allergy in regions where they grow abundantly. They are monoecious, and the male catkins open in the spring, releasing large quantities of pollen grains. *Betula occidentalis (fontinalis)* is a common shrubby stream-side birch throughout much of the Rocky Mountains, extending eastward into northwestern Ontario. Sweet/black birch *(B. lenta)* occurs in cove sites with hardwoods and white pine; its range extends from Maine to Alabama along the Appalachians. The river birch *(B. nigra)* is a large, common floodplain tree along creekbeds of eastern deciduous forests alongside maples, elms, and sycamore. Tag alder *(Alnus rugosa)* forms swamp thickets. The red alder *(A. rubra)* attains heights above 100 feet (30 m) and is an important hardwood tree in the Pacific Northwest; its range extends from the southern Yukon to southern California, in a narrow band within 100 miles (160 km) of the Pacific Coast. The American hazel *(Corylus americana)* is an abundant shrub throughout the eastern USA and can occur as dense stands in wet sites. The pollen grains are 20–30 μm and generally triporate, occasionally with four and up to seven pores equatorially arranged. The intine is thickened below the pores, forming onci that resemble pollen from members of Myricaceae (Fig. 32.7).

Oaks

The oak family (Fagaceae) contains five genera found in North America, of which only the beeches *(Fagus)* and the oaks *(Quercus)* are anemophilous and of allergenic importance. The pollen grains of *Fagus* and *Quercus* are similar: spheroidal or suboblate with a 'warty' granular

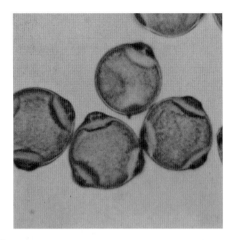

Fig. 32.7. Typical triporate birch *(Betula)* pollen grains (25–28 µm) with protruding domes extending around apertures (aspidate) and large onci (thickened intine below pores).

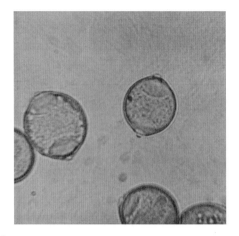

Fig. 32.9. Diporate mulberry *(Morus)* pollen (16–18 µm) with apertures slightly aspidate and with onci.

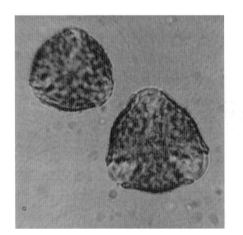

Fig. 32.8. Tricolporate oak *(Quercus)* pollen grains (25–30 µm) with large, bulging furrows and 'warty' surface.

exine, 30–40 µm, triangular in outline, and tricolporate or tricolpate (Fig. 32.8). The American beech *(Fagus grandifolia)* ranges from Nova Scotia to Florida and westward to Missouri and Texas but is of only minor allergenic importance.

In contrast, the oaks shed enormous amounts of pollen and are one of the most important aeroallergens in areas where they are found in abundance. The genus *Quercus* is highly diverse because of its variability and tendency to form natural hybrids. The oaks are native to all 48 contiguous states with the exception of Idaho. Black oak *(Quercus velutina)* and red oak *(Q. rubra)* are widely distributed throughout the eastern and central USA and extreme southwestern Ontario, Canada. In the USA, black oak occurs from southwestern Maine, west to southern Wisconsin and southeastern Minnesota, south through Iowa to eastern Nebraska, eastern Kansas, central Oklahoma, and eastern Texas, and east to northwestern Florida and Georgia. The California black oak *(Q. kelloggii)* is distributed along foothills and lower mountains of California

and southern Oregon. The California 'live' oak *(Q. agrifolia)* is abundant in the coastal regions of California.

The white oak *(Quercus alba)* is one of the largest and most valuable US forest trees, ranging throughout the eastern states from southwest Maine to northern Florida, Alabama, and Georgia. It extends westward throughout southern Ontario and Quebec into central Michigan, northern Wisconsin, and southeastern Minnesota and south to southwestern Iowa, eastern Kansas, Oklahoma, and Texas. The typical 'live' oak *(Q. virginiana)* is a white oak, occurring on the lower southeastern Coastal Plain from southeast Virginia to Florida, including the Florida Keys, and west to southeast Texas. Bur oak is widely distributed throughout much of northern-central USA and the eastern Great Plains.

Mulberries

The mulberry family (Moraceae) comprises some 70 genera of mostly tropical to subtropical trees and shrubs. Some members of this family are entomophilous, but pollen from the mulberries *(Morus)* is regularly trapped in air samplers. The pollen grains are small, 11–20 µm, and possess two to four pores, and the intine is slightly thickened below the pores (Fig. 32.9). The white mulberry *(Morus alba)* was introduced from China in the attempt to establish a silk industry in the USA. Currently it is mainly a 'weedy' species of urban environments. The red mulberry *(M. rubra)* of the eastern USA may grow to 60 feet (18 m) or more and occurs in bottomlands, including coves and lower slopes, on a wide range of soil types. The paper mulberry *(Broussonetia papyrifera)* is still a source of high-quality pulp used for lens paper and cosmetic tissues. The ornamental tree of the central USA, Osage orange *(Maclura)*, and the fig *(Ficus)* belong to the same family but are entomophilous and thus are not important aeroallergens.

Hickories and walnuts

The walnuts and hickories belong to the family Juglandaceae. Of the 15 species of walnuts *(Juglans)*, three are common in North America. The largest orchards of English walnuts *(Juglans regia)* are in California (>125 000 acres). The California black walnut *(J. californica)* occurs at Walnut Creek and in the coastal ranges of southern California, hills of

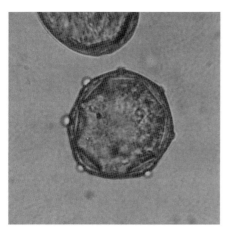

Fig. 32.10. Periporate walnut *(Juglans)* pollen (35 µm) with heteropolar distribution of pores (on equator and one hemisphere) and with onci.

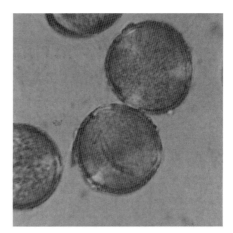

Fig. 32.11. Tricolpate box elder *(Acer negundo)* pollen (24 µm) with long, tapering furrows.

Los Angeles, and Santa Monica. Trees produce pollen in abundance during April and May, but it is not carried far from the trees. The black walnut *(J. nigra)* is a valuable timber tree in eastern states. In northeastern states, its pollen is conspicuous on pollen slides during May and early June. *Carya*, or the hickories, with 12 species in eastern North America, mostly produce small, hard nuts. The notable exception is the pecan *(Carya illinoensis)* from the southern USA, growing principally in the bottomlands of the Mississippi River Valley. Shagbark hickory *(C. ovata)* occurs throughout most of the eastern North America but is largely absent from the southeastern and Gulf coastal plains and the lower Mississippi Delta. The pollen grains are 30–45 µm, rounded, triangular or polygonal, and triporate or tetraporate *(Carya)* or periporate *(Juglans)*. Pores are slightly aspidate or flattened conical and located on the equator. The intine is thickened beneath the pores, forming a lens-shaped oncus (Fig. 32.10).

Maples and box elder

More than 100 species of maple (Aceraceae) are found in North America, and many are significant sources of aeroallergens. The most widely distributed species, *Acer negundo*, or box elder, is a prolific producer of pollen and thus one of the most allergenically important maples. Box elder is widespread throughout most of the contiguous USA and flowers from March through May with or before the appearance of the leaves. The red *(Acer rubrum)*, silver *(A. saccharinum)*, and sugar *(A. saccharum)* maples are widely distributed in eastern North America. The sugar maple, as with box elder, produces an abundance of pollen and is also considered to be an important allergen source. The maples are one of the first trees to flower in early spring. Specific flowering dates largely depend on weather conditions, latitude, and elevation. The pollen grains are 20–30 µm, spheroidal with slightly convex sides, and tricolpate or tricolporate, with long tapering furrows (Fig. 32.11).

Olives and ashes

The olive family (Oleaceae) comprises about 20 genera of trees and shrubs, most of which are entomophilous and of limited importance. The allergenically important genera of this family are *Olea*, *Ligustrum*,

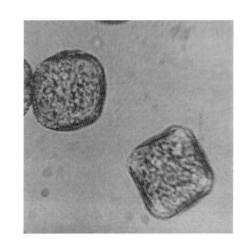

Fig. 32.12. Quadrangular and tetracolpate ash *(Fraxinus)* pollen (28–30 µm).

and *Fraxinus*. The pollens grains are 15–25 µm and spheroidal, triangular, or quadrangular with a coarsely reticulate exine and have three to five furrows (Fig. 32.12). Green ash *(Fraxinus pennsylvanica)* is the most widely distributed; its range extends from Cape Breton Island and Nova Scotia to southeastern Alberta and Montana and southward to central Texas and northern Florida. White ash *(F. americana)* is found mainly in eastern North America. The majority of ashes in the USA are entirely anemophilous, and their pollen is among the most abundant identified in pollen slides during the early-spring season. *Olea europaea* is a small spreading tree and primarily entomophilous but is known to produce large amounts of pollen that become air-borne. It can be an important cause of pollinosis in California, Arizona, and in the Mediterranean areas where the trees are extensively grown for their fruit. The privets are primarily evergreen shrubs bearing small, white, fragrant flowers. The common privet *(Ligustrum vulgare)* is grown as a hedge plant because it tolerates shearing and grows 12–15 feet high and spreads 12–15 feet

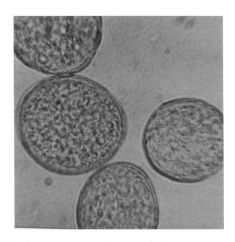

Fig. 32.13. Inaperturate pollen (30–35 μm) from poplar *(Populus)* with thin exine and 'warty' surface.

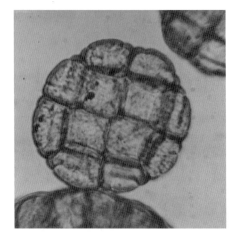

Fig. 32.14. Acacia pollen (50 μm) is a polyad of 16 roughly quadrangular individual grains.

(3.6–4.5 m). It is primarily entomophilous but its pollen, similar in morphology to the other members of the family, becomes air-borne when the plants are shaken.

Poplars and willows

The willows *(Salix)* and poplars *(Populus)* belong to the family Salicaceae. The willows are entomophilous and are not considered important aeroallergen sources. The poplars are diecious and anemophilous and produce spherical pollen grains, 25–35 μm in diameter, with thick intines and thin exines (Fig. 32.13). Eastern cottonwood *(Populus deltoides)* is the fastest growing native tree in North America. It commonly increases 5 feet (1.5 m) in height each year for the first 10–15 years and grows at only a slightly slower rate up to 30–35 years of age. Eastern cottonwood occurs from southern Quebec and Ontario south to Florida. It extends west to North Dakota and through the eastern parts of Nebraska, Kansas, Oklahoma, and Texas. Plains cottonwood is found throughout the Great Plains region to the foothills of the Rocky Mountains, northeastern New Mexico, and northern Texas. Rio Grande cottonwood *(P. wislizenii)* occurs along the Colorado River from southern Colorado to southeastern Utah and northeastern Arizona, extending to the Rio Grande drainage in western Texas, New Mexico, and northwestern Mexico. Where the western limit of eastern cottonwood and the eastern limit of plains cottonwood overlap, plants display intermediate morphologic characteristics. Fremont cottonwood occurs in riparian habitats from western Texas through New Mexico, Arizona, and California and northward into Nevada, Utah, and Colorado.

Mimosas, acacias, locusts, and mesquites

The mimosas, acacias, locusts, and mesquites are leguminous plants and can be grouped to form the plant family Leguminosae, which contains slightly less than one-twelfth of the world's flowering plants. Many species are important as crop plants (e.g., soybeans, peanuts), and their pollens are not allergenically important. They are responsible for much of the world's soil fertility through nitrogen fixation. Among the genera

potentially important in pollinosis are *Acacia, Robinia, Prosopis*, and *Mimosa*. The acacias are primarily tropical and subtropical trees found in the hot and arid regions of America and cultivated as ornamental trees. The common name 'acacia' is also applied to *Robinia pseudoacacia*, or the black locust, ranging in the central Appalachian Mountains from central Pennsylvania and southern Ohio to northern Alabama, Georgia, and South Carolina. The locust tree has been successfully planted in every state. The mesquites *(Prosopis)* occur throughout most of Texas, southern New Mexico, Arizona, Colorado, and Kansas. Mesquites hybridize naturally, and thus many intermediate forms exist, making identification difficult at the species level. The pollen grains may be monads (single pollen) or polyads (aggregation of more than four pollens), with a bilateral diameter ranging from 35 to 140 μm. The monads *(Prosopis* and *Robinia)* are prolate to subprolate, 30–50 μm, and tricolporate with long and narrow furrows. The polyads have four *(Mimosa)* or usually 16 *(Acacia)* roughly quadrangular grains (Fig. 32.14).

THE WEEDS

The general category of 'weeds' is used to group those invasive, undesirable plants that are not trees or grasses (Table 32.5).

Pigweeds, saltbrushes, and chenopods

The pigweeds (Amaranthaceae) and chenopods (Chenopodiaceae) are closely related but generally not similar in appearance. Their pollen grains, however, are similar: spheroidal, 20–35 μm in diameter, and periporate with a thin, granular exine (Fig. 32.15). The genus *Amaranthus* is represented by the ubiquitous *A. retroflexus*, or rough pigweed, found in cultivated or waste soil throughout North America. It is also found throughout Europe, South America, Eurasia, and Africa. Redroot pigweed is a native of tropical America. *A. palmeri* (careless weed) is distinguished by its long, slender terminal flowering spikes, shedding much more pollen than other species of this genus. This species is abundant in Missouri, Kansas, Oklahoma, and eastern Texas. The western water hemp *(A. tuberculatus)* is abundant

Table 32.5 Common allergenic weeds

Family	Genus/species	Common name
Amaranthaceae (incl. Chenopodiaceae)	*Allenrolfea occidentalis*	Iodine bush
	Amaranthus retroflexus	Rough pigweed
	Amaranthus spinosus	Spiny pigweed
	Amaranthus hybridus	Careless weed
	Atriplex wrightii	Annual saltbush
	Atriplex polycarpa	Allscale
	Atriplex lentiformus	Lenscale
	Chenopodium album	Lamb's quarter
	Chenopodium botrys	Jerusalem oak
	Kochia scoparia	Burning bush
	Salsola kali	Russian thistle
Asteraceae	*Ambrosia artemisiifolia*	Short ragweed
	Ambrosia trifida	Giant ragweed
	Ambrosia psilostachya	Western ragweed
	Artemisia tridentata	Sagebrush
	Artemisia vulgaris	Mugwort
	Baccharis spp	Groundsel-tree
	Eupatorium capillifolium	Dog fennel
	Iva xanthifolia	Burweed marsh elder
	Xanthium strumarium	Cocklebur
Plantaginaceae	*Plantago lanceolata*	English plantain
Polygonaceae	*Rumex acetosella*	Red sorrel
	Rumex crispus	Curly dock
Urticaceae	*Urtica dioica*	Nettle
	Parietaria spp	Pellitory

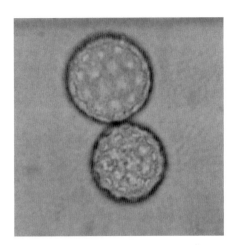

Fig. 32.15. Saltbush *(Atriplex)* pollen (23–28 μm) is typical of periporate pollen grains of pigweed and chenopod families.

The saltbushes *(Atriplex)* are primarily found in western USA and shed large amounts of pollen (Fig. 32.15). *Atriplex canescens* (wingscale) is by far the most widely distributed of the genus, ranging from Alberta to Kansas, western Texas, Mexico, Baja California, Washington, and Montana. *Kochia*, or 'firebush', named for its red leaves of autumn, was introduced from Europe and Asia primarily as a garden plant. It has escaped cultivation and is now naturalized throughout North America, except the southeast USA. Native to Eurasia, the Russian thistle *(Salsola kali)* is distributed throughout most arid and semiarid regions of the world. In North America, Russian thistle is most common in central and western regions of Canada and the USA, as well as along the Atlantic and Gulf coasts. It flowers from June to September, and among the chenopods, *S. kali* is probably the most important cause of 'hay fever'.

The composites

The Asteraceae ('composites') comprises a family of 13 000 species in 900 genera and forms one of the largest flowering-plant families. They are mainly herbaceous plants and are distributed over most of the world and grown for their attractive flowers. The most important among the anemophilous species are the ragweeds, sagebrushes, mugworts, and wormwoods of the genera *Ambrosia* and *Artemisia*.

Ragweeds

The ragweeds are some of the most important allergenic weeds in North America. The giant ragweed *(Ambrosia trifida)* can reach a height of 15 feet (4.5 m). Short ragweed *(A. artemisiifolia)* and other species *(A. bidentata, A. psilostachya)* grow to about 4 feet (1.2 m) in height and shed enormous amounts of pollen. The ragweeds are highly invasive pioneer plants. Introduced from North America, the ragweeds have invaded Hawaii, Europe, and Japan. The pollen grains are spheroidal (15–25 μm) with small (<3 μm) spines and typically tricolporate or tetracolporate (Fig. 32.16).

in the prairie region from South Dakota, Nebraska, and Kansas southward through eastern Texas and Oklahoma, where it is most abundant.

The chenopods comprise about 75 genera of worldwide distribution and are represented by the summer-blooming *Chenopodium album* (lamb's quarter), introduced from Europe and naturalized throughout North America. *C. ambrosioides* (Mexican tea) was introduced from tropical America and is also naturalized throughout North America and flowers from August to October. *C. botrys* (Jerusalem oak) is occasionally cultivated in the northern USA and Canada and flowers from July to September.

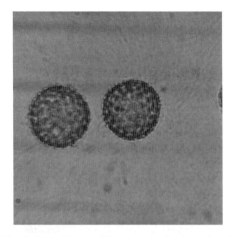

Fig. 32.16. Spheroidal ragweed *(Ambrosia)* pollen (20 μm) with outer surface of exine sculptured with short, broad-based spines.

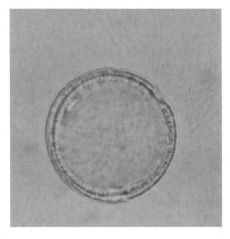

Fig. 32.18. Equatorial view of *Xanthium strumarium* pollen (25 μm) showing spine vestiges and two apertures.

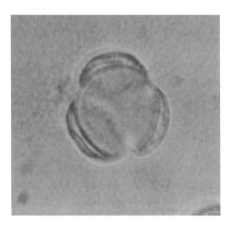

Fig. 32.17. Polar view of tricolporate pollen (25 μm) of *Artemisia* showing exine significantly thicker between furrows, creating three-lobed appearance.

Sagebrush and mugwort

Artemisia tridentata, or common sagebrush, is one of the most widespread shrubs in western North America. Various times of flowering have been reported, including periods from August through December and year-round. *A. vulgaris*, or common mugwort, is found mainly on the East Coast and Midwest. The pollen grains of sagebrush and mugwort are indistinguishable, being 20–30 μm in diameter, with three furrows, central pores, a thick exine with no spines (Fig. 32.17). The pollen allergens of the two species are highly cross-reactive.

Cockleburs

The cockleburs *(Xanthium)* can also be a major cause of pollinosis. The pollen grains range from 20 to 30 μm in diameter with spine vestiges that are scarcely apparent (Fig. 32.18). Common cocklebur *(Xanthium strumarium, X. commune)* has a nearly worldwide distribution. In North America it is widespread across southern Canada, over the contiguous

USA with the exception of northeastern New York and Maine, and in mountainous terrain. It grows in cultivated fields and waste areas and on beaches and sand dunes. The plant will not flower or will flower only poorly when day length exceeds 14 h, so flowering does not occur until late summer in most regions.

Nettles

The Urticaceae, or nettle family, is widely dispersed in tropical and temperate regions of the world. In North America, this family is best known for the stinging nettle *(Urtica)*, which is the most common genus in temperate North America and occurs throughout Canada and much of the USA. In the East and Midwest, *Urtica dioica* occurs as far south as Virginia and in Missouri and Kansas, and in the West it occurs along the coast south to central California and in the Rocky Mountains to Mexico. Stinging nettle is characterized by leaves, stems, and flowers that are sparsely to moderately covered with stinging hairs. It occurs in moist sites along streams, coulees, and ditches; on mountain slopes; in woodland clearings; and in disturbed areas. *U. dioica* flowers from late May–October, although it may flower as early as January or February in southern latitudes. In northern areas, flowering is condensed into a shorter period, ending in late August.

In the Mediterranean regions of Europe, the nettle family is best known for the wall pellitory *(Parietaria)*, a plant similar to the nettles but lacking hairs that sting. The pellitory's thin-walled and nearly smooth pollen grains, 12–16 μm in diameter with three or four pores, are almost indistinguishable from nettle *(Urtica)* pollen (Fig. 32.19). Three or four species of *Parietaria* are established in some regions of the USA, but they have not yet been established as important aeroallergens.

Plantains

Plantago lanceolata, or English plantain, is the only allergenic member of the family Plantaginaceae. *P. lanceolata* is found throughout the USA and southern Canada, with the greatest concentration from the eastern Rocky Mountains to the Appalachian Mountains. It pollinates during the grass pollen season, and its pollen (20–40 μm in diameter) can

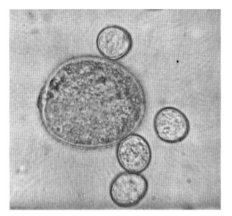

Fig. 32.19. Nettle *(Urtica)* pollen grains (12–14 μm) are dwarfed by grass pollen (40 μm); nettle and grass pollen are frequently found together in air samples.

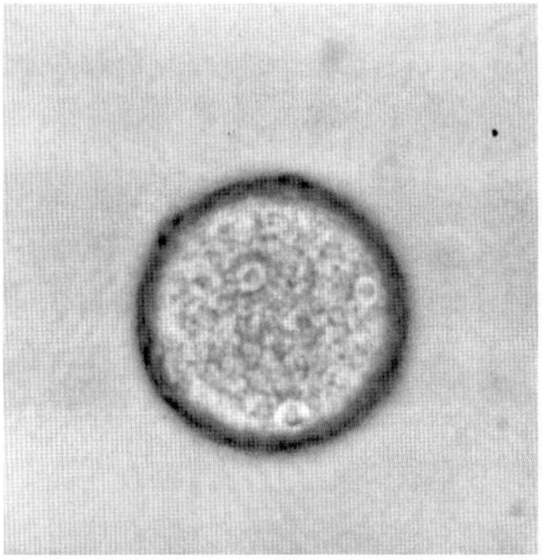

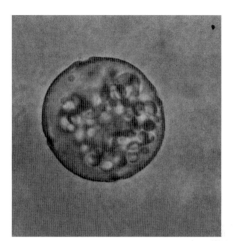

Fig. 32.21. Sheep sorrel *(Rumex acetosella)* pollen (25 μm) with characteristic starch inclusion bodies.

throughout North America, sheds its pollen during the summer months and is a common weed in dry, acidic fields. *R. crispus* is similar in appearance to *R. acetosella* but is taller with broader, curly leaves. The two species are known to hybridize naturally. The pollen grains are spheroidal, 20–30 μm, and colporate, with characteristic starch inclusion bodies (Fig. 32.21).

PLANTS OF REGIONAL OR LIMITED IMPORTANCE

Australian pine

Australian pine was introduced to the USA at about the turn of the twentieth century from Australia, the Philippines, and Pacific islands. *Casuarina equisetifolia*, a medium to tall evergreen tree resembling pine trees, is the most common species, planted in southern Florida as a windbreak and also found in California, Arizona, and Hawaii. It is anemophilous and sheds large amounts of pollen in late summer, although *C. equisetifolia* can flower year-round. Australian pine can colonize nutrient-poor soils. It can grow in sloughs, glades, and wet prairies; along rocky coasts; on sandbars and dunes; and in water-logged clay or brackish tidal areas. The pollen grains are suboblate, 19–30 μm, and triporate or tetraporate, and the outer exine surface is transgressed by narrow, irregular ridges (Fig. 32.22).

Bayberry

North American species of the Myricaceae include bayberry *(Myrica cerifera)*, the source of myrtle wax, and *M. californica*, which is distributed from Washington to California. The diminutive flowers are unisexual, diecious, and borne on catkin-like axillary spikes. The pollens resemble those of the birches and *Casuarina*. Pollen grains are suboblate, 20–30 μm, and triporate or tetraporate, with the intine conspicuously thickened beneath the pores and forming an *oncus* (Fig. 32.23). *M. cerifera* grows in thickets near swamps and marshes and is common in a variety of habitats and plant communities in the southeastern USA. It grows

Fig. 32.20. Operculi of periporate plantain *(Plantago)* pollen (25 μm) give apertures a characteristic 'doughnut' appearance.

be distinguished by its multiple (6–10) scattered pores of variable size (1.5–3.0 μm) and a pluglike operculum (Fig. 32.20). *P. lanceolata* is an acaulescent perennial with flowers in a terminal spike. Flowering progresses from the base to the tip of the spike over a period of weeks.

Dock and sorrel

The Polygonaceae, or the buckwheat family, is a diverse group of about 40 genera, including herbs, shrubs, and a few trees, characterized by their swollen nodes and with a membranous collar or sheath *(ocrea)*. All members of the family are entomophilous with the exception of the rhubarb *(Rheum rhaponticum)* and the docks *(Rumex)*. The rhubarb has long been cultivated for culinary use in pies and desserts, but there are no reports of rhubarb pollen as a cause of pollinosis. The genus *Rumex* is the only known allergenic member of this family. *Rumex acetosella* (sheep sorrel) and *R. crispus* (dock) are the most important species. *R. acetosella*, found

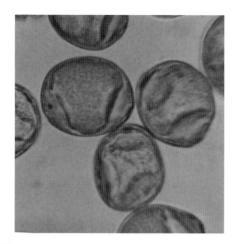

Fig. 32.22. *Casuarina* pollen grains (22–28 µm) with narrow, irregular ridges on exine surface.

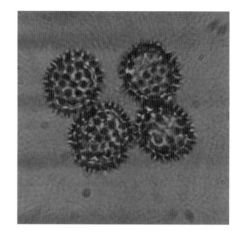

Fig. 32.24. Surface sculpturing of *Baccharis* pollen (22–25 µm) resembles that of ragweed; *Baccharis* spines are longer than those of ragweed pollen.

in moist, sunny streambeds, ditches, and desert oases. *B. sarothroides* is a prolific producer of pollen and has been identified as an important aeroallergen in Arizona and New Mexico. The pollen grains resemble that of ragweed, except the spines are longer: 3–4 µm (Fig. 32.24).

NORTH AMERICAN FLORISTIC ZONES

Although sharp boundaries are shown in the spatial and seasonal prevalence of allergenic pollens in distinctive areas of North America, these 'life zones' regularly overlap in broad transition areas (Fig. 32.25 and Table 32.6). Pollen prevalence may also vary predictably within regions.

POLLEN EXPOSURE OUTSIDE NORTH AMERICA

Grasses are the most common cause of pollen allergy outside the USA, including both temperate grasses and Bermuda grass. Birch and alder pollens are major causes of spring hay fever in the Scandinavian countries, and Japanese red cedar pollen is a major offender in Japan. Short ragweed can be found in eastern France and the Balkans, but mugwort is a more widespread weed allergen in Europe. Russian thistle pollen is a major weed allergen in the Middle East. Wall pellitory *(Parietaria officinalis)* pollen is an important aeroallergen in the Mediterranean basin. D'Amato et al[42] and Roth[43] list allergenic pollens present in Europe and elsewhere in the world.

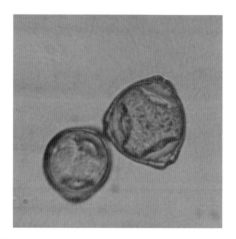

Fig. 32.23. Triporate bayberry *(Myrica)* pollen (22–25 µm) with narrow ridges resembling those of *Casuarina* pollen and with onci resembling birch pollen.

equally well with the subtropical vegetation of southern Florida. Bayberry is planted as an ornamental on a variety of sites but seems to be restricted to climates with mild winters and long, hot, humid summers and to elevations below 500 feet (150 m).

Groundsel-tree

Baccharis, or groundsel-tree, grows along the Atlantic and Gulf coasts of North America from Mexico, through Texas, and peninsular Florida to Massachusetts. *Baccharis halimifolia* is most common on the southeastern coastal plain, growing as far inland as Arkansas and the central Piedmont Plateau. The trees grow in moist sites with a high organic content, including pond and bay margins, swamps, wet prairies, marshes, and Everglades hammocks. They pollinate from August to October and reportedly are an important 'hay fever' plant in parts of Florida. In the western states, *Baccharis* species, commonly named 'mulefat' and 'desert broom,' are found

FUNGI AS AEROALLERGENS

Fungal spores and other fungal particles are widely distributed throughout the world except over the polar regions. These particles often form the majority of suspended biologic particles in the air. Fungi can cause a number of human diseases. They can act as pathogens and cause HP,

*The term 'mold' is often used as a synonym for fungi. More precisely, mold denotes types of fungi that lack macroscopic reproductive structures but may produce visible colonies or other growth.

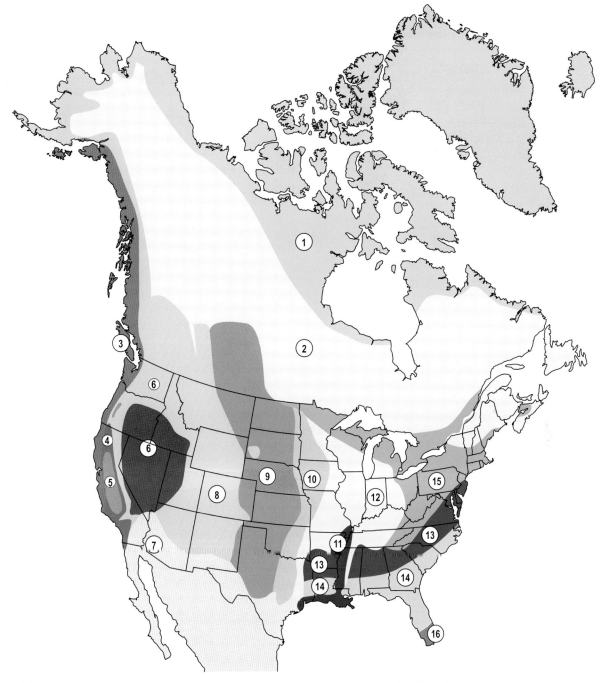

Fig. 32.25. Distribution and prevalence of allergenic pollens in North American Floristic Zones (see Table 32.6 on the next page).

AEROBIOLOGY AND ALLERGENS

Table 32.6 Allergenic pollens in North American floristic zones[a]

Zone	Grasses	Weeds	Trees
Northern Region			
1. Tundra	Phleum, Poa, Agrostis		
2. Boreal Forests	Phleum, Lolium, Poa, Festuca, Dactylis, Agrostis	Rumex, Artemisia	Pinus, Betula, Alnus, Populus, Salix
3. Pacific Coast Maritime Forest	Phleum, Lolium, Poa	Chenopodium, Amaranthus, Ambrosia, Rumex, Artemisia	Betula, Alnus, Ulmus, Acer, Quercus, Populus, Salix
Western Region			
4. California	Phleum, Lolium, Poa, Festuca, Cynodon, Sorghum	Chenopodium, Amaranthus, Ambrosia, Rumex, Artemisia, Salsola	Alnus, Ulmus, Acer, Quercus, Olea, Populus, Fraxinus, Salix, Platanus
5. California Prairie	Phleum, Lolium, Poa, Festuca, Cynodon, Sorghum	Chenopodium, Amaranthus, Atriplex, Ambrosia, Rumex, Salsola	Ulmus, Acer, Quercus, Olea, Populus, Fraxinus
6. Great Basin/ Columbia Plateau	Phleum, Lolium, Poa, Dactylis, Cynodon, Sorghum	Chenopodium, Amaranthus, Atriplex, Ambrosia, Rumex, Artemisia, Salsola, Xanthium	Ulmus, Populus, Juniperus
7. Hot Desert Region	Cynodon, Sorghum	Chenopodium, Amaranthus, Atriplex, Ambrosia, Baccharis, Rumex, Artemisia, Salsola, Xanthium	Ulmus, Quercus, Populus, Juniperus, Acacia, Fraxinus, Tamarix
8. Western Cordillera	Festuca, Phleum, Dactylis, Lolium, Cynodon, Sorghum	Chenopodium, Amaranthus, Atriplex, Ambrosia, Rumex, Plantago, Artemisia, Salsola, Xanthium	Pinus, Ulmus, Quercus, Populus, Acer, Juniperus, Alnus
Central Region			
9. Short-Grass Prairie	Festuca, Phleum, Poa, Dactylis, Lolium, Cynodon, Sorghum	Chenopodium, Kochia, Amaranthus, Ambrosia, Rumex, Plantago, Artemisia, Salsola, Xanthium	Quercus, Populus, Ulmus, Fraxinus
10. Tall-Grass Prairie	Festuca, Phleum, Poa, Dactylis, Lolium, Cynodon, Sorghum	Chenopodium, Kochia, Amaranthus, Ambrosia, Rumex, Plantago, Artemisia, Salsola, Xanthium	Quercus, Populus, Acer, Ulmus, Carya, Fraxinus
11. Lower Mississippi Valley Flood Plain	Phleum, Poa, Dactylis, Lolium, Cynodon, Sorghum, Paspalum	Chenopodium, Kochia, Amaranthus, Ambrosia, Rumex, Plantago, Artemisia, Xanthium	Quercus, Populus, Acer, Ulmus, Salix, Taxodium, Carya
12. Central Hardwoods	Phleum, Poa, Dactylis, Lolium, Cynodon, Sorghum	Chenopodium, Kochia, Amaranthus, Ambrosia, Rumex, Plantago, Artemisia, Xanthium	Quercus, Populus, Acer, Ulmus, Carya, Celtis
Eastern Region			
13. Upland Southeastern Forests	Phleum, Poa, Dactylis, Lolium, Cynodon, Sorghum	Chenopodium, Amaranthus, Ambrosia, Rumex, Plantago, Artemisia, Xanthium	Quercus, Populus, Acer, Ulmus, Carya, Pinus
14. Lowland Southeastern Forests	Phleum, Poa, Dactylis, Lolium, Cynodon, Sorghum, Paspalum	Chenopodium, Kochia, Amaranthus, Ambrosia, Rumex, Plantago, Artemisia, Salsola, Xanthium, Baccharis	Quercus, Populus, Acer, Ulmus, Carya, Myrica, Pinus, Liquidambar
15. Northern Hardwood Forests	Phleum, Poa, Dactylis, Lolium, Cynodon, Sorghum	Chenopodium, Amaranthus, Ambrosia, Rumex, Plantago, Artemisia, Xanthium	Quercus, Populus, Acer, Ulmus, Betula, Pinus
16. Southern Florida	Cynodon, Sorghum, Paspalum	Chenopodium, Amaranthus, Ambrosia	Quercus, Casuarina, Myrica, Schinus, Taxodium

[a]See Figure 32.25.

allergic bronchopulmonary mycoses, allergic fungal sinusitis, allergic rhinitis, and allergic asthma. Respiratory allergies in individuals exposed to various fungi have long been recognized. However, effects of fungi on individuals are difficult to judge, and many common organisms have not been studied.

Environmental exposures to fungi are often assessed by direct microscopic sampling of air-borne materials. Because of their diverse and often small size, fungal emanations present special challenges. Problems of particle viability and requirements for selective media present challenges to culture-based studies. Indeed, it has proven quite difficult to quantitate exposure to fungal allergens. The methods used to estimate exposure to other allergens and that use immunoassays for major allergens (e.g., house-dust mite, cockroach, cat) are not readily available for fungal allergens or are early in their development.

Several international studies have demonstrated that immunoglobulin E (IgE)-mediated sensitivity to fungal allergens, particularly *Alternaria alternata*, is common among patients with allergic rhinitis or allergic asthma.[44,45] Also, up to 80% of subjects with confirmed asthma may have positive skin test reactions to one or more fungi.[46] Several epidemiologic studies have established a role for fungal sensitivity in the development of symptomatic asthma. An accumulating body of evidence suggests that sensitization to fungi, particularly *Alternaria*, is associated with asthma.[47–51]

A relationship has been demonstrated between increased fungal spore count levels in the patient's environment and the presence of allergic symptoms. In a study of children 9–18 years of age in San Diego, fungal spore exposure resulted in a 10–30% increase in symptoms for every 1000 spores/m³ of air.[52] In addition, seasonal epidemics of asthma have been reported in England and New Zealand during periods of high fungal spore counts,[53] and high levels of the ascomycete *Didymella* have been associated with epidemic asthma in England.[54] An increased volume of hospitalizations for asthma have been reported in New Orleans during periods of high basidiospore counts.[55]

Emergency department (ED) visits have been prompted by high levels of ascospores.[56] Others have reported that ED visits for asthma in children is associated with sensitivity to a variety of allergens, including *A. alternata*.[57,58] Severity of asthma has been linked to sensitivity to *Alternaria*.[59,60] *Alternaria* sensitivity has also been found to correlate with persistence of asthma in children who were skin test positive at age 6 years.[61]

Finally, fungal sensitivity has been linked to severe and potentially fatal episodes of asthma.[62–64] In addition to these epidemiologic studies, direct inhalation of spores of *Penicillium* and *Alternaria* has been shown to precipitate acutely decreased pulmonary function in patients sensitive to these fungi.[65]

FUNCTIONAL ANATOMY OF FUNGI

Despite the large numbers of fungi, they exhibit only two basic types of structures. The minority of species, termed yeasts, grow as single cells by central division or by budding to form 'daughter' cells. Most other fungi are composed of branching threads, 3–10 μm in width, termed *hyphae*. Hyphae have well-defined walls, reinforced with cellulose or chitin, and true nuclei that are unapparent. Hyphal strands often show septa at intervals, whereas in other forms, such as Zygomycetes, cross-walls are few or absent, which allows for the free streaming of cytoplasm. A *mycelium* is a collection of hyphae, although some of these produce buds sequentially, forming a linear *pseudomycelium*. Hyphae are modified to bear the reproductive parts of many fungi and also form the structural tissues

of the 'fleshy fungi' (e.g., mushrooms, puffballs). Importantly, mycelia in their natural environment seem to be a single physiologic and ecologic unit but in reality are a genetic mosaic.[66]

SPORE STRUCTURE AND DEVELOPMENT

Fungi reproduce by sexual and asexual spores (although hyphal fragments can also proliferate), and spore-bearing parts provide one basis for the classification of fungi. Two basic types of asexual spores are recognized: *sporangiospores*, which are formed in enclosed sacs or *sporangia*, and *conidia*, which are not formed in this way. Most conidia form on specialized hyphae or *conidiospores*; others arise from undifferentiated hyphae. In addition, many fungi produce thick-walled *chlamydophores* as a result of the rounding and condensation of intercalary hyphal segments. The modes of conidial formation have been examined and a series of categories described.[67] Some of these processes, such as the formation of *arthrospores* by simple segmentation and wall formation of hyphae are obvious (Fig. 32.26); others require minute, sequential observation. Mature spores are described by their color, size, shape, and surface texture. A further characteristic, septation, defines categories as having no septa *(amerospores)*, one septum *(didymospores)*, two or more transverse septa *(phragmospores)*, and transverse and longitudinal septa *(dictyospores)*.

FUNGAL TAXONOMY

Fungal taxonomy is a dynamic and evolving discipline that consequently requires frequent changes in the nomenclature of organisms, which can lead to confusion among clinicians. In general, most allergenic fungi reproduce asexually. However, in the life cycle, fungal organisms typically produce both sexual and asexual spores from morphologically different structures, termed *perfect* and *imperfect* stages, respectively. Often these reproductive forms require different growth conditions and may not occur together, although in certain instances they may coexist. As a result, different life cycle stages have been named as separate organisms when, in fact, they may be the same organism. Most clinicians are familiar with only one stage of the fungus, the stage that develops by

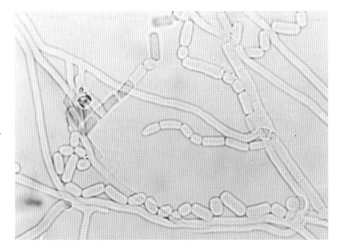

Fig. 32.26. Culture mount of *Geotrichum candidum* showing hyphae generally forming arthrospores; individual spores are 6–10 μm in length.

asexual reproduction. However, the sexual stages are the basis of fungal taxonomy and nomenclature. The development of molecular techniques (see Chapter 35) should allow for most of the allergenic fungi to be connected to their corresponding sexual stages and integrated into more understandable taxonomic relationships.

The basic rank in taxonomy is the species. However, different mycologists disagree as to what may be considered a 'species'. With different approaches for delineating species, attempts to reach consensus for a universal definition of species have been unsuccessful. Nonetheless, several basic processes have been applied. In the classic morphologic approach, species are defined on the basis of morphologic characteristics and by differences among them. On the other hand, concepts based on combinations of characteristics are now increasingly utilized, with molecular techniques helping to resolve some of these differences. Currently, the nomenclature of fungi (including yeasts) is governed by the International Code of Botanical Nomenclature (ICBN).[68] Any proposed changes to the code are published in *Taxon*, the official journal of the International Association for Plant Taxonomy, then debated for final approval.[69]

Because fungi may have a dual modality of propagation (sexual and asexual), a dual nomenclature exists for these different stages of the same organism. Many fungi, as a whole, comprise a *teleomorph* (sexual stage) and one or more *anamorphs* (asexual stages), developing at different times and on different substrates. In many cases, each stage was described as a species in total ignorance of the other. The term Deuteromycetes has been applied to anamorphs, which are widely recognized as common allergenic fungi.

Because different life cycle stages were named as separate organisms when their true relationships were not apparent, some organisms have two different names when in fact they are derived from the same organism.[69] The ascomycete *Neurospora sitophila* has an asexual stage, *Monilia sitophila* ('red bread mold'), and the ascomycete *Eurotium herbariorum* has an imperfect stage, *Aspergillus glaucus*. To add to the confusion, organisms classified separately because of their perfect stages may have similar asexual forms. For example, members of several genera besides *Eurotium* have *Aspergillus* imperfect stages. Because the classification of fungi that produce asexual spores does not necessarily reflect the natural affinity to the sexual stage (or may not be known), and for historical reasons, its members are grouped as form genera. These taxa in turn comprise form families, form orders, and so forth, in the *form class* 'Fungi Imperfecti' or Deuteromycetes. Unfortunately, these sets of names may have little association with the allergenic relationships between and among form taxa and the organism's sexual stage.

FUNGAL GROUPS IMPLICATED AS AEROALLERGENS

Fungi have traditionally been placed in the context of five kingdoms: animals, plants, fungi, protista, and monera.[70,71] Five major phyla, or groups that contain recognized allergenic fungi, are Zygomycota, Ascomycota, Basidiomycota, Oomycota, and the form genera known as Deuteromycetes, which are members of the fungal kingdom.

Zygomycota

The most important class in this phylum are the Zygomycetes. Species of genera within the order Mucorales, such as *Mucor, Rhizopus*, and *Absidia*, have been implicated as allergenic. Members of this class include common bread and sugar molds and have thick-walled (although seldom seen) zygospores that form after the meeting of two specialized hyphal branches. Characteristics of Zygomycetes are broad hyphae (up to $10 \mu m$), often with few or absent septae (i.e., 'coenocytic'), and sporangia, typically stalked and containing numerous sporangiospores (rarely only one). These spores generally are unicellular, $4–8 \mu m$, and bear no evident landmarks on their smooth, spiny, or reticulated surfaces. Species of *Rhizopus, Mucor*, and *Absidia* are especially prominent in composting plant litter, soil, and food residues.

Ascomycota

Ascomycota is the largest phylum of fungi and composes almost 50% of all known fungal species. Characteristic of this phylum is the *ascus*, a saclike cell in which sexual spores *(ascospores)* develop without wall attachments. In typical species, each ascus forms eight spores that are actively expelled at maturity; however, both spore number and mode of dispersion may vary. Asci form 'naked' or more often in specialized fruiting bodies *(ascocarps)*. These structures may appear as minute dots on stem and leaf surfaces but reach appreciable size, as found in truffles, morels, and many 'cup fungi'. Many ascospores have well-recognized imperfect (asexual) stages.

Five classes of Ascomycota are recognized: basal Ascomycetes, unitunicate Pyrenomycetes, bitunicate Pyrenomycetes, Plectomycetes, and budding yeasts. In the unitunicate Pyrenomycetes, four orders have recognized allergenic fungi. In the order Microscales, the species *Pseudoallescheria boydii* has been identified as allergenic and has the anamorph (asexual stage) *Graphium aumorphium*. In the order Sordariles, *Chaetomium globosum* is recognized as an allergen. As previously mentioned, *Neurospora sitophila* has the anamorph *Monilia sitophila*. In the order Hypocreales, several genera have well-recognized allergenic anamorphs, including *Gibberella* with the *Fusarium* anamorphs and *Hypocrea* with the anamorph *Trichoderma*.

The class Pyrenomycetes has several families with species implicated as allergens, including the family Mycosphaerellaceae and the genus *Mycosphaerella*, which contains the anamorphs of several form species of *Cladosporium*. The family Dothideaceae contains the asexual stage of *Aureobasidium pullulans*. The family Pleosporaceae contains a number of well-recognized imperfect stages, including *Drechslera (Bipolaris), Stemphylium, Curvularia, Alternaria*, and *Ulocladium*.

The class Plectomycetes contains orders that also have recognized allergenic potential. The imperfect forms such as *Penicillium* are in this group. In the order Eurotiales, *Neuosartorya* genera contain the anamorph *Aspergillus fumigatus*, and as mentioned previously, *Eurotium* genera are telomorphs (sexual stages) of *Aspergillus glaucus*. *Thermoascus* has recognizable anamorphs in *Paecilomyces*. In the order Onygenales, *Arthroderma* genera include the anamorph *Trichophyton rubrum*, as well as the anamorphs *Nannizzla* and *Microsporum*.

In the class of budding yeasts and the order Saccharomycetales, the genus *Saccharomyces* has anamorphs, including *Candida* species.

Basidiomycota

The subphylum Basidiomycota comprises almost 23 000 fungal species divided into three classes, two of which have relevance to allergy. The class Basidiomycetes (Holobasidiomycetes) contains the order Agaricales. The genus *Coprinus* produces well-recognized allergens within this

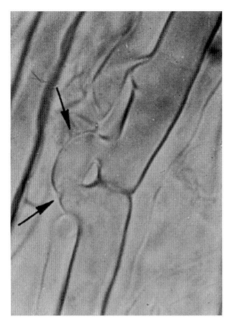

Fig. 32.27. Clamp connection between two adjacent hyphal segments, a prominent microscopic feature of many basidiomycetes.

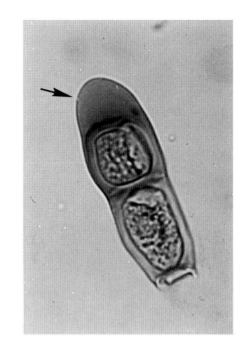

Fig. 32.28. Typical large, dark-brown, septate teliospore of rust (*Puccinia* species) 45 μm in length; arrow points to minute germinal pore.

group, and additional types are strongly suspected. The order Tremellales contains form genera, such as *Malassezia furfur* and 'jelly fungi' on natural substrates.

The class Teliomycetes contains the orders Ustilaginales (smuts) and Uredinales (rusts). Species of *Rhodosporidium* have anamorphs in the form of *Rhodotorula*, and the genus *Sporidiobolus* contains *Sporobolomyces* form species.

The Basidiomycetes includes diverse forms such as puffballs, mushrooms, rust, and smuts. These organisms grow poorly as teleomorphs on laboratory medium, and of those producing mycelium, an even smaller number produce identifiable sexual spores. Basidiomycetes often present arcuate structures (clamp connections) peripheral to the septa, joining attached hyphosegments (Fig. 32.27). Basidiospores typically develop in groups of four on specialized tissues called *basidia*, from which spores are often actively discharged. Most basidiospores show a short, eccentric projection *(apiculus)* marking a prior point of attachment to the basidium (Figs 32.28–32.30).

Deuteromycetes *(Fungi Imperfecti)*

All the fungi that do not have any known connection with any ascomycetous or basidiomycetous taxa are included in the broad artificial group of Deuteromycetes. At present, Deuteromycetes is the second largest group of fungi after the Ascomycota. Because the relationship between the sexual and asexual stages allows for more precise classification, generally a single name will be given to the organism. However, because of historical use, the original designation of many organisms will undoubtedly persist. These organisms produce only sterile mycelium or mycelia with conidia. Four form orders are usually distinguished.

Moniliales

Conidia are present and are not associated with the *pycnidia* or *acervuli* that distinguish Sphaeropsidales and Melaconiales. By far, Moniliales is the largest and most important group of Deuteromycetes and contains most of the recognized and suspected allergenic fungi.

Sphaeropsidales

These organisms have conidia that form on short hyphae within globular or flask-shaped organs *(pycnidia)* and extrude in a mucinous mass through an orifice or ostiole. The *pycnidia* often superficially resemble the fruiting bodies of ascomycetes. In the form order Sphaeropsidales, *Phoma* form species are recognized as allergen sources. In some species an *Alternaria* life stage also occurs.

Melaconiales

Conidia are borne on cushion-like masses of erect hyphae *(acervuli)* that burst through the substrate or host tissues. Although important as plant pathogens, Melaconiales genera have not been definitely implicated as allergens.

Mycelia sterilia

This form order encompasses a few fungi that appear to lack any type of spore, and some may be infertile forms of higher fungi, but these exact relationships are unknown. Many additional organisms fail to sporulate on various culture media despite significant hyphal growth. Many of these isolates are derived from ascospores and basidiospores. Sterile

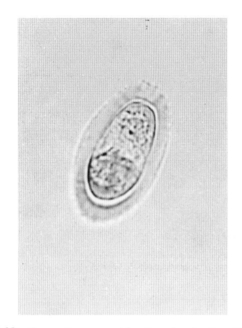

Fig. 32.29. Rust ureidospore; particles often minutely spiny with yellow or orange granules (28–40 μm).

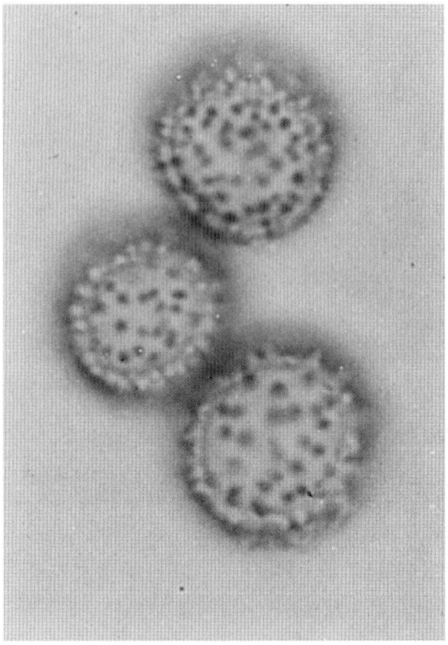

Fig. 32.30. Brown, spiny spores of corn smut *(Ustilago maydis)* 9–13 μm in diameter.

growth should be termed *Mycelia sterilia* only when their specific genera, such as *Pythium* and *Rizoctonia*, are indicated.

Oomycota

Members of this phylum are rarely reported as allergens. Because of fundamental differences between these fungi and those of the Ascomycota, Basidiomycota, and Zygomycota, Oomycota organisms have been assigned to the kingdom Chromista. The downy mildews (family Peronosporaceae) have been reported to be allergenic. Where local infection of grass or crops (e.g., grapes, onions) occurs, the spores may appear abundantly during dry, breezy weather.

GROWTH CONDITIONS

Fungi have developed remarkable diversity in form and metabolic requirements (Table 32.7).[72] Fungi require elemental oxygen during growth. Traces of carbohydrate are also essential, although many, especially Deuteromycetes, need only inorganic nitrogen sources. Most fungi grow best between 18 and 32°C, and although most become dormant at subfreezing temperatures, a few may even sporulate below 0°C. Many species are able to survive prolonged storage at –45° to –56°C or lower. At the other extreme, 71°C is generally lethal, although certain types thrive just below this point. Thermophilic forms will not grow below 45°C. Thermotolerant organisms flourish over a broad (including quite warm) range and include *Aspergillus fumigatus*, *A. niger*, and *Paecilomyces varioti*. Moisture is critical to fungal growth, although many terrestrial types can survive prolonged drying. When substrate moisture is limited, relative humidity above 65% is essential. Even with dryer air, however, fungi may find free

---

*A preference for this temperature range distinguishes mesophilic organisms.

water in deep shade, on moist soil, on leaf surfaces, and in cool areas of condensation.

Atmospheric moisture affects not only the growth of fungi but also spore dispersal and resulting prevalence. Many ascospores and basidiospores, collectively termed 'ballistospores', are shot from their points of origin by processes that require free water.[73] High ballistospore levels occur with rainfall, fog, and typically damp nighttime conditions. Rain and dew splash also foster dispersal of 'slime' spores, exposed in mucoid masses. As a consequence, atmospheric recoveries of *Fusarium*, *Phoma*, *Cephalosporium*, and *Trichoderma* form species peak with precipitation. In addition, the tapping of rain drops on puffballs effectively releases spores by a miniature bellows effect.[73] In typical wet-weather, air spora, ascospores and basidiospores predominate (Fig. 32.31). In contrast, reproductive units of many fungi are detached by wind or wind-induced substrate motion. Such dry-weather spore dispersal increases as the air speed increases and relative humidity falls, often peaking during the sunny afternoon periods. At such times, typical spores of *Cladosporium*, *Alternaria*, *Epicoccum*, and *Helminthosporium* form species rise dramatically, as do those of rusts, smuts, and other fungi (Fig. 32.32). Dry spore dispersal is also seen in *Rhizopus* species and form species of *Aspergillus* and *Penicillium*, although the resulting peaks are much lower. A subset of 'xerophytic' Deuteromycetes are not deterred by relatively dry conditions. Once air-borne, spores are cleared from the atmosphere by the same processes that affect pollen, such as rain and gravitational fallout.

Circadian rhythms, temperature, humidity, and air speed frequently interact to promote a diurnal air spora, primarily dark-spored Deuteromycetes, rusts, and smuts (a nocturnal pattern is predominantly ballistospores). Light intensity and duration also affect the production of spores; in certain *Cladosporium* form species, for example, a dark interval is required for spore crop formation in each 24-h period.[74] Naturally occurring ultraviolet (UV) radiation often promotes spore formation but can

Table 32.7 Prevalence and habitat of common allergenic fungi (Reproduced from Esch RE. Selection of allergen products for skin testing. Immunology and Allergy Clinics of North America 2001; 21:251).

Fungus	Prevalence/habitat
Alternaria alternata (Alternaria tenuis)	Cosmopolitan; isolated from variety of plants and from soil
Aspergillus amstelodami (Aspergillus glaucus)	Cosmopolitan; isolated primarily from soil, plants, and house dust
Aspergillus flavus	Cosmopolitan; isolated mainly from plants and soil; found on peanuts
Aspergillus fumigatus	Ubiquitous; peaks during high humidity and warm weather; often found in humidifiers, dehumidifiers, basements, attics, plants, and food
Aspergillus niger	Ubiquitous; common 'black bread mold'; isolated from soil and decomposing plant material
Aureobasidium pullulans (Pullularia pullulans)	Cosmopolitan; found in bark of sequoia trees and on plant leaves
Bipolaris sorokiniana (Helminthosporium sativum)	Cosmopolitan; isolated from soil and plants; found more in tropical/subtropical areas
Botrytis cinerea	Cosmopolitan; often found in regions of high humidity; can be found indoors on decaying fruits and vegetable matter
Candida albicans	Common; normal flora on mucous membranes of warm-blooded animals
Chaetomium globosum	Common; isolated from soil and decomposing plant materials, especially straw and mulch, and from herbivore dung
Cladosporium cladosporoides	Ubiquitous; found frequently in air, soil, and plant debris
Cladosporium herbarum	Ubiquitous; found frequently in air, soil, and plant debris
Cladosporium sphaerospermum (Hormodendrum hordei)	Ubiquitous; found frequently in air, soil, and plant debris
Drechslera spicifera (Curvularia spicifera)	Cosmopolitan; isolated from soil and plants; found more in tropical/subtropical areas
Epicoccum nigrum	Cosmopolitan; isolated from soil and plants
Fusarium moniliforme	Cosmopolitan; isolated from soil and plants
Mucor spp	Cosmopolitan; isolated from soil and decaying organic material
Penicillium chrysogenum	Ubiquitous; found on food products; spores often air-borne
Penicillium digitatum	Cosmopolitan; found on citrus fruits
Phoma betae	Common; parasitizes sugar beets
Puccinia graminis	Common; rusts; produces rust-colored spores on leaves and stems of primary host (oats, wheat)
Rhizopus stolonifer (Rhizopus nigricans)	Ubiquitous; causes spoilage of refrigerated foods; found on cereal grains
Saccharomyces cerevisiae	Common; common bread yeast (baker/brewer's yeast)
Stemphylium solani	Common; plant pathogen; causes leaf spot on tomatoes
Trichophyton mentagrophytes (Trichophyton interdigitale)	Common; causes athlete's foot and inflammatory skin lesions
Ustilago spp	Common; smuts spp: *cynodontis* (Bermuda grass), *maydis* (corn), *avenae* (oat), *tritici* (wheat)

From Esch.[72]

also impair spore viability and independently affects recoveries of fungi in culture-based recovery techniques. Regional vegetation strongly affects the local air spora. In the grasslands and grain-growing areas, *Alternaria, Cladosporium, Helminthosporium-Drechslera*, and *Epicoccum* spores predominate. High local levels of rust and smut spores can result from heavily infected crops. In forests, dark Deuteromycetes, rust, and smuts are fewer, but wood-rotting basidiomycetes (e.g., *Ganoderma* species) often predominate. Similarly, orchards can raise autumn levels of air-borne yeast cells.

Total air-borne fungi in North America range from extremely low levels during snow cover to peak levels usually in late summer and early autumn. This pattern reflects the variations in the dominant *Cladosporium* and *Alternaria* form species in many areas; however, other taxa can show distinctive trends. Near the Great Lakes, certain ascospores appear during favorable periods in the early spring and disappear by midsummer; others persist, with basidiospores of *Coprinus* species occurring throughout the growing season. Ballistospores of many mushrooms as well as

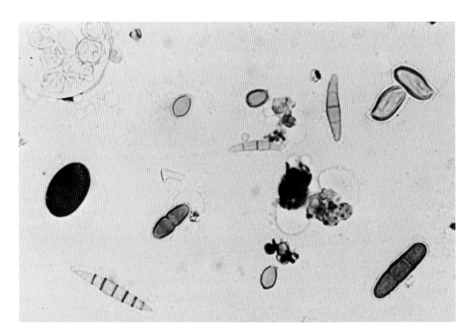

Fig. 32.31. Montage showing typical wet-weather air spora dominated by ascospores and basidiospores of many types.

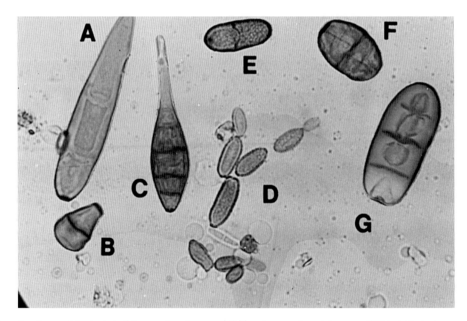

Fig. 32.32. Montage showing particles typical of dry-weather air spora. (A) Tapering pseudoseptate spore of *Helminthosporium* species. (B) Spore of parasitic species, *Polythrincium trifolii*. (C) Beaked, brown dictospore of *Alternaria* species. (D) Spore cluster of *Cladosporium cladosporioides*. (E) Single conidium of *Cladosporium herbarum*. (F) Brown dictyospore of *Stemphylium botryosum*. (G) Pseudoseptate spore of *Drechslera* species. In addition, at least one hyaline ascospore and (below) several ash spheres (fused silica) are present.

those of yeasts, such as *Sporobolomyces* species, favor autumn months. In many areas, levels of *Penicillium* form species lack a defined annual pattern; *Aspergillus* species may be more prominent from December to April or may be quite unpredictable. Because a 'mold season' does not occur even in eastern North America, it is difficult to identify fungal sensitivity in individual patients. However, symptoms that last throughout the warm months peaking in midsummer and persisting well after a killing frost may suggest fungal sensitization. Many fungus-sensitive patients report no relief of symptoms between local grass and ragweed pollen seasons.

The recognition of situations where heavy fungus exposures occur can provide diagnostic clues and help the physician recommend practical avoidance strategies. Physical activity can promote liberation of spores. For example, walking in old fields causes spore levels of deuteromycetes and smut fungi to increase 10–20-fold.[75] More vigorous disturbances of natural materials can induce even more striking effects. Field cutting, threshing, and baling operations by farmers often create spore clouds that are visible to the naked eye. Similar risks occur with silage operations and composting as well as the use of straw and leaf for mulches. Lawn cutting and leaf raking often will provoke symptoms in fungus-sensitive subjects, although other aeroallergens may contribute as well.

Fungi readily colonize indoor surfaces and may contribute to perennial allergic symptoms (see Chapter 33). Many fungi recovered indoors enter from the outdoor environment. However, certain species are thought to arise from indoor sources, particularly if their levels are higher than outdoor levels. These species are often dominated by small-spored Deuteromycetes, especially *Penicillium* and *Aspergillus* form species plus yeast, and rarely *Rhizopus* and *Mucor* species. Food storage areas, soiled upholstery, and garbage containers are frequent sites of fungal growth in the indoor environment. Flooded basement carpeting is also a major source. Other organic substrates can be colonized, and cellulose–splitting organisms can attack a variety of substances. Rubber and synthetic foams retain moisture and promote colonization. Other surfaces, although providing marginal nutrition, can allow for growth if there is sufficient moisture. Basement and 'outside' walls, windowsills, shower curtains, and plumbing fixtures are common sites. Poorly maintained cool-mist vaporizers can emit dense aerosols during operation.

ASSESSMENT OF FUNGAL EXPOSURE

Exposure to fungi, and presumably to fungal allergens, has traditionally been assessed by microscopically identifying and quantitating the number of fungal spores in air samples or by using semiquantitative cultures obtained from air or settled dust samples. The total spore counts for individual genera that can be identified microscopically are typically collected by volumetric samplers (e.g., Rotorod, Sampling Technologies; Burkard Sampler, Burkard Manufacturing; Sampler MK-3, Allergenco). Generally, suction samplers such as the Burkard are more efficient over a broader range of particle sizes (particularly for small fungal spores) than impaction samplers such as the Rotorod. Volumetric samplers can be used to conduct repeated samples at various intervals because they can be programmed to obtain samples over a specific period. Typically, suction samplers collect air-borne spores by directing air at an adhesive-coated surface where particles impact and are captured. Air can also be drawn through membranes or into small fluid volumes for subsequent analysis or onto culture media for determinations of viable colony-forming units (CFUs). The latter approach often favors the single-stage Andersen sampler, which collects viable CFUs on a single plate, but multistage samplers can also be used to separate spores by size for particular investigations.

For microscopic identification, unstained specimens are usually mounted in an aqueous medium such as hard glycerine jelly. Stains, such as phenosafranin or cotton blue, serve special purposes. Unfortunately, no authenticated spore samples are readily available, and no single manual for identification exists. However, illustrations in several references are helpful.[76–79]

Some fungal spore types can easily be identified by their appearance; other spores, however, such as those of *Penicillium* and *Aspergillus* species, are not distinctive, making analysis by cultural growth essential. Culture sampling techniques complement direct particle counts. For these minute particles, efficient volumetric collectors are especially needed. For general purposes of culturing fungi, several agar media may suffice, including Sabouraud's dextrose, potato dextrose, and malt extract. However, certain organisms, such as *Stachybotrys* species, grow slowly or not at all on common substrates. Other fungal types, such as *Wallemia*, require selected media (e.g., DG18). Additional agar substrates (e.g., tap water, cornmeal, V-8 juice) have been valuable for inducing sporulation, and some initially sterile colonies may be stimulated to sporulate by the use of near-UV irradiation. Colonies can often be identifiable to the genus level by gross appearance, although many require scanning or high-power microscopy. The fine structural details are best observed in slide cultures, unmounted or prepared in lactophenol (popular mounting medium made by combining 10 g phenol, 10 g lactic acid syrup, 20 g glycerol, and 10 g distilled water; adding 50 mg cotton blue to each 100 ml of medium allows staining of many fungal structures). Reference to some basic mycologic techniques may be helpful.[67,80–82]

The most direct way to assess the level of fungal allergen exposure is by direct measurement of allergen concentrations in air-borne or settled dust samples. However, the technology as applied to fungi is not as highly developed as the widely used approaches for house-dust mite, cockroach, or cat allergens.

Several fungal allergens have been purified and molecularly cloned (see Chapter 35). The purification of fungal allergens is important for the development of immunoassays to quantitate fungal allergen exposure. Direct immunostaining using human IgE antibodies or double-immunostaining using human IgE antibodies in combination with allergen-specific rabbit antibodies can be used to detect aerosolized fungal conidia, hyphae, and fragments.[83,84] Other approaches employ dual monoclonal antibody-based immunoassays that rely on binding of two different sites of the molecule under study. Such assays have been reported for the measurement of the major *Alternaria alternata* allergen (Alt a 1) and the major *Aspergillus fumigatus* allergen (Asp f 1).[85–88] Because of limitations in the measurement of allergens by these techniques, including the requirement for active growth of an organism for allergen secretion into the medium, a combination of assays may be necessary to assess fungal allergen exposure adequately.

In addition to morphologic techniques, a variety of biochemical and immunochemical markers of fungal presence have been developed. Such indicators include assays of ergosterol, extracellular polysaccharides (EPSs), 1→3-β-glucan, volatile organic compounds (VOCs), phylogenetic markers, and fungal mycotoxins. Although these markers do not measure specific allergen exposure, they can accurately indicate the presence of fungal growth. Their use in quantitating fungal exposure and its relationship to human allergic disease is still largely investigational. Ergosterol is a primary cell membrane sterol of most fungi, useful as a marker for total fungal biomass. The quantity produced by a particular fungus isolate depends on the surface area and growth conditions. Levels of ergosterol correlate well with total spore counts[89] but are not helpful indicators of individual taxa.[90]

Extracellular polysaccharides are carbohydrates that are secreted or shed during fungal growth. They have antigenic specificity, usually at the (form) genus level. EPSs may serve as a marker for fungal exposure[91] but seem to play no direct pathogenic role in fungal-related disease.

The $1\rightarrow3$-β-glucans are glucose polymers found in filamentous fungal cell walls and in other sources, including yeast, some bacteria, and many plants. The polymer can be used as a marker of total fungal biomass[92] in samples eluted from membrane filters by using the Limulus amebocyte lysate assay with factor G. Again, a role in the pathogenesis of fungal-related illnesses is suggested but not clearly established.

Volatile organic compounds are produced by a number of fungi and generally include simple organic metabolites such as alcohols, aldehydes, ketones, and carbonyl sulfite-like compounds.[93] VOCs are often noticeable in fungus-contaminated environments as the 'moldy', 'earthy', or 'musty' smells. VOCs have diverse fungal sources, although some may be more specific for individual taxa and can serve as a marker for their presence.[94] Generally, the presence of VOCs indicates buildings with air quality problems. Although VOCs serve as markers for fungi, many of these compounds may have other sources.

Molecular analysis of phylogenetic markers have been applied to the detection of specific fungal taxa. A variety of DNA probes can be designed for PCR assays. Universal primers based on the 18 S rRNA gene sequences of fungi were used to develop a fungus-specific PCR assay,[95] while species-specific PCR primers were used to detect *Penicillium roquefortii* in environmental samples.[96]

Mycotoxins are biologically active, heat-stable, low-molecular-weight compounds produced during fungal growth. Although mycotoxins are not directly related to allergic disease, as allergens they have been implicated in carcinogenesis, neurotoxicity, and teratogenesis.[97] More often, mycotoxin levels are measured once fungi have been identified through cultural or microscopic techniques. Mycotoxins may be produced by *Aspergillus* and *Penicillium* species, which are common contaminants of indoor environments.[98] However, their role in the exposed individual's overall health is not clear. Most cases of air-borne mycotoxin exposure causing disease are described in farm workers exposed to moldy materials.

COMMON AIRBORNE FUNGI

The allergenic importance of many common fungi remains difficult to assess because of the many different fungal spores that may occur in air samples, all of which may have the potential to cause allergic disease. The importance of fungal allergy is often based on skin test reactivity to extracts of common fungi. At present, however, these extract preparations are not standardized. The extracts, often prepared from submerged growth, can elicit IgE-mediated skin test responses, but it is uncertain whether the materials are also widely encountered in the spores that appear to dominate air samples. Molecular cloning techniques have allowed the identification of a number of important fungal allergens, and further investigation may lead to better diagnostic materials.

Alternaria

Spores of *Alternaria* species are predominant in temperate, particularly grain-growing, regions. Typically, levels of 500–1000 spores/m^3 of air occur on dry days in the late summer and fall; *A. alternata* and *A. tenuissima* are especially common. Extracts of these fungi frequently produce skin test reactivity in fungus-allergic individuals, and symptoms have been provoked experimentally with fungal spores.[65] Spores are variable in form but typically have a beaked appearance (Fig. 32.33). Species of *Stemphylium* and *Pithomyces* produce similar-appearing dark dictyospores and must be distinguished from one another. Other Deuteromycetes

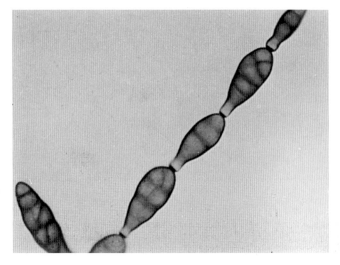

Fig. 32.33. Chain of beaked dictyospores typical of *Alternaria alternata*.

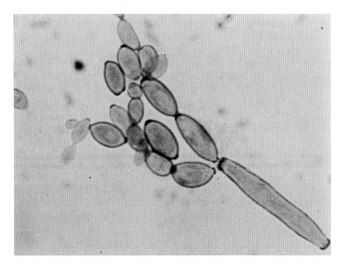

Fig. 32.34. Spore cluster of *Cladosporium* species recovered intact in Hirst trap collection; note strongly refractile points of attachment.

(e.g., *Ulocladium*) must also be distinguished, as well as certain multiseptate ascospores. The *Stemphylium* spores do not have the beaklike elongated chains of *Alternaria* spores and are borne singly with a constricting, central transverse septum. Several allergens have been isolated from *Alternaria* (see Chapter 35).

Cladosporium

Spores from this form genus usually outnumber all other outdoor bioaerosols, and their sources are prominent saprophytes and parasites of various crops. Two form species, *Cladosporium herbarum* and *C. cladosporoides*, are widespread in temperate North America and often attain daily mean levels of 5000 or more spores/m^3 (Fig. 32.34). Additional types,

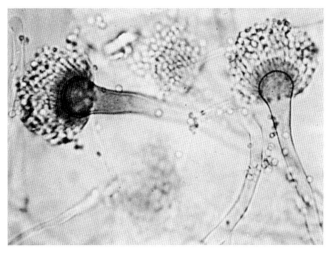

Fig. 32.35. Culture mount of *Aspergillus fumigatus* showing characteristic bulbous enlargement of terminal conidiophore into 'vesicle'. Spores in this form species arise from sterigmata that develop on distal half of vesicle.

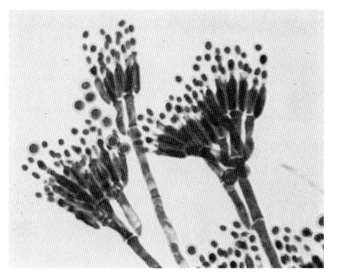

Fig. 32.36. Stained culture mount of a *Penicillium* form species. Conidiophore shows branches (metulae), each bearing one or more spore-producing structures termed sterigmata or phialides. In some penicillia, phialides arise directly from the terminal conidiophore.

including *C. macrocarpum* and *C. sphaerospermum*, are less abundant. Several *Cladosporium* allergens have been purified (see Chapter 35).

Aspergillus

Aspergillus form species are widely prevalent spoilage organisms. Sensitivity to these species not only causes allergic rhinitis and asthma, but is also associated with allergic fungal sinusitis and bronchopulmonary mycoses, particularly with *A. fumigatus* (Fig. 32.35). At least 18 allergens of *A. fumigatus* have now been identified (see Chapter 35). Secreted proteins appear to play a role in allergic asthma, whereas non-secreted internal allergens may be important in the development of allergic bronchopulmonary aspergillosis (ABPA).

On selected media, aspergilli form typical conidial heads. In general, distinguishing isolated conidia aspergilli from those of other taxa (e.g., *Penicillium, Rhizopus*) that produce similar spores cannot be done with confidence.

Recovery of *Aspergillus* colonies from interior environments may exceed that from the outdoor air. Thus, these organisms are often considered to be indoor allergen exposures, although outdoor exposure occurs as well. In addition to spoilage organisms, *A. oryzae* is used to produce soy sauce and commercial enzymes. Specific allergens from this species have been identified.[99]

Penicillium

Penicillium form species have a broad distribution, are often found indoors, and have commercial uses, such as the production of cheeses. As with *Aspergillus, Penicillium* species vary but can be found regionally or in specific interiors. Individual penicillia are highly variable, making identification of strains tedious although feasible[100] (Fig. 32.36). At least 20 different allergens have been isolated from various *Penicillium* species[99] (see Chapter 35). An alkaline serine proteinase has been isolated from *P. citrinum* that is cross-reactive with similar allergens from *Aspergillus*

species.[101] It is noteworthy that mutant forms of *P. chrysogenum*, rather than *P. notatum*, are the common commercial source of penicillin substrate.

Helminthosporium

Dark, tapering spores with predominant septi or pseudosepti that are often 50–100 µm in length are typical of *Helminthosporium* species (Fig. 32.32A). Emanations of *Drechslera* and *Bipolaris* are strongly similar. Levels of *Helminthosporium*-like spores generally are lower than for *Alternaria*, although skin test reactivities may be similar in Midwestern populations. Spores of *Drechslera spicifera* (formerly *Curvularia*) have three to five septa and are strongly curved with one enlarged central cell. These species are found more often in warmer regions, including the southern USA, and with aspergilli are prominent agents of allergic fungal sinusitis.

Epicoccum

Epicoccum nigrum is widespread, especially in grassland and agricultural areas, and levels can reach 100–200 spores/m^3 or higher during dry fall periods in the Midwest. *E. nigrum* forms a distinctive orange or rust-colored pigment on culture, and many strains require near-UV light for sporulation. The conidia are brown and multiseptate and covered with verrucae after *E. purpurascens* spore production (Fig. 32.37).

Fusarium

Fusarium is an important spoilage organism and plant pathogen. *Fusarium* often secretes soluble pigments and forms large, sickle-shaped septate spores with pointed ends *(macroconidia)* (Fig. 32.38). Occasionally, spores may be small and oval or comma shaped. Several forms of

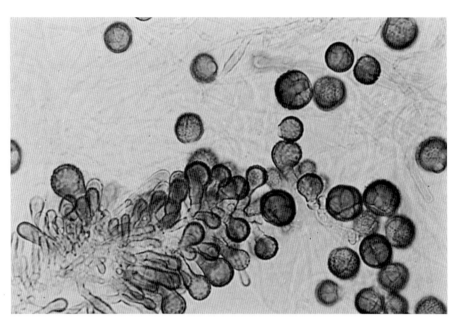

Fig. 32.37. Culture mount of *Epicoccum purpurascens* showing spore production by cluster of upright hyphae (sporodochium) at lower left. Mature multiseptate, brown, warty spores generally measure 18–26 μm in diameter.

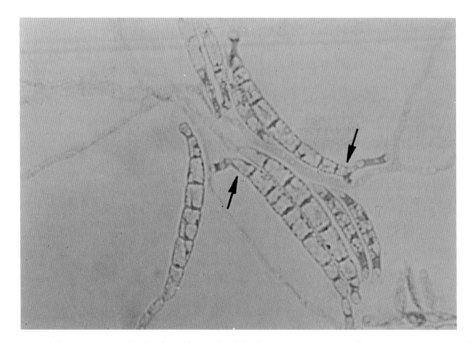

Fig. 32.38. Culture mount of *Fusarium* species showing long (about 40 μm) fusiform macrospores, as well as several microspores at lower right. Basal cells (arrow) will be evident on most *Fusarium* macroconidia if they are scrutinized carefully.

Fusarium are known to have ascomycete sexual stages (e.g., *Gibberella, Nectria*). Extracts from *F. vasoinfectium* frequently cause skin test reactivity, but other taxa lack test materials.

Aureobasidium

This taxon is represented by *Aureobasidium pullulans* (formerly *Pullularia pullulans*). This organism colonizes paper, lumber, and painted surfaces. Although widely prevalent, air-borne levels are less than for *Cladosporium* species. In culture, colonies change from creamy, mucoid form to black, leathery disks with radial striations (Fig. 32.39). About 8–12% of atopic patients in the Midwest show skin test reactivity to *A. pullulans*.

Phoma

Phoma organisms produce dark, flask-shaped pycnidia and are prominent during wet periods. Recovery levels of *Phoma* species in the air rarely exceed 20 spores/m^3, but sharing of allergens with *Alternaria* form species is suggested.

Ascomycetes

Ascospore concentrations reach thousands of particles/m^3 in temperate and tropical areas, especially with high humidity. Many species remain unidentified. Human sensitivity to a few obtainable spore types has been demonstrated, especially in Great Britain.[54,102] In central North America, *Leptosphaeria* species are especially prominent. Common types include *Nectria* and others that remain unidentified. These organisms, which are the sexual stages of many Deuteromycetes, have not been examined for allergenic cross-reactivity.

Basidiomycetes

Rusts and smuts are parasitic Basidiomycetes that affect many crops, including cereal grains. In urban environments, rust levels rarely exceed 100 spores/m^3, but much higher concentrations occur in agricultural areas (Fig. 32.29). Smut spores, by contrast, are abundant, particularly in areas of extensive agriculture. Many recoveries suggest the genus *Ustilago* (Fig. 32.30). Skin test reactivity rates are relatively low, <10% of atopic subjects. Spores of mushrooms (fungi, puffballs) contribute to the air spora during the night and wet weather. The peak concentrations and diversity of air-borne basidiospores occur during the late summer and fall. Spores of *Coprinus* are predominant throughout the growing season. *Ganoderma* species are abundant throughout the summer months in the Great Lakes states and elsewhere. Skin test reactivity has been demonstrated to *Agaricus, Calvatia, Pleurotus,* and *Psilocybe* species.[53] Commercial extracts for skin testing, however, are not available.

Zygomycetes

Species of *Rhizopus, Mucor,* and *Absidia* are extremely common on decaying leaves and other substrates, where their white-gray spreading growth often occurs. Usually, spores of these groups are not prominent in free air but can be found in abundance in damp indoor areas, particularly where there is seepage of soil water and around composting vegetation. Skin test reactivity to *Rhizopus stolonifer* and *Mucor racemosus* has been demonstrated.[72]

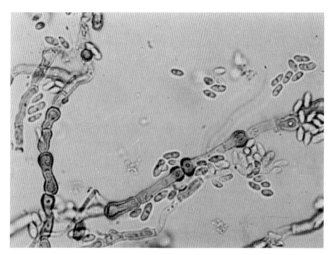

Fig. 32.39. *Aureobasidium pullulans* showing dark, septate chlamydospores and abundant hyaline blastospores.

Yeasts

Yeast fungi share a unicellular growth form that can lead to mucoid bacteria-like colonies on culture media. The group is heterogenous; some types, such as *Saccharomyces cerevisiae* (brewer/baker's yeast), form ascospores, whereas others, such as *Rhodotorula*, show only budding and rarely fission. An additional group of genera, including *Sporobolomyces*, form bean-shaped spores on short projections and are discharged forcefully similar to basidiospores. Many yeast cells are dispersed by rain and are prominent in nighttime and wet-weather collections. In the central USA, the atmospheric levels peak during rainy fall seasons, especially where food crops are grown.

Yeasts can tolerate acidic and hypertonic conditions and therefore may be found in fluid reservoirs of humidifiers and cold-mist vaporizers.

The role of *Candida albicans* as an aeroallergen is controversial, although IgE skin test reactivity is well documented. Besides being cultured from humans, *C. albicans* is rarely found in air samples, although other *Candida* species are recovered in small numbers. *Monilia sitophila* is especially common in tropical localities, but elsewhere only occurs in bakeries and flour mills.

OTHER FUNGAL SPECIES

Additional imperfect fungi are frequently recovered in culture-based surveys, and specific locations may be of particular interest. Genera include *Trichoderma, Wallemia,* and *Botrytis*.

◼ OTHER PLANT AND MICROBIAL PARTICLES AS ALLERGEN SOURCES ◼

Sensitivity to algae has been implicated in respiratory symptoms among lake swimmers. In addition, algae may also act as possible inhalant allergens. Using this approach, large numbers of green and blue-green algae have been recovered from the air, particularly where soil is disturbed. Green algae, including *Chlorella* and *Chlorococcum* species, have been found in house-dust samples. Skin test reactivity to green algae has been demonstrated, with symptoms provoked in sensitive individuals by nasal challenge.[103] Because of the toxic components in these extracts, however, further studies have not been done.

Actinomycetes (especially thermophilic species) are known causes of hypersensitivity pneumonitis (see Chapter 54). Allergic rhinitis and asthma have not been demonstrated despite heavy occupational exposure. Home humidifiers and commercial ventilating systems that contain thermophilic actinomycetes have led to outbreaks of allergic alveolitis (HP), and other sources (e.g., silage, dry sugar cane) are widely recognized.

Acknowledgement

We acknowledge the assistance of William R Solomon, MD, in the preparation of this chapter, and CJ Hartsell of Greer Laboratories for preparing the pollen photographs.

References

Aeroallergens and sources

1. Gregory PH. Microbiology of the atmosphere. 2nd edn. New York: Wiley; 1973.

Factors influencing clinical significance of aeroallergens

2. Faegri K, van der Pijl L. The principles of pollination ecology. Oxford: Pergamon; 1979.
3. Agarwal MK, Swanson MC, Reed CE, et al. Air-borne ragweed allergens: association with various particle sizes and short ragweed plant parts. J Allergy Clin Immunol 1984; 74:687.
4. Schumacher MJ, Griffith RD, O'Rourke MK. Recognition of pollen and other particulate aeroantigens by immunoblot microscopy. J Allergy Clin Immunol 1988; 82:608.
5. Suphioglu C. Thunderstorm asthma due to grass pollen. Int Arch Allergy Immunol 1998; 116:253.
6. Grote M, Vrtala S, Niederberger V, et al. Release of allergen-bearing cytoplasm from hydrated pollen: a mechanism common to a variety of grass (Poaceae) species revealed by electron microscopy. J Allergy Clin Immunol 2001; 108:109.
7. Baraniuk JN, Bolick M, Esch R, et al. Quantification of pollen solute release using pollen grain column chromatography. Allergy 1992; 47:411.
8. Mitakakis TZ, Barnes C, Tovey ER. Spore germination increases allergen release from Alternaria. J Allergy Clin Immunol 2001; 107:388.

Detection of aeroallergens

9. Lacey J, Venette J. Outdoor air sampling techniques. In: Cox CS, Wathes CM, eds. Bioaerosols handbook. Boca Raton: CRC Press; 1995:407.
10. Wilken-Jensen K, Gravesen S. Atlas of moulds in Europe causing respiratory allergy. Copenhagen: Foundation for Allergy Research in Europe; 1984.
11. Smith EG. Sampling and identifying allergenic pollens and molds: an illustrated identification manual for air samplers. San Antonio: Blewstone; 1990.
12. Colloff MJ, Spieksma FTM. Pictorial keys for the identification of domestic mites. Clin Exp Allergy 1992; 22:823.
13. Jensen J, Poulsen LK, Mygind K, et al. Immunochemical estimations of allergenic activities from outdoor aero-allergens, collected by a high-volume air sampler. Allergy 1989; 44:52.
14. Kimura JY, Matsuoka H, Ishii A. ELISA inhibition method in detection of mite and chironomid antigens in environmental samples of dust, soil and air. Allergy 1990; 45:167.
15. Andersen AA. New sampler for the collection, sizing, and enumeration of viable air-borne particles. J Bacteriol 1958; 76:471.
16. Durham OC. The volumetric incidence of atmospheric allergens. IV. A proposed standard method of gravity sampling, counting and volumetric interpolation of results. J Allergy 1944; 17:79.
17. Grinnell SW, Perkins WA, Vaughn LM. Sampling apparatus and method. Patent No 2,973,642. Washington, DC: US Patent Office; 1961.
18. Frenz DA. Comparing pollen and spore counts collected with the Rotorod sampler and Burkard spore trap. Ann Allergy Asthma Immunol 1999; 83:341.
19. Hirst JM. An automatic volumetric spore trap. Ann Appl Biol 1952; 39:257.
20. Portnoy J, Landuyt J, Pacheco F, et al. Comparison of the Burkard and Allergenco MK-3 volumetric collectors. Ann Allergy Asthma Immunol 2000; 84:19.

21. May KR. Multistage liquid impinger. Bacteriol Rev 1966; 30:559.
22. Muilenberg ML. Aeroallergen assessment by microscopy and culture. Immunol Allergy Clin North Am 1989; 9:245.
23. Kenny LC, Bowry A, Crook B, et al. Field testing of a personal size-selective bioaerosol sampler. Ann Occup Hyg 1999; 43:393.
24. Gordon S, Tee RD, Lowson D, et al. Reduction of air-borne allergenic urinary protein from laboratory rats. Br J Ind Med 1992; 49:416.
25. Swanson MC, Agarwal MK, Reed CE. An immunochemical approach to indoor aeroallergen quantitation with a new volumetric air sampler: studies with mite, roach, cat, mouse, and guinea pig antigens. J Allergy Clin Immunol 1985; 76:724.
26. Wynn SR, Swanson MC, Reed CE, et al. Immunochemical quantitation, size distribution, and cross-reactivity of Lepidoptera (moth) aeroallergens in southeastern Minnesota. J Allergy Clin Immunol 1988; 82:47.
27. Gautam M, Sreenath A. Performance of a respirable multi-inlet cyclone sampler. J Aerosol Sci 1997; 28:1265.
28. Wodehouse RP. Hayfever plants: their appearance, distribution, time of flowering, and their role in hayfever. 2nd edn. New York: Haefner; 1971.
29. Lewis WH, Vinay P, Zenger VE. Air-borne and allergenic pollen of North America. Baltimore: Johns Hopkins University Press; 1984.
30. Jelks M. Allergy plants. Tampa: World-Wide Publications; 1977.
31. Burge HA. Aerobiology of the indoor environment. Occup Med 1995; 10:27.
32. Rogers C, Muilenberg M. Comprehensive guidelines for the operation of Hirst-type suction bioaersol samplers. Standardized Protocol, Pan-American Aerobiology Association.
33. Steriling M, Rogers C, Levetin E. An evaluation of two methods used for microscopic analysis of air-borne fungal spore concentrations from the Burkard spore trap. Aerobiologia 1999; 15:9.
34. Burge HP, Solomon WR, Boise JR. Comparative merits of eight popular media in aerometric studies of fungi. J Allergy Clin Immunol 1977; 60:199.
35. Morring KL, Sorenson WG, Attfield MD. Sampling for air-borne fungi: a statistical comparison of media. Am Ind Hyg Assoc J 1983; 44:662.
36. Hocking AD, Pitt JI. Dichloran-glycerol medium for enumeration of xerophilic fungi from low moisture foods. Appl Environ Microbiol 1980; 39:488.
37. Verhoeff AP, van Wijnen JH, Boleij JS, et al. Enumeration and identification of air-borne viable mould propagules in houses: a field comparison of selected techniques. Allergy 1990; 45:275.
38. Rantio-Lehtimaki A, Viander M, Koivikko A. Air-borne birch pollen antigens in different particle sizes. Clin Exp Allergy 1994; 24:23.
39. Stewart GA, Holt PG. Submicronic air-borne allergens. Med J Aust 1985; 143:426.
40. Cruz MJ, Rodrigo MJ, Anto JM, et al. An amplified ELISA inhibition method for the measurement of air-borne soybean allergens. Int Arch Allergy Immunol 2000; 122:142.
41. Moreno-Grau S, Elvira-Rendueles B, Moreno J, et al. Correlation between Olea europeae and Parietaria judaica pollen counts and quantitative of their major allergens Ole e 1 and Par j 1-Par j 2. Ann Allergy Asthma Immunol 2006; 196:764.

Pollen aeroallergens

42. D'Amato G, Spieksma F, Liccardi G, et al. Pollen-related allergy in Europe. Allergy 1998; 53:567.
43. Roth A. Allergy in the world. Honolulu: University of Hawaii Press; 1978.

Fungi as aeroallergens

44. Nolles G, Hoekstra MO, Schouten JP, et al. Prevalence of immunoglobulin E for fungi in atopic children. Clin Exp Allergy 2001; 31:1564.
45. Gergen PJ, Turkeltaub PC, Kovar MG. The prevalence of allergic skin test reactivity to eight common aeroallergens in the U.S. population: results from the Second National Health and Nutrition Examination Survey. J Allergy Clin Immunol 1987; 80:669.
46. Lopez M, Salvaggio JE. Mould sensitive asthma. Clin Rev Allergy 1985; 3:183.
47. Gergen PJ, Turkeltaub PC. The association of individual allergen reactivity with respiratory disease in a national sample: data from the Second National Health and Nutrition Examination Survey, 1976–1980 (NHANES II). J Allergy Clin Immunol 1992; 90:579.
48. Peat JK, Tovey E, Mellis CM, et al. Importance of house dust mite and Alternaria allergies in childhood asthma: an epidemiological study in two climatic regions of Australia. Clin Exp Allergy 1993; 23:812.
49. Halonen M, Stern DA, Wright AL, et al. Alternaria as a major allergen for asthma in children raised in a desert environment. Am J Respir Crit Care Med 1997; 155:1356.
50. Henderson FW, Henry MM, Ivins SS, et al. Correlates of recurrent wheezing in school-age children. Physicians of Raleigh Pediatric Association. Am J Respir Crit Care Med 1995; 151:1786.
51. Perzanowski MS, Sporik R, Squillace SP, et al. Association of sensitization to Alternaria allergens with asthma among school-age children. J Allergy Clin Immunol 1998; 101:626.
52. Delfino RJ, Coate BD, Zeiger RS, et al. Daily asthma severity in relation to personal ozone exposure and outdoor fungal spores. Am J Respir Crit Care Med 1996; 154:633.
53. Horner WE, O'Neil CE, Lehrer SB. Basidiospore aeroallergens. Clin Rev Allergy 1992; 10:191.
54. Frankland AW, Gregory PH. Allergenic and agricultural implications of air-borne ascospore concentrations from a fungus, Didymella exitialis. Nature 1973; 245:336.
55. Salvaggio J, Seabury J, Schoenhardt FA, New Orleans asthma V. Relationship between Charity Hospital asthma admission rates, semiquantitative pollen and fungal spore counts, and total particulate aerometric sampling data. J Allergy Clin Immunol 1971; 48:96.
56. Rosas I, McCartney HA, Payne RW, et al. Analysis of the relationships between environmental factors (aeroallergens, air pollution, and weather) and asthma emergency admissions to a hospital in Mexico City. Allergy 1998; 53:394.

57. Nelson RP Jr, DiNicolo R, Fernandez-Caldas E, et al. Allergen-specific IgE levels and mite allergen exposure in children with acute asthma first seen in an emergency department and in non-asthmatic control subjects. J Allergy Clin Immunol 1996; 98:258.
58. Dales RE, Cakmak S, Burnett RT, et al. Influence of ambient fungal spores on emergency visits for asthma to a regional children's hospital. Am J Respir Crit Care Med 2000; 162: 2087.
59. Neukirch C, Henry C, Leynaert B, et al. Is sensitization to Alternaria alternata a risk factor for severe asthma? A population-based study. J Allergy Clin Immunol 1999; 103:709.
60. Downs SH, Mitakakis TZ, Marks GB, et al. Clinical importance of Alternaria exposure in children. Am J Respir Crit Care Med 2001; 164:455.
61. Halonen M, Stern DA, Lohman C, et al. Two subphenotypes of childhood asthma that differ in maternal and paternal influences on asthma risk. Am J Respir Crit Care Med 1999; 160:564.
62. O'Hollaren MT, Yunginger JW, Offord KP, et al. Exposure to an aeroallergen as a possible precipitating factor in respiratory arrest in young patients with asthma. N Engl J Med 1991; 324:359.
63. Targonski PV, Persky VW, Ramekrishnan V. Effect of environmental molds on risk of death from asthma during the pollen season. J Allergy Clin Immunol 1995; 95:955.
64. Black PN, Udy AA, Brodie SM. Sensitivity to fungal allergens is a risk factor for life-threatening asthma. Allergy 2000; 55:501.
65. Licorish K, Novey HS, Kozak P, et al. Role of Alternaria and Penicillium spores in the pathogenesis of asthma. J Allergy Clin Immunol 1985; 76:819.
66. Burnett JH. Fundamentals of mycology. 2nd edn. London: Arnold; 1976.
67. Baron GL. The genera of Hyphomycetes from soil. Baltimore: Williams & Wilkins; 1968.
68. Greuter W, Barrie FR, Burdet HM, et al. International Code of Botanical Nomenclature (Tokyo Code). Fifteenth International Botanical Congress, Yokohama; Regnum Veg 131. Königstein: Koeltz Scientific Books; 1994.
69. Guarro J, Gené J, Stchigel AM. Developments in fungal taxonomy. Clin Microbiol Rev 1999; 12:454.
70. Margulis L, Schwartz KV. Five kingdoms. San Francisco: Freeman; 1982.
71. Hawksworth DL, Kirk PM, Sutton BC, et al. Ainsworth and Bisby's dictionary of the fungi, 8th edn. Egham: International Mycological Institute; 1995.
72. Esch RE. Selection of allergen products for skin testing. Immunol Allergy Clin North Am 2001; 21:251.
73. Ingold CT. Fungal spores: their liberation and dispersal. Oxford: Clarendon; 1971.
74. Rich S, Waggoner PE. Atmospheric concentration of Cladosporium spores. Science 1962; 137:962.
75. McDonald JL, Solomon WR. Effects of outdoor activity on the aeroallergens in human microenvironment. J Allergy Clin Immunol 1975; 55:89.
76. Gregory PH. Microbiology of the atmosphere. 2nd edn. New York: Wiley; 1973.
77. Smith EG. Sampling and identifying allergenic pollens and molds, San Antonio: Blewstone; 1984.
78. Ellis MB. Dematiaceous Hyphomycetes. Surrey: Commonwealth Mycology Institute; 1971.
79. Dennis RWG. British ascomycetes. 3rd edn. Forestburgh: Lubrecht & Cramer; 1981.
80. Smith D, Onions HS, The preservation and maintenance of living fungi. Forestburgh: Lubrecht & Cramer; 1983.
81. Barnett HL, Hunter BB. Illustrated genera of imperfect fungi. 4th edn. New York: Macmillan; Burgess 1987.
82. Von Arx JA. The genera of fungi sporulating in pure culture. 3rd edn. Forestburgh: Lubrecht & Cramer; 1981.
83. Green B.J., Sercombe J.K., Tovey E.R.. Fungal fragments and undocumented conidia function as aeroallergen sources. J Allergy Clin Immunol 2005; 115:1043.
84. Green BJ, Schmechel D, Tovey ER. Detection of aerosolized Alternaria alternaria conidia, hyphae, and fragments using a novel double-immunostaining technique. Clin Diag Lab Immunol 2005; 12:1114.
85. Portnoy J, Brothers D, Pacheco F, et al. Monoclonal antibody based assay for Alt a 1, a major Alternaria allergen. Ann Allergy Asthma Immunol 1998; 81:59.
86. Aden E, Weber B, Bossert J, et al. Standardization of Alternaria alternata: extraction and quantification of Alt a 1 by using an mAb-based 2-site binding assay. J Allergy Clin Immunol 1999; 103:128.
87. Barnes C, Schreiber K, Pacheco F, et al. Comparison of outdoor allergenic particles and allergen levels. Ann Allergy Asthma Immunol 2000; 84:47.
88. Sporik RB, Arruda LK, Woodfolk, et al. Environmental exposure to Aspergillus fumigatus allergen (Asp f 1). Clin Exp Allergy 1993; 23:326.
89. Dharmage S, Bailey M, Raven J, et al. A reliable and valid home visit report for studies of asthma in young adults. Indoor Air 1999; 9:188.
90. Miller JD, Young JC. The use of ergosterol to measure exposure to fungal propagules in indoor air. Am Ind Hyg Assoc J 1997; 58:39.
91. Douwes J, van der Sluis B, Doekes G, et al. Fungal extracellular polysaccharides in house dust as a marker for exposure to fungi: relations with culturable fungi, reported home dampness, and respiratory symptoms. J Allergy Clin Immunol 1999; 103:494.
92. Rylander R. Indoor air-related effects and air-borne $(1\to3)$-β-D-glucan. Environ Health Perspect 1999; 107:501.
93. Ahearn DG, Crow SA, Simmons RB, et al. Fungal colonization of air filters and insulation in a multi-story office building: production of volatile organics. Curr Microbiol 1997; 35:305.
94. Fischer G, Schwalbe R, Moller M, et al. Species-specific production of microbial volatile organic compounds (MVOC) by air-borne fungi from a compost facility. Chemosphere 1999; 39:795.
95. Zhou G, Whong W, Ong T, et al. Development of a fungus-specific PCR assay for detecting low-level fungi in an indoor environment. Mol Cell Probes 2000; 14:339.
96. Williams RH, Ward E, McCartney HA. Methods for integrated air sampling and DNA analysis for detection of air-borne fungal spores. Appl Environ Microbiol 2001; 67:2453.
97. Samson RA. Mycotoxins: a mycologist's perspective. J Med Vet Mycol 1992; 30:9.
98. Dillon HK, Miller JD, Sorenson WG, et al. Review of methods applicable to the assessment of mold exposure to children. Environ Health Perspect 1999; 107:473.
99. Kurup VP, Shen H-D, Banerjee B. Respiratory fungal allergy. Microbes Infect 2000; 2:1101.
100. Ramirez C. Manual and atlas of penicillia. New York: Elsevier; 1982.
101. Shen H-D, Lin W-L, Tam MF, et al. Alkaline serine proteinase: a major allergen of Aspergillus oryzae and its cross-reactivity with Penicillium citrinum. Int Arch Allergy Immunol 1998; 116:29.
102. Herxheimer H, Hyde HA, Williams DA. Allergic asthma caused by basidiospores. Lancet 1969; 2:131.

Other plant and microbial particles as allergen sources

103. Bernstein IL, Safferman RS. Clinical sensitivity to green algae demonstrated by nasal challenge and in vitro tests of immediate hypersensitivity. J Allergy Clin Immunol 1973; 51:22.

Indoor Allergens

33

Thomas A E Platts-Mills

CONTENTS

- Introduction 539
- History 539
- Relevance to allergic diseases 541
- Sources of indoor allergens 541
- Molecular biology 546
- Indoor allergen exposure and sensitization or disease 546
- Air-borne indoor allergens 547
- Avoidance measures for indoor allergens 549
- Immune responses to allergens from different sources 551
- Conclusions 552

SUMMARY OF IMPORTANT CONCEPTS

>> The average child or adult spends at least 23 h/day indoors, at home, in a school, or at work

>> Allergens carried on smaller particles (e.g., cat and dog) stay air-borne and, as a result, larger quantities are inhaled

>> With some allergens (e.g., cat and dog), the highest levels of exposure are *not* associated with the highest prevalence of sensitization and may induce tolerance

>> Many different allergens are found indoors, but dust mite, cat, cockroach, mouse, and dog appear to be the most important

>> Allergen avoidance is front-line treatment for asthma, perennial rhinitis, and atopic dermatitis; but in order to be successful, avoidance needs to be both comprehensive and specific for those allergens to which the patient has demonstrable sensitization.

INTRODUCTION

Individuals predisposed to become allergic make immunoglobulin E (IgE) antibody responses to a wide range of proteins found inside houses. Although there are some pollen antigens in which a specific HLA type is linked to responsiveness, allergic individuals generally have an increased probability of responding to several different indoor and outdoor allergens. At the beginning of the twenty-first century, normal behavior patterns include spending 23 h/day indoors and correspondingly little time outdoors. This pattern has consequences for many chronic diseases but has special significance for allergic disease.

Families who spend many hours a day sitting prefer homes that are warmer, more fully furnished, and tighter. Increased temperatures can increase the population of mites or cockroaches, and furnishings will become reservoirs of accumulated allergens inside the home. Conversely, if humidity is marginal, increased heat can dry the house and decrease both mold and mite growth. When indoor air is very still, the critical factor determining the quantity of allergen air borne is the settling velocity of the particles carrying allergen. Typically, particles larger than 10 µm in diameter will fall rapidly in still air, whereas even pollen grains that are 20–30 µm in diameter will remain air-borne in a breeze outdoors. The still air indoors may also explain why indoor allergens, unlike outdoor pollens, are not a major cause of conjunctivitis. In addition, because of the length of time spent indoors, cumulative allergen exposure inside may be more important than outdoor exposure. For example, the presence of one-tenth of the number of fungal spores per cubic meter of air indoors may represent a larger number inhaled indoors than outdoors.

HISTORY

The significance of house dust as an allergen was first recognized by Kern in 1921, when he reported that many patients with asthma or rhinitis gave positive wheal-and-flare skin responses to extracts of dust obtained from their own house (autologous dust).[1] Subsequently, commercial 'house-dust' extracts were made using dust from vacuum cleaner bags obtained through church and other groups. These extracts were used for both diagnosis and immunotherapy; not surprisingly, they had widely different concentrations of allergens and could not be standardized.

Before 1960, several sources of allergens in house dust had been recognized, including animal danders, insects, fungi, and horse hair (Box 33.1).[2] However, dust from some houses, particularly in geographic areas that were consistently humid, caused large skin responses in allergic individuals, although there was no apparent source of allergen. In 1967, Spieksma and Voorhorst provided definitive evidence that the dust mite, *Dermatophagoides pteronyssinus*, was an important source of house-dust allergens in the Netherlands.[3] They also developed techniques for growing this mite so that dust mite extracts could be marketed. In studies conducted at that time (i.e., 1960–1980) it was shown that mite allergic children with asthma improved when they spent 6 months or more in a mountain sanatorium.[3,4] The association between positive skin tests to mite extracts and asthma was confirmed in many different countries, including the UK, Australia, Japan, and Brazil.[5–8] In some of those studies, dust mites were so important that other sources of allergens in house dust appeared to be insignificant.

Attempts to purify allergens from house dust were uniformly unsuccessful. By contrast, purification of allergens from specific extracts has formed the basis for understanding the role of indoor allergens. The first indoor allergen to be purified was Fel d 1 from the cat, *Felis domesticus*.[9] The terminology for allergens uses the first three letters of the genus followed by the first letter of the species name and a number that in general indicates the order in which the allergen was identified (see Chapter 35). In 1980 the first mite allergen, Der p 1, was purified using classical protein purification techniques.[10] As with Fel d 1, this protein was initially identified and measured using polyclonal rabbit antisera.[11]

A major advance in defining and measuring indoor proteins came with the development of monoclonal antibodies (mAbs) to allergens. These reagents play an important role because mAbs can provide a sensitive and specific method of measuring the allergen in extracts, reservoir dust samples, and air-borne particulates,[12] which in turn has provided a basis for assessing methods of allergen avoidance.[13] In addition, mAbs can be used to purify allergens using affinity chromatography which made it possible to obtain partial amino acid sequence data. Several approaches can be used to measure allergens, but the most widely used one is a mAb-based two-site immunometric assay, using enzyme-labeled second antibodies.[12,13]

The next breakthrough came when Chua and her colleagues cloned Der p 1 and obtained the full sequence.[14] The Der p 1 sequence revealed a striking homology with cysteine proteases. Cloning of other allergens followed, including many other dust mite allergens, Fel d 1, and German cockroach allergens, including Bla g 2 (see www.allergen.org).[15,16] Cloning proteins not only simplifies sequencing but also opens the way to production of recombinant proteins. The production of recombinant allergens has several problems because the ability to interact with IgE antibody depends on the tertiary structure, including glycosylation. A recombinant protein may have the same amino acid sequence as the natural protein but may be significantly different antigenically. The problem is that most of the cell lines used to produce recombinant proteins are either bacterial (*Escherichia coli*) or fungal (*Pichia pastoris*) in origin. However, progress is being made by using sequence variants that are better expressed by a specific vector and also by using different vectors. It is important to remember that recombinant proteins must be purified, and they may still contain traces of proteins that are produced by the vector or used in the purification. The availability of purified proteins

---

BOX 33.1   SOURCES OF ALLERGENS IN HOUSE DUST

Acarids
Dust mites/domestic mites
Dermatophagoides pteronyssinus
Dermatophagoides farinae
Euroglyphus maynei
Blomia tropicalis
Storage mites

Others
Spiders
Silverfish

Mammals
Cats (*Felis domesticus*)
Dogs (*Canis familiaris*)
Rabbits
Ferrets

Rodents
Pets (mice, gerbils, guinea pigs, chinchilla, etc.)
Pests
➤➤   Mice (*Mus musculus*)
➤➤   Rats (*Rattus norvegicus*)

Insects
Cockroaches
Blattella germanica (German)
Periplaneta americana (American)
Blatta orientalis (Oriental)

Others
Harmonia axyridis – Asian lady beetles
Crickets
Flies
Fleas
Moths
Midges

Fungi
Derived from inside house
Penicillium
Aspergillus
Cladosporium (growing on surfaces of rotting wood)
Other species

Derived from outside house
Multiple species from entry with incoming air

Pollens
Derived from outside house

Sundry
Horse hair in furniture
Kapok (insulation, filling; silky fibers from ceiba tree)
Food dropped by residents

has made major contributions to research on the structure, biology, and immunology of allergens. Whether recombinant allergens will replace natural allergen extracts in clinical practice is not clear.[17]

RELEVANCE TO ALLERGIC DISEASES

In population-based, cross-sectional, and prospective studies, subjects with a positive skin test or detectable IgE antibody to one or more of the major indoor allergens are significantly more likely to have asthma (Table 33.1).[5–8,18–20] On the other hand, in all studies a significant proportion (up to 15%) of asymptomatic individuals are sensitized to an indoor allergen. Thus, there are at least two issues: why some individuals become sensitized and why some of these subjects develop symptoms (Fig. 33.1).

Although exposure plays a significant role in both the acute and the chronic effects of indoor allergens, in some comparisons a large part of the increase in asthma prevalence can be explained by increased wheezing among the allergic individuals. The only diseases that have been associated statistically with exposure to dust mite or the other indoor allergens are chronic rhinitis, asthma, and atopic dermatitis. Rarely, cases of conjunctivitis, urticaria, and even anaphylaxis are associated with dust mite sensitization. For atopic dermatitis, the epidemiologic evidence is almost all about dust mite sensitization.[26] In one study, having high titre IgE antibody to dust mite, i.e. >30 IU/mL, was very strongly associated with atopic dermatitis (OR ~30).[27] For cockroach allergens, the published evidence is almost entirely related to asthma.[18,19,28–30] Very few patients present with nasal symptoms that appear to be related to cockroach sensitization. Differences in the association between allergens and diseases are primarily explained by exposure. The importance of cockroach sensitization among inner city populations reflects the fact that a large proportion of houses are infested with these insects. In some inner city studies mites appear to be unimportant, but those studies were conducted in Northern cities where, because of low humidity, mites do not flourish.[30] By contrast, in Atlanta, GA; Dallas, TX; Wilmington, DE; or Seattle, WA, dust mites are found in all types of housing and the inner city or poor populations are as allergic to dust mites as suburban populations in the same region.[31] For cat and dog allergens, the relationship to exposure is strikingly different. First, because the allergens remain air-borne, estimates of inhaled allergen are higher than for other allergens. Second, the proteins may have different biological properties, e.g., no enzymic activity, as well as different glycosylation patterns (see Chapter 36). Third, the allergens of cat and dog become widely distributed and are consistently present in homes that do not have animals.[32]

SOURCES OF INDOOR ALLERGENS

ARTHROPODS

Acaridae

Many different species of mites have been reported in house dust, but in most parts of the world the so-called pyroglyphid mites dominate. These include *D. pteronyssinus*, *D. farinae*, and *Euroglyphus maynei* (Fig. 33.2). In tropical areas (e.g., Brazil, Florida) the mite species include *Blomia tropicalis*. Occasionally, houses may have a large number of storage mites (e.g., *Lepidoglyphus destructor*, *Tyrophagus putrescentior*), predator mites of the genus Cheyletidae, and the smaller *Tarsonemus* (Tarsonemidae).[3,33–35] It is probably best to reserve the term 'dust mites' for pyroglyphid mites and use the term 'domestic mites' to cover any species of mites when they are found in houses.[36]

Pyroglyphid mites are eight-legged and sightless. They live on skin scales and other debris. They have a very precarious water balance,

Table 33.1 Sensitization to indoor allergens and asthma

Country	Study	Dominant allergen(s)	Odds ratio[a]	Pollen	Author
UK	Prospective	Mite (cat)	19.7	NS	Sporik et al (1990)[7]
New Zealand	Prospective	Mite (*Aspergillus*)	6.6	NS	Sears et al (1989)[20]
Sweden	Population	Cat, dog	3.9	Birch[b]	Rönmark et al (1998)[21]
Australia	School(s)	Mite	>10	NS	Peat et al (1996)[8]
Germany	Birth cohort	Mite, cat		NS	Illi et al (2006)[22]
USA (Virginia)	School(s)	Mite (cat, cockroach)	6.6	NS	Sporik et al (1999)[100]
Georgia (Atlanta)	Emergency room	Mite, cockroach	8.2	NS	Call et al (1992)[23]
Arizona	Prospective	*Alternaria*	<0.01	NS	Halonen et al (1997)[24]
New Mexico	School	Cat, dog	6.2	NS	Sporik et al (1995)[25]
Massachusetts (Boston)	Birth cohort	Mite, cat	3.8	NS	Lewis et al (2001)[c]

[a]p <0.001 [b]p <0.05. NS, not significant. [c]Lewis SA, Weiss ST, Platts-Mills TA et al. Association of specific allergen sensitization with socioeconomic factors and allergic disease in a population of Boston women. J Allergy Clin Immunol 2001; 107:615.

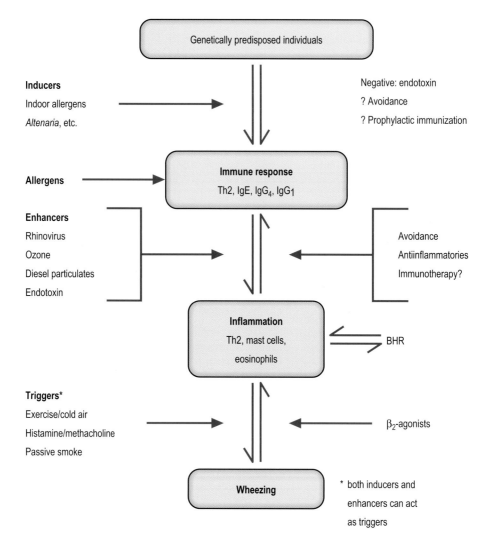

Fig. 33.1. Role of indoor allergens in asthma. Th2, T helper type 2 cells; Ig, immunoglobulin; BHR, bronchial hyperresponsiveness.

absorbing water through a hygroscopic substance extruded from their leg joints. Mites are not capable of searching for or drinking liquids and are thus entirely dependent on ambient humidity. In addition, they have a fairly tight optimal growth temperature between 65 and 80°F. Although it is common practice to measure ambient humidity, it is the humidity within carpets, sofas, mattresses, or clothing that is relevant. As humidity falls, mites will withdraw from the surface, so that even in very dry conditions, it may take months for mites to die and longer for allergen levels to decrease in carpets, sofas, or mattresses (Fig. 33.3).[37] Mites excrete partially digested food and digestive enzymes as a fecal particle surrounded by a chitinous peritrophic membrane.[35,38] Some species of mites are coprophagic, which may also be true of the genus *Dermatophagoides*.[38] Large numbers of fecal particles are found in mite cultures, and they represent a major form in which mite allergens accumulate in house dust. Presumably because of the peritrophic membrane, the particles tend to remain intact; however, this 'membrane' is not waterproof, and allergens elute from fecal particles rapidly.[38] Thus, mite fecal pellets are similar to

pollen grains in size (10–35 μm in diameter), in the quantity of allergen they carry (~0.2 ng), and in their rapid release of proteins (Fig. 33.4).

Dust mites are approximately 0.3 mm in length and difficult to see with the naked eye. When examining dust under an incident light microscope, it is possible to see moving mites. However, dead or motionless mites cannot be identified without preliminary flotation on a sucrose gradient and filtration onto filter paper.[11,35,36] The identification of mites is time-consuming and requires skill, which has led to a demand for simpler measures to quantify the presence of mites in house dust. However, counting mites under a microscope remains important to define the species of mites present, particularly in new environments.[33,36]

Mite allergens

Purification of mite allergens became possible once the technique for large-scale cultures was developed. The first major allergen purified was *Dermatophagoides pteronyssinus* allergen I (Der p I), now Der p 1.[10]

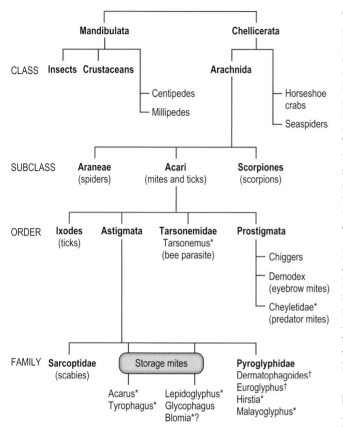

*All mites found in house dust are collectively referred to as domestic mites.
† The term "dust mites" is generally restricted to Dermatophagoides and Euroglyphus.

Fig. 33.2. Classification of the phylum Arthropoda.

This 24-kDa glycoprotein has both sequence homology with cysteine proteinases and functional enzymatic activity.[39–43] Monoclonal antibodies to Der p 1 were reported in 1984. The protein was sequenced from a clone in 1988.[14] A second major allergen was first identified by Lind[44] and was initially called DpX because it could not be identified on crossed immunoelectrophoresis. However, mAbs developed by Heymann et al[45] allowed purification and subsequent cloning of the protein, Der p 2.[44] Further studies established that homologous cross-reacting allergens are produced by D. farinae and also by a third species, D. microceras.[46,47] These mite allergens are now referred to as group 1 (Der p 1 and Der f 1) and group 2 (Der p 2 and Der f 2). The group 2 allergens are very similar to each other in structure, having >90% sequence homology, and are strongly cross-reacting; indeed, no mAbs currently available can distinguish Der p 2 from Der f 2. Sensitive immunoassays are widely used to measure Der p 1 and Der f 1 separately, and the group 2 mite allergens can also be measured in dust samples.[13,48]

The 'tropical' dust mite *Blomia tropicalis* is present in many houses in Florida, Puerto Rico, Venezuela, and Brazil. Antibodies to *B. tropicalis* cross-react partially with other dust mites. However, patient sera from Brazil contain significant quantities of IgE antibodies that do not cross-react with *D. pteronyssinus*, strongly suggesting that *B. tropicalis* is a significant cause of symptoms. The first allergen identified and clone from *B. tropicalis* was designated Blo t 5 because it has sequence homology with Der p 5. This protein causes positive skin tests in mite-allergic individuals, and a large proportion of sera from asthmatic patients in Brazil have IgE antibody to this allergen.[49]

Dust and dust mite extracts

House-dust extracts formerly were collected from vacuum cleaner bags. In general, dust was collected outside the pollen season and from houses without animals. The quantity of dust mite allergen in house-dust extracts varied widely, from 0.05 to 2.0 μg/mL Der p 1. Other allergens in these extracts also varied widely; in particular, cat allergen ranged from less

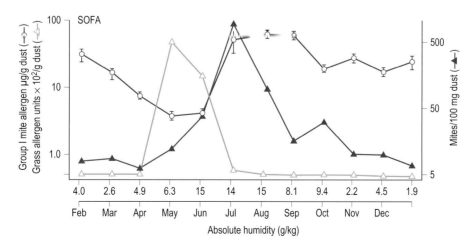

Fig. 33.3. Seasonal variation in mite, mite allergen (group 1), and grass pollen allergen in a sofa followed over 1 year in central Virginia. A sharp rise in mite numbers (▲-▲) follows the rise in outdoor absolute humidity. Mite allergen levels rise during the summer but remain high until after Christmas (○-○). Allergen from ryegrass pollen (△-△) was only detected in May, June, and July. (Adapted from Plat-Mills TA, Hayden ML, Chapman MD, et al. Seasonal variation in dust mite and grass-pollen allergens in dust from the houses of patients with asthma. J Allergy Clin Immunol 1987; 79:781.[37])

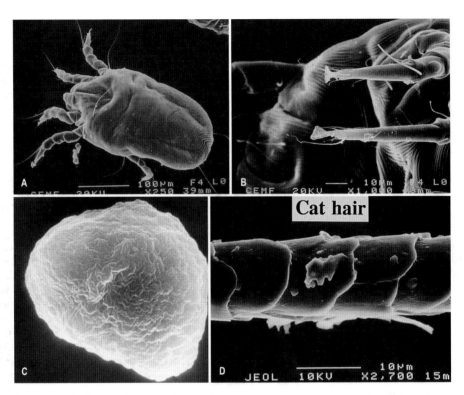

Fig. 33.4. (A) Dust mite of the species *Dermatophagoides farinae*, showing legs and mouth parts; these acarids are sightless but are sensitive to light, so they are not normally present on the surface of carpets or upholstered furniture. (B) Details of the legs of a dust mite, showing the pads on the end that allow the mite to hold on to surfaces. (C) Mite fecal particle, which has a chitinous peritrophic membrane that prevents it from breaking up. (D) Scanning electron micrograph of a cat hair, showing the size and presence of adherent particles of dander/skin scales that carry antigen. (A–C, courtesy of John Vaughan; D, courtesy of Judith Woodfolk.)

Table 33.2 Concentrations of major allergens in aqueous extracts of selected samples of dust from houses of asthmatic patients[18,19,23,75,77]

US State	Source	Der p 1, mite (µg/g)	Der f 1, mite (µg/g)	Fel d 1, cat (µg/g)	Bla g 2, cockroach (U/g)	Lol p 1, grass (µg/g)
Virginia	Floor	<0.2	<0.2	472	<1.0	<0.2
Ohio	Bedding	1.7	240	<0.2	<1.0	<0.2
Virginia	Carpet	26.5	0.4	20.6	<1.0	1.9
Virginia	Carpet	0.8	0.2	<0.2	<1.0	1.3
California	Carpet	1.9	0.2	2.2	<1.0	148
California	Bedding	20.5	59.3	6.7	<1.0	33.4
Delaware	Kitchen	0.43	0.2	<0.2	296	–
Atlanta	Mixed	0.7	5.9	<0.2	210	–

than 0.01 to 10.0 µg/mL Fel d 1 (Table 33.2). In the author's experience, commercially available house-dust extracts contain no detectable cockroach allergen (by immunoassay) and little detectable fungal allergen (by skin testing patients who are selectively allergic to fungi). Commercial dust mite extracts are made from either whole-mite culture or from isolated mite bodies; this creates a different ratio of group 1 to group 2 allergens. Thus, extracts made from bodies of *D. pteronyssinus* may contain 40 µg/mL Der p 1 and 30 µg/mL Der p 2, whereas a whole culture extract typically contains at least 10-fold more group 1 than group 2. In the USA, all extracts are made from isolated mite bodies, whereas in

Europe, both types of extracts are available. Mite cultures contain fungi which appear to be necessary for reproduction. They may also contain bacteria. As judged by endotoxin content, there can be big differences in bacteria between cultures. In the USA, $D.$ $farinae$ extracts (and cultures) contain large quantities of endotoxin, while the levels are much lower in $D.$ $pteronyssinus$ extracts.[50] Recent studies have shown that in addition to endotoxin, mite fecal particles contain both mite DNA and bacterial DNA. Given the role of these substances in binding Toll-like receptors (TLR), the presence of these substances may be highly relevant to explain why dust mites are such a potent allergen.

DOMESTIC ANIMALS

Cat allergens

Most patients who are allergic to cats are aware of symptoms on entering a house with a cat or if they touch their face after contact with an animal. Purification of the main cat allergen Fel d 1 from cat washings or pelt extract is difficult, partly because it is expensive to keep a large number of cats. The details of the structure of this allergen were not known until mAbs made it possible to obtain the N-terminal sequence and then to clone and sequence the molecule.[15,51] At one point it seemed likely that Fel d 1 was a salivary protein, and that it accumulated on the fur, in part because cats licked themselves. However, when cats were restrained from licking themselves, Fel d 1 still accumulated on shaved skin, and it became clear that the primary site of synthesis of this allergen was in the skin.[15,52,53] On crossed radioimmunoelectrophoresis (CRIE) or on Western blotting, other proteins produced by cats can be shown to be allergens for some patients. Three of these have been purified and characterized, cat albumin (Fel d 2), cystatin (Fel d 3), and a lipocalin (Fel d 4); however, each of these are less important than Fel d 1 (see Table 35.8).[54] Sensitization to the other allergens is only found in a minority of cat-allergic patients.

Cat extracts are manufactured either from washings or from pelt. Pelt extracts are thought to be less representative of natural exposure because they contain a large relative concentration of serum proteins (e.g., albumin). Because washing cats is used as a method of making commercial cat extracts, it is obvious that this procedure can remove allergens from the cat. When cats are washed repeatedly, the allergen recovered decreases progressively.[55] This observation led to the investigation of washing as a method of controlling exposure.[56] Additional studies showed that cat allergen can be removed from a cat by washing, and that the animal will subsequently release less allergen.[56,57] However, this effect lasts for less than 1 week,[58] so that washing of cats or dogs would need to be repeated frequently to be effective.[57]

Dog allergens

Dogs can be a potent source of allergen, although in most studies, dog allergy appears to be less common than cat allergy as a cause of asthma. Many dogs are kept outside, or at least out of bedrooms, and some dogs are washed regularly, which may explain this lower prevalence. However, studies on patients with asthma from New Mexico and Arizona have found a high prevalence of IgE antibodies to dog allergens.[59,60] In 1991, a major dog allergen was purified, and mAbs have been developed to Can f 1 so that specific assays are possible.[59,61] High levels of Can f 1 can accumulate in house dust, and significant levels of both cat and dog allergens can be found in dust from schools.[62–64] In several studies it has been possible to confirm the presence of air-borne Can f 1 and to demonstrate that the use of high-efficiency particulate air (HEPA) filters in a room or the washing of dogs can significantly decrease air-borne allergen.[65]

Rodents

Rodents are an important source of occupational allergens.[66,67] Proteins present in the urine of rats and mice can induce both IgE and immunoglobulin G (IgG) antibodies in animal handlers and scientists who work with these animals.[68,69] Rodents are present in domestic houses both as pets and as pests. Occasional cases of rhinitis and asthma related to pet animals (e.g., rabbits, chinchillas, ferrets, mice) are well recognized. Rats as well as mice can become a significant problem inside houses. Questionnaire data from Harlem Hospital suggested that the presence of rats in the home was a significant determinant of severe asthma. More specifically, evidence from the National Cooperative Inner City Asthma Study (NCICAS) showed that the presence of mouse allergens in dust correlated with IgE antibodies to the allergens and with asthma.[70] Although it seems certain that rodents can be a significant source of indoor allergens among patients living in cities or rural areas, there appear to be major differences between areas of the USA.[71] In addition, it is well established that occupational exposure can induce IgG and IgG4 antibodies to rodent antigens without IgE ab responses.[68,72,73]

INSECTS

Many different insects have been identified as sources of inhalant allergens in case reports or small outbreaks, including moths, crickets, locusts, beetles, nimitti flies, lake flies, and houseflies.[74,75] However, the insect that has been recognized most commonly as a source of indoor allergen is the cockroach.[28,75–77] For domestic cockroaches, allergens can be derived from feces, saliva, or debris from dead animals. Large quantities of cockroach allergens can accumulate in homes and may remain for years after cockroaches have been eradicated.[78–81] The recent epidemic of imported Asian lady beetles (*Harmonia axyridis*) on the east coast and mid-west USA, has provided further evidence that any insect growing in large numbers within a house can become a significant source of allergens.[82–85] The epidemic is an important reminder that the constituents of the indoor environment are not fixed. Surprisingly, few cases of allergy to houseflies, moths, spiders or other common insects are recognized, which may reflect the lack of routine testing for these allergens.

Cockroaches

Several species of cockroaches are common in houses, but the best known are *Blattella germanica* and *Periplaneta americana*. The German cockroach is common in cities where the climate is hot enough or where heating is maintained in houses or apartment buildings. However, these insects are particularly common in inner-city apartments in the USA. As early as 1964, it was recognized that many patients presenting with asthma to indigent care clinics had positive skin tests to cockroach. Positive results were reported in clinic populations from Boston, New York, Kansas City, Detroit, Chicago, and Washington, DC.[28–31] In most cases, suburban clinics have found few or no positive skin tests to cockroach extracts. Asthmatic patients from inner cities demonstrated positive IgE antibodies, positive bronchial provocation tests, and good responses to immunotherapy with cockroach extract.[23,28] Enrolling random adult patients presenting with asthma to a hospital emergency room and random controls confirmed the significant association of cockroach sensitivity with asthma.[18,23] Furthermore, in a subsequent study in Wilmington, Delaware, the risk of asthma associated with sensitization to cockroach allergens was restricted to the inner-city area; that is, that area where cockroach allergens were found in the houses.[19]

Several studies have reported partial or complete purification of allergens derived from German cockroaches.[76] Specific mAbs have enabled measurements of Bla g 2 in house dust.[16,19,23,79–81] Three studies have measured air-borne cockroach allergen, and the results are consistent.[78,80,81] As with dust mite allergen, little or no allergen was detected in the air of undisturbed houses. By contrast, both Bla g 1 and Bla g 2 can be measured in the air of infested houses during vacuum cleaning.[80,81] The implication is that *B. germanica* allergens become air-borne on particles that are aerodynamically large, $>10\,\mu m$ in diameter, and that consequently fall rapidly. However, the nature of the particles carrying air-borne cockroach allergens has not been resolved. A direct parallel with mite allergens should not be assumed, because the highest levels of cockroach allergens are found in kitchens, whereas the highest levels of mite allergen are often found in bedding. In the NCICAS study, however, it was the concentration of cockroach allergen in children's bedrooms that correlated with the risk of hospitalization.[30]

■ MOLECULAR BIOLOGY ■

The amino acid sequence of proteins can be determined by Edman degradation or mass spectroscopy; however, this is very time-consuming and was not achieved with any of the indoor allergens before these proteins were cloned. Once the deoxyribonucleic acid (DNA) for a protein has been cloned, it is relatively simple to obtain the sequence of the gene and thus the protein. It is also simple to compare the sequence to other known sequences in the published databases (e.g., Genebank). Homologies identified in this way provide important clues about the possible function of the proteins and may also help to define their tertiary structure. In at least one case, understanding the sequence homologies has provided information that may be important in understanding the reasons why the protein is such a potent allergen. In other cases, structural information has provided clues about cross-reactivity (see also Chapter 35).[17] In the case of Der p 1, the sequence data confirmed that the allergen is an enzyme. This information has also been used to investigate the relevance of the enzymic activity to immunogenicity of the mite protein.[86] By contrast, the sequence data on Fel d 1 identified homology with uteroglobin or Clara cell secretory protein and suggested ways in which the protein might be an immunomodulator.[87] Finally in several cases sequence data has helped to understand cross-reactivity (see Chapter 35).

USE OF PEPTIDES TO INVESTIGATE IMMUNE RESPONSE TO INDOOR ALLERGENS

Overlapping peptides have been used extensively to investigate the responses of circulating T cells to Der p 1, Der p 2, Fel d 1, and also the *Trichophyton* allergen, Tri r 2.[88–90] Peptides can only be derived once the amino acid sequence is known, and the responses in vitro may involve a different form of antigen processing than occurs with the whole molecule. Using peptides allows the identification of major epitopes and detailed investigation of cytokine responses.[89,90] The proliferative and cytokine response in vitro is influenced by the number of responses occurring, as well as by the nature of the antigen, the medium, and the concentration of cells.[90] Thus, responses to whole allergens may give a different cytokine pattern than responses to peptides.

Peptides derived from Fel d 1 have also been used for immunotherapy. Initial trials using three peptides from chain 1 established that the peptides could produce a therapeutic benefit.[89,91] More recently, Haselden and his colleagues in London have shown that intradermal injections of peptides can produce late reactions in the lungs of patients with asthma. These reactions were followed by decreased proliferative responses of circulating T cells and prolonged decreased reactivity of the lungs.[92] The results suggest that there is potential for a therapeutic strategy using peptides; however, it is not yet clear whether the peptides used should focus on epitopes that induce Th2 cytokines in vitro or those that induce IL-10 and or IFNγ.[93] The in vitro results argue strongly that there are Fel d 1-specific T cells in the lungs of patients with asthma.

RECOMBINANT INDOOR ALLERGENS

After the cloning of Der p 1, it became possible to express the protein in vitro. However, expressing the correct amino acid sequence does not ensure the same tertiary structure, and recombinant Der p 1 was initially poorly reactive with IgE antibodies or in skin tests.[14] By contrast, some other allergens, including Der p 2, can be expressed in a form that is very similar to the native allergen.[47] The expression of recombinant protein depends on the folding of the molecule and glycosylation. These factors are influenced both by the expression system used (e.g., *E. coli, P. pastoris*) and by the vector used (e.g., pPIC9, pBlue Bac III). In addition, many of the vectors use different codons to express a particular amino acid. Thus, modifying codon use in the recombinant DNA for an allergen may improve expression of the protein in vitro.[94] Detailed studies of this type may be necessary for many of the allergens.

In addition, it is necessary to decide how many different recombinant proteins would be needed to 'replace' the natural extract. For example, how many of the currently identified 14 different allergens from *D. pteronyssinus* need to be included in a diagnostic reagent? The potential for recombinant proteins is obvious; there are still many practical problems to be solved. It has also been established that minor changes to a molecule using site-directed mutagenesis can produce a molecule with dramatically reduced reactivity with IgE antibody, but no change in T cell reactivity.[95] With Der p 2, a simple change in a disulfide bond can produce a major effect.[47,95] However, the practicality of using modified molecules for immunotherapy remains to be established.

■ INDOOR ALLERGEN EXPOSURE AND SENSITIZATION OR DISEASE ■

Once immunoassays for dust mite allergens were available, it was possible to analyze the relationship between exposure in houses and sensitization (Table 33.3).[7,36,96–98] The evidence provided strong support for

Table 33.3 Specific levels of dust mite exposure in houses of asthmatic patients regarded as risk factors for sensitization and asthma

Study	Country	Threshold level
Dust mites		
Voorhorst and Spieksma (1967)[3]	The Netherlands	500 mites/g
Peat et al (1996)[8]	Australia	100 mites/g
Dowse et al (1985)[96]	Papua New Guinea	1000 mites/g
Mite allergens (Der p 1/Der f 1)		
Platts-Mills et al (1982)[97]	England (London)	13.5 μg/g
Charpin et al (1991)[99]	France (Marseilles)	2 μg/g
Sporik et al (1990)[7]	England	10 μg Der p 1/g
Kuehr et al (1994)[98]	Germany	2 μg Der p 1/g
Platts-Mills et al (1987)[37]	USA (Virginia)	2 μg group 1/g
Sporik et al (1999)[100]	USA (Virginia)	2–10 μg/g

a threshold level of exposure (2-μg group 1 mite allergen, or about 100 mites/g of dust), above which sensitization of genetically at-risk individuals becomes increasingly common. Furthermore, a dose–response relationship exists between the mean concentration of mite allergen in houses and the importance of this sensitization to asthma.[36,37,96,99] In a large cohort of children followed prospectively for 2 years, 2 μg/g was the threshold for sensitization for allergic children (i.e., those who had a positive skin test to another allergen such as pollen), but the 'threshold' for sensitization of non-allergic children was closer to 20 μg/g or higher.[98] In a prospective study involving 68 children, exposure to high levels of allergen at age 1 year increased the risk of asthma at age 10 years and was related to early onset of asthma.[7] In addition, studies on children admitted to the hospital in southern England showed that approximately 80% were both sensitized and exposed to high levels of relevant allergen at home.

In studies from the UK, Australia, USA, and Japan, where a majority of houses (>80%) contain high levels of mite allergen (>2 μg/g dust), sensitization to mite allergens is consistently an important risk factor for asthma.[36,54] This appears to be true both for chronic symptomatic bronchial hyperreactivity (BHR) and for admission to hospital.[19] For allergens other than dust mite, much less data are available on the levels of exposure associated with sensitization or disease. For cockroach allergen, evidence indicates a dose–response relationship between exposure and sensitization.[30,31,100] This finding comes from analysis of data from NCICAS participants and comparison of sensitization rates in suburban areas of Virginia or Georgia with rates in children living in the cities.[29–31,100] Thus, a Bla g 2 concentration greater than 10 U/g dust is associated with sensitization and disease. Such high concentrations are most unusual in suburban houses. Similar but less well-defined thresholds have been suggested for rodent urine. By contrast, for allergens associated with fungal spores that can grow outdoors or indoors, it would be difficult to make any statement about the concentrations or quantities present in a house that create a risk of sensitization.

SENSITIZATION TO CAT AND DOG ALLERGENS

Evidence about dose–response relationships between indoor allergen exposure and sensitization depends on the measurement of these proteins in house dust being a 'valid index of exposure'. Although the measurement of proteins in dust is well standardized and accurate, the relationship between floor dust and allergen inhaled is less well defined. For domestic animal allergens the evidence is complex, both for practical reasons related to the behavior of air-borne particles and because the highest levels of exposure do not correlate with the highest prevalence of sensitization.

First, cat allergen remains air-borne in 'undisturbed' conditions, and estimates of the quantity inhaled are much higher than for mite or cockroach. Second, cat and dog allergens are distributed widely beyond homes with domestic animals. Concentrations of allergen that are considered sufficient to sensitize are found in schools, other public buildings, and in homes without an animal.[25,63,64,101] Third, in some studies, children raised in a house with a cat are less likely to become sensitized and less likely to develop asthma.[102,103] Collectively, these three factors suggest that the highest exposure to cat allergen must induce a different response or some form of tolerance and also that the concentrations of cat allergen that are passively transferred are sufficient to sensitize. In some studies, as many as 75% of children who develop IgE antibodies to cat have never lived in a house with a cat.[104] Thus, the dose–response relationship between cat allergens and sensitization is not linear. In some studies, the relationship has a plateau, but in other studies, it is bell-shaped.[105] Several factors could contribute to the complexity of the relationship between cat exposure and, sensitization or asthma, as follows:

- Allergic families can choose whether they own cats, while they are less able to 'choose' to avoid other allergens. However, population-based studies in New Zealand and the USA make it unlikely that choice explains more than a small part of the effect.[20,106]
- High exposure can induce a different form of immune response, which includes IgG and IgG4 antibodies to Fel d 1 without IgE antibodies, which should be regarded as a form of tolerance.[106]
- Continuous exposure can lead to a form of 'clinical tolerance' in which symptoms are not apparent, even though the patient remains skin-test positive.
- Biologic differences exist between allergens derived from cats and those of mites or cockroaches, including the lack of enzymatic activity in Fel d 1 or cat albumin and the heavy glycosylation of Fel d 1.

■ AIR-BORNE INDOOR ALLERGENS ■

The major outdoor allergens are carried on well-defined particles that are 'designed' to remain air-borne to aid fertilization or dispersal of the species, and in most cases these particles can be identified microscopically. By contrast, indoor allergens are carried on a variety of amorphous particles. Thus, all measurements of air-borne indoor allergens depend on immunoassays for the allergens derived from a given source. Sampling air-borne allergens can be achieved by drawing air through a filter or a cascade impactor or by collecting charged particles on steel plates.[11,78,107–110] There are advantages and disadvantages to each approach. Although in many cases the nature of the particles carrying a specific indoor allergen is not known, distinct differences exist in the aerodynamic behavior of these particles that are important in defining the exposure of allergic individuals. Particle size will influence not only deposition in the lung but also (1) the quantity of allergen on each particle, (2) the time that the particles remain air-borne, and (3) the quantities that become air-borne during disturbance.

HOUSE-DUST MITE

Shortly after mite fecal particles were first recognized as an important source of house-dust allergens, it was demonstrated that these particles are the form in which Der p 1 becomes air-borne.[11] However, air-borne mite allergen was only detected during or shortly after disturbance of a house.[11,111] Little or no air-borne allergen (e.g., $<1\,ng/m^3$) is present in undisturbed conditions. Subsequent studies using artificial disturbance of dust in a laboratory demonstrated that air-borne mite allergen fell rapidly after disturbance. Thus, the following support the view that mite allergen is predominantly air-borne on particles $>10\,\mu m$ in diameter: evidence from sizing of particles on an Anderson or a cascade impactor; the fact that allergen is only air-borne during and shortly after disturbance; and the rate of fall after disturbance. For particles of 20-μm diameter, 5–10% would be expected to enter the lung during gentle mouth breathing.[112,113] Given that the particles contain 0.2 ng Der p 1, an air-borne level of $20\,ng/m^3$ implies that a maximum of 100 fecal particles would be inhaled per hour, suggesting that as few as 5–10 particles per hour would enter the lung. This natural exposure is different from bronchial provocation, which generally involves approximately 10^8 droplets about $2\,\mu m$ in diameter, with each droplet containing 10^{-6} ng per droplet (a positive bronchial provocation test in a sensitive patient generally requires 10–1000 ng of allergen).

A major problem with any assessment of exposure to dust mite antigens is that patients often sleep or sit with their heads very close to mite-infested material (e.g., sofas, blankets, pillows, carpet). This creates a distinction between dust mite allergens and allergens such as those derived from cockroaches, where the highest levels are found on kitchen floors. The use of personal monitors close to the breathing zone is theoretically the way to gather accurate information. Recent studies using a nasal sampler have shown that individuals inhale allergens while in bed; however, these results relate to the nose rather than the mouth and it is still difficult to quantitate the allergen inhaled or to relate the results to other sampling techniques.[100]

AIR-BORNE CAT ALLERGEN

Patients who are allergic to cats often report rapid onset of eye and respiratory tract symptoms when they enter a house in which a cat lives. This phenomenon (which is unusual with mite-allergic patients) strongly suggests that cat allergen can be air-borne in an undisturbed house. When sensitive assays for Fel d 1 became available, the presence of air-borne cat allergen was confirmed, and it became clear that a proportion of the air-borne allergen (10–40%) was being carried on smaller particles ($<5\,\mu m$ in diameter).[107,111,114,115] The size of these particles has some important consequences. First, small particles fall

slowly and can be kept air-borne by any movement in the house. Second, increased ventilation helps to remove small particles from a house (ventilation has less effect on large particles). Third, air filtration with a room air cleaner may be a useful method of reducing exposure to allergen on small particles. Because cat allergen remains air-borne, the quantity inhaled may be much higher than the quantities of those allergens that are only transiently air-borne, such as mite or cockroach. Indeed, recent estimates suggest that the quantity of cat allergen inhaled may be 10–100 times as high as mite allergen.[115] The evidence for the small size of cat allergen particles has been obtained from experiments using a variety of different samplers, including a Casella cascade impactor, an Andersen impactor, and a liquid impinger. These sampling techniques actually provide evidence about the aerodynamic behavior of these particles which is *equivalent* to that of spheres of $1–7\,\mu m$ in diameter. Some particles carrying cat allergen have been visualized and it is important to realize that a flat 'flake' of dander could have an aerodynamic size *smaller* than its real mass. Because high ventilation rates, or more than two air changes per hour (ACH), will decrease air-borne small particles, increasingly airtight housing over the last 20 years may have led to progressively higher levels of cat allergen in houses.[56] There is a dramatic contrast between a laboratory animal vivarium, which has a ventilation rate of 10 ACH (by federal regulation), and domestic houses, with 0.2–0.5 ACH.[107]

OTHER AIR-BORNE ALLERGENS AND AIR-BORNE ENDOTOXIN

Although it is reasonable to assume that the other allergens that can contribute to house dust become air-borne, only a few have been measured in indoor air, including cockroach, rat urine, and dog allergens.[78] In most cases a variety of particle sizes have been reported, but it is possible to classify cat and dog allergens as one group, characterized by small particles that remain air-borne, and mite and cockroach allergens as a second group, characterized by particles that do not remain air-borne for more than a few minutes after disturbance. Researchers have also studied air-borne allergen derived from laboratory animals, particularly guinea pigs and rats. In experiments on rat urinary protein, the quantity becoming air-borne was dependent both on disturbances and on the condition of the litter. Litter in rodent cages contains very large quantities of rat, mouse, rabbit, or guinea pig protein derived from the urine. When the litter is wet, very little allergen becomes air-borne, even when the cages are disturbed. By contrast, as the litter dries, much larger quantities become air-borne with the same level of disturbance. We assume that smaller particles become free as they dry and can then become air-borne. At present, very little is known about comparable effects within the home. Changes in the absolute water content of a carpet or sofa or in the ambient humidity at the surface of a carpet may change the rate at which allergen-containing particles are released into the room air during vacuum cleaning or other activity. More research is needed on the form in which different allergens become air-borne and on the factors that influence release of different particles from surfaces in the home. Air-borne endotoxin is not easy to measure and some published results have implied measurements below the detection limits of the assays.[110] Part of the problem is that sampling techniques are noisy and therefore cannot be left running in a patient's home. Using a novel ion charging technique, it a possible to sample much larger quantities of air.[108] The results confirm the presence of air-borne endotoxin in most houses. However, there was no effect of cat ownership and only a modest positive effect of dog ownership on air-borne endotoxin.

■ AVOIDANCE MEASURES FOR INDOOR ALLERGENS ■

Reducing exposure to obvious 'trigger factors' has always been a standard part of the treatment of allergic disease. Furthermore, it was normal practice to recommend avoidance measures for patients who were skin test positive to house dust. This practice was strongly supported by the experiments of Storm van Leeuwen et al[116] and Rost,[117] who demonstrated benefit to patients with asthma and atopic dermatitis, respectively, from living in a climate chamber. However, several factors limited the clinical use of avoidance measures. Many patients, despite being skin test positive, were not aware that dust related to their symptoms. Also, because allergens were not regarded as a 'cause' of asthma, avoidance measures were not thought to help control the underlying bronchial reactivity. Finally, because the sources and nature of indoor allergens were not well understood, advice offered on avoidance was often inadequate or even wrong.

It is now well established that full avoidance of allergens (e.g., changing homes, moving to a sanatorium or hospital room) can reduce both symptoms and BHR.[4,13,97] The measurement of specific allergens has also provided simple methods for evaluating avoidance measures[13,118] and has strongly reinforced the view that the measures recommended should be different for each allergen source. The primary reason for testing the sensitivity of a patient by skin test or in vitro test is to provide education about the effects of exposure and allergen-specific avoidance advice.

DUST MITE

When the importance of dust mites was first appreciated, it was difficult to convince patients about the cause of their problem because mites cannot be seen and do not have a specific smell. Even with public awareness, it still requires considerable effort to explain the methods necessary to decrease mite exposure. There are several issues in evaluating the available data about controlling exposure. The evidence from sanatoria or hospital rooms shows that a change that includes a >90% decrease in allergen is consistently effective at reducing symptoms and BHR.[36,97,118] Where studied, these sites have had very low numbers of mites (e.g., <20/g) or mite allergen (<0.4 μg Der p 1/g). Controlled trials in patients' homes have generally been less effective both in decreasing allergen and in clinical outcome. A meta-analysis applied to all published trials concluded that avoidance of mite allergens was not an effective treatment for asthma.[119] However, the meta-analysis was deeply flawed in that multiple studies were included that did not decrease mite allergen or were very short in duration (3 months or less). In addition, by including those ineffective studies, the clinical outcomes relevant to the successful studies were excluded. The controlled trials that have achieved decreased allergen for longer than 6 months have consistently reported a decrease in symptoms and BHR (Table 33.4).[13,36,54,120,121] In addition, an excellent controlled trial of mite avoidance in the treatment of atopic dermatitis reported highly significant improvement in symptoms and skin rash.[122]

Current views on mite avoidance are based on the results of the successful controlled trials and detailed studies on specific measures.[13] Avoidance measures can be divided into those in the bedroom and those for the rest of the house (Box 33.2). In the bedroom, covering mattresses and pillows with impermeable covers is effective; washing bedding at 130°F once weekly is effective; and removing carpets is more effective in

Table 33.4 Controlled trials of allergen avoidance achieving prolonged decrease in mite allergen

Study	Duration	Avoidance	n	Decrease in mite allergen	Primary outcome(s)
Murray and Ferguson (1983)[d]	1 year	Physical barriers	10/10	++	BHR[a]
Carswell et al (1996)[e]	6 month	Physical barriers and Acarosan	24/25	+	PEFR,[b] BHR
Ehnert et al (1992)[120]	1 year	Physical barriers and tannic acid	8/16	++	BHR[a]
Walshaw and Evans (1986)[f]	1 year	Physical barriers	22/20	++	PEFR/BHR[a]
Htut et al (2001)[121]	12 months	Heat treatment	10/10/10	++	BHR[c]
Morgan et al (2004)[143]	12 months	Multiple measures	425/441	++	Symptoms[a]

BHR, bronchial hyperreactivity; PEFR, peak expiratory flow rate.
[a]Highly significant improvement.
[b]Improvement, but not significant.
[c]Significant improvement.
[d]Murray AB, Ferguson AC. Dust-free bedrooms in the treatment of asthmatic children with house dust or house dust mite allergy: a controlled trial. Pediatrics 1983; 71:418.
[e]Carswell F, Birmingham K, Oliver J, et al. The respiratory effects of reduction of mite allergy in the bedrooms of asthmatic children – a double-blind controlled trial. Clin Exp Allergy 1996; 26:386.
[f]Walshaw MJ, Evans CC. Allergen avoidance in house-dust mite sensitive adult asthma. Q J Med 1986; 58:199.

BOX 33.2 AVOIDANCE MEASURES FOR MITE ALLERGENS

Bedrooms
1. Cover mattresses and pillows with impermeable covers.*
2. Wash bedding regularly at 130°F.
3. Remove carpets, stuffed animals, and clutter from bedroom.
4. Vacuum weekly (wearing a mask) using vacuum cleaner with double-thickness bag or high-efficiency particulate air (HEPA) filter.

Rest of house
1. Minimize carpets† and upholstered furniture.
2. Reduce humidity below 45% relative humidity (or 6 g H_2O/kg air).
3. Treat carpets with benzyl benzoate or tannic acid.

*For pillow cases or duvets, covers should be 'fine woven'; for mattress covers, plastic or other impermeable fabric can be used together with a mattress 'pad'.
†Carpets on unventilated floors (e.g., in basements) are difficult to keep dry.

BOX 33.3 AVOIDANCE MEASURES FOR CAT ALLERGENS

Remove cat from the house.*

Measures to reduce allergen with cat in situ
1. Reduce reservoirs for cat allergen (e.g., carpets, sofas).
2. Use vacuum cleaners with effective filtration system.
3. Increase ventilation or use air filtration (HEPA) to remove small air-borne particles.
4. Wash cat weekly; if possible.

*Reducing allergen levels requires about 12–16 weeks after cat is removed.

the long term than any currently available carpet cleaning measure.[121–124] The remaining details for the bedroom are designed to eliminate sites where mites can grow and to reduce dust collectors so as to make cleaning easier. In the remainder of the house, the greatest problem is with carpets and sofas. Three different approaches are possible, as follows:

1. Designing the house with polished floors and wooden or vinyl/leather furniture so as to limit the sites where mites can grow.
2. Controlling humidity so that indoor relative humidity is kept below 50% (absolute humidity below 6 g/kg). In some areas of the world this can be done by increasing ventilation; in other areas it is necessary to use air conditioning during the most humid months of the summer. In temperate climates, whole-house dehumidification can effectively control mite growth.[125] However, air conditioning as a routine measure is too expensive to be realistic in subtropical areas such as Florida, the Gulf Coast, or Brazil.
3. Chemical treatment of carpets and furniture to control mite growth or denature mite allergens. A variety of acaricides have been used to treat carpets or furniture, including pyrethroids, natamycin (an antifungal), pirimiphos methyl, and benzyl benzoate.[13] In each case the chemicals are effective in killing mites, so the problem is to achieve sufficient effect in a carpet. In addition to acaricides, 1% or 3% tannic acid has been recommended as a method of denaturing mite allergens.[123] Again, reduction of mite allergen can be achieved, but tannic acid does not kill mites, so the effect can only be temporary, approximately 6 weeks to 3 months. Either benzyl benzoate powder or 3% tannic acid for carpets and sofas may be recommended when it is not possible to remove the carpets or change the furniture.

A special problem is posed by carpets fitted onto unventilated floors, as in basements or the ground floor of houses built on concrete slabs.[37] Under these circumstances, water can accumulate either because of condensation onto the cold surface of the concrete or because of leakage (either domestic or rain water from outside). In either case, once the carpet is wet, it will stay wet, and if the temperature rises, it will become an excellent environment for the growth of both fungi and mites. Using measurement of allergen in the carpets or in the air during disturbance, several treatments produced 60–90% reduction of mite levels in a basement, but the residual levels were still well above the levels in comparable rooms with a polished floor.[123]

DOMESTIC ANIMALS

Traditional wisdom is that removing the cat is the only effective way to control exposure to cat allergen.[126] However, it is usually difficult to persuade a family to give away their cat. Removal of the cat(s) from a home leads to progressive reductions in the concentration of Fel d 1 in the house, although it may take as long as 4 months for the levels in carpet dust to fall below 8 μg/g.[123] Thus, it is not surprising that most cat allergic patients develop symptoms when they move into a house where a cat had resided. Keeping the cat outdoors is an alternative and will reduce cat allergen; however, if the family plays with the cat, there is likely to be significant allergen brought into the house by passive transfer. On the other hand, some patients maintain that cats do not cause symptoms if they have polished floors and air filtration and wash the cat regularly. The possibility that washing a cat is helpful was first suggested by experiments showing that the recovery of allergen from a cat decreased progressively with regular washing.[55] Detailed experiments on cats showed that the combination of polished floors, air filtration, vacuum cleaning, and regular washing of the cat could dramatically reduce air-borne cat allergen (Box 33.3).[56]

Subsequent experiments were not as successful and it now appears that it would be necessary to wash the cat twice a week in order to maintain a decrease in air-borne allergen. Nonetheless, washing a cat can remove 5–30 mg of Fel d 1 and this may be an effective method of decreasing accumulation of cat allergen in the house. Up to 40% of air-borne cat allergen is associated with particles that are similar in size to those generated by a nebulizer which makes it possible to make comparisons between natural exposure and bronchial provocation. Inhaling 10 ng of Fel d 1 on droplets of approximately 2 μm in diameter in a provocation experiment will produce a measurable fall in 1-s forced expiratory volume (FEV_1) in sensitive patients.[127] Thus, if such a patient was in a house with an air-borne level of 40 ng/m^3, the onset of lung symptoms would be predicted to occur within 15 min. If this level were reduced to ≤2 ng/m^3 (which appears to be possible), the same dose would be inhaled in approximately 5 h. Thus, measurement of air-borne cat allergen could theoretically be used as a true index of exposure, although these measurements are technically difficult. At present, reservoir measurements remain the standard for assessing both exposure and the effectiveness of avoidance measures.

Avoidance measures for dogs appear to be similar in general to those for cats: that is, keeping the dog out of the house and controlling accumulation in reservoirs. In addition, using HEPA room filters and washing the animal have each been shown to decrease air-borne dog allergen.[65]

COCKROACH AND OTHER ALLERGENS

For most other allergens, there are only case reports of benefit from avoidance measures. For domestic or wild rodents, the measures are obvious, and the primary problems may be persuading the family to admit to the presence of a caged animal or agree to remove it. Although the best-recognized source of allergens related to inner-city asthma is the German cockroach, other allergens are also important. In Atlanta (Georgia), Delaware, and Charlottesville (Virginia), both dust mite and cockroach allergens were shown to be significant to patients residing in the poorest areas of the town, which is probably true throughout the south and south-east.[19,23,29,79] In the mid-west and north-east, mice and rats may also be an important source of allergens, and skin testing with rodent extracts should be routine in clinics that treat patients living in these cities.

Avoidance measures for cockroach allergens have been shown to be effective when applied as part of an overall avoidance plan.[29,128] The primary strategies are: (1) poison bait, (2) careful housekeeping to enclose all sources of food for the insects, (3) cleaning to remove any accumulated allergen, and (4) sealing all possible access points to the house. Bait for killing cockroaches ranges from boric acid, which can kill mites by damaging the foregut, to a variety of chemicals including hydramethylnon, abamectin, and fipronil.[128] Baits can be applied as traps or as paste. Spraying with insecticides is generally ineffective and has the additional problem that the volatile organic substances used are often irritating to patients with asthma.

For indoor fungi, the situation is confusing. It is not clear that spore counts are consistent from day to day or that they relate to allergen exposure.[129,130] Simple assays for allergens derived from *Aspergillus* (Asp f 1) and *Alternaria* (Alt a 1) have been developed, but the use of these assays to measure allergens derived from these fungi indoors has been disappointing. Many spores are not viable, and some allergens may only be expressed after the spore germinates.[131] Thus, it is very difficult to evaluate proposed procedures to reduce fungal allergen exposure. Carpet dust usually contains fungal spores, and carpets can become overtly mildewed. However, conditions in a carpet that would be optimal for mite growth (i.e., 75% relative humidity) are still dry for mold spore germination. At present, it is reasonable to recommend controlling humidity, removing sites for fungal growth, avoiding basements, and cleaning surfaces with fungicides. Accurate methods for evaluating fungal exposures indoors are still needed.

Although the importance of bacteria as a source of allergens is generally discounted, this is largely because of the lack of good evidence in favor of the concept rather than clear evidence against their role. By contrast, extensive evidence shows that endotoxins produced by Gram-negative bacteria can influence allergic disease. The endotoxins produced by bacteria are a complex group of lipids. Most available data relate to measurements inside houses and from buildings using the *Limulus amoebocyte* assay, which is a non-specific assay for endotoxin.[132,133] In different studies, endotoxin has been proposed to reduce or increase allergic disease. In farming villages, children who are exposed to cow barns early

in life appear to be protected against both sensitization and asthma. In keeping with this, children raised in houses with high levels of endotoxin had lower prevalence of sensitization to allergen.[133] However, the 'high' levels of endotoxin in houses in the USA are much lower than the levels reported from bedrooms of farm houses in southern Germany or Austria.[133] In complete contrast, a series of studies from Belgium found that endotoxin exposure in the homes of mite-allergic children predicts the severity of asthma better than mite exposure.[134] The mechanisms of these positive and negative effects of endotoxin are not known, but evidence suggests that polymorphisms of the endotoxin receptor influence allergic responses. Cows are certainly not the only animals that produce large quantities of endotoxin. Some studies suggest that the paradoxical effects of domestic animals could be caused by an increase in endotoxin. However, direct measurements of air-borne endotoxin in homes with cats have not confirmed this.[108,109] Exposure to endotoxin or some other bacterial products probably influences the onset of allergic disease (decrease) and the symptoms of established disease (increase).[134,135]

Air coming into the house from outside can carry either pollen grains or fungal spores into the house. With fungal spores found inside the house, it is often difficult to tell whether they arise from inside or outside the house because many species can grow in either environment.[136] For pollen grains, the source is obvious. During the spring in Virginia, it is not unusual to see large numbers of very distinctive (but probably non-allergenic) pine pollen grains in house dust. More significant, in areas such as northern California or Oregon, grass pollen can become a major component of house dust and has been found in high levels in dust from the houses of grass pollen-sensitive patients with asthma.[37,137] Controlling entry of pollens could be achieved by filtering incoming air, but very few domestic houses have a defined site of entry for outside air. Keeping doors and windows closed will decrease the amount of outside air and pollen or fungal spores entering the house. Certainly, pollen-allergic individuals should be advised not to have a window fan blowing into their bedroom, which can maintain outdoor levels of pollen exposure all night.

■ IMMUNE RESPONSES TO ALLERGENS FROM DIFFERENT SOURCES ■

The first suggestion that all allergens are not created equal came from the finding that children raised in a house with a cat were less likely to be sensitized to cat allergens. This observation was confirmed in several studies and extended to dogs. Several explanations were proposed including parental choice not to keep animals, the effect of domestic animals on endotoxin, and the induction of tolerance by Fel d 1. More recently, it had become clear that many children and adults raised in a house with a cat have made an IgG and IgG4 ab response to Fel d 1 without becoming allergic.[106] This response has been called a 'modified Th2 response' because the expression of the gene for IgG4 is dependent on the Th2 cytokine IL-4. Initially, we proposed that cat and dog allergens should be regarded as a separate class of indoor allergens. We would now put this together with evidence that a similar response can occur in animal handlers who are exposed to high levels of mouse or rat allergens.[71–73] This leads to the hypothesis that the immune response to

Table 33.5 Differences between mammalian and non-mammalian allergens that could be relevant to the immune response

	Mammalian	**Non-mammalian**
Allergen source	Cat, dogs, mice, etc.	Mite, cockroach, grass, trees, and, fungi
Size of air-borne particles	Small (2–15 µm)	Large (10–30 µm)
Exposure	Air-borne continuously 0.2–1 µg/day	Air-borne with disturbance 1–10 ng/day
Specific proteins	Not enzymes	Often enzymes
	Fel d1 (CSSP, uteroglobulin)	Der p 1 (cysteine protease)
	Can f 1	Der p 2 (no homology)
Tolerance, i.e., IgG ab without sensitization	Common among children raised with high exposure	Rare

mammalian allergens is different from the response to insect-, acarid-, or plant-derived proteins (Table 33.5).[138,139] There are many differences between different groups of allergens. All estimates show that exposure to allergens derived from mammalian dander is *higher* than for other allergens. Nonetheless, these allergens are associated with *lower* prevalence, and lower titer of, IgE ab.

Dust mite exposure differs from cat exposure in several additional ways: first, the proteins of mites are more foreign as judged by evolutionary distance; second, the DNA of mites, but not cats, is unmethylated and would therefore stimulate Toll-like receptor 9 (TLR9); third, the carbohydrate determinants on mammalian proteins differ from those on non-mammalian proteins; and finally, mite fecal particles also contain both endotoxin and DNA derived from bacteria. From this list, it is clear that the explanation for the different responses to these allergens is not likely to be simple. However, the differences may have important epidemiological effects. The prevalence and severity of asthma is lower in those countries where cat exposure is the primary source of allergens as compared to those countries where high concentrations of mite allergens are common.[139]

■ CONCLUSIONS ■

The evidence that asthma, rhinitis, and atopic dermatitis are inflammatory diseases in which a major cause of the inflammation is exposure to indoor allergens is now overwhelming.[140–142] The logical conclusion is that controlling exposure to these foreign proteins should be a first-line antiinflammatory treatment for diseases related to indoor allergens.[143] All models used to study the mechanisms of inflammation in the human lung use allergen challenge of allergic patients to induce influx of inflammatory cells into the lung. The evidence for an increase in asthma is unequivocal, but it appears that this increase has been associated with many different indoor allergen: i.e., dust mite in NZ, Australia, UK, and southern States of the USA; cat and dog in Scandinavia and the mountain states; and cockroach in the American inner city.[142] For the increase in asthma to be attributed to increased exposure, one would have to propose that several different allergens had increased in parallel. Many authors find this difficult to believe.

The alternative explanation is that, in addition to spending more time indoors, some other aspect of modern civilization has increased the immunologic, inflammatory, or physiologic response to indoor allergens. The possible candidates are dietary changes, extensive use of broadspectrum antibiotics in children, and dramatic decreases in outdoor physical activity that have accompanied the increase in indoor entertainment.[144,145] However, none of these changes alone are thought to give rise to asthma and they would need to act selectively on children who were allergic to indoor allergens.

References

History

1. Kern RA. Dust sensitization in bronchial asthma. Med Clin North Am 1921; 5:751.
2. Spivacke CA, Grove EF. Studies in hypersensitiveness. XIV. A study of the atopen in house dust. J Immunol 1925; 10:465.
3. Voorhorst R, Spieksma FTM, Varekamp H, et al. The house-dust mite (Dermatophagoides pteronyssinus) and the allergens it produces: identity with the house-dust allergen. J Allergy 1967; 39:325.
4. Kerrebijn KF. Endogenous factors in childhood CNSLD: methodological aspects in population studies. In: Orie NG, van der Lende R, eds. Bronchitis, Vol III. The Netherlands: Royal Vangorcum Assen; 1970:38.
5. Smith JM, Disney ME, Williams JD, et al. Clinical significance of skin reactions to mite extracts in children with asthma. Br Med J 1969; 1:723.
6. Miyamoto T, Oshima S, Ishizaka T, et al. Allergenic identity between the common floor mite (Dermatophagoides farinae Hughes, 1961) and house dust as a causative antigen in bronchial asthma. J Allergy 1968; 42:14–28.
7. Sporik R, Holgate ST, Platts-Mills TA, et al. Exposure to house-dust mite allergen (Der p I) and the development of asthma in childhood: a prospective study. N Engl J Med 1990; 323:502.
8. Peat JK, Tovey E, Toelle BG, et al. House-dust mite allergens: a major risk factor for childhood asthma in Australia. Am J Respir Crit Care Med 1996; 153:141.
9. Ohman JL Jr. Lowell FC, Bloch KJ. Allergens of mammalian origin. III. Properties of a major feline allergen. J Immunol 1974; 113:1668.
10. Chapman MD, Platts-Mills TA. Purification and characterization of the major allergen from Dermatophagoides pteronyssinus-antigen P1. J Immunol 1980; 125:587.
11. Tovey ER, Chapman MD, Wells CW, et al. The distribution of dust mite allergen in the houses of patients with asthma. Am Rev Respir Dis 1981; 124:630.
12. Luczynska CM, Arruda LK, Platts-Mills TA, et al. A two-site monoclonal antibody ELISA for the quantification of the major Dermatophagoides spp. allergens, Der p I and Der f I. J Immunol Methods 1989; 118:227.
13. Platts-Mills TA, Vaughan JW, Carter MC, et al. The role of intervention in established allergy: avoidance of indoor allergens in the treatment of chronic allergic disease. J Allergy Clin Immunol 2000; 106:787.
14. Chua KY, Stewart GA, Thomas WR, et al. Sequence analysis of cDNA coding for a major house-dust mite allergen, Der p 1: homology with cysteine proteases. J Exp Med 1988; 167:175.
15. Morgenstern JP, Griffith IJ, Bauer AW, et al. Amino acid sequence of Fel d I, the major allergen of the domestic cat: protein sequence analysis and cDNA cloning. Proc Natl Acad Sci U S A 1991; 88:9690.
16. Arruda LK, Vailes LD, Mann BJ, et al. Molecular cloning of a major cockroach (Blatella germanica) allergen, Bla g 2: sequence homology to the aspartic proteases. J Biol Chem 1995; 270:19563.
17. Chapman MD, Pomes A, Breiteneder H, et al. Nomenclature and structural biology of allergens. J Allergy Clin Immunol 2007; 119:414–420.

Relevance to allergic diseases

18. Pollart SM, Chapman MD, Fiocco GP, et al. Epidemiology of acute asthma: IgE antibodies to common inhalant allergens as a risk factor for emergency room visits. J Allergy Clin Immunol 1989; 83:875.
19. Gelber LE, Seltzer LH, Bouzoukis JK, et al. Sensitization and exposure to indoor allergens as risk factors for asthma among patients presenting to hospital. Am Rev Resp Dis 1993; 147:573.
20. Sears MR, Herbison GP, Holdaway MD, et al. The relative risks of sensitivity to grass pollen, house-dust mite and cat dander in the development of childhood asthma. Clin Exp Allergy 1989; 19:419.
21. Rönmark E, Lundbäck B, Jönsson E, et al. Asthma, type-1 allergy and related conditions in 7- and 8-year-old children in northern Sweden: prevalence rates and risk factor pattern. Respir Med 1998; 92:316.
22. Illi S, von Mutius E, Lau S, et al; Multicentre Allergy Study (MAS) group. Perennial allergen sensitisation early in life and chronic asthma in children: a birth cohort study. Lancet 2006; 368:763–770.
23. Call RS, Smith TF, Morris E, et al. Risk factors for asthma in inner city children. J Pediatr 1992; 121:862.
24. Halonen M, Stern DA, Wright AL, et al. Alternaria as a major allergen for asthma in children raised in a desert environment. Am J Respir Crit Care Med 1997; 155:1356.
25. Sporik R, Ingram JM, Price W, et al. Association of asthma with serum IgE and skin test reactivity to allergens among children living at high altitude: tickling the dragon's breath. Am J Respir Crit Care Med 1995; 151:1388.
26. Mitchell EB, Crow J, Rowntree S, et al. Cutaneous basophil hypersensitivity to inhalant allergens in atopic dermatitis patients: elicitation of delayed responses containing basophils following local transfer of immune serum but not IgE antibody. J Invest Dermatol 1984; 83:290.
27. Scalabrin DM, Bavbek S, Perzanowski MS, et al. Use of specific IgE in assessing the relevance of fungal and dust mite allergens to atopic dermatitis: a comparison with asthmatic and nonasthmatic control subjects. J Allergy Clin Immunol 1999; 104:1273.
28. Kang B, Vellody D, Homburger H, et al. Cockroach cause of allergic asthma: its specificity and immunologic profile. J Allergy Clin Immunol 1979; 63:80.
29. Carter MC, Perzanowski MS, Raymond A, et al. Home intervention in the treatment of asthma among inner-city children. J Allergy Clin Immunol 2001; 108:732.
30. Rosenstreich DL, Eggleston P, Kattan M, et al. The role of cockroach allergy and exposure to cockroach allergen in causing morbidity among inner-city children with asthma. N Engl J Med 1997; 336:1356.
31. Gruchalla RS, Pongracic J, Plaut M, et al. Inner city asthma study: relationships among sensitivity, allergen exposure, and asthma morbidity. J Allergy Clin Immunol 2005; 115:479–485.
32. Custovic A, Green R, Taggart SC, et al. Domestic allergens in public places. II: Dog (Can f 1) and cockroach (Bla g 2) allergens in dust and mite, cat, dog and cockroach allergens in the air in public buildings. Clin Exp Allergy 1996; 26:1246–1252.

Sources of indoor antigens

33. Hughes AM. The mites of stored food and houses. London: Her Majesty's Stationery Office, 1976.
34. Van Hage-Hamsten M, Johansson SG, Hoglund S, et al. Storage mite allergy is common in a farming population. Clin Allergy 1985; 15:555.
35. Wharton GW. House-dust mites. J Med Entomol 1976; 12:577.
36. Platts-Mills TA, Vervloet D, Thomas WR, et al. Indoor allergens and asthma: report of the Third International Workshop. J Allergy Clin Immunol 1997; 100:S2.
37. Platts-Mills TA, Hayden ML, Chapman MD, et al. Seasonal variation in dust mite and grass-pollen allergens in dust from the houses of patients with asthma. J Allergy Clin Immunol 1987; 79:781.
38. Tovey ER, Chapman MD, Platts-Mills TA. Mite faeces are a major source of house-dust allergen. Nature 1981; 289:592.
39. Arlian LG, Bernstein D, Bernstein IL, et al. Prevalence of dust mites in the homes of people with asthma living in eight different geographical areas of the United States. J Allergy Clin Immunol 1992; 90:292.
40. Stewart GA, Thompson PJ. The biochemistry of common aeroallergens. Clin Exp Allergy 1996; 26:1020.
41. Hewitt CR, Brown AP, Hart BJ, et al. A major house-dust mite allergen disrupts the immunoglobulin E network by selectively cleaving CD23: innate protection by antiproteases. J Exp Med 1995; 182:1537.
42. Schulz O, Sewell HF, Shakib F. Proteolytic cleavage of CD-25, the alpha subunit of the human T cell interleukin 2 receptor, by Der p 1, a major mite allergen with cysteine protease activity. J Exp Med 1998; 187:271.
43. Wan H, Winton HL, Soeller C, et al. Quantitative structural and biochemical analyses of tight junction dynamics following exposure of epithelial cells to house-dust mite allergen Der p 1. Clin Exp Allergy 2000; 30:685.
44. Lind P. Purification and partial characterization of two major allergens from the house-dust mite Dermatophagoides pteronyssinus. J Allergy Clin Immunol 1985; 76:753.
45. Heymann PW, Chapman MD, Aalberse RC, et al. Antigenic and structural analysis of group II allergens (Der f II and Der p II) from house-dust mites (Dermatophagoides spp). J Allergy Clin Immunol 1989; 83:1055.
46. Yuuki T, Okumura Y, Ando T, et al. Cloning and sequencing of cDNAs corresponding to mite major allergen Der f II. Jpn J Allergol 1990; 39:557.
47. Smith AM, Benjamin DC, Hozic N, et al. The molecular basis of antigenic cross-reactivity between the group 2 mite allergens. J Allergy Clin Immunol 2001; 107:977.
48. Chapman MD, Vailes LD, Ichikawa K. Immunoassays for indoor allergens. Clin Rev Allergy Immunol 2000; 18:285.
49. Arruda LK, Vailes LD, Platts-Mills TA, et al. Sensitization to Blomia tropicalis in patients with asthma and identification of allergen Blo t 5. Am J Respir Crit Care Med 1997; 155:343.
50. Trivedi B, Valerio C, Slater JE. Endotoxin content of standardized allergen vaccines. J Allergy Clin Immunol 2003; 111:77–83.
51. Chapman MD, Aalberse RC, Brown MJ, et al. Monoclonal antibodies to the major feline allergen Fel d I. II. Single step affinity purification of Fel d I, N-terminal sequence analysis, and development of a sensitive two-site immunoassay to assess Fel d I exposure. J Immunol 1988; 140:812.
52. Charpin C, Mata P, Charpin D, et al. Fel d I allergen distribution in cat fur and skin. J Allergy Clin Immunol 1991; 88:77.
53. Wang SZ, Rosenberger CL, Espindola TM, et al. CCSP modulates airway dysfunction and host responses in an ova-challenged mouse model. Am J Physiol Lung Cell Mol Physiol 2001; 281:L1303.
54. Ichikawa K, Iwasaki E, Baba M, et al. High prevalence of sensitization to cat allergen among Japanese children with asthma, living without cats. Clin Exp Allergy 1999; 29:754.
55. Ohman JL, Baer H, Anderson MC, et al. Surface washes of living cats: an improved method of obtaining clinically relevant allergen. J Allergy Clin Immunol 1983; 72:288.
56. De Blay F, Chapman MD, Platts-Mills TA. Air-borne cat allergen (Fel d I): environmental control with the cat in situ. Am Rev Respir Dis 1991; 143:1334.
57. Avner DB, Perzanowski MS, Platts-Mills TA, et al. Evaluation of different techniques for washing cats: quantitation of allergen removed from the cat and the effect on airborne Fel d 1. J Allergy Clin Immunol 1997; 100:307.
58. Klucka CV, Ownby DR, Green J, et al. Cat shedding of Fel d 1 is not reduced by washings, Allerpet-C spray, or acepromazine. J Allergy Clin Immunol 1995; 95:1164.
59. Ingram JM, Sporik R, Rose G, et al. Quantitative assessment of exposure to dog (Can f 1) and cat (Fel d 1) allergens: relationship to sensitization and asthma among children living in Los Alamos, NM. J Allergy Clin Immunol 1995; 96:449.
60. Remes ST, Castro-Rodriguez JA, Holberg CJ, et al. Dog exposure in infancy decreases the subsequent risk of frequent wheeze but not of atopy. J Allergy Clin Immunol 2001; 108:509.
61. Wood RA, Eggleston PA, Lind P, et al. Antigenic analysis of household dust samples. Am Rev Respir Dis 1988; 137:358.
62. Munir AK, Einarsson R, Dreborg SK. Indirect contact with pets can confound the effect of cleaning procedures for reduction of animal allergen levels in house dust. Pediatr Allergy Immunol 1994; 5:32.
63. Perzanowski MS, Ronmark E, Nold B, et al. Relevance of allergens from cats and dogs to asthma in the northernmost province of Sweden: schools as a major site of exposure. J Allergy Clin Immunol 1999; 103:1018.
64. Almqvist C, Larsson PH, Wickman M, et al. School as a risk environment for children allergic to cats and a site for transfer of cat allergens to homes. J Allergy Clin Immunol 1999; 103:1012.
65. Custovic A, Green R, Fletcher A, et al. Aerodynamic properties of the major dog allergen, Can f 1: distribution in homes, concentration and particle size of allergens in the air. Am J Respir Crit Care Med 1997; 155:94.
66. Cockcroft A, Edwards J, McCarthy P, et al. Allergy in laboratory animal workers. Lancet 1981; 1:827.
67. Sjostedt L, Willers S. Predisposing factors in laboratory animal allergy: a study of atopy and environmental factors. Am J Ind Med 1989; 16:199.
68. Platts-Mills TA, Longbottom J, Edwards J, et al. Occupational asthma and rhinitis related to laboratory rats: serum IgG and IgE antibodies to rat urinary allergen. J Allergy Clin Immunol 1987; 79:505.
69. Wood RA. Laboratory animal allergens. ILAR J 2001; 42:12.
70. Phipatanakul W, Eggleston PA, Wright EC, et al. Mouse allergen. II. The relationship of mouse allergen exposure to mouse sensitization and asthma morbidity in inner-city children with asthma. J Allergy Clin Immunol 2000; 106:1075.
71. Platts-Mills TAE, Naccara L, Satinover SM, et al. Prevalence and titer of IgE antibodies to mouse allergens. J Allergy Clin Immunol 2007; 120:1058–1064.
72. Matsui EC, Diette GB, Krop EJ, et al. Mouse allergen specific immunoglobulin G and immunoglobulin G4 and allergic symptoms in immunoglobulin E-sensitized laboratory animal workers. Clin Exp Allergy 2005; 35:1347.
73. Jeal H, Draper A, Harris J, et al. Modified Th2 responses at high-dose exposures to allergen: using an occupational model. Am J Respir Crit Care Med 2006; 174:21.
74. Koshte VL, Kagen SL, Aalberse RC. Cross-reactivity of IgE antibodies to caddis fly with Arthropoda and Mollusca. J Allergy Clin Immunol 1989; 84:174.
75. Twarog FJ, Picone FJ, Strunk RS, et al. Immediate hypersensitivity to cockroach: isolation and purification of the major antigens. J Allergy Clin Immunol 1977; 59:154.
76. Pollart SM, Smith TF, Morris EC, et al. Environmental exposure to cockroach allergens: analysis with monoclonal antibody-based enzyme immunoassays. J Allergy Clin Immunol 1991; 87:505.
77. Kang BC, Wilson M, Price KH, et al. Cockroach-allergen study: allergen patterns of three common cockroach species probed by allergic sera collected in two cities. J Allergy Clin Immunol 1991; 87:1073.
78. Swanson MC, Agarwal MK, Reed CE. An immunochemical approach to indoor aeroallergen quantitation with a new volumetric air sampler: studies with mite, roach, cat, mouse, and guinea-pig antigens. J Allergy Clin Immunol 1985; 76:724.
79. Platts-Mills TA, Sporik RB, Chapman MD, et al. The role of domestic allergens. In: CIBA eds. The rising trends in asthma. London: CIBA Foundation, 1996.
80. Mollet JA, Vailes LD, Avner DB, et al. Evaluation of German cockroach (Orthoptera: Blattellidae) allergen and seasonal variation in low-income housing. J Med Entomol 1997; 34:307.
81. De Blay F, Sanchez J, Hedelin G, et al. Dust and air-borne exposure to allergens derived from cockroach (Blatella germanica) in low-cost public housing in Strasbourg (France). J Allergy Clin Immunol 1997; 99:107.
82. Yarbrough JA, Armstrong JL, Blumberg MZ, et al. Allergic rhinoconjunctivitis caused by Harmonia axyridis (Asian lady beetle, Japanese lady beetle, or lady bug). J Allergy Clin Immunol 1999; 104:704.

83. Nakazawa T, Satinover SM, Naccara L, et al. Asian ladybugs (Harmonia axyridis): a new seasonal indoor allergen. J Allergy Clin Immunol 2007; 119:421.
84. Albright DD, Jordan-Wagner D, Napoli DC, et al. Multicolored Asian lady beetle hypersensitivity: a case series and allergist survey. Ann Allergy Asthma Immunol 97:521, 2006.
85. Sharma K, Muldoon SB, Potter MF, et al. Ladybug hypersensitivity among residents of homes infested with ladybugs in Kentucky. Ann Allergy Asthma Immunol 2006; 97:521.

Molecular biology

86. Kikuchi Y, Takai T, Kuhara T, et al. Crucial commitment of proteolytic activity of a purified recombinant major house-dust mite allergen Der p 1 to sensitization toward IgE and IgG responses. J Immunol 2006; 177:1609.
87. Kaiser L, Gronlund H, Sandalova T, et al. The crystal structure of the major cat allergen Fel d 1, a member of the secretoglobin family. J Biol Chem 2003; 278:37730–37735.
88. Jarnicki AG, Tsuji T, Thomas WR Inhibition of mucosal and systemic T(h)2-type immune responses by intranasal peptides containing a dominant T cell epitope of the allergen Der p 1. Int Immunol 2001; 13:1223.
89. Oldfield WL, Kay AB, Larche M. Allergen-derived T cell peptide-induced late asthmatic reactions precede the induction of antigen-specific hyporesponsiveness in atopic allergic asthmatic subjects. J Immunol 2001; 167:1734.
90. Woodfolk JA, Platts-Mills TA. Diversity of the human allergen-specific T cell repertoire associated with distinct skin test reactions: delayed-type hypersensitivity-associated major epitopes induce Th1- and Th2-dominated responses. J Immunol 2001; 167:5412.
91. Norman PS, Ohman JL Jr, Long AA, et al. Treatment of cat allergy with T-cell reactive peptides. Am J Respir Crit Care Med 1996; 154:1623.
92. Haselden BM, Kay AB, Larche M. Immunoglobulin E-independent major histocompatibility complex-restricted T cell peptide epitope-induced late asthmatic reactions. J Exp Med 1999; 189:185.
93. Reefer AJ, Carneiro RM, Custis NJ, et al. A role of IL-10 mediated HLA-DR7 restricted T cell-dependent events in development of the modified Th2 response to cat allergen. J Immunol 2004; 172:2763–2772.
94. Shoji H, Shibuya I, Hirai M, et al. Production of recombinant Der f 1 with the native IgE-binding activity using a baculovirus expression system. Biosci Biotechnol Biochem 1997; 61:1668.
95. Smith AM, Chapman MD, Taketomi EA, et al. Recombinant allergens for immunotherapy: a Der p 2 variant with reduced IgE reactivity retains T-cell epitopes. J Allergy Clin Immunol 1998; 101:423.

Indoor allergen exposure and desensitization or disease

96. Dowse GK, Turner KJ, Stewart GA, et al. The association between Dermatophagoides mites and the increasing prevalence of asthma in village communities within the Papua New Guinea highlands. J Allergy Clin Immunol 1985; 75:75.
97. Platts-Mills TA, Tovey ER, Mitchell EB, et al. Reduction of bronchial hyperreactivity during prolonged allergen avoidance. Lancet 1982; 2:675.
98. Kuehr J, Frischer T, Meinert R, et al. Mite exposure is a risk factor for the incidence of specific sensitization. J Allergy Clin Immunol 1994; 94:44.
99. Charpin D, Birnbaum J, Haddi E, et al. Altitude and allergy to house-dust mites: a paradigm of the influence of environmental exposure on allergic sensitization. Am Rev Respir Dis 1991; 143:983.
100. Sporik R, Squillace SP, Ingram JM, et al. Mite, cat and cockroach exposure, allergen sensitization and asthma in children: a case-control study of three schools. Thorax 1999; 54:675.
101. Bollinger ME, Eggleston PA, Flanagan E, et al. Cat antigen in homes with and without cats may induce allergic symptoms. J Allergy Clin Immunol 1996; 97:907.
102. Hesselmar B, Aberg N, Aberg B, et al. Does early exposure to cat or dog protect against later allergen development? Clin Exp Allergy 1999; 29:611.
103. Rönmark E, Jönsson E, Platts-Mills T, et al. Incidence and remission of asthma in schoolchildren: report from the obstructive lung disease in northern Sweden studies. Pediatrics 2001; 107:E37.
104. Perzanowski MS, Rönmark E, Platts-Mills TA, et al. Effect of cat and dog ownership on sensitization and development of asthma among preteenage children. Am J Respir Crit Care Med 2002; 166:696.
105. Platts-Mills TA, Perzanowski M, Woodfolk JA, et al. Relevance of early or current pet ownership to the prevalence of allergic disease. Clin Exp Allergens 2002; 32:335.
106. Platts-Mills TA, Vaughan J, Squillace S, et al. Sensitization, asthma and a modified Th2 response in children exposed to cat allergen: a population-based cross-sectional study. Lancet 2001; 357:752.

Air-borne indoor allergens

107. Luczynska CM, Li Y, Chapman MD, et al. Air-borne concentrations and particle size distribution of allergen derived from domestic cats (Felis domesticus): measurements using cascade impactor, liquid impinger and a two-site monoclonal antibody assay for Fel d I. Am Rev Resp Dis 1990; 141:361.
108. Custis NJ, Woodfolk JA, Vaughan JW, et al. Quantitative measurement of air-borne allergens from dust mites, dogs, and cats using an ion-charging device. Clin Exp Allergy 2003; 33:986–991.
109. Sohy C, Lieutier-Colas F, Cassett A, et al. Dust and airborne endotoxin exposure in dwellings in the Strasbourg metropolitan area (France). Allergy 2005; 60:541–542.

110. Rabinovitch N, Liu AH, Zhang L, et al. Importance of the personal endotoxin cloud in school-age children with asthma. J Allergy Clin Immunol 2005; 116:1053–1057.
111. De Blay F, Heymann PW, Chapman MD, et al. Airborne dust mite allergens: comparison of group II allergens with group I mite allergen and cat-allergen Fel d I. J Allergy Clin Immunol 1991; 88:919.
112. Bates DV, Fish BR, Hatch DF, et al. Deposition and retention models for internal dosimetry of the human respiratory tract. Task group on lung dynamics. Health Phys 1966; 12:173.
113. Svartengren M, Falk R, Linnman L, et al. Deposition of large particles in human lung. Exp Lung Res 1987; 12:75.
114. Razmovski V, O'Meara TJ, Taylor DJ, et al. A new method for simultaneous immunodetection and morphologic identification of individual sources of pollen allergens. J Allergy Clin Immunol 2000; 105:725.
115. Platts-Mills JA, Custis NJ, Woodfolk JA, et al. Air-borne endotoxin in homes with domestic animals: implications for cat specific tolerance. J Allergy Clin Immunol 2005; 116:384.

Avoidance measures for indoor allergens

116. Storm van Leeuwen W, Einthoven W, Kremer W. The allergen-proof chamber in the treatment of bronchial asthma and other respiratory diseases. Lancet 1927; i:1287.
117. Rost GA. Ueber erfagrungen mit der allergenfreien kammer nach Storm van Leeuwen: insbesondere n der spatperiode der exsudativen diasthese. Arch Dermatol Syphilis 1932; 155:297.
118. Wood RA, Flanagan E, Van Natta M, et al. The effect of a HEPA room air cleaner on cat-induced asthma and rhinitis. J Allergy Clin Immunol 1997; 99:S388 (abstract).
119. Gotzsche PC, Hammarquist C, Burr M. House-dust mite control measures in the management of asthma: meta-analysis. Br Med J 1998; 317:1105.
120. Ehnert B, Lau-Schadendorf S, Weber A, et al. Reducing domestic exposure to dust mite allergen reduces bronchial hyperreactivity in sensitive children with asthma. J Allergy Clin Immunol 1992; 90:135.
121. Htut T, Higenbottam TW, Gill GW, et al. Eradication of house-dust mite from homes of atopic asthmatic subjects: a double-blind trial. J Allergy Clin Immunol 2001; 107:55.
122. Tan BB, Weald D, Strickland I, et al. Double-blind controlled trial of the effect of housedust mite allergen avoidance on atopic dermatitis. Lancet 1996; 347:15.
123. Woodfolk JA, Hayden ML, Couture N, et al. Chemical treatment of carpets to reduce allergen: comparison of the effects of tannic acid and other treatments on proteins derived from dust mites and cats. J Allergy Clin Immunol 1995; 96:325.
124. McDonald LG, Tovey E. The role of water temperature and laundry procedures in reducing house-dust mite populations and allergen content of bedding. J Allergy Clin Immunol 1992; 90:599.
125. Arlian LG, Neal JS, Morgan MS, et al. Reducing relative humidity is a practical way to control dust mites and their allergens in homes in temperate climates. J Allergy Clin Immunol 2001; 107:99.
126. Wood RA, Chapman MD, Adkinson NF Jr, et al. The effect of cat removal on allergen content in household-dust samples. J Allergy Clin Immunol 1989; 83:730.
127. Sicherer SH, Wood RA, Eggleston PA. Determinants of airway responses to cat allergen: comparison of environmental challenge to quantitative nasal and bronchial allergen challenge. J Allergy Clin Immunol 1997; 99:798.
128. Wood RA, Eggleston PA, Rand C, et al. Cockroach allergen abatement with extermination and sodium hypochlorite cleaning in inner-city homes. Ann Allergy Asthma Immunol 2001; 87:60.
129. Burge HA. Fungus allergens. Clin Rev Allergy 1985; 3:319.
130. Bush RK, Portnoy JM. The role and abatement of fungal allergens in allergic diseases. J Allergy Clin Immunol 2001; 107:S430.
131. Arruda LK, Platts-Mills TA, Fox JW, et al. Aspergillus fumigatus allergen I, a major IgE-binding protein, is a member of the mitogillin family of cytotoxins. J Exp Med 1990; 172:1529.
132. Reed CE, Milton DK. Endotoxin-stimulated innate immunity: a contributing factor for asthma. J Allergy Clin Immunol 2001; 108:157.
133. Gereda JE, Leung DY, Thatayatikom A, et al. Relation between house-dust endotoxin exposure, type 1 T-cell development, and allergen sensitization in infants at high risk of asthma. Lancet 2000; 355:1680.
134. Michel O, Ginanni R, Duchateau J, et al. Domestic endotoxin exposure and clinical severity of asthma. Clin Exp Allergy 1991; 21:441.
135. Eisenbarth SC, Piggott DA, Huleatt JW, et al. Lipopolysaccharide-enhanced, toll-like receptor 4-dependent T helper cell type 2 responses to inhaled allergen. J Exp Med 2002; 196:1645.
136. Meldrum JR, O'Rourke MK, Pleskett PR, et al. Fungal spores in the indoor and outdoor environment. Proc Indoor Air 1993; 4:189.
137. Pollart SM, Reid MJ, Fling JA, et al. Epidemiology of emergency room asthma in northern California: association with IgE antibody to ryegrass pollen. J Allergy Clin Immunol 1988; 82:224.

Immune responses to allergens from different sources

138. Platts-Mills TA. The role of indoor allergens in chronic disease. J Allergy Clin Immunol 2007; 119:297.
139. Erwin EA, Ronmark E, Wickens K, et al. Contribution of dust mite and cat specific IgE and total IgE: relevance to asthma prevalence. J Allergy Clin Immunol 2007; 119:359.

Conclusions

140. Pope AM, Patterson R, Burge H, eds. Indoor allergens: assessing and controlling adverse health effects. Washington, DC: National Academy Press; 1993. .

141. Institute of Medicine. Impact of ventilation and air cleaning on asthma. In: Institute of Medicine, eds. Clearing the air: asthma and indoor air exposures. Washington, DC: Institute of Medicine; 2000:327.
142. Platts-Mills TA, Sporik RB, Wheatley LM, et al. Is there a dose-response relationship between exposure to indoor allergens and symptoms of asthma? J Allergy Clin Immunol 1995; 96:435.
143. Morgan WJ, Crain EF, Gruchalla RS, et al. Results of a home-based environmental intervention among urban children with asthma. N Engl J Med 2004; 351:1068–1080.
144. Camargo CA Jr, Weiss ST, Zhang S, et al. Prospective study of body mass index weight change, and risk of adult-onset asthma in women. Arch Intern Med 1999; 159:2582.
145. Crater DD, Heise S, Perzanowski M, et al. Asthma hospitalization trends in Charleston, South Carolina, 1956 to 1997: twentyfold increase among black children during a 30-year period. Pediatrics 2001; 108:E97.

REFERENCES

Preparation and Standardization of Allergen Extracts

Jay E Slater, Robert E Esch, and Richard F Lockey

CONTENTS

SUMMARY OF IMPORTANT CONCEPTS

>> Allergenic extracts are derived from a variety of biological source materials and contain a wide range of substances that may or may not be allergenic in individual patients

>> All extracts for skin testing and allergen immunotherapy vaccines should be standardized to define allergenic potency to assure accurate interpretation of skin test results and effective allergen immunotherapy

>> There are 19 standardized allergen extracts available in the USA. For each of these extracts, there is a *US standard of potency* to which each lot of the extract is compared before release for sale to the public

>> In Europe, manufacturers ensure batch-to-batch consistency using an *in-house standard*, which may be characterized by a number of physiochemical and immunologic assays, with demonstration of the presence of individual allergens preferred. There are no external reference standards to ensure consistency among manufacturers

The views expressed in this article are the personal opinions of the authors and are not the official opinion of the US Food and Drug Administration (FDA) or the Department of Health and Human Services.

INTRODUCTION

Allergen avoidance, pharmacotherapy, and allergen immunotherapy are accepted and effective treatments for allergic diseases and asthma. *Allergen avoidance* is difficult to achieve in an increasingly urban society in which both parents may work, fur-bearing animals may be 'part of the family', and 'spring cleaning' may be rarely, if ever, done. *Pharmacotherapy* improves but does not eliminate symptoms and does not result in long-term improvement. *Allergen immunotherapy* may be the best option for prevention of the onset of asthma in an atopic individual or for achieving long-term improvement, especially when the patient has both allergic rhinitis and allergic asthma or insect allergy.

The World Health Organization (WHO) recommends that the term 'allergy extract' be replaced by 'allergen vaccine'.[1,2] In recognition of this recommendation, the term *allergen vaccine* is used in this chapter to denote FDA approved preparations of therapeutic allergens used to treat allergic diseases. The term *allergen extract* is used for preparations of allergens that are not yet FDA-approved, are FDA-approved but not yet incorporated into a therapeutic vaccine for an individual patient, or are used for experimental purposes. Allergen vaccines are used therapeutically to downregulate the mechanism mediated by immunoglobulin E (IgE) that causes allergic diseases. To accomplish this, allergen vaccines immunologically modify the heightened allergic response to allergens that cause these diseases. *Diagnostic allergens* are FDA-approved allergen extracts used for diagnostic purposes and are used to confirm a suspected clinical allergy in patients with allergic diseases. This is accomplished by doing appropriate immediate skin testing.

Standardization is the process by which a reference extract is selected, and methods and procedures are developed to quantitatively compare a test extract with a reference extract to establish equivalence.[3-5] Allergen standardization became a reality in the USA in the late 1970s when the first allergen extracts were produced to meet FDA criteria for potency and composition. 'The goals of standardization are to assure that the assayed property of the extract is clinically relevant for defining potency, the test methods are accurate and precise for estimating the clinically relevant property, and the standard extract is clinically relevant to assure that standardization will result in safe and effective products'.[6]

Currently in the USA and throughout the world, more extracts are being standardized. This chapter outlines the nature of the process for manufacturing extracts as well as the methods by which they are biologically standardized.

SOURCE MATERIALS

POLLENS

Pollen extracts derived from more than 300 plant species are manufactured in the USA and represent the most diverse group of allergen products used in medical practice. Common grasses, trees, and 'weeds' cause allergy in humans (Table 34.1). The general category of weeds is used to group those invasive, undesirable plants that are not trees or grasses. (The tables in Chapter 32 provide a more extensive listing of allergenic plants.) Approximately 60–75% of seasonal rhinitis patients have positive skin test reactions to weed pollens, 40% to grass pollens, and 10% to tree pollens. Climatic factors influence the pollination patterns, and variations are seen from year to year within a given locale as well as between geographic areas.[7–9] For example, an early frost can abruptly end the weed pollen season, or an unusually mild winter may initiate an early tree pollen season. Thus, pollen collection is a highly seasonal activity, and the inventory of pollen source materials for allergen extracts has always been regarded a critical asset for manufacturers.

Pollen source materials may be collected in the field by vacuum collection or in a greenhouse by water setting, or the flower heads may be cut, dried, ground, and sieved in the laboratory. *Vacuum collection* is the most efficient method and is widely used in cultivated fields or pure stands during pollination. For *water setting*, the freshly cut stems and flowers of the plant are placed in water in a greenhouse shortly before pollination. The plant is allowed to pollinate over days onto paper surrounding the plants, and the pollen is collected. Finally, mature flowering heads of the plant may be collected just before pollination, dried, and ground to release the pollen. The pollen grains are separated from the plant parts by sifting through different types of sieves. Contamination by plant parts is usually limited to <1%. In contrast, the cut-dry-grind-and-sieve method yields pollens contaminated with plant parts at a level of 5–10% and may require additional separation steps. If necessary, the pollen is purified by additional sieving, perchloroethylene flotation, or centrifugal density separation. The identity and purity of each lot of pollen is verified microscopically before extraction. Dried pollens stored at less than 0°C are known to maintain their allergenic activity for more than 10 years.[10] The allergen contents of pollens may vary depending on the location and year during which they were collected (Table 34.2). To minimize variability of allergen content in the final allergen extracts, manufacturers may combine lots from different locations and collection years.

FUNGI

Air-borne fungal spores can exceed those of pollen by 1000-fold depending on meteorologic conditions. Outdoor spore levels tend to be higher than those measured indoors, and the outdoor spore levels have

a significant influence on indoor levels. The 10 most common allergenic fungi, based on prevalence and on skin sensitization among allergic subjects in the southeastern USA, are *Alternaria, Helminthosporium, Cladosporium, Aspergillus, Penicillium, Epicoccum, Fusarium, Rhizopus, Mucor,* and the Basidiomycetes (smuts and rusts).[11,12]

Progress in the standardization of fungal extracts has been impeded by the limited information available on fungal allergens. Apart from *Alternaria, Aspergillus,* and *Cladosporium* species, minimal data are available on the identity and characteristics of clinically important allergens (see Chapter 35).

Fungal source materials are produced from laboratory cultures using well-defined seed cultures derived from established culture collections, such as the American Type Culture Collection (ATCC) and the Centraalbureau voor Schimmelcultures (CBS). Growth conditions, such as the culture medium, temperature, pH, photoperiod, aeration, and cultivation time, are known to affect the allergenic composition of an individual species or strain of fungi. In addition, the allergen composition of different strains of the same species grown under identical conditions will vary widely.[13,14]

Information on the ideal culture conditions required for fungal allergen extracts and the relative importance of the spores, mycelia, and spent culture medium as source materials is scarce and contradictory. Studies identifying spore-specific allergens suggest the need for spores as a source material for allergen extracts from these species.[15,16] In contrast, some allergens are secreted and may require the extraction of actively growing mycelia or the processing of the culture medium.[17] Most commercial fungal source materials contain spores and mycelia in varying proportions, and analytic methods to establish specifications are lacking.

Different manufacturers use different culture conditions and different strains. No fungal allergen extracts have been standardized in the USA. Thus, it is reasonable to assume that fungal allergen products manufactured by different companies with identical labeling are not quantitatively or qualitatively similar. The maintenance of stable strains without repeated subculturing and the use of standardized culture conditions are minimum requirements for batch-to-batch uniformity. The purity and identity assessments of fungal source materials are more difficult than for other allergen sources because fungi display a high degree of genetic variability among strains. Successful quality control procedures usually require a combination of methods, including examination of the cultural and morphologic characteristics under varying growth conditions, metabolic characteristics determined by the ability to assimilate various substrates, and specific allergen measurement. Culture conditions for strains that are capable of producing mycotoxins should be validated to ensure that mycotoxins are not produced.

More than 200 fungal allergen extracts are produced by nine manufacturers, and none has been standardized in the USA. The only candidate reference available is an *Alternaria alternata* extract prepared by an international collaborative study[18] but awaits acceptance by regulatory authorities.

ACARIDS (MITES)

A number of mite genera and species are responsible for allergic reactions. The house-dust mites, *Dermatophagoides farinae* and *D. pteronyssinus,* are the most important worldwide.[19] In tropical and subtropical regions of the world, *Blomia tropicalis* may be found in homes at densities equal to that of *Dermatophagoides* species.[20] Storage mites, which belong

Table 34.1 Common allergenic pollens and sources

	Cross-reacting groups	Representative genera[a]
Grasses	Pooideae	*Poa* (bluegrass), *Dactylis* (orchard), *Festuca* (fescue), *Lolium* (perennial rye), *Agrostis* (redtop), *Anthoxanthum* (vernal), *Phleum* (timothy)
	Chloridoideae	*Cynodon* (Bermuda)
	Panicoideae	*Paspalum* (Bahia), *Sorghum* (Johnson)
Trees	Aceraceae	*Acer* (maples, box elder)
	Betulaceae	*Alnus* (alder), *Betula* (birches), *Corylus* (hazelnut)
	Cupressaceae	*Cupressus* (cypress), *Juniperus* (junipers, cedars), *Taxodium* (bald cypress)
	Fabaceae	*Acacia* (mimosa), *Robinia* (locust), *Prosopsis* (mesquite)
	Fagaceae	*Quercus* (oaks), *Fagus* (beech)
	Juglandaceae	*Carya* (hickory, pecan), *Juglans* (walnut)
	Moraceae	*Morus* (mulberry)
	Oleaceae	*Olea* (olive), *Fraxinus* (ash), *Ligustrum* (privet)
	Pinaceae	*Pinus* (pines)
	Platanaceae	*Platanus* (sycamore)
	Salicaceae	*Populus* (cottonwood, poplars), *Salix* (willows)
	Ulmaceae	*Ulmus* (elms)
'Weeds'	Chenopodiaceae	*Atriplex* (scales, saltbush), *Chenopodium* (lamb's quarter), *Salsola* (Russian thistle), *Kochia* (firebush)
	Asteraceae	*Artemisia* (mugworts, wormwood, sages)
		Ambrosia (ragweeds), *Xanthium* (cocklebur)
	Amaranthaceae	*Amaranthus* (careless weed, pigweeds), *Acnida* (Western water hemp)
	Plantaginaceae	*Plantago* (plantain)
	Polygonaceae	*Rumex* (dock, sorrel)

[a]Representative genera are members of the same botanical family or subfamily. Manufacturers currently offer allergen products derived from one or more species of each listed genus.

to a wide range of taxonomic groups, are found in stored grain, barn dust, and hay. Mite allergens can be detected in house dust samples collected from beds, carpets, furniture, and clothing. Until the licensing of house-dust mite extracts in 1985, the primary source of house-dust mite allergens was house dust itself.

D. farinae and *D. pteronyssinus* allergen extracts are standardized and at present are the only extracts derived from mites that are commercially available in the USA. Although highly cross-reactive, both species are used individually or as a mixture in allergen vaccines. Their life cycle, growth conditions, and allergenic composition have been extensively studied, and production-scale cultures of *Dermatophagoides* mites have been established at several facilities. The allergen content of extracts may vary depending on whether the purified mite bodies or total spent culture is used as the source material. Mite bodies can be separated from cultures to >99% purity and are almost exclusively used in the USA. Spent cultures containing adult mites, eggs, larvae, fecal particles, and culture medium have been shown to be suitable source materials and are often used in Europe as source materials for mite extracts. With spent cultures, it is critical that residual proteins derived from the culture medium are reduced below defined limits, especially when culture components contain potentially allergenic proteins from yeast, soy, wheat, or shrimp.

MAMMALS

Many domesticated animals live and work in close contact with humans as companions or livestock. More than 100 million domestic animals reside in the USA. Cats and dogs are the most common cohabitants and are found in more than one-third of all US homes. Occupational exposure to rodents (rats, mice, guinea pigs, rabbits) among laboratory animal technicians and to cattle, horses, sheep, and pigs among farmers and veterinarians can result in sensitization and allergic symptoms. Animals raised for fur production (mink, fox, raccoons) can also pose an occupational risk for sensitization. Positive skin test reactions to animal allergens occur in about 20–30% of the atopic population, but the relationship between sensitization as demonstrated by skin test reactivity and clinical reactivity is not known.

One reason for this limited knowledge is the lack of well-characterized or standardized diagnostic allergen preparations. At this time, only products derived from cat source materials are standardized. Cat extracts are standardized on the basis of the major allergen, Fel d 1, and are labeled as 'cat hair' or 'cat pelt extract', depending on the source material used for their manufacture. Standardized cat hair and pelt extracts contain equivalent concentrations of Fel d 1, but cat pelt extracts contain

Table 34.2 Content (Amb a 1) of short ragweed pollen lots

Collection year	Amb a 1 content[a]
1980	5860–7880
1981	8790–10230
1984	4670–6230
1985	3500–3620
1986	4150–5300
1987	1120–2290
1988	3000–4670
1989	3290–4360
1990	3580–5360
1991	4950–5120
1992	3230–3900
1995	5680–6220
1996	4700–6560
1997	5940–6460
1998	6120–8420
1999	3990–4330
2000	4660–5550
2002	2234–3050
2004	1974–2951

Data from Greer Laboratories.

[a]Results reported as Amb a 1 units/g of defatted ragweed pollen determined by radial immunodiffusion assay.

10- to 100-fold higher concentrations of cat albumin than cat hair extracts. The relative clinical utility of the two types of cat extracts has not been thoroughly investigated.[21]

Several allergenic source materials have been identified from mammals, including hair or dander, pelt, saliva, and urine. Most known animal allergens, including the rodent allergens (Mus m 1 and Rat n 1), the dog allergens (Can f 1 and Can f 2), the cat allergen (Fel d 1), the bovine allergen (Bos d 2), and the horse allergens (Equ c 1 and Equ c 2), belong to a family of small extracellular proteins called *lipocalins* (see Chapter 35).[22,23] The lipocalin allergens of rodents can be recovered in high concentrations from their urine or saliva; however, allergen extracts are almost exclusively produced from their hair or pelt. As it becomes increasingly apparent that the allergens derived from animals do not always arise primarily from the skin, alternative source materials for the manufacture of animal extracts should be considered.

There is conflicting evidence on the existence of breed-specific allergens among dogs. The industry practice is to include source materials from multiple breeds and mixed breeds. The health of the animals used for source materials must be verified by veterinarians, and cattle must originate from sources documented to be free of bovine transmissible spongiform encephalopathies.

INSECTS

Insect source materials are derived from varying parts of the insect anatomy depending on the type of insect allergen extract. For stinging insect allergens, the most common source is the venom sac. Venom proteins are extracted from the sacs of hornets (*Dolichovespula* species), paper wasps (*Polistes* species), and yellow jackets (*Vespula* species) for the manufacture of venom protein extracts. Recoveries of the major allergenic components – hyaluronidase, phospholipase, and vespid antigen 5 – are monitored by their enzyme or immunochemical activities. It is possible to collect venom in a relatively pure form by electrical stimulation of honeybees or by 'milking' individual wasps or fire ants. These materials are relatively free of non-venom proteins but with the exception of honeybees, the use of these techniques is too tedious and inefficient for commercial application. Fire ant venom proteins have been found to be present in sufficient concentrations in whole-body extracts to be suitable for use as diagnostic allergens and therapeutic vaccines.[24–26] The disadvantage of whole-body fire ant extract is that it contains significant concentrations of non-allergenic proteins in addition to the venom.

For insects that are a cause of inhalant allergy, the whole body may serve as suitable source materials.[27–30] Respirable emanations from caddis fly, midge, and cockroach species are established sources of potent aeroallergens. The predominant caddis fly (Trichoptera) allergen is a 13-kDa hemocyanin-like protein that cross-reacts with other invertebrate allergens found in arthropods and mollusks.[31] The allergenic activity of midges, or lake flies, resides in the hemoglobin (erythrocruorin) molecules produced by the midge larvae and excreted by the adult flies while air-borne.[32] The two dominant species responsible for cockroach allergy are *Blattella germanica* (German cockroach) and *Periplaneta americana* (American cockroach). Cockroach allergy has received attention in recent years because of its link to the increase in the prevalence of fatal asthma in inner-cities.[33] A variety of source materials have been used to identify and isolate cockroach allergens, including whole bodies, cast skins, and fecal pellets.[29,30,34] Some preparations contain high concentrations of protease activity, which may lead to the reduced stability of extracts.

For biting insects, the optimal allergen source may be the salivary glands.[35] Direct recovery of saliva from fleas and mosquitoes has been possible in the laboratory, but these processes have not yet been developed for commercial distribution.

FOODS

More than 170 foods have been documented in the scientific literature as causing allergic reactions, and extracts of most are commercially available for diagnostic use. Cow's milk, eggs, peanut, wheat, soy, fish, shellfish, and tree nuts account for up to 90% of the serious allergic food reactions. Food source materials vary in composition, extent of processing, and allergenic activity. Food allergens are predominantly water-soluble glycoproteins with molecular weights ranging from 10 to 60 kDa.[36] They are generally resistant to heat, acid, and proteolytic digestion. Some manufacturers initiate the extraction process immediately after receiving fresh foods and before any signs of degradation are observed. Others may pretreat the source materials by defatting in acetone, drying, freeze-drying, or milling. The pretreated source materials may be stored for several years before extraction. The portions of the food used (e.g., seeds, skin), whether the food source is cooked or uncooked, the cultivar, and the country of origin all may influence the allergen content of food source materials.

Allergen extracts derived from some food sources, especially fruits and vegetables, are highly unstable and difficult to prepare.[37] In these cases, direct use of the unprocessed fresh fruit in skin tests ('prick and prick' method) has been proposed.[38] The great variety of source materials, manufacturing methods, and the lack of information about relevant food allergens have impeded progress in standardization. There are no standardized food allergen products available commercially.

MANUFACTURE OF ALLERGEN EXTRACTS

AQUEOUS AND GLYCERINATED EXTRACTS

The extraction ratio, buffer, temperature, and time are the critical process parameters and can be optimized for maximum recovery of allergenic activity. Non-standardized allergen extracts are manufactured and labeled on the basis of the *protein nitrogen unit* (PNU) or on the weight of source material extracted with a given volume of extracting fluid (*w/v*). Standardized allergen vaccines are manufactured and labeled on the basis of specific allergen content or overall allergenic activity (Table 34.3).

The extraction processes employed for non-standardized and standardized products are essentially the same; the major difference is in the quality control procedures (Fig. 34.1). In general, the manufacture of standardized allergen extracts requires stricter controls of source materials, in-process testing, and potency adjustments of final products. In the USA, standardized allergen extracts are tested and released by regulatory authorities before commercial distribution. Optimal conditions for extraction must consider the presence of heat-labile and protease-sensitive allergens. Thus, extractions are either performed at reduced temperatures or in the presence of additives that suppress microbial growth (e.g., 0.4% phenol, 50% glycerin). Slightly alkaline buffers such as bicarbonate buffer pH 8.4 are generally preferred for increasing protein and allergen yields. Dialysis or ultrafiltration may be used to remove low-molecular-weight (<5 kDa) non-antigenic substances. Prolonged processing times may increase total protein recovery from source materials but may denature the allergens and may not lead to concomitant increases in allergenic potency. *In-process testing* for specific allergen content or marker proteins can be used to monitor the processing steps and ensure a reproducible and high-quality product. The bulk intermediate may be freeze-dried to maximize stability and consistency of the final products.

All allergen extracts must be sterile, which is accomplished by filtration through a sterilizing filter with a nominal 0.2 μm pore size. Sterility

Table 34.3 Standardized allergen extracts currently licensed in the USA

Allergen vaccine	Current lot release tests	Labeled unitage
Dust mite *(Dermatophagoides farinae)*	Competition ELISA Protein[a]	AU/mL (equivalent to BAU/mL)
Dust mite *(Dermatophagoides pteronyssinus)*		
Cat pelt *(Felis domesticus)*	Fel d 1 (RID)	BAU/mL
Cat hair *(Felis domesticus)*	IEF	5–9.9 Fel d 1 U/mL = 5000 BAU/mL
	Protein	10–19.9 Fel d 1 U/mL = 10 000 BAU/mL
Bermuda grass *(Cynodon dactylon)*	Competition ELISA	BAU/mL
Red top grass *(Agrostis alba)*	IEF	
June (Kentucky blue) grass *(Poa pratensis)*	Protein[a]	
Perennial ryegrass *(Lolium perenne)*		
Orchard grass *(Dactylis glomerata)*		
Timothy grass *(Phleum pratense)*		
Meadow fescue grass *(Festuca elatior)*		
Sweet vernal grass *(Anthoxanthum odoratum)*		
Short ragweed *(Ambrosia artemisiifolia)*	Amb a 1 (RID)	Amb a 1 units
Yellow hornet *(Vespa* species)	Hyaluronidase and phospholipase activity	μg protein
Wasp *(Polistes* species)		
Honey bee *(Apis mellifera)*		
White faced hornet *(Vespa* species)		
Yellow jacket *(Vespula* species)		
Mixed vespid *(Vespa + Vespula* species)		

ELISA, enzyme-linked immunosorbent assay; AU, allergy units; BAU, bioequivalent allergy units; IEF, isoelectric focusing; RID, radial immunodiffusion.

[a]Test for informational purposes only.

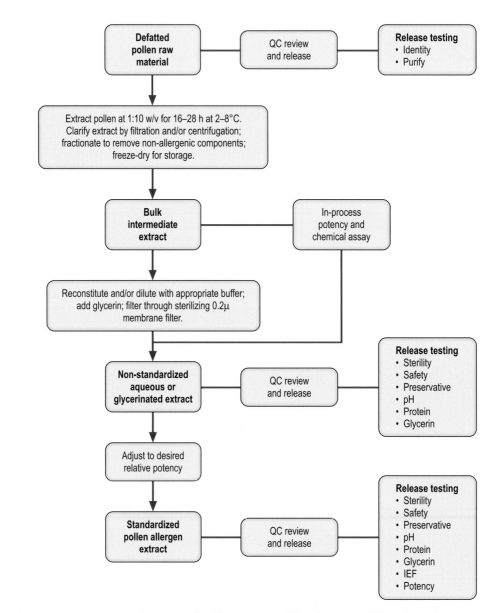

Fig. 34.1. Typical extraction and quality control steps for pollen allergen extracts. QC, quality control; IEF, isoelectric focusing.

testing is carried out according to the *US Pharmacopeia*. All extracts prepared in multiple-dose vials must also contain a preservative that is bacteriostatic and fungistatic. Most manufacturers use phenol at a concentration of 0.2–0.5% with or without 50% glycerin.

The characterization and standardization of allergen extracts are required to ensure the identity, purity, potency, and batch-to-batch consistency of the final products. Total protein content, specific allergen content, protein and allergen profile, and allergenic activity as determined by skin testing or IgE enzyme-linked immunosorbent assay (ELISA) inhibition, all contribute to the quality control process. Different methods may be employed by different manufacturers depending on the characteristics of

their product and regulatory requirements. For example, certain assays may be suitable for validation or revalidation studies when changes occur in packaging, formulation, equipment, or processes that could impact product effectiveness or product characteristics. Other assays may be well suited for stability verification or lot release testing. In the USA, lot release testing for standardized extracts is performed using a single national potency standard or reference preparation (see later discussion). In contrast, lot release testing in the European countries employs the manufacturer's *in-house reference* (IHR) preparation derived from a production run after the validated and licensed manufacturing process.

This difference reflects the real problem of whether interchangeability can be expected between vaccines produced by different manufacturers. For example, standardized extracts in the USA are labeled solely on the basis of *bioequivalent allergy units* (BAUs), whereas in Europe, alternatives can be used, including major allergen content or various arbitrary relative potency units. Both approaches ensure batch-to-batch uniformity with a single company's product, and the BAU labeling attempts to reduce the risk associated with switching between different manufacturers' products.

NAMED-PATIENT PRODUCTS

Named-patient products are the allergy treatment vaccines formulated specifically for individual patients. These products are mixtures and dilutions of the manufacturers' bulk concentrates. In the USA, the vast majority of named-patient products are formulated in the clinic or pharmacy under the direction of the practicing allergist. In contrast, licensed manufacturers produce the majority of treatment formulations in Europe. The optimal therapeutic dose of immunotherapy may vary among patients, and this may require adjusting the number and proportion of allergen products included in named-patient products. For example, dilution limits the number of individual allergen vaccines that can be included if a therapeutic effective dose is to be delivered. Knowledge of allergen cross-reactivity may offer practical information in reducing the number of allergens used for immunotherapy and helps in attaining therapeutic effective doses with fewer treatment vials or injections.

STABILITY OF ALLERGEN EXTRACTS

The shelf life of allergen extracts varies depending on the formulation, dilution, composition, and storage conditions.[39,40] The stability of some allergens may differ depending on whether they are stored as individual extracts or as mixtures with other allergen extracts.[41,42]

The potency of allergen extracts decreases when stored at room temperature or higher. In general, aqueous stock concentrates (e.g., 1:10 to 1:100 w/v or 10000–100000 BAU/mL) may lose potency within weeks of storage at room temperature (20–25°C) and within days at higher temperatures (30–35°C). To minimize this effect, allergen extracts should be stored under refrigeration (2–8°C). Glycerinated extracts are more resistant to the deleterious effect of temperature than aqueous formulations and thus have a longer shelf life.

Diluted extracts may lose their potency by adsorption of active components to the surfaces of glass vials and syringes. The use of diluting buffers containing 0.05% human serum albumin or 0.005% Tween-80 reduces adsorption of allergens and should be used for extract dilutions >1:1000.[43]

Information about the stability of allergen extracts is primarily based on studies performed on single products. In practice, however, allergen vaccines are frequently stored as mixtures formulated for individual patients. Studies conducted on vaccine mixtures have showed that the stability of mixtures may be significantly different from that of the individual vaccines. Interactions between components of different vaccines and the presence of enzymes, especially proteases from fungal-derived

and insect-derived vaccines, may have detrimental effects on some vaccines.[41,42] For this reason, it is recommended that mixing fungal and cockroach vaccines with pollen or dander vaccines should be avoided.[44] The presence of glycerin at 10% or higher concentration has a protective effect against protease activity, which may explain why glycerinated vaccines such as those derived from house-dust mites (*Dermatophagoides* species) had little or no effect on other vaccines.[42]

The expiration dating of standardized allergen extracts is based on stability study results ensuring that the biologic potency of the extract is maintained throughout the labeled dating period. This requirement does not extend to non-standardized extracts or to vaccine mixtures lacking standards of potency. In these cases, the dating periods are assigned in accordance with FDA regulations (21 CFR 610.53). For extracts in final containers with 50% or more glycerin stored at 2–8°C, the dating period is 3 years after the product leaves the manufacturer's storage. For extracts in final containers with less than 50% glycerin and for alum-precipitated vaccines, the period is 18 months after the product leaves the manufacturer's storage.

US STANDARDIZATION OF EXTRACTS

CENTER FOR BIOLOGICS EVALUATION AND RESEARCH

Allergen extracts and other biologics were first regulated by the Hygienic Laboratory of the Public Health and Marine Hospital Service. In 1930, the Hygienic Laboratory was renamed the National Institute *(singular)* of Health (NIH). Beginning in 1955, through its Division of Biologics Standards, the NIH continued to regulate biologics for more than 40 years. In 1972, regulatory authority over biologics was transferred to the FDA Bureau of Biologics. In 1982, the FDA merged the Bureau of Biologics and the Bureau of Drugs into a single Center for Drugs and Biologics; 5 years later, the entities that regulated drugs and biologics were once again separated, and the Center for Biologics Evaluation and Research (CBER) assumed responsibility for allergen extract regulation.[45,46]

CBER authority to regulate allergen extracts derives from two laws enacted by Congress, the Food, Drug and Cosmetic Act of 1938 and the Public Health Service Act of 1944. The specific regulations that govern CBER regulation of allergens appear in part 680 of Title 21 of the Code of Federal Regulations (21 CFR 680), although other parts of 21 CFR also apply to allergen regulation. Over the past 20 years, two features of the CBER regulatory program have had a significant impact on allergen manufacturers and enhanced the safety of allergen vaccines marketed to the American public. The first feature is the enforcement of *current good manufacturing practice* (cGMP) standards (21 CFR 210, 211, and 600–680) on the manufacture of allergen products. The cGMP standards include requirements regarding organization and personnel, buildings and facilities, equipment, control of components and drug product containers and closures, production and process controls, holding and distribution, quality control, laboratory controls, and records and reports. These standards have been in effect since the 1960s.

A second feature is *allergen standardization*. The 21 CFR 680.3(e) standard specifies that when a potency test exists for a specific allergenic product, and when CBER has notified manufacturers that the test exists, manufacturers are required to determine the potency of each lot of the product before release. Since the 1980s, 19 allergen extracts have been standardized (Table 34.3). The following discussions focus primarily on these standardized products and the tests used to ascertain vaccine potency.

MARKETED ALLERGEN EXTRACTS

Allergen extracts are manufactured and sold worldwide for the diagnosis and treatment of IgE-mediated allergic disease. These extracts are complex vaccines of natural biomaterials. Each extract contains proteins, carbohydrates, enzymes, and pigments, of which the allergens – presumably the active ingredients – may constitute only a small proportion.[47] As mentioned previously, allergen extracts have been labeled either with a designation of extraction ratio (w/v) or with a protein unit designation determined using the Kjeldahl method (PNU/mL). However, little correlation exists between these two designations and biologic measures of allergen potency.[48,49]

In the absence of a concerted effort to maintain product consistency, lot-to-lot variations in allergen content may be considerable. Product consistency may be enhanced by the inherent nature of the raw materials; for example, pollen and pure mite extracts generally have greater lot-to-lot consistency than mold and insect extracts. In addition, manufacturers can increase the consistency of their products by controlled collection, storage, and processing of the raw materials; by reproducible and optimized extraction and manufacturing techniques; and by expiration dating based on real-time stability data. However, consistency can only be ensured by measuring the potency of each lot of extract and by marketing only those lots whose potency falls within an acceptable range.

FDA allergen standardization regulation mandates that when an appropriate potency test exists, manufacturers must test each lot of an allergen extract for potency before sale. This regulation takes product consistency one step further by establishing a US standard of potency for each standardized product. The purpose of allergen standardization is to ensure that the extracts are well characterized in terms of allergen content and that variation between lots is minimized even among different manufacturers.[50] Because standardized extracts are compared to a single, national potency standard, patients and their physicians can switch from one manufacturer's product to another with minimized risk of adverse reaction.

Currently, 19 standardized allergen extracts are available from US manufacturers (Table 34.3). For each of these extracts, there is a US standard of potency to which each lot of the extract is compared before release for sale to the public. The potency measures and the assays used to determine these measures are specified in the approved product license applications of each manufacturer for each product. Manufacturers may use the methods described in CBER's *Methods of the Allergen Products Testing Laboratory* or may seek CBER approval to use alternative test methods that provide equally reliable measures of product potency and meet regulatory requirements.

The level of quality control for the 19 standardized allergen extracts is the exception rather than the rule. In vitro potency tests that correlate with in vivo clinical responses have not been developed for the hundreds of non-standardized extracts available in US product lines. Thus, for most allergen extracts manufactured in the USA, consistency cannot be ensured by potency testing.

BASIS FOR ALLERGEN STANDARDIZATION

Allergen standardization comprises two important components: the selection of a reference preparation of an allergenic extract and the selection of the procedures to compare manufactured products to the reference preparation.[4,5,51] In the USA, the use of a biologic model of allergen standardization has permitted the assignment of bioequivalent allergy units (BAUs) for most standardized allergens.[5] Once a specific unitage is assigned to a reference, all allergen extracts from the same source can be assigned units based on the *relative potency* (RP) with respect to the reference using the established quantitative in vitro potency method.[52]

In theory, standardizing an allergen extract might involve purifying each allergen in the extract and establishing with precision the importance of these allergens. However, most allergen extracts are complex mixtures of several relevant allergens of uncertain immunodominance. In addition, an individual allergen may be less 'allergenic' in a particular lot due to instability or denaturation. The choice of the best potency test depends on the allergen extract to be standardized.

In the absence of data supporting the safety of potency designations based on single allergen content, a measure of overall allergenicity may be a better predictor of safe dosing. For two allergen extracts, short ragweed and cat hair, data have supported the use of single allergen determinations, Amb a 1 and Fel d 1, respectively. For cat pelt and Hymenoptera venoms, the presence of two allergens, Fel d 1 and albumin for cat pelt and hyaluronidase and phospholipase A2 for Hymenoptera venoms, is verified for each lot. For dust mites and grass pollens, overall allergenicity is determined.

For initial overall allergenicity assessment, CBER has developed a method using erythema size after serial intradermal testing of highly allergic individuals. *Intradermal* testing was chosen over prick/puncture testing to achieve greater dosing accuracy; *erythema* size was chosen over wheal size to achieve greater accuracy in reaction measurements. This method, called *intradermal dilution for 50 mm sum of erythema determines the bioequivalent allergy units* ($ID_{50}EAL$), can be used to compare the allergenicity of extracts regardless of source. Subsequent comparisons of extracts from the same source material are made by a variant analysis called the *parallel-line bioassay*. Both these methods are described in CBER's *Methods of the Allergenics Testing Laboratory* and are discussed briefly here.

In the $ID_{50}EAL$ method, allergenic extracts are evaluated in subjects maximally reactive to the respective reference concentrates. Each subject is tested with serial three-fold dilutions of the reference. After 15 min, the sum of the longest and midpoint orthogonal diameters of erythema (ΣE) is determined at each dilution, and the log dose producing a 50 mm ΣE response (D_{50}) is calculated.[52] The mean D_{50} for 15 highly allergic individuals is used to determine the D_{50} for the extract. Extracts that produce similar D_{50} responses can be considered bioequivalent and are assigned similar units, the bioequivalent allergy unit (BAU). Because the modal D_{50} of a series of extracts was 14 (3^{-14}, or 1:4.8 million dilution), extracts with a mean D_{50} of 14 were arbitrarily assigned the value of 100 000 BAU/mL.[4]

By a similar technique and analysis, bioequivalent doses of test extracts from the same source as the reference can be determined by the *parallel-line bioassay*.[51] The inverse ratio of the doses of test extract required to produce identical D_{50} responses to a reference is the RP of that extract. This analysis requires that the log dose-response curves of the test extract and the reference be parallel; if the two dose-response lines are not parallel, the ratio of skin test doses for identical responses – and the RP – will vary with the dose. In this situation, which strongly suggests compositional differences between the two extracts, the distance between the two lines is different at each dose, and a meaningful RP cannot be determined (Fig. 34.2).[3,52]

Although skin testing is an essential component of the allergen standardization program, it is not intended for routine use in the testing of manufactured lots of extracts before release. In vitro potency assays that accurately predict the in vivo activity of extracts have been developed.[52] Once an in vivo assay has been used to assign unitage to a reference, an appropriate surrogate in vitro assay can be used to assign units to test extracts from the same sources. These methods can be based on quantitation of the total protein content (e.g., Hymenoptera venoms), the specific allergen content within the allergen extract (e.g., short ragweed, cat pelt), or the inhibition of the binding of IgE from pooled allergic sera to reference allergen (e.g., grasses, mites).[53] For the Hymenoptera venom allergens, the potency determination is also based on the content of the known principal allergens within the extracts, hyaluronidase and phospholipase, which are determined by enzyme activity (Table 34.3).

The potency units for short ragweed extracts were originally assigned based on their Amb a 1 content. Subsequent data suggested that 1 unit of Amb a 1 is equivalent to 1 μg of Amb a 1 and that 350 Amb a 1 units/mL is equivalent to 100 000 BAU/mL. However, the Amb a 1 unitage has been retained. Grass pollen extracts are labeled in BAU/mL, based on $ID_{50}EAL$ testing. In some cases, the assignment of potency units to standardized allergenic extracts in the USA has changed as better bioequivalence data have become available.[6] Cat extracts were originally standardized based on their Fel d 1 content, with arbitrary unitage (allergy units, or AU) tied to the Fel d 1 determinations. Subsequent $ID_{50}EAL$ testing suggested that the 100 000 AU/mL cat extracts, which contained 10–19.9 Fel d 1 U/mL, should be relabeled as 10 000 BAU/mL.[54] In addition, 20% of individuals allergic to cat were found to have antibody to non-Fel d 1 proteins,[55] and the identification of a cat albumin band on IEF was added as a requirement for cat pelt extracts. In the mid-1980s, dust mite extracts were standardized (in AU/mL) by inhibition radioimmunoassays. Subsequent $ID_{50}EAL$ testing indicated that the arbitrary unitage was statistically bioequivalent to BAU/mL[56]; in this case, the original AU designation was retained.[57]

The identity of an allergen extract may be verified by visualizing the separated allergen proteins based on their size and isoelectric points.[17] The *isoelectric focusing* (IEF) assay is an important safety test in the lot release of grass pollen and cat extracts. The patterns produced by the crude allergen mixtures are reproducible enough to indicate consistently the presence of known allergens, to identify possible contaminants present in the extracts, and to check lot-to-lot variation in the extracts.[58] In addition, IEF is used to verify the presence of cat albumin in cat pelt extracts.

TESTS WITH STANDARDIZED ALLERGENS

Several in vitro tests have been established for testing the potency and identity of standardized allergens (Table 34.3). Tests for potency include assays for the specific allergen content, for the RP, and for the enzyme activity of allergenic extracts. In addition, the identity of standardized extracts may be tested by the qualitative assessment of allergen content.

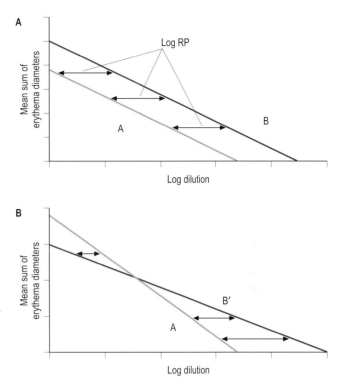

Fig. 34.2. Hypothetic parallel-line bioassay curves. (A) Curves are parallel, and the difference of log dilutions resulting in the same diameters is constant at all diameters. The log relative potency *(log RP)* of test sample *B* compared with reference *A* is represented by the difference. (B) Curves are not parallel, and the differences vary with the strength of the reaction; thus, the log RP of *B'* compared with *A* cannot be calculated.

The *specific allergen content* of certain allergen extracts can be measured by *radial immunodiffusion* (RID) *assay*. This assay is currently applied to two standardized allergenic extracts, short ragweed and cat pelt, in which the immunodominant allergens (Amb a 1 and Fel d 1, respectively) have been identified and defined. In RID, monospecific antiserum is added to an agar solution, which is allowed to solidify. Wells are then cut into the agar, and test allergen is placed in the wells. As the specific allergen diffuses out into the agar, a precipitin ring forms, which delineates the equivalence zone for antigen-antibody binding. The radius of the precipitin ring can then be measured. Because the antibody concentration in the agar is constant, the antigen concentration decreases with increasing distance from the well and is proportional to the log of the concentration of the applied test allergen in comparison to the reference preparation.

The *potency* of those standardized allergen extracts for which the immunodominant components have not been identified with certainty may be estimated using assays for IgE-antigen binding that compare the overall IgE-binding properties of test and reference extracts, using pooled sera from several allergic persons. Initially, an inhibition radioimmunoassay (RIA) was used for this purpose; CBER adopted the competition ELISA as its standard assay because of its greater precision and convenience. After coating the wells of a polystyrene microtiter plate with the reference allergen and blocking the wells with bovine albumin, a mixture of the allergen extract to be tested and a reference serum pool is added to the wells. The greater the amount of immunoreactive allergen in the mix, the less free IgE antibody will be available from the serum pool to bind to the immobilized allergen on the plate. Once again, the concentration of the allergens in the allergen extract is determined by comparison to the reference allergen preparation. However, because this assay does not explicitly measure a specific allergen, the allergen concentration is expressed as RP, with the reference assigned an arbitrary RP of 1.0. Early studies showed good or excellent correlation between RP assigned by titration skin testing and RP determined by inhibition RIA;[4] subsequent studies showed the competitive ELISA to be equivalent as well.[59]

Since its introduction as the major potency assay for mite and grass pollen allergen extracts in the USA, the competition ELISA has proven to be a highly useful regulatory tool. In a recent re-evaluation,[60] several of the assay procedures were re-optimized, and the performance characteristics were confirmed. In another study, investigators were able to demonstrate that the competition ELISA could be engineered to detect the loss of specific allergens as well as overall potency.[61]

Hymenoptera venoms contain multiple glycoprotein enzymes, the most important of which are hyaluronidase and phospholipases A1 and A2. Venom allergen extracts are standardized using enzymatic assays that estimate hyaluronidase and phospholipase content based on their enzymatic activity. An agar solution is prepared with the appropriate enzymatic substrate, and test samples are then added to cut wells. As the enzyme present in the sample diffuses into the agar, the enzyme digests the substrate, forming clearing zones around the wells. The radius of the clear zones is then measured and calculated as the log of the concentration of the enzyme present in the sample.

In addition to determining the potency of these allergen extracts, manufacturers are expected to confirm the *identity* of certain standardized extracts (Table 34.3) by IEF. This technique separates the proteins in the test extract based on their isoelectric points. The profile obtained in this technique is compared with the CBER standard to confirm the stated identity of the allergen extract.[58]

In the past, manufacturers were required to perform *ninhydrin protein assays* on most standardized allergen extracts. CBER developed and adopted a modification of the more cumbersome ninhydrin technique for protein determination[62] in response to concerns about the inaccuracy of the more standard protein estimation techniques. However, release limits were not established for the total protein content of standardized allergen extracts. Rather, the results of the ninhydrin assay were required 'for information only'. When the results were checked as part of CBER's lot release program, CBER required that the results of the CBER assay be within 40% of the manufacturer's result.

In effect, the protein assay requirement was a quality control test; in this phase of the allergen standardization program, CBER did not have data on the protein content of the standardized allergens or the effect of the protein content on potency assays. The requirement that manufacturers perform the ninhydrin assay on their standardized allergen extracts was re-examined.[60] As a result of these considerations, CBER no longer requires the use of the ninhydrin assay for standardized mite and grass allergen extracts. However, manufacturers continue to perform a validated protein assay on each lot of material, and CBER continues to require this information as part of its lot release program. The choice of protein assay is left to the manufacturer. Currently approved protein assay methods for other allergens (standardized cat, short ragweed, Hymenoptera venoms) are unchanged.

LOT RELEASE LIMITS

Fundamental to the standardization process is establishing an acceptable range of comparability or equivalence. Limits that are too broad lead to unacceptable risk to patients (e.g., anaphylaxis when the physician changes from one bottle to another or changes to a different manufacturer), whereas limits that are too narrow lead to unacceptable risk for manufacturers (e.g., rejection of a large percentage of safe and effective lots of product).

In the competition ELISA, potency limits have been set according to the precision of the test. The candidate extracts are expected to be statistically equivalent to the reference preparation, at a specified level of confidence with a specified test. Mite and grass pollen extracts are currently expected to be identical to reference at the 98% confidence level, using three replicates of a validated competition ELISA; the standard deviations in log (RP) for a single replicate is 0.1375.[59] The 98% confidence interval is given by $10^{\pm 2.326\sigma/\sqrt{3}}$. Consequently, a lot with an RP that falls in the range of 0.654–1.530 is within the 98% confidence interval and is approved for release. This criterion also implies that, on average, 2% of lots submitted to CBER will fall outside of the release limits even if they are identical to the reference preparation. Lots that are not identical to the reference would fail at predictably higher rates, while a small fraction of lots with RP outside the limits (as could be established by more exhaustive testing) will pass release testing.

An alternative approach would be to base the potency limits on *acceptable ranges* established in clinical studies. The following three criteria would be important:

1. *Therapeutic equivalence* addresses the efficacy of allergen vaccines for immunotherapy. Thus, an RP range will have the property of therapeutic equivalence if, for the allergen vaccine in question, lots with RPs anywhere in that range have an equal likelihood of effecting clinical improvement in an immunotherapy trial.
2. *Diagnostic equivalence* addresses the efficacy of allergen extracts for in vivo diagnostics.
3. *Safety equivalence* reflects the likelihood of the safe administration of the extract for either diagnostic or therapeutic indications.

The acceptable limits should fall within the narrowest of the equivalence ranges established by these criteria.

The aggregate consistency of manufactured lots might also be taken into account when developing testing methods and limits. For example, if typical lot-to-lot consistency is very high and well within clinical limits, testing protocols could be adjusted to eliminate outliers while rarely failing lots whose RP is close to 1.0. At the other extreme, if the distribution of lots is broad, equivalence to the reference would be imposed. This would narrow the distribution, but at a cost: at 95% equivalence, 5% of lots whose RP = 1.0 would fail release.

An analysis of studies using ragweed and dust mite allergens found that the range of therapeutic equivalence was at least tenfold and the ranges of diagnostic equivalence and safety equivalence approximately fourfold.[63] This study also analyzed the lot-to-lot consistency of 412 lots of grass pollen extracts and 91 lots of dust mite extracts. The variability of the samples was comparable to the assay variability. Furthermore, it was postulated that the mean ratio (in RP) of two randomly selected lots of allergen would be 1.12 (for mites) and 1.18 (for grass pollen). The calculated 95th percentile ratio was 1.48 and 1.80. Thus the equivalence ranges appear to be considerably broader than the current lot release limits (twofold) and the expected variations in product potency using current manufacturing and quality control practices. Based on these estimates, CBER broadened the release limits for standardized dust mite and grass pollen allergen extracts to 0.5–2.0.[64]

FUTURE STANDARDIZATION EFFORTS

The effort to standardize allergens in the USA has resulted in the development of a core group of often-used allergen vaccines that are better characterized and more consistent than their non-standardized predecessors. Standardized allergens also facilitate accurate and informative scientific studies of the efficacy, safety, and mechanisms of allergen immunotherapy, and they will be essential for the study of novel immunotherapeutic products in the future. Despite these clear advantages, most allergens marketed in the USA remain non-standardized. At a minimum, all allergen extracts should be subject to potency testing and compared to a reference preparation, whether manufacturer specific, industry wide, national, or international. CBER continues to work with the allergen extract manufacturers to establish and maintain US standards of potency for an increasing number of allergen extracts and to improve the consistency of those products that are not standardized.

Future standardization targets will be selected to maximize the public health benefit of greater allergen consistency. Criteria for allergen selection include the following:

1. Availability of stable, preferably lyophilized material for use as long-term reference preparations.
2. Consistency of currently marketed product.
3. Widespread use as a diagnostic or therapeutic reagent in the USA.
4. Number of manufacturers producing the product.
5. Potential use in immunotherapy or diagnostics.
6. Public health impact of correct diagnosis or adequate treatment.

These impact criteria are meant to help establish priorities and are not intended to be exclusionary. Thus, for example, an extract produced by only one manufacturer might still be a standardization target if other impact criteria are met. Likewise, CBER might decide to move forward with a little-used product of great public health importance, the standardization of which might enhance its availability and quality in the USA.

Once an allergen standardization target is selected, the marketed products that contain the allergen will be examined and compared with the best products available worldwide. Biologic potency will be established using the $ID_{50}EAL$ method, and a surrogate test will be identified for lot release purposes. CBER intends to pursue these goals with the full knowledge and, ideally, active participation of the allergen extract industry and scientific investigators. When a test for a standard of potency exists, FDA notifies manufacturers under 21 CFR 680.3(e). The regulation requires that manufacturers comply with the standard and test each lot of the specified extract before release for sale.

ALLERGEN EXTRACTS IN EUROPE

In Europe, the Committee for Proprietary Medicinal Products issued a 'Note for Guidance on Allergen Products' that was revised in 1996.[65] The European system for standardizing allergens and determining allergen extract potency[66] is different from the US system, as follows:

1. Manufacturers ensure batch-to-batch consistency using an *in-house standard*, which may be characterized by a number of physicochemical and immunologic assays, with demonstration of the presence of individual allergens preferred.
2. No external reference standards exist to ensure consistency among manufacturers.
3. Potency may be determined by any validated measure of in vitro IgE binding or other immunoassay. A skin test technique may be used to test the potency of the in-house standard.

One method for testing European products is called the *Nordic technique*.[6] The Nordic skin test method differs from the CBER $ID_{50}EAL$ method in Nordic's use of prick skin tests, its focus on wheal size rather than erythema, its choice of study subjects, and its use of a histamine dose-response curve to determine unitage. The method likely provides a reasonable estimate of extract potency. In theory, the comparison of the skin test reactivity of all allergens to a single standard (histamine dihydrochloride, 10 mg/mL) allows the assignment of universal unitage without the development or maintenance of specific allergen reference standards. However, the 'Note for Guidance' does not prescribe the specifics of the skin test technique to be used, and manufacturers are free to modify it as needed, as long as the test is validated. Thus, as applied in Europe, this method cannot provide a level of standardization among the different manufacturers that market products in the European Union.

Recently, the European Union funded an ambitious project to generate large quantities of well-characterized natural and recombinant allergens to be used for standardization in Europe and elsewhere.[67] This project is ongoing.

SUMMARY

Many pollens, fungi, acarids, mammals, insects, and foods are capable of producing IgE-mediated human allergic diseases. Extracts of these allergens are useful as diagnostic skin test reagents and as immunotherapeutic vaccines. Most of these extracts are not standardized and are marketed with PNU or w/v labeling. However, to better ensure identity, purity, potency, and consistency from batch to batch and from one manufacturer to another, 19 of the extracts most widely used in the USA are standardized. Standardization techniques use national reference extracts of known biologic activity provided by the FDA and include quantitation of major individual allergens, measurement of total allergen content by competition ELISA, and confirmation of protein-banding profiles by IEF. In Europe, allergen standardization is accomplished using manufacturers' in-house reference preparations and either in vitro IgE-binding assays or titration skin prick testing using histamine dose-response curves to determine allergen unitage.

References

Introduction

1. Bousquet J, Lockey RF, Malling HJ, eds. Allergen immunotherapy: therapeutic vaccines for allergic diseases. World Health Organization position paper. Allergy 1998; 44:S1.
2. Bousquet J, Lockey RF, Malling HJ, eds. Allergen immunotherapy: therapeutic vaccines for allergic diseases. World Health Organization position paper. J Allergy Clin Immunol 1998; 102:558.
3. Turkeltaub PC. In vivo standardization. In: Middleton E Jr, Reed CE, Ellis EF, et al. eds. Allergy: principles and practice. 3rd edn. St. Louis: Mosby; 1988:388.

4. Turkeltaub PC. Biological standardization of allergenic extracts. Allergol Immunopathol 1989; 17:53.
5. Turkeltaub PC. Biological standardization. Arb Paul Ehrlich Inst 1997; 91:145.
6. Turkeltaub PC. Allergen vaccine unitage based on biological standardization: clinical significance. In: Lockey RF, Bukantz SC, ed. Allergens and allergen immunotherapy. 2nd edn. New York: Marcel Dekker; 1999:321.

Source materials

7. Samach A, Coupland G. Time measurement and the control of flowering in plants. Bioessays 2000; 22:38.
8. Emberlin J, Jones S, Bailey J, et al. Variation in the start of the grass pollen season at selected sites in the United Kingdom: 1987–1992. Grana 1994; 33:94.
9. Kosisky SE, Carpenter GB. Predominant tree aeroallergens of the Washington DC area: a six year survey (1989–1994). Ann Allergy Asthma Immunol 1997; 78:381.
10. Esch RE. Personal observation. Greer Laboratories, Inc.
11. Lehrer SB, Aukrust L, Salvaggio JE. Respiratory allergy induced by fungi. Clin Chest Med 1983; 4:23.
12. Lehrer SB, Lopez M, Butcher BT, et al. Basidiomycete mycelia and spore-allergen extracts: skin test reactivity in adults with symptoms of respiratory allergy. J Allergy Clin Immunol 1986; 78:478.
13. Portnoy J, Pacheco F, Barnes C, et al. Selection of representative Alternaria strain groups on the basis of morphology, enzyme profile, and allergen content. J Allergy Clin Immunol 1993; 91:773.
14. Esch RE. Manufacturing and standardizing fungal allergen products. J Allergy Clin Immunol 2004; 113:210.
15. Weissman DN, Halmepuro L, Salvaggio JE, et al. Antigenic/allergenic analysis of basidiomycete cap. mycelia, and spore extracts. Int Arch Allergy Appl Immunol 1987; 84:56.
16. Aukrust L, Borch SM, Einarsson R. Mold allergy – spores and mycelium as allergen sources. Allergy 1985; 40:43.
17. Arruda LK, Mann BJ, Chapman MD. Selective expression of a major allergen and cytotoxin, Asp f 1, in Aspergillus fumigatus. J Immunol 1992; 149:3354.
18. Helm RM, Squillace DL, Yuninger JW. Production of a proposed international reference standard Alternaria extract. II. Results of a collaborative trial. J Allergy Clin Immunol 1988; 81:651.
19. Arlian LG, Platts-Mills TAE. The biology of dust mites and the remediation of mite allergens in allergic disease. J Allergy Clin Immunol 107:S406, 2001.
20. Fernandez-Caldas E, Puerta L, Mercado D, et al. Mite fauna, Der p I, Der f I and Blomia tropicalis allergen levels in a tropical environment. Clin Exp Allergy 1993; 23:292.
21. Esch RE. Allergen source materials and quality control of allergenic extracts. Methods 1997; 13:2.
22. Flower DR. A structural signature characteristic of the lipocalin protein family. Prot Pep Lett 1995; 2:341.
23. Virtanen T, Zeiler T, Mantyjarvi R. Important animal allergens are lipocalin proteins: why are they allergenic? Int Arch Allergy Immunol 1999; 120:247.
24. Freeman TM, Hylander R, Ortiz A, et al. Imported fire ant immunotherapy: effectiveness of whole body extracts. J Allergy Clin Immunol 1999; 90:210.
25. Nordvall SL, Johansson SGO, Ledford DK, et al. Allergens of the imported fire ant. J Allergy Clin Immunol 1988; 82:567.
26. Stafford CT, Wise SL, Robinson DA, et al. Safety and efficacy of fire ant venom in the diagnosis of fire ant allergy. J Allergy Clin Immunol 1992; 90:653.
27. Gupta S, Jain S, Chaudhry S, et al. Role of insects as inhalant allergens in bronchial asthma with special reference to the clinical characteristics of patients. Clin Exp Allergy 1990; 20:519.
28. Reisman RE, Hale R, Wypych JI. Allergy to honeybee body components: distinction from bee venom sensitivity. J Allergy Clin Immunol 1983; 71:18.
29. Richman PG, Khan HA, Turkeltaub PC, et al. The important sources of German cockroach allergens as determined by RAST analyses. J Allergy Clin Immunol 1984; 73:590.
30. Menon P, Menon V, Hilman B, et al. Skin test reactivity to whole body and fecal extracts of American (Periplaneta americana) and German (Blattella germanica) cockroaches in atopic asthmatics. Ann Allergy 1991; 67:573.
31. Kagen S, Muthiah R. Insect allergens: Characterizations and partial sequencing of a caddis fly hemoglobin aeroallergen. J Allergy Clin Immunol 1990; 85:152.
32. Baur X, Aschauer H, Mazur G, et al. Structure, antigenic determinants of some clinically important insect allergens: chironomid hemoglobins. Science 1986; 233:351.
33. Rosenstreich DL, Eggleston PA, Kattan M, et al. The role of cockroach allergy and exposure to cockroach allergen in causing morbidity among inner-city children with asthma. N Engl J Med 1997; 336:1356.
34. Yun YY, Ko SH, Park JW, et al. Comparison of allergenic components between German cockroach whole body and fecal extracts. Ann Allergy Asthma Immunol 2001; 86:551.
35. Peng Z, Li H, Simons FE. Immunoblot analysis of salivary allergens in 10 mosquito species with worldwide distribution and the human IgE responses to these allergens. J Allergy Clin Immunol 1998; 101:498.
36. Lemanske RF Jr, Taylor SL. Standardized extracts, foods. Clin Rev Allergy 1987; 5:23.
37. Veiths S, Hoffmann A, Holzhauser T, et al. Factors influencing the quality of food extracts for in vitro and in vivo diagnosis. Allergy 53:65, 1998.
38. Dreborg S, Foucard T. Allergy to apple, carrot, and potato in children with birch-pollen allergy. Allergy 1983; 38:167.

Stability of allergen extracts

39. Anderson MC, Baer H. Antigenic and allergenic changes during storage of a pollen extract. J Allergy Clin Immunol 1982; 69:3.
40. Nelson HS. Effect of preservatives and conditions of storage on the potency of allergy extracts. J Allergy Clin Immunol 1981; 67:64.
41. Nelson HS, Ikle D, Buchmeier A. Studies of allergen extract stability: the effects of dilution and mixing. J Allergy Clin Immunol 1996; 98:382.
42. Esch RE. Role of proteases on the stability of allergenic extracts. Arb Paul Ehrlich Inst; 1992; 85:171.
43. Norman PS, Marsh DG. Human serum albumin and Tween-80 as stabilizers of allergen solutions. J Allergy Clin Immunol; 1978; 62:314.
44. Nelson HS. Preparing and mixing allergen vaccines. In: Lockey RF, Bukantz SC, eds. Allergens and allergen immunotherapy. 2nd edn. New York: Marcel Dekker; 1999:401.

US standardization of extracts

45. Harden V.A. A short history of the National Institutes of Health, 2000. Online. Available: http://www.nih.gov/od/museum/exhibits/history
46. Milestones in US food and drug law history, 2000. Online. Available: http://www.fda.gov/opacom/backgrounders/miles.html
47. Yunginger JW. Allergenic extracts: Characterization, standardization and prospects for the future. Pediatr Clin North Am 1983; 30:795.
48. Baer H, Maloney CJ, Norman PS, et al. The potency and Group I antigen content of six commercially prepared grass pollen extracts. J Allergy Clin Immunol 1974; 54:157.
49. Baer H, Godfrey H, Maloney CJ, et al. The potency and antigen E content of commercially prepared ragweed extracts. J Allergy 1970; 45:347.
50. Yunginger JW. Allergens: recent advances. Pediatr Clin North Am 1988; 35:981.
51. Turkeltaub PC, Rastogi SC, Baer H, et al. A standardized quantitative skin-test assay of allergen potency and stability: studies on the allergen dose-response curve and effect of wheal erythema, and patient selection on assay results. J Allergy Clin Immunol 1982; 70:343.
52. Turkeltaub PC. In vivo methods of standardization. Clin Rev Allergy 1986; 4:371.
53. Platts-Mills TAE, Rawle F, Chapman MD. Problems in allergen standardization. Clin Rev Allergy 1985; 3:271.
54. Matthews J, Turkeltaub PC. The assignment of biological allergy units (AU) to standardized cat vaccines. J Allergy Clin Immunol 1992; 89:151.
55. Turkeltaub PC, Matthews J. Determination of compositional differences (CD) among standardized cat vaccines by in vivo methods. J Allergy Clin Immunol 1992; 89:151.
56. Turkeltaub PC, Anderson MC, Baer H. Relative potency (RP), compositional differences (CD), and assignment of allergy units (AU) to mite vaccines (Dp and Df) assayed by parallel line skin test (PLST). J Allergy Clin Immunol 1987; 79:235.
57. Turkeltaub PC. Use of skin testing for evaluation of potency, composition, and stability of allergenic products. Arb Paul Ehrlich Inst 1994; 87:79.
58. Yunginger JW, Adolphson CR. Standardization of allergens. In: Rose N, Conway de Macario E, Fahey JL, eds, Manual of clinical laboratory immunology. 4th edn. Washington, DC: American Society for Microbiology; 1992:678.
59. Lin Y, Miller CA. Standardization of allergenic extracts: an update on CBER's standardization program. Arb Paul Ehrlich Inst 1997; 91:127.
60. Slater JE, Gam AA, Solanki MD, et al. Statistical considerations in the establishment of release criteria for allergen vaccines in the USA. Arb Paul Ehrlich Inst 1999; 93:47.
61. Dobrovolskaia E, Gam A, Slater JE. Competition ELISA can be a sensitive method for the specific detection of small quantities of allergen in a complex mixture. Clin Exp Allergy 2006; 36:525–530.
62. Richman PG, Cissel DS. A procedure for total protein determination with special application to allergenic extract standardization. J Biol Stand 16:225, 1988.
63. Slater JE, Pastor RW. The determination of equivalent doses of standardized allergen vaccines. J Allergy Clin Immunol 2000; 105:468.
64. Slater, JE. Guidance for reviewers: potency limits for standardized dust mite and grass allergen vaccines: a revised protocol, 2000. Online. Available: http://www.fda.gov/cber/gdlns/mitegrasvac.htm

Allergen extracts in Europe

65. Note for Guidance on Allergen Products (Committee for Proprietary Medicinal Products, Human Medicines Evaluation Unit, European Agency for the Evaluation of Medicinal Products). Online. Available: http://www.emea.eu.int/pdfs/human/bwp/024396en.pdf (accessed 13 Mar 1996).
66. Spangfort MD, Larsen GD. Standardization of allergen-specific immunotherapy vaccines. Immunol Allergy Clin North Am 2006; 26:191–206.
67. Van Ree R. The CREATE project: EU support for the improvement of allergen standardization in Europe. Allergy 2004; 59:571–574.

The Structure and Function of Allergens

35

Geoffrey A Stewart, Jihui Zhang, and Clive Robinson

CONTENTS

- Introduction 569
- Allergen nomenclature 570
- Allergens and allergen sources 570
- Aeroallergens – pollens 570
- Aeroallergens – fungi 576
- Aeroallergens – animal-derived 581
- Aeroallergens – arthropod-derived 583
- Aeroallergens – occupational 585
- Ingested allergens 590
- Injected insect allergens 591
- Pathogen-derived allergens and autoallergens 595
- Three-dimensional structures of allergens 597
- Allergen biochemistry, immunogenicity, and inflammation 599
- Conclusions 607

SUMMARY OF IMPORTANT CONCEPTS

>> Allergen exposure may occur within and outside the home as well as in the workplace

>> The major sources of allergens include herbaceous dicotyledons, tree and grass pollens, fungi, animal danders, house-dust mites, cockroaches, and foods such as fruit, vegetables, nuts, fish, and shellfish

>> Each of these sources will contain several individual allergens, most of which will be proteins and have physiological importance for the source itself

>> Some of these allergens will be classified as major or minor based on their recognition by an allergic population, with a major allergen being recognized by 50% or more of the population

>> Phylogenetically related species will produce similar spectra of allergens which may be recognized by individuals sensitized to a single species in that group

>> Several of the clinically relevant allergens possess biochemical properties such as protease activity that may facilitate the sensitization process, for example, by enhancing epithelial permeability or stimulating proinflammatory cytokine release

INTRODUCTION

The impact of molecular biology and genomics on our understanding of allergen structure and function over the past 25 years has been enormous, and the data obtained during this period have made major contributions to the study of allergic diseases as well as other branches of science. The majority of clinically significant allergens have now been sequenced and their endogenous biochemical activities determined. More recently, the complete genomes of allergy-associated organisms such as *Aspergillus fumigatus*, the honey bee, and rice have been determined and it is anticipated that others will be soon completed. These advances have facilitated the determination of the three-dimensional structures of a significant number of allergens, the determination of allergen T cell-and B cell-reactive epitopes, and the construction of hypoallergenic variants for use

in the treatment of allergic disease (protein or DNA vaccines). In this chapter, the major and minor allergens from diverse sources associated with allergic disease will be catalogued in a manner reflecting the route of exposure usually associated with the allergen source in question. Not only will their basic physicochemical, biochemical and immunological properties be described but also the possibility that the inherent biochemical properties of allergens contribute to allergenicity will also be explored.

The reader is referred to previous reviews on the molecular and biochemical characteristics of allergens[1,2] as these provide additional and complementary data. In this way, the reader will be able to appreciate the history of allergen discovery. In addition, these reviews will also be a useful source of specific references that could not be included, due to space restraints. The reader is also referred to the Allergen Nomenclature Subcommittee of the International Union of Immunological Societies (IUIS) website (http://www.allergen.org) and the Allergome website (http://www.allergome.org), both of which maintain a list of characterized allergens. The IUIS Subcommittee also plays a central role in advising the scientific community on naming recently characterized allergens according to specific criteria. This system has served the allergen characterization community well and will be used throughout this chapter, although allergens yet to receive the IUIS imprimatur will also be described.

◼ ALLERGEN NOMENCLATURE ◼

Before the advent of detailed sequence information, the IUIS Allergen Nomenclature Subcommittee introduced guidelines to facilitate the consistent naming of purified allergens from complex sources. The naming procedure is based on using the first three letters (although four are sometimes used to avoid confusion e.g., 'Cand' and 'Can' for *Candida* and *Canis*, respectively) of the genus source (e.g., *Der*matophagoides) and combining it with the first one or two letters of the species name (e.g., *p*teronyssinus) and an Arabic numeral reflecting either the order in which the allergen was isolated or its clinical importance, or both. Allergens from different species within a genus or across phylogenetically related genera but similar on the basis of sequence identity, use the same numbering arrangement. For example, the related house-dust mite cysteine protease allergens from mites such as *Dermatophagoides pteronyssinus, D. farinae, Euroglyphus maynei,* and *Blomia tropicalis* are individually referred to as Der p 1, Der f 1, Eur m 1, and Blo t 1, or collectively as the Group 1 mite allergens. Where isoallergens from the same species have been characterized (>67% sequence identity), they are given a suffix (00–99), e.g., Amb a 1.01, Amb a 1.02. Where allergens from the same species differ by only a few residues, an additional two digits are used (e.g., Amb a 1.101) to differentiate them.

◼ ALLERGENS AND ALLERGEN SOURCES ◼

Individuals are exposed to a range of foreign substances in a variety of settings, both at home and at work. The term 'allergen' is used to describe any substance stimulating the production of immunoglobulin IgE in a genetically disposed individual but is synonymous with 'antigen', a term usually used to describe a substance that generates immunoglobulin responses other than IgE, or a cellular immune response. Although recent data suggest that the glycan part of a glycoprotein may be allergenic, e.g., that associated with *Cupressus arizonica* pollen allergens and the bee venom phospholipase A_2, IgE is usually produced against the proteinaceous part. About 20% of allergic patients may however, produce IgE to allergen glycan moieties with the potential to contribute to cross-reactivity. Most allergens, therefore, are proteins ranging in molecular weight from 5000 to 100000 Da.

Allergens are usually found in mixtures of (glyco) proteins comprising a particular source, and the most complex of these are pollens, fungi, and mites; with the least complex being animal danders and urine, and the

occupational allergens. The number of proteins from any given source that may be allergenic will vary, but sensitized patients producing IgE to a source will usually recognize more than one allergenic protein. The capacity of a susceptible individual to produce allergen-specific IgE will reflect both their genetic capability, the complexity of the source, the concentration of specific allergen in a source, the sensitivity of the assay used to determine allergenicity and, possibly, the inherent biochemical activity associated with the allergen (see later sections). Those allergens in a source recognized by more than 50% of allergic individuals are operationally termed 'major' but some of those considered 'minor' on a population basis may, of course, be of clinical significance at an individual level.

Potential allergens enter the body via a number of routes such as the respiratory and gastrointestinal tracts but they may also be injected (both natural, e.g., venoms as well as iatrogenically), although, the respiratory route is the most clinically important. The route of exposure will influence the types of allergic symptoms subsequently occurring, with exposure to aeroallergens giving rise to respiratory symptoms, in contrast to those ingested or injected which give rise to localized gastrointestinal or dermal symptoms, or more generalized systemic symptoms. In addition, individuals may be exposed to allergens resulting from gastrointestinal or respiratory infections due to fungal, bacterial, or helminthic pathogens. Finally, certain host proteins may also be allergenic (autoallergens).

◼ AEROALLERGENS – POLLENS ◼

Aeroallergens are considered to be the most common cause of allergic disease and are derived from a variety of complex sources, usually particulate, present in the environment. They include pollens, fungal spores, insect and mite feces, animal danders and dusts, and exposure may be perennial or seasonal. For example, exposure to pollen occurs in spring and summer, and symptoms generally correspond to atmospheric pollen concentrations, although perennial exposure may occur since pollen allergens have been detected in house dust. Fungal and mite allergen exposure may also be seasonal due to the effects of domestic microclimates on reproductive processes but is often perennial as allergens in the form of fecal pellets or spores accumulate in dust. Exposure to dander allergens, as well as occupational aeroallergens, is also likely to be perennial unless the precipitating source is removed.

Exposure to pollen allergens is dependent on the pollination process occurring in wind-pollinated (anemophilous) angiosperms and gymnosperms, including trees, herbaceous dicotyledons (weeds), and grasses, rather than insect-pollinated plants, and usually occurs in the temporal order listed. Exposure to pollen aeroallergens will be dependent on the types of plants growing in a particular location, as well as pollen-specific characteristics, such as buoyant density, ease of dispersion, and profusion. In addition, exposure will also be influenced by whether or not plants produce submicronic particles since they too contain allergens. Pollen grains range in size from about 5 to >200 µm, whereas submicronic particles vary from 0.5–2 µm, and studies suggest that approximately 20–100 grains/m^3 are sufficient to provoke disease. However, the concentrations of specific pollen-derived allergens, or submicronic particles required to initiate symptoms are presently unknown.

Thus far, most studies have been directed at allergens contained within pollens since they are primary sources of allergen but, attention is now turning to submicronic allergens in submicronic vectors originating either from within the pollen cytoplasm such as starch granules (amyloplasts;

approximately 700/pollen and each approximately 3 μm in diameter) and polysaccharide-containing wall-precursor bodies (P-particles),[3] or from pollen-related plant structures, such as orbicules or Ubisch bodies (<4 μm).[4] Starch granules and P-particles are released from pollen grains which land on the stigma of the receiving plant and, if genetically compatible, activation occurs. For example, the pollen grains from angiosperms hydrate on contact and pollen components either diffuse (e.g., pollen coat proteins, brassinosteroids) or are expelled from the grains after which pollen tube development occurs through the style, leading to fertilization. It is this process that is thought to account for allergen exposure in humans when grains land on mucosal surfaces. In contrast, pollen from gymnosperms (which lack stigma) is either trapped by a pollination drop (a secretion arising from the ovula per se), which is absorbed into the micropyle chamber, or engulfed by the ovula extensions. After this has occurred, pollen tube development begins. Angiosperm pollen grains may also encounter environmental water and it has been shown that when this occurs, cytoplasmic particles are expelled from the grains, thus releasing submicronic allergen particles into the atmosphere. This process is thought to contribute to thunderstorm-related outbreaks of asthma in the community,[5] since submicronic particles, in contrast to whole pollen, are capable of entering sufficiently deep into the respiratory tree to precipitate symptoms. In contrast to amyloplasts and P-particles, which are derived from pollen grains per se, orbicules are granules of plant sporopollenin that take up proteins, carbohydrates, and lipids in the anthers during pollen development. They are produced by secretory tapetal cells, accumulate in the locules of the anthers, and are released during anthesis. Although their specific function is unclear, they have been shown to contain major allergens in, for example, some clinically important angiosperm trees, herbaceous dicotyledons, and grasses as well as gymnosperm trees.[6] They are numerically superior compared with pollen, suggesting an important role in pollen-induced allergic disease, although there is little direct evidence to support this.

GRASS POLLEN ALLERGENS

Allergens from the pollens of several grass species have been described at the molecular level and include species belonging to the clinically important subfamilies Pooideae and Panicoideae. There is significant sequence similarity and, hence, immunological cross-reactivity between allergens from botanically-related pollens which has made it possible to group allergens from related species together (Table 35.1). This has resulted in the description of more than 13 distinct groups of proteins with diverse biochemical properties. Most of the available information on grass pollen allergens has been derived from the study of grass species belonging to the subfamily Pooideae such as rye (*Lolium perenne*), timothy (*Phleum pratense*), and Kentucky blue grass (*Poa pratensis*), but significant data from Bermuda grass *(Cynodon dactylon)* and maize *(Zea mays)* belonging to the subfamily Panicoideae have been generated.

The Group 1 (e.g., Lol p 1, Phl p 1) and related Group 2 and 3 allergens (e.g., Lol p 2, Lol p 3) are β-expansins present in most grass species in the two subfamilies, and are located in the anther cuticexine and intine wall layers, pollen cytoplasm, orbicules, and anther locules. The Group 4 and 13 allergens (e.g., Lol p 4, Phl p 4, Phl p 13) are enzymes involved in pectin degradation (as are some of the major allergens from tree pollen), whereas the Group 5 allergens (e.g., Lol p 5, Ph1 p 5, Poa p 5) and the related Group 6 allergens are ribonucleases. The function of the Group 11 allergens is presently unknown although they share sequence

homology with the Lamiales Group 1 allergens and soybean trypsin inhibitor. The Cyn d Bd 46K and the BG60 allergens show homology with cytochrome C oxidase and berberine bridge enzyme, respectively. The minor pollen allergens include the Group 7 calcium-binding proteins, the Group 10 cytochrome C proteins, and the Group 12 profilins. The clinical significance of the Group 14 (non-specific lipid transfer protein, LTP), 24 (antifungal, pathogenesis-related protein, PR-1), and 25 (thioredoxin) allergens in grass pollen, in general, is yet to be determined as they have only been described in the context of Bermuda grass pollen or maize pollen.

HERBACEOUS DICOTYLEDON SPECIES POLLEN ALLERGENS

The aeroallergens associated with pollens from Asteraceae, Urticaceae, Chenopodiaceae, and the Brassicaceae species are shown in Table 35.2. The most clinically important species from Asteraceae are ragweed, mugwort, sunflower, and feverfew, whereas the most important Urticaceae and Brassicaceae species are the wall pellitory, and oilseed rape and turnip, respectively. Several allergens from each of these species have been characterized. The major allergens in the Asteraceae group include pectin lyases (e.g., Amb a 1, 2), electron transport-related proteins (e.g., Amb a 3) and β-extensins (e.g., Par h 1), or are of unknown function (e.g., Art v 1, although related to the anther-specific SF18 protein from sunflower). In Urticaceae, Chenopodiaceae, and the Euphorbiaceae, the major allergens are lipid transfer proteins (LTP; e.g., Par o 1, 2) profilins (e.g., Mer a 1, Che a 3) and an olive-related allergen (Che a 1). The minor allergens in the Asteraceae and Brassicaceae families include cystatin, profilin (e.g., Hel a 2, Par j 3, Mer a 1), calcium-binding proteins (e.g., Bra j 1, 2), a berberine bridge enzyme, a receptor-like protein kinase, a cobalamin-independent methionine synthetase, a putative electron transfer associated proteins (e.g., Amb a 7), thioredoxin (e.g., PEC-2), and pollen coat proteins (e.g., PCP-1) and a ragweed protein of unknown function (Amb a 5). In contrast to that seen with the Urticaceae, the LTP from Asteraceae and Brassicaceae are minor allergens (e.g., Amb a 6, PEC-1, Art v 3). Several of the herbaceous dicotyledon pollen allergens correspond to those present in both grass and tree pollen and are, therefore, likely to function in the same way (see Tables 35.1, 35.3, 35.4, 35.6). The LTP allergens (which also represent important cross-reacting fruit allergens in the oral allergy syndrome [OAS][7]), are a ubiquitous group of low molecular weight proteins possessing a common hydrophobic core that can bind a variety of molecules such as lipids, and are likely to play a transport role within pollen. Interestingly, this role may involve binding to receptors since LTP within the plant per se bind to receptors on plasma membranes, known as elicitin receptors, suggesting a role in initiating plant defense mechanisms.[8]

TREE POLLEN ALLERGENS

The clinically important tree pollens described thus far are derived from both angiosperms (flowering trees, e.g., the Fagales and Lamiales) (Table 35.3) and gymnosperms (non-flowering conifers, e.g., the Taxoidiaceae and Cupressaceae) (Table 35.4). As for the grasses, pollens from species within the same family, for example, olive, lilac, ash and privit (Oleaceae), possess similar allergens and can, therefore, be grouped together, but there is limited similarity between divisions. The major angiosperm tree pollen allergens include the Fagales Group 1 pathogenesis-related

B

AEROBIOLOGY AND ALLERGENS

AEROALLERGENS – POLLENS

Table 35.1 Physicochemical and biochemical characteristics of grass pollen aeroallergens

Allergen	Frequency[a] of reactivity (%)	Mol. weight (kDa)	Function
Poaceae. Subfamily: Pooideae (i.e., rye, timothy, orchard, rice) and Panicoideae (e.g., Bermuda, Johnson, maize)			
Group 1 (e.g., Lol p 1)	>90	30	β-Expansins involved in cell wall loosening; shows homology with groups 2 and 3 allergens
Group 2 (e.g., Lol p 2)	>60	11	Shows homology with groups 1 and 3 grass allergens
Group 3 (e.g., Lol p 3)	70	11	Shows homology with groups 1 and 2 grass allergens
Group 4 (e.g., Lol p 4)	50–88	57	Pectate lyase
Group 5 (e.g., Lol p 5)	>90	29–31	Ribonuclease
Group 6 (e.g., Phl p 6)	76	12	Shows homology with Group 5 allergens
Group 7 (e.g., Cyn d 7)	10	9	Calcium-binding proteins
Group 10 (e.g., Lol p 10)	0–nd	12	Cytochrome C
Group 11 (e.g., Lol p 11)	65	15	Function unknown; shows homology with tree allergen Ole e 1, Che a 1 and soybean trypsin inhibitor
Group 12 (e.g., Phl p 12)	20–35	12	Profilin
Group 13 (e.g., Phl p 13)	50–100	55–60	Polygalacturonase
Group 14 (e.g., Zea m 14)	86	9	Non-specific lipid transfer protein
Group 24 (e.g., Cyn d 24)	29	21	Pathogenesis-related protein, PR-1
Group 25 (e.g., Zea m 25)	nd	14	Thioredoxin
Cyn d Bd46K	64	46	Shows homology with cytochrome c oxidase III from corn pollen
Cyn d BG60	nd	60	Berberine bridge enzyme

[a]Frequency data presented in each of these tables have been derived from many sources and will be dependent on a variety of factors. In addition, the data presented may reflect immediate hypersensitivity diseases including atopic dermatitis and allergic bronchopulmonary aspergillosis (ABPA) as well as delayed-type hypersensitivity disease.

[b]The Ph1 p 4 allergen is classified as a berberine bridge enzyme showing homology with the celery allergen Api 5.

nd, no data.

proteins (PR-10), which possess the ribonuclease activity (e.g., Bet v 1) (Table 35.5), pectin methyl esterase, the globulin-protein like proteins and LTP allergens. The Group 1 Fagales allergens are associated with starch granules and are extruded on contact with water in a manner similar to that described for grass pollen allergens. The important Lamiales allergens include the Group 1 soybean trypsin inhibitor-related allergens (Ole e 1; which share sequence similarity with grass pollen allergens, e.g., Lol p 11), the Group 3 calcium-binding proteins, the Group 7 LTP allergens, and the Group 4/9 β1,3-glucanases. A number of minor allergens have also been described in Angiosperm pollen, which are either common between the Fagales and the Lamiales, or specific. They include profilins (e.g., Bet v 2, Ole e 2), isoflavone reductase (e.g., Bet v 5), peptidyl-prolyl isomerase (e.g., Bet v 7), superoxide dismutase (e.g., Ole e 5), the cytosolic calcium-binding proteins (e.g., Bet v 3, 4, Ole e 8), LTP (e.g., Ole e 7), and a cysteine-rich allergen (e.g., Ole e 6).

In contrast to the angiosperm tree pollens, the majority of the clinically significant gymnosperm tree pollen allergens in both the Taxoidiaceae and Cupressaceae families (Table 35.4) are associated with pectin degradation, e.g., pectate lyase (e.g., Cry j 1, Jun a 1, Cha o 1) and polymethylgalacturonase (e.g., Cry j 2, Jun a 2, Cha o 2). Both enzyme types show sequence identities with the corresponding allergens in pollens derived from Asteraceae and Brassicaceae species (Table 35.2). Chitinase and isoflavone reductase are also clinically significant in Japanese cedar pollen. In addition to these allergens, several minor tree pollen allergens have been described and include calcium-binding proteins (e.g., Jun o 4) gymnosperm and thaumatin-like proteins (e.g. Jun a 3).

POLLEN PROTEINS AND FUNCTION

The functions of many of the allergens within pollen are now being delineated and this process is being helped enormously by proteomic analyses of pollen and pollen tube development.[9,10] So far, four analyses have been published (rice, Eastern white pine, Arabidopsis, and *Picea meyeri* pollen) and these studies show that pollen contain several hundred proteins with a significant proportion (about 40%) associated with the cytoplasm and involved in signal transduction, protein synthesis, and cell wall

572

Table 35.2 Physicochemical and biochemical characteristics of herbaceous dicotyledon pollen aeroallergens

Allergen	Frequency of reactivity (%)	Mol. weight (kDa)	Function
Asteraceae			
Short ragweed (*Ambrosia artemisiifolia*)			
Amb a 1	>90	40	Pectate lyase
Amb a 2	>90	41	Pectate lyase
Amb a 3	51	11	Plastocyanin; shows homology with electron transport proteins
Amb a 5	17	5	Function unknown
Amb a 6	21	11	Lipid transfer protein
Amb a 7	20	12	Shows homology with electron transport proteins
Amb a 8	nd	14	Profilin
Cytochrome c	nd	12	Cytochrome c
Cystatin	30	10	Cysteine protease inhibitor
Mugwort (*Artemisia vulgaris*)			
Art v 1	>70	47–60	Shows homology with *Helianthus* anther specific protein SF18
Art v 2	33	20	Shows homology with pathogenesis-related protein PR-1 from tomato, potato and the venom allergen Ves v 5
Art v 3	70	10	Lipid transfer protein
Art v 4	36	14	Profilin
Art v 5	nd	10	Polycalcin
Art v 6	nd	44	Pectate lyase
Feverfew (*Parthenium hysterophorus*)			
Par h 1	>90	31	β-Extensin
Sunflower (*Helianthus annus*)			
Hel a 1	57	34	Function unknown
Hel a 2	31	14	Profilin
Hel a 3	nd	9	Lipid transfer protein
Urticaceae			
Wall pellitory (*Parietaria officinalis/judaica*)			
Group 1 (e.g., Par o 1)	100	14	Lipid transfer protein
Group 2 (e.g., Par o 2)	82	11	Lipid transfer protein
Group 3 (e.g., Par j 3)	nd	14	Profilin
Chenopodiaceae			
Pigweed (*Chenopodium album*)			
Che a 1	77	17	Function unknown; shows homology with Ole e 1, Group 11 grass pollen allergens
Che a 2	55	14	Profilin
Che a 3	46	10	Polycalcin

(Continued)

Table 35.2 Physicochemical and biochemical characteristics of herbaceous dicotyledon pollen aeroallergens—cont'd

Allergen	Frequency of reactivity (%)	Mol. weight (kDa)	Function
Brassicaceae			
Oilseed rape (Brassica napus)			
Bra n 1	nd	9	Calcium-binding protein; shows homology with grass Cyn d 7 allergen
Bra n 2	nd	9	Calcium-binding protein
6/8 kDa protein	50	6/8	Calcium-binding protein
14 kDa protein	34	14	Profilin
27–69 kDa cluster	80	27–69	Shows homology with grass pollen Group 4 allergens
40 kDa protein	nd	40	Receptor-like protein kinase
70 kDa protein	nd	70	Berberine bridge protein
80 kDa protein	nd	80	Cobalamin-independent methionine synthetase
TRX-H-1	nd	14	Thioredoxin
PCP-1	nd	9	Pollen coat protein
Turnip (Brassica rapa)			
Bra r 1	nd	9	Calcium-binding protein; shows homology with grass Cyn d 7 allergen
Bra r 2	nd	9	Calcium-binding protein
PEC-1	>30	13	Lipid transfer protein
PEC-2	nd	14	Thioredoxin
PCP-1	nd	9	Pollen coat protein
Euphorbiaceae			
Mercurialis annua			
Mer a 1	>59	14	Profilin, actin-binding protein

remodeling. In this regard, it can be seen (Table 35.5) that the majority of allergens from grass, herbaceous dicotyledons, and tree pollens belong to those proteins involved in cell wall remodeling required for such processes as pollen tube growth. For example, the Group 1 allergens belong to the β group of plant proteins known as the expansins. These proteins are thought to play a central role in this process since they are involved in the cell wall loosening[11] required for the pollen tube to penetrate the stigma and grow through the style and into the ovary. The biochemical mechanism(s) involved in β-expansin-mediated cell wall loosening is yet to be determined. In this regard, although they show sequence homology with the family-45 glucosidases, they lack an essential aspartate residue necessary for catalytic activity.[11] In addition to the β-expansins, recent data also suggest a cell wall loosening-role for the lipid transfer protein (LTP) allergen. Pollen tube growth is also dependent on calcium ions and it can be seen that several of the allergens from grass, herbaceous dicotyledons, and tree pollen are calcium-binding proteins.

In addition, calcium-binding allergens are also thought to be involved in pollen tube growth and it is possible that the pollen-derived calcium-binding allergens are similarly involved. The process of pollen tube growth per se, as well as its progress through the style transmitting tract, may also involve degradation of pectin, a major plant cell wall polymer of α-linked galacturonic acid.[12] Grass pollens as well as Asteraceae, Brassicaceae, and tree pollens, comprise several enzymes necessary for its degradation, including pectate lyase and polymethylgalacturonase, all of which are allergenic. Pectin methylesterase, which is required to demethylate pectin prior to degradation, is also allergenic in the Fagales but its allergenicity in grass, herbaceous dicotyledons, Lamiales, and gymnosperms is unknown. Other allergens thought to be important in pollen tube growth are the profilins, a ubiquitous group of proteins involved in actin polymerization due to their ability to bind to proline residues. In pollen, these proteins are found in the pollen tube cytoplasm where they play a role in cytoskeletal actin streaming. The roles of the other major allergens in pollen biology, such as the grass Group 5 and the related Group 6 ribonuclease allergens are unclear, despite the former allergen being shown to be single-stranded nucleases with unusual topoisomerase activity. Similarly, the functions of the cytochrome oxidase allergen (Cyn d Bd46K), and the

Table 35.3 Physicochemical and biochemical characteristics of angiosperm tree pollen aeroallergens

Allergen	Frequency of reactivity (%)	Mol. weight (kDa)	Function
Fagales (birch, alder, hornbeam, oak)			
Group 1 (e.g., Bet v1)	>95	17	Ribonuclease, pathogenesis–related protein, PR-10
Group 2 (e.g., Bet v 2)	22	14	Profilin
Group 3 (e.g., Bet v 3)	<10	23	Calcium-binding protein
Group 4 (e.g., Bet v 4)	20	9	Calcium-binding protein
Group 5 (e.g., Bet v 5)	32	35	Isoflavone reductase
Group 7 (e.g., Bet v 7)	21	18	Peptidyl-prolyl isomerase (cyclophilin)
Group 8 (e.g., Cor a 8)	77	9	Lipid transfer protein
Group 9 (e.g., Cor a 9)	86	40	Globulin-like protein
Group 10 (e.g., Cor a 10)	nd	70	Luminal binding proteins
Group 11 (e.g., Cor a 11)	47	48	7S vicilin-like protein
Pectin methylesterase	66	65	Pectin methylesterase
Lamiales (olive, lilac, privet, ash, English plantain)			
Group 1 (e.g., Ole e 1)	>90	19, 20	Shows limited homology with soybean trypsin inhibitor and Lol p 11
Group 2 (e.g., Ole e 2)	>40	14	Profilin
Group 3 (e.g., Ole e 3)	20->50	9	Calcium-binding protein
Group 4 (e.g., Ole e 4)	80	32	Possibly Group 9 allergen
Group 5 (e.g., Ole e 5)	35	16	Superoxide dismutase
Group 6 (e.g., Ole e 6)	5–20	6	Cysteine-rich protein
Group 7 (e.g., Ole e 7)	>60	10	Lipid transfer protein
Group 8 (e.g., Ole e 8)	3–4	19	Calcium-binding protein
Group 9 (e.g., Ole e 9)	65–80	32–46	β-1,3-glucanase
Group 10 (e.g., Ole e 10)	nd	11	Shows homology with mosquito allergen Aed a 3 and Ascaris allergen Asc s 1; binds to laminarin. The allergen is homologous to the C-terminal domain of Ole e 9. Belongs to the CBM43 family of carbohydrate-binding proteins

berberine bridge allergen which, in other plant tissues, is involved in the synthesis of antimicrobial, alkaloid biosynthesis, are unclear.

Pollen allergens may also be involved in stress or defense responses. For example, several belong to the plant pathogenesis-related (PR) proteins (Table 35.6), which are constitutively expressed or produced in response to developmental signals, physical stress or infection by fungal, viral, and bacterial pathogens, and other elicitors. Currently, there are about 14 families of PR proteins (Table 35.6), comprising enzymes (glucanases, chitinases, peroxidases, ribonucleases, and proteases), enzyme inhibitors, defensins, thionins, LTP, and thaumatin-like proteins. They are found in a variety of plant tissues including fruit and nuts, and some are recognized as cross-reacting pan-allergens, which

play a role in OAS.[13,14] Thus far, allergens belonging to PR groups 1, 2, 3, 4, 5, 6, 9, 10, 11, and 14 have been described (Table 35.6)[15] and it is likely that they play a role in protecting the plant as the pollen tube breaches innate defense barriers as it grows towards the ovum. Other allergens likely to be involved in defense include the isoflavone reductases, which show about 60–80% sequence identity to plant-derived enzymes involved in the biosynthesis of lignins and isoflavones and the peptidyl-prolyl isomerases, also known as cyclophilins. The latter enzymes are a ubiquitous and highly conserved group of cytosolic enzymes whose role within cells is still unclear. However, they are known to play a role in protein folding and may also be important in stress responses in other plant tissue.

Table 35.4 Physicochemical and biochemical characteristics of gymnosperm tree pollen aeroallergens

Allergen	Frequency of reactivity (%)	Mol. weight (kDa)	Function
Taxodiaceae			
Japanese cedar (*Cryptomeria japonica*)			
Cry j 1	>85	39	Pectate lyase; shows homology with bacterial pectate lyase and Amb a 1 and 2
Cry j 2	76	37	Polymethylgalacturonase; shows homology with the Group 13 allergens from grasses
CJP-4	100	34	Class 1P chitinases; shows homology with Class I chitinase allergens from Per S a 1 and Mus a 1 Class I chitinases, latex allergen Hev b 11
CJP-6	76	30	Shows homology to isoflavone reductase, birch Bet v 6, and pear Pyr c 5 allergens
Cupressaceae			
Japanese juniper (*Juniperus rigida*)			
70 kDa allergen	100	70	Function unknown
Mountain cedar (*Juniperus ashei*)			
Jun a 1	71	40	Pectate lyase
Jun a 2	100	43	Polymethylgalacturonase
Jun a 3	43	30	Shows homology with thaumatin, osmotin, and amylase/trypsin inhibitor
Eastern red cedar (*Juniperus virginiana*)			
Jun v 1	46–92	43	Pectate lyase
Jun v 4	85	145	Function unknown
Prickly juniper (*Juniperus oxycedrus*)			
Jun o 1	nd	40	Pectate lyase
Jun o 4	15	18	Calcium-binding protein
Cypress (*Cupressus sempervirens*)			
Cup s 1	81	42	Pectate lyase
Cypress (*Cupressus arizonica*)			
Cup a 1	57	43	Pectate lyase
Japanese cypress (*Chamaecyparis obtusa*)			
Cha o 1	>50	38	Pectate lyase
Cha o 2	83	46	Polymethylgalacturonase

AEROALLERGENS – FUNGI

Spores from several fungal species have been shown to be important sources of indoor and outdoor allergens, and may even be found in space stations.[16] Of the many fungal species, the most clinically important are those derived from the Ascomycota (e.g., *Aspergillus fumigatus, Cladosporium herbarum, Penicillium chrysogenum, Alternaria alternata, Trichophyton rubrum,* and *Candida albicans*) and the Basidiomycota (e.g., *Malassezia furfur, Psilocybe cubensis,* and *Coprinus conatus*). All of these species use air-borne spore dispersal, and spores are often produced in concentrations exceeding those seen with pollens. In addition to spores, allergens may also be released from mycelia and yeast forms, and such sources will be particularly relevant in fungi which cause conditions such as allergic bronchopulmonary aspergillosis (ABPA), and immediate and delayed-type dermal infections involving *A. fumigatus, C. albicans, Trichophyton* species, and *M. furfur.* As with other allergen sources, the majority of

Table 35.5 Distribution of different functional types of protein in pollen/pollen tube and correlation with allergenicity

	Percent of proteome			[a]Allergen/homologue identified in pollen from:		Tree	
Function	Angiosperm	Gymnosperm	Grass	Herbaceous dicotyledon	Angiosperm	Gymnosperm	
Signal transduction	6–10	9–12	None	None	None	None	
Vesicle trafficking	3	–	None	None	None	None	
Transcriptional regulation-related	2	10	None	None	None	None	
Storage proteins	8	4	None	None	Group 9 fagales; Group 11 fagales	None	
Transposition	1	–	None	None	None	None	
Cytoskeleton dynamics	2–3	6	Profilin	Profilin	Profilin	None	
Protein synthesis, assembly, and degradation	14–15	16	None	None	Luminal binding protein	None	
Stress response and/or defence	4–7	16	Cyn d 24; Cyn d Bd 60 kDa; cyclophilin	Legumin-like protein; cyclophilin	Endo-β-1,3-1 glucanase; ribonuclease; isoflavone reductase; cyclophilin	Thaumatin-like proteins; isoflavone reductase	
Wall remodeling and metabolism	11–15	12	β-expansins; polygalacturonase; pectin methylesterase; pectate lyase; calcium-binding proteins; lipid transfer proteins	Pectate lyase; calcium-binding protein	Calcium-binding protein; lipid transfer protein; pectin-methylesterase	Polygalacturonase; pectate lyase; pectin-methylesterase; calcium-binding proteins	
Carbohydrate and energy metabolism	16–25	18–30	None	None	None	None	
Ion/electron transport	4	–	Group 10	Plastacyanin; Amb a 7	None	None	
Metabolism	8–21	17	None	Cobalamin-independent methionine synthetase	None	None	
Miscellaneous	2	–	Thioredoxin	Thioredoxin	None	None	
Unknown function	8–11	12	Group 11	Group 5; Amb a 5; Art v 1; Art v 2; Hel a 1; Che a 1	Group 1 lamiales; Group 5 lamiales	70 kDa cypress allergen; Jun v 4	

[a]Categorization based on homologue or allergen found in proteomic studies or in allergen characterization studies. Percent proteins in a particular category reflect recent data from rice, *Arabidopsis*, *Picea meyeri*, and *Pinus strobe* pollen. Categorization may vary between different proteomes.

AEROALLERGENS – FUNGI

allergens are proteins or glycoproteins but recent evidence indicates that mannans from fungi such as *C. albicans* and *M. furfur* may be allergenic.

Although fungal allergens can be found in both mycelia and spores, some of the spore-derived allergens may be absent in mycelial extracts. At present, it is not clear whether atopic individuals are initially sensitized to spore- or to mycelial-derived allergens. However, many of the fungal allergens described below appear to be cytoplasmic and involved in protein synthesis or energy metabolism, although secretory and cell wall allergens also feature. These functions would, therefore, be consistent with observations that the concentrations of certain spore-derived allergens increase with germination,[17] a process requiring the synthesis of a range of proteins for structural and metabolic purposes.

The most clinically important sources of aeroallergens are *Aspergillus*, *Penicillium*, *Cladosporium*, and *Alternaria* species. Of these species, there is a relatively low degree of allergenic cross-reactivity between *A. alternata* and the rest. The major allergens from the three clinically important species (either with regard to respiratory disease or ABPA) include Alt a 1, 2, and 13, Asp f 1, 2, and 4, and Cla h 1, respectively (Table 35.7). The functions of Alt a 1 and Cla h 1 are unknown at present; however, Alt a 2 is a low molecular weight, alkaline protein which has eukaryote-2 initiation factor (EIF) α kinase activity and, therefore, may play a role in protein synthesis, and Alt a 13 is a glutathione-S-transferase. Asp f 1 is homologous to the fungal cytotoxin mitogillin (from *A. restrictus*) and alpha-sarcin (from *A. gigantus*), and is found in both spores and mycelium. These low molecular weight proteins are non-glycosylated, cytotoxic enzymes with purine specific ribonuclease activity. The Asp f 2 allergen is a protein showing homology with the *C. albicans* 54 kDa mannoprotein, which has been shown to bind to human fibrinogen. The Asp f 4 is a

binding protein associated with peroxisomes which are self-replicating organelles similar in size to lysosomes and play an important metabolic role in removing toxic substances from cells due to their specific collection of enzymes.

The major allergens from *Penicillium*, *Candida*, and *Trichophyton* species are serine proteases, dipeptidyl peptidases, aspartate proteases, enolases, peroxisomal membrane proteins, or are of unknown function. With regard to the serine proteases, they are similar in structure to the bacterial subtilisins and two types have been identified. They include the secreted 33 kDa alkaline proteases (e.g., Asp f 13, Asp fl 13, Pen c 13, Pen ch 13, Tri r/t 2) and the 39 kDa vacuolar proteases (e.g., Pen ch 18) involved in protein processing within vacuoles. The dipeptidyl peptidase from *Trichophyton* species (Tri r 4) is also a secretory protein but shares sequence similarity with enzymes from *Aspergillus* species implicated in aspergilloma. The function of the 30 kDa *Trichophyton* Tri t 1 allergen is unknown, although it may be an exo-β-1,3-glucanase, given limited sequence homology data. The peroxisomal membrane protein allergens (e.g., Asp f 3, Pen c 3, Mala f 2, 3, 5) possess thiol-dependent peroxidase activity. The enolases, glycolytic enzymes involved in the dehydration of glycerate-2-phosphate to produce phosphoenolpyruvate, represent a major group of cross-reacting allergens from a variety of fungal species (e.g., Cla h 6, Asp f 22w, Alt a 11).[18]

In addition to these allergens, several minor allergens have been described which are associated with specific cellular functions and, therefore, share significant sequence identity with proteins in many diverse species, including humans. For example, several belong to the group of proteins termed molecular chaperones which play a role in protein assembly and include protein disulfide isomerases (e.g., Alt a 4), peptidyl-prolyl

Table 35.6 Relationship between plant pathogenesis-related proteins and allergens

Family	Description or characteristics	Allergen or source
PR-1	Antifungal, mechanism unknown	Cyn d 24
PR-2	Endo-β-1,3-glucanase	Hev b 2, Ole e 4/9
PR-3[a]	Endochitinase	Per s a 1, Hev b 11, Mus a 1
PR-4[a]	Chitin-binding proteins	Turnip prohevein, Hev b 6, wheat germ agglutinin
PR-5	Thaumatin-like proteins, antifungal, may have endo-β-1,3-glucanase activity	Pru av 2, Mal d 2, Jun a 3
PR-6	Protease inhibitor	nd
PR-7	Protease	nd
PR-8[a]	Endochitinase	nd
PR-9	Peroxidase	Wheat, barley allergens
PR-10	Ribonuclease	Bet v 1, Mal d 1, Pru av 1, Pyr c 1, Api g 1, Dau c 1, etc.
PR-11[a]	Chitinase	Pru av 1, Pyr c 1, Api g 1
PR-12	Plant defensins	nd
PR-13	Thionins	nd
PR-14	Lipid transfer proteins	Pru p 3, Mal d 3, Gly m 1

[a]PR-3 – type I (basic), II (acidic), IV, V, VI, VII chitinases; PR-4 – type I, II chitinases; PR-11 – type I chitinase. nd, indicates that allergens belonging to a particular group have yet to be described.

Table 35.7 Physicochemical and biochemical characteristics of fungal allergens

Allergen	Frequency of reactivity (%)	Mol. weight (kDa)	Function
Ascomycota			
Alternaria alternata			
Alt a 1	>80	14	Function unknown
Alt a 2	61	20	EIF-2α kinase
Alt a 3	5	70	Heat shock protein 70
Alt a 4	42	57	Protein disulfide isomerase
Alt a 5	8–14	11	Ribosomal P2 protein, shows homology with Cla h 4
Alt a 6	50	46	Enolase
Alt a 7	7	22	YCP4 protein
Alt a 8	41	29	Mannitol dehydrogenase
Alt a 10	2	54	Aldehyde dehydrogenase, shows homology with Cla h 3
Alt a 12	nd	12	Ribosomal P1 protein
Alt a 13	100	26	Glutathione-S-transferase
Aspergillus fumigatus			
Asp f 1	85	17	Ribonuclease; shows homology with mitocillin
Asp f 2	96	36	Shows homology with *Candida albicans* fibrinogen-binding protein
Asp f 3	84	19	Peroxisomal membrane protein, belongs to the peroxiredoxin family, thiol-dependent peroxidase
Asp f 4	78–83[a]	40	Shows homology with bacterial ABC transporter binding protein, associated with peroxisome
Asp f 5	74	40	Metalloprotease
Asp f 6	42–56[a]	27	Manganese superoxide dismutase, shows homology with Hev b 10
Asp f 7	29	12	Shows homology with fungal riboflavin, aldehyde-forming enzyme
Asp f 8	8–15	11	Ribosomal P2 protein
Asp f 9	31	34	Shows homology with plant and bacterial endo-β-1,3–1,4 glucanases
Asp f 10	3	34	Aspartic protease
Asp f 11	nd	24	Peptidyl-prolyl isomerase
Asp f 12	nd	90	Heat shock protein 90
Asp f 13	>60	34	Alkaline serine protease
Asp f 15	nd	16	Shows homology with a serine protease antigen from *Coccidioides immitis*
Asp f 16	70	43	Shows homology with Asp f 9
Asp f 18	79	34	Vacuolar serine protease
Asp f 22w	nd	46	Enolase

(Continued)

Table 35.7 Physicochemical and biochemical characteristics of fungal allergens—cont'd

Allergen	Frequency of reactivity (%)	Mol. weight (kDa)	Function
Cladosporium herbarium			
Cla h 1	>60	13	Function unknown
Cla h 2	43	19	Function unknown
Cla h 5	22	11	Ribosomal P2 protein
Cla h 6	20	48	Enolase
Cla h 7	nd	22	YCP4 protein
Cla h 8	57	29	Mannitol dehydrogenase
Cla h 9	nd	nd	Vacuolar serine protease
Cla h 10	36	53	Aldehyde dehydrogenase
Cla h 12	nd	11	Ribosomal P1 protein
HSP 70	nd	70	Heat shock protein
Penicillium chrysogenum/notatum			
Pen ch 13	>80	34	Alkaline serine protease
Pen ch 18	>80	28–34	Vacuolar serine protease
Pen ch 20	56	62	Shows homology with β-N-acetylglucosaminidase from *Candida albicans*
Penicillium citrinum			
Pen c 3	46	18	Peroxisomal membrane protein, belongs to the peroxiredoxin family, thiol-dependent peroxidase
Pen c 13	100	33	Alkaline serine protease
Pen c 19	41	70	Show homology with hsp 70 heat shock protein
Pen c 22	nd	46	Enolase
Pen c 24	8	25	Elongation factor 1-beta
Candida albicans			
Cand a 1	77	40	Alcohol dehydrogenase
Cand a 3	nd	nd	Peroxisomal protein
37 kDa allergen	nd	37	Aldolase
43 kDa allergen	nd	43	Phosphoglycerate kinase
48 kDa allergen	50	46	Enolase
Acid protease	75	35	Aspartate protease
Trichophyton tonsurans			
Tri t 1	54	30	Function unknown, possible
Tri t 2	42	30	Subtilisin-like protease, shows homology with Pen ch 13, Pen c 13
Tri t 4	61	83	Dipeptidyl peptidase
Trichophyton rubrum			
Tri r 1/2	nd	30	Subtilisin-like protease, shows homology with Pen ch 13, Pen c 13
Tri r 4	nd	83	Dipeptidyl peptidase
Rhodoturala mucilaginosa			
Rho m 2	57	31	Vacuolar serine protease

Table 35.7 Physicochemical and biochemical characteristics of fungal allergens – cont'd

Allergen	Frequency of reactivity (%)	Mol. weight (kDa)	Function
Basidiomycota			
Malassezia furfur			
Mala f 1	61	36	Function unknown
Mala f 2	72	21	Peroxisomal membrane protein, belongs to the peroxiredoxin family, thiol-dependent peroxidase
Mala f 3	70	20	Peroxisomal membrane protein, belongs to the peroxiredoxin family, thiol-dependent peroxidase, shows homology with Asp f 3 and Mala f 2
Mala f 4	83	36	Mitochondrial malate dehydrogenase
Mala f 5	nd	18	Peroxisomal membrane protein, belongs to the peroxiredoxin family, thiol-dependent peroxidase, shows homology with Mala f 2/3 and Asp f 3
Mala f 6	nd	17	Peptidyl-prolyl isomerase (cyclophilin)
Mala f 7	89	16	Function unknown
Mala f 8	nd	19	Shows homology with immunoreactive mannoprotein from *Cryptococcus neoformans*
Mala f 9	44	14	Function unknown
Coprinus comatus			
Cop c 1	25	9	Function unknown
Cop c 2	19	12	Thioredoxin
Cop c 3	nd	37	Function unknown
Cop c 5	nd	16	Function unknown
Cop c 7	nd	16	Function unknown
Psilocybe cubensis			
Psi c 1	>50	46	Function unknown
Psi c 2	>50	16	Peptidyl-prolyl isomerase (cyclophilin)

[a]Frequency determined in ABPA patients.

isomerases (e.g., Asp f 11, Psi c 2, Mala f 6), and heat shock proteins (e.g., Alt a 3, Asp f 12, Pen c 19). Some of these proteins work in concert to facilitate the folding of proteins after they are synthesized, e.g., heat shock proteins and peptidyl-prolyl isomerases.[19] Such pairs of proteins are found in spores from *Aspergillus* and *Alternaria* species, and one or other of these have been shown to be allergenic in other species (e.g., *C. herbarium*), suggesting that the corresponding member yet to be isolated, will also be allergenic.

Other common groups of fungal allergens include the 60S P1 and P2 ribosomal proteins involved in protein chain elongation (e.g., Cla h 3/4, Alt a 6, Asp f 8, Alt a 12, Cla h 12), superoxide dismutase (e.g., Asp f 6), dehydrogenases (e.g., Alt a 10, Cla h 3, Cand a 1), aldehyde-forming enzyme (e.g., Asp f 7), 1,4-benzoquinone reductase (e.g., Alt a 7, Cla h 5), aldolase (a 37kDa allergen from *Candida*), thioredoxin (Cop c 2), proteins showing homology with the 88kDa mannoprotein from *Filobasidiella* (*Cryptococcus*) *neoformans* (e.g., Mala f 8), and a possible serine protease (e.g., Asp f 15) showing homology with *Coccidioides immitis* 19kDa antigen. The functions of some of the other minor fungal allergens that have been described remain to be determined (e.g., Asp f 16, Cla h 2, Mala f 7, 9, Cop c 1, 3, 5, 7).

■ AEROALLERGENS – ANIMAL-DERIVED ■

The clinically important animal allergens in both domestic and occupational settings are derived from cats, dogs, cows, rats, mice, horses, rabbits, mice, gerbils, and guinea pigs (Table 35.8), which accumulate in dusts in both settings. The allergens are derived from either dander, epithelium,

Table 35.8 Physicochemical and biochemical characterization of animal and dander allergens

Allergen	Frequency of reactivity (%)	Mol. weight (kDa)	Function
Cat (Felix domesticus)			
Fel d 1	>80	33–39	Heterodimer, function unknown; chain 1 shows homology with 10 kDa secretory protein from human Clara cells, mouse salivary androgen-binding protein subunit; rabbit uteroglobin and a Syrian hamster protein
Fel d 2	15–22	69	Serum albumin
Fel d 3	60–90	11	Cystatin
Fel d 4	nd	22	Lipocalin
Fel d 5W	nd	400	IgA
Fel d 6W	nd	800–1000	IgM
Fel d 7W	nd	150	IgG
Dog (Canis familiaris)			
Can f 1	>70	19–25	Lipocalin; shows homology with Von Ebner's gland protein which has cysteine protease inhibitory activity
Can f 2	70	27	Lipocalin; shows homology with other lipocalin allergens
Can f 3	35–77	69	Serum albumin
IgG	88	150	Immunoglobulin G
Horse (Equus caballus)			
Equ c 1	100	22	Lipocalin; shows homology with rodent urinary proteins
Equ c 2	100	16	Lipocalin; shows homology with rodent urinary proteins
Equ c 3	nd	67	Serum albumin
Equ c 4	nd	19	Shows homology with rat mandibular gland protein A
Equ c 5	nd	17	Function unknown
Cow (Bos domesticus)			
Bos d 2^a	97	18	Function; shows homology to the rodent lipocalin allergens
Bos d 3	nd	11	S100 calcium-binding protein
AS1	31	21	Oligomycin sensitivity-conferring protein of the mitochondrial adenosine triphosphate synthase complex
BDA 11	nd	12	Shows homology with human calcium-binding psoriasin protein
Mouse (Mus musculus)			
Mus m 1	>80	19	Major urinary protein; shows homology with lipocalins such as β-lactoglobulin, odorant-binding proteins, Rat n 2 Rat (Rattus norvegicus)

(Continued)

Table 35.8 Physicochemical and biochemical characterization of animal and dander allergens—cont'd

Allergen	Frequency of reactivity (%)	Mol. weight (kDa)	Function
Rat (Rattus norvegicus)			
Rat n 1	>80	21	Lipocalin; shows homology with lipocalins such as β-lactoglobulin, odorant-binding proteins, Mus m 1
Albumin	24	69	Serum albumin
Rabbit (Oryctolagus cuniculi)			
Ory c 1	nd	18	Odorant-binding protein, lipocalin; shows homology with Ory c 2
Ory c 2	nd	21	Odorant-binding protein
8 kDa allergen	nd	8	Shows homology with rabbit uteroglobin
Albumin	<50	69	Serum albumin

[a]See also Table 35.13 for cows' milk-derived allergens.

fur, urine, or saliva. However, it is possible that the allergens originate from the same source, e.g., saliva or urine, and are then distributed to other sites by grooming. The major mammalian dander allergens include the lipocalins (also referred to as calycines)[20] which play a role in the binding and/or transport of small hydrophobic molecules and comprise proteins such as β-lactoglobulin, bilin-binding proteins, α_1-microglobin and odorant-binding proteins, cystatins, immunoglobulins, and albumins. Allergens in the lipocalin superfamily group include those from horse (e.g., Equ c 1, 2), cow (e.g., Bos d 2, Bos d 5 – β-lactoglobulin), dog (e.g., Can f 1, 2; which may also have cysteine protease inhibitory activity), rabbit (e.g., Ory c 1, 2), mouse (e.g., Mus m 1), and rat (e.g., Rat n 1) dander or urine. These proteins may exist as monomers (Bos d 2 and Mus m 1) or homodimers (Equ c 1 and Bos d 5). The nature of the ligands bound by the mammalian lipocalin allergens is unclear although the mouse allergen is thought to bind pheromones, and there are data to suggest that the horse allergen may bind histamine. Recently however, it has been shown that the Bos d 5 lipocalin allergen, along with other non-allergenic lipocalins, possesses non-specific endonuclease activity. In this regard, the catalytically important glutamic acid at position 134 in Bos d 5 necessary for phosphodiester bond cleavage is also conserved in Bos d 2, Equ c 1, Can f 1 (but not Can f 2), and Mus m 1, as well as the cockroach Bla g 4 lipocalin allergen, suggesting that they, too, may possess such activity.[21]

In addition to the major allergens described above, several minor mammalian allergens have been demonstrated and include the serum albumins (e.g., Fel d 2, Equ c 3, Can f 3, rat, mouse, and rabbit albumin), immunoglobulins (e.g., Fel d 5–7), an oligomycin sensitivity-conferring protein (e.g., AS1) of the mitochondrial adenosine triphosphate synthase complex, a calcium-binding psoriasin-like allergen (e.g., BDA 11), a horse allergen showing homology to rat mandibular gland protein A (e.g., Equ c 4), and a protein of unknown function (e.g., Equ c 5). The sequence identities observed between similar proteins from different species, for example, the albumins account for the marked allergenic cross-reactivity observed in clinical studies.

In contrast to the above animal-derived allergens, the major cat allergens appear to be non-lipocalin proteins. In this regard, Fel d 1 is a heterodimeric protein comprising two distinct peptides, designated chains 1 and 2, where chain 1 shows sequence homology with proteins belonging to the uteroglobin family thought to play a role in inflammation. Recent crystallographic studies indicate structural homology with uteroglobin. Allergens corresponding to Fel d 1 appear to be restricted to cat and dog species and to the lagomorphs, such as rabbit. The function of this group of proteins is unclear, but recent data[22] suggest that they may be closely associated with protease activity. The other major cat allergen is the cystatin allergen, Fel d 3, which is a cysteine protease inhibitor. Finally, cat dander has been shown to contain a minor serum albumin allergen (Fel d 2).

■ AEROALLERGENS – ARTHROPOD-DERIVED ■

The main arthropod allergen sources are to be found in *Insecta* (e.g., midges, cockroaches, moths, butterflies, flies, silverfish, locusts) and *Arachnida* (mites),[23] and allergy may arise either in the home or in scientific institutions where many arthropods are reared or studied. Of the arthropods, house-dust mites and cockroaches are the most clinically important sources and atopy results from exposure to allergens derived from whole bodies, salivary secretions, and fecal pellets which accumulate in house-dust or in dusts generated by the rearing of insects in occupational settings.

MITE AEROALLERGENS

Mite species are ubiquitous but the most clinically important species belong to the Pyroglyphidae (e.g., *Dermatophagoides pteronyssinus, D. farinae, Euroglyphus maynei*), Acaridae (e.g., *Acarus siro, Tyrophagus putrescentiae, T. longior*), Glycyphagidae (e.g., *Glycyphagus domesticus, Lepidoglyphus destructor*), and Echimyopodidae (e.g., *Blomia tropicalis*). The major allergens from different mite species are either enzymes, actin-binding proteins, ligand-binding proteins or proteins of unknown function (Table 35.9). The mite enzymes include those involved in digestion such as cysteine protease (e.g., Der p 1, Der f 1, Eur m 1), trypsin (e.g., Der p 3), chymotrypsin (e.g., Der p 6), a collagenase-like enzyme (e.g., Der p 9), and amylase (e.g., Der p 4), as well as a chitinase that has been shown to be an allergen for humans (Der f 18) and dogs (Der p 15) with atopic dermatitis. In this regard, the region comprising residues 505–543 shows limited homology with the C-terminal third of Blo t 12 allergen suggesting that the latter is enzymatically similar although of lower molecular weight.

The actin-binding allergens include tropomyosin (e.g., Der p 10) and paramyosin (e.g., Der f 11), both of which form part of the cytoskeleton of most cells, suggesting that cellular debris is a significant source of

allergen, and derived either from the whole body or from fecal pellets. The mite tropomyosin allergens show marked sequence identity with similarly allergenic proteins from other invertebrates (see Table 35.13 below). In addition to the above allergens, the Group 2 allergens (e.g., Der p 2, Lep d 2, Gly d 2) are also classified as major allergens, although their function in mites is still to be determined. It has been proposed that the Group 2 allergens play a role in reproduction since they show significant sequence similarity with a group of phylogenetically conserved mammalian epididymal proteins. However, this role has been difficult to reconcile on the basis of data showing that the allergen is restricted to the mite gut and fecal pellets rather than reproductive organs. Despite this, recent studies have shown that the mammalian epidymal-equivalent proteins bind cholesterol and that Der p 2 binds to liposomes suggesting that the Group 2 allergens are involved in the transfer of this or similar ligands in either the mite gut or reproductive system. More recently, mites have been shown to produce the high molecular weight Group 14 allergen

Table 35.9 Physicochemical and biochemical characteristics of mite aeroallergens

Allergen	Frequency of reactivity (%)	Mol. weight (kDa)	Function
Pyroglyphidae/Glycyphagidae/Acaridae/Echimyopodidae			
Group 1 (e.g., Der p 1)	>90	25	Cysteine protease
Group 2 (e.g., Der p 2)	>90	14	Shows homology with putative human epididymal protein, possible cholesterol-binding protein
Group 3 (e.g., Der p 3)	90	25	Trypsin
Group 4 (e.g., Der p 4)	25–46	56	Amylase
Group 5 (e.g., Der p 5)	9–70	13	Function unknown
Group 6 (e.g., Der p 6)	39	25	Chymotrypsin
Group 7 (e.g., Der p 7)	53–62	11–29	Function unknown
Group 8 (e.g., Der p 8)	40	26	Glutathione transferase
Group 9 (e.g., Der p 9)	>90	28	Collagenase-like serine protease
Group 10 (e.g., Der p 10)	81	33	Tropomyosin
Group 11 (e.g., Der f 11)	82	98	Paramyosin
Group 12 (e.g., Blo t 12)	50	16	May be a chitinase; shows homology with Der f 15
Group 13 (e.g., Lep d 13)	11–23	15	Fatty acid-binding protein
Group 14 (e.g., Der f 14)	84	190	Vitellogenin or lipophorin
Group 15 (e.g., Der f 15)	95	63/98[a]	Chitinase; shows homology with Blo t 12 allergen
Group 16 (e.g., Der f 16)	35	53	Gelsolin
Group 17 (e.g., Der f 17)	35	30	Calcium-binding protein
Group 18 (e.g., Der f 18)	nd	60	Chitinase
Group 20 (e.g., Der p 20)	nd	40	Arginine kinase
Mag29	nd	67	Heat shock protein

[a]Glycosylated and non-glycosylated form. Frequency determined in dogs with atopic dermatitis.

which encompasses two previously described allergens (Mag 1 and 3) which show sequence identity with a number of lipid-binding proteins including lipophorins and vitellogenin. Finally, mites have been shown to possess two major groups of allergens of unknown function (e.g., Der p 5 and 7). Mites also produce a number of minor allergens (Table 35.9), including gelsolin (e.g., Der f 16), fatty acid-binding protein (e.g., Lep d 13, Aca s 13, Blo t 13), glutathione S-transferase, heat shock protein, and an EF-hand calcium-binding protein (e.g., Der f 17).

INSECT AEROALLERGENS

A number of insect-derived proteins have been shown to be clinically significant aeroallergens.[23] In this regard, allergens from midges (e.g., *Chironomus thummi thummi*; bloodworms), *Cladotanytarsus lewisi*, *Polypedium nubifer* and *Chironomus kiiensis*, cockroaches (e.g., *Blattella germanica* and *Periplaneta americana*) and moths (e.g., *Plodia interpunctella*) have been described (Table 35.10). These allergens may be derived from whole insect bodies or from feces, and there is evidence to indicate that the spectrum and concentrations of specific allergens in these different sources may vary. In midges, the major allergens are hemoglobins (e.g., Chi t 1, Cla l 1, Pol n 1), whereas in cockroach, the major allergens are enzymes, such as glutathione S-transferase (e.g., Bla g 5) and an inactive aspartate protease (e.g., Bla g 2), lipocalin (e.g., Bla g 4), troponin C, a calcium-binding protein (e.g., Bla g 6), tropomyosin (e.g., Per a 7), hexamerin (an insect storage protein belonging to the hemocyanin superfamily (e.g., Per a 3), or proteins of unknown function (e.g., Bla g 1, Per a 1; structurally related to a group of mosquito proteins induced in the gut after a blood meal).

The Bla g 2 allergen shows marked sequence similarity to porcine pepsin, although it appears to be proteolytically inactive due to amino acid substitutions in the catalytic region. However, the allergen is related to a large group of pregnancy-associated glycoproteins of unknown function found in the mononuclear and invasive binucleate cells of the epithelial layer of the trophectoderm in artiodactyl species, such as cow and sheep. These aspartate protease-related proteins possess the characteristic bilobed aspartate protease structure with a cleft capable of binding peptide ligands. However, in the cockroach, just as in the case of the mite Group 2 allergens, which show homology with proteins present in the mammalian reproductive system, the allergen is expressed solely in the gut. In addition to cockroach and midges, an arginine kinase allergen from the Indian meal moth has been described (Plo i 1),[24] which possesses an actin-binding site and is involved in energy storage. It shows marked homology with similar enzymes from various invertebrates, including an ingested allergen from the shrimp, *Parapenaeus fissures*.[25]

■ AEROALLERGENS – OCCUPATIONAL ■

The major occupational allergens include fungal, bacterial, and mammalian hydrolytic enzymes, egg powder, latex products, and flours derived from rice, wheat, barley and rye seeds, castor bean and mustard seeds, green coffee beans, Ispaghula and soybeans (Table 35.11). Allergy results from exposure to such materials in industries where they are produced, used or added to other products such as washing detergents, pancreatic

supplements and doughs and, particularly with regard to the latter, are associated with the clinical condition known as Baker's asthma.[26] Although the respiratory tract is the major route, exposure may also occur via the skin as, for example, with latex allergens present in latex gloves and other materials used in spina bifida and other patients undergoing multiple surgical procedures[27] (Table 35.12). It should also be noted, however, that many of these aeroallergens are also important as ingested allergens.

FUNGAL, BACTERIAL, MAMMALIAN, AND PLANT-DERIVED HYDROLYTIC AEROALLERGENS

The major enzymatic aeroallergens include the bacterial subtilisins and amylases used in the detergent industry, mammalian serine proteases (e.g., trypsin, chymotrypsin, and pepsin) used in pancreatic supplements in the treatment of cystic fibrosis patients, the plant cysteine proteases (e.g., Car p 1, Ana c 2) used in the pharmaceutical industry, fungal amylases (e.g., Asp o 21) and various other carbohydrases, such as β-xylosidase (Asp f 14), cellulase, and glucoamylase used in the baking industry (Table 35.11).

EGG AEROALLERGENS

The major egg allergens in egg powder are derived from either the white or yolk (Table 35.11).[28] Those contained within egg white include ovomucoid (Gal d 1), ovalbumin (Gal d 2), conalbumin (Gal d 3), and lysozyme (Gal d 4), whereas that in yolk is α-livitin (chicken albumin, Gal d 5). However, the most frequently recognized egg allergens are Gal d 3 and Gal d 5. The biochemical activities of each of these proteins, with the exception of ovalbumin, is known and, in this regard, ovomucoid, conalbumin (also known as ovotransferrin), lysozyme, and α-livitin are protease inhibitors, an iron transport protein, a bacteriostatic agent, a carbohydrase with bacteriolytic properties, and a ligand transport protein, respectively. Many of the egg (and flour)-derived allergens will also be important as ingested allergens and will be described below.

LATEX AEROALLERGENS

The major allergens from latex include the rubber-associated proteins prohevein (Hev b 1, 3), prohevein (Hev b 6), and a protein of unknown function (Hev b 5) (Table 35.12).[29] The minor allergens include a patatin-like protein (Hev b 7), enolase (Hev b 9), manganese superoxide dismutase (Hev b 10), profilin (Hev b 8), and carbohydrases (Hev b 2, 11w). Exposure to these allergens occurs due to their absorption into the starch powder used to facilitate the donning of gloves or leach from latex-derived materials used in surgical procedures.

SEED-DERIVED AEROALLERGENS

The major seed-derived aeroallergens are proteins that play important roles in defense, storage, or metabolism (Table 35.11). The major defense-related proteins include 12–15 kDa amylase/trypsin inhibitory albumin proteins (e.g., Hor v 15, Ory s 1, Sec c 1), the 2S seed storage albumins (napins; e.g., Sin a 1, Ric c 1), vicilin-related proteins (which may possess chitin-binding activity with consequent antifungal

Table 35.10 Physicochemical and biochemical characteristics of insect aeroallergens

Allergen	Frequency of reactivity (%)	Mol. weight (kDa)	Function
Chironomidae			
Bloodworm (Chironomus thummi thummi)			
Chi t I-9	>50	15	Hemoglobin
Midges			
Cladotanytarsus lewisi			
Cla l 1	>50	17	Hemoglobin
Polypedium nubifer			
Pol n 1	>50	17	Hemoglobin
Chironomus kiiensis			
Chi k 10	nd	33	Tropomyosin
Blattidae			
German cockroach (Blattella germanica)			
Bla g 1	50	25	Shows homology with Per a 1 allergen, CrPII, and with ANG12 secretory mosquito protein
Bla g 2	58	36	Aspartate protease (inactive)
Bla g 4	40–60	21	Lipocalin
Bla g 5	70	23	Glutathione transferase
Bla g 6	50	18	Troponin C
Bla g 7	nd	31	Tropomyosin C
Bla g 8	nd	nd	Myosin , light chain
Trypsin	nd	35	Trypsin
American cockroach (Periplaneta americana)			
Per a 1	>70	24	Shows homology with Bla g 1 allergen, CrPII and ANG12 secretory mosquito protein
Per a 3	83	78	Hexamerin, subunit protein; shows homology with larval insect storage proteins
Per a 6	nd	17	Tropomin C
Per a 7	50	33	Tropomyosin
Arginine kinase	100	41	Arginine kinase
Indian meal moth (Plodia interpunctella)			
Plo i 1	25	40	Arginine kinase

properties) and the glycinins, or are enzymes involved in essential plant biochemical processes such as amylases (e.g., Hor v 16, 17), peroxidase, fructose biphosphate-aldolase, glyoxalase, and lipoxygenase (Table 35.11).[30] The types of seed proteins involved in allergic disease will vary according to the source. For example, the amylase/trypsin inhibitors are characteristic of the Poaceae, the 2S storage albumins are prominent in the Brassicaceae and Euphorbiaceae, and the vicilin, conglutin, and glycinin storage proteins as well as the Leguminoseae allergens associated with soybean husks (Gly m 1, 2; see also Table 35.14). These abundant, hydrophobic, and cysteine-rich, seed surface proteins reduce the wettability of surfaces and are, therefore, thought to play a role in defense. They and the 2S storage albumins described earlier are similar to plant LTP. The gliadins (e.g., Tri a 19, rye gliadins) and the related secalins (rye), and hordeins (e.g., Hor v 21) are characteristic of the Poaceae, as are glyoxalase, acyl-CoA oxidase, peroxidase (a PR protein) and fructose biphosphate-aldolase.

Table 35.11 Physicochemical and biochemical characteristics of occupational aeroallergens

Allergen	Frequency of reactivity (%)	Mol. weight (kDa)	Function
Fungal allergens			
Aspergillus niger			
Pectinase	nd	35	Poly(1,4)-α-D-galacturonidase
Cellulase	8	26	1,4-(1,3;1,4)-β-D-glucan glucanhydrolase
Glucoamylase	5	66	1,4-α-D-glucan glucanhydrolase
Phytase	>50	50	Histidine acid phosphatase
Asp n 14	14	105	β-Xylosidase
Aspergillus oryzae			
Asp o 13	nd	34	Alkaline serine protease; belongs to subtilase family
Asp o 21	56	52	α-Amylase
Lactase	nd	nd	1,4-β-D-Galactoside galactohydrolase
Cryphonectira parasitica			
Renin	nd	34	Aspartate protease; shows homology with mammalian and cockroach pepsins
Bacterial proteases			
Bacillus subtilis			
Alcalase	>50	28	Subtilisin serine protease
Bacillus licheniformis			
Esperase	>50	28	Subtilisin serine protease
Clostridium histolyticum			
Collagenase[b]	>50	68–125	Metalloprotease
Streptomyces grisens	nd	36	Chymotrypsin-type protease
Caricaceae			
Pawpaw (*Carica papaya*)			
Car p 1	nd	23	Papain, cysteine protease
Kiwi fruit (*Actinidia chinensis*)			
Act c 1	100	30	Actinidin, cysteine protease
Act c 2	nd	24	Thaumatin-like protein
Bromelaceae			
Pineapple (*Ananas comosus*)			
Ana c 1	42	15	Profilin
Ana c 2	nd	23	Bromelain, cysteine protease

(Continued)

Table 35.11 Physicochemical and biochemical characteristics of occupational aeroallergens—cont'd

Allergen	Frequency of reactivity (%)	Mol. weight (kDa)	Function
Mammalian proteases			
Trypsin (porcine)	nd	24	Serine protease; shows homology with mite groups 3, 6, and 9 allergens
Chymotrypsin (bovine)	nd	25	Serine protease; shows homology with mite groups 3, 6, and 9 allergens
Pepsin (porcine)	nd	35	Aspartate protease; shows homology with Bla g 2 and rennin
Amylase (porcine)	nd	55	Amylase
Chicken egg allergens			
Chicken *(Gallus domesticus)*			
Egg white			
Gal d 1	34–38	20	Ovomucoid, protease inhibitor
Gal d 2	32	43	Ovalbumin, function unknown but protein shows homology with serine protease inhibitors
Gal d 3	47–53	76	Conalbumin (ovotransferrin), iron transport protein
Gal d 4	15	14	$1,4\text{-}\beta\text{-N-acetylmuramidase}$ (lysozyme)
Egg yolk			
Gal d 5	>50	65–70	Serum albumin (α-livetin)
Brassicaceae			
Yellow mustard seed *(Sinapis alba* L.*)*			
Sin a 1	100		Napin, 2S albumin
Short chain		4	
Long chain		10	
Oriental mustard seed *(Brassica juncea)*			
Bra j 1	64		Napin, 2S albumin
Short chain		4	
Long chain		10	
Oilseed rape *(Brassica napus)*			
Bra r 1	80		Napin, 2S albumin
Short chain		4	
Long chain		10	
Euphorbiaceae			
Castor bean *(Ricinus communis)*			
Ric c 1	96		Napin, 2S albumin
Short chain		4	
Long chain		7	

Table 35.11 Physicochemical and biochemical characteristics of occupational aeroallergens—cont'd

Allergen	Frequency of reactivity (%)	Mol. weight (kDa)	Function
Ric c 2	nd	47	11 S crystalloid protein
Ric c 3	nd	47–51	Function unknown
Leguminoseae			
Seed husk allergens			
Soybean			
(Glycine max)			
Gly m 1^d	95	8	Cysteine-rich, hydrophobic seed protein, member of lipid transfer protein family
Gly m 2	95	8	Function unknown
Flour			
Soybean^a (Glycine max)			
Trypsin-inhibitor (B)	86	20	Kunitz protease inhibitor
Lipoxygenase	nd	94	Lipoxygenase
Poaceae			
Barley (Hordeum vulgare)			
Hor v 15	nd	14	α-Amylase/trypsin inhibitor; shows homology with wheat allergens and 2S albumin allergens
Hor v 16	>96	64	α-Amylase (1,4-α-D-glucan glucanohydrolase)
Hor v 17	>96	60	β-Amylase (1,4-α-D-glucan maltohydrolase)
Hor v 21	91^c	34	Hordein; shows homology with rye secalins and wheat gliadins
Rice (Oryza sativa)			
Ory s 1	>90	15	α-Amylase inhibitor; shows homology with wheat and barley α-amylase/trypsin inhibitor allergens
33 kDa protein	nd	33	Glyoxalase I
Wheat (Triticum spp)			
Tr I a 3	nd	nd	Function unknown, found in wheat ovaries; shows homology with pollen allergens
Tri a 12	nd	14	Profilin
Tri a 18	nd	17	Lectin
Tri a 19	100	65	ω-Gliadin; shows homology with rye secalins and barley hordein
Tri a 25	nd	nd	Thioredoxin
Tri a 26	nd	88	Glutenin
Gliadin	72	40	α-Gliadin
37 kDa allergen	nd	37	Fructose biphosphate-aldolase

AEROALLERGENS – OCCUPATIONAL

(Continued)

Table 35.11 Physicochemical and biochemical characteristics of occupational aeroallergens—cont'd

Allergen	Frequency of reactivity (%)	Mol. weight (kDa)	Function
CM16	>50	13	Wheat α-amylase/trypsin inhibitor; shows homology with barley allergens and 2S albumin allergens
WMAI-1	nd	13	Wheat α-amylase/trypsin inhibitor; shows homology with barley allergens and 2S albumin allergens
27 kDa allergen	nd	27	Shows homology with acyl-CoA oxidase from barley and rice
35 kDa allergen	60	35	Peroxidase
Rye *(Secale cereale)*			
Sec c 1	>50	14	α-Amylase/trypsin inhibitor; shows homology with wheat allergens and 2S albumin allergens
Sec c 20	91[c]	70	Rye gamma-70 secalin; shows homology with wheat gliadins and barley hordeins
34 kDa protein	83[c]	34	Rye gamma-35 secalin; shows homology with wheat gliadins and barley hordeins

[a]See Table 35.14 for ingested allergens from this source.
[b]Represents a mixture of proteases.
[c]Frequency based on patients with wheat-dependent, exercise-induced anaphylaxis.
[d]Note that this designation has also been used for the ingested cysteine protease allergen from soybean.[3]

■ INGESTED ALLERGENS ■

A variety of food sources contain allergens provoking IgE-mediated symptoms but seven appear to be most clinically important, accounting for >90% of food-induced allergy.[31] They include, in decreasing order of frequency, eggs, peanut, milk, nuts, soy, fish, and wheat. However, more recently, allergens from animal meats have been shown to be clinically important (see Table 35.13).[32] Allergy to ingested food proteins may result in a range of symptoms such as dermatitis, asthma, anaphylaxis, angioedema, and abdominal symptoms and, in this regard, certain sources are often associated with a particular allergic manifestation. For example, peanuts, fish, and crustaceans are associated with anaphylaxis, whereas egg and milk are associated with atopic dermatitis, and wheat allergens may be associated with the exercise-induced anaphylaxis.

ANIMAL AND FISH-DERIVED ALLERGENS

The ingested mammalian meat allergens include the serum albumins (e.g., Bos d 6), immunoglobulins (e.g., Bos d 7), and transferrin (Bos d 8) in raw meat, whereas in cow's milk, the allergens are principally α-lactalbumin (Bos d 4), β-lactoglobulin (Bos d 5; a lipocalin), and casein (Bos d 8), with the latter being particularly important (Table 35.13). In fish, the major allergens are the calcium-binding parvalbumins (e.g., Gal c 1), whereas in shellfish and mollusks, such as shrimp,

crab, and snails, the major allergens are tropomyosins (e.g., Pen a 1, Met e 1, Cha f 1) or actin-associated arginine kinases (Table 35.13). Similar allergens from different species show high sequence similarity and are, therefore, immunologically cross-reactive. With regard to the tropomyosins, this cross-reactivity extends to allergens from invertebrates, such as cockroaches and dust mites, and the nematode parasite, *Anisakis simplex.*[33]

SEED-DERIVED ALLERGENS

The major ingested seed-derived allergens are similar to those described previously as occupational aeroallergens (Table 35.11). As ingested allergens, however, the most clinically important are those derived from peanuts and include the major vicilin storage protein (Ara h 1), conglutin (Ara h 2), and peanut agglutinin allergens (Table 35.14). The minor peanut allergens include profilin (Ara h 5), the glycinin allergens (Ara h 4, 5) and proteins similar to conglutins (Ara h 6, 7). The most important ingested allergens from soybean include Gly m 1, Gly m Bd 28K and Gly m 3. Gly m 1 is a cysteine protease which shows homology with members of the papain family including the house-dust mite allergen Der p 1. This enzyme may play a role in mobilizing seed storage proteins during germination. In contrast, Gly m 3 is a profilin and Gly m Bd 28K shows homology with a range of vicilin-related storage proteins including Ara h 1 and may possess chitin-binding properties. Allergens

Table 35.12 Physicochemical and biochemical characteristics of latex allergens

Allergen	Frequency of reactivity (%)	Mol. weight (kDa)	Function
Euphorbiaceae: Rubber tree (latex; *Hevea brasiliensis*)			
Hev b 1	22–82	15	Rubber elongation factor, exists as homotetramer with mol wt of 58 kDa and pI of 8.5
Hev b 2	20–61	30	Endo-1, 3-β-glucosidase
Hev b 3	79	24	Shows some homology with rubber elongation factor
Hev b 4	65–77	50–57	Microhelix component
Hev b 5	56–92	16[a]	Shows homology with an acidic protein from kiwifruit and potato
Hev b 6	83	20	Prohevein; chitin-binding lectin, causes latex agglutination; native hevein exists as 5 kDa protein
Hev b 7	23–49	43	A patatin-like protein with lipid acyl-hydrolase and PLA_2 activity, shows cross-reactivity with Sol t 1
Hev b 8	24	14	Profilin, plays role in actin polymerization
Hev b 9	15	51	Enolase
Hev b 10	4	26	Manganese superoxide dismutase, shows homology with Asp f 6
Hev b 11	3	30	Class I chitinase
Hev b 12	24	9	Lipid transfer protein
Hev b 13	63	42	Esterase

[a]Hevein is a 4.7 kDa chitin-binding domain from this precursor.

belonging to the vicilin family are also present in walnut (Jug r 2) and coconuts. Interestingly, profilins are usually regarded as minor allergens but, in both soybean (Gly m 3) and *Mercurialis annua* pollen (Mer a 1), they are recognized by >50% of sensitized individuals.[34] The soybean minor allergens include members of the glycinin family (G1 and G2 glycinins), which share homology with Ara h 3 and the α-subunits of β-conglycinin. Seed proteins belonging to a group of methionine-rich 2S albumins have been described in walnut (Ber e 1) and brazil nuts (Jug r 1) as well as sunflower and sesame seeds.

FRUIT- AND VEGETABLE-DERIVED ALLERGENS

A range of allergens have been described from fruits and vegetables such as banana, pear, cherry, kiwi fruit, apple, peach, plum, apricot, mango, avocado, tomato, potato, celery, zucchini, and carrot (Table 35.14). However, sensitivity to these allergens is thought to arise from prior sensitization to pollen allergens. This syndrome, as indicated earlier, is referred to as OAS and arises due to the cross-reactivity between proteins in the respiratory allergen and those in food.[35] The condition is associated predominantly with uncooked food rather than cooked food, since processing results in protein denaturation, and symptoms range from mild oropharyngeal symptoms, to severe, systemic reactions. The allergens involved are biochemically and, therefore, immunologically related to several pollen allergens described previously. They include the Fagales

tree pollen Groups 1 and 2 allergens, the Asteraceae, Brassicaceae, and Urticaceae herbaceous dicotyledon pollen LTP, the 34 kDa and 60 kDa allergens of unknown function from pellitory, the thaumatin-like allergens, and endochitinases. The allergens associated with exposure to kiwi fruit and fig include cysteine proteases, as well as others yet to be characterized. The allergens from potato include patatin (Sol t 1) and several protease inhibitors that inhibit the activities of three of the major classes of proteases (Sol t 2, 3, 4) (Table 35.14).

OAS reactions may also be specifically classified by reference to the respiratory sensitizer and oral elicitors other than fruit and vegetables.[36] For example, 'bird–egg', 'egg–egg', 'latex–fruit', 'latex–mold', 'pork–cat', and 'mite–crustacean mollusk' syndromes have been described (Table 35.15). The latex allergens associated with fruit allergies are proheveins, chitinase, and those associated with mold, including manganese superoxide dismutase and enolase. Allergens associated with mites and crustaceans are the tropomyosins, whereas those associated with eggs and meat are the corresponding serum albumins.

■ INJECTED INSECT ALLERGENS ■

The most important injected insect allergens are derived from the stinging or biting insects and include venoms from bees (*Apis* and *Bombus* spp), wasps (yellow jackets; *Vespula* spp), hornets (*Dolichovespula* spp),

Table 35.13 Physicochemical and biochemical characteristics of ingested, animal-derived food allergens

Allergen	Frequency of reactivity (%)	Mol. weight (kDa)	Function
Animal			
Mammal-derived			
Cow *(Bos domesticus)*			
Bos d 4[a]	6	14	α-Lactalbumin, lactose synthase
Bos d 5	13	18	β-Lactoglobulin, lipocalin
Bos d 6	29	67	Serum albumin
Bos d 7	83	160	Immunoglobulin
Bos d 8	100	20–30	Casein
75 kDa allergen	16	75	Transferrin
Fish-derived			
Atlantic salmon *(Salmo salar)*, cod *(Gadus callarias)*			
Group 1	100	12	Parvalbumin, calcium-binding protein
Crustacean-derived			
Shrimp *(Metapenaeus* spp, *Penaeus* spp)			
Group 1 (e.g., Met p 1)	>50	34–36	Tropomyosin
	70	39	Arginine kinase
Crab *(Charybdis feriatus)*			
Group 1	>50	34	Tropomyosin
Group 2 (e.g., Pen m 2)			
Squid *(Todarodes pacificus)*			
Group 1	>50	38	Tropomyosin

[a]See also Table 35.18.

paper wasps (*Polistes* spp) and ants (*Solenopsis* spp),[37,38] and salivary proteins from mosquitoes (human allergens)[39] and fleas (dog allergens)[40] (Table 35.16). Venoms contain a number of proteins as well as low molecular mass peptides, and several venom allergens show homology with proteins associated with mammalian reproduction. They include cysteine-rich secretory proteins found in epididymis, testis, and salivary gland, sperm hyaluronidase, and prostatic-like acid phosphatase. On this basis, it has been suggested that since the allergens are derived from stingers which represent modified ovipositors, venom allergens may have evolved from proteins associated with insect reproduction.

VENOM ALLERGENS

The major allergens in venoms from bees, wasps, and hornets include phospholipase A_1 (e.g. Dol m 1, Pol a 1), phospholipase A_2 (e.g., Api m 1, Bom p 1), hyaluronidase (e.g., Api m 2, Dol m 2), acid phosphatase (e.g., Dol m 3, Api m 3), and a protein of unknown

function from bee venom (Api m 6). In the ants, the major venom allergen is the group 2 (e.g., Sol i 2) allergen of unknown function (Table 35.16). A range of minor allergens are also present and include proteins of unknown function such as the related Group 5 and 3 allergens from vespids and ants, respectively, which also show homology with plant pathogenesis-related proteins, fungal proteins, and nematode proteins (e.g., Ac-avp-2), a serine protease allergen (e.g., Bom p 4), with homology to the sperm head acrosin protease and melittin (e.g., Api m 4).

SALIVARY ALLERGENS

With regard to the biting insects, flea and mosquito saliva have been shown to contain a variety of minor and major allergens. They include apyrase, an enzyme that catalyzes the breakdown of ATP to release phosphate, a Vespidae Group 5 homologue (e.g., Cte f 2), and a procalin (kissing bug allergen),[41] together with proteins of unknown function. The major silverfish allergen is tropomyosin.

Table 35.14 Physicochemical and biochemical characteristics of ingested seed and fruit allergens

Allergen	Frequency of reactivity (%)	Mol. weight (kDa)	Function
Leguminoseae			
Peanut (*Arachis hypogaea*)			
Ara h 1	>90	70	Vicilin seed storage protein
Ara h 2	>90	18	Conglutin seed storage protein
Ara h 3	44	60	Glycinin seed storage protein
Ara h 4	43	36	Glycinin seed storage protein
Ara h 5	16	14	Profilin
Ara h 6	38	16	Conglutin
Ara h 7	43	15	Conglutin
Ara h 8	85	17	Pathogenesis-related protein, PR-10
Peanut agglutinin	50*	27	Lectin
Soybean[a]			
(*Glycine. max*)			
Gly m Bd 30K	90	34	Seed vacuolar protein; cysteine protease; shows homology with mite group 1 allergen, papain, and bromelain
Gly m Bd 28K	>50	22	Vicilin-like glycoprotein; shows homology with Ara h 1
Gly m 3	67	14	Profilin
Gly m 4	nd	17	Pathogenesis-related protein, PR-10
21 kDa allergen	nd	22	A member of the G2 glycinin family
G1 glycinin	nd	40	A member of the G1 glycinin family; shows homology with Ara h 3
Gly m Bd 60K	25	60	β-Conglycinin seed storage protein
Juglandaceae			
Brazil nut (*Bertholletia excelsa*)			
Ber e 1	100	9	2S albumin
Ber e 2	nd	29	11S globulin seed storage protein
Lecythidaceae			
English walnut (*Juglans regia*)			
Jug r 1	nd	15–16	2S albumin
Jug r 2	60	47	Vicilin-like glycoprotein
Jug r 3	91	9	Lipid transfer protein
Polygonaceae			
Buckwheat (*Fagopyrum esculentum Moench*)			
Fag e 1	>50	26	β-Chain of 11S globulin
19 kDa protein	78	19	2S albumin
16 kDa protein	<50	16	2S albumin
9 kDa protein	50	9	Trypsin inhibitor

(Continued)

INJECTED INSECT ALLERGENS

Table 35.14 Physicochemical and biochemical characteristics of ingested seed and fruit allergens—con'd

Allergen	Frequency of reactivity (%)	Mol. weight (kDa)	Function
Heliantheae			
Sunflower *(Helianthus annus)*			
16kDa allergen	66	16/17	2S albumin
Apiaceae			
Celery *(Apium graveolens)*			
Api g 1	100	16	Pathogenesis-related protein Pr-10; ribonuclease
Api g 3	nd	nd	Chlorophyll a-b binding protein
Api g 4	23	14	Profilin
Api g 5	100	58	FAD–containing oxidase
Rosaceae			
Apple *(Malus domestica)*			
Mal d 1	100	18	Pathogenesis-related protein PR-10; ribonuclease
Mal d 2	nd	23	Thaumatin-like protein
Mal d 3	90	9	Non-specific lipid transfer protein
Mal d 4	nd	14	Profilin
60kDa allergen	nd	60	Phosphoglyceromutase
Prunoideae			
Cherry *(Prunus avium)*			
Pru av 1	96	18	Pathogeneric-related protein PR-10; ribonuclease; shows homology with Bet v1
Pru av 2	100	30	Thaumatin-like protein
Pru av 3	3	10	Non-specific lipid transfer protein
Pru av 4	16	14	Profilin
Solanaceae			
Potato *(Solanum tuberosum)*			
Sol t 1	74	43	Patatin, defense-related storage protein; has PLA_2 activity
Sol t 2	51	20	Cathepsin D protease inhibitor; Kunitz-type protease inhibitor
Sol t 3	43	20	Cysteine protease inhibitor
Sol t 4	58	20	Aspartate protease inhibitor

[a]See also Table 35.10.

Table 35.15 Allergens involved in cross-reactivity syndromes

Sensitizing source	Provoking source	Cross-reacting allergen(s)
Plant-derived allergens		
Pollen-fruit		
Birch pollen	Apple, carrot, cherry, pear, peach, plum, fennel, walnut, potato, spinach, wheat, buckwheat, peanut, honey, celery, kiwi fruit	Profilin, Bet v 1 analogues
Japanese ceder pollen	Melon, apple, peach, kiwi fruit	Pectate lyase
Mugwort pollen	Celery, carrot, spices, melon, watermelon, apple, camomile, hazelnut, chestnut	Lipid transfer proteins, profilins, 34 and 60 kDa allergens, Art v 1 analogues
Grass pollen	Melon, tomato, watermelon, orange, cherry, potato	Profilins
Ragweed pollen	Melon, camomile, honey, banana, sunflower seeds	Pectate lyase
Latex-fruit		
Latex	Avocado, potato, banana, tomato, chestnut, kiwi fruit, herbs, carrot	Patatin (e.g. Sol t 1), profilin, class I chitinases, Hev b 6, Pers a 1
Latex-mold		
Latex	*Aspergillus fumigatus*	Manganese superoxide dismutase
Animal-derived allergens		
Bird–egg		
Bird material	Egg yolk	Serum albumin (Gal d 5)
Egg–egg		
Egg white powder	Egg-containing foods	Lysozyme (Gal d 4)
Pork–cat		
Animal meat	Animal danders	Serum albumin
Arthropod–shellfish		
Mites	Shellfish, snails	Tropomyosin
Mites	*Anisakis simplex*	Tropomyosin
Cockroach	Shellfish, snails	Tropomyosin
Wasp–mosquito		
Vespula venom	Mosquito	Hyaluronidase

■ PATHOGEN-DERIVED ALLERGENS AND AUTOALLERGENS ■

A number of potentially pathogenic organisms may also be associated with allergic diseases due to their capacity to stimulate the production of IgE. These include fungi such as *C. albicans* and *A. fumigatus*, which may colonize patients with pre-existing conditions including asthma, allergic bronchopulmonary aspergillosis, and cystic fibrosis; bacteria such as *Staphylococcus aureus*, which are associated with atopic dermatitis; and helminthic parasites such as *Anisakis simplex*, *Ascaris lumbricoides*, and *Schistosoma mansoni*. The allergens associated with the fungal diseases are usually the same as those associated with allergic diseases (see Table 35.7) but the allergens from *S. aureus* include the enterotoxins SAE,

SEB, SEC, SED, and toxic shock syndrome toxin (TSST-1) (Table 35.17). The *S. aureus* enterotoxins are superantigens that bind MHC class II molecules with the potential to stimulate T-cell proliferation in a non-antigen specific manner. They stimulate IgE production in patients with asthma and atopic dermatitis. Whether other bacterial species produce allergens is unclear at present.

By far the most studied pathogenic organisms associated with allergenicity are the helminthic parasites. A number of allergens have been described and include the polyprotein lipid-binding allergens from *Ascaris* species and *Dirofilaria immitis*, the serine proteases from *Trichinella spiralis*, cyclophilin from *Echinococcus granulosus*, and a range of protease inhibitors from *Anisakis simplex*, *E. granulosus*, and *Schistosome* species. Many, if not all, of these proteins are found in secretions

Table 35.16 Physicochemical and biochemical characteristics of stinging and biting insect allergens

Allergen	Frequency of reactivity (%)	Mol. weight (kDa)	Function
Venom allergens			
Aidae			
Honey bee (*Apis mellifera*)			
Api m 1	>90	15	Phospholipase A_2
Api m 2	95	41	Hyaluronidase
Api m 3	>50	49	Acid phosphatase prostatic
Api m 4	<50	3	Melittin
Api m 6	>42	8	Function unknown
Api m 7	nd	39	CUB serine protease
Bumble bee (*Bombus pennsylvanicus/terrestris*)			
Bom p 1	82	16	Phospholipase A_2
Bom p 4	82	27	Protease
Bom t 1	nd	49	Acid phosphatase
Vespidae			
White faced and yellow hornets (*Dolichovespula* spp), paper wasps (*Polistes* spp), and yellow jackets (*Vespula* spp)			
Group 1	66	34	Phospholipase A_1
Group 2	64	39	Hyaluronidase
Group 3	nd	49	Acid phosphatase
Group 4	nd	33	Serine protease
Group 5	100	26	Shows homology with cysteine-rich secretory protein found in epididymis, testis, and salivary gland
Formicoidea			
Fire ant (*Solenopsis invicta*)			
Sol i 1	87	18	Phospholipase A_1
Sol i 2	61	13	Function unknown
Sol i 3	61	24	Shows homology with the vespids Group 5 allergens
Sol i 4	74	13	Shows homology with Sol i 2
Australian jumper ant (*Myrmecia pilosula*)			
Myr p 1	>50	9	Pilosulin 1, function unknown
Myr p 2	35	5	Function unknown
Salivary allergens			
Culicidae			
Mosquito (*Aedes aegypti*)			
Aed a 1	29–43	68	Apyrase
Aed a 2	11	37	Salivary protein; function unknown
Aed a 3	32	30	Function unknown; shows homology with olive pollen allergen Ole e 10

Table 35.16 Physicochemical and biochemical characteristics of stinging and biting insect allergens—cont'd

Allergen	Frequency of reactivity (%)	Mol. weight (kDa)	Function
Pulicidae			
Flea (Ctenocephalides felis felis)			
Cte f 1	80	20	Function unknown
Cte f 2	nd	30	Salivary protein; shows homology with ant Sol i 3 allergen, and vespid Group 5 allergens
Reduviidae			
Kissing bug (Triatoma protracta)			
19 kDa allergen	89	19	Procalin, a member of the lipocalin family; shows homology with triabin, a thrombin inhibitor
Lepismatidae			
Silverfish (Lepisma saccharina)			
Lep s 1	nd	36	Tropomyosin

and are likely to be essential in protecting the parasite from host defense mechanisms. In addition to the allergens associated with bacteria and parasites, IgE production may be stimulated by certain host-derived proteins, particularly in atopic dermatitis. The majority of allergens appear to be of intracellular origin and are not associated with any particular cell type, although it is speculated that exposure arises due to cell damage. However, at least one autoallergen – namely, prostate-specific antigen – is a secreted protein which plays a role in females sensitized to seminal fluid.

THREE-DIMENSIONAL STRUCTURES OF ALLERGENS

The structures of many allergens (Table 35.18) have been determined experimentally using X-ray diffraction or nuclear magnetic resonance, or modeled on structures determined for homologous proteins. Of particular interest is the structure of the Birch pollen allergen, Bet v 1 complexed to the Fab fragment of a mouse IgG monoclonal antibody which is known to block the binding of allergen-specific IgE. On this basis, the epitope bound by the monoclonal Fab fragment is likely to represent an IgE epitope with obvious relevance.

Of the indoor allergens, the house-dust mite allergen Der p 1 is arguably the one with the greatest clinical significance. The three-dimensional structure of Der p 1 has recently been reported in both its proenzyme and mature forms[42,43] These studies confirm the impression that Der p 1 is a papain-like enzyme of the C1 family in the CA clan of cysteine proteases, but highlight a number of significant differences that distinguish it from the C1 archetype, notably in the size of the non-prime binding pockets, especially S2. These differences also demarcate the active site of Der p 1 from human cysteine proteases, which, although showing conserved sequence identity around the catalytic triad

(Fig. 35.1), have significant differences in the size of their substrate-binding pockets. Structural data obtained for proDer p1 suggest that the remnant and surrogate residues of the propiece ERFNIN motif probably serves to stabilize the tertiary structure of the 80 residue propiece, enabling correct interaction with the catalytic site of the enzyme. This is akin to the situation in cathepsins L and K, which have been studied in more detail. Correct orientation allows two of the propiece α-helices to interact with one end of the binding cleft, while its other two β-helices cover the prime and non-prime substrate binding pockets. In addition to inhibiting enzymatic activity by steric hindrance of the catalytic site, the bound propiece also serves to mask some Der p 1 epitopes.[43] How the propiece is removed is presently unknown, but generation of mature Der p 1 creates fully immunogenic Der p 1 and reveals its powerful catalytic activity.

Structural analysis of the mature protein indicates it has the ability to dimerize, especially under conditions of high concentration and alkaline pH.[42] To what extent this influences the behavior of Der p 1 in causing allergy is unknown, although the conditions favoring association seem unlikely to support extensive dimer formation on the respiratory mucosa.

X-ray diffraction data for Der p 1 are valuable additions to knowledge gained from homology modeling and studies of its cleavage specificity in peptide substrate libraries. The structure–action relationships of Der p 1 have also been explored using novel peptoid inhibitors created by appending warheads to the non-prime targeting sequence of a substrate peptide. A number of these irreversible inhibitors show high reactivity with Der p 1 ($K_{obs}/[I] > 10^8$ M^{-1} s^{-1}) but are limited as experimental tools due to the metabolic liabilities of the peptide backbone. In the quest to unravel the contribution of proteolytic activity to the development of allergy, biochemical, structural and modeling approaches have enabled *in silico* docking studies to probe more fully the nature of the Der p 1 catalytic site using substrates and inhibitors (Fig. 35.2).

Table 35.17 Physicochemical and biochemical characteristics of pathogen-derived allergens and autoallergens

Allergen	Frequency of reactivity (%)	Mol. weight (kDa)	Function
Helminthic parasites			
Ascaridida			
Anisakis simplex			
Ani s 1	85	24	Function unknown
Ani s 2	nd	97	Paramyosin
Ani s 3	nd	41	Tropomyosin
Ani s 4	75	9	Function unknown
Ani s 5	25	15	SXP/RAL-2 protein
Ani s 6	nd	8	Shows homology with mammalian serine protease inhibitors
Ascaris suum[a]			
Asc c -1	>80	14	Nematode polyprotein lipid-binding protein
Cyclophyllidae			
Echinococcus granulosus			
EA21	80	7	Peptidyl-prolyl isomerase (cyclophilin) shows homology with Mal f 6 and Asp f 11
EgEF-1β/λ	56–90	14	Elongation factor; shows homology with 25 kDa *P. citrinum* allergen
EgHSP70	57	70	Heat shock protein
AgB	nd	12	Protease inhibitor
Antigen 5	nd	67	Dimer, 22 kDa chain and 38 kDa chain with trypsin-like similarity although not active
Spirurida			
Brugia malayi			
58 kDa allergen	100	58	γ-Glutamyl transpeptidase
Bm 23–25	nd	23–25	Function unknown
Dirofilaria immitis			
DiAg	nd	nd	Polyprotein lipid-binding antigen
Enoplidae			
Trichinella spiralis			
Serine proteases	nd	18, 40, 50	Serine proteases
Strigeatida			
Trichostrongylus colubriformis (sheep parasite)			
31 kDa allergen	nd	31	Aspartyl protease inhibitor homologue (Aspin)
Necator americanus			
60 kDa protein	nd	60	Calreticulin
Schistosoma mansoni			
Sm22.6	10 (children); 36 (adults)	22.6	α- and γ-thrombin inhibitor
Schistosoma japonicum			
23 kDa protein	>50	23	Function unknown

Table 35.17 Physicochemical and biochemical characteristics of pathogen-derived allergens and autoallergens—cont'd

Allergen	Frequency of reactivity (%)	Mol. weight (kDa)	Function
Schistosoma haematobium			
90 kDa protein	nd	90	Serine protease inhibitor
Strongylidae			
Strongyloides stercoralis			
NIE antigen	90	31	Function unknown; shows homology with vespid Group 5 allergens
Atopic dermatitis-associated bacteria and autoallergens			
Staphylococcus aureus			
SEA	15–46	24	Superantigen, enterotoxin A
SEB	15–46	28	Superantigen, enterotoxin B
TSST-1	23	22	Toxic shock syndrome toxin-1
Human autoallergens			
Hom s 1	nd	55–60	Squamous cell carcinoma antigen SART
Hom s 2	nd	nd	Nascent polypeptide-associated complex α-subunit
Hom s 3	40	22–23	BCL7B oncogen protein
Hom s 4	54	46	Calcium-binding protein; shows homology with Ph1p 7, Cyp c p 1
Hom s 5	2	nd	Type II cytoskeletal keratin
MnSOD	43	24	Manganese superoxidase dismutase
Prostate-specific antigen	nd	33	Chymotrypsin-like protease

[a]A pig parasite used on a surrogate for *A. lumbricoides*.

ALLERGEN BIOCHEMISTRY, IMMUNOGENICITY, AND INFLAMMATION

Comparatively little attention has been directed at the question of why and how allergens evoke the immunological responses that result in allergic disease. Attempts to define the nature of allergens have been directed largely towards a description of their physicochemical properties in the hope that the secrets of allergenicity will be revealed by the identification of shared structural features. While being an entirely reasonable approach, it will be apparent that allergens represent a highly diverse collection of molecules in which a common structural motif is unlikely to provide a universal explanation of allergenicity. The probability is that sensitization and disease are likely to be determined by a complex interplay of functional and structural properties of allergens, as well as the genetic susceptibility of individuals. Table 35.19 lists the biochemical activities that may contribute towards enhanced immunogenicity and the reader is referred to several reviews that discuss these possibilities in detail.[1,44,45]

Immunogenicity is thought to be dependent on factors such as molecular size and the amount and duration of allergen exposure but, more recently, route of delivery and inflammatory events occurring in the vicinity of allergen deposition have been recognized as playing similarly important roles. Recognition of this has given rise to the concept of the 'danger signal', which hypothesizes that immune responses do not occur unless accompanying inflammation signals are provided, particularly from the host tissue.[46] Numerous cell types may have the capacity to provide danger signals and thus contribute to the generation of both innate and adaptive immunity. The most important cell types likely to interact with aeroallergens in the respiratory tract and generate the appropriate signals include epithelial cells, mast cells, macrophages, and dendritic cells. These interactions may occur directly, via specific receptors, or indirectly via humoral factors, such as surfactant and protease inhibitors. The outcome of allergen exposure may additionally be dictated by functional interactions between different allergens or between allergens and adjuvants found among the many poorly characterized components that coexist with established allergens in biological matrices such as dust.

Table 35.18 Clinically important allergens of known three-dimensional structure

Allergen	Function	Technique used to determine structure	PDB number
Pollens			
Birch			
Bet v 1	Ribonuclease	X-ray diffraction	1BV1
Bet v 1-Fab complex		X-ray diffraction	1FSK
Bet v 2	Profilin	X-ray diffraction	IG5U
Timothy grass			
Phl p 2	Unknown	X-ray diffraction	1WHO
Ragweed			
Amb t 5	Unknown	NMR	2BBG
Mountain cedar			
Jun a 3	PR-5 protein	Modeling	Based on 1AVN, structure of mouse urinary protein, Mus m 1
Latex			
Heb v 8	Profilin	X-ray diffraction	1BV1
Seed			
Soybean			
Gly m 1	Lipid transfer protein	X-ray diffraction	1HYP
Wheat			
CM16	2S Trypsin/amylase inhibitor	X-ray diffraction	1HSS
Fruit			
Cherry			
Pru av 1	Ribonuclease	NMR	1EO9
Peach			
Pru p 3	Lipid transfer protein	X-ray diffraction	2B5S
Fungi			
Aspergillus fumigatus			
Asp f 6	Manganese superoxide dismutase	X-ray diffraction	
Malassezia sympodialis			
Mala s 6	Cyclophilin	X-ray diffraction	2CFE
Mala s 13	Thioredoxin	X-ray diffraction	2J23

Table 35.18 Clinically important allergens of known three-dimensional structure—cont'd

Allergen	Function	Technique used to determine structure	PDB number
Stinging insect venom			
Bee			
Api m 2	Hyaluronidase	X-ray diffraction	1FCQ
Wasp			
Ves v 2	Hyaluronidase	X-ray diffraction	2ATM
Ves v 5	Unknown	X-ray diffraction	IQNX
Mammalian dander			
Horse			
Equ c 1	Lipocalin	X-ray diffraction	1EW3
Cow			
Bos d 2	Lipocalin	X-ray diffraction	1BJ7
Mouse			
Mus m 1	Lipocalin	X-ray diffraction	1MUP
Cat			
Fel d 1	Secretoglobulin	X-ray diffraction	1ZKR
Fel d 3	Cystatin, cysteine protease inhibitor	Modelling	Based on human cystatin A (1CYU), stefin A (1DVC), stefin B (1STF)
Dust mites			
D. pteronyssinus			
Der p 1	Cysteine protease	X-ray diffraction	1XKG (proDer p 1) 2AS8 (mature, active Der p 1)
Der p 2	Unknown	NMR	1A9V
D. farinae			
Der f 2	Unknown	NMR/X-ray diffraction	1AHK/2F08
Cockroach			
Bla g 2	Unknown	X-ray diffraction	1YG9
Milk			
α-Lactalbumin	Lactose synthase	X-ray diffraction	1F6S
β-Lactoglobulin	Lipocalin	X- ray diffraction	1J8W
Egg			
Ovalbumin	Unknown	X-ray diffraction	1OVA
Lysozyme	Carbohydrase	X- ray diffraction	1DPX
Ovotransferrin	Iron transporter	X-ray diffraction	1AIV

PDB, Protein data base.

```
CATH    136 GACGSCWTFSTTG 148
Papain  153 GSCGSCWAFSAVV 165
CATS    134 GSCGACWAFSAVG 146
CATK    134 GQCGSCWAFSSVG 146
CATL    133 GQCGSCWAFSATG 145
DERP1   127 GGCGSCWAFSGVA 139
DERG1   128 GGCGSCWAFSGVA 140
CATF    290 GMCGSCWAFSVTG 302
CATB    103 GSCGSCWAFGAVE 115
            * **:**:*. .
```

```
CATB    278 KVNHAVLAVGYGEKNG---IP-YWIVKNSWGPQWGMNGYFLIERGK- 319
Papain  289 KVDHAVAAVGYG-PN-------YILIKNSWGTGWGENGYIRIKRGTGN 328
CATS    275 NVNHGVLVVGYGDL----NGKEYWLVKNSWGHNFGEEGYIRMARNKG 317
CATK    273 NLNHAVLAVGYGIQ----KGNKHWIIKNSWGENWGNKGYILMARNKN 315
CATL    273 DMDHGVLVVGYGFESTESDNNKYWLVKNSWGEEWGMGGYVKMAKDRR 319
DERP1   265 PNYHAVNIVGYSNAQ----GVDYWIVRNSWDTNWGDNGYGYFAANID 307
DERG1   266 PNYHAVNIVGYGSTQ----GDDYWIVRNSWDTTWGDSGYGYFOAGNN 308
CATF    428 LIDHAVLLVGYGNRS----DVPFWAIKNSWGTDWGEKGYYLHRGSG 470
CATB    275 MGGHAIRILGWGVEN---GTPYWLVANSWNTDWGDNGFFKILRGQD 317
            *.: :*:. . : ***. :* *: . .
```

Fig. 35.1. Sequence alignments of the regions containing the catalytic residues of Der p 1, Der f 1, the archetypal C1 protease, papain, and human cathepsins most closely related by sequence identity. Arrows denote positions of the catalytic triad residues. Asterisks denote identical residues. Double dots and single dots denote strong similarity and similarity of residues, respectively. Compared to the whole length mature sequence of Der p 1, the human cathepsins show sequence identity as follows: cathepsin H (CATH, 31%); cathepsin S (CATS, 27%); cathepsin K (CATK, 32%); cathepsin L (CATL, 30%); cathepsin F (CATF, 29%); cathepsin B (CATB, 23%). Der p 1 and Der f 1 are 82% identical. In each case, sequence identity was calculated using alignments made by CLUSTALW.

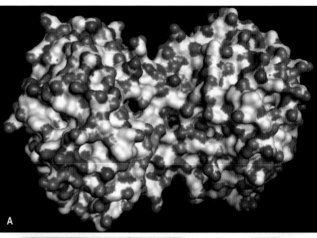

The potential significance of interactions between enzymatic and non-enzymatic allergens has been studied in mice. Compared with other strains, C57BL/6 mice typically develop weak Th2 responses, and model allergens, such as ovalbumin, induce tolerance when delivered to their airways. However, the addition of enzyme-rich allergen mixtures from *Aspergillus fumigatus* or *Aspergillus oryzae* to ovalbumin converts tolerance to a vigorous allergic reaction.[47] Supporting the concept that proteases are critical factors in driving allergic sensitization, the alkaline serine protease allergen Asp f 13 has been shown to facilitate the IgE responses and inflammation of the non-protease allergen Asp f2 in BALB/c mice.[48] The reasons why enzymatic allergens, especially proteases, are notable in their ability to override tolerance and unmask potent allergenicity in a model non-enzymatic allergen are not fully established, but several potential mechanisms, which might collectively contribute to this effect are discussed in the next section. In broad terms, these mechanisms concern allergen detection by antigen-presenting cells and the creation of a signaling environment that favors Th2 immunity.

BIOLOGICAL ACTIONS OF PROTEASES – TRANSEPITHELIAL ALLERGEN DELIVERY

Dendritic cells (DCs) are the major antigen-presenting cells of the respiratory tract and thus a vital component in the development of allergy. In the process of sensitization, inhalant allergens must penetrate the barrier formed by the epithelial cells lining the airways to contact

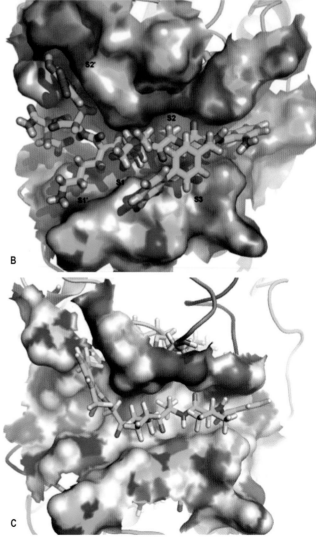

Fig. 35.2. Der p 1 and its catalytic site. (A) Three-dimensional structure of mature Der p 1 in its dimeric form as obtained by X-ray diffraction at 1.9 Å resolution. Docking of a synthetic substrate peptide with the catalytic site of Der p 1 showing (B) prime and (C) non-prime side interactions.

Table 35.19 A summary of the potential consequences of the biochemical properties of allergens

Property of allergen	Potential consequence
Protease activity	Epithelial permeability due to:
	Mast cell degranulation
	Tight junction degradation
	Kinin generation
	Apoptosis
	Macrophage/monocyte receptor interaction
	Cytokine release
	Adhesion molecule upregulation
	Complement activation
	Receptor interaction
	T helper cell polarization
Protease inhibitor	Macrophage/monocyte receptor interaction
Lipocalin	Epithelium receptor interactions
Glycosylation	Macrophage/DC receptor interaction
High focal concentration	Epithelial permeability due to osmotic effects

dendritic antigen-presenting cells that lie beneath it. Paracellular pathways offer a potential route for the delivery of inhaled allergens, particularly as DCs are thought to intercalate into paracellular spaces. However, access to paracellular spaces is restricted by tight junctions (TJs) that occlude the paracellular channels apically. TJs have been identified as key targets in the transepithelial delivery of these allergens. These discoveries suggest that the IgE-independent effects of allergens are significant factors in the development of allergy in the genetically predisposed.[44,49,50]

Small numbers of fecal pellets from *D. pteronyssinus* cleave TJs and increase the permeability of airway epithelial barriers. This effect is subtle, occurs without gross derangement of the epithelium and, at least in its early stages or mildest forms, can only be observed with specialized imaging techniques or use of sensitive permeability probes. The action of hydrated fecal pellets is replicated by protease allergens, notably the Group 1 cysteine protease,[51,52] the Group 3 tryptic serine protease, the Group 6 chymotryptic serine protease, and the Group 9 collagenolytic serine proteases.[53] In all cases, cleavage involved proteolysis of the extracellular domains of the TJ adhesion proteins. Transepithelial delivery of mite allergen occurred in proportion to the extent of TJ cleavage, both of which were reduced when the protease activity was inhibited. In the case of fully inactive protease allergen, transepithelial delivery could not be detected.

TIGHT JUNCTIONS AS TARGETS OF PROTEASE ALLERGENS

TJs are supramolecular assemblies situated apically in the lateral membrane of epithelial cells, where they occlude the paracellular space between adjacent cells. They are composed of proteins that span the cell membrane and others that are localized at the cytoplasmic face of the junction where it interacts with the cytoskeleton (Fig. 35.3). The transmembrane proteins have roles in intercellular adhesion and the regulation of paracellular permeability, whereas the cytoplasmic face proteins transduce 'inside-out' and 'outside-in' intercellular signalling.[54] The transmembrane (TM) proteins of TJs are occludin, claudins and the junctional adhesion molecules (JAMs) (Fig. 35.3). Occludin and claudins share similar membrane topography in having four TM α-helices, which create two extracellular domains.[54] The extracellular domains of claudins contain notable sequence similarity indicative of conserved function, whereas the regions of difference possibly create operational diversity within the family. The first extracellular domain of occludin is rich in Tyr and Gly residues, but the second is compositionally more diverse. The amino- and carboxy- termini of occludin and claudins are intracellular, these domains being longer in occludin than in claudins. The carboxy-termini of occludin and claudins are established as sites of interaction with ZO-1, ZO-2, and ZO-3. These are related membrane-associated guanylate kinase-like proteins (MAGUKs) and are cytoplasmic components of the TJ plaque. Occludin interacts with the GUK domain of these proteins, whereas claudins and JAMs interact at their PDZ domains.[54]

Claudins are adhesive and create the distinctive anastomosing strands that characterize the appearance of TJ when viewed as freeze-fracture replicas.[54] Occludin is adhesive, associates with claudins, and regulates paracellular permeability and cell migration. JAM differs from the other TM proteins in being a 40kDa member of the immunoglobulin superfamily with a single membrane-spanning domain and two Ig-like extracellular domains. Several different JAMs may exist, but their role in TJs remains less clear. Although it is unlikely that JAMs contribute greatly to the appearance of TJ strands, they may have a significant role in TJ (re)assembly, because direct and indirect interactions can occur with the cytoplasmic TJ proteins cingulin and ZO-1, respectively.

At concentrations that mimic daily exposures to these allergens, mite proteases attack the extracellular domains of occludin and claudins[51–53] (Fig. 35.4). This cleaves TJs and initiates the proteolytic processing of the TJ plaque protein ZO-1.[51,52] The consequence of TJ cleavage is an increased epithelial permeability that enables allergens to cross the epithelial barrier. When TJ cleavage is blocked, transepithelial delivery of allergen does not occur.[51] The increase in epithelial permeability is nonspecific, increasing the transepithelial delivery of any solute (including other allergens), provided it is smaller than the diameter of the paracellular channels at the cleaved junctions. This might account for allergic reactivity to allergens from diverse sources being common and provides a simple explanation of how non-protease allergens gain access to DCs. It has been proposed that in addition to facilitating transepithelial allergen delivery, the cleavage of TJs might provide some of the danger signals that drive DCs into orchestrating adaptive immune responses.[46,55] If correct, this potentially interesting idea suggests novel ways in which allergy prophylaxis might be achieved. More recently, an alkaline serine protease allergen from *Penicillium chrysogenum*, Pen ch 13, has been reported to have similar effects on TJs as the mite allergens.[56]

The effects of mite protease allergens on TJs can be subtle and are potentially reversible.[51] Pulse-chase labeling of occludin has established that de novo synthesis occurs rapidly after TJ cleavage is initiated and that the acute repair process is largely independent of changes in occludin gene expression.[52] The process of TJ reassembly occurs in an ordered manner with a reticular scaffold of ZO-1 being established before rings of occludin are reinstated.[51]

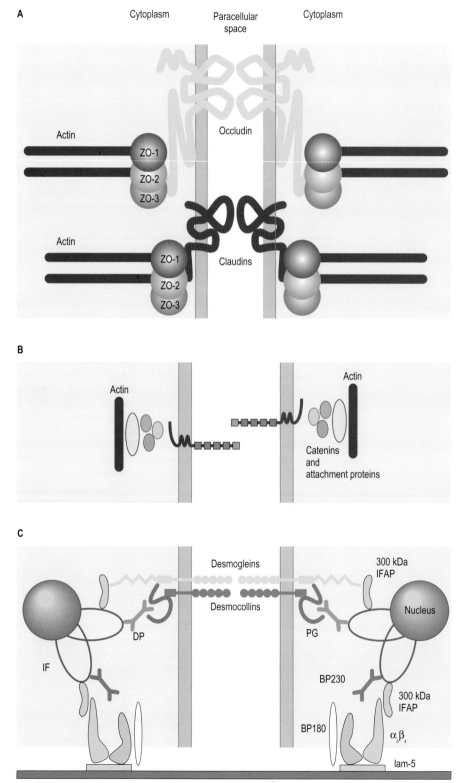

Fig. 35.3. Simplified representation of the major components of the epithelial adhesion complex in adjoining epithelial cells. (A) depicts a tight junction (TJ) which occludes the entrance to the paracellular space and shows the relationship of the transmembrane adhesion proteins (occludin and claudins) with components of the TJ plaque and the actin cytoskeleton. Other intracellular components of TJs and the transmembrane protein JAM have been omitted for clarity. (B) depicts the adherens junction, showing the probable arrangement of the extracellular domains of E-cadherin, with the calcium-binding adhesion domain EC1 shown in red. Intracellular attachments to the actin cytoskeleton via catenins and attachment proteins are shown. In (C) a schematic depiction of desmosomal adhesion shows the adhesion proteins (desmocollins and desmogleins) and their attachment to intermediate filaments (IF) via plakoglobin (PG) and desmoplakin (DP). Also shown is the probable IF-dependent relationship to hemidesmosomal adhesion to the biomatrix, e.g., laminin-5 (lam-5) via integrins, e.g., $\alpha_6\beta_4$.

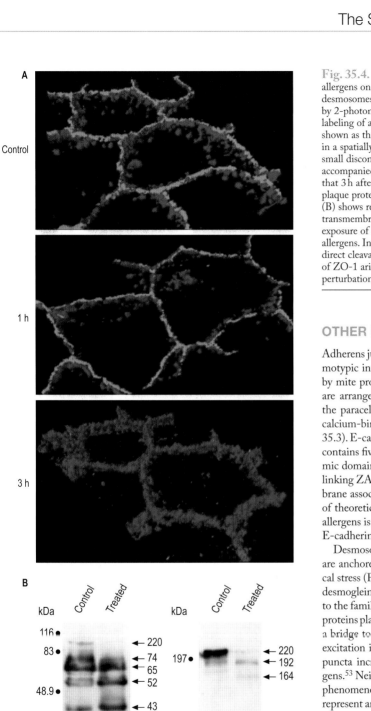

A
Control
1 h
3 h

B
kDa   Control Treated   kDa   Control Treated
116 ●
83 ●   ← 220   197 ●   ← 220
                    ← 74   ← 192
                    ← 65   ← 164
                    ← 52
48.9 ●   ← 43   115 ●

                    ← 34
33.1 ●   89 ●

       Occludin   ZO-1

Fig. 35.4. (A) illustrates the effect of house dust mite serine protease allergens on epithelial tight junctions (depicted by green fluorescence) and desmosomes (depicted by red fluorescence). Cell images were acquired by 2-photon molecular excitation microscopy after fluorescent antibody labeling of appropriate proteins from the interepithelial junctions and are shown as three-dimensional isosurface reconstructions to illustrate changes in a spatially meaningful way. Note that 1 h after exposure to the allergens, small discontinuities become evident as the TJ rings break down. This is accompanied by an increase in epithelial permeability (not illustrated). Note that 3 h after allergen exposure, loss of TJs is total and the desmosomal plaque protein desmoplakin shows an increased staining intensity. (B) shows representative immunoblots that reveal proteolytic processing of a transmembrane TJ protein (occludin) and a plaque protein (ZO-1) following exposure of bronchial epithelial cells to house dust mite serine protease allergens. In the case of occludin the proteolytic processing is initiated by direct cleavage of residues in the extracellular domains, whereas cleavage of ZO-1 arises by activation of intracellular processing pathways following perturbation by the protease allergens.

OTHER INTEREPITHELIAL JUNCTION TARGETS

Adherens junctions (zonulae adherentes, ZAs) encircle cells forming homotypic interactions with neighboring cells[57] and can also be attacked by mite proteases.[52] Although ZAs are closely associated with TJs and are arranged contiguously at lateral cell surfaces, they do not occlude the paracellular channel. In the airways, ZAs consist of E-cadherin, a calcium-binding protein with a single transmembrane domain (Fig. 35.3). E-cadherin is a classical cadherin in which the extracellular region contains five repeating domains with internal homology.[57] The cytoplasmic domain of E-cadherin forms complexes with α-, β- and γ-catenins, linking ZAs to the actin cytoskeleton and thus, indirectly, to other membrane associated proteins, such as those of TJs.[58] Despite an abundance of theoretical cleavage sites, proteolysis of E-cadherin by mite protease allergens is less extensive than that of occludin, suggesting that access to E-cadherin is sterically hindered until TJs are cleaved.[52]

Desmosomes constitute a third type of interepithelial adhesion and are anchored to intermediate filaments to confer resilience to mechanical stress (Fig. 35.3).[59,60] Desmosomes are adhesive because they contain desmogleins and desmocollins, single-pass TM glycoproteins belonging to the family of desmosomal cadherins. These interact with the phosphoproteins plakoglobin and desmoplakin in the desmosomal plaque, forming a bridge to keratin intermediate filaments.[60] Using 2-photon molecular excitation imaging it has been shown that the intensity of desmosomal puncta increases as other cell adhesions are cleaved by protease allergens.[53] Neither the molecular basis nor the functional significance of this phenomenon is known. It is tempting to propose that this process might represent an acute adaptation to the focal disruption of interepithelial adhesion produced by protease allergens, especially because it accompanies potentially adaptive changes in the actin cytoskeleton.

PROTEASE ALLERGENS AND APOPTOSIS

Mite protease allergens exert a gradual and reversible effect on the intercellular adhesions of epithelia. When only TJs are cleaved, an effect which can be extremely localized and subtle, resynthesis of junctional proteins and TJ reassembly is rapid and complete. When cleavage is more extensive, other adaptational changes occur. These adaptations may be insufficient to maintain epithelial integrity and apoptosis may result.[55]

During the exfoliation of apoptotic cells, the permeability of the epithelial barrier may be very high in the immediate vicinity of these events, further facilitating allergen delivery. This apoptotic response is activated through a mechanism that is independent of TJ cleavage.[61] Although the events are not consequential, there may nevertheless be biochemical linkage between TJ cleavage and apoptosis. During the proteolysis of occludin by protease allergens, we have consistently observed a C-terminal intracellular cleavage that is reminiscent of its caspase-mediated processing in staurosporine-induced apoptosis.[62]

PROTEASE ALLERGENS AND PROINFLAMMATORY CYTOKINE AND MEDIATOR PRODUCTION

In addition to enhancing the presentation of any allergen, the proteolytic activity of certain major allergens has other aspects of potential importance to the initiation of allergy. These range from the inactivation of mucosal defense mechanisms to the activation of signal transduction pathways, which create a cell signaling environment that favors allergy development in the genetically predisposed.

Mite protease allergens (usually Der p 1), and increasingly protease allergens from other sources, have been implicated in a variety of events at the airway interface. These effects range from the production of inflammatory mediators by epithelial cells to actions on molecules present in epithelial lining fluid. For example, α_1-antitrypsin, a serpin that protects the airways from injury by serine proteases, is attacked at its reactive center loop and proximal to its NH_2 terminus, causing its inactivation.[63] This interaction is potentially significant because it is expected to potentiate the activity of serine protease allergens from dust mites and other sources.

The presence of protease inhibitor gene defects may have significant effects on the predisposition to allergy. Several mutations have been identified in serpins (LETKI-1, PAI-1, C1 esterase inhibitor, α_1-antichymotrypsin), which appear to be associated with the expression of allergic disease.[64] These gene polymorphisms confirm data from functional studies that have been accrued over the past 25 years. It has been proposed that the existence of such defects may cause the host susceptible to the effects of protease allergens, although formal proof is awaited.

Mite proteases stimulate the release of various cytokines and PGE_2, as well as initiating the IgE-independent degranulation of mast cells.[65,66] For example, both Der p 1 and Der p 3 elicit a net release of histamine and IL-4 from human lung mast cells.[66] Similarly, both Der p 1 and Der p 9 upregulate cytokine gene transcription and cytokine production (IL-6, IL-8, and GM-CSF) in bronchial epithelial cells.[67] Protease-containing extracts of *Aspergillus fumigatus* or purified fungal allergens elicit responses that share similar features,[56,68] suggesting that major allergens from diverse sources converge on the same effector pathways. Therefore, the signaling mechanisms that underlie the secreted mediator responses of protease allergens are now being studied.

Interpretation of apparently conflicting data from studies of protease allergen signal transduction is dogged by problems common to many investigations of the IgE-independent actions of allergens. The nascent literature contains studies performed with crude allergen extracts, native proteins of varying purity and their recombinant counterparts which may be folded incorrectly or contaminated with endotoxin. It is unsurprising that a comparison of studies conducted with this miscellany of stimuli

sometimes results in a confusing picture. However, general conclusions may be drawn even though elucidation of the finer details and a full understanding of this protease-mediated signaling in allergy requires more research.

Unlike the actions on TJs, the liberation of cell-derived mediators by mite protease allergens is due, at least in part, to the activation of signal transduction pathways that are linked to protease-activated receptors.[69,70] PARs are G-protein coupled receptors (GPCRs), typically stimulated by serine proteases, which cleave the N terminus of the latent receptor. This creates a new N terminus, which behaves as a tethered ligand, binding to the receptor and activating it. Der p 1, Der p 3, and Der p 9 all cleave the NH_2 terminus of the PAR-2 receptor. Suitable cleavage of PAR-2 can lead to an increase in phosphoinositide turnover, an increase in intracellular Ca^{2+} and release of eotaxin and GM-CSF by cultured epithelial cells.[71,72] More chronically, protease allergen-induced cytokine release might involve the phosphorylation of I-κBα, a cytoplasmic inhibitor of the transcription factor NF-κB.[73]

Downstream effects of protease allergens involve the mitogen activated protein kinase (MAPK) pathways. MAPK signaling plays a central role in orchestrating inflammatory responses from their initiation to their resolution. The involvement of MAPK signaling in transducing at least some of the responses of protease allergens is therefore anticipated. MAPKs phosphorylate a variety of cytoplasmic and nuclear targets, modification of the latter altering gene expression to promote cell growth, differentiation, apoptosis, inflammation, and adaptation to environmental stress. Multiple MAPK pathways exist, the three major groups being the extracellular signal-related kinases (ERKs),[74] the c-Jun N-terminal kinases (JNKs), and the p38 kinases. These groups of MAPKs are hierarchically activated by upstream kinases known as MAPK kinases (MAP2Ks), which in turn are activated by families of MAPK kinase kinases (MAP3Ks). The MAP3Ks are ultimately coupled to the detection of extracellular stimuli through kinase-linked receptors and GPCRs, such as the PAR family, normally resident within the cell membrane.

Crude extracts of house-dust mite and cockroach have been shown to activate the ERK1/2 MAPK pathway in airway epithelial cells,[75] which is involved in signaling from various GPCR-linked receptors. Similarly, ERK1/2 activation and NF-κB activation have been implicated in IL-8 production by stimulation of airway epithelial cells with Der p 1. However, the ERK1/2-mediated response was found to be largely independent of PAR-2 activation. In contrast, HDM serine protease allergens signaled effectively via PAR-2 activation, inducing responses via the p38 and JNK kinases and the transcription factors NF-κB and AP-1.[76] These results contrast with earlier work which demonstrated PAR-2-dependent release of IL-8 by Der p 1.[70] ERK1/2 signaling is an activation stimulus for cytosolic phospholipase A_2 and is thus an enabling step in eicosanoid biosynthesis. It is currently unclear if ERK1/2 activation is entirely responsible for transducing the protease-dependent production of eicosanoids by dust mite allergens, or that evoked by the fungal serine protease Pen ch 13.[56]

PROTEASES AND IMMUNE RESPONSES

The proteolytic action of Der p 1 can skew immune responses towards an allergic phenotype, as demonstrated in mice sensitized to *Schistosoma mansoni*.[77] Additionally, a number of studies show that catalytically active protease allergens produce heightened allergic responses compared with their enzymatically inactive forms[78] and responses to a non-protease bystander allergen are also increased by the protease activity of Der p 1[79] or crude *Aspergillus* extracts or purified Asp f 13.[47] Several investigations have attempted to determine whether protease allergens might skew adaptive responses. Initially, it was suggested that IgE production might be enhanced by Der p 1 cleaving the low-affinity IgE receptor, CD23 on B lymphocytes,[80,81] but in vivo evidence to support the initial cell culture observations is lacking.[82] Skewing might also occur by cleavage of the α-subunit of the IL-2 receptor (CD25) by Der p 1, thereby suppressing IL-2-dependent proliferation of T cells into the Th1 phenotype, and possibly favoring the development or persistence of Th2 responses.[83] This is a potentially interesting mechanism in view of current thinking regarding neonatal programming of adaptive responses. However, the differences between commitment to Th1 and Th2 responses are more clearly distinguishable in mice than in humans and it, therefore, remains to be established whether protease allergens do actually skew the responses in people as predicted from animal and in vitro studies.

■ CONCLUSIONS ■

In this chapter, the structure and function of the many aero-, ingested, and injected allergens have been described. We now know much about the allergens associated with allergic disease, and these data continue to complement those emerging from many other scientific disciplines. It can be seen that the protein allergens fall, not unexpectedly, into previously delineated protein groups. Thanks to efforts directed towards the identification, purification, and characterization of clinically important allergens, it has become possible to appreciate some of the reasons why these substances lead to disease. While it is clear that allergens are functionally and structurally diverse, the application of molecular techniques has revealed important clues and relationships between certain major allergens. These approaches have led to the first mechanism-based description of how one important group of allergens may modulate immune function, such as facilitating contact with DC, a step essential to allergic sensitization. Similarly, studies have revealed how their IgE-independent effects could create conditions that promote allergy in the genetically predisposed. There are several lessons from these findings. The obvious ones relate specifically to mite allergy in asthma and rhinitis, where proteases appear to dictate key steps in transepithelial allergen delivery and inflammation. However, they also serve as an important reminder that interactions between allergens and with adjuvants are likely to be important in defining the outcome of sensitization. The striking ability of at least some protease allergens to override the tolerance and unmask the potent allergenicity of comparatively innocuous proteins suggests that there may now be a simple and instructive way of categorizing allergens in a way that transcends the traditional classification based on groupings from a particular biological origin. A small cadre of allergens with enzymatic activity, especially proteases, appear to represent a category which contains all of the attributes to drive the development of allergy. In contrast, the majority of allergens would fall within a separate category, distinguished by their reliance on the former category for them to cause allergy. This simple categorization is suggested by experimental evidence, but much work will be necessary to confirm its validity. However, an approach based on the IgE-independent actions, particularly enzymatic activity, of allergens may allow us to understand more fully the roots of allergy and the links that

explain its diversity. Through such an understanding, the prospects for improved treatment and even prevention of allergy will be possible.

Acknowledgments

The authors' work described in this chapter was supported by the Australian NHMRC, the Asthma Foundation of WA, Asthma UK, The Medical Research Council (UK), and The Wellcome Trust. We thank Dr Martha Ludwig for reviewing the botanical section of this chapter.

References

Introduction

1. Stewart GA. Molecular biology of allergens. In: Busse WW, Holgate ST, eds. Asthma and rhinitis. Oxford: Blackwell; 2000:1107–1142.
2. Aalberse RC. Structural biology of allergens. J Allergy Clin Immunol 2000; 106:228–238.

Aeroallergens – pollens

3. Vrtala S, Fischer S, Grote M, et al. Molecular, immunological, and structural characterization of Phl p 6, a major allergen and P-particle-associated protein from Timothy grass (Phleum pratense) pollen. J Immunol 1999; 163:5489–5496.
4. Vinckier S, Smets E. The potential role of orbicules as a vector of allergens. Allergy 2001; 56:1129–1136.
5. Suphioglu C, Singh MB, Taylor P, et al. Mechanism of grass-pollen-induced asthma. Lancet 1992; 339:569–572.
6. Vithanage HI, Howlett BJ, Jobson S, et al. Immunocytochemical localization of water-soluble glycoproteins, including group 1 allergen, in pollen of ryegrass, Lolium perenne, using ferritin-labelled antibody. Histochem J 1982; 14:949–966.
7. Pastorello EA, Pompei C, Pravettoni V, et al. Lipid transfer proteins and 2S albumins as allergens. Allergy 2001; 56 Suppl 67:45–47.
8. Buhot N, Douliez J, Jacquemard A, et al. A lipid transfer protein binds to a receptor involved in the control of plant defence responses. FEBS Lett 2001; 509:27–30.
9. Dai S, Chen T, Shen S, et al. Proteomic analyses of Oryza sativa mature pollen reveal novel proteins associated with pollen germination and tube growth. Proteomics 2006; 6: 2504–2529.
10. Chen Y, et al. Differential display proteomic analysis of Picea meyeri pollen germination and pollen-tube growth after inhibition of actin polymerization by latrunculin B. Plant J 2006; 47:174–195.
11. Li LC, Cosgrove DJ. Grass group I pollen allergens (beta-expansins) lack proteinase activity and do not cause wall loosening via proteolysis. Eur J Biochem 2001; 268:4217–4226.
12. Lenartowska M, Rodriguez-Garcia MI, Bednarska E. Immunocytochemical localization of esterified and unesterified pectins in unpollinated and pollinated styles of Petunia hybrida Hort. Planta 2001; 213:182–191.
13. Midoro-Horiuti T, Brooks EG, Goldblum RM. Pathogenesis-related proteins of plants as allergens. Ann Allergy Asthma Immunol 2001; 87:261–271.
14. Ebner C, Hoffmann-Sommergruber K, Breiteneder H. Plant food allergens homologous to pathogenesis-related proteins. Allergy (Suppl) 2001; 67:5643–44.
15. Breiteneder H, Ebner C. Molecular and biochemical classification of plant-derived food allergens. J Allergy Clin Immunol 2000; 106:27–36.

Aeroallergens – fungi

16. Makimura K, Hanazawa R, Takatori K, et al. Fungal flora on board the Mir-Space Station, identification by morphological features and ribosomal DNA sequences. Microbiol Immunol 2001; 45:357–363.
17. Mitakakis TZ, Barnes C, Tovey ER. Spore germination increases allergen release from Alternaria. J Allergy Clin Immunol 2001; 107:388–390.
18. Breitenbach M, Simon B, Probst G, et al. Enolases are highly conserved fungal allergens. Int Arch Allergy Immunol 1997; 113:114–117.
19. Nadeau K, Das A, Walsh CT. Hsp90 chaperonins possess ATPase activity and bind heat shock transcription factors and peptidyl prolyl isomerases. J Biol Chem 1993; 268:1479–1487.

Aeroallergens – animal-derived

20. Mantyjarvi R, Rautiainen J, Virtanen T. Lipocalins as allergens. Biochim Biophys Acta 2000; 1482:308–317.
21. Stewart GA, McWilliam AS. Endogenous function and biological significance of aeroallergens: an update. Curr Opin Allergy Clin Immunol 2001; 1:95–103.
22. Ring PC, Wan H, Schou C, et al. The 18-kDa form of cat allergen Felis domesticus 1 (Fel d 1) is associated with gelatin- and fibronectin-degrading activity. Clin Exp Allergy 2000; 30:1085–1096.

Aeroallergens – arthropod-derived

23. Arlian LG. Arthropod allergens and human health. Annu Rev Entomol 2002; 47:395–433.
24. Binder M, Mahler V, Haye KB, et al. Molecular and immunological characterization of arginine kinase from the Indianmeal moth, Plodia interpunctella, a novel cross-reactive invertebrate pan-allergen. J Immunol 2001; 167:5470–5477.
25. Lin RY, Shen HD, Han SH. Identification and characterization of a 30 kd major allergen from Parapenaeus fissurus. J Allergy Clin Immunol 1993; 92:837–845.

Aeroallergens – occupational

26. Baur X, Degens PO, Sander I. Baker's asthma: still among the most frequent occupational respiratory disorders. J Allergy Clin Immunol 1998; 102:984–997.
27. Posch A, Chen Z, Dunn MJ, et al. Latex allergen database. Electrophoresis 1997; 18: 2803–2810.
28. Bernstein DI, Smith AB, Moller DR, et al. Clinical and immunologic studies among egg-processing workers with occupational asthma. J Allergy Clin Immunol 1987; 80:791–797.
29. Kurup VP, Fink JN. The spectrum of immunologic sensitization in latex allergy. Allergy 2001; 56:2–12.
30. Menendez-Arias L, Moneo L, Dominguez R, et al. Primary structure of the major allergen of yellow mustard (Sinapis alba L.) seed, Sin a I. Eur J Biochem 1988; 177:159–166.

Ingested allergens

31. Ring J, Brockow K, Behrendt H. Adverse reactions to foods. J Chromatogr B Biomed Sci Appl 2001; 756:3–10.
32. Han GD, Matsuno M, Ito G, et al. Meat allergy: investigation of potential allergenic proteins in beef. Biosci Biotechnol Biochem 2000; 64:1887–1895.
33. Pascual CY, Crespo JF, San Martin S, et al. Cross-reactivity between IgE-binding proteins from Anisakis, German cockroach, and chironomids. Allergy 1997; 52:514–520.
34. Vallverdu A, Asturias JA, Arilla MC, et al. Characterization of recombinant Mercurialis annua major allergen Mer a 1 (profilin). J Allergy Clin Immunol 1998; 101:363–370.
35. Ortolani C, Ispano M, Pastorello E, et al. The oral allergy syndrome. Ann Allergy 1988; 61:47–52.
36. Aalberse RC, J. Akkerdaas, van Ree R, Cross-reactivity of IgE antibodies to allergens. Allergy 2001; 56:478–490.

Injected insect allergens

37. Hoffman DR. Allergens in Hymenoptera venom XIII: Isolation and purification of protein components from three species of vespid venoms. J Allergy Clin Immunol 1985; 75: 599–605.
38. King TP, Spangfort MD. Structure and biology of stinging insect venom allergens. Int Arch Allergy Immunol 2000; 123:99–106.
39. Wu CH, Lan JL. Immunoblot analysis of allergens in crude mosquito extracts. Int Arch Allergy Appl Immunol 1989; 90:271–273.
40. Lee SE, Johnstone IP, Lee RP, et al. Putative salivary allergens of the cat flea, Ctenocephalides felis felis. Vet Immunol Immunopathol 1999; 69:229–237.
41. Paddock CD, McKerron JH, Hansell E, et al. Identification, cloning, and recombinant expression of procalin, a major triatomine allergen. J Immunol 2001; 167:2694–2699.

Three-dimensional structures of allergens

42. de Halleux S, Stura E, Vander Elst L, et al. Three-dimensional structure and IgE-binding properties of mature fully active Der p 1, a clinically relevant major allergen. J Allergy Clin Immunol 2006; 117:571–576.
43. Meno K, Thorsted PB, Ipsen H, et al. The crystal structure of recombinant proDer p 1, a major house dust mite proteolytic allergen. J Immunol 2005; 175:3835–3845.

Allergen biochemistry, immunogenicity, and inflammation

44. Robinson C, Kalsheker NA, Srinivasan N, et al. On the potential significance of the enzymatic activity of mite allergens to immunogenicity. Clues to structure and function revealed by molecular characterization. Clin Exp Allergy 1997; 27:10–21.
45. Stewart GA, Thompson PJ, McWilliam AS. Biochemical properties of aeroallergens: contributory factors in allergic sensitization? Pediatr Allergy Immunol 1993; 4:163–172.
46. Gallucci S, Matzinger P. Danger signals: SOS to the immune system. Curr Opin Immunol 2001; 13:114–119.
47. Kheradmand F, Kiss A, Xu J, Lee SH, et al. A protease-activated pathway underlying Th cell type 2 activation and allergic lung disease. J Immunol 2002; 169:5904–5911.
48. Kurup VP, Xia JQ, Shen HD, et al. Alkaline serine proteinase from Aspergillus fumigatus has synergistic effects on Asp-f-2-induced immune response in mice. Int Arch Allergy Immunol 2002; 129:129–137.
49. Herbert CA, Holgate ST, Robinson C, et al. Effect of mite allergen on permeability of bronchial mucosa. Lancet 1990; 336:1132.
50. Herbert CA, King CM, Ring PC, et al. Augmentation of permeability in the bronchial epithelium by the house dust mite allergen Der p1. Am J Respir Cell Mol Biol 1995; 12: 369–378.

51. Wan H, Winton HL, Soeller C, et al. Der p 1 facilitates transepithelial allergen delivery by disruption of tight junctions. J Clin Invest 1999; 104:123–133.
52. Wan H, Winton HL, Soeller C, et al. Quantitative structural and biochemical analyses of tight junction dynamics following exposure of epithelial cells to house dust mite allergen Der p 1. Clin Exp Allergy 2000; 30:685–698.
53. Wan H, Winton HL, Soeller C, et al. The transmembrane protein occludin of epithelial tight junctions is a functional target for serine peptidases from faecal pellets of Dermatophagoides pteronyssinus. Clin Exp Allergy 2001; 31:279–294.
54. Tsukita S, Furuse M, Itoh M. Multifunctional strands in tight junctions. Nat Rev Mol Cell Biol 2001; 2:285–293.
55. Winton HL, Wan H, Cannell MB, et al. Class specific inhibition of house dust mite proteinases which cleave cell adhesion, induce cell death and which increase the permeability of lung epithelium. Br J Pharmacol 1998; 124:1048–1059.
56. Tai HY, Tam MF, Chou H, et al. Pen ch 13 allergen induces secretion of mediators and degradation of occludin protein of human lung epithelial cells. Allergy 2006; 61:382–388.
57. Takeichi M. Cadherin cell adhesion receptors as a morphogenetic regulator. Science 1991; 251:1451–1455.
58. Rajasekaran AK, Hojo M, Huima T, et al. Catenins and zonula occludens-1 form a complex during early stages in the assembly of tight junctions. J Cell Biol 1996; 132:451–463.
59. Garrod DR. Desmosomes and hemidesmosomes. Curr Opin Cell Biol 1993; 5:30–40.
60. Green KJ, Jones JC. Desmosomes and hemidesmosomes: structure and function of molecular components. FASEB J 1996; 10:871–881.
61. Baker SF, Runswick SK, Stewart GA, et al. Peptidase allergen Der p 1 initiates apoptosis of epithelial cells independently of tight junction proteolysis. Mol Membr Biol 2003; 20:71–81.
62. Bojarski C, Weiske J, Schoneberg T, et al. The specific fates of tight junction proteins in apoptotic epithelial cells. J Cell Sci 2004; 117:2097–2107.
63. Kalsheker NA, Deans S, Chambers L, et al. The house dust mite allergen Der p1 catalytically inactivates alpha 1-antitrypsin by specific reactive centre loop cleavage: a mechanism that promotes airway inflammation and asthma. Biochem Biophys Res Commun 1996; 221:59–61.
64. Smith PK, Harper JI. Serine proteases, their inhibitors and allergy. Allergy 2006; 61: 1441–1447.
65. Stewart GA, Boyd SM, Bird CH, et al. Immunobiology of the serine protease allergens from house dust mites. Am J Ind Med 1994; 25:105–107.
66. Machado DC, Horton D, Harrop R, et al. Potential allergens stimulate the release of mediators of the allergic response from cells of mast cell lineage in the absence of sensitization with antigen-specific IgE. Eur J Immunol 1996; 26:2972–2980.
67. King C, Brennan S, Thompson PJ, et al. Dust mite proteolytic allergens induce cytokine release from cultured airway epithelium. J Immunol 1998; 161:3645–3651.
68. Kauffman HF, Tomee JF, van de Riet MA, et al. Protease-dependent activation of epithelial cells by fungal allergens leads to morphologic changes and cytokine production. J Allergy Clin Immunol 2000; 105:1185–1193.
69. Hong PW, Flummerfelt KB, Nguyen S, et al. Human immunodeficiency virus envelope (gp120) binding to DC-SIGN and primary dendritic cells is carbohydrate dependent but does not involve 2G12 or Cyanovirin binding sites: implications for structural analyses of gp120-DC-SIGN binding. J Virol 2002; 76:12855–12865.
70. Asokananthan N, Graham PT, Fink J, et al. Activation of protease-activated receptor (PAR)-1, PAR-2, and PAR-4 stimulates IL-6, IL-8, and prostaglandin E_2 release from human respiratory epithelial cells. J Immunol 2002; 168:3577–3585.
71. Asokananthan N, Graham PT, Stewart DJ, et al. House-dust mite allergens induce proinflammatory cytokines from respiratory epithelial cells: the cysteine protease allergen, Der p 1, activates protease-activated receptor (PAR)-2 and inactivates PAR-1. J Immunol 2002; 169:4572–4578.
72. Sun G, Stacey MA, Schmidt M, et al. Interaction of mite allergens Der p3 and Der p9 with protease-activated receptor-2 expressed by lung epithelial cells. J Immunol 2001; 167:1014–1021.
73. Stacey MA, Sun G, Vassalli G, et al. The allergen Der p1 induces NF-kappaB activation through interference with IkappaB alpha function in asthmatic bronchial epithelial cells. Biochem Biophys Res Commun 1997; 236:522–526.
74. Nieuwland J, Feron R, Huisman BA, et al. Lipid transfer proteins enhance cell wall extension in tobacco. Plant Cell 2005; 17:2009–2019.
75. Kuderer NM, San Juan Vergara HG, Kong X, et al. Mite and cockroach proteases activate p44/p42 MAP kinases in human lung epithelial cells. Clin Mol Allergy 2003; 1:1.
76. Adam E, Hansen KK, Astudillo Fernandez O, et al. The house-dust mite allergen Der p 1, unlike Der p 3, stimulates the expression of interleukin-8 in human airway epithelial cells via a proteinase-activated receptor-2-independent mechanism. J Biol Chem 2006; 281:6910–6923.
77. Comoy EE, Pestel J, Duez C, et al. The house dust mite allergen, Dermatophagoides pteronyssinus, promotes type 2 responses by modulating the balance between IL-4 and IFN-gamma. J Immunol 1998; 160:2456–2462.
78. Gough L, Schultz O, Sewell HF, et al. The cysteine protease activity of the major dust mite allergen Der p 1 selectively enhances the immunoglobulin E antibody response. J Exp Med 1999; 190:1897–1902.
79. Gough L, Sewell HF, Shakib F. The proteolytic activity of the major dust mite allergen Der p 1 enhances the IgE antibody response to a bystander antigen. Clin Exp Allergy 2001; 31:1594–1598.
80. Hewitt CR, Brown AP, Hart BJ, et al. A major house dust mite allergen disrupts the immunoglobulin E network by selectively cleaving CD23: innate protection by antiproteases. J Exp Med 1995; 182:1537–1544.
81. Schulz O, Laing P, Sewell HF, et al. Der p I, a major allergen of the house dust mite, proteolytically cleaves the low-affinity receptor for human IgE (CD23). Eur J Immunol 1995; 25:3191–3194.
82. Shakib F, Schulz O, Sewell H. A mite subversive: cleavage of CD23 and CD25 by Der p 1 enhances allergenicity. Immunol Today 1998; 19:313–316.
83. Schulz O, Sewell HF, Shakib F. Proteolytic cleavage of CD25, the alpha subunit of the human T cell interleukin 2 receptor, by Der p 1, a major mite allergen with cysteine protease activity. J Exp Med 1998; 187:271–275.

section C

PHYSIOLOGY

Structural and Functional Cutaneous Immunology

Douglas A Plager and Mark R Pittelkow

36

CONTENTS

SUMMARY OF IMPORTANT CONCEPTS

>> The stratified cellular epidermis, including its outermost cornified layer, and the underlying relatively acellular dermis contain the immune cells common to epithelial surfaces and the specialized sweat and sebaceous glands; both layers are highly innervated, and the dermis is abundantly vascularized

>> Epidermal barrier defects caused by filaggrin mutations have been associated with development of atopic skin and lung disease

>> Various constitutive and inducible innate immune mechanisms function in the skin to fight infection and to direct acquired immunity – these include keratinocyte–derived molecules such as IL-1, antimicrobial peptides, TSLP, and RANKL (induced by ultraviolet light), as well as more broadly expressed pattern-recognition receptors

>> Immune functions attributed to cutaneous mast cells and dendritic cells (DCs) (including Langerhans' cells, dermal DCs, and DCs infiltrating during inflammatory disease) are increasing in number and being redefined

>> Skin homing of memory, effector, and regulatory T-cell subtypes is programmed by skin-derived DCs and prominently directed by CLA, CCR4/CCL17, and CCR10/CCL27

■ INTRODUCTION ■

The skin is the largest organ of the human body. In the average adult, it covers an area of $1.5–2.0\,m^2$. It comprises two principal layers, the epidermis and the dermis (Fig. 36.1). The epidermal cells are modified epithelial cells and rest on a basement membrane that separates them from the underlying mesenchymal layer or dermis. Vital interactions occur between the cells of the epidermis, dermis, and peripheral blood (Table 36.1) as a mechanism for maintaining the skin's structure and homeostatic and protective functions. In addition, blood vessels, lymphatics, nerve tissue, and specialized epidermal appendages (i.e., hair follicles and sweat and sebaceous glands) maintain various skin functions (Fig. 36.1). Recognized activities include thermoregulation, sensation, metabolism (e.g., vitamin D synthesis), physical barrier function (e.g., prevention of desiccation; protection from ultraviolet light, mechanical trauma, and chemical irritants or toxins), and immunologic barrier function. Although each of these functions is critical to an individual's health, the main focus of this chapter is on the structural and cellular aspects of the skin as they relate to cutaneous immune function.

■ CELLS AND STRUCTURE OF THE SKIN ■

CELLS OF THE EPIDERMIS

The epidermis is composed primarily of cells; it is approximately $150\,\mu m$ thick and is schematically represented in Figure 36.2. The projections of the epidermis into the underlying papillary dermis are referred to as rete pegs. The most abundant epidermal cell type is the keratinocyte (approximately 90% of cells). Keratinocytes are continually renewing cells that are roughly divided into four types: basal (*stratum germinativum*), spinous (*stratum spinosum*), granular (*stratum granulosum*), and cornified (*stratum corneum*) keratinocytes.[1] The keratinocytes of the different epidermal layers characteristically express pairs of various acidic (type I) and basic-neutral (type II) keratin proteins, for which an updated consensus nomenclature has been proposed.[2,3] Several elements control keratinocyte proliferation, differentiation, and apoptosis-like cornification, including

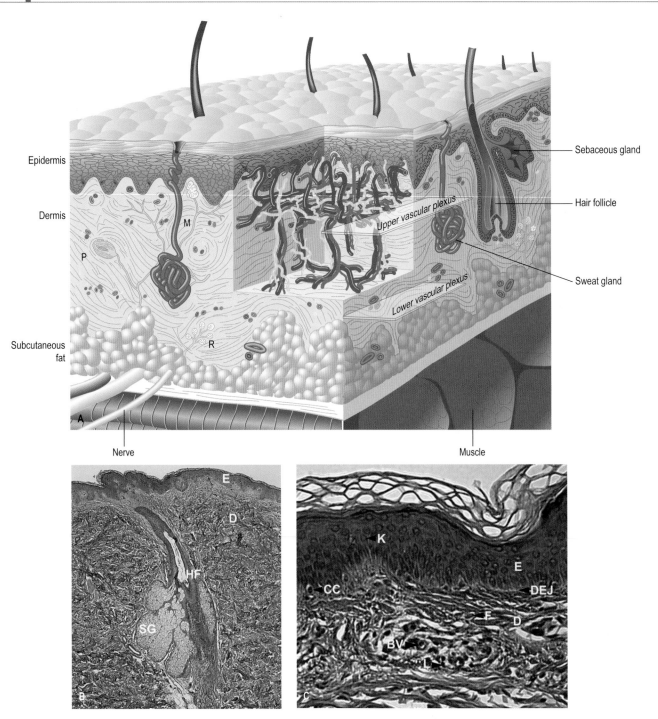

Fig. 36.1. Structure of human skin. (**A**) Schematic representation of skin cross-section. The two major layers of human skin, the epidermis and the dermis, overlie subcutaneous fat and muscle. Arterioles (red), venules (blue), and lymph vessels (yellow) of the dermis form a lower and an upper vascular plexus. Capillary loops extend towards the epidermis from the upper plexus of blood vessels into the dermal papillae – approximately one loop per dermal papilla. Sensory and autonomic nerves (orange fibers) are also arranged in a lower and upper plexus at the junction of the dermis and subcutaneous fat and in the upper dermis, respectively (not explicitly shown). Specialized sensory structures, including Meissner's (M), Pacinian (P), and Ruffini (R) corpuscles, and free nerve endings, which extend into the epidermis, arise from these nerve plexuses. Sweat glands and hair follicles and associated sebaceous glands are also integral components of the skin. (**B**) Skin histology, showing epidermis (E), dermis (D), hair follicle (HF), and sebaceous gland (SG). (Hematoxylin and eosin stain, ×50.) (**C**) Skin histology, showing keratinocyte (K), clear cell (CC, representing melanocyte, Langerhans' cell, or Merkel cell) of the epidermis, dermal-epidermal junction (DEJ), and dermal fibroblast (F), lymphocyte (L), and blood vessel (BV). (Hematoxylin and eosin stain, ×250.) Other cellular and structural components of the skin require special staining or immunomarkers for identification.

Table 36.1 Cells of human skin

Resident cells of healthy skin			
Epidermis	**Dermis**	**Specialized structure**	**Recruited cells**
Keratinocyte (~92%)[a]	Fibroblast	Endothelial cell	Neutrophil
Langerhans' cell (~3%)	Mast cell	Pericyte and smooth muscle cell	Eosinophil
Melanocyte (~3%)	Macrophage	Schwann cell and nerve axon	Basophil
Merkel cell	Dermal dendritic cell[b]	Hair follicle cell	T lymphocyte[c]
Epidermal T lymphocyte	Dermal T lymphocyte	Sebocyte	B lymphocyte (?)
	Natural killer cell (?)	Eccrine gland cell	Natural killer cell (?)[c]
		Apocrine gland cell	Natural killer T cell (?)
			Monocyte[c]
			Blood dendritic cell[c]
			Mast cell precursor[c]

[a]Percentage of epidermal cells.
[b]Used here to denote all non-macrophage dendritic cells normally present in the dermis.
[c]Corresponds to a resident cell type.

growth factors, cytokines, neuropeptides, adrenergic and cholinergic signaling, calcium, and cell–cell and cell–matrix interactions.[1,4] Recently, key roles for p63 and caspase-14 in epidermis development have been identified.[5,6] Some of the critical signals regulating keratinocyte development also originate from the dermis.[7,8] Most importantly, keratinocytes are key participants in host defense against environmental exposures via both physical and immunologic barrier functions.

Non-migrating basal keratinocytes rest on the basement membrane, a structure that divides the epidermis from the dermis. They are tethered to the basement membrane by protein structures called hemidesmosomes; known proteins in hemidesmosomes are listed in Figure 36.3.[9,10] Basal keratinocytes form a single layer of columnar-shaped cells expressing keratins K5 (basic–neutral) and K14 (acidic), and their three recognized subtypes are distinguished by mitotic activity.[1] One subtype includes the so-called epidermal stem cells that constitute approximately 5–10% of basal keratinocytes, with multipotent epidermal stem cells apparently residing in the bulge region of hair follicles.[11,12] Epidermal stem cells retain radiolabeled thymidine because of infrequent cell division, and they appear to express high levels of β_1-integrin.[11] Transient amplifying cells are a second subtype and constitute the majority of basal keratinocytes. These cells divide to produce the third subtype, postmitotic keratinocytes, which progressively differentiate and migrate toward the surface of the skin. During migration, postmitotic keratinocytes gradually flatten, lose their cellular organelles, dehydrate, and modify their protein and lipid composition toward a more impermeable, cornified composition.[13] The postmitotic basal keratinocyte requires 14 days to migrate to the stratum corneum and another 14 days before desquamation from the surface of healthy skin.

Suprabasal spinous keratinocytes are named for their abundant spine-like desmosomes. Desmosomes serve to attach adjacent keratinocytes to one another – in contrast to hemidesmosomes, which attach keratinocytes to the basement membrane – and to provide resistance to mechanical stress. Known proteins in desmosomes are listed in Figure 36.3.[14] Adherens junctions,[15] gap junctions,[16,17] and tight junctions[18] further mediate interkeratinocyte attachment and communication. Changes in

keratin composition also accompany the conversion to a spinous cell. For example, K1 (basic–neutral) and K10 (acidic) keratins are newly synthesized in spinous keratinocytes.[2] Lamellar granules containing precursors of stratum corneum lipids are first evident in the cytoplasm of upper spinous cells as well.[19] These granules contain glucosylceramides that are the precursors for ceramides, the principal lipid of stratum corneum.[19] Lamellar granules also contain a variety of other lipids, including sterols and triglycerides, glycoproteins, and enzymes, including lipases, glycosidases, proteases, acid hydrolases, and phosphatases.

Granular keratinocytes are identified by their basophilic keratohyalin granules, which contain mostly profilaggrin, loricrin, and keratin intermediate filaments.[1] Granular keratinocytes are the penultimate differentiation stage before cornification. Their lamellar granule contents are released into the intercellular space between the stratum granulosum and stratum corneum.[19] This process forms a hydrophobic lipid seal at the interface between the granular and cornified layers that impedes transepidermal water loss.[19] Proper formation of this lipid barrier requires a variety of enzymatic proteins and host intake of essential fatty acids.

The programmed conversion of granular keratinocytes to cornified keratinocytes of the stratum corneum involves numerous degradative enzymes that break down cell organelles and nuclei; these enzymes include DNases, RNases, proteases, phosphatases, esterases, acid hydrolases, and plasminogen activator.[1] This conversion includes profilaggrin proteolysis to filaggrin (filament aggregation protein) monomeric subunits.[13] Filaggrin serves as the matrix protein that embeds and promotes aggregation and disulfide bonding of keratin filaments.[13] Both prevalent and rare loss-of-function mutations in the filaggrin (FLG) gene recently have been linked to ichthyosis vulgaris and a predisposition to develop eczema (Fig. 36.4).[20] Interestingly, some of these filaggrin mutations have also been associated with the 'atopic march' towards eczema-associated asthma and also with asthma severity independent of eczema status.[21,22] The cornified cell envelope, a proteinaceous layer just below the plasma membrane, also develops during cornification and involves interprotein disulfide formation and N-(γ-glutamyl) lysine cross-linking by transglutaminases.[13] Proteins detected in the cornified cell envelope include

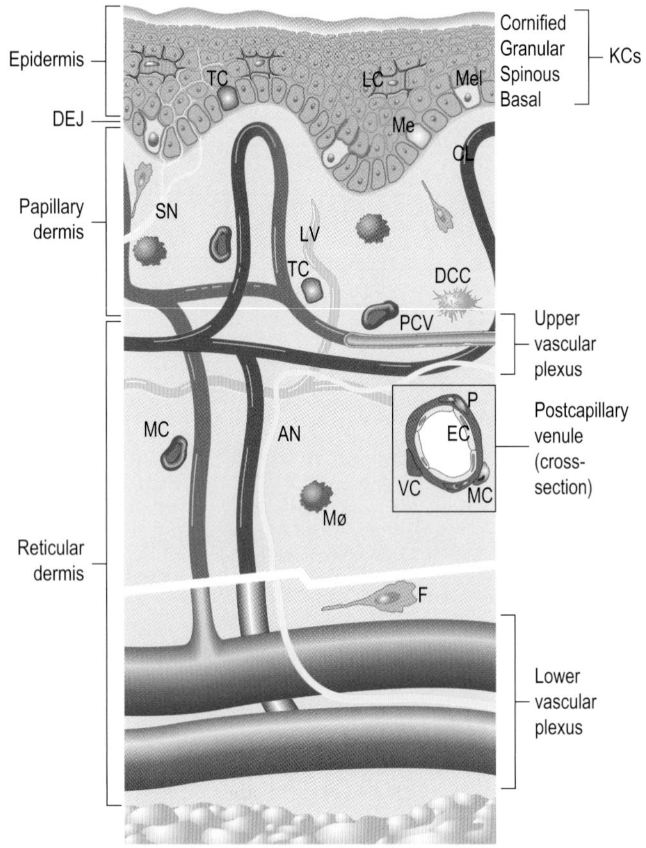

Epidermis

DEJ

Papillary dermis

Reticular dermis

TC · LC · Mel

Cornified
Granular
Spinous
Basal

KCs

Me

CL

SN

LV

TC

DCC

PCV

Upper vascular plexus

P
EC
VC · MC

Postcapillary venule (cross-section)

MC · AN

MØ

F

Lower vascular plexus

Fig. 36.2. Cellular and vascular organization of normal human skin. Keratinocytes (KCs) are the most abundant of epidermal cells and they are typically categorized from the skin surface to the dermal–epidermal junction (DEJ) as cornified, granular, spinous, and basal keratinocytes. Suprabasal Langerhans' cells (LC) and basal level melanocytes (Mel), T cells (TC), and Merkel cells (Me) are also widely distributed in normal epidermis. Sensory nerve (SN) endings innervate all vital layers of the epidermis. The DEJ separates the epidermis from the papillary dermis, which extends down to the upper vascular plexus. Capillary loops (CL), approximately one loop per dermal papilla, project upward towards the epidermis. The postcapillary venule (PCV), important in inflammatory cell extravasation into the skin, is shown partially in cut-edge section and in an enlarged cross-section (*inset*). Endothelial cells (EC) form the inner surface of the postcapillary venule, and they are surrounded by a lamellar basement membrane. Pericytes (P) reside within the layers of the venule basement membrane while veil cells (VC) and mast cells (MC) often contact the outer surface of the venule basement membrane. Lymph vessels (LV) and nerves, including autonomic nerves (AN) controlling cutaneous involuntary muscle contraction, track with blood vessels. The remainder of the dermis down to the subcutaneous fat is referred to as the reticular dermis. Fibroblasts (F), mast cells (MC), and macrophages (MØ) are relatively more abundant in the papillary dermis than the reticular dermis. Perivascular dermal T cells (TC) and dermal dendritic cells (DDC, e.g. dermal dendrocytes) also normally reside in the papillary dermis. The lower vascular plexus lies just above the subcutaneous fat layer 2–4 mm below the surface of the skin.

loricrin (75% of protein mass of the cornified cell envelope), involucrin (transglutaminase cross-linked), keratolinin, small proline-rich proteins, elafin (a serine protease inhibitor), and envoplakin. Many of the genes associated with cornified envelope formation are found in a 2.5 Mbp region of chromosome 1q21 referred to as the epidermal differentiation complex (EDC)[13] and genetic linkage to this chromosome location for both atopic dermatitis and psoriasis has been reported.[23] Mutations and polymorphisms in protease (stratum corneum chymotryptic enzyme; encoded by the *KLK7* gene) or protease inhibitor genes (Lymphoepithelial Kazal-type 5 serine protease inhibitor (LEKTI); encoded by the *SPINK5* gene) that influence epidermal integrity have also been associated with an atopic dermatitis/eczematous phenotype.[24] Specific mutations in SPINK5 are associated with Netherton syndrome and the accompanying, more severe manifestations of atopy. Ultimately, flat, polyhedral cornified keratinocytes of the stratum corneum lose their nuclei, and eventually their desmosomal connections, and form a barrier via their high molecular weight, intermolecular disulfide-bonded keratins (up to 80%) and cornified cell envelopes interlayered with lipid lamellae (primarily ceramides, cholesterol, and free fatty acids) derived from lamellar granules. The thickness of the stratum corneum can vary from as low as 15–25 cornified cell layers (approximately 15 μm thick) on many body areas to hundreds of cornified cell layers on the palms and soles.

Keratinocytes have the potential to express a wide variety of small molecule and peptide mediators. These will be described in greater detail as they relate to the innate and acquired cutaneous immune system later in this chapter. A number of interleukins, chemokines, growth factors, and neuropeptides have been demonstrated to be expressed by resting or stimulated keratinocytes. For example, ultraviolet B (UVB) or inflamed skin expresses receptor activator of NK-κB ligand (RANKL), which, in turn, functionally alters epidermal dendritic cells and increases regulatory T cells (CD4+, CD25+). A second epidermal cell type interspersed among the living keratinocytes of the substratum corneum layers is the Langerhans' cell (Fig. 36.2 and Table 36.1). These bone marrow-derived cells comprise 2–4% of epidermal cells and are a major histocompatibility class II (MHC II)-bearing dendritic cell subset.[25] Mouse studies suggest a key role for transforming growth factor-beta (TGF-β) in Langerhans' cell development.[26] Under non-inflammatory conditions, Langerhans' cells appear to be long-lived and/or locally repopulated by replicating Langerhans' cells or differentiating skin-resident precursors (possibly dermal CD14+ cells).[26–28] Most recently, repopulation of Langerhans' cells in inflamed skin has been reported to occur via classical CD14+CD16− monocytes in a colony stimulating factor-1 receptor dependent manner.[27] However, other cell populations have been proposed as Langerhans' cell precursors. Thus, the molecular signals mediating epidermal localization and/or development of Langerhans' cells are incompletely understood, although it has been shown that E-cadherin mediates Langerhans' cell adhesion to keratinocytes.[29] The highly dendritic structure of Langerhans' cells allows efficient antigen sampling of virtually the entire surface of the skin. The density of Langerhans' cells varies somewhat over the surface of the body from 200 to 1000 cells/mm2, with the face being most heavily populated at 600 to 1000 Langerhans' cells/mm2.[25,30] Langerhans' cells can be recognized by electron microscopy, which demonstrates their unique rod- and racket-shaped cytoplasmic Birbeck granules (Lag antibody-reactive), and by immunohistochemical staining with antibodies recognizing langerin/CD207, adenosine triphosphatase (ATPase), or CD1a.[25] Immature Langerhans' cells are phagocytic cells, and the calcium-dependent (C-type) lectin,

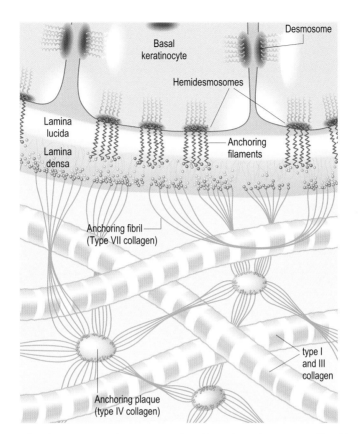

Fig. 36.3. Dermal-epidermal junction (DEJ). Desmosomes function to attach and laterally stabilize juxtaposed basal keratinocytes. Proteins important in desmosome formation include intermediate filaments (e.g., keratins), desmoplakins, desmogleins, desmocollins, plakophilins, and plakoglobin. Basal keratinocytes attach to the lamina densa (basement membrane) via hemidesmosomes which are composed of bullous pemphigoid antigen 1 (BPAg1), plectin, BPAg2 (i.e., collagen XVII), and $\alpha_6\beta_4$-integrin. Hemidesmosome-associated BPAg2 and $\alpha_6\beta_4$-integrin extend down to interact with laminin 5 (i.e., laminin 332) that extends up from the lamina densa into the lamina lucida. As such, these are the primary components of anchoring filaments. Laminin 6 is also present in the lamina lucida. The lamina densa is composed of type IV collagen, laminin 1, entactin (i.e., nidogen), and heparan sulfate proteoglycan. Anchoring fibrils attach to the dermalside of the lamina densa and interweave with type I and III collagen fibrils prior to attaching to anchoring plaques within the dermis or reattaching to the lamina densa. Note that exact locations, interactions, and identities of all DEJ proteins are actively being defined.

langerin/CD207, functions in antigen capture and subsequent Birbeck granule formation.[31] Notably, with respect to allergic disease, a unique high-affinity immunoglobulin E (IgE) receptor, Fc epsilon receptor type I (FcεRI), with an $\alpha\gamma_2$ subunit composition is expressed on Langerhans' cells and can greatly 'facilitate' presentation of IgE-bound antigen.[32] The antigen-presentation capabilities of Langerhans' cells are only revealed after interleukin-1β (IL-1β)- and tumor necrosis factor-α (TNF-α)-induced migration toward skin-draining lymph nodes.[33,34] After this cytokine-induced migration, Langerhans' cells are thought to prime naive T cells in the lymph node and initiate antigen-specific T cell immunity, as well as possibly present antigen intracutaneously to previously activated effector or memory T cells.[35] However, this paradigm of Langerhans' cell-mediated antigen presentation and immune activation is being re-evaluated.[26] For instance, migrating Langerhans' cells may transport and pass antigen to lymph node dendritic cells rather than directly presenting antigen to naive T cells themselves.[36] A role for Langerhans' cells in maintaining tolerance to damaged skin antigens has also been proposed.[26]

Intraepidermal T lymphocytes within normal human skin predominantly express αβ T cell receptors (TCRs) and a restricted V_α and V_β TCR repetoire.[37,38] They are irregularly distributed,[37] constitute fewer than 1% of epidermal cells and only about 2% of all normal skin T cells, and reside within the basal and suprabasal layers of the epidermis. In contrast, mouse skin contains >1% intraepidermal T lymphocytes expressing primarily γδ TCRs of limited diversity and exhibiting a much more dendritic morphology.[37,39] These murine γδ T cells are predominantly CD4-CD8- (double-negative) and seem to exhibit qualities of both natural killer cells and regulatory T cells, and they also appear to recognize stress-induced cutaneous ligands as a means of maintaining skin integrity.[39] A majority of intraepidermal T cells in normal human skin are CLA+ and CD8+CD45RO+.[37,38] CLA and CD45RO expression are indicative of prior activation via cutaneous antigen exposure and a memory cell phenotype, respectively, suggesting that they are not naive T cells; however, the precise functions of these and other intraepidermal T cells of normal skin await further clarification.

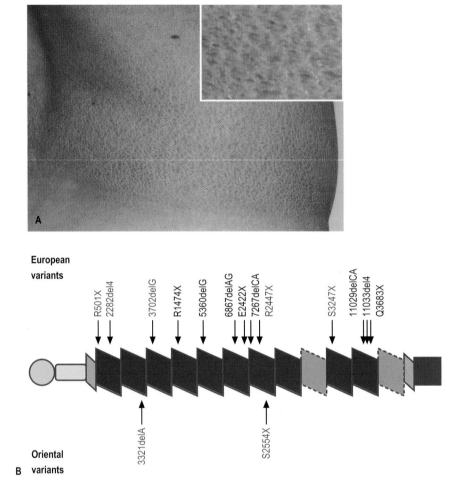

Fig. 36.4. Ichthyosis vulgaris, profilaggrin protein structure, and reported loss-of-function mutations and size variants of the *FLG* gene. (**A**) Characteristic dry and scaly skin of the lower back and side of an ichthyosis vulgaris patient; inset is ×4. Note the epidermal separations. (**B**) Diagram of profilaggrin protein structure with its S100 calcium-binding domain (light blue circle), B-domain (orange rectangle), partial filaggrin repeats (purple parallelograms), 10–12 filaggrin repeats (red parallelograms), and C-terminal domain (dark blue square). Prevalent (red) and rare (black) genetic loss-of-function mutations in *FLG* as they relate to standard filaggrin repeats 1–10 (numbered left to right and colored solid red) are indicated by arrows. Three size variants have been identified and involve duplication of filaggrin repeat 8, repeat 10, or both (potential duplicate repeats are shown in light red with a dashed border). (Adapted with permission of Macmillan Publishers Ltd from: Sandilands A, Smith FJ, Irvine AD, et al. Filaggrin's fuller figure: a glimpse into the genetic architecture of atopic dermatitis. J Invest Dermatol 2007; 127:1282–1284.)

Melanocytes and Merkel cells make up the remaining cell types of the normal epidermis, and they reside primarily in the basal layer.[40,41] As with the dermal mast cell (discussed later), melanocyte development and survival depend heavily on the cell-surface tyrosine kinase receptor, c-kit, and its ligand, stem cell factor. However, melanocytes arise from embryonic neural crest cells, whereas mast cells originate from bone marrow CD34+ stem cells. Melanosomes are the distinctive cytoplasmic organelles of melanocytes and are the site of melanin formation, part of the tanning response to ultraviolet radiation exposure. The melanocortin system, which includes proopiomelanocortin (POMC)-derived peptides (e.g. α-melanocyte-stimulating hormone (α-MSH)), is a key regulator of cutaneous pigmentation, and α-MSH has potent immunomodulatory activity.[42] Each minimally proliferating melanocyte interacts with

approximately 36 basal or suprabasal keratinocytes via its dendritic extensions; however, no direct junctions form between these two cell types. Still, by an incompletely understood mechanism, the melanocyte transfers pigment to its associated keratinocytes.[43] Similar to Langerhans' cells, melanocytes utilize E-cadherins to adhere to keratinocytes.

Merkel cells perform a very different function than melanocytes, apparently augmenting slow-adapting, type I mechanoreceptors.[1,44] They are closely associated with nerves via synaptic contacts (i.e., the Merkel cell–axon complex) and are located in sites of high tactile sensitivity, including the so-called tactile discs or touch domes. These neuroendocrine epithelial cells also contain neurotransmitter-like substances in cytoplasmic granules, and these granules often localize in proximity to adjacent unmyelinated axons that innervate the dermis and epidermis.

Keratin 20 and villin are reliable markers for the Merkel cell. Interestingly, Merkel cells appear to develop directly from precursor epidermal cells, possibly keratinocytes, and may reside in the dermis of adult skin as well.[44]

DERMAL–EPIDERMAL JUNCTION

The dermal–epidermal junction (DEJ) functions to join the epidermis to the dermis. It can be subdivided into three layers visible by electron microscopy after glutaraldehyde fixation: hemidesmosome-anchoring filament (including the lamina lucida), basement membrane (lamina densa), and anchoring fibril layers (Fig. 36.3).[45,46] The DEJ is composed mainly of basal keratinocyte products, with a minor contribution from dermal fibroblasts. In addition to connecting the epidermis and dermis, it functions to protect against mechanical shear, to orientate cell growth, and to serve as a semipermeable barrier. The various proteins present in each of these layers are indicated in Figure 36.3.[9,10,46] Within the hemidesmosomes are several macromolecules that attach the plasma membrane of the basal keratinocyte to the basement membrane. These include antigens initially recognized by serum from patients with bullous pemphigoid (BP) and designated BPAg230 (BPAg1) and BPAg180 (BPAg2 or type XVII collagen). BPAg230 resides within the basal keratinocyte but is exposed to the extracellular environment after trauma or ultraviolet radiation exposure. BPAg180 is a transmembrane protein, with the major portion extracellular and located within the lamina lucida. Additional hemidesmosome proteins include plectin and $\alpha_6\beta_4$-integrin. CD151 and $\alpha_3\beta_1$-integrin also appear to be expressed in basal keratinocytes and to function in hemidesmosome formation and stability.[9] The lamina lucida is the layer most easily disrupted, as demonstrated by its susceptibility to separation by heat, suction, saline solutions, proteolytic enzymes, and autoimmune disease.

The lamina lucida is composed of laminin 1 (laminin 111) and laminin 5 (laminin 332)-cruciform, non-collagenous glycoproteins composed of a large α-chain intertwined with a β- and a γ-chain. Laminin 6 (laminin 311) is a Y-shaped isoform composed of β- and γ-chains that complexes with laminin 5 by disulfide bonding. BPAg180 is also located within the lamina lucida. The new three digit identification nomenclature of the laminins is based on the specific numeric subunit (α, β, γ) designation of each of the chains composing the trimer. The basement membrane proper, or lamina densa, is composed primarily of type IV collagen, which, along with heparan sulfate proteoglycan (e.g., perlecan) and entactin (i.e., nidogen), is present in both DEJ and dermal blood vessel basement membranes.[45,46] Interestingly, a recently characterized protein, extracellular matrix protein-1 (ECM-1), which is expressed in both the epidermis and dermis, appears to interact with perlecan and has been associated with two skin diseases, one a rare genodermatosis, lipoid proteinosis, and the other a more common acquired inflammatory disorder, lichen sclerosus.[47] The lamina densa restricts passage of cationic molecules, facilitated by associated anionic sulfated proteoglycans, and molecules with a molecular mass >40 kDa. However, various cell types and neurites penetrate the lamina densa, most likely by use of cellular type IV collagenase and metalloproteases. Type IV collagen also makes up the anchoring plaques to which anchoring fibrils, comprised of relatively skin-restricted type VII collagen, attach. Instead of attaching to an anchoring plaque, anchoring fibrils can also attach to another location on the lamina densa, forming a loop through which dermal collagen fibers may traverse.

EXTRACELLULAR MATRIX AND CELLS OF THE DERMIS

Unlike the epidermis, the normal dermis is relatively acellular. It is divided into the papillary dermis and the reticular dermis (Fig. 36.2). The papillary dermis is about twice the depth of the epidermis, approximately 300 μm, and contains dermal papillae that interdigitate with epidermal rete pegs. The papillary dermis contains relatively fine extracellular matrix fibers and extends from the lamina densa to the upper (subpapillary) vascular plexus within the dermis. The remaining dermis, approximately 2500 μm in depth, contains thicker extracellular matrix fibers and is called the reticular dermis.

The relatively few cells within the dermis are interspersed in an extracellular matrix that is composed mainly of collagen, approximately 72% of dry weight.[48] There are currently 21 recognized 'types' of cutaneous collagen; type I and type III collagens are the most abundant in adult dermis.[48] Collagen 'molecules,' each composed of three individual polypeptides containing the characteristic repeating Gly-X-Y amino acid triplets, are arranged in various configurations – designated staggered, chicken wirelike, and antiparallel – that are intermolecularly cross-linked to produce collagen 'fibers'. These fibers provide mechanical strength to the dermis.

A successive network of elastic fibers are also part of the extracellular matrix of the dermis, approximately 4% of dry weight.[49] There are three main 'types' of elastic fibers: oxytalan fibers, elaunin fibers, and mature elastic fibers. They contain as much as 90% elastin, with lesser amounts of various other proteins including fibrillin, vitronectin, decay accelerating factor, and fibronectin. The elastic fiber network extends from the lamina densa through the dermis, with oxytalan fibers extending vertically from the DEJ to the interface between the papillary and reticular dermis, then converting to horizontally distributed elaunin fibers and, finally, to mature elastic fibers in the reticular dermis.[1] The elastic fiber network allows the skin to return to its original shape after stretching or deformation.

Dermal collagen fibers and elastic fibers are embedded in a hydroscopic 'ground substance' formed by large proteoglycans of approximately 100 to 2500 kDa that account for up to 0.2% of the dry weight of the dermis.[1,50] Each proteoglycan has a core protein (e.g., versican and decorin), with one or more covalently attached glycosaminoglycan (GAG) polysaccharides, such as chondroitin sulfate, heparan sulfate, keratan sulfate, and dermatan sulfate or hyaluronic acid as a free GAG. Proteoglycan nomenclature depends on both the core protein amino acid sequence and the identity of the disaccharide subunits forming the attached GAG or GAGs.[50] Proteoglycans influence dermal volume and compressibility through their substantial capacity to bind water. They also influence dermal cell activity by binding growth factors, such as basic fibroblast growth factor (bFGF) and vascular endothelial growth factor (VEGF), their receptors, and various cytokines.[50,51] Similarly, different forms of hyaluronic acid appear capable of modulating Langerhans' cell maturation and T-cell activation, with high and low molecular weight forms generally being anti- and pro-inflammatory, respectively.[52] Besides their presence in the extracellular matrix, proteoglycans can be found intracellularly (e.g., a serglycin core protein-containing proteoglycan in mast cell secretory granules) and on membrane surfaces (e.g., a syndecan-2 core protein-containing proteoglycan on fibroblasts) of dermal cells. Proteoglycans are expressed in the DEJ and epidermis of the skin as well.[50] Fibronectin, thrombospondin, vitronectin, and tenascin are dermal glycoproteins (i.e., proteins glycosylated with non-GAG polysaccharides) that also influence dermal cell functions such as cell activation, migration, and differentiation. For example, Langerhans' cell migration involves the interaction of cellular β_1-integrin with basement membrane laminin and extracellular matrix fibronectin.

The sparsely distributed cells of the dermis are relatively more abundant in the papillary dermis than the reticular dermis of normal skin. Mesenchyme-derived dermal fibroblasts (Table 36.1) synthesize and degrade extracellular matrix proteins, including collagen, elastin, proteoglycans, and fibronectin.[1] Their activity is increased during wound healing. However, fibroblasts also secrete various soluble mediators involved in an immune response when stimulated by cytokines. For example, eotaxin is produced by fibroblasts in response to IL-4 stimulation. Stem cell factor expression by fibroblasts may also contribute to normal cutaneous mast cell development.[53]

Mast cells are present in subepithelial connective tissues throughout the body.[1,54,55] Mast cells occur in normal skin at a density of approximately 7000 to 10 000/mm³ and are often found in close proximity to cutaneous appendages, blood vessels, and nerves. Metachromatically staining cationic dyes and avidin conjugates are used to identify human mast cells in sectioned tissues.[54] Cutaneous and intestinal submucosal mast cells have granules containing both tryptase and chymase (designated MC_{TC}). In contrast, lung and intestine mucosal mast cells primarily express only tryptase (designated MC_T), and mast cell populations that express only chymase (designated MC_C) have also been reported. By electron microscopy, human mast cells are identified by their villous cell surface projections and numerous dark-staining cytoplasmic granules.[1] Lattice-like and scroll-like structures within granules predominate in MC_{TC} and MC_T, respectively. Additional functional heterogeneity of mast cells also exists. Their development in peripheral tissues from bone marrow-derived stem cells depends primarily on c-kit receptor and its ligand, stem cell factor (also known as c-kit ligand), and possibly on IL-3.[54,56] In general, type 2 cytokines (e.g. IL-5 and IL-9) favor, while the type 1 cytokine interferon-γ inhibits, human mast cell development.[56] Mast cell involvement in the immediate allergic reaction is well documented and is exerted via its stores of histamine, various other mediators, and surface FcϵRI-bound IgE.[57] Interestingly, mast cells may be directly linked to induction of IgE synthesis by B cells; however, whether this is relevant in skin is uncertain because B cells are typically absent.[58] More recently, there is evidence that certain forms of IgE can modulate mast cell function independent of antigen[59] and that mast cells have a role in other diseases such as autoimmunity (MS, rheumatoid arthritis) and arteriosclerosis. In addition to numerous preformed mediators stored in their granules, mast cells synthesize and release growth factors, cytokines including TNF-α (also preformed) and IL-4, and lipid mediators such as leukotrienes, prostaglandins, and platelet-activating factor. Furthermore, mast cells participate in microbial defense against parasites and bacteria, in control of vascular tone and permeability via histamine and leukotriene release, in tissue repair and angiogenesis, and in sensation and response to a variety of immunologic (C5a, TNF-α, and IgE) and non-immunologic (physical and chemical) stimuli.[54,55,60] The importance of cutaneous mast cells in directing acquired immunity[61–63] and as regulators of neurogenic inflammation during physical (e.g., heat and UV exposure) and psychological stress responses has also been proposed.[64,65] Besides expression of a variety of activation receptors, mast cells also express a range of inhibition receptors[66] and they can mediate local immune suppression in a skin transplantation model.[67] Thus, important and diverse mast cell functions continue to be recognized.

Dermal macrophages are bone marrow-derived, phagocytic cells that differentiate from blood monocytes after entering peripheral tissues.[1,68] The functions of macrophages in skin are numerous and include effector phase processing and presentation of antigen, wound healing activities, microbicidal/tumoricidal activity, and general phagocytic and secretory activities. Furthermore, macrophages appear capable of mediating irritant-induced (sodium lauryl sulfate) and psoriasis-like cutaneous inflammation.[69,70] The CD68 surface marker distinguishes and identifies the macrophage within skin.

Dermal dendritic cells, which include dermal dendrocytes, represent a fourth, heterogeneous cell population of the normal dermis.[1,25,71] Careful histologic evaluation allows distinctions to be made among macrophages, dermal dendrocytes, and the other dermal dendritic cells; however, distinguishing these cell types can be difficult in the presence of an inflammatory reaction because of increased heterogeneity and cellular activity among them (including the presence of plasmacytoid DCs and inflammatory dendritic epidermal cells, IDECs).[72,73] Human dermal dendritic cells are characterized by DC-SIGN/CD209 expression and a greater role in antigen presentation relative to Langerhans' cells has recently been reported.[25,26] Dermal dendrocytes are often present in close proximity to mast cells[74] and blood vessels and, like other dermal dendritic cells, express markers common to antigen-presenting cells. The precise functions of the various dermal dendritic cells and their relationships to cutaneous macrophages are still being elucidated.

Dermal T lymphocytes, often located near postcapillary venules, comprise the vast majority (over 90%) of T cells present in normal skin.[37] An estimated 70 000 lymphocytes are present in a 4-mm punch biopsy of normal skin.[75,76] Natural killer T (NKT) lymphocytes, B lymphocytes, and natural killer (NK) lymphocytes have generally been thought to be absent from normal skin,[37,77] although NK cells have recently been reported in normal skin[78] and their presence in inflamed skin has been observed (Table 36.1).[79–81] Dermal T lymphocytes in normal skin are typically CLA⁺CCR4⁺CD45RO⁺ memory cells expressing a highly diverse TCR repertoire with the majority appearing to be CD4⁺ helper cells.[76] Unlike their absence in normal human epidermis, T cells expressing $\gamma\delta$ TCRs of limited diversity have been reported in normal human dermis.[78,82] Interestingly, recent enumeration of T cells indicate that under normal conditions nearly twice as many T cells reside in skin as in the circulation, and this includes 98% of the CLA⁺ effector memory cells.[76] So-called natural T regulatory cells (nTregs; CD4⁺CD25⁺FoxP3⁺) are among these cells and such Tregs appear to maintain tolerance in normal skin.[83,84] Overall, normal skin appears to contain a wide range of memory T cells with both effector and regulatory function.

SPECIALIZED STRUCTURES AND ASSOCIATED CELLS

Beyond the normal cellular constituents that have been elaborated, the skin includes an extensive network of blood and lymphatic vessels (Fig. 36.1).[85–87] The myriad of cutaneous blood vessels, consisting of arterioles, capillaries, venules, and anastomoses, is indicative of the skin's important thermoregulatory role. Blood and lymph vessels are typically present together, but they never anastomose. Both are arranged into an upper and a lower plexus, and capillary loops and deeper open-ended lymphatic vessels extend into the dermal papillae (Fig. 36.2). Vessels extending vertically connect the upper and lower plexus vessels of both the blood and the lymphatic vasculature. Each day, half of the total circulating protein escapes from blood vessels, and the lymphatic vessels return the extravasated fluid and macromolecules into the bloodstream via the thoracic duct, thus maintaining plasma volume and preventing increased tissue pressure. Both lymphatics and blood vessels have a continuous endothelial cell lining (Fig. 36.2), although the respective endothelial cells exhibit distinct phenotypes.[86] In general, lymphatic vessels tend to be less densely distributed, have wider and more irregular lumens, and have thinner vessel walls. Perivascular veil cells of unknown function and smooth muscle cells (bordering arterioles) or pericytes (bordering capillaries and venules) are intimately associated with dermal blood vessels (Fig. 36.2). Both smooth muscle cells and pericytes have contractile function, while fine cytoplasmic and extracellular anchoring filaments serve a contractile function for separating overlapping lymphatic endothelial cells in response to increased interstitial fluid pressure. Integration of elastic fibers into the lymphatic vessel wall also facilitates fluid collection by shuttling interstitial fluid toward the vessels. Finally, tight and adherens junctions are more frequently seen in blood vessels than in lymphatics. Notably, higher-molecular-weight molecules and particles, such as fluorescein-5-isothiocyanate-labeled dextran and cell debris, more readily enter lymphatic vessels than blood vessels.

Blood vessel endothelial cells participate in inflammation and coagulation regulation via their expression of such molecules as chemokines, prostaglandins, von Willebrand factor, and tissue factor.[88] They also allow entry of cells and molecules into the dermis (typically at postcapillary venules) (Fig. 36.2). Cellular entry involves the expression of endothelial cell-surface adhesion molecules such as P-selectin (also sequestered in endothelial cell Weibel–Palade bodies), E-selectin, intercellular adhesion molecule 1 (ICAM-1), vascular cell adhesion molecule 1 (VCAM-1), and chemokines.[36,89,90] These interact with their counterligands on the surface of circulating leukocytes (e.g., E-selectin binding to T-cell CLA) to allow the extravasation of these cells.[91–93] However, few adhesion molecules appear to be expressed on lymphatic endothelial cells.[86] Therefore, it is unclear whether the exit of cells (e.g., activated Langerhans' cells) from the skin via open-ended lymphatic vessels is actively mediated by similar ligand-counterligand interactions.[87] Nonetheless, the chemokine CCL21 (a ligand for CCR7) is preferentially secreted by lymphatic endothelial cells and this appears to mediate migration of maturing dendritic cells from the surrounding tissue into lymphatic vessels, analogous to its role in directing lymphocytes into lymph nodes.[86] Immunostaining readily distinguishes blood vessels from lymph vessels based on expression of several mutually exclusive endothelial cell markers, such as PAL-E (blood vessels), LYVE-1 (lymph vessels), and podoplanin (D2–40).[86] Recent comparative microarray analyses of cultured lymphatic and blood vessel endothelial cells have demonstrated the similarity of these two endothelial cell types but also identified several additional lineage-specific markers. This includes the Prox1 transcription factor and VEGF-C, either of which when knocked out in mice leads to the absence of lymphatic vessels.[86] Microscopic dermal lymphatics perform critical functions of lymph circulation and extracellular fluid transit through the skin, including the transport of T cells, various antigen-presenting cells as well as cellular host and microbial breakdown products and potential antigens. Tumors may also usurp the normal functional properties of lymphatics. For example, primary melanomas associated with increased lymphangiogenesis appear to be more metastatic.[86]

Skin is also extensively innervated (Fig. 36.1, 36.5).[94–96] Cutaneous innervation consists of two classes of nerve fibers: afferent sensory and efferent autonomic axons. Sensory and postganglionic autonomic nerve

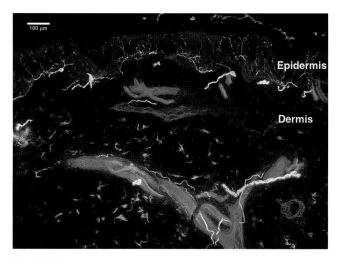

Fig. 36.5. Cutaneous innervation. Nerve fibers (*yellow–green*) stained with antibody recognizing a general nerve marker, protein gene product 9.5 (PGP9.5), are often closely associated with blood vessels (*orange–red*) stained with antibody against type IV collagen of the vessels' basement membrane. Fine nerve fibers also reside just beneath and traverse into the epidermis as marked by the dermal-epidermal junction basement membrane that also stains orange-red with type IV collagen antibody. (Courtesy of WR Kennedy.)

fibers are co-distributed by large cutaneous branches of musculocutaneous nerves that arise segmentally from spinal nerves or, for the face, from branches of the trigeminal cranial nerve. The main subcutaneous nerve trunks branch to form a deep nerve plexus at the subcutaneous–dermal junction and a superficial nerve plexus in the papillary dermis. Sensory nerve fibers innervating non-facial skin, as many as $1000/cm^2$, travel as individual continuous axons bundled within peripheral nerves that extend from a single dorsal root ganglion of the spinal column. This leads to segmental sensory innervation of the skin (dermatomes). In contrast, the autonomic nervous system typically uses two synaptically coupled neurons, the preganglionic and the postganglionic neurons, to connect the central nervous system with peripheral organs. This is the case for skin where, consistent with their functional classification, autonomic nerves innervate involuntary vascular smooth muscle, arrector pili muscles of hair follicles, sweat glands, and, possibly, sebaceous glands.[94,96] Individual nerve axons in the skin can be either myelinated (i.e., Schwann cell membrane repeatedly wrapped around the axon) or non-myelinated (i.e., axon sheathed by fenestrated invagination of the Schwann cell membrane). In general, these cutaneous nerve axons include myelinated A-β (~10 μm wide) and A-δ fibers and non-myelinated C-fibers (~1 μm wide). Nerve impulse conduction velocity, fiber diameter, sensitivity to anesthetics, and function (e.g., sensing touch, vibration, temperature, or itch) are variables used to distinguish the various cutaneous nerve fibers.

Autonomic activities in skin appear to be mediated by non-myelinated postganglionic C-fibers, although other C-fibers also have an important role in sensory function. These autonomic fibers are classified as adrenergic (containing catecholamines), cholinergic (containing acetylcholine), or purinergic (containing ATP or related purines). Notably, all three subclasses of autonomic C-fibers innervate the microcirculation, with adrenergic fibers mediating vasoconstriction and cholinergic fibers mediating vasodilation.

Afferent sensory nerves perceive the external environment. An important terminal sensory nerve structure is the so-called 'free nerve ending' of A-δ and C-fibers. These nerve fibers are ensheathed by Schwann cells and a basal lamina. They are present in the dermis and are particularly abundant in the papillary dermis. However, they lose much of their protective sheath upon penetrating into the epidermis, thus acquiring the designation of free nerve endings, and they are generally categorized as peptidergic (containing calcitonin gene-related peptide (CGRP)) or non-peptidergic (identified by their binding sites for lectin IB4, a subpopulation of which appears exclusively present in skin and expresses the Mrgprd marker).[94] A-δ and polymodal C-fiber free nerve endings innervate all vital layers of the epidermis and appear capable of sensing pain, itch,[97] noxious stimuli, temperature, and pressure. In the case of itch, the small axon, large innervated territory, C-fibers serving this sensation are very slowly conducting and had not been recognized as a distinct functioning neural population in the past. Only recently, therefore, have itch fibers been distinguished from pain and other sensory afferent input from the skin. With regard to temperature, multiple non-voltage-gated cation channels of the transient receptor potential (TRP) superfamily preferentially activate in specific temperature ranges to allow thermoreception.[94] A variety of TRP channels (particularly TRPV1) and neuromediators (including acetylcholine, cytokines (e.g., IL31), histamine, kinins, eicosanoids, neuropeptides, neurotrophins, proteases (e.g., via protease-activated receptor-2 activation), and opioids) have also been implicated in the modulation of itch. Several forms of dedicated peripheral C-itch fibers within skin appear to convey the sensation of itch.[94,97] Free nerve endings can also innervate specialized skin structures (e.g., hair follicles). Other terminal nerve structures innervated primarily by A-β nerve fibers include Merkel cell-associated 'touch spots' and Meissner's, Pacinian, and Ruffini's corpuscles, which are believed to sense different modes of deformation of the skin-touch, vibration, and stretch, respectively. Efferent activities of sensory nerves in cutaneous inflammation and wound healing are also recognized. For example, sensory nerves release neuropeptides, which lead to vasodilation and increased vasopermeability.[94,98] These neuropeptides, such as CGRP and substance P, can modulate Langerhans' cell activity, induce mast cell TNF-α synthesis and release, and induce endothelial cell adhesion molecule expression as well.[98] Efferent homeostatic activity is also demonstrated by reduced keratinocyte mitosis and subsequent thinning of the skin in denervated areas.[94]

Hair follicles, sebaceous glands, and apocrine and eccrine sweat glands are composed of differentiated cell types. Knowledge of the hair follicle's role in cutaneous immunology is limited.[99] However, secretions from sebaceous glands (e.g., free fatty acids) and from sweat glands (lactic acid, dermcidin, and immunoglobulin) contribute to innate and acquired immunity (see later discussion).

■ CUTANEOUS IMMUNOLOGY ■

INNATE IMMUNITY

A vital function of the cutaneous immune system[100–103] is to defend against pathogenic organisms (bacteria, viruses, fungi, and parasites). Passage of a pathogenic organism beyond the skin's surface can occur after physical, chemical, radiant energy, or direct pathogen insult to healthy skin (Fig. 36.6). The first-line defense against such an insult is the innate immune system. Innate immunity of the skin can be roughly divided into two separate categories: constitutive innate immunity, involving an anatomic and physiologic barrier, and inducible innate immunity, involving an acute inflammation and cellular infiltration barrier. Neither constitutive nor inducible innate immunity of the skin demonstrates acquired specificity or memory for an invading pathogen. Therefore, the immune protection provided by these two functional barriers is essentially unchanged regardless of the number of previous encounters with a particular pathogen.

Cutaneous constitutive innate immunity consists of (1) normal skin flora, (2) cornified keratinocytes, (3) constitutively expressed antimicrobial polypeptides and lipids, (4) low pH, and (5) normal body temperature (Fig. 36.6). The currently recognized normal flora of the skin includes various bacteria (primarily coryneforms and staphylococci) and, to a much lesser extent, fungi (primarily *Malassezia*).[104] These microorganisms assist the host by competing with other, more pathogenic organisms for resident status.[103] Interlocking cornified keratinocytes form a relatively impenetrable surface, and the outward growth and shedding of cornified keratinocytes help to eliminate superficially bound pathogens. The reduced water content of these cells and the underlying lipid layers of the stratum corneum reduce the relative humidity at the skin surface, providing a less-than favorable environment for pathogenic organisms. The constitutive presence of protective antimicrobial polypeptides includes β-defensin-1 and -2, dermcidin, iron-binding proteins, lysozyme, RNases, DNases, and natural IgM on the skin from sweat and from keratinocytes entering their final stages of cornification. Similarly, some epidermal lipids such as sphingosine and keratinocyte- and sebum-derived fatty acids, via their ability to reduce skin surface pH, exhibit antibacterial activity. Lactic acid excreted in eccrine sweat also lowers skin surface pH, and normal body temperature inhibits the growth of some pathogens.

A key initiator of cutaneous inducible innate immunity and a distinguishing feature of skin is the abundant preformed IL-1α stored in the cytoplasm of keratinocytes.[105] If skin integrity is disturbed with concurrent disruption or stimulation of epidermal keratinocytes, IL-1α is directly liberated into the skin. Even mechanical deformation appears sufficient to induce IL-1α liberation and this may contribute to the itch/scratch-associated changes that often accompany allergic skin disease. Release of IL-1α (a so-called 'primary' cytokine, along with TNF-α, based on their early and broad inflammatory and immunologic activities) appears to be key in initiating a cascade of events (Fig. 36.6), in part mediated by cellular nuclear factor-κB (NF-κB).[35,105] These events contribute to the classic signs of acute inflammation: redness, heat, swelling, and pain. Important among these events is the induced expression of inflammatory cytokines, chemokines, mediators (e.g. eicosanoids, histamine, neuropeptides, and reactive oxygen species), and adhesion molecules (Fig. 36.6). For example, although the precise molecular response to different antigens and pathogens varies,[106] the principal IL-1α-induced molecules of a typical cutaneous inflammatory response include additional IL-1α, IL-1β, TNF-α, IL-8 (i.e., CXCL8), nitrous oxide synthase, and prostaglandin-producing cyclooxygenase.[105] IL-1α also induces postcapillary venule endothelial cell expression of ICAM-1, VCAM-1, and E-selectin.[90,105] Moreover, IL-1α and the other induced molecules activate most cell types of the skin, alerting and preparing them for further host defense functions including additional cytokine and chemokine secretion, wound repair, release of antimicrobial products, phagocytosis, and initiation of acquired immune responses.[103,105] Thus, IL-1α is an important contributor to the inducible acute inflammation

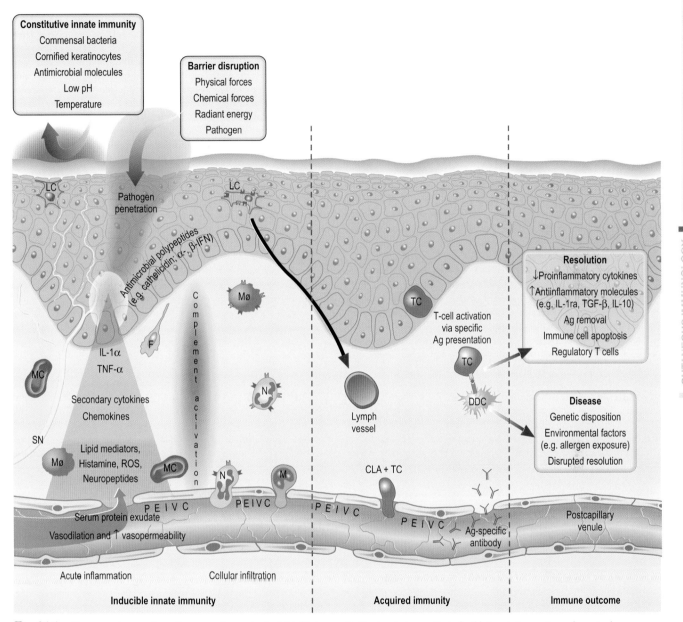

Fig. 36.6. Cutaneous immunology. Cutaneous immunity is divided into constitutive innate immunity, inducible innate immunity, and acquired immunity. Upon disruption of the skin barrier (upper left), an inflammatory response ensues marked by the early release of primary cytokines (e.g. IL-1α and TNF-α). These cytokines activate a broad variety of cell types (including fibroblasts (F), mast cells (MC), macrophages (MØ), and endothelial cells lining the postcapillary venule), and additional cytokines, chemokines, and mediators are released. Vasodilation and increased vasopermeability, characteristic of an inflammatory response, result. Subsequent inducible events such as increased antimicrobial polypeptide expression and complement activation contribute to the early neutralization of invading pathogens. The pattern of endothelial adhesion molecule expression (e.g. P-selectin (P), E-selectin (E), intercellular adhesion molecule-1 (I), vascular cell adhesion molecule-1 (V), and surface-presented chemokines (C)) also responds to favor extravasation of neutrophils (N), monocytes (M), and, eventually, effector T cells (TC). Pathogen-recognition receptors constitutively expressed on a wide variety of cell types (red and green cell surface shapes – only shown on neutrophils and a single macrophage and Langerhans' cell) also contribute to pathogen clearance and help direct the acquired immune response. Following activation and antigen uptake, epidermal Langerhans' cells can migrate to a lymph vessel and then to a draining lymph node and present antigen-derived peptides to naive T cells. The resulting antigen-specific CLA+ effector T cells can then home back to the site of cutaneous inflammation and extravasate into the skin. Subsequent antigen presentation in the skin can activate these T cells to perform their programmed function (e.g., cytolysis or cytokine production). Plasma cell-derived antigen-specific antibody also develops during the acquired immune response and infiltrates the inflammatory site to neutralize and mark an invading pathogen for destruction. Clearance of and heightened immunity against the invading pathogen followed by resolution of the inflammatory response with concurrent wound healing is the desired outcome; however, development of disease can also occur.

barrier of cutaneous innate immunity. Together with other triggers such as plasma-derived kinins, neuropeptides, and mast cell-derived histamine and eicosanoids, the cutaneous inflammatory response ultimately leads to vasodilation and increased vasopermeability, which allow serum protein exudate and leukocytes to enter the injured tissue (Fig. 36.6).

Keratinocytes, as well as other epithelial cells, such as those in the gut, express specific cytokines and growth factors that likely represent novel members of the innate immune system. For example, overexpression of amphiregulin (a member of the epidermal growth factor (EGF) family of growth factors) within the epidermis induces a unique inflammatory-immune reaction mimicking psoriasis by engaging and targeting restricted T-cell responses to the skin. Moreover, recent findings implicate expression of amphiregulin by Th2 cells as an important mechanism to clear intestinal helminth infestations through epithelial shedding. Injury-induced innate immune responses in skin also have been shown to be mediated, via transactivation, by the EGF receptor. Thus, epidermal injury or loss of barrier function (via inherited alteration or by acquired disruption) may play critical roles to signal the innate (and by secondary mechanisms, the adaptive) immune responses as part of the re-epithelialization and repair processes in skin.

Under certain circumstances, cutaneous injury occurs without overtly exceeding the inherent capacity of constitutive immunity, such that inflammation followed by tissue repair is sufficient to manage the damage. However, if disruption of the constitutive skin barrier allows significant penetration of commensal microorganisms or pathogens, innate immunity molecules with broad specificity and relatively targeted activity against intruding microbes prevent dissemination of infection and, when necessary, guide acquired immunity (see later discussion). These pathogen-targeted molecules can be broadly divided into soluble molecules (i.e., secreted and cytosolic pattern-recognition receptors (PRRs)) and cell-surface molecules (i.e., endocytic and signaling PRRs), both of which are discussed later. Each represents a component of inducible innate immunity, as do early infiltrating leukocytes that express some of these molecules (Fig. 36.6).

Important inducible pathogen-targeted soluble innate immunity molecules of the skin include (1) inducible antimicrobial polypeptides, (2) complement-activating and/or opsonin proteins, and (3) complement proteins. Included among the inducible antimicrobial polypeptides are the so-called 'antimicrobial peptides,' β-defensin-2 and -3 and cathelicidin LL-37. Several antimicrobial polypeptides are distinct to epithelial surfaces and are produced by keratinocytes in skin.[107,108] Interestingly, a novel relationship between toll-like receptors (a form of PRR; see below), vitamin D (synthesized in human skin upon ultraviolet light exposure), cathelicidin expressed by human macrophages, and tuberculosis susceptibility was recently reported.[109] Antimicrobial peptides also demonstrate other biologic properties, such as chemotactic activity for various immune cells.[110] Interferon-α (IFN-α), IFN-β, and IFN-κ are members of another class of antimicrobial polypeptides (type I interferons) that are important in antiviral defense.[111] Unlike the antimicrobial peptides, the protective activities of type I interferons are apparently related to antiviral effects on host cells rather than direct toxicity toward a pathogen.

The complement-activating/opsonin molecules of the innate immune system include members of the acute phase proteins (C-reactive protein and serum amyloid protein), members of the collectin (e.g., mannan-binding lectin) and ficolin lectin protein families, the C3b fragment of complement component C3, and possibly natural IgM.[112] The acute phase proteins are produced by the liver and supplied to the skin via

the blood. Substantial (1000-fold) increases in serum concentrations of acute phase proteins occur in response to IL-1, IL-6, and TNF-α from activated macrophages at inflammatory sites. The collectins and ficolins recognize unique carbohydrates on bacteria, fungi, and viruses and mark them for destruction. Initial availability of the C3 complement component, as well as other complement proteins, is provided by the minor but significant quantities produced by resident cells of the skin. These complement proteins are rapidly supplemented by an influx of additional complement proteins from blood, following vasodilation and increased vasopermeability resulting from the acute inflammatory response. Ultimately, complement activation in skin, as in other parts of the body, leads to generation of the opsonin C3b (which targets a pathogen for phagocytosis via binding to complement receptor-1), the anaphylatoxins C3a and C5a (which have relevant keratinocyte activating,[113] chemoattractant,[114] and mast cell degranulating functions), and the membrane attack complex composed of C5b, C6, C7, C8, and C9 (which assembles to form a lethal pore in a target pathogen's external membrane; the complement system is discussed in Chapter 6). Pathogen-targeted molecules, such as antimicrobial peptides and complement-related proteins, represent soluble components of the inducible innate immunity barrier that function in skin to counter pathogen invasion.

A group of innate immunity molecules called PRRs are host molecules that recognize pathogen-associated molecular patterns (PAMPs)[115,116] – that is, molecules that are distinct to certain pathogens. PAMPs include unmethylated CpGs of bacterial DNA, double-stranded RNA (e.g., of influenza), mannans (on a wide range of microorganisms), Gram-positive bacterial lipoteichoic acids, Gram-negative bacterial lipopolysaccharide (LPS), bacterial peptidoglycan and N-terminal formyl-methionine, parasitic phosphoglycans, and fungal glucans/zymosan. PRRs have been subcategorized further as secreted, cytosolic, endocytic, or signaling type. Soluble PRRs include the secreted pathogen-targeted acute phase proteins, collectins, and ficolins, and the cytosolic nucleotide-binding oligomerization domain (NOD) 1 and NOD2 proteins, the latter of which recognize degradation products of bacterial peptidoglycans.[116] The endocytic and signaling PRRs are cell-surface pathogen-targeted innate immunity molecules. The macrophage mannose receptor (present on dendritic cells and human dermal microvascular endothelial cells)[117] and the macrophage scavenger receptor are examples of endocytic PRRs that function to enhance microorganism uptake and lysosomal degradation. The LPS-binding CD14 molecule, the zymosan-binding Dectin-1 receptor, and members of the toll-like receptor (TLR) family, which currently comprises 10 distinct molecules, are vitally important and evolutionarily conserved signaling PRRs that lead to host cell activation, including the proinflammatory NF-κB and type I interferon pathways, after recognition of various pathogens.[118,119] Together, these secreted, cytosolic, endocytic, and signaling PRRs allow host cells to respond more effectively and with enhanced specificity to invading pathogens.

Resident macrophages and dendritic cells, activated during a cutaneous inflammatory response, are among the first phagocytic host cells capable of utilizing their cell-surface PRRs (e.g., various cell-surface lectins such as the mannose receptor[25]) to capture and destroy intruding pathogens. Moreover, inflammation-associated increases in chemotactic factors (e.g., chemokines), likely produced in part by keratinocytes stimulated via their TLRs,[120] and postcapillary venule endothelial cell adhesion molecules (P- and E-selectin, ICAM-1, and VCAM-1) synergistically mediate integrin-dependent extravasation of PRR-expressing leukocytes (Fig. 36.6).[89,90] In a typical cutaneous inflammatory response, neutrophils are the earliest infiltrating leukocytes, as expected, due to early expression of neutrophil active CXC chemokines such as IL-8.[103,114] Later, monocytes begin to extravasate into the inflammatory site (Fig. 36.6). After entering the tissue, opsonizing PRRs and cell surface PRRs on neutrophils and monocytes/macrophages assist in phagocytosis and intracellular destruction of pathogens with cell-derived products such as lysozyme, defensins, and reactive oxygen intermediates. CD14 is a classic PRR expressed by neutrophils and tissue macrophages that mediates LPS-sensitive killing of bacteria. However, different pathogens and antigens lead to different patterns of host gene expression and influence the degree and composition of immune cell infiltration. For example, effective elimination of pathogens that are not easily phagocytosed, such as fungi and parasites, may require mechanisms that target excretion of toxic leukocyte products directly onto the pathogen. Thus, signals generated by 'frustrated' phagocytes,[103] and presumably by PRRs recognizing PAMPs of pathogens that are difficult to phagocytose, such as the glycoprotein ES-62 from the filarial nematode *Acanthocheilonema vitae* or soluble extracts from the eggs of *Schistosoma mansoni*,[115] direct the immune response toward more effective pathogen clearance. Functional differences between eosinophils and neutrophils may be relevant here. Although eosinophils are less phagocytic than neutrophils, they produce reactive oxygen species at the plasma membrane surface, not intracellularly,[121] and they have been shown to readily degranulate and deposit toxic cationic proteins onto the surface of parasites.[122] Therefore an immune response favoring eosinophil infiltration over neutrophil infiltration may be a more effective defense against parasitic infection. Furthermore, specific cell types other than neutrophils and monocytes and/or increased numbers of a particular cell type can preferentially enter skin under circumstances of chronic inflammation or disease (Table 36.1). These include eosinophils,[123] basophils,[124] blood dendritic cell precursors and/or inflammatory dendritic epidermal cells (IDECs),[125] mast cells,[126] and T cells[114] (see later discussion). Only occasionally have B cells,[79] natural killer T (NK-T) cells,[81] and natural killer (NK) cells[80] been reported in non-cancerous skin disease (Table 36.1). Overall, the acute inflammatory response, leading to resident cell activation and increased accessibility of blood components and leukocytes to the site of pathogenic incursion, together with various subclasses of PRRs, works synergistically to enhance direct killing and phagocytic pathogen clearance as part of inducible innate immunity in skin.

ACQUIRED IMMUNITY

Acquired (i.e. adaptive) immunity has often been considered distinctly separate from innate immunity. However, more recent studies are elucidating the impact that components of the innate immune system have on acquired immunity.[115] Some examples include the chemotactic activity of β-defensin-2[127] and C5a[128] for dendritic cells and/or T cells of the acquired immune system. In addition, tissue injury 'danger' signals or engagement of PRRs (e.g., LPS receptor, mannose binding receptor, TLRs, and CD1a), expressed on cutaneous antigen-presenting cells such as Langerhans' cells, dermal dendritic cells, and macrophages, can promote increased co-stimulatory molecule expression (e.g., CD80 and CD86) and modulate cytokine expression patterns.[25,26,129,130] For instance, LPS binding to cell surface CD14 of macrophages induces IL-12 secretion that favors type 1 helper T-lymphocyte (Th1) development.[131] Likewise, mast cell-produced cytokines, such as IL-4 and histamine,[132] and keratinocyte-derived thymic stromal lymphopoietin (TSLP),[133] particularly in atopic

dermatitis, direct subsequent acquired immune responses toward a Th2 profile. A new class of T-helper cell, Th17 cells, has also been reported, although a role for these cells in cutaneous immunity is only beginning to be explored.[134] Initiators of inducible innate immunity such as IL-1 and TNF-α are also important in activating Langerhans' cells to migrate to lymphatic vessels within the papillary dermis, while other inflammation-associated molecules such as keratinocyte-produced MIP-3α (i.e., CCL20) lead to influx of additional Langerhans' cells into skin.[135,136] Therefore the potential for cutaneous innate immunity to direct acquired immunity, such as generating a polarized Th1 or Th2 cytokine profile, is an investigative area of great interest.[137] The ability of acquired immunity to influence innate immunity (e.g., pathogen-specific antibodies directing Fc receptor-mediated phagocytosis and Th2 cytokines suppressing keratinocyte antimicrobial peptide production[138]) has also been recognized.

Migrating Langerhans' cells that have endocytosed antigen and have been activated by the inducible innate immune response may directly present antigen in the skin to previously generated skin-resident memory T cells, or they may exit the skin via lymph vessels (Fig. 36.6) and proceed to the draining lymph node by modulating their adhesion molecule (e.g., α₆ integrin, CD44, and E-cadherin) and matrix metalloprotease (e.g., MMP-9 and -2) expression.[25] In the lymph node, Langerhans' cells have been thought to process and present antigenic peptide to naive T cells in an initial step to develop acquired immunity.[139] As mentioned previously, however, the in vivo role of Langerhans' cells in presentation of cutaneous antigens is being re-evaluated.[26] For example, dermal dendritic cells, not Langerhans' cells, appear to induce protective Th1 responses to HSV2 and leishmania, and another report suggests that CD8+ T cell priming or tolerization to viral or self-antigen, respectively, is mediated by secondary lymphoid CD8α+ DCs, not Langerhans' cells or dermal dendritic cells.[27] Finally, in contrast to immune activation, it was recently proposed that Langerhans' cells can induce tolerance to self-antigens.[140] Another interesting observation is that Langerhans' cells and dermal dendritic cells apparently migrate to different areas of draining lymph nodes.[141] Regardless of these recent ambiguities, cutaneous dendritic cell antigen presentation can presumably involve either interaction of MHC class II-antigenic peptide with CD4+ T cell TCR (typically extracellular antigen presented) or MHC class I-antigenic peptide with CD8+ T cell TCR (typically intracellular antigen presented), as well as antigen presentation via CD1 molecules (non-peptide microbial antigens presented).[26,142] Cross presentation of extracellular antigen-derived peptide by cutaneous dendritic cells developing from rapidly recruited circulating monocytes appears to be another mechanism for generating antigen-specific CD8+ T-cell responses.[135,143] The resulting activated antigen-specific effector or memory T cells (CD4+, CD8+, and perhaps CD4-CD8- natural killer T cells[26]) expressing CLA are targeted to and infiltrate the inflammatory site, in part via the interaction of CLA with E-selectin (CD62E) that is upregulated during cutaneous inflammation (Fig. 36.6). Interestingly, in a contact sensitivity model, cutaneous infiltration by a minor population of CD4+ lymphocytes within the first 2 h after topical antigen challenge was necessary for subsequent late-phase leukocyte infiltration at 24 h.[114] The mechanism(s) inducing T-cell expression of CLA (a carbohydrate epitope displayed on a modified form of P-selectin glycoprotein ligand-1 and on CD43)[144,145] are still being elucidated, but IL-12 and properties unique to cutaneous dendritic cells seem to be contributors.[93,146,147] Notably, CLA is also expressed on most epidermal Langerhans' cells and some other cell types.[77,148] Chemokines, such as TARC/CCL17 and CTACK/CCL27, and their receptors, CCR4 and CCR10, respectively, are also critical to extravasation of effector or memory T cells into the skin.[35,89,93] Under these circumstances, an effector or memory T cell infiltrates an inflammatory site and is reactivated to perform its particular function (e.g., cytokine secretion, cell killing) via intracutaneous presentation of its specific antigenic peptide.[35] However, whether Langerhans' cells or other antigen-presenting cells of the dermis (e.g., dermal dendritic cells, macrophages) represent the principal antigen-presenting cells in this subsequent elicitation phase remains debatable. Similarly, intraepidermal T cells that express the putative memory marker CD45RO may also contribute to the cutaneous immune response.[103] Overall, CLA+ T cells (both CD4+ or CD8+ and effector or memory) are critical in cutaneous acquired immunity and disease.[35,149]

In addition to antigen-presenting cells and T cells, B cells are the other key cells of acquired immunity. Differentiated B-cell (plasma cell)-derived antigen-specific antibody, particularly that of the IgE isotype, has a strong association with allergic diseases of the skin. B cells recognize relatively intact antigens, in contrast to T cells, whose activation involves antigenic peptide recognition. Thymus-dependent protein antigens do not induce antibody responses in the absence of T cells. This is in contrast to thymus-independent polysaccharide and lipid antigens, which do induce antibody production with little or no T cell help. Antigen recognition occurs via surface immunoglobulins, all with identical specificity on a given B cell. In general, plasma cell precursor and memory B-cell development, immunoglobulin class switching (from IgM or IgD to the other classes of IgA, IgE, or IgG), and somatic hypermutation all occur in secondary lymphoid germinal centers such as skin-draining lymph nodes. Thus the apparent absence of cutaneous B cells and the necessity for relatively intact antigen suggests a need for antigens that enter the skin to be transported to B cells, as opposed to B cells' migrating to antigen in the skin. One possibility is that a relatively intact antigen enters the lymph fluid (either free in solution or in association with a migrating skin cell) for transport to an antigen-specific B cell residing in a skin-draining lymph node; however, the exact mechanism of B-cell activation induced by an antigen entering through the skin remains unclear. Nonetheless, all five classes of immunoglobulin have been detected in normal human sweat.[150] This includes secretory IgA (sIgA), which appears to arise from secretory epithelia of eccrine glands.[150] Sebum may also contain IgA.[150] However, unlike gut mucosa, antibody-producing B cells (plasma cells) do not appear to reside in the skin,[37] although detection of CD21+ cells (suggestive of mature B cells) and a potential increase in IgE mRNA in atopic dermatitis skin have recently been reported.[79,151] Thus, the exact source of cutaneously secreted immunoglobulins remains unresolved. One known source is from the circulation; antigen-specific antibody can enter a cutaneous inflammatory site as part of the serum protein exudate (Fig. 36.6). Perhaps periglandular plasma cells are a source of cutaneous immunoglobulin as well.

Antigen-specific immunoglobulins of the IgG1 and IgA isotypes appear capable of contributing to clearance of pathogenic organisms from the skin via typical Fcγ receptor-mediated immune mechanisms (e.g., antibody-dependent cell cytotoxicity and complement fixation) and sIgA-coating of bacteria.[150] However, individuals with selective IgA deficiency do not have an inordinate number of cutaneous infections, although reduced sIgA on the skin of atopic dermatitis patients, who often present with cutaneous infections, has been reported.[152] The relative lack of cutaneous infections associated with selective IgA deficiency may be attributable to compensatory protection via secretory IgM.[153]

Other immunoglobulin isotypes such as IgE and IgG4 have long been associated with allergic disease, and the so-called type 2 cytokines, IL-4

and IL-13, appear critical for class switching to IgE and IgG4 in humans. Furthermore, like other epithelial surfaces, the skin appears biased toward mounting a Th2 response to epicutaneous administration of intact protein antigens.[154,155] Therefore, unless tolerance develops or Th1-skewing signals are effectively transmitted during an immune response, Th2 costimulatory 'help' to B cells appears to be the default response and will lead to IgE production. Subsequently, antigen-specific IgE, presumably supplied via the blood (although for respiratory mucosa, local IgE production appears possible), can bind to cutaneous FcεRI-bearing cells (i.e., Langerhans' cells, mast cells, and infiltrating basophils) and contribute to various forms of allergic skin disease. Antibodies specific for FcεRI receptor may contribute to cutaneous diseases such as urticaria; antibodies against desmosomal and hemidesmosomal proteins may provoke immunobullous disease. Thus, like other aspects of the immune response, B-cell-derived antibodies typically maintain health but, when inappropriately directed, produce disease.

As mentioned previously, neurotransmitters/neuropeptides can contribute to cutaneous inflammation. A dynamic dialog exists between the nervous system and the cutaneous immune system.[95,156] For instance, immune cells liberate factors influencing neural tissue (e.g., neurotrophic factors produced by eosinophils[157] and Langerhans' cells[158]) in concert with neural tissue influencing immune cells (e.g., neuropeptide regulation of dendritic cell activity and mast cell degranulation).[65,159] Clinically, stress can adversely influence symptoms of several cutaneous inflammatory diseases,[64] and lymphocyte expression of adrenergic and cholinergic receptors suggest the potential for immune modulation by both non-neuronal (i.e. epidermal) and neuronal sources of catecholamines and acetylcholine.[6] This includes atopic dermatitis, in which stress-induced changes in immune cells have been identified. Therefore, the nervous and immune systems reciprocally balance and modulate one another, implicating neural input as an important component of cutaneous immunology that is only beginning to be understood. Overall, unlike the rapid mobilization of innate immunity, a 'primary' acquired immune response after the encounter of an antigen for the first time requires several days for fully functional antigen-specific T and B cells to develop. A 'secondary' response (i.e., an immune response to a previously encountered antigen) begins more quickly, with full mobilization of memory T cells in approximately 1 day, and it is more robust, with substantially increased antigen-specific antibody titers produced by memory B cells. In toto, the cutaneous innate immune system controls an initial pathogenic assault while directing the more specific recognition and destruction of the pathogen via the acquired immune system. Modulation of skin immunity or disease via pathogen insult to organs other than the skin (e.g., gut, airways) is an additional level of complexity that is not well understood but warrants consideration.

RESOLUTION OF IMMUNE REACTION

To control an infection, a sufficiently vigorous immune response involving innate and, if necessary, acquired immune mechanisms is required. However, clearance of the pathogen and reestablishment of the cutaneous barrier function (e.g., via hemostasis, granulation tissue formation, and re-epithelization) must be accompanied by eventual downregulation of the immune reaction to avoid continued, untoward damage to host cells and to allow complete wound repair (Fig. 36.6).[160] The waning levels of inflammatory cytokines (e.g., IL-1α, TNF-α) and pathogen-derived antigens are principal pathways toward resolution of the inflammatory immune response; that is, with no antigen, there is no triggering of innate immune system PRRs or activation of acquired immune system cells. A proportional increase in antiinflammatory molecules such as IL-1ra (from keratinocytes) and TGF-β (from macrophages phagocytosing apoptotic cells[160] and from regulatory T cells[161]) also contributes to downregulation of the inflammatory response. In mice, a 'decoy receptor' named D6 contributes to lymphatic endothelial cell uptake and degradation of β-chemokines, thus reducing proinflammatory cell infiltration into skin.[162] Similarly, accumulation of extracellular adenosine,[163] lipoxins and resolvins,[164] and stress proteins[165] in inflamed tissue are implicated in downregulation of an inflammatory response. Reciprocal regulation of Th1 and Th2 responses, as exemplified by IFN-γ inhibition of a Th2 response and IL-10 inhibition of a Th1 response (possibly via induction of increased TGF-β[161]), has also been demonstrated. Therefore, effective removal of the pathogen and a shift from a proinflammatory to an antiinflammatory molecular milieu are important components of immune reaction resolution.

Apoptosis also contributes to immune reaction resolution – for example, through controlled elimination of activated neutrophils and T cells. Increased expression of CCR5 on apoptotic neutrophils and T cells further controls inflammation by sequestering its counterligand chemokines and targeting them for elimination.[166] Langerhans' cells also undergo apoptosis after successful antigen presentation to CD4+ T cells, and this appears capable of controlling cutaneous immune responses.[167] In general, apoptotic cell death occurs when a cell exceeds its natural lifespan, but it can be induced via specific cell–cell interactions such as cell-surface Fas and Fas ligand binding and the interaction of tumor necrosis factor-related apoptosis-inducing ligand (TRAIL) with its receptor.[168,169] Inhibitory receptor-ligand pairs may also contribute to cutaneous immune regulation. For instance, CD200 (recently detected on a subpopulation of murine keratinocytes and on murine Langerhans' cells) can bind to its relatively leukocyte-restricted CD200 receptor and induce an immunoregulatory signal capable of reducing cutaneous immune responses, such as that leading to alopecia.[170] Soluble TLRs and intracellular suppressor of cytokine signalling (SOCS) molecules are regulators of TLR-mediated responses.[171] The nervous system, via neuropeptides such as CGRP and α-MSH, may also help temper inflammation, as suggested by delayed wound healing of denervated skin.[98] Overall, various antiinflammatory (i.e. inhibiting inflammation before it starts) and pro-resolution (i.e. shutting down inflammation after it has begun) mechanisms[164] have been identified in recent years. Delineating the precise roles of these interrelated mechanisms and how they lead to the desired outcome of effective pathogen control and/or tissue injury repair while avoiding disease will continue to be an important topic of research.

Ideally, after exposure to a pathogen and resolution of the inflammatory immune response, the host will have developed appropriate and effective acquired immunity to the invading pathogen. Under these circumstances, a second exposure will result in more rapid and effective elimination of the offending pathogen. Memory T and B cells mediate this secondary response. However, an exaggerated inflammatory immune response is undesirable if it is directed against a commonly encountered and relatively innocuous antigen or autoantigen. In this instance, beyond thymic clonal deletion (central tolerance), peripheral anergic and suppressive mechanisms (peripheral tolerance) may be critical for avoiding atopic and/or autoimmune responses. For example, induction of T-cell anergy (i.e., unresponsiveness) via antigen presentation by an 'amateur' antigen-presenting cell such as a keratinocyte is suggested as a method

to control allergic contact dermatitis.[172] Alternatively, IL-10-producing regulatory T cells have also been shown to moderate allergic contact dermatitis and the blistering diseases, pemphigus vulgaris and bullous pemphigoid.[173,174] IL-10 appears to play a beneficial role in effective specific immunotherapy as well. Other members of a tentative IL-10 cytokine family exist (IL-19, IL-20, IL-22, IL-24, and IL-26), but their potential immunoregulatory function(s) in skin awaits further study.[175] Natural regulatory T cells (nTregs; CD4+CD25+FoxP3+ T cells), which appear to be distinct from contact-independent regulatory T cells that produce IL10, also likely control cutaneous inflammation. For instance, a mutation in the FoxP3 transcription factor that is critical to nTreg development occurs in immune dysregulation, polyendocrinopathy, enteropathy X-linked syndrome (IPEX) patients who exhibit skin manifestations similar to atopic dermatitis, and a lack of functional nTregs in skin of atopic dermatitis patients has been reported.[176,177] Therefore, mechanisms leading to immune tolerance toward non-infectious agents also appear to be important in avoiding, and possibly treating, atopy and autoimmunity. Clinically, immunosuppression of cutaneous immune reactions is a mainstay of dermatology and includes the use of topical corticosteroids, tacrolimus, pimecrolimus, and ultraviolet radiation. Interestingly, a recent study indicates that exposure of skin keratinocytes to ultraviolet light (or viral infection) upregulates keratinocyte surface expression of receptor activator of NF-κB ligand (RANKL), and subsequent interaction of RANKL with its counterligand, RANK, which is expressed on cutaneous dendritic cells, stimulates increased proliferation of nTregs.[178] Thus, this mechanism may participate in ultraviolet light immune suppression. Much remains to be learned about the body's natural mechanisms for terminating or controlling both desirable and undesirable cutaneous inflammatory immune reactions, but increased understanding in these areas holds great promise.

DYSREGULATION AND DISEASE

The skin has remarkable generative, homeostatic, and reparative properties. However, disturbances in these highly regulated states occur, and skin disease results. Under certain circumstances, acquired hypersensitivity develops to a substance that does not normally cause a reaction. In its broadest definition, this acquired hypersensitivity is referred to as allergy, and the offending substance is termed the allergen. A different definition of allergy derives from the pathophysiologic response: an allergic reaction involves histamine release, eosinophilia, and elevated IgE as a consequence of Th2 reactivity. Allergens may be proteins or other biologic antigens. They include substances such as autoantigens (FcεRI), animal products, infectious agents, foods, drugs, chemical contactants, and physical agents. The pathologic consequences of allergy are varied and dependent on the organs involved. The Gell and Coombs classification has been a commonly used means of categorizing hypersensitivity reactions, but many diseases do not fit the classification well. For example, atopic dermatitis appears to be a combination of type I and type IV reactivity. Other cutaneous diseases cross hypersensitivity types or are not able to be categorized into any specific type.

The more recent delineation of T-helper cell types into Th1 and Th2 provides another way to define cutaneous immunologic disease. Classic cell-mediated reactivity (Gell and Coombs type IV), as found in contact dermatitis, graft rejection, granulomatous diseases such as sarcoidosis, and intracellular infections such as tuberculosis, is associated with Th1 activation. On the other hand, atopic dermatitis, urticaria, and angioedema are

Table 36.2 Immunobullous skin diseases

Immunobullous disease	Clinical presentation	Serum autoantibodies	Targeted protein/structure	Tissue immunofluorescence[a]
Pemphigus				
Pemphigus vulgaris	Flaccid bullae on non-inflamed skin, crusting, Nikolsky sign[b] present, commonly affects scalp, chest, intertriginous areas and oral mucosa	IgG epithelial cell surface; correlate with disease activity	Desmoglein 3, also desmoglein 1/desmosome	Epidermal IgG and C3 cell surface (intercellular substance) staining
Pemphigus foliaceous	Superficial bullae, erosions, and scale with crusting, Nikolsky sign[b] present	IgG epithelial cell surface; correlate with disease activity	Desmoglein 1/desmosome	Epidermal IgG and C3 cell surface staining
Paraneoplastic pemphigus	Flaccid bullae, lichenoid or erythema multiforme-like, usually involves mucosa, often extensively including esophageal and respiratory	IgG epithelial cell surface and basement membrane zone (staining on rodent bladder epithelium is characteristic); correlate with disease activity	Desmoglein 3, desmoplakin 1, desmoplakin 2, BP230, envoplakin, periplakin, other/desmosome and hemidesmosome	Epidermal IgG and C3 cell surface and basement membrane zone staining
IgA pemphigus	Flaccid bullae, similar to pemphigus vulgaris	IgA epithelial cell surface; correlate with disease activity	Desmocollin 1/desmosome	Epidermal IgA cell surface staining
Pemphigoid				
Bullous pemphigoid	Tense bullae, often on urticarial base, prominent pruritus	IgG basement membrane zone, epidermal	BP180, BP230/ hemidesmosome and lamina lucida	Linear basement membrane zone IgG and C3
Cicatricial pemphigoid	Tense bullae and erosions, scarring sequelae	IgG basement membrane zone, epidermal	BP180, laminin V/ hemidesmosome and lamina lucida	Linear basement membrane zone IgG and C3
Herpes gestationis	Tense bullae, similar to bullous pemphigoid, onset during or immediately after pregnancy	Complement fixing, basement membrane zone, epidermal	BP180, BP230/ hemidesmosome and lamina lucida	Linear basement membrane zone C3

Epidermolysis bullosa acquisita	Tense bullae, commonly occur in areas of trauma and in oral mucosa	IgG basement membrane zone, dermal	Type VII collagen/anchoring fibrils	Linear basement membrane zone IgG and C3, may show linear IgA and IgM
Linear IgA bullous dermatosis and chronic bullous disease of childhood	Tense bullae, similar to bullous pemphigoid; oral involvement common in adult disease	IgA basement membrane zone, epidermal (rarely dermal)	97 kDa portion of BP180/hemidesmosome and lamina lucida	Linear basement membrane zone IgA
Dermatitis herpetiformis	Small bullae on extensor surfaces (elbows and knees); markedly pruritic; associated with intestinal gluten sensitivity	IgA endomysial and transglutaminase antibodies; transglutaminase activity correlate with disease activity and compliance with gluten-free diet	Epidermal transglutaminase	Granular basement membrane zone IgA with stippling in dermal papillae
Bullous lupus erythematosus (see Table 36.3 for information on other connective tissue diseases)	Tense bullae, photodistributed	IgG basement membrane zone, dermal	Type VII collagen/anchoring fibrils	Linear basement membrane zone IgG, also may show granular IgM and C3 basement membrane zone as in lupus band

[a]In all suspected immunobullous disease, it is best to obtain biopsy for diagnosis from perilesional tissue because immunoreactants may not be present in lesional tissue; perilesional is defined as an area of skin immediately adjacent to but not involving a lesion. Serum studies are also essential to distinguish diseases.

[b]Nikolsky's sign is the formation of a new blister or extension of a blister from shearing pressure applied on normal-appearing skin or at the edge of an existing blister.

BP230, BP Ag1; BP180, BP Ag2; cell surface, intercellular substance; epidermal and dermal refer to localization of antibodies on human split skin by indirect immunofluorescence of serum.

the result of Th2 activation and the production of cytokines that lead to IgE production and/or other antibody elaboration. Drug reactions (reviewed in Chapter 68), insect bites and stings (reviewed in Chapter 57), eosinophil-associated skin diseases (reviewed in Chapter 49), and immunobullous diseases are also in this group. The immunobullous diseases are autoreactive diseases characterized by antibody production to various skin components, as summarized in Table 36.2.[179] Immunofluorescence tests of both tissue (biopsy specimens) and serum can be particularly helpful diagnostically in these disorders. Other autoreactive diseases include the various types of lupus erythematosus, cutaneous vasculitis, and the so-called connective tissue diseases in which antibodies to self-antigens (nuclear antigens) most likely play a pathogenic role, including scleroderma, dermatomyositis, and connective tissue disease overlap syndromes. Indirect immunofluorescence and serologic testing to detect circulating antibodies is diagnostically important (Table 36.3).[180,181] The pathomechanisms leading to the development of these diseases are complex, and the molecular distinctions and similarities among these diseases are under intense investigation.

Deviations in the skin's ability to generate and maintain its structural and compositional integrity also result in cutaneous disease. Here, the best examples are malignancies of the skin. Basal cell and squamous cell carcinomas result from dysregulated malignant growth of basaloid-follicular cells or of squamous cells of the epidermis, respectively. Less commonly, malignant melanoma and, very rarely, Merkel cell (neuroendocrine) carcinomas result from dysregulated malignant growth of melanocytes and Merkel cells in skin, respectively. Langerhans' cell histiocytosis (histiocytosis-X) is a complex disorder with several different presentations resulting from neoplastic growth of Langerhans' cells. Mastocytosis (reviewed in Chapter 60) also shows many different presentations. Virtually every cutaneous compartment may proliferate excessively, lose proliferative activity and atrophy, or overproduce or underproduce cell products that result in disease. Examples include various types of vascular proliferations, keratodermas, lymphedemas, and dermal mucinoses. As noted, any change in cutaneous structural or immunologic homeostasis may result in skin disease, and aberration in structure or immunology triggers a compensatory response. For example, cutaneous malignancies (basal cell carcinoma, squamous cell carcinoma, and melanoma) are often associated with an immunologic response that may, in some circumstances, control the malignant state and form the basis for new vaccine strategies and immunotherapies. Conversely, chronic antigenic exposure may lead to cutaneous T-cell lymphoproliferative disorders. Lymphomas may involve the skin, including B-cell, T-cell and NK-cell types. T cells expressing CLA are found in cutaneous T-cell lymphomas, which usually are limited to skin for long periods. Ultraviolet exposure, both acute and chronic, induces changes in skin composition and immunology that may provoke a variety of photodermatoses, in addition to the acute inflammation associated with sunburn.

Inherited or spontaneous genetic mutations also give rise to skin diseases. Genodermatoses are those cutaneous diseases that result from genetic alterations affecting skin composition. A group of inherited blistering diseases called epidermolysis bullosa (distinct from epidermolysis bullosa acquisita, which is an acquired autoimmune disorder with some similar features to the inherited forms) is a good example.[182] Various mutations in type VII collagen result in dystrophic epidermolysis bullosa, which may be inherited as an autosomal dominant or recessive disease. Patients with epidermolysis bullosa simplex, a distinct type

of mechanobullous disease, show severe intraepidermal blistering and ultrastructural evidence for tonofilament clumping. Dominant forms of epidermolysis bullosa simplex have mutations in keratin genes 5 and 14. Mutations in genes that code for proteins involved in the insertion of keratin filaments into hemidesmosomes may also be present in epidermolysis bullosa simplex, but these mutations have not yet been delineated. Mutations in genes coding for all three subunits of laminin 5 are associated with the lethal form of junctional epidermolysis bullosa. Mutations of the gene coding for the hemidesmosomal component, BPAg2 or BP180, have been demonstrated in individuals with the less severe generalized atrophic benign form of junctional epidermolysis bullosa. Interestingly, structural mutations of LAMB3, one of the genes encoding laminin 5 (laminin 332), have also been demonstrated in individuals with this less severe form. Mutations of the gene coding for the β_4-integrin subunit have been demonstrated in a form of junctional epidermolysis bullosa associated with pyloric atresia. Many parallels exist between these inherited genetic diseases that lead to cutaneous blistering and acquired immunobullous diseases in which autoantibody production to the same skin components results in blistering. The mutations resulting in epidermolysis bullosa are only a small sample of many genodermatoses. Much of skin structure has been defined in the pursuit of explaining cutaneous dysfunction, either through analyses of what inherited mutations mediate as genetic diseases or in determining what targets antibodies are directed toward in various autoimmune skin diseases.

■ SUMMARY ■

The skin provides protective immunity against pathogenic organisms. To perform this function, the outermost layer of the skin (i.e., the stratum corneum) forms a 'brick and mortar'-like structure of cornified keratinocytes within layers of lipids as a physical barrier to prevent penetration of potential pathogens. Underlying this outer layer are developing keratinocytes (containing large quantities of preformed IL-1α and expressing various PRRs) and nerve fibers that act together as an early warning system to signal disruption of the overlying barrier. In response to the cascade of signals indicating barrier disruption, other resident cells including Langerhans' cells, macrophages, dermal dendritic cells, mast cells, and fibroblasts are activated to express antimicrobial polypeptides, to phagocytose invading pathogens, to produce additional warning signals, and/or to stimulate vasodilatation and vasopermeability, allowing effective recruitment of soluble PRRs and leukocytes expressing cell-surface PRRs from the highly vascularized dermis. If needed to contain pathogens, the immune response persists with Langerhans' cell and/or dermal dendritic cell migration via draining lymphatic vessels to establish antigen-specific acquired immunity involving both T cells and B cells and antibody production. T-cell-surface CLA and expression of relatively skin-specific chemokines such as CCL17 and CCL27 appear particularly critical in T-cell homing to the skin. Ideally, this response completely eliminates an invading pathogen, then subsides and remains poised to respond to a future re-encounter with that pathogen.

The normally fine-tuned processes of skin function can become misregulated and lead to skin disease. This results from underproduction or overproduction of cell products, production of defective cell products,

Table 36.3 Autoimmune cutaneous connective tissue diseases[a]

Autoimmune disease	Indirect immunofluorescence pattern of antinuclear antibody staining in serum	Nuclear antigens to which autoantibodies are directed	Direct immunofluorescence of tissue
Lupus erythematosus (LE)			
Systemic LE	Peripheral (rim), homogeneous, nucleolar, speckled	nDNA or double-stranded DNA, single-stranded DNA, histones, nucleolar RNA, various ribonucleoproteins, cardiolipin, Sm (Smith), U1-snRNP, HMG-17	Two or more granular immunoglobulin and complement deposits at BMZ, IgG, IgM, and/or IgA with C3 in involved and uninvolved skin (lupus band); lichenoid changes with numerous cytoids and shaggy fibrinogen staining of BMZ also found
Discoid LE	Usually no circulating antibodies	Usually none detected	Two or more granular immunoglobulin and complement deposits at BMZ, IgG, IgM, and/or IgA with C3 in involved skin; lichenoid changes with numerous cytoids and shaggy fibrinogen staining of BMZ also found
Subacute cutaneous LE	Fine speckled or speckled, may be negative	SS-A/Ro, SS-B/La	Particulate intercellular staining with or without granular immune deposits at BMZ or lichenoid changes
Neonatal LE	Fine speckled or speckled, may be negative	SS-A/Ro, SS-B/La	Granular IgG (transplacental) at BMZ
Drug-induced LE	Peripheral, homogeneous	Histones	Granular immune deposits at the BMZ
Scleroderma			
Cutaneous scleroderma (localized and generalized morphea)	Peripheral	Scl-70, SS-A/Ro, SS-B/La	No characteristic changes; vascular staining may be observed
Limited disease (acrosclerosis, CREST)	Centromere	Centromere, Scl-70, U1-snRNP, HMG-17	No characteristic changes; vascular staining may be observed
Diffuse disease (systemic sclerosis)	Nucleolar, speckled	Scl-70, U1- and U3-snRNP, RNA pol I, II, and III	No characteristic changes; vascular staining may be observed
Dermatomyositis, polymyositis	Speckled, nucleolar	Jo-1, PM-Scl, Mi-2, U1-snRNP, SS-A/Ro s	No characteristic changes; lichenoid features and vascular staining may be observed
Sjögren's syndrome	Fine speckled, nucleolar	SS-A/Ro, SS-B/La, histones, U1-snRNP	No characteristic changes; vascular staining may be observed
Mixed connective tissue disease	Speckled	U1-snRNP, PM-scl	No characteristic changes; granular immune deposits at the BMZ lichenoid features and vascular staining may be observed
Overlap and undifferentiated connective tissue disease	Any single or combination pattern	Any one or multiple, PM-Scl	May show granular immune complex deposition at BMZ (lupus band), vascular staining, and/or lichenoid changes

Indirect immunofluorescence on substrates with nucleated cells was the original means of testing for circulating antibodies in these diseases; with the identification of the antigens to which antibodies are directed, immunoassay has replaced indirect immunofluorescence in most diagnostic laboratories.
[a]BMZ, basement membrane zone; CREST, calcinosis, Raynaud's syndrome, esophageal dysmotility, sclerodactyly, telangiectasia; Rim, peripheral staining pattern; Scl-70, DNA topoisomerase I.

and/or excessive or deficient proliferation of skin cells including malignant proliferation. Abnormal immunologic reactivity, potentially due to an imbalance in effector and regulatory signals, leads to the inappropriate recognition of and response to otherwise benign environmental allergens or autoallergens. Additional mechanisms and individual patient complexities probably contribute to the clinical manifestations of allergic skin disease as well.

References

Cells and structure of the skin

1. Chu DH, Haake AR, Holbrook K, et al. The structure and development of skin. In: Freedberg IM, Eisen AZ, Wolff K, et al, eds. Fitzpatrick's dermatology in general medicine, 6th edn. New York: McGraw-Hill; 2003:58–88.
2. Fuchs E. Keratins and the skin. Annu Rev Cell Dev Biol 1995; 11:123–153.
3. Schweizer J, Bowden PE, Coulombe PA, et al. New consensus nomenclature for mammalian keratins. J Cell Biol 2006; 174:169–174.
4. Grando SA, Pittelkow MR, Schallreuter KU. Adrenergic and cholinergic control in the biology of epidermis: physiological and clinical significance. J Invest Dermatol 2006; 126:1948–1965.
5. Lippens S, Denecker G, Ovaere P, et al. Death penalty for keratinocytes: apoptosis versus cornification. Cell Death Differ 2005; 12:S1497–S1508.
6. Raj D, Brash DE, Grossman D. Keratinocyte apoptosis in epidermal development and disease. J Invest Dermatol 2006; 126:243–257.
7. Werner S, Smola H. Paracrine regulation of keratinocyte proliferation and differentiation. Trends Cell Biol 2001; 11:143–146.
8. Olivera-Martinez I, Thelu J, Dhouailly D. Molecular mechanisms controlling dorsal dermis generation from the somitic dermomyotome. Int J Dev Biol 2004; 48:93–101.
9. Litjens SH, de Pereda JM, Sonnenberg A. Current insights into the formation and breakdown of hemidesmosomes. Trends Cell Biol 2006; 16:376–383.
10. Ghohestani RF, Li K, Rousselle P, et al. Molecular organization of the cutaneous basement membrane zone. Clin Dermatol 2001; 19:551–562.
11. Morasso MI, Tomic-Canic M. Epidermal stem cells: the cradle of epidermal determination, differentiation and wound healing. Biol Cell 2005; 97:173–183.
12. Kaur P. Interfollicular epidermal stem cells: identification, challenges, potential. J Invest Dermatol 2006; 126:1450–1458.
13. Candi E, Schmidt R, Melino G. The cornified envelope: a model of cell death in the skin. Nat Rev Mol Cell Biol 2005; 6:328–340.
14. Kottke MD, Delva E, Kowalczyk AP. The desmosome: cell science lessons from human diseases. J Cell Sci 2005; 119:797–806.
15. Vasioukhin V, Fuchs E. Actin dynamics and cell-cell adhesion in epithelia. Curr Opin Cell Biol 2001; 13:76–84.
16. Wiszniewski L, Limat A, Saurat JH, et al. Differential expression of connexins during stratification of human keratinocytes. J Invest Dermatol 2000; 115:278–285.
17. Richard G. Connexin disorders of the skin. Clin Dermatol 2005; 23:23–32.
18. Brandner JM, Kief S, Wladykowski E, et al. Tight junction proteins in the skin. Skin Pharmacol Physiol 2006; 19:71–77.
19. Madison KC. Barrier function of the skin: 'la raison d'etre' of the epidermis. J Invest Dermatol 2003; 121:231–241.
20. Sandilands A, Terron-Kwiatkowski A, Hull PR, et al. Comprehensive analysis of the gene encoding filaggrin uncovers prevalent and rare mutations in ichthyosis vulgaris and atopic eczema. Nat Genet 2007; 39:650–654.
21. Marenholz I, Nickel R, Ruschendorf F, et al. Filaggrin loss-of-function mutations predispose to phenotypes involved in the atopic march. J Allergy Clin Immunol 2006; 118:866–871.
22. Palmer CN, Ismail T, Lee SP, et al. Filaggrin null mutations are associated with increased asthma severity in children and young adults. J Allergy Clin Immunol 2007; 120:64–68.
23. Bowcock AM, Cookson WO. The genetics of psoriasis, psoriatic arthritis and atopic dermatitis. Hum Mol Genet 2004; 13:R43–R55.
24. Cork MJ, Robinson DA, Vasilopoulos Y, et al. New perspectives on epidermal barrier dysfunction in atopic dermatitis: gene-environment interactions. J Allergy Clin Immunol 2006; 118:3–21.
25. Valladeau J, Saeland S. Cutaneous dendritic cells. Semin Immunol 2005; 17:273–283.
26. Larrengina AT, Falo LD. Changing paradigms in cutaneous immunology: adapting with dendritic cells. J Invest Dermatol 2005; 124:1–12.
27. Ginhoux F, Tacke F, Angeli V, et al. Langerhans cells arise from monocytes in vivo. Nat Immunol 2006; 7:265–273.
28. Koch S, Kohl K, Klein E, et al. Skin homing of Langerhans cell precursors: adhesion, chemotaxis, and migration. J Allergy Clin Immunol 2006; 117:163–168.
29. Tang A, Amagai M, Granger LG, et al. Adhesion of epidermal Langerhans cells to keratinocytes mediated by E-cadherin. Nature 1993; 361:82–85.
30. Chen H, Yuan J, Wang Y, et al. Distribution of ATPase-positive Langerhans cells in normal adult human skin. Br J Dermatol 1985; 113:707–711.
31. Valladeau J, Dezutter-Dambuyant C, Saeland S. Langerin/CD207 sheds light on formation of Birbeck granules and their possible function in Langerhans cells. Immunol Res 2003; 28:93–107.
32. Novak N, Bieber T, Kraft S. Immunoglobulin E-bearing antigen-presenting cells in atopic dermatitis. Curr Allergy Asthma Rep 2004; 4:263–269.
33. Cumberbatch M, Dearman RJ, Kimber I. Langerhans cells require signals from both tumour necrosis factor-alpha and interleukin-1 beta for migration. Immunology 1997; 92:388–395.
34. Jakob T, Ring J, Udey MC. Multistep navigation of Langerhans/dendritic cells in and out of the skin. J Allergy Clin Immunol 2001; 108:688–696.
35. Robert C, Kupper TS. Inflammatory skin diseases, T cells, and immune surveillance. N Engl J Med 1999; 341:1817–1828.
36. Iezzi G, Frohlich A, Ernst B, et al. Lymph node resident rather than skin-derived dendritic cells initiate specific T cell responses after Leishmania major infection. J Immunol 2006; 177:1250–1256.
37. Foster CA, Elbe A. Lymphocyte subpopulations of the skin. In: Bos JD, ed. Skin immune system, 2nd edn. Boca Raton: CRC Press LLC; 1997:85.
38. Spetz AL, Strominger J, Groh-Spies V. T cell subsets in normal human epidermis. Am J Pathol 1996; 149:665–674.
39. Girardi M, Lewis JM, Filler RB, et al. Environmentally responsive and reversible regulation of epidermal barrier function by gammadelta T cells. J Invest Dermatol 2006; 126:808–814.
40. Halaban R, Hebert DN, Fisher DE. Biology of melanocytes. In: Freedberg IM, Eisen AZ, Wolff K, et al, eds. Fitzpatrick's dermatology in general medicine, 6th edn. New York: McGraw-Hill; 2003:127–148.
41. Nordlund JJ, Boissy RE: The biology of melanocytes. In: Freinkel RK, Woodley DT, eds. The biology of the skin. New York: Parthenon; 2001:113.
42. Bohm M, Luger TA, Tobin DJ, et al. Melanocortin receptor ligands: new horizons for skin biology and clinical dermatology. J Invest Dermatol 2006; 126:1966–1975.
43. Van Den Bossche K, Naeyaert JM, Lambert J. The quest for the mechanism of melanin transfer. Traffic 2006; 7:769–778.
44. Sidhu GS, Chandra P, Cassai ND. Merkel cells, normal and neoplastic: an update. Ultrastruct Pathol 2005; 29:287–294.
45. Burgeson RE. Basement membranes. In: Freedberg IM, Eisen AZ, Wolff K, et al, eds. Fitzpatrick's dermatology in general medicine, 5th edn. New York: McGraw-Hill; 1999:271.
46. Masunaga T. Epidermal basement membrane: its molecular organization and blistering disorders. Connect Tissue Res 2006; 47:55–66.
47. Chan I. The role of extracellular matrix protein 1 in human skin. Clin Exp Dermatol 2004; 29:52–56.
48. Uitto J, Pulkkinen L, Chu ML. Collagen. In: Freedberg IM, Eisen AZ, Wolff K, et al, eds. Fitzpatrick's dermatology in general medicine, 6th edn. New York: McGraw-Hill; 2003:165–179.
49. Uitto J, Chu ML. Elastic fibers. In: Freedberg IM, Eisen AZ, Wolff K, et al, eds. Fitzpatrick's dermatology in general medicine, 6th edn. New York: McGraw-Hill; 2003:180–189.
50. Gallo RL, Trowbridge JM. Proteoglycans and glycosaminoglycans of skin. In: Freedberg IM, Eisen AZ, Wolff K, et al, eds. Fitzpatrick's dermatology in general medicine, 6th edn. New York: McGraw-Hill; 2003:210–216.
51. Taylor KR, Gallo RL. Glycosaminoglycans and their proteoglycans: host-associated molecular patterns for initiation and modulation of inflammation. FASEB J 2006; 20:9–22.
52. Cantor JO, Nadkarni PP. Hyaluronan: the Jekyll and Hyde molecule. Inflamm Allergy Drug Targets 2006; 5:257–260.
53. Yamamoto T, Hartmann K, Eckes B, et al. Role of stem cell factor and monocyte chemoattractant protein-1 in the interaction between fibroblasts and mast cells in fibrosis. J Dermatol Sci 2001; 26:106–111.
54. Tharp MD. Skin mast cells. In: Freinkel RK, Woodley DT, eds. The biology of the skin. New York: Parthenon; 2001:265.
55. Hsieh FH, Bingham CO III, Austen KF. The molecular and cellular biology of the mast cell. In: Freedberg IM, Eisen AZ, Wolff K, et al, eds. Fitzpatrick's dermatology in general medicine, 6th edn. New York: McGraw-Hill; 2003:330–335.
56. Okayama Y, Kawakami T. Development, migration, and survival of mast cells. Immunol Res 2006; 34:97–115.
57. Galli SJ, Kalesnikoff J, Grimbaldeston MA, et al. Mast cells as 'tunable' effector and immunoregulatory cells: recent advances. Annu Rev Immunol 2005; 23:749–786.
58. Gauchat JF, Henchoz S, Mazzei G, et al. Induction of human IgE synthesis in B cells by mast cells and basophils. Nature 1993; 365:340–343.
59. Kawakami T, Kitaura J. Mast cell survival and activation by IgE in the absence of antigen: a consideration of the biologic mechanisms and relevance. J Immunol 2005; 175:4167–4173.
60. Marshall JS, Jawdat DM. Mast cells in innate immunity. J Allergy Clin Immunol 2004; 114:21–27.
61. Galli SJ, Nakae S, Tsai M. Mast cells in the development of adaptive immune responses. Nat Immunol 2005; 6:135–142.
62. Kitawaki T, Kadowaki N, Sugimoto N, et al. IgE-activated mast cells in combination with pro-inflammatory factors induce Th2-promoting dendritic cells. Int Immunol 2006; 18:1789–1799.
63. Mazzoni A, Siraganian RP, Leifer CA, et al. Dendritic cell modulation by mast cells controls the Th1/Th2 balance in responding T cells. J Immunol 2006; 177:3577–3581.
64. Arck PC, Slominski A, Theoharides TC, et al. Neuroimmunology of stress: skin takes center stage. J Invest Dermatol 2006; 126:1697–1704.
65. Peters EM, Ericson ME, Hosoi J, et al. Neuropeptide control mechanisms in cutaneous biology: physiological and clinical significance. J Invest Dermatol 2006; 126:1937–1947.
66. Li L, Yao Z. Mast cell and immune inhibitory receptors. Cell Mol Immunol 2004; 1:408–415.
67. Lu LF, Lind EF, Gondek DC, et al. Mast cells are essential intermediaries in regulatory T-cell tolerance. Nature 2006; 442:997–1002.
68. Lu KQ, McCormick TS, Gilliam AC, et al. Monocytes and macrophages in human skin. In: Bos JD, ed. Skin immune system, 3rd edn. Boca Raton: CRC Press LLC; 2004:183–209.
69. Thepen T, van Vuuren AJ, Kiekens RC, et al. Resolution of cutaneous inflammation after local elimination of macrophages. Nat Biotechnol 2000; 18:48–51.
70. Clark RA, Kupper TS. Misbehaving macrophages in the pathogenesis of psoriasis. J Clin Invest 2006; 116:2084–2087.
71. Headington JT. The dermal dendrocyte. Adv Dermatol 1986; 1:159–171.
72. Kiekens RC, Thepen T, Oosting AJ, et al. Heterogeneity within tissue-specific macrophage and dendritic cell populations during cutaneous inflammation in atopic dermatitis. Br J Dermatol 2001; 145:957–965.
73. Novak N, Bieber T. The role of dendritic cell subtypes in the pathophysiology of atopic dermatitis. J Am Acad Dermatol 2005; 53:S171–S176.

74. Sueki H, Telegan B, Murphy GF. Computer-assisted three-dimensional reconstruction of human dermal dendrocytes. J Invest Dermatol 1995; 105:704–708.

75. Ellingsen AR, Sorensen FB, Larsen JO, et al. Stereological quantification of lymphocytes in skin biopsies from atopic dermatitis patients. Acta Derm Venereol 2001; 81:258–262.

76. Clark RA, Chong B, Mirchandani N, et al. The vast majority of CLA+ T cells are resident in normal skin. J Immunol 2006; 176:4431–4439.

77. Hunger RE, Yawalkar N, Braathen LR, et al. The HECA-452 epitope is highly expressed on lymph cells derived from human skin. Br J Dermatol 1999; 141:565–569.

78. Ebert LM, Meuter S, Moser B. Homing and function of human skin gammadelta T cells and NK cells: relevance for tumor surveillance. J Immunol 2006; 176:4331–4336.

79. Simon D, Vassina E, Yousefi S, et al. Reduced dermal infiltration of cytokine-expressing inflammatory cells in atopic dermatitis after short-term topical tacrolimus treatment. J Allergy Clin Immunol 2004; 114:887–895.

80. Ottaviani C, Nasorri F, Bedini C, et al. CD56brightCD16(-) NK cells accumulate in psoriatic skin in response to CXCL10 and CCL5 and exacerbate skin inflammation. Eur J Immunol 2006; 36:118–128.

81. Bonish B, Jullien D, Dutronc Y, et al. Overexpression of CD1d by keratinocytes in psoriasis and CD1d-dependent IFN-gamma production by NK-T cells. J Immunol 2000; 165: 4076–4085.

82. Holtmeier W, Pfander M, Hennemann A, et al. The TCR-delta repertoire in normal human skin is restricted and distinct from the TCR-delta repertoire in the peripheral blood. J Invest Dermatol 2001; 116:275–280.

83. Hirahara K, Liu L, Clark RA, et al. The majority of human peripheral blood CD4+CD25highFoxp3+ regulatory T cells bear functional skin-homing receptors. J Immunol 2006; 177:4488–4494.

84. Cavani A, Nasorri F, Ottaviani C, et al. Human CD25+ regulatory T cells maintain immune tolerance to nickel in healthy, nonallergic individuals. J Immunol 2003; 171:5760–5768.

85. Braverman IM. Cutaneous microvasculature. In: Freedberg IM, Eisen AZ, Wolff K, et al, eds. Fitzpatrick's dermatology in general medicine, 5th edn. New York: McGraw-Hill; 1999:299.

86. Cueni LN, Detmar M. New insights into the molecular control of the lymphatic vascular system and its role in disease. J Invest Dermatol 2006; 126:2167–2177.

87. Randolph GJ, Angeli V, Swartz MA. Dendritic-cell trafficking to lymph nodes through lymphatic vessels. Nat Rev Immunol 2005; 5:617–628.

88. Petzelbauer P, Schechner JS, Pober JS. Endothelium. In: Freedberg IM, Eisen AZ, Wolff K, et al, eds. Fitzpatrick's dermatology in general medicine, 6th edn. New York: McGraw-Hill; 2003:216–229.

89. Mackay CR. Chemokines: immunology's high impact factors. Nat Immunol 2001; 2:95–101.

90. Bochner BS, Beck LA. Adhesion molecules and their role in allergic skin diseases. In: Leung DY, Greaves MW, eds. Allergic skin disease: a multidisciplinary approach. New York: Marcel Dekker; 2000:87.

91. Luster AD, Alon R, von Andrian UH. Immune cell migration in inflammation: present and future therapeutic targets. Nat Immunol 2005; 6:1182–1190.

92. Issekutz AC, Issekutz TB. The role of E-selectin, P-selectin, and very late activation antigen-4 in T lymphocyte migration to dermal inflammation. J Immunol 2002; 168:1934–1939.

93. Mora JR, von Andrian UH. T-cell homing specificity and plasticity: new concepts and future challenges. Trends Immunol 2006; 27:235–243.

94. Oaklander AL, Siegel SM. Cutaneous innervation: form and function. J Am Acad Dermatol 2005; 53:1027–1037.

95. Roosterman D, Goerge T, Schneider SW, et al. Neuronal control of skin function: the skin as a neuroimmunoendocrine organ. Physiol Rev 2006; 86:1309–1379.

96. Ruocco I, Cuello AC, Parent A, et al. Skin blood vessels are simultaneously innervated by sensory, sympathetic, and parasympathetic fibers. J Comp Neurol 2002; 448:323–336.

97. Steinhoff M, Bienenstock J, Schmelz M, et al. Neurophysiological, neuroimmunological, and neuroendocrine basis of pruritus. J Invest Dermatol 2006; 126:1705–1718.

98. Peters EM, Ericson ME, Hosoi J, et al. Neuropeptide control mechanisms in cutaneous biology: physiological and clinical significance. J Invest Dermatol 2006; 126:1937–1947.

99. Paus R. Immunology of the hair follicle. In: Bos JD, ed. Skin immune system, 2nd edn. Boca Raton: CRC Press LLC; 1997:377.

Cutaneous immunology

100. Bos JD, ed. Skin immune system, 3rd edn. Boca Raton: CRC Press LLC; 2004:3–11.

101. Kim J, Modlin RL. Innate immunity and the skin. In: Freedberg IM, Eisen AZ, Wolff K, et al, eds. Fitzpatrick's dermatology in general medicine, 6th edn. New York: McGraw-Hill; 2003:247–252.

102. Stingl G, Maurer D, Hauser C, et al. The skin: an immunologic barrier. In: Freedberg IM, Eisen AZ, Wolff K, et al, eds. Fitzpatrick's dermatology in general medicine, 6th edn. New York: McGraw-Hill; 2003:253–273.

103. Spellberg B. The cutaneous citadel: a holistic view of skin and immunity. Life Sci 2000; 67:477–502.

104. Noble WC. Ecology and host resistance in relation to skin disease. In: Freedberg IM, Eisen AZ, Wolff K, et al, editors: Fitzpatrick's dermatology in general medicine, 5th edn. New York: McGraw-Hill; 1999:184.

105. Murphy JE, Robert C, Kupper TS. Interleukin-1 and cutaneous inflammation: a crucial link between innate and acquired immunity. J Invest Dermatol 2000; 114:602–608.

106. Huang Q, Liu D, Majewski P, et al. The plasticity of dendritic cell responses to pathogens and their components. Science 2001; 294:870–875.

107. Braff MH, Gallo RL. Antimicrobial peptides: an essential component of the skin defensive barrier. Curr Top Microbiol Immunol 2006; 306:91–110.

108. Kisich KO, Leung DYM. Defensins and cathelicidins. In: Bos JD, ed. Skin immune system, 3rd edn. Boca Raton: CRC Press LLC; 2004:315–326.

109. Liu PT, Stenger S, Li H, et al. Toll-like receptor triggering of a vitamin D-mediated human antimicrobial response. Science 2006; 311:1770–1773.

110. Yang D, Chertov O, Oppenheim JJ. Participation of mammalian defensins and cathelicidins in anti-microbial immunity: receptors and activities of human defensins and cathelicidin (LL-37). J Leukoc Biol 2001; 69:691–697.

111. Steinhoff M, Luger TA. The skin cytokine network. In: Bos JD, ed. Skin immune system, 3rd edn. Boca Raton: CRC Press LLC; 2004:349–372.

112. Asghar SS, Timar KK, Pasch MC. Complement as a part of the skin immune system. In: Bos JD, ed. Skin immune system 3rd edn. Boca Raton: CRC Press LLC; 2004:327–348.

113. Purwar R, Wittmann M, Zwirner J, et al. Induction of C3 and CCL2 by C3a in keratinocytes: a novel autocrine amplification loop of inflammatory skin reactions. J Immunol 2006; 177:4444–4450.

114. Hwang JM, Yamanouchi J, Santamaria P, et al. A critical temporal window for selectin-dependent CD4+ lymphocyte homing and initiation of late-phase inflammation in contact sensitivity. J Exp Med 2004; 199:1223–1234.

115. Clark R, Kupper T. Old meets new: the interaction between innate and adaptive immunity. J Invest Dermatol 2005; 125:629–637.

116. McGirt LY, Beck LA. Innate immune defects in atopic dermatitis. J Allergy Clin Immunol 2006; 118:202–208.

117. Groger M, Holnthoner W, Maurer D, et al. Dermal microvascular endothelial cells express the 180-kDa macrophage mannose receptor in situ and in vitro. J Immunol 2000; 165: 5428–5434.

118. Gross O, Gewies A, Finger K, et al. Card9 controls a non-TLR signalling pathway for innate anti-fungal immunity. Nature 2006; 442:651–656.

119. Kang SS, Kauls LS, Gaspari AA. Toll-like receptors: applications to dermatologic disease. J Am Acad Dermatol 2006; 54:951–983.

120. Miller LS, Modlin RL. Human keratinocyte Toll-like receptors promote distinct immune responses. J Invest Dermatol 2007; 127:262–263.

121. Lacy P, Moqbel R: Redistribution of human eosinophil NADPH oxidase components is associated with a predominantly extracellular production of superoxide. J Allergy Clin Immunol 2002; 109:S118.

122. Kephart GM, Gleich GJ, Connor DH, et al. Deposition of eosinophil granule major basic protein onto microfilariae of Onchocerca volvulus in the skin of patients treated with diethylcarbamazine. Lab Invest 1984; 50:51–61.

123. Leiferman KM, Peters MS, Gleich GJ. Eosinophils in cutaneous diseases. In: Freedberg IM, Eisen AZ, Wolff K, et al, eds. Fitzpatrick's dermatology in general medicine, 6th edn. New York: McGraw-Hill; 2003:959–966.

124. Plager DA, Weiss EA, Kephart GM, et al. Identification of basophils by a mAb directed against pro-major basic protein 1. J Allergy Clin Immunol 2006; 117:626–634.

125. Novak N, Bieber T. The role of dendritic cell subtypes in the pathophysiology of atopic dermatitis. J Am Acad Dermatol 2005; 53:S171–S176.

126. Damsgaard TE, Olesen AB, Sorensen FB, et al. Mast cells and atopic dermatitis. Stereological quantification of mast cells in atopic dermatitis and normal human skin. Arch Dermatol Res 1997; 289:256–260.

127. Yang D, Chertov O, Bykovskaia SN, et al. Beta-defensins: linking innate and adaptive immunity through dendritic and T cell CCR6. Science 1999; 286:525–528.

128. Tsuji RF, Kawikova I, Ramabhadran R, et al. Early local generation of C5a initiates the elicitation of contact sensitivity by leading to early T cell recruitment. J Immunol 2000; 165:1588–1598.

129. Kadowaki N, Ho S, Antonenko S, et al. Subsets of human dendritic cell precursors express different toll-like receptors and respond to different microbial antigens. J Exp Med 2001; 194:863–869.

130. Flacher V, Bouschbacher M, Verronese E, et al. Human Langerhans cells express a specific TLR profile and differentially respond to viruses and Gram-positive bacteria. J Immunol 2006; 177:7959–7967.

131. Fearon DT, Locksley RM. The instructive role of innate immunity in the acquired immune response. Science 1996; 272:50–53.

132. Mazzoni A, Siraganian RP, Leifer CA, et al. Dendritic cell modulation by mast cells controls the Th1/Th2 balance in responding T cells. J Immunol 2006; 177:3577–3581.

133. Liu YJ, Soumelis V, Watanabe N, et al. TSLP: An epithelial cell cytokine that regulates T cell differentiation by conditioning dendritic cell maturation. Annu Rev Immunol 2007; 25: 193–219.

134. Weaver CT, Hatton RD, Mangan PR, et al. IL-17 Family cytokines and the expanding diversity of effector T cell lineages. Annu Rev Immunol 2007; 25:821–852.

135. Le Borgne M, Etchart N, Goubier A, et al. Dendritic cells rapidly recruited into epithelial tissues via CCR6/CCL20 are responsible for CD8+ T cell crosspriming in vivo. Immunity 2006; 24:191–201.

136. Kimber I, Cumberbatch M, Dearman RJ, et al. Cytokines and chemokines in the initiation and regulation of epidermal Langerhans cell mobilization. Br J Dermatol 2000; 142:401–412.

137. Jankovic D, Liu Z, Gause WC. Th1- and Th2-cell commitment during infectious disease: asymmetry in divergent pathways. Trends Immunol 2001; 22:450–457.

138. Howell MD, Gallo RL, Boguniewicz M, et al. Cytokine milieu of atopic dermatitis skin subverts the innate immune response to vaccinia virus. Immunity 2006; 24:341–348.

139. He Y, Zhang J, Donahue C, et al. Skin-derived dendritic cells induce potent CD8(+) T cell immunity in recombinant lentivector-mediated genetic immunization. Immunity 2006; 24:643–656.

140. Romani N, Ebner S, Tripp CH, et al. Epidermal Langerhans cells – changing views on their function in vivo. Immunol Lett 2006; 106:119–125.

141. Kissenpfennig A, Henri S, Dubois B, et al. Dynamics and function of Langerhans cells in vivo: dermal dendritic cells colonize lymph node areas distinct from slower migrating Langerhans cells. Immunity 2005; 22:643–654.

142. Mueller SN, Jones CM, Smith CM, et al. Rapid cytotoxic T lymphocyte activation occurs in the draining lymph nodes after cutaneous herpes simplex virus infection as a result of early antigen presentation and not the presence of virus. J Exp Med 2002; 195: 651–656.

REFERENCES

143. Stoitzner P, Tripp CH, Eberhart A, et al. Langerhans cells cross-present antigen derived from skin. Proc Natl Acad Sci U S A 2006; 103:7783–7788.

144. Fuhlbrigge RC, Kieffer JD, Armerding D, et al. Cutaneous lymphocyte antigen is a specialized form of PSGL-1 expressed on skin-homing T cells. Nature 1997; 389:978–981.

145. Fuhlbrigge RC, King SL, Sackstein R, et al. CD43 is a ligand for E-selectin on CLA+ human T cells. Blood 2006; 107:1421–1426.

146. Biedermann T, Lametschwandtner G, Tangemann K, et al. IL-12 instructs skin homing of human Th2 cells. J Immunol 2006; 177:3763–3770.

147. Dudda JC, Simon JC, Martin S. Dendritic cell immunization route determines CD8+ T cell trafficking to inflamed skin: role for tissue microenvironment and dendritic cells in establishment of T cell-homing subsets. J Immunol 2004; 172:857–863.

148. Kieffer JD, Fuhlbrigge RC, Armerding D, et al. Neutrophils, monocytes, and dendritic cells express the same specialized form of PSGL-1 as do skin-homing memory T cells: cutaneous lymphocyte antigen. Biochem Biophys Res Commun 2001; 285:577–587.

149. Santamaria Babi LF, Picker LJ, Perez Soler MT, et al. Circulating allergen-reactive T cells from patients with atopic dermatitis and allergic contact dermatitis express the skin-selective homing receptor, the cutaneous lymphocyte-associated antigen. J Exp Med 1995; 181:1935–1940.

150. Metze D, Gebhart W. Secretory immunoglobulins. In: Bos JD, ed. Skin immune system, 2nd edn. Boca Raton: CRC Press LLC; 1997:255.

151. Plager DA, Leontovich AA, Henke SA, et al. Early cutaneous gene transcription changes in adult atopic dermatitis and potential clinical implications. Exp Dermatol 2007; 16:28–36.

152. Imayama S, Shimozono Y, Hoashi M, et al. Reduced secretion of IgA to skin surface of patients with atopic dermatitis. J Allergy Clin Immunol 1994; 94:195–200.

153. Norhagen G, Engstrom PE, Hammarstrom L, et al. Immunoglobulin levels in saliva in individuals with selective IgA deficiency: compensatory IgM secretion and its correlation with HLA and susceptibility to infections. J Clin Immunol 1989; 9:279–286.

154. Bellinghausen I, Enk AH, Mohamadzadeh M, et al. Epidermal cells enhance interleukin 4 and immunoglobulin E production after stimulation with protein allergen. J Invest Dermatol 1996; 107:582–588.

155. Herrick CA, MacLeod H, Glusac E, et al. Th2 responses induced by epicutaneous or inhalational protein exposure are differentially dependent on IL-4. J Clin Invest 2000; 105:765–775.

156. Lambrecht BN. Immunologists getting nervous: neuropeptides, dendritic cells and T cell activation. Respir Res 2001; 2:133–138.

157. Kobayashi H, Gleich GJ, Butterfield JH, et al. Human eosinophils produce neurotrophins and secrete nerve growth factor on immunologic stimuli. Blood 2002; 99:2214–2220.

158. Torii H, Yan Z, Hosoi J, et al. Expression of neurotrophic factors and neuropeptide receptors by Langerhans cells and the Langerhans cell-like cell line XS52: further support for a functional relationship between Langerhans cells and epidermal nerves. J Invest Dermatol 1997; 109: 586–591.

159. Botchkarev VA, Yaar M, Peters EM, et al. Neurotrophins in skin biology and pathology. J Invest Dermatol 2006; 126:1719–1727.

160. Karin M, Lawrence T, Nizet V. Innate immunity gone awry: linking microbial infections to chronic inflammation and cancer. Cell 2006; 124:823–835.

161. Terui T, Sano K, Shirota H, et al. TGF-beta-producing CD4+ mediastinal lymph node cells obtained from mice tracheally tolerized to ovalbumin (OVA) suppress both Th1- and Th2-induced cutaneous inflammatory responses to OVA by different mechanisms. J Immunol 2001; 167:3661–3667.

162. Jamieson T, Cook DN, Nibbs RJ, et al. The chemokine receptor D6 limits the inflammatory response in vivo. Nat Immunol 2005; 6:403–411.

163. Ohta A, Sitkovsky M. Role of G-protein-coupled adenosine receptors in downregulation of inflammation and protection from tissue damage. Nature 2001; 414:916–920.

164. Serhan CN, Brain SD, Buckley CD, et al. Resolution of inflammation: state of the art, definitions and terms. FASEB J 2007; 21:1–8.

165. Willoughby DA, Moore AR, Colville-Nash PR, et al. Resolution of inflammation. Int J Immunopharmacol 2000; 22:1131–1135.

166. Ariel A, Fredman G, Sun YP, et al. Apoptotic neutrophils and T cells sequester chemokines during immune response resolution through modulation of CCR5 expression. Nat Immunol 2006; 7:1209–1216.

167. Pradhan S, Genebriera J, Denning WL, et al. CD4 T cell-induced, bid-dependent apoptosis of cutaneous dendritic cells regulates T cell expansion and immune responses. J Immunol 2006; 177:5956–5967.

168. De Panfilis G. 'Activation-induced cell death': a special program able to preserve the homeostasis of the skin? Exp Dermatol 2002; 11:1–11.

169. Vassina E, Leverkus M, Yousefi S, et al. Increased expression and a potential anti-inflammatory role of TRAIL in atopic dermatitis. J Invest Dermatol 2005; 125:746–752.

170. Rosenblum MD, Yancey KB, Olasz EB, et al. CD200, a 'no danger' signal for hair follicles. J Dermatol Sci 2006; 41:165–174.

171. Liew FY, Xu D, Brint EK, et al. Negative regulation of toll-like receptor-mediated immune responses. Nat Rev Immunol 2005; 5:446–458.

172. Gaspari AA. Mechanisms of resolution of allergic contact dermatitis. Am J Contact Dermat 1996; 7:212–219.

173. Cavani A, Nasorri F, Ottaviani C, et al. Human CD25+ regulatory T cells maintain immune tolerance to nickel in healthy, nonallergic individuals. J Immunol 2003; 171:5760–5768.

174. Hertl M, Eming R, Veldman C. T cell control in autoimmune bullous skin disorders. J Clin Invest 2006; 116:1159–1166.

175. Kunz S, Wolk K, Witte E, et al. Interleukin (IL)-19, IL-20 and IL-24 are produced by and act on keratinocytes and are distinct from classical ILs. Exp Dermatol 2006; 15:991–1004.

176. Verhagen J, Akdis M, Traidl-Hoffmann C, et al. Absence of T-regulatory cell expression and function in atopic dermatitis skin. J Allergy Clin Immunol 2006; 117:176–183.

177. Ou LS, Goleva E, Hall C, et al. T regulatory cells in atopic dermatitis and subversion of their activity by superantigens. J Allergy Clin Immunol. 2004; 113:756–763.

178. Loser K, Mehling A, Loeser S, et al. Epidermal RANKL controls regulatory T-cell numbers via activation of dendritic cells. Nat Med 2006; 12:1372–1379.

179. Mutasim DF, Adams BB. Immunofluorescence in dermatology. J Am Acad Dermatol 2001; 45:803–822.

180. Mutasim DF, Adams BB. A practical guide for serologic evaluation of autoimmune connective tissue diseases. J Am Acad Dermatol 2000; 42:159–174.

181. Kavanaugh A, Tomar R, Reveille J, et al. Guidelines for clinical use of the antinuclear antibody test and tests for specific autoantibodies to nuclear antigens. American College of Pathologists. Arch Pathol Lab Med 2000; 124:71–81.

182. Fine JD, Eady RA, Bauer EA, et al. Revised classification system for inherited epidermolysis bullosa: Report of the Second International Consensus Meeting on diagnosis and classification of epidermolysis bullosa. J Am Acad Dermatol 2000; 42:1051–1066.

Airway Smooth Muscle and Related Extracellular Matrix in Normal and Asthmatic Lung

37

R Robert Schellenberg and Chun Y Seow

SUMMARY OF IMPORTANT CONCEPTS

>> Excessive airway smooth muscle (ASM) shortening in asthma can be achieved by:
  – changes in muscle contractile properties
  – decreasing tissue resistance to contraction
  – adaptation to abnormally short lengths

>> Muscle contractile properties are dynamic and can adapt to the microenvironment of the airway and optimize contractility at virtually any muscle lengths through rearrangement and reassembly of the contractile filaments

>> Airway inflammation damaging extracellular matrix elements within the airway wall or those tethering airways to parenchymal components would produce excessive ASM shortening

>> The immediate proximity of mast cells to ASM suggests that mast cell mediators and cytokines may be critically important in altering ASM function

INTRODUCTION

Asthma symptoms and the related abnormal lung function are caused, at least in part, by the exaggerated airway narrowing due to excessive shortening of the smooth muscle cells lining the airway wall.[1–3] The exact role of airway smooth muscle (ASM) in asthma, however, is not clear. There are several scenarios under which excessive airway narrowing could occur: (1) an enhanced intrinsic ability of airway smooth muscle to generate force and shorten; (2) hypertrophy or hyperplasia of airway smooth muscle; (3) a weakened extracellular tethering and/or matrix stiffness that allow airway smooth muscle to adapt to a shortened length and become refractory to the relaxing effect of mechanical perturbation associated with tidal breathing and deep inspiration; (4) a combination of the above scenarios. In this chapter, the elements associated with each scenario are examined separately, with an emphasis placed on airway smooth muscle and its interaction with the microenvironment of the airway wall.

Recent advances in our understanding of airway smooth muscle in terms of its structural plasticity and functional dynamics has fundamentally altered our view on how the muscle interacts with other airway components, how it responds to mechanical perturbation, and how the dynamic lung environment modifies the muscle properties. The traditional view on what determines the extent of airway narrowing has been based on a *static* balance of forces. That is, the airway should stop narrowing when the force generated by the encircling smooth muscle cells is exactly counterbalanced by the tethering force of the lung parenchyma,[4,5] the force necessary to accomplish mucosal folding and compression,[6–8] the axial and radial constraints of the extracellular matrix,[9–11] and the force arising from the transmural pressure difference. This static model has been challenged by the recent reports that the *dynamic* environment of the breathing lung plays an important role in modulating ASM contractility.[12–14] Although useful in elucidating several important mechanisms in determining airway caliber,[15,16] the static model failed to predict accurately the extent of airway narrowing during broncho-provocation in normal subjects.[17,18] Furthermore, in vitro studies of ASM mechanics suggest that airway smooth muscle, under static conditions, has the potential to completely close all airways in the lung when stimulated.[19,20] Although complete closure can occur in some maximally stimulated airways,[21,22] most airways remain open in a healthy lung even when the muscle is maximally activated.[17,18,23] The discrepancies appear to be due to the oscillatory stress and strain imposed on the ASM cells by the constant tidal action of spontaneous breathing interposed by deep inspirations.

The cytoskeleton of airway smooth muscle and the extracellular matrix in which the muscle cells are embedded have increasingly been viewed as dynamic structures that have an actively supportive role in force generation. In altering their mechanical properties, these structures modulate the load against which the muscles shorten, and regulate the degree of airway narrowing caused by ASM contraction. Therefore, a better understanding of the function of airway smooth muscle in vivo, and dysfunction under diseased conditions, has to be linked to the mechanically dynamic lung environment.

STRUCTURE AND FUNCTION OF AIRWAY SMOOTH MUSCLE

Compared with striated muscle, the structure and function of smooth muscle is poorly understood. Although many of the proteins (e.g., myosin and actin) associated with the contractile apparatus of striated muscle are found in smooth muscle (in different isoforms), how these proteins are assembled in smooth muscle is not entirely clear. In striated muscle, functional properties can be deduced from the structure of the contractile units (i.e., sarcomeres). For example, the length–tension relationship of striated muscle can be delineated from the dimensions of the sarcomere and the lengths of the actin and myosin filaments.[24] In smooth muscle, the structure of the contractile units and their assembly are often postulated based on incomplete structural data[25] and functional data.[26,27] Although there are similarities in functional characteristics between striated and smooth muscles, there are fundamentally different properties that differentiate these muscles, primarily due to the unique plastic properties associated with smooth muscle.

ULTRASTRUCTURE OF AIRWAY SMOOTH MUSCLE

Despite their difference in embryonic origin, all smooth muscle cell types share a very similar ultrastructure.[28] Besides the obvious structures like plasmalemma and nucleus, they all possess the myosin-containing (thick) filaments and the actin-containing (thin) filaments, intermediate filaments, microtubules, dense bodies and plaques, mitochondria, caveolae, sarcoplasmic reticulum, Golgi apparatus, and endoplasmic reticulum. These structures can be readily identified in a cross-section of airway smooth muscle (Fig. 37.1). The thin filaments have a diameter of about 6 nm. The intermediate filaments have a diameter of about 10 nm. The microtubules have a diameter of about 25 nm with an electron-translucent center. All these filaments have circular cross-sections. The thick filaments, on the other hand, have an irregular cross-sectional profile, due to the presence of cross-bridges along the length of the filament. The average diameter of thick filaments is about 15–20 nm. The dense

bodies also have an irregular cross-sectional profile, and their 'diameters' vary greatly. The dense bodies are anchorage sites for the thin and intermediate filaments, much like the Z-disks of striated muscle. The dense plaques are also anchorage sites for the thin and intermediate filaments. The network of thin and intermediate filaments connected through the dense bodies and plaques is thought to form the scaffold of cytoskeleton. Dense plaques in adjacent cells also form intermediate junctions (circle, Fig. 37.1) for transmission of force between cells.

STRUCTURE AND FUNCTION OF SMOOTH MUSCLE CONTRACTILE UNIT

Although the structure of a contractile unit in smooth muscle has never been clearly delineated based on solid structural data, it is believed that it consists of three basic components: a myosin thick filament, actin thin filaments, and dense bodies or plaques. These elements can be seen to occupy most of the cytoplasmic space in airway smooth muscle (Fig. 37.1). The thick filaments in smooth muscle are believed to be side-polar.[25,29] This means that the cross-bridges on one side of a thick filament can only interact with a thin filament possessing the 'right' polarity and pull the thin filament (causing it to slide) in one direction, while the cross-bridges on the other side of the thick filament interact with another thin filament with opposite polarity and cause it to slide in the opposite direction. Although the exact structure of a contractile unit in smooth muscle has yet to be established, a model has been proposed;[25] this is shown schematically in Figure 37.2. The side-polar thick filament is different from the bi-polar thick filament found in striated muscle (Fig. 37.2B). A sarcomere-like contractile unit is therefore not likely to exist in smooth muscle because of the side-polar thick filaments.

Cyclic interaction of the cross-bridges with the thin filaments produces sliding of thick and thin filaments relative to each other. Because the thin filaments are anchored to dense bodies (or dense plaques on the cell membrane), which in turn are connected to the cytoskeletal filament network, sliding of the contractile filaments brings the dense bodies closer to each other and thus shortening of the muscle cell. When cell shortening is prevented by external force, the cross-bridge-actin interaction produces tension in the cell that can be transmitted through mechanical junctions to adjacent cells or extracellular matrix.

Within a bundle of smooth muscle cells, the contractile units are organized in series and in parallel in a trans-cellular syncytium[30] so that the force generated by or transmitted through the muscle bundle is uniform despite the non-uniform cell cross-sections within a single cell, as depicted in Figure 37.3. Studies of single cell mechanics of smooth muscle therefore have to be aware of the possible artifacts stemming from severing mechanical connections between cells in an intact tissue bundle.

ADAPTATION OF AIRWAY SMOOTH MUSCLE TO LENGTH CHANGE

Airway smooth muscle is able to adapt to large changes in cell length and maintain its capability to generate maximal force.[31,32] This property originates from the cell's ability to restructure plastically its contractile apparatus[27] and cytoskeleton,[33,34] in order to maintain the optimal overlap of the contractile filaments. This adaptability to length change is essential for proper function of smooth muscles lining the wall of hollow organs that regularly undergo large changes in volume (such as urinary

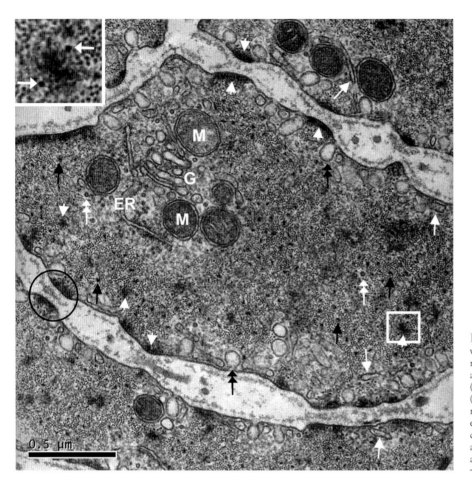

Fig. 37.1. Electron micrograph of transverse section of porcine trachealis showing myosin thick filaments (arrows) surrounded by actin thin filaments, dense bodies and plaques (white arrowheads), sarcoplasmic reticulum (white arrows), caveolae (double-arrows), and microtubules (white double-arrows). A rough endoplasmic reticulum (ER) with ribosomes can also be seen. M, mitochondria; G, Golgi apparatus. Inset: A dense body with intermediate filaments (arrows).

bladder); however, it presents a problem for maintaining airway patency, especially in previously narrowed airways. Understanding length adaptability of airway smooth muscle is therefore important for understanding obstructive airway diseases such as asthma.

One essential feature of length adaptation in airway smooth muscle is the addition and deletion of contractile units in series and parallel as the muscle adapts to different lengths. It has been shown that muscle cells adapted to a longer length can shorten faster and produce more power.[26,31] The increase in power is matched by an increase in the rate of ATP utilization in the muscle.[26] Accompanying all these changes in muscles adapted to a longer length is an increase in the amount of thick filaments per muscle cell.[26,35] All these experimental observations can be summarized quantitatively in a mathematical model[36] based on the assumption that the number of contractile units in smooth muscle cells is variable.

As in striated muscle, the length–force relationship in smooth muscle is determined by the amount of overlap of the thin and thick filaments at various muscle lengths. Because the structure of the contractile apparatus in striated muscle is stable (i.e., the assembly of sarcomeres are relatively permanent), the length–force relationship is fixed (i.e., the structural change resulting in different amounts of filament overlap due to muscle length change predetermines the force). In smooth muscle, this is

true only when length adaptation is prevented. As shown in Figure 37.4, a length–force curve can be obtained from a muscle adapted at a certain length. To prevent adaptation from occurring during the time of measurement, a muscle is allowed to shorten from its adapted length under various loads, and the loads in turn determine the extents to which the muscle can shorten.[27] To obtain each data point in Figure 37.4, isotonic contraction is elicited and each contraction lasts for a few seconds. The linear relationship reflects the linear decrease in the amount of overlap between the thin and thick filaments during the brief shortening. This length–force curve, however, is only unique to the muscle adapted at one particular length. When the same muscle is adapted to a different length, a different linear relationship is obtained (Fig. 37.4). This change in the length–force relationship likely reflects the changes in the organization of the contractile units that have occurred during the process of length adaptation, which takes at least 30 minutes.

Regardless of the mechanism, the ability of airway smooth muscle to adapt and maintain maximal force production in a wide range of length creates a potential risk for airway closure due to muscle contraction. From Figure 37.4, it is clear that a muscle adapted at a shorter length can shorten further than a muscle adapted at a longer length, at any loads. Pre-shortening in partially activated airway smooth muscle also potentiates the muscle's ability to shorten further when fully activated.[37]

DETERMINANTS OF AIRWAY NARROWING

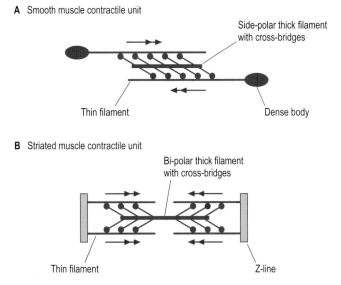

A Smooth muscle contractile unit

Side-polar thick filament with cross-bridges

Thin filament

Dense body

B Striated muscle contractile unit

Bi-polar thick filament with cross-bridges

Thin filament

Z-line

Fig. 37.2. Contractile units of smooth (A) and striated (B) muscles showing basic components and how side-polar and bi-polar thick filaments may influence contractile unit design. Double arrows indicate direction of thin filament sliding relative to thick filament.

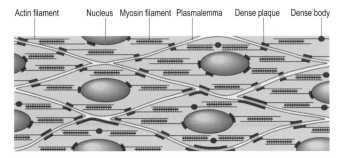

Actin filament   Nucleus   Myosin filament   Plasmalemma   Dense plaque   Dense body

Fig. 37.3. Illustration of contractile unit organization in a bundle of smooth muscle cells. (Reproduced from Kuo and Seow 2004, J Cell Sci,[30] with permission.)

Prevention of airway smooth muscle to adapt at a shortened length may be a key step in preventing airway hyperresponsiveness.

DETERMINANTS OF AIRWAY NARROWING

To what extent a stimulated airway can narrow depends on the force generated by the airway smooth muscle and all the forces that oppose the constriction due to muscle contraction. As mentioned above, this is not a static balance of forces; rather, the modulation of muscle contractility by the dynamic lung environment must be factored into the equation.

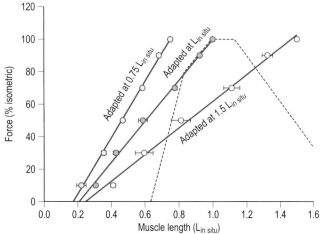

Fig. 37.4. Length–force relationships obtained from airway smooth muscle (trachealis) adapted at different lengths. The symbols are data from experiments and the solid lines are linear fits to the data. The dotted lines depict the same relationship in striated muscle (based on data from Gordon et al, 1966[24]). The in situ length of the trachealis ($L_{in\ situ}$) is used as a reference length.

COUPLINGS BETWEEN AIRWAY SMOOTH MUSCLE, AIRWAY WALL, AND LUNG PARENCHYMA

As discussed later in this chapter, in the extracellular matrix where ASM cells are embedded, there are intercellular proteins and proteoglycans that form various fibers and structures. The mechanical properties of these various structures in the matrix directly influence the muscle's ability to constrict the airways. There is in vivo evidence that airway diameter varies in proportion to lung volume,[38–42] at least in healthy lungs. This suggests that airway smooth muscle, airway wall, and lung parenchyma are mechanically coupled. For a deep inspiration to open an airway, the parenchymal tethers on the airway wall have to be sufficiently stiff, and at the same time, the airway wall has to be sufficiently compliant. If the parenchymal tethering is too weak or the airway wall is too stiff, uncoupling of airways from the rest of the lung will occur, and changes in lung volume will have no influence on airway diameter or ASM contractility. Effective mechanical coupling between the adventitial layer of the airway wall and the ASM layer will also depend on an optimal stiffness of the airway components for proper transmission of strain to the ASM cells due to expansion of the outer airway wall. Uncoupling of the ASM layer from the rest of the lung therefore could occur at various locations within the lung structure due to any disease process.

DYNAMIC STRAIN ASSOCIATED WITH LUNG VOLUME CHANGE

The importance of coupling between airway and parenchyma is in the maintenance of airway patency. Besides providing a tethering force on the airways during lung inflation, the undulating strain applied to the airway smooth muscle due to tidal breathing and deep inspirations is likely a potent bronchodilator. In vitro studies of isolated and activated airway smooth muscle have shown dramatic effects of length and force oscillation on reducing ASM contractility.[13,23,43–45] Deep inspirations taken by healthy subjects have also been shown to be effective in reversing experimentally induced bronchoconstriction.[46–51] The bronchodilating effect of deep inspiration could stem from mechanical perturbation of airway smooth muscle, as suggested by the in vitro experiments. When taken before bronchoprovocation, deep inspirations have also been shown to reduce the severity of bronchoconstriction.[52–55] In isolated and relaxed airway smooth muscle, length oscillation is known to reduce the force generated by the muscle in subsequently induced contraction.[14] This in vitro observation may explain the bronchoprotective effect of deep inspiration taken before bronchoprovocation. Effective transmission of dynamic strain (due to lung volume change) to airway smooth muscle therefore is likely very important for maintenance of airway patency.

CYTOSKELETAL ELEMENTS OF AIRWAYS MODULATE MUSCLE CONTRACTION

Because myocytes are physically linked to each other and to the neighboring structures, the elements forming the cytoskeleton of the myocyte, intercellular connections, and matrix components between and around myocytes will directly modulate the extent of muscle contraction. Inflammation may have greater effects on components outside the myocyte than within, leading to altered muscle function. Extracellular matrix (ECM) surrounding and between individual myocytes as well as muscle bundles structural and adhesive properties. The fibrillar collagens I, II, and III contribute to the tensile modulus of tissues, elastin gives tissue elasticity, and aggregating proteoglycans contribute to compressive and hysteretic properties of the tissue.

The inflammatory processes lead to changes in the matrix, including altered synthesis and local extracellular matrix degradation. Serine proteinases such as elastase and cathepsin G are released by granulocytes early in inflammation, and macrophages and connective tissue cells release a number of powerful matrix metalloproteinases including MMP-1, MMP-3, and MMP-7 (macrophages), and MMP-2, MMP-3, and MMP-9 (connective tissue cells) in inflammation and remodeling conditions that have been studied. This combination of enzymes has the capacity to degrade fibrillar collagens (MMP-1), elastin (elastase, cathepsin G, and MMP-7), gelatinized collagen (MMP-2, -9 and -7) and matrix glycoproteins and proteoglycan core proteins (MMP-2, -3, -7, -9, elastase, and cathepsin G). Matrix degradation is considered an unwanted side-effect of a limited proteolytic process that is required for immune and phagocytic cells to be able to enter inflammatory sites and destroy microorganisms, but unwanted consequences on tissue integrity may result.

INTRACELLULAR CYTOSKELETON – DYNAMICS AND ALTERATIONS WITH MECHANICAL LOADS

Phosphorylation of intracellular cytoskeletal proteins alters the mechanics of muscle contraction. The importance of proteins associated with focal adhesion kinase in the region of plasma membrane dense plaques, presumably by orienting actin molecules and linking them to the cell surface where they interact with extracellular matrix elements and neighboring myocytes, has been demonstrated. Contractile activation was found to induce phosphorylation of talin, paxillin, and focal adhesion kinase.[56,57] Depletion of paxillin by an antisense oligonucleotide inhibited smooth muscle contraction[58] and inducing mutations at the two tyrosine-phosphorylation sites on paxillin inhibited smooth muscle force production without altering myosin light-chain phosphorylation.[59] Using muscle strips with a different paxillin mutant rendered incapable of localizing to focal adhesions, force generation and recruitment of vinculin to the cell membrane.[60] These studies demonstrate the importance of 'anchoring' contractile proteins to the cell surface for transmission of force between cells.

BASAL LAMINA AND INTERCELLULAR PROTEINS

The basal lamina provides a foundation upon which is attached the continuous epithelium of the nose, airways, and alveoli. The principal constituents of the basal lamina are type IV collagen,[61] laminin,[61,62] and the proteoglycan perlecan,[63] which are contained in the lamina densa, the electron-dense middle layer of basal lamina as detected by electron microscopy. The basal lamina can be considered a mat of adhesive glycoproteins including laminin and heparan sulfate proteoglycans, associated with a structural network of type IV collagen.[64,65] The basal lamina appears to impart fundamental positional information to the cells of the lung, which may be mediated by integrins and promotes cell growth through the presentation of basal lamina proteoglycan-bound growth factors to cell surface receptors, as is the case for basic fibroblast growth factor.[66] An intact basal lamina was shown to be critical for injury repair.[67] Even after epithelial and endothelial desquamation, regeneration and function were completely restored if basal laminae remained intact. Of interest, electron microscopy studies by Dr David Walker (personal communication) have demonstrated a thickened basal lamina layer around airway myocytes of asthmatics. The mechanical consequences of this are unclear.

An area that has not been well explored to date is whether alterations of proteins forming mechanical junctions between myocytes, such as the cadherins, are altered in conditions of excessive airway narrowing. Clearly, the alignment of contractile proteins with those of the neighboring myocytes through these unique areas on the plasma membrane is critical for optimal force generation and shortening of the muscle.

EXTRACELLULAR MATRIX

The airways from the trachea to the alveoli are dynamic structures, always in motion, some areas in particular undergoing large changes in distention and deformation. Elastic fibers and smooth muscle cells maintain tissue mechanics over a range of distension, while preserving the integrity of the system. Fibrillar collagen composed primarily of type I and III collagen, although capable of rearrangement within the connective tissue, provides the ultimate high tensile modulus to the tissue when fully extended.

Elastic fibers

Elastic fibers have been subdivided into three types: elastic, elaunin, and oxytalin,[68] which can be distinguished both histochemically[69] and ultrastructurally.[70] There is an intimate association between smooth muscle cells and elastic fibers with oxytalan and elaunin fibers present among the smooth muscle cells. While oxytalan fibers may terminate at smooth muscle basal lamina, elastic fibers may terminate at smooth muscle cell plasma membranes. Leick-Maldonado and Lemos[71] have shown that elastic fibers penetrate from the lamina propria between the smooth muscle bundles into the deeper submucosa and adventitia and suggest that they play a role in epithelial folding during bronchoconstriction.

Collagen

Collagens are the most abundant proteins in the body. The best understood collagens are the fibril-forming collagens types I, II, III, V, and XI,[72] and these form the major matrix element that resists tensile stresses. Fibers containing principally type I collagen constitute the major fibrous elements of dense connective tissue while fibers in the lamina propria[73] and surrounding smooth muscle cells contain more type III. These type III collagen fibrils constitute the extracellular matrix element reticulin, as defined by histochemical and ultrastructural observations,[74] and are smaller in diameter than type I fibrils[75] and less closely packed, a phenomenon attributed to the greater abundance of fibril-associated proteoglycans.[74] The arrangement of collagen and elastic fibers in the airway wall and parenchyma reflects and is adapted to resist the dynamic forces experienced by each tissue. In the case of the airway, these include airway smooth muscle contraction.

ROLE OF EXTRACELLULAR MATRIX IN AIRWAY REMODELING IN ASTHMA

A renewed emphasis on the structural changes that occur in asthma has led to the term 'remodeling' to suggest that injury and repair processes cause functional alterations of asthmatic airways, including excessive airway narrowing to a contractile agonist, decreased bronchodilator responses to physiological stimuli as a big breath or to a smooth muscle relaxant such as a β-agonist, and persistent irreversible airway obstruction in some cases. Although this concept of functional alterations due to injury, and in some cases to overexuberant repair processes, forms a helpful framework, it is limited by a multitude of factors, some beyond our present ability to adequately evaluate, and there are considerable conflicting data regarding parameters that we can measure.[76,77] Correlations between a specific structural property and in vivo determinants of pulmonary function are of limited benefit in understanding the pathophysiologic processes involved and, as a result, it is not surprising that conflicting results arise when evaluating a complex disease at different time points and disease severity. However, these studies provide valuable information and suggest that alterations in extracellular matrix elements are key factors in pathophysiologic changes, as outlined below.

ECM-INTEGRIN INTERACTIONS

The importance of interactions of matrix proteins such as fibronectin and tenascin with integrin receptors in alterations of asthma has been highlighted in studies dealing especially with epithelial integrity. Human epithelial cells from nasal polyps cultured on type I collagen

were shown to be dependent on fibronectin and α_5/β_1 integrin for wound repair.[78] Using a similar system with the human epithelial cell line 16HBE145, other investigators demonstrated that antibodies to α_2, α_3 or α_6 blocked wound repair of cells grown on type IV collagen but not if grown on laminin-1 or -2.[79] This may be relevant to the disease state, since epithelial cells express integrins for laminin-1 and fibronectin present in basement membranes[80–82] but laminin-2 has been found to be expressed only in airways of subjects with chronic asthma.[83] Blocking the β_1 integrin VLA-4 inhibited both early and late allergic reactions plus airways hyperresponsiveness in animals.[84–87] This did not affect eosinophilic infiltration as would be anticipated. Further studies demonstrated that an antibody to VLA-4 strikingly inhibited mast cell mediator release,[88] raising the possibility that mediators altering ECM, possibly mast cell tryptase, may be important in induction of airway hyperresponsiveness. The complexity of integrin interactions is highlighted by the demonstration that TGF-β_1 latency-associated protein binds α_V/β_6, restricting activation of TGF-β_1.[89] Mice lacking this integrin develop exaggerated inflammation but are protected from developing fibrosis. Relatively little information is available for asthmatic tissues but one study did demonstrate increased tenascin in airway basement membrane of asthmatics, a change that was decreased on treatment with inhaled steroid.[90]

SUBEPITHELIAL COLLAGEN DEPOSITION

A thickening of the layer below the basal lamina consisting of collagens type I, III, and V plus fibronectin[91] is a hallmark of remodeling in asthma. Some studies have correlated the degree of thickening with airway hyperresponsiveness or disease severity but others have not and thickness is not altered by duration of asthma.[92]

The primary factor implicated in subepithelial fibrosis is transforming growth factor beta (TGF-β), in particular the β_1 isotype. In situ hybridization has demonstrated that a major source of TGF-β_1 is the eosinophil[93,94] and eosinophilia correlated with subepithelial fibrosis.[94,95] Electron microscopy evaluation suggests that this layer in asthmatics is not in normal fibrillar array but is a disorganized reticulin mesh. Whereas a thickened layer of fibrillar collagen might be expected to limit bronchoconstriction, a disorganized reticulin layer would be expected to be more compliant in compression and could additionally increased airway narrowing for a given degree of smooth muscle contraction, due to its thickness alone.

COLLAGEN WITHIN MUSCLE BUNDLES

Human airway myocytes are intimately associated with fibrillar collagen as shown in Figure 37.5.[96] Collagen degradation would decrease the load on the muscle, thereby allowing greater shortening. This was demonstrated in our study of the mechanical properties of human airway smooth muscle prior to and following treatment with 20 U/ml collagenase.[10] This treatment could also decrease the radial constraint to myocyte expansion and allow greater shortening and force generation as suggested by studies of rabbit trachea.[11]

ELASTIN

Elastic fibers are present in the subepithelium as well as in the smooth muscle layer of airways. Studies of asthmatic airways have suggested a disruption and loss of the thinner fibers that normally lie perpendicular to

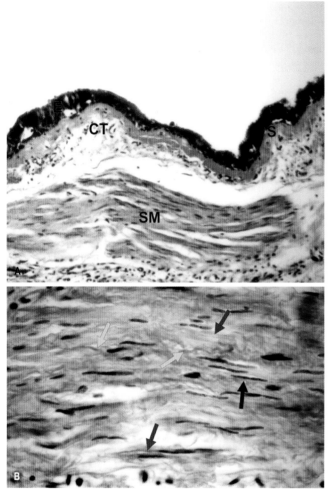

Fig. 37.5. A Masson's trichrome-stained 5 μm-thick cross-section of non-asthmatic large airway. Upper panel: low magnification view demonstrating the epithelium (E), connective tissue (CT), and smooth muscle (SM) layers. The aqua-staining collagen can be appreciated below the epithelial basement membrane as well as within the smooth muscle layer. Lower panel: higher magnification of the smooth muscle bundle demonstrating the red/brown staining muscle cells (red arrows) with elongated, dark brown-staining nuclei and the abundant aqua-staining collagen (black arrow) between myocytes. (Reported from Thomson RJ, Bramley AM, Schellenberg RR. Airway muscle sterology: implications for increased shortening in asthma. Am J Resp Crit Care Med 1996; 154:749–757.[96])

the smooth muscle and appear anchored to the basement membrane.[97,98] Loss of this normal structure may allow the development of excessive inward folding of the inner wall into the lumen. Loss of these elastic fibers might also dissociate the inner airway structures from the smooth muscle so that relaxation of the muscle would have less effect on dilating the lumen. Increased levels of elastase have been detected in induced sputum samples of asthmatics,[99] which suggests that even transient neutrophil infiltration in asthmatics may be more detrimental than the far greater numbers of eosinophils present.

PROTEOGLYCANS

Matrix proteoglycans influence tissue mechanics, matrix assembly, cell growth, and maturation, and they also influence the biological activities of growth factors.[100,101] Increased amounts of a number of proteoglycans have been found in human asthmatic airways. Deposition of versican, biglycan, and hyaluronan were greater in autopsy samples from fatal asthma cases[100] and versican, biglycan, and lumican were increased in the submucosa of asthmatic airway biopsies with the amount correlating with the degree of airway hyperresponsiveness.[102] Although always difficult to define changes due to underlying pathology vs treatment effects, one study comparing airways of moderate vs severe asthmatics found relatively enhanced deposition of lumican in the subepithelial layer in severe asthmatics, whereas moderate asthmatics had greater proteoglycan deposition in the smooth muscle layer.[103] Such increase in the smooth muscle layer could represent a protective effect by increasing the load-limiting shortening. In large airways, the loss of proteoglycan (primarily aggrecan) from airway cartilage as noted in fatal asthma[100,104] would decrease the load on ASM, allowing excessive shortening. Perichondrial thickening in asthmatics and chronic lung diseases was found to correlate with the degree of eosinophilia,[105] in keeping with the previously mentioned studies of TGF-β_1. This study also evaluated the proportion of degenerated cartilage which was increased in airways of asthmatics and chronic bronchitics and this parameter correlated with the number of neutrophils in the airway. This is of specific interest in light of the findings of increased neutrophils in severe asthmatics refractory to steroid therapy[95] – consistent with neutrophilic proteases degrading matrix elements and eosinophil TGF-β_1-inducing collagen production.

ASTHMATIC AIRWAY SMOOTH MUSCLE MORPHOLOGY AND MECHANICAL PROPERTIES

Many investigators have suggested that asthmatics have increased smooth muscle on the basis of evaluation of autopsy material.[106–112] Rather surprisingly, we did not demonstrate an increase in muscle in airways of two asthmatic subjects, whose airway tissue showed striking 2–3-fold increases in force and shortening.[96] This has major implications regarding the defect in asthma, since it clearly shows that increased muscle is not required for the unique mechanical properties of these airways as the muscle stress (kg/cm^2) in these asthmatic tissue samples was 2–3 times greater than that for non-asthmatic tissues.

Our findings of unique mechanical properties of human airway preparations should be emphasized. Under the restraints of the normal surrounding tissue in larger airways, muscle shortening is very limited, with maximal shortening averaging about 10%.[113] This compares with shortening of 80% for pig trachealis.[114] A comparison of airway smooth muscle responses from different species revealed that the degree of shortening is inversely correlated with the amount of ECM present in the tissue preparation.[115] These differences highlight the importance of external loads in limiting muscle shortening. For this reason (and the finding that we could not explain increased muscle shortening on the basis of increased amount of muscle in asthmatic tissues), we hypothesized that decreasing the load imposed on the smooth muscle by ECM elements could induce the changes noted in asthma.[116] Figure 37.6 shows a schematic diagram representing this.

639

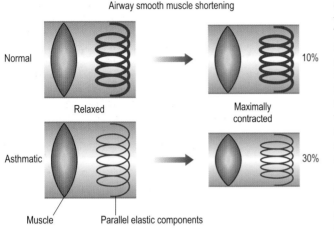

Fig. 37.6. Schematic diagram illustrating how a decrease in the stiffness of extracellular elements composing parallel elastic elements leads to increased smooth muscle shortening without a requirement for any change in the muscle itself. (Reproduced from Bramley AM, Thomson RJ, Roberts CR, et al. Hypothesis: excessive bronchoconstriction in asthma is due to decreased airway elastance. Eur Resp J 1994; 7:337–341.[116])

A host of studies have evaluated the proliferation and secretory properties of isolated airway smooth muscle cells (beyond the scope of this discussion). Such studies are helpful in defining intracellular signalling mechanisms and cell surface determinants but have limitations in terms of modulating factors present in the normal tissue milieu. This is due to the rapid differentiation of cultured cells to a non-contractile phenotype with loss of muscle myosin and α-smooth muscle actin.[117,118] Although conceivable that this might happen in asthma to increase muscle mass, these cells would have to later redifferentiate to a contractile phenotype.

Extracellular matrix elements may limit smooth muscle proliferation and degradation of these elements would then allow increases in muscle. Matrix metalloproteinase-1 (MMP-1), but not MMP-2, -3, or -9, was shown to be increased in asthmatic smooth muscle by immunocytochemistry and biological activity.[119] In addition to cleaving collagen, which surrounds smooth muscle cells in vivo, MMP-1 has proteolytic activity for IGF binding proteins which inhibit cell growth. In isolated smooth muscle cell cultures, leukotriene D_4 is mitogenic[120] and modulates the IGF axis by inducing MMP-1.[121] Therefore the increased MMP-1 activity could lead to increased amount of smooth muscle. Whether this occurs in vivo remains to be demonstrated. In studies which we have performed with airway explants, factors shown to induce proliferation of isolated airway cells (including leukotrienes) have had no effect on the amount of muscle measured morphometrically or by BrdU incorporation, nor had increases in muscle force generation.[122] This emphasizes the importance of the normal cellular milieu including extracellular matrix elements in modulating myocyte proliferation as well as function.

MATRIX-DEGRADING ENZYMES

A major interest in asthma has been the role played by matrix metalloproteinases (MMPs) and the tissue inhibitors of MMPs (TIMPs). The regulation of these enzymes which are secreted as zymogens is very complex and it is likely that our measurements of activities provide us with limited information. As a result, some of the data are conflicting. The most striking elevations in MMP-9 (10–160-fold increases) were noted in BAL from ventilated subjects with status asthmaticus[123] who also had elevated MMP-3 levels. No increases in these were determined in BAL of mild asthmatics. Another study found higher TIMP-1 levels in untreated asthmatics which correlated with IL-6 levels and numbers of alveolar macrophages.[124] Sputum MMP-9/TIMP-1 molar ratios were lower in asthmatics with a correlation with FEV_1, neutrophil, and macrophages[125] in one study and serum MMP-9/TIMP-1 ratio correlated with a response to oral corticosteroids in a group of severe asthmatics in another.[126]

The finding that several ADAM 33 single-nucleotide polymorphisms and their haplotypes are associated with asthma and airway hyperresponsiveness[127] has made this metalloproteinase an appealing candidate as a critical enzyme in the pathology of asthma. However, it has not been shown to be overly expressed in asthmatic airways[128] and its function in mature airways remains to be determined.

Mast cells have been demonstrated to be increased within the smooth muscle layer in asthmatic airways[129,130] and these contain a number of proteases such as tryptase, chymase, and cathepsin G. Tryptase has striking effects on the ECM of human airways. In preliminary experiments in our laboratory, the addition of mast cell tryptase to human airway explants leads to a three-fold increase in the shortening ability of the smooth muscle, comparable with the changes found in asthmatic tissues. Smaller changes have been reported with shorter incubations with guinea pig tissue.[131] Using the selective tryptase inhibitor 1,5-bis-{4-[(3-carbamimidoyl-benzenesulfonylamino)-methyl]-phenoxyl}-pentane, Wright et al[132] demonstrated inhibition of allergen-induced early and late phase bronchoconstriction as well as airway hyperresponsiveness in sheep. This inhibitor has more selective activity on tryptase than the naturally produced secretory leukocyte protease inhibitor (SLPI) which is a potent inhibitor of cathepsin G, elastase, chymotrypsin, and trypsin as well as mast cell tryptase. Its broader action may be preferable in light of evidence for neutrophil-mediated changes in asthmatic airways. That mast cell tryptase may also influence collagen deposition in airways is suggested by the study by Cairns and Walls,[133] showing that it stimulates collagen synthesis in a fibroblast cell line. Whether this effect is seen in whole airway tissue remains to be determined.

These studies highlight the difficulty in determining primary vs secondary events in a pathophysiologic process involving simultaneous inflammatory injury and tissue repair. Although most studies have concentrated on the deposition of new collagen as a detrimental component of remodeling (largely because this is a relatively easy parameter to evaluate with bronchial biopsies), the mechanical consequences of this are unknown. The relative contributions of geometric factors, quality of matrix, and structural changes in matrix to increased airway narrowing are as yet difficult to assess.

IMPLICATIONS REGARDING THERAPY FOR ASTHMA

Alterations in extracellular matrix components in allergic diseases, such as asthma, involve both degradation and new synthesis. Both processes are ongoing simultaneously by the time the disease state is recognized and treatments with agents such as corticosteroids may alter many different elements, some limiting ECM degradation and some limiting repair. If one accepts that the initial injury in allergic disease, causing structural changes, is the release of proteolytic enzymes from mast cells and recruited inflammatory cells, then inhibition of enzymatic activities would be important therapeutic goals. Inhibition of protease release by agents inhibiting mast cell mediator release or IgE induction of release is discussed in other chapters in this volume. We await data on whether monoclonal anti-IgE antibodies can reverse the structural changes of the asthmatic airway.

One potential target is tumor necrosis factor alpha (TNFα), which is synthesized and released from isolated mast cells[134] and from alveolar macrophages following antigenic challenge[135] and stimulates the release of numerous proteolytic enzymes from inflammatory cells. Recent evaluation of etanercept and infliximab in asthma is encouraging.[136,137] Inhibitors of matrix metalloproteinases may also be of value in limiting the initial injury. A number of specific inhibitors have been developed and await testing in animal models and human allergic disease. It is likely that therapy for remodeling processes in chronic inflammatory lung disease will continue to center on corticosteroids, despite the fact that these affect multiple components of airway inflammation, injury, and repair. More specific agents that antagonize cytokines and growth factors generated in the inflammatory process are in development, as are agents that may have the capacity to repress mesenchymal cell proliferation or matrix synthesis. Long-term suppression of extracellular matrix remodeling will be central to future therapeutic approaches to chronic inflammatory lung diseases.

UNIFYING HYPOTHESIS: ALTERED MECHANICAL RESTRAINTS AND MUSCLE PLASTICITY INDUCE EXCESSIVE AIRWAY SMOOTH MUSCLE SHORTENING IN ASTHMA

To answer the question posed in the Introduction of this chapter regarding possible mechanisms maintaining normal airway patency, it will be helpful to list all factors contributing or limiting narrowing of the airways. The dominant factor contributing to airway narrowing is force generated by the muscle cross-bridges. The force constricting the airways is opposed extracellularly by tethers that connect the force generators (muscle cells) to the extracellular matrix, and intracellularly by cytoskeleton. Together this network of protein filaments provides elastic loads and radial constraints on shortened cells. Tidal breathing and deep inspiration reduces the force generated by the cross-bridges by disrupting the equilibrium of cross-bridge binding and assembly of contractile filaments. This is possible only if mechanical perturbation associated with the lung volume change can be transmitted to the muscle cells; that is, it requires effective tethering between muscle cells and their dynamic physical environment. Enzymes and mediators that disrupt mechanical coupling between muscle cells and extracellular matrix will therefore constitute limiting factors to muscle shortening. As defined by a conventional length–tension relationship, the ability of smooth muscle to generate force is reduced when the muscle shortens beyond its optimal length. This, under normal circumstances, provides a brake on muscle shortening. Adaptation of the shortened muscle to its new length, however, will occur if the muscle is

allowed to remain at the short length for a prolonged period of time; the ability of the shortened muscle to generate force will increase and the braking effect will be offset. It appears that muscle adaptation to short length should be avoided if airway patency is to be maintained.

We propose that the initial insult to the airway allowing excessive muscle shortening is proteolytic damage to extracellular matrix caused by inflammatory cells. Once the muscle is allowed to reach a shorter length, its innate capability to optimize force generation at this new shorter length (plasticity) accentuates airway narrowing.

Acknowledgment

This chapter was supported by grants from the Canadian Institutes for Health Research (MOP 13271).

References

Introduction

1. Macklem PT. Mechanical factors determining maximum bronchoconstriction. Eur Respir J Suppl 1989; 6:516–519.
2. Sterk PJ, Bel EH. Bronchial hyperresponsiveness: The need for a distinction between hypersensitivity and excessive airway narrowing. Eur Respir J 1989; 2:267–274.
3. King GG, Paré PD, Seow CY. The mechanics of exaggerated airway narrowing in asthma: the role of smooth muscle. Resp Physiol 1999; 118:1–13.
4. Okazawa M, Bai TR, Wiggs BR, et al. Airway smooth muscle shortening in excised canine lung lobe. J Appl Physiol 1993; 74:1613–1621.
5. Okazawa M, Vedal S, Verburgt L, et al. Determinants of airway smooth muscle shortening in excised lung lobe. J Appl Physiol 1995; 78:608–614.
6. Lambert RK, Wiggs BR, Kuwano K, et al. Functional significance of increased airway smooth muscle in asthma and COPD. J Appl Physiol 1993; 74:2771–2781.
7. Lambert RK, Paré PD. Lung parenchymal shear modulus, airway wall remodeling, and bronchial hyperresponsiveness. J Appl Physiol 1997; 83:140–147.
8. Seow CY, Wang L, Paré PD. Airway narrowing and internal structural constraints. J Appl Physiol 2000; 88:527–533.
9. Stephens NL, Kong SK, Seow CY. Mechanisms of increased shortening of sensitized airway smooth muscle. Prog Clin Biol Res 1988; 263:231–254.
10. Bramley AM, Roberts CR, Schellenberg RR. Collagenase increases shortening of human bronchial smooth muscle in vitro. Am J Respir Crit Care Med 1995; 152:1513–1517.
11. Meiss RA. Influence of intercellular tissue connections on airway muscle mechanics. J Appl Physiol 1999; 86:5–15.
12. Shen X, Gunst SJ, Tepper RS. Effect of tidal volume and frequency on airway responsiveness in mechanically ventilated rabbits. J Appl Physiol 1997; 83:1202–1208.
13. Fredberg JJ, Inouye DS, Mijailovich SM, et al. Perturbed equilibrium of myosin binding in airway smooth muscle and its implications in bronchospasm. Am J Respir Crit Care Med 1999; 159:1–9.
14. Wang L, Paré PD, Seow CY. Effects of length oscillation on the subsequent force development in swine tracheal smooth muscle. J Appl Physiol 2000; 88:2246–2250.
15. Macklem PT. The clinical relevance of respiratory muscle research. A J. Burns Amberson lecture. Am Rev Respir Dis 1986; 134:812–815.
16. Macklem PT. A theoretical analysis of the effect of airway smooth muscle load on airway narrowing. Am J Respir Crit Care Med 1996; 153:83–89.
17. Woolcock A, Solome CM, Yan K. The shape of the dose-response curve to histamine in asthmatic and normal subjects. Am Rev Respir Dis 1984; 130:71–75.
18. Ding DJ, Martin JG, Macklem PT. Effects of lung volume on maximal methacholine-induced bronchoconstriction in normal humans. J Appl Physiol 1987; 62:1330–1324.
19. Stephens NL, Van Niekerk W. Isometric and isotonic contractions in airway smooth muscle. Can J Physiol Pharmacol 1977; 55:833–838.
20. Seow CY, Stephens NL. Velocity-length-time relations in canine tracheal smooth muscle. J Appl Physiol 1988; 64:2053–2057.
21. Martin C, Uhlig S, Ullrich V. Videomicroscopy of methacholine-induced contraction of individual airways in precision-cut lung slices. Eur Respir J 1996; 9:2479–2487.
22. Brown RH, Mitzner W. The myth of maximal airway responsiveness in vivo. J Appl Physiol 1998; 85:2012–2017.
23. Gunst SJ, Stropp JQ, Service J. Mechanical modulation of pressure-volume characteristics of contracted canine airways in vitro. J Appl Physiol 1990; 68:2223–2229.

Structure and function of airway smooth muscle

24. Gordon AM, Huxley AF, Julian FJ. The variation in isometric tension with sarcomere length in vertebrate muscle fibres. J Physiol 1966; 184:170–192.
25. Hodgkinson JL, Newman TM, Marston SB, et al. The structure of the contractile apparatus in ultrarapid frozen smooth muscle: freeze fracture, deep-etch, and freeze-substitution studies. J Struct Biol 1995; 114:93–104.

26. Kuo KH, Herrera AM, Wang L, et al. Structure-function correlation in airway smooth muscle adapted to different lengths. Am J Physiol Cell Physiol 2003; 285:C384–C390.
27. Herrera AM, McParland BE, Bienkowska A, et al. 'Sarcomeres' of smooth muscle: functional characteristics and ultrastructural evidence. J Cell Sci 2005; 118(Pt 11):2381–2392.
28. Bagby, RM. Organization of contractile/cytoskeletal elements. In: Stephens NL, ed. Biochemistry of smooth muscle, Boca Raton: CRC Press; 1983.
29. Cooke PH, Kargacin G, Craig R, et al. Molecular structure and organization of filaments in single, skinned smooth muscle cells. In: Siegman MJ, Somlyo AP, Stephens NL, eds. Regulation and contraction in smooth muscle. New York: Alan R Liss; 1987:1–25.
30. Kuo KH, Seow CY. Contractile filament architecture and force transmission in swine airway smooth muscle. J Cell Sci 2004; 117(Pt 8):1503–1511.
31. Pratusevich VR, Seow CY, Ford LE. Plasticity in airway smooth muscle. J Gen Physiol 1995; 105:73–94.
32. Wang L, Paré PD, Seow CY. Effect of chronic passive length change on airway smooth muscle length-tension relationship. J Appl Physiol 2001; 90:734–740.
33. Gunst SJ, Meiss RA, Wu MF, et al. Mechanisms for the mechanical plasticity of tracheal smooth muscle. Am J Physiol 1995; 268: C1267–1276.
34. Bursac P, Lenormand G, Fabry B, et al. Cytoskeletal remodelling and slow dynamics in the living cell. Nat Mater 2005; 4:557–561.
35. Smolensky AV, Ragozzino J, Gilbert SH, et al. Length-dependent filament formation assessed from birefringence increases during activation of porcine tracheal muscle. J Physiol 2005; 563(Pt 2):517–527.
36. Lambert RK, Pare PD, Seow CY. Mathematical description of geometric and kinematic aspects of smooth muscle plasticity and some related morphometrics. J Appl Physiol 2004; 96:469–476.
37. McParland BE, Tait RR, Pare PD, et al. The role of airway smooth muscle during an attack of asthma simulated in vitro. Am J Respir Cell Mol Biol 2005; 33:500–504.

Determinants of airway narrowing

38. Brown RH, Scichilone N, Mudge B, et al. HRCT Evaluation of airways distensibility and the effects of lung inflation on airway caliber in healthy and asthmatic individuals. Am J Respir Crit Care Med 2001; 163:989–993.
39. Brown RH, Scichilone N, Mudge B, et al. High-resolution computed tomographic evaluation of airway distensibility and the effects of lung inflation on airway caliber in healthy subjects and individuals with asthma. Am J Respir Crit Care Med 2001; 163:994–1001.
40. Klingele TG, Staub NC. Terminal bronchiole diameter changes with volume in isolated, air-filled lobes of cat lung. J Appl Physiol 1971; 30:224–227.
41. Hughes JM, Hoppin FG Jr. Mead J. Effect of lung inflation on bronchial length and diameter in excised lungs. J Appl Physiol 1972; 32:25–35.
42. Hahn HL, Watson A, Wilson AG, et al. Influence of bronchomotor tone on airway dimensions and resistance in excised dog lungs. J Appl Physiol 1980; 49:270–278.
43. Gunst SJ. Contractile force of canine airway smooth muscle during cyclical length changes. J Appl Physiol 1983; 55:759–769.
44. Gump A, Haughney L, Fredberg JJ. Relaxation of activated airway smooth muscle: relative potency of isoproterenol vs. tidal stretch. J Appl Physiol 2001; 90:2306–2310.
45. Fredberg JJ, Inouye D, Miller B, et al. Airway smooth muscle, tidal stretch, and dynamically determined contractile state. Am J Resp Critical Care Med 1997; 156:1752–1759.
46. Nadel JA, Tierney DF. Effect of a previous deep inspiration on airway resistance in man. J Appl Physiol 1961; 16:717–719.
47. Fish JE, Peterman VI, Cugell DW. Effect of deep inspiration on airway conductance in subjects with allergic rhinitis and allergic asthma. J Allergy Clin Immunol 1977; 60:41–46.
48. Burns CB, Taylor WR, Ingram RH Jr. Effects of deep inhalation in asthma: relative airway and parenchymal hysteresis. J Appl Physiol 59:1590–1596, 1985.
49. Skloot G, Permutt S, Togias A. Airway hyperresponsiveness in asthma: a problem of limited smooth muscle relaxation with inspiration. J Clin Invest 1995; 96:2393–2403.
50. Lim TK, Pride NB, Ingram RH Jr. Effects of volume history during spontaneous and acutely induced air-flow obstruction in asthma. Am Rev Respir Dis 1987; 135:591–596.
51. Lim TK, Ang SM, Rossing TH, et al. The effects of deep inhalation on maximal expiratory flow during intensive treatment of spontaneous asthmatic episodes. Am Rev Respir Dis 1989; 140:340–343.
52. Malmberg P, Larsson K, Sundblad BM, et al. Importance of the time interval between FEV1 measurements in a methacholine provocation test. Eur Respir J 1993; 6:680–686.
53. Scichilone N, Kapsali T, Permutt S, et al. Deep inspiration-induced bronchoprotection is stronger than bronchodilation. Am J Respir Crit Care Med 2000; 162:910–916.
54. Scichilone N, Permutt S, Togias A. The lack of the bronchoprotective and not the bronchodilatory ability of deep inspiration is associated with airway hyperresponsiveness. Am J Respir Crit Care Med 2001; 163:413–419.
55. Kapsali T, Permutt S, Laube B, et al. Potent bronchoprotective effect of deep inspiration and its absence in asthma. J Appl Physiol 2000; 89:711–720.

Cytoskeletal elements of airways modulate muscle contraction

56. Pavalko FM, Adam LP, Wu MF, et al. Phosphorylation of dense-plaque proteins talin and paxillin during tracheal smooth muscle contraction. Am J Physiol Cell Physiol 1995; 268:C563–C571.
57. Tang D, Mehta D, Gunst SJ. Mechanosensitive tyrosine phosphorylation of paxillin and focal adhesion kinase in tracheal smooth muscle. Am J Physiol Cell Physiol 1999; 276:C250–C258.
58. Tang DD, Gunst SJ. Depletion of focal adhesion kinase by antisense depresses contractile activation of smooth muscle. Am J Physiol 2001; 280: C874–C883.
59. Tang DD, Wu MF, Opazo Saez AM, et al. The focal adhesion protein paxillin regulates contraction in canine tracheal smooth muscle. J Physiol 2002; 542:501–513.
60. Opazo Saez AM, Tang D, Turner C, et al. Recruitment of paxillin to the membrane is necessary for contraction in response to acetylcholine (Ach) in airway smooth muscle (SM). Am J Respir Crit Care Med 2002; 165:A118.
61. Scott PG. Macromolecular constituents of basement membranes: a review of current knowledge on their structure and function. Can J Biochem Cell Biol 1983; 61:942–948.
62. Sage H. Collagens of basement membranes. J Invest Dermatol 1982; 79:51–59.
63. Murdoch AD, Dodge GR, Cohen I, et al. Primary structure of the human heparan sulfate proteoglycan from basement membrane. J Biol Chem 1992; 267:8544–8557.
64. Yurchenco PD, Ruben GC. Basement membrane structure in situ: evidence for lateral associations in the type IV collagen network. J Cell Biol 1987; 105:2559–2568.
65. van der Rest M, Garrone R. Collagen family of proteins. FASEB J 1991; 5:2814–2823.
66. Yayon A, Klagsbrun M, Esko JD, et al. Cell surface heparin-like molecules are required for binding basic fibroblast growth factor to its high affinity receptor. Cell 1991; 64:841–848.
67. Vracko R. Significance of basal lamina for regeneration of injured lung. Virchows Arch A Path Anat 1972; 355:264–274.
68. Montes GS. Distribution of oxytalan, elaunin and elastic fibres in tissues. J Brazil Ass Adv Sci 1992; 44:224–233.
69. Gawlik Z. Morphological and morphochemical properties of the elastic system in the motor organ of man. Folia Histochem Cytochem 1965; 3:223–251.
70. Böck P, Stockinger L. Light and electron microscopic identification of elastic, elaunin and oxytalan fibers in human tracheal and bronchial mucosa. Anat Embryol 1994; 170:145–153.
71. Leick-Maldonado EA, Lemos M. Differential distribution of elastic system fibers in control and bronchoconstricted intraparenchymatous airways in the guinea-pig lung. J Submicrosc Cytol Pathol 1997; 29:427–434.
72. Olsen BR, Ninomiya Y. Basement membrane collagens (Type IV). In: Kreis T, Vale R, eds. Guidebook to the extracellular matrix and adhesion proteins. Oxford: Oxford University Press, 1993:32–48.
73. Junqueira LCU, Montes GS, Martins JEC, et al. Dermal collagen, distribution. A histochemical and ultrastructural study. Histochemistry 1983; 79:397–403.
74. Montes GS, Krisztan RM, Shigihara KM, et al. Histochemical and morphological characterization of reticular fibers. Histochemistry 1980; 65:131–141.
75. Montes GS, Bezerra MSF, Junqueira LCU. Collagen distribution in tissues. In: Ruggeri A, Motta, PM eds. Ultrastructure of the connective tissue matrix. Boston: Martinus Nijhoff; 1984: 65–88.

Role of extracellular matrix in airway remodeling in asthma

76. Fish JE, Peters SP. Airway remodeling and persistent airway obstruction in asthma. J Allergy Clin Immunol 1999; 104:509–516.
77. Busse W, Elias J, Sheppard D, et al. Airway remodeling and repair. Am J Respir Crit Care Med 1999; 160:1035–1042.
78. Herard A-L, Pierrot D, Hinnrasky J, et al. Fibronectin and its $\alpha_5\beta_1$-integrin receptor are involved in the wound-repair process of airway epithelium. Am J Physiol 1996; 271:L726–L733.
79. White SR, Dorsheid DR, Rabe KF, et al. Role of very late adhesion integrins in mediating repair of human airway epithelial cell monolayers after mechanical injury. Am J Respir Cell Mol Biol 1999; 20:787–796.
80. Jeffrey PK, Godfrey RW, Adelroth E, et al. Effects of treatment on airway inflammation and thickening of the basement membrane reticular collagen in asthma: a quantitative and electron microscopic study. Am Rev Respir Dis 1992; 145:890–899.
81. Albelda SM. Endothelial and epithelial cell adhesion molecules. Am J Respir Cell Mol Biol 1995; 4:195–203.
82. Pilewski JM, Latoche JD, Arcasoy SM, et al. Expression of integrin cell adhesion receptors during human airway epithelial repair in vivo. Am J Physiol 1997; 273: L256–L263.
83. Altraja A, Laitinen A, Virtanen I, et al. Expression of laminins in various types of asthmatic patients: a morphometric study. Am J Respir Cell Mol Biol 1996; 15:482–488.
84. Rabb HA, Olivenstein R, Issekutz TB, et al. The role of leukocyte adhesion molecules VLA-4, LFA-1, and Mac-1 in allergic airway responses in the rat. Am J Respir Crit Care Med 1994; 149:1186–1191.
85. Laberge S, Rabb H, Issekutz TB, et al. The role of VLA-4 and LFA-1 in allergen-induced airway hyperresponsiveness and lung inflammation in the rat. Am J Respir Crit Care Med 1995; 151:822–829.
86. Abraham WM, Sielczak MW, Ahmed A, et al. Alpha 4-integrins mediate antigen-induced late bronchial responses and prolonged airway hyperresponsiveness in sheep. J Clin Invest 1994; 93:776–787.
87. Pretolani M, Ruffie C, Lapa e Silva JR, et al. Antibody to very late antigen 4 prevents antigen-induced bronchial hyperreactivity and cellular infiltration in the guinea pig airways. J Exp Med 1994; 180:795–805.
88. Hojo M, Maghni K, Issekutz TB, et al. Involvement of α_4 integrins in allergic airway responses and mast cell degranulation in vivo. Am J Respir Crit Care Med 1998; 158:1127–1133.
89. Munger JS, Huang X, Kawakatsu H, et al. The integrin $\alpha_\nu\beta_6$ binds and activates latent TGFB₁: a mechanism for regulating pulmonary inflammation and fibrosis. Cell 1999; 96:319–328.
90. Laitinen A, Altaja A, Kampe M, et al. Tenascin is increased in airway basement membrane of asthmatics and decreased by an inhaled steroid. Am J Respir Crit Care Med 1997; 156:951–958.
91. Roche WR, Beasley R, Williams JH, et al. Sub-epithelial fibrosis in the bronchi of asthmatics. Lancet 1989; 1:520–524.
92. Bai TR, Cooper J, Koelmeyer T, et al. The effect of age and duration of disease on airway structure in fatal asthma. Am J Respir Crit Care Med 2000; 162:663–669.
93. Ohno I, Lea RG, Flanders KC, et al. Eosinophils in chronically inflamed airway tissues express transforming growth factor β_1 gene (TGF-β_1). J Clin Invest 1992; 89:1662–1668.
94. Minshall EM, Leung DYM, Martin RJ, et al. Eosinophil-associated TGF-β_1 mRNA expression and airways fibrosis in bronchial asthma. Am J Respir Cell Mol Biol 1997; 17:326–333.

95. Wenzel SE, Szefler SJ, Leung DYM, et al. Bronchoscopic evaluation of severe asthma: persistent inflammation associated with high dose glucocorticoids. Am J Respir Crit Care Med 1997; 156:737–743.
96. Thomson RJ, Bramley AM, Schellenberg RR. Airway muscle stereology: implications for increased shortening in asthma. Am J Respir Crit Care Med 1996; 154:749–757.
97. Bousquet J, Lacoste J, Chanez P, et al. Bronchial elastic fibers in normal subjects and asthmatic patients. Am Respir Care Med. 1996; 153:1648–1653.
98. Mauad T, Xavier ACG, Saldiva PHN, et al. Elastosis and fragmentation of fibers of the elastic system in fatal asthma. Am J Respir Crit Care Med 1999; 160:968–975.
99. Vignola AM, Bonanno A, Mirabella A, et al. Increased levels of elastase and α_1-antitrypsin in sputum of asthmatic patients. Am J Respir Crit Care Med 1998; 157:505–511.
100. Roberts CR. Is asthma a fibrotic disease? Chest 1995; 107:111S–117S.
101. Iozzo RV. Matrix proteoglycans: from molecular design to cellular function. Ann Rev Biochem 1998; 67:609–652.
102. Huang J, Olivenstein R, Taha R, et al. Enhanced proteoglycan deposition in the airway wall of atopic asthmatics. Am J Respir Crit Care Med 1999; 160:725–729.
103. Pini L, Hamid Q, Shannon J, et al. Differences in proteoglycan deposition in the airway of moderate and severe asthmatics. Eur Respir J: 2006; 28.
104. Roberts CR, Okazawa M, Wiggs BR, et al. Airway Wall thickening. In: Barnes PJ, Grunstein MM, Leff AR, et al. Asthma. London: Lippincott-Raven; 1997: 925–935.
105. Haraguchi M, Shimura S, Shirato K. Morphometric analysis of bronchial cartilage in chronic obstructive pulmonary disease and bronchial asthma. Am J Respir Crit Care Med 1999; 159:1005–1013.

Asthmatic airway smooth muscle morphology and mechanical properties

106. Huber HL, Koessler KK. The pathology of bronchial asthma. Arch Intern Med 1922; 30:689–760.
107. Dunnill MS, Massarella GR, Anderson JA. A comparison of the quantitative anatomy of the bronchi in normal subjects, in status asthmaticus, in chronic bronchitis and in emphysema. Thorax 1969; 24:176–9.
108. Hossain, S. Quantitative measurement of bronchial muscle in men with asthma. Am Rev Respir Dis 1973; 107:99–109.
109. Heard BE, Hossain S. Hyperplasia of bronchial muscle in asthma. J Pathol 1973; 110:319–331.
110. Carroll N, Elliot J, Morton A, et al. The structure of large and small airways in nonfatal and fatal asthma. Am Rev Respir Dis 1993; 147:405–410.
111. Ebina M, Takahashi T, Chiba T, et al. Cellular hypertrophy and hyperplasia of airway smooth muscles underlying bronchial asthma. A 3D morphometric study. Am Rev Respir Dis 1993; 48:720–726.
112. Kuwano K, Bosken CH, Pare PD, et al. Small airways dimensions in asthma and in chronic obstructive pulmonary disease. Am Rev Respir Dis 1993; 148:1220–1225.
113. Ishida K, Pare PD, Hards J, et al. Mechanical properties of human bronchial smooth muscle in vivo. J Appl Physiol 1992; 73:1481–1485.
114. Ishida K, Pare PD, Blogg T, et al. Effects of elastic loading on porcine trachealis smooth muscle mechanics. J Appl Physiol 1990; 69:1033–1039.
115. Opazo Saez AM, Schellenberg RR, Ludwig M, et al. Tissue elastance influences airway smooth muscle shortening: comparison of mechanical properties among different species. Can J Physiol Pharmacol 2002; 80:1–7.
116. Bramley AM, Thomson RJ, Roberts CR, et al. Hypothesis: excessive bronchoconstriction in asthma is due to decreased airway elastance. Eur Respir J 1994; 7:337–341.
117. Halayko AJ, Salari H, Ma X, et al. Markers of airway smooth muscle phenotype. Am J Physiol 1996; 270:L1040–L1051.
118. Halayko AJ, Rector E, Stephens NL. Characterization of molecular determinants of smooth muscle cell heterogeneity. Can J Physiol Pharmacol 1997; 75:917–929.
119. Rajah R, Nachajon RV, Collins MH, et al. Elevated levels of the IGF-binding protein protease MMP-1 in asthmatic airway smooth muscle. Am J Respir Cell Mol Biol 1999; 20:199–208.
120. Cohen P, Bhala A, Herrick D, et al. The effects of leukotriene D_4 on the proliferation of airway smooth muscle cells are mediated by modulation of the IGF axis. Am J Physiol 1995; 269:L151–L157.
121. Rajah R, Nunn S, Herrick D, et al. Leukotriene D_4 induces MMP-1, which functions as an IGFBP protease in airway smooth muscle cells. Am J Physiol 1996; 271:L1014–L1022.
122. Loewen DAJ, Pare PD, Schellenberg RR. Prolonged effects of epithelial injury and repair on the mechanical properties and proliferation of airway smooth muscle (ASM). Am J Respir Crit Care Med 1997; 155:A369.
123. Lemjabbar H, Gosset P, Lamblin C, et al. Contribution of 92 kDa gelatinase/type IV collagenase in bronchial inflammation during status asthmaticus. Am J Respir Crit Care Med 1999; 159:1298–1307.
124. Mautino G, Oliver N, Chanez P, et al. Increased release of matrix metalloproteinase-9 in bronchoalveolar lavage fluid and by alveolar macrophages of asthmatics. Am J Respir Cell Mol Biol 1997; 17:583–592.
125. Vignola AM, Riccobono L, Mirabella A, et al. Sputum metalloproteinase-9/tissue inhibitor of metalloproteinase-1 ratio correlates with airflow obstruction in asthma and chronic bronchitis. Am J Respir Crit Care Med 1998; 158:1945–1950.
126. Bosse M, Chakir J, Rouabhia M, et al. Serum matrix metalloproteinase-9: tissue inhibitor of metalloproteinase-1 ratio correlates with steroid responsiveness in moderate to severe asthma. Am J Respir Crit Care Med 1999; 159:596–602.
127. Van Eerdewegh P, Little RD, Dupuis J, et al. Association of the ADAM 33 gene with asthma and bronchial hyperresponsiveness. Nature 2002; 418:426–430.
128. Haitchi HM, Powell RM, Shaw TJ, et al. ADAM 33 expression in asthmatic airways and human embryonic lung. Am J Respir Crit Care Med 2005; 171:958–965.
129. Carroll NG, Mutavdzic S, James AL. Distribution and degranulation of airway mast cells in normal and asthmatic subjects. Eur Respir J 2002; 19:879–885.
130. Brightling CE, Bradding P, Symon FA, et al. Mast-cell infiltration of airway smooth muscle in asthma. N Engl J Med 2002; 346:1699–1705.
131. Barrios VE, Middleton SC, Kashem MA, et al. Tryptase mediates hyperresponsiveness in isolated guinea pig bronchi. Life Sci 1998; 63:2295–2303.
132. Wright CD, Havill AM, Middleton SC, et al. Inhibition of allergen-induced pulmonary responses by the selective tryptase inhibitor 1,5-bis-[4-[(3-carbamimidoyl-benzenesulfonylamino)-methyl]-phenoxyl]-pentane (AMG-126737). Biochem Pharmacol 1999; 58:1989–1996.
133. Cairns JA, Walls AF. Mast cell tryptase stimulates the synthesis of type I collagen in human lung fibroblasts. J Clin Invest 1997; 99:1313–1321.

Implications regarding therapy for asthma

134. Gordon JR, Galli SJ. Mast cells as source of both preformed and immunologically inducible TNFα/cachectin. Nature 1990; 346:274–276.
135. Gosset P, Tsicopoulos A, Wallaert B et al. Increased secretion of tumor necrosis factor α and interleukin-6 by alveolar macrophages consecutively to the late asthmatic reaction after bronchial allergen challenge. J Allergy Clin Immunol 1991; 88:561–571.
136. Howarth PH, Babu KS, Arshad HS, et al. Tumor necrosis factor (TNFα) as a novel therapeutic target in symptomatic corticosteroid dependent asthma. Thorax 2005; 60:1012–1018.
137. Erin EM, Leaker BR, Nicholson C, et al. The effects of a monoclonal antibody directed against tumor necrosis factor-α in asthma. Am J Respir Crit Care Med 2006; 174:753–762.

REFERENCES

Development, Structure, and Physiology in Normal Lung and in Asthma

38

Anne E Dixon and Charles G Irvin

CONTENTS

SUMMARY OF IMPORTANT CONCEPTS

>> Rapid and intricate changes in growth and architecture of the lung render it prone to injury from insults such as cigarette smoke and viral infections

>> Several structural changes characterize the asthmatic airway, the most striking of which are those of the epithelium and airways smooth muscle. The functional impact of airway remodeling is less well characterized

>> Characteristic abnormalities of pulmonary function that define the asthmatic patient can be explained by airway narrowing and enhanced airway closure

>> Physiological assessment of the asthmatic patient with spirometry is a necessary part of the diagnostic workup as well as an important part of therapeutic monitoring

INTRODUCTION

Alterations in structure of the asthmatic lung are central to the pathophysiology of asthma. Structural changes underlie the clinical manifestations of asthma, which include dyspnea, wheezing, cough, excess mucus production, airflow limitation, and hyper-responsiveness. To understand how structural changes produce the symptoms of asthma, it is first necessary to understand the normal development and structure of the lung. We will review the normal development and structure of the lung, and discuss how this development and structure is altered in patients with asthma; this leads to changes in pathophysiology of the lung, which are responsible for the clinical manifestations of asthma.

LUNG DEVELOPMENT

The lung develops in a series of defined stages. The *embryonic* stage begins approximately day 24–26 after fertilization, and is complete by 7 weeks' gestation. Lung sacs develop from the ventral wall of the esophagus, which accounts for some of the common features between the two structures such as patterns of anatomical innervation, and the major airways and lobes are formed by a series of successive budding. The *pseudoglandular* stage occurs during the 15th–17th week of gestation; the bronchial tree first develops as solid tubes, which bud to form bronchi, bronchioles, and terminal bronchioles. In the *canalicular* stage, 16–26 weeks of gestation, lumens begin to form in the bronchial tree, the peripheral epithelium differentiates into type I and II pneumatocytes, and capillaries arrange into sleeves around the bronchioles. The saccal period, 24–38 weeks of gestation, is characterized by the formation of alveolar ducts and air sacs, though the majority of the alveoli develop postnatally.[1]

In a term baby, the lung volume doubles by 6 months, and triples by a year; this requires a phenomenal rate of growth. Growth that occurs in the first year of life is accompanied by other developments in respiratory physiology, including changes in shape, and compliance of the rib cage.

The rapid rate of embryonic and postnatal lung growth is likely to predispose the lung to damage from inflammatory insults.[2] Other factors that are implicated in alteration of structure and function of lung in development include fetal nutrition, maternal smoking during pregnancy, environmental allergens, respiratory infections during infancy, and genetics.[3]

The structure of the lungs in the infant and young child differs from the adult; airways are relatively large in relation to lung volume in fetal life and infancy. Thus, airway edema and mucus secretion associated with lower respiratory infections are more likely to produce wheezing in the lung of a child than in an adult. This may account for why FEV_1 does not predict asthma exacerbation[4] and may not even be an appropriate measure in asthmatic children[5] In addition, the infant chest wall is highly compliant, which leads to an increased tendency for peripheral airways to close during tidal breathing.[6]

There are gender differences in airway development; longitudinal studies of airway parenchymal size demonstrate that the airways of boys are smaller than girls.[7] Over time, boys demonstrate more pronounced airway growth compared with girls; as a result the airway/ lung volume ratios in males are equal to or greater than females after puberty. As smaller airways are more likely to develop critical airway narrowing that results in airflow limitation and wheezing, gender differences in airway development and lung anatomy have been proposed as the explanation for the increased prevalence of asthma in prepubertal boys compared with girls.[8]

Normal lung development is a complex process that may be affected by various environmental and genetic factors; insults during normal development will affect lung structure – structural changes will lead to changes in lung function. The structure of the lung in early childhood makes it particularly susceptible to developing airway narrowing, and asthmatic-type symptoms. Understanding how developmental insults affect structure and function is an area of intense investigation.

■ AIRWAY REMODELING ■

Asthmatic patients have structural changes in their airways compared with non-asthmatic patients and these structural changes are thought to contribute to the pathogenesis of asthma, but exactly how is unclear. Structural changes in the airway walls of asthmatics are referred to as 'airway remodeling'. The airway wall of asthmatics is thickened or remodeled compared with non-asthmatics in studies with high-resolution chest computed tomography (HRCT) scans that show thickening in both large and small airways.[9,10] The physiological significance of this observation is the subject of intense investigation, since studies suggest that airway thickening is related to clinical measures of asthma severity.[11] Airway wall thickness is inversely related to lung function as measured by the FEV_1,[12] and large airway luminal diameter after bronchodilator therapy correlates directly with the ratio of FEV_1/FVC.[9] Central airway wall thickening can be decreased with inhaled corticosteroid treatment.[13] Airway wall thickening is a characteristic of asthma and, at least by some measures, related to asthma severity; at the microscopic level airway wall thickening involves changes in all components of the airway wall.

The airway epithelium can also be profoundly abnormal and is hyperplastic and injured in asthma (Fig. 38.1). James et al demonstrated that the airway epithelium is hyperplastic in both central and peripheral airways in asthma.[14] Some biopsy studies show that the airway epithelium is also damaged,[15] while others have found no damage;[16] this led to speculation that biopsy forceps may cause artifactual epithelial damage.[17] However, autopsies clearly show epithelial sloughing in patients who have died from status asthmaticus (Fig. 38.1), and studies with induced sputum[18] and bronchoalveolar lavage[19] show increased epithelial cells in asthma. These observations support the concept that epithelial integrity is reduced in asthmatics but the functional significance of these changes in the epithelium are not well defined. Recent data suggest that the epithelium is an important source of cytokines regulating the immune response to environmental stimuli in asthma.[20]

The airway epithelial cells lie on a basement membrane that is thickened in asthma because of subepithelial fibrosis in the region of the laminar reticularis. Thickening reflects increased deposition of type I, III, and IV collagen,[21] proteoglycans and other elements of the extracellular matrix;[22] this fibrosis is a result of both increased synthesis, and decreased breakdown of extracellular matrix.[23] Subepithelial fibrosis is seen in asthma of all severity, and has been detected even in patients with rhinitis,[24] suggesting that it is a feature of atopic airway disease. The degree of thickening does not clearly correlate with asthma severity, but rather is a characteristic of all asthma.[25,26] The effect of treatment with inhaled corticosteroids on this subepithelial fibrosis has been inconsistent across studies,[27] though long-term treatment targeted to reducing airways hyper-responsiveness may be effective in reducing subepithelial fibrosis.[28]

The submucosal layer of the airway is also altered in asthma; the submucosal layer of asthmatic airways exhibits both hyperplasia and hypertrophy of mucus-secreting cells[29] – this will produce increased mucus secretion into the airway, with an increased productive cough and airway plugging by secretions. Epidemiological studies show that mucus hypersecretion is a marker of asthma severity.[30] Case series report that excess mucus secretion with increased goblet cells is a feature of status asthmaticus;[31] airway plugging with mucus has been frequently observed in postmortem examinations of patients who died of asthma[32] and mucus gland hyperplasia has also been associated with sudden death in asthma.[33] These changes have obvious effects on airway obstruction and loss of lung function.

The airway wall of asthmatic patients has increased vascularity compared with non-asthmatics; this likely contributes to airway narrowing from vascular engorgement and edema.[34] Increases in vascularity appear to be related to increased local expression of the angiogenic factors such as vascular endothelial growth factor.[35] The functional role of the increased vascularity of the airway wall is unknown.

Increased smooth muscle in the airway wall is a characteristic of asthma; increased smooth muscle may arise from hypertrophy and/or hyperplasia of smooth muscle in the airway.[36] Smooth muscle is not simply the effector of bronchoconstriction in asthma because smooth muscle cells also elaborate pro-inflammatory cytokines and extracellular matrix proteins.[37]

The functional consequences of airway wall thickening are complex. Certainly increased thickening could contribute to the pathogenesis of an asthma phenotype, with narrowed airways predisposing to airflow limitation, but recent studies suggest that airway wall thickening may also be protective and reduce airway hyperreactivity[12] – stiffer airways may constrict less well in response to a stimulus than a thinner-walled airway. Studies of structure and function that use sophisticated imaging techniques are one way to improve our understanding of the functional consequences of remodeling in asthmatics.[9] Thus the impact of structural remodeling can be potentially both causative and ameliorating on lung function and airways hyper-responsiveness.

■ AIRFLOW LIMITATION ■

Reversible and variable airflow limitations are also key features of asthma. Indeed, perhaps the most characteristic features of asthma are variability or periodicity of lung dysfunction, which is an aspect that distinguishes

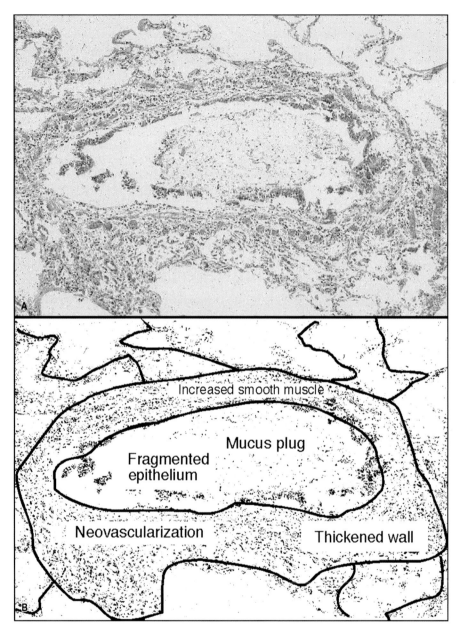

Fig. 38.1. (A) An airway of the lung of a patient who died from asthma (status asthmaticus). There are profound changes in the structure of the airways and lungs (remodeling). (B) The airway wall is thickened by cellular infiltration, extracellular matrix deposition, and expansion of airways smooth muscle. There is also pronounced neovascularization. The epithelium is clearly friable and disintegrating, and a mucus plug occupies the airway lumen. (×100, stained with H&E).

asthma from chronic obstructive pulmonary disease (COPD). While some severe asthmatic subjects have persistent airflow limitation and some patients with COPD have reversible airflow limitation, the presence of widely variable airflow limitation generally distinguishes asthma from COPD. Asthma is often categorized as an 'obstructive' disease. The term 'obstructive' denotes the complete absence of flow when in reality airflow may simply be reduced but not absent, so a more generic term is

airflow limitation,[38] although, as we will see, 'obstruction' may turn out to be the best term after all.

Spirometry is the easiest and perhaps most clinically useful method of measuring airflow limitation in most clinical situations. Spirometry correlates well with airway cross-sectional area and has been shown to be more sensitive than a patient's report of symptoms and physical examination.[39] In addition, spirometry predicts mortality in patients with chronic airway disease;[40] in fact, low spirometric values predict mortality due to all causes.[41] These facts make spirometry the test of choice to be performed in an office setting.

Spirometry is based on the notion that forceful expiration results in effort-independent maximal flow, the magnitude of which is determined in part by airway physiology. Airways are essentially flexible tubes in a box of air (the thoracic cavity). In order to expire, respiratory muscles contract and increase the pressure both within the box and within the airways at the same time. As the airways are a tube, pressure drops because energy is lost due to overcoming resistance of the tube and the Bernoulli effect, where pressure drops as velocity increases. Meanwhile, the pressure within the box remains roughly uniform. At a point along the tube, the pressure inside the tube becomes less than that of the air in the box (thoracic cavity), at which point the airways narrow, thus limiting flow (Fig. 38.2). This physical event is commonly known as the equal pressure point.[42] The physical variables that most profoundly affect expiratory flow are airway caliber, airway wall compliance, and elastic recoil. Airflow limitation occurs when one or all of these factors decrease, contrary to the common assumption that a reduced FEV_1 is due simply to a decrease in airway caliber. As outlined below, FEV_1 is also dependent on the FVC.

A clinically useful way to present these relationships is the flow-volume loop (Fig. 38.3). The flow-volume loop consists of flow on the y-axis and volume on the x-axis measured as the individual forcefully exhales following maximal inspiration. Even in normal individuals, flow limitation is evident on the flow-volume loop during much of maximal expiration, known as the flow-limiting envelope (Fig. 38.3). If the airway is narrowed, either by bronchoconstriction, mucus plugging, airway remodeling or edema, the increased resistance effectively moves the flow-limiting envelope leftward, due to hyperinflation and/or downward because of flow limitation. Characteristic changes occur in the flow-volume loop with different etiologies of flow limitation (Fig. 38.4); accordingly, it is important to plot the entire flow volume loop.

The FEV_1 is the most reproducible pulmonary function test with a coefficient of variation of 2–3% in normal individuals, but as asthma is characterized by variable airflow limitation, it can be normal even in a patient with significant disease.[39] FEF_{25-75} is typically determined as the middle fraction of the FVC and, consequently, is sensitive to changes in FVC (effort) or changes in the shape of the flow-volume curve[43] – as such, the FEF_{25-75} is much more variable and less reproducible than the FEV_1.[44] Moreover, it has been shown that FEV_1/FVC is a considerably better measure of subtle airflow limitation; so for all the above reasons, the use of the FEF_{25-75} is strongly discouraged.

Peak expiratory flow (PEF) is also very effort-dependent; even so, frequent determinations of PEF can be helpful in documenting the variable nature of a patient's airflow limitation, one of the central features of asthma. It is important to understand that the PEF and FEV_1 are not equivalent measures of airflow limitation. The greatest expiratory flow, the PEF, occurs early in expiration and therefore reflects the discharge of air from large central airways, whereas air that is more distal in the lung is discharged later in a forced exhalation. Thus, measuring flow later in the time course of exhalation (1 second) is more representative of distal airflow limitation. In individuals with an upper airway obstruction, PEF and FEV_1 are often equally diminished, whereas FEV_1 tends to be diminished to a larger degree than PEF in asthma, probably as a result of small airway closure.[45]

Measurement of lung volume is an important component of the physiologic assessment of asthma. The most useful lung volumes are the forced vital capacity (FVC), total lung capacity (TLC), functional residual capacity (FRC), and residual volume (RV) (Fig. 38.5). The FVC is measured by spirometry, while TLC, FRC, and RV are measured either by helium dilution or body plethysmography. In the helium dilution technique the volume required to dilute an inhaled concentration of helium is used to determine the lung volume at FRC. The drawback of the helium dilution technique is that it only assesses the volume of lung that is communicating with the airway opening; in a patient with severe airflow limitation, airway closure or mucus plugging can result in a falsely low FRC by helium, as the helium mixture is unable to dilute the air that is 'trapped' behind a closed or markedly narrowed airway. This often leads to the erroneous conclusion that the patient has a mixed picture of an airflow limitation and lung volume restriction, when in fact the patient may only have airflow limitation and obstructed airways.

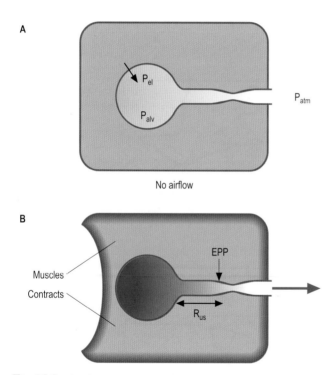

Fig. 38.2. Model of airflow limitation. (A) The simple model consists of an airway/alveolus unit within a box (thorax). At the end of expiration during tidal volume breathing, the pressure within the box is zero and there is no pressure gradient between the alveolus (P_{alv}) and atmosphere (P_{atm}) – at this point the recoil pressure of the alveolus (P_{el}) is equal, and opposite, to the pleural pressure (determined by the tendency of the chest wall to recoil outwards). (B) When the diaphragm contracts, the pleural pressure exerts a positive pressure on the outside of the alveolus and airways. Pressure in the alveolus is then the sum of the elastic recoil (P_{el}) and pleural pressure; together this now exceeds atmospheric pressure, and air flows out of the lungs. There is now a pressure gradient from the alveolus to more proximal parts of the airway. Because of energy loss due to resistive forces and the Bernoulli effect, at some point the pressure outside the airway equals the pressure inside the airway – the equal pressure point (EPP arrow). Beyond this point the airways narrow and airflow is limited. R_{us}, resistance of the upstream segment.

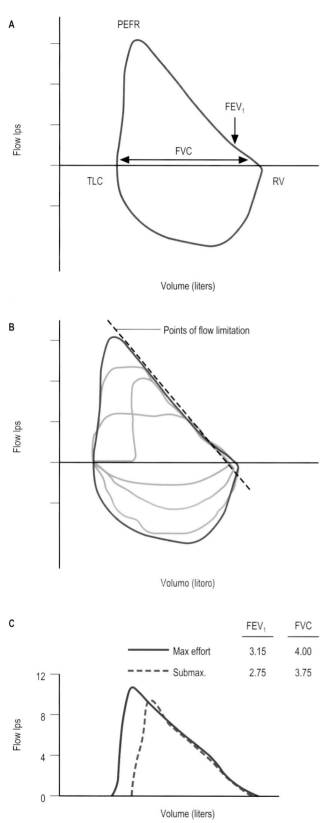

Fig. 38.3. Basic flow-volume relationships. (A) Flow (lps) plotted against volume during forced expiration produces a characteristic flow-volume 'loop'. The FEV_1 occurs in a normal person at approximately 80% of the forced vital capacity. FEV_1, (forced expiratory volume in 1 s); FVC, forced vital capacity; RV, residual volume; TLC, total lung capacity; PEFR, peak expiratory flow rate. (B) When expiratory maneuvers are performed at different TLCs or effort, a family of loops is created. While the inspiratory loops are all effort-dependent, the expiratory loops are clearly flow limited even when expiratory is less than maximal (effort-independent) or when a lower TLC is achieved. (C) The effect of failing to inspire maximally to TLC on the measurement of FEV_1. The maximal effort is shown by solid line; the submaximal effort is shown by the dotted line. When the patient inhales to a lower TLC <0.5 L, the FEV_1 falls by 0.4 L, or 12.7%. FVC also fallls.

A more useful approach is to use body plethysmography, which relies upon Boyle's law and gas compression, to determine the volume of air in the lung whether or not it communicates with the main airways. Determination of lung volume with body plethysmography is not subject to the risk of underestimation in the setting of air trapping, and thus body plethysmography is the preferred technique.

Any disease process that diminishes lung volume or results in muscle weakness will also diminish the FEV_1, which is an important cause of false-positive results (Fig. 38.3C). One way to determine if a diminished FEV_1 is the result of airflow limitation is to determine the FEV_1/FVC ratio. A percent predicted FEV_1/FVC ratio of <0.7 is the most sensitive indicator of airflow limitation, although a ratio <0.8 is often considered to be indicative of airflow limitation. A normal FEV_1/FVC does not rule out airflow limitation. If the defect involves air trapping due to closure of lung units, then FVC may also fall, thereby preserving the FEV_1/FVC ratio. In this setting, determination of lung volumes (TLC, FRC) or airway conductance by body plethysmography can be particularly helpful.

Determining the degree of air trapping due to airway closure is an established index of airway disease. While the TLC of an asthmatic should be normal or slightly increased, the RV is invariably elevated (Fig. 38.5) and may be the first abnormality observed in the patient with mild disease. Air trapping can also be observed on HRCT by comparing inspiratory and expiratory scans (Fig. 38.6), although the sensitivity and specificity of such findings in the absence of bronchoprovocation are unclear.[46] In the setting of marked air trapping, chest radiographs will demonstrate visibly increased lung volumes and flattened diaphragms. These increases in lung volume contribute to the symptoms of asthma, and in the case of a severe exacerbation, increased intrathoracic pressure can impair blood return to the heart, resulting in cardiovascular compromise, or can result in the development of pneumomediastinum or pneumothorax.

A recent study by Brown and associates[9] where lung volume, spirometry and CT were performed before and after bronchodilator treatment illustrates these points. In mild patients, there is a rise in RV, but the TLC rises in concert, resulting in a preserved FEV_1. As the RV rises further, the TLC reaches a presumed limit, where after the FVC falls, the FEV_1 decreases as a consequence. The FEV_1/FVC ratio was also shown to relate to large but not smaller airway thickness.[9,47]

Body plethysmography also allows for the determination of *airway resistance* and *specific conductance*, which are measures of airflow that are both complementary yet different from spirometry. Ohm's law is stated as voltage (pressure drop) = current (flow) × resistance. In like fashion, airway resistance can be determined from lung volume, airway pressure,

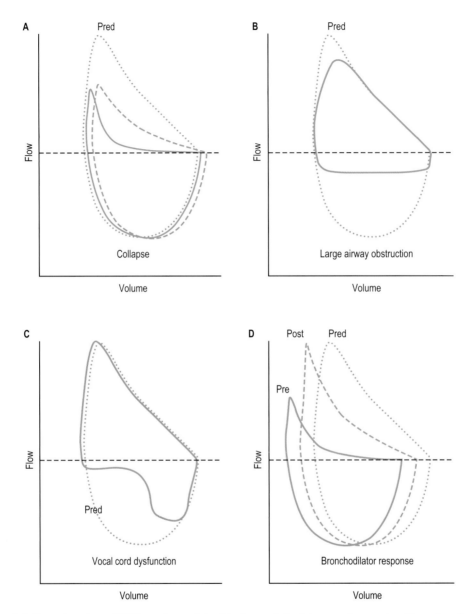

Fig. 38.4. Characteristic flow-volume loops. (A) Flow-volume relationship characteristic of airways collapse and an illustration of negative effort dependence. The first (higher flow-volume) occurs when the patient makes a submaximal effort. The second loop occurs when the patient exhales maximally, i.e., flow falls with increased effort or negative effort dependence. Pred, predicted flow-volume relationship. (B) A consistent truncation of the inspiratory loop is indicative of a large airway obstruction or an extrathoracic lesion. (C) Partial truncation of the type usually associated with vocal cord dysfunction shown by the solid line. Where there is initial preservation of flow and then flow truncation as the vocal cords appose. (D) Bronchodilator responses can be quite varied. In this example, the patient shows marked improvement in airflow and an increase in FVC. (Compare solid line, pre-bronchodilation, with dashed lines, post-bronchodilation). However, the flow-volume relationship is still not normal, suggesting further treatment is warranted.

and flow. These values can be easily obtained from a body box by having the patient breathe while the shutter is open and then again when it is closed (Fig. 38.7). Normal is approximately 1.5 cmH$_2$O/L per second. As the resistance varies significantly with lung volume, one has to express airways resistance in terms of the specific conductance, which takes volume at which the airway resistance was determined into account. For

these reasons, specific conductance, not airway resistance, is the most useful measure to be obtained.

Reversibility of airflow limitation, if present, is a common feature of all but the most severe asthmatic patients. The post-bronchodilator FEV$_1$ is the best determinant of airflow limitation over time as it is less susceptible to day-to-day variability and, as such, is used as a measure of

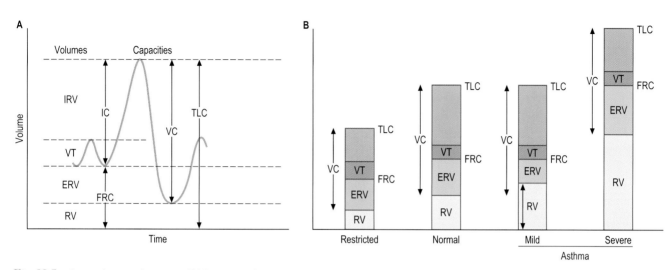

Fig. 38.5. Lung volumes and capacities. (A) Spirogram of maximal lung volume excursion. There are four lung volumes (IRV, VT, ERV, and RV) and four lung capacities (TLC, IC, FRC, and VC). A lung capacity is made up of more than one lung volume. (B) Lung volumes of various patients. Restrictive lung disease is, by definition, a reduction in total lung capacity. In asthma, or other obstructive lung disorders, lung volume(s) rises. In mild asthma, the first change is a rise in RV; more severe cases show rises in FRC and TLC. RV, residual volume; ERV, expiratory reserve volume; VT, tidal volume; IRV, inspiratory reserve volume; TLC, total lung volume; VC, vital capacity; IC, inspiratory capacity; FRC, functional reserve capacity.

the more permanent effects of inflammation.[48,49] Some individuals will have an isolated change in FVC as a result of the release of trapped air with bronchodilation, resulting in a shift of the flow-volume curve that maintains the FEV_1 at the same level pre- and post-bronchodilator, which is called the isovolume shift. Isovolume shifts are a rare occurrence in isolation but may contribute to asthma symptoms, especially chest tightness.[50,51] Response to a bronchodilator has been linked to the presence of airway inflammation,[52] and as such it is an important adjunct to office spirometry.

AIRWAY HYPER-RESPONSIVENESS

Airways of asthmatic subjects are hyper-responsive; the airways of asthmatics will react to a lower dose, and constrict more, in response to a bronchoconstrictor than the airways of normal individuals. In other words, a hyper-responsive airway is one that reacts too readily and too much. Hyper-responsiveness is most commonly demonstrated by a methacholine challenge. This form of bronchial challenge involves delivering methacholine (a chemical analogue of acetylcholine) in increasing concentrations, via nebulization and determining the FEV_1 after each dose. Individuals with hyper-responsive airways will react to a lower dose of methacholine and have a larger drop in FEV_1 than normals (Fig. 38.8). The main outcome variable assessed is the PC_{20}, which is a provocative concentration of methacholine that causes the FEV_1 to fall 20% from baseline.[53] Treatment with inhaled steroids leads to a reduction in bronchial reactivity, beginning as early as 6h after the first dose of inhaled steroid and peaking at 6 weeks.[54] If treatment with inhaled corticosteroids is delayed, the benefit in terms of improved bronchial reactivity is reduced,[55,56] which suggests that inhaled corticosteroids are

preventing an irreversible change – perhaps airway remodeling. It has been shown that intensive treatment with inhaled corticosteroids and careful monitoring can completely normalize the PC_{20}.[28]

Why are asthmatic airways hyper-responsive? All of the structural changes that are observed in the asthmatic lung, as outlined above, likely contribute to altered responsiveness. Airway wall thickening and a subsequent decreased airway intraluminal diameter alone have been thought to result in hyper-responsiveness.[14,28] Epithelial damage has also been suggested as a cause of airway hyper-responsiveness mostly through its effects on mediators that relax and keep control of the smooth muscle, but in humans, a functional link between epithelial damage and hyper-responsiveness has not be established.[57] Smooth muscle is also a likely contributor given that it is the contraction of airway smooth muscle, which narrows airways in both asthma exacerbations and during methacholine challenge. However, it is important to note that there has been no clear link between in vivo smooth muscle hyper-responsiveness and in vitro smooth muscle hyper-responsiveness.[58,59] Taken together, this suggests that airways hyper-responsiveness is due to the ensemble of changes in airway structure and not to changes in just one component or mechanism.

LUNG PARENCHYMA

Once it was a commonly held notion that the parenchyma is spared in asthma, but more recent evidence suggests that this is probably not the case. Inflammatory cells, notably eosinophils, can be found in the alveolar tissue of asthmatic patients; the presence of these eosinophils correlates with changes in lung function.[60] This is of potentially major importance; resistance of the lung is not entirely generated by airway resistance, but also has a significant tissue component (tissue resistance), which is thought to arise as a result of inhomogeneous viscoelastic properties.

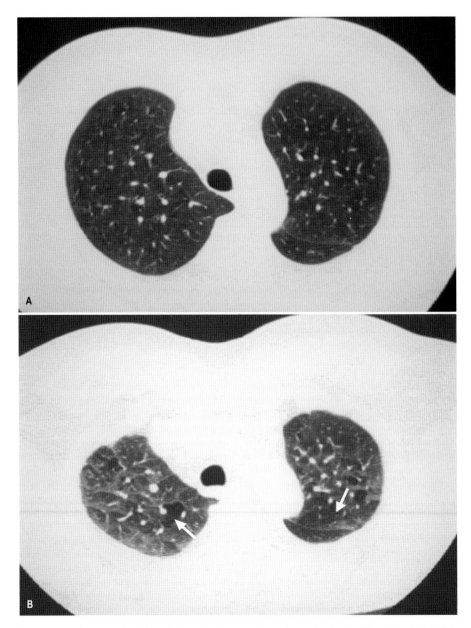

Fig. 38.6. High-resolution computed tomography (HRCT) through the upper thorax during inspiration (A) and expiration (B). On expiration, the HRCT should demonstrate homogenous increase in radiodensity in the lung parenchyma; instead, areas of persistent radiolucency are visible (white arrows), demonstrating the retention of trapped gas behind obstructed small airways. (Figures courtesy of Jeffery Klein, MD.)

It is important to note that even patients with mild asthma, and normal spirometry, have peripheral airflow resistance that is 10-fold greater than normal.[61,62] There is evidence that tissue resistance is a major contributor to the increased resistance and hyper-responsiveness observed during airway inflammation.[63] Elastic recoil of the parenchyma, as measured by pressure-volume curves, is decreased in some asthmatic patients;[64,65] this contributes to air trapping and hyperinflation as less volume will be expelled with each breath. Newer formulations of inhaled medications that

utilize hydrofluoroalkane instead of chlorofluorocarbons have a much smaller particle size and are therefore likely to reach the parenchyma.[66] It is widely speculated that such improvements in aerosol delivery will potentially more effectively treat distal lung inflammation. There is some indication that this is true,[67] but benefit has only been shown in terms of quality of life and not improved lung function. Oral delivery of therapeutics has the virtue of better delivery to the distal lung as they reach the lung through the pulmonary circulation. Unlike treatments that cannot

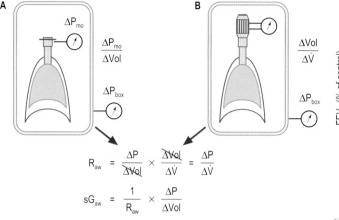

Fig. 38.7. Determination of airway resistance (R_{aw}) and specific conductance (sG_{aw}) by the body plethysmograph. (A) Patient (lung within the box) pants against a closed shutter to obtain the mouth (alveolar) pressure/box volume relationship. (B) Next, the shutter opens and the patient continues to pant. The box volume and airflow relationships are obtained. R_{aw} is calculated as shown and then 'corrected' for lung volume to obtain sG_{aw}.

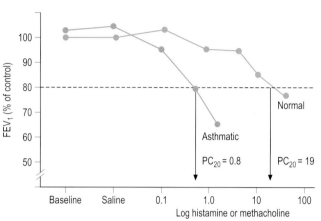

Fig. 38.8. Bronchial responsiveness. The responsiveness of the airways is determined by measuring lung function, e.g., FEV_1, as a function of the concentration of an inhaled bronchoactive agonist, either histamine or, more commonly, methacholine. FEV_1 is expressed as a percentage of control, either baseline or following saline inhalation, and is plotted for a normal (solid line) or an asthmatic patient (dotted line). Responsiveness is determined as the interpolated dose of agonist that causes the FEV_1 to fall 20% (PC_{20}). The asthmatic responds early and at a lower dose than the normal (left shift dose-response curve).

pass beyond a closed airway, oral medications may be more effective in reversing inflammation in the distal lung. A recent study with the oral medication montelukast suggests this may be the case.[68]

AIRWAY AND PARENCHYMAL INTERDEPENDENCE

The parenchyma is physically linked to the airway by means of the attachment of alveolar septae to the airway wall. During normal tidal breathing these 'tethers' are thought to be relatively slack, but when lung volume increases, they become taut – this applies radial traction to the airway, causing airway resistance to fall (Fig. 38.9). In other words, the parenchyma and the airways are interdependent.[69] These tethers work to oppose airway narrowing unless they are effectively broken by subepithelial fibrosis, inflammation, and airway wall thickening as occurs with airway remodeling.

The concept of airway-parenchyma interdependence is strongly supported by the observed effects of deep inspiration on airway hyper-responsiveness. When normal persons are prohibited from taking a deep breath, they demonstrate a similar degree of hyper-responsiveness to that of asthma (Fig. 38.10), which resolves when they are allowed to take a deep breath. On the other hand, deep breaths do not alter hyper-responsiveness in asthma; this suggests that the bronchodilating effect of a deep breath is lost,[70] with the loss of parenchyma-airway interdependence the asthmatic lung is unable to effectively 'pull' open the airways. Further evidence is provided by the observation that patients with nocturnal asthma have acute and transient changes in airway resistance which are uncoupled from changes in lung volume,[71] coinciding with the migration of inflammatory cells into the airway;[60] accordingly, inflammation is uncoupling the parenchyma from the airway. Alternatively, this effect has been attributed to the effects of mediators such as nitric oxide, changes in the physical properties of smooth muscle with deep inspiration,[72] or changes in vagal tone.[73] Overall, the importance of all these factors is supported by modeling approaches[74] which suggest that airway wall thickening and the loss of parenchyma-airway interdependence may be some of the most important factors in determining airway hyper-responsiveness.

AIRWAY CLOSURE

While complete airway closure, mostly due to mucus plugging, has been recognized for some time as part of the pathophysiology of status asthmatics, evidence is mounting that airway closure occurs in most asthmatic subjects, including those with mild disease.[75-77] This enhanced tendency towards airway closure is of an unknown etiology, but it stands to reason that an important contribution comes from airway secretions.

Animal studies have shown that peripheral resistance increases with bronchoconstriction in a heterogeneous manner,[78,63] presumably in part because of small airways closure. More recent studies in mice show that airway closure accounts for airways hyper-responsiveness[79] and that dissolution of fibrin-induced airway closure will reverse this effect.[79] Bronchoscopic studies have shown that small collateral channels, alveolar ducts, and terminal bronchi react to methacholine and, indeed, in all likelihood, close.[76,62] In patients with nocturnal asthma, distal lung airway closure was assessed as increased RV and correlated to airways hyper-responsiveness.[62] The most convincing evidence of airway closure in asthma is provided by imaging the lung with polarized helium or techniques that make ventilation defects due to airway closure visibly apparent (Fig. 38.11).[80] This paradigm shift has important ramifications on our notions of how asthma therapeutics actually work.

PFT INTERPRETATION

The structure and function of the lung takes on practical importance in the interpretation of lung function testing results. The greatest insight from pulmonary function tests (PFTs) occurs when they are associated

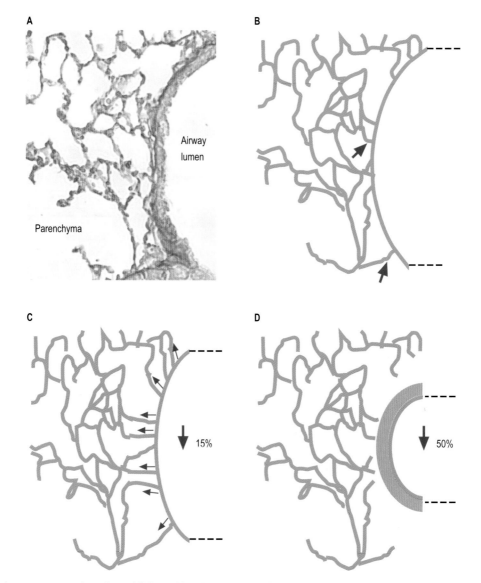

Fig. 38.9. Parenchyma-airway interdependence. (A) Stained histological section of a lung with the airway and parenchyma readily apparent. Attachments of the alveolar septae to the outer portion of the airway wall (red arrows, B) function as tethers applying outward tension (red arrows, C) when a normal (un-remodeled) airway constricts. When an airway is remodeled (shaded area, D), the tethers are effectively, although not literally, broken, allowing the airway to constrict more than is seen with an un-remodeled airway.

with clinical history and radiological (CT) studies, though considerable insight is obtained even if read in isolation from other clinical information. However, full advantage of PFTs is best obtained with a clear and complete understanding of the foregoing discussion of the basic structure and function of the respiratory system. The following approach is suggested and is based on our clinical experience in view of the paucity of guidance provided for interpretation of pulmonary function tests in the medical literature; however, the interested reader is referred to a few references that will provide some additional guidance.[81,82] What is presented below is a basic 'step-by-step' approach to integrate common

questions with the interpretation of data derived from standard PFTs (Table 38.1). Further detail can be obtained from another discussion of the subject.[83]

It is assumed, for this discussion, that a complete set of lung function tests have been ordered: lung volumes, flow-volume loops, diffusion capacity, and an acute response to bronchodilator. Additional tests to be considered are a methacholine or an exercise challenge. Other studies, such as pressure-volume curves or cardiopulmonary stress tests, could and, if indicated, should be considered in the individual case as guided by the clinical picture.

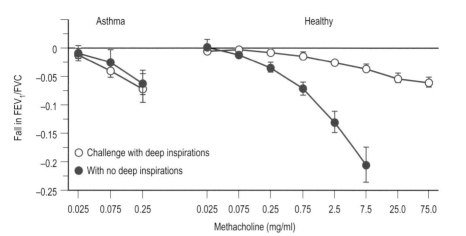

Fig. 38.10. Effects of deep inspiration. Ten subjects with asthma and 11 healthy controls undergoing two methacholine bronchoprovocations. On one occasion, conventional spirometry is performed (full expiratory maneuvers, from total lung capacity to residual volume), which involves deep inspirations. The slope of the reduction in the forced expiratory volume in 1 s/forced vital capacity (FEV_1/FVC) ratio is much steeper in the asthmatic patient compared with the healthy subjects, who received up to 75 mg/mL of methacholine with minimal effect. On second occasion, methacholine provocation is performed in the absence of deep inspirations (partial expiratory maneuvers, from end-tidal inspiration to residual volume). The slope of the reduction in the partial FEV_1/FVC ratio is similar in both groups because, in the absence of deep inspirations, healthy controls demonstrate significant loss of lung function at concentrations of methacholine that are within the asthmatic range (<7.5 mg/mL). In contrast, the presence or absence of deep inspirations does not appear to influence airway responsiveness of the asthmatic subjects. If the two groups are compared with respect to the slope of the reduction in FEV_1/FVC, in the absence of deep inspiration the difference is very small. The challenge does not progress to higher doses of methacholine in the asthma group because baseline lung function is already low (data not shown) and the reduction induced by methacholine drops lung function to a point that is the cutoff point for safety concerns. (Modified from Skloot et al,[70] data courtesy of Alkis Togias, Johns Hopkins University.)

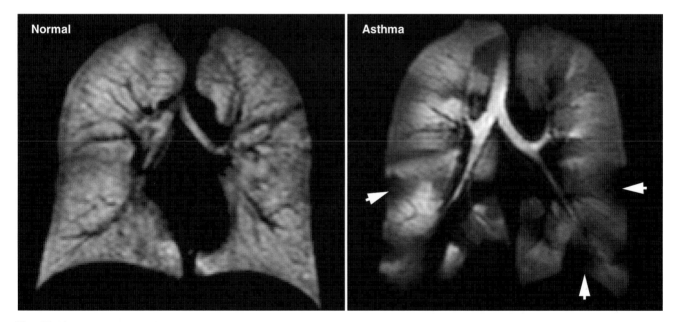

Fig. 38.11. Ventilation defect. Magnetic resonance scan of healthy individual (A) who inhaled polarized helium shows homogeneous distribution of the gas. In asthma (B) the polarized helium distribution is heterogeneous, demonstrating multiple ventilation defects (arrowheads), presumably from airway closure. (Courtesy of John P Mulger III, Center for In-vivo Hyperpolarized Gas MR Imaging, University of Virginia.)

Table 38.1 Questions to be addressed – PFT interpretation

1. Was patient effort acceptable? What was overall test quality?

2. Assess patient demographics; how useful are the reference equations in this case?

3. Review flow-volume loops and/or spirograms, are there characteristic findings?

4. Assess FEV_1, FVC, and then the FEV_1/FVC; what is the degree of airflow limitation?

5. Is there a significant bronchodilator response and is there residual obstruction?

6. Is the TLC low (restriction), normal, or elevated (obstruction)? Is FRC low, normal, or high? Is the RV elevated? Are the lung volumes consistent with asthma and its severity?

7. Is the D_{LCO} elevated? Is VA low or similar to TLC?

8. Is the PC_{20} below 8 mg/mL?

9. Do the patterns of PFT results confirm the clinical impression or are they at odds?

QUALITY OF TEST RESULTS AND CONCEPTS OF NORMALCY

The first step in assessing lung function is to determine test quality.[84] While it may stand to reason that tests of poor quality have limited usefulness, it is known that even poor tests often can be helpful.[41,84] The guidelines for test quality are well known, so will not be repeated here in detail,[44,53] but some key elements include reproducibility and good patient performance. Spirometry should be reproducible (+150 mL), and good patient performance is best assessed by direct observation, or at least by careful annotations by the person performing the test. In a situation where poor test performance is suspected, increased reliance should then be placed on those endpoints that are less effort-dependent: functional residual capacity (FRC), specific conductance, DLCO, and evidence of a flow-volume envelope even if it occurs at the point of mid vital capacity flows (Fig. 38.3B).

The next step is to assess the applicability of the so-called predicted equations for the specific patient in question. For some patients, e.g., a 30-year-old white male who is 5 feet 10 inches high, the equations for FEV_1 and FVC are probably a fairly good estimate of normalcy. For others, e.g., a very short Asian boy of 13 years, the 'predictions' are much less accurate because there are fewer Asian-specific equations available. Short stature leads to false positives, and persons during growth spurts have more variable lung functions. Nevertheless, age, gender, race, and height explain only 70% of the variance,[44,85] which means that 30% of the variance in lung function is simple biology; it is for these reasons that some prefer to use the term 'reference equations' rather than 'predicted equations'. While many equations for FEV_1/FVC exist, it is recommended that the study of NHANES III[86] be used, as these are currently the most complete values,[84] covering a large age range and include race-specific equations. The availability of current data for other endpoints, e.g., lung volumes (see below), is even less reliable; accordingly, it is recommended that one should observe the changes with time or follow the response to therapy.

While most interpretations simply comment on the presented values for FEV_1 and FVC, it is important to first review each of the flow-volume curves looking for reproducibility and characteristic patterns (Fig. 38.4); while physicians in practice can correctly identify airflow limitation and a significant response to bronchodilation, many fail to observe a fixed, or variable, intra/extrathoracic lesion. Mixed disease patterns are particularly problematic. Some common variants are the shape of the inspiratory flow-volume loop caused by vocal cord dysfunction (VCD) – a known co-morbid condition of asthma. A probable diagnosis of VCD can be made only if the shape of the inspiratory limb is abnormal and not limited to just one or two loops.

ASSESS AIRFLOW LIMITATION AND BRONCHODILATOR RESPONSES

The response to bronchodilators is a critical addition to PFT testing in asthma (Fig. 38.4D). The current recommendations state[44,84] that only a 12% and at least a 200 mL change is to be considered clinically significant. A change of 8% or 150 mL may be due to inherent variability of testing,[44,87] and forms the rationale for current 12% and 200 mL index.

However, failure to achieve this magnitude of a bronchodilator response does not preclude the prescribing of bronchodilators, as the response will vary with the activity of the disease. Moreover, bronchodilator responses are often taken as a measure of underlying inflammation.[49] The addition of specific conductance is also warranted as this measure is notably different from flow-volume determinants[88] and certainly is different in a subset of patients presenting with reversible airways disease.[51] Incomplete reversal of airflow limitation (Fig. 38.4D) is also an indication of lung remodeling and the need for additional therapy.[48,49,89]

LUNG VOLUMES: RESTRICTION VERSUS OBSTRUCTION

Measurement of lung volumes promises critical insight into the function of the lung, for it is the size of the lung that determines the overall gas exchange capacity. As FVC is the major predictor of morbidity,[41] it is reasonable to assume that this is because a temporal decrease in FVC represents the loss of gas exchange units, placing the patient at risk.

The measurements of TLC, FRC, and RV are the most useful indices of lung volume to obtain (Fig. 38.5). Falls in TLC (<80% of predicted) are interpreted as a restrictive processes, whereas rises in the TLC (>120% of predicted) are indicative of obstruction such as observed in more chronic or persistent asthma. The rise in TLC is greatest in the most severe cases and, if not readily reversed with acute treatment with a bronchodilator, would indicate that remodeling of the lung has occurred. Elevations in RV (>150% of predicted) are usually the first alteration in lung volume and are also a sensitive measure of small airways function[62] because RV is a function of airway closure.[38] In lieu of measurements of RV, the difference between slow vital capacity (SVC) and the forced vital capacity (FVC) may provide an alternative estimate of airway closure and gas trapping. The obese patient presents a particular, and common, problem in interpretation. The effect of body weight when the patient weighs above 0.5 kg/cm is to cause FRC to fall and above 1.0 kg/cm can cause TLC to fall.[90] Lastly, it is important to note that the studies most commonly used for lung volumes were made years ago, and people in general are now taller so that the predictions for lung volume generally run about 10% low (C Irvin, personal observations).

CLASSIFICATION OF AIRFLOW LIMITATION WITH DLCO

Measurement of the diffusing capacity of carbon monoxide (DLCO)[91] can be quite useful in two regards. First, the DLCO contributes to the assessment of airway disease. In the patient with emphysema, the DLCO is reduced in proportion to the loss of lung tissue.[91,92] This is important as patients who smoke will often present with a self-diagnosis of asthma – a disease they know to be more socially acceptable and, more importantly, treatable. In the case of COPD, the DLCO will be diminished, while in patients with asthma, DLCO is normal or elevated. The elevated DLCO is suggestive of active inflammation and the uptake of CO by red blood cells that are known to be present in the bronchoalveolar lavage fluid of asthmatic subjects; thus an elevated DLCO will be found in asthma that is uncontrolled. Another useful aspect of the DLCO is that one typically determines the alveolar volume (VA) as part of determining the DLCO. Alveolar volume is determined by a single breath measurement of a gas dilution, and, as such, measures gas volume that is communicating with the airway opening. In normal subjects the VA should equal TLC ($+200\,mL$), but in the setting of air trapping, the VA will be less than the TLC since the trapped air is not communicating with the airway opening. Hence, the TLC – VA difference can be used to detect the presence of air trapping. Lastly, it is important to note that the DLCO has little correlation to gas exchange (e.g. PaO_2) per se, and that the DLCO is, in essence, a measurement of the potentially available lung for gas exchange.

BRONCHIAL CHALLENGE

Details of bronchial challenge are found in professional society publications[53] and elsewhere within this textbook. Probably the most important aspect of bronchial challenge, from an interpretation point of view, is the fact that, for the diagnosis of asthma, bronchial challenge is a sensitive but not specific determinant. Patients with many other diseases, COPD, ARDS and cystic fibrosis, will present with bronchial hyper-responsiveness. Although, if the PC_{20} is less than $1\,mg/mL$, then the specificity of the test increases considerably, and it has been suggested that the PC_{20} can also be used to stage the severity of the disease.[53] Like the response to acute treatment with bronchodilation, changes in the measures of bronchial challenge can be used to assess inflammatory activity.[28] Probably the single most important point to make is that bronchial challenge results must be linked to current symptoms to be useful. In addition, in some patients (e.g., following antigen challenge), the PC_{20} falls and then resolves very quickly, making the connection to current clinical presentation difficult, which is important to recognize.

Assessment of a bronchial response to exercise is less often indicated[53] but can be useful to assess airway responsiveness in the child or athlete. It is important to understand that there is not a complete overlap in hyper-responsiveness in patients who are methacholine and exercise positive.[93] This finding suggests that the mechanisms involved may not be the same and also indicates that, in some cases, both tests may need to be performed.

▨ INTERPRETATION SUMMARY ▨

Knowledge of the physiology and structure of the lung is clinically useful. Asthma is the most significant disease in this regard, as the syndrome is defined by a pattern of lung dysfunction that characterizes the disorder. In fact, asthma is the only lung disease that is diagnosed solely on the basis of clinical presentation and pulmonary function tests. Interpretation of pulmonary function tests requires an in-depth knowledge of both the structures and function of the lung. Interpretation of a battery of lung function tests should include elements of test quality, lung volume considerations, presence of airflow limitation, and the response to bronchodilation. DLCO and bronchial challenge provide further clarification of the nature of the airflow limitation present. In addition to diagnosis, lung function tests provide an invaluable guide to the progress of the disease or its resolution to successful treatment.

References

Lung development

1. Chinoy MR. Lung growth and development. Front Biosci 2003; 8:d392–d415.
2. Irvin CG. Interaction between the growing lung and asthma: role of early intervention. J Allergy Clin Immunol 2000; 105:S540–S546.
3. Dezateux C, Stocks J, Wade AM, et al. Airway function at one year: association with premorbid airway function, wheezing, and maternal smoking. Thorax 2001; 56:680–686.
4. McCoy K, Shade DM, Irvin CG, et al. Predicting episodes of poor asthma control in treated patients with asthma. J Allergy Clin Immunol 2006; 118:1226–1233.
5. Spahn JD, Cherniack R, Paull K, et al. Is forced expiratory volume in one second the best measure of severity in childhood asthma? Am J Respir Crit Care Med 2004; 169:784–786.
6. Papastamelos C, Panitch HB, England SE, et al. Developmental changes in chest wall compliance in infancy and early childhood. J Appl Physiol 1995; 78:179–184.
7. Merkus PJ, Borsboom GJ, Van Pelt W, et al. Growth of airways and air spaces in teenagers is related to sex but not to symptoms. J Appl Physiol 1993; 75:2045–2053.
8. Wright AL. Epidemiology of asthma and recurrent wheeze in childhood. Clin Rev Allergy Immunol 2002; 22:33–44.

Airway remodeling

9. Brown RH, Pearse DB, Pyrgos G, et al. The structural basis of airways hyper-responsiveness in asthma. J Appl Physiol 2006; 101:30–39.
10. de Jong PA, Muller NL, Pare PD, et al. Computed tomographic imaging of the airways: relationship to structure and function. Eur Respir J 2005; 26:140–152.
11. Little SA, Sproule MW, Cowan MD, et al. High resolution computed tomographic assessment of airway wall thickness in chronic asthma: reproducibility and relationship with lung function and severity. Thorax 2002; 57:247–253.
12. Niimi A, Matsumoto H, Amitani R, et al. Airway wall thickness in asthma assessed by computed tomography. Relation to clinical indices. Am J Respir Crit Care Med 2000; 162:1518–1523.
13. Niimi A, Matsumoto H, Amitani R, et al. Effect of short-term treatment with inhaled corticosteroid on airway wall thickening in asthma. Am J Med 2004; 116:725–731.
14. James AL, Pare PD, Hogg JC. The mechanics of airway narrowing in asthma. Am Rev Respir Dis 1989; 139:242–246.
15. Laitinen LA, Heino M, Laitinen A, et al. Damage of the airway epithelium and bronchial reactivity in patients with asthma. Am Rev Respir Dis 1985; 131:599–606.
16. Lozewicz S, Wells C, Gomez E, et al. Morphological integrity of the bronchial epithelium in mild asthma. Thorax 1990; 45:12–15.
17. Ordonez C, Ferrando R, Hyde DM, et al. Epithelial desquamation in asthma: artifact or pathology? Am J Respir Crit Care Med 2000; 162:2324–2329.
18. Hallstrand TS, Moody MW, Aitken ML, et al. Airway immunopathology of asthma with exercise-induced bronchoconstriction. J Allergy Clin Immunol 2005; 116:586–593.
19. Oddera S, Silvestri M, Balbo A, et al. Airway eosinophilic inflammation, epithelial damage, and bronchial hyper-responsiveness in patients with mild-moderate, stable asthma. Allergy 1996; 51:100–107.
20. Bleck B, Tse DB, Jaspers I, et al. Diesel exhaust particle-exposed human bronchial epithelial cells induce dendritic cell maturation. J Immunol 2006; 176:7431–7437.
21. Beasley R, Roche WR, Roberts JA, et al. Cellular events in the bronchi in mild asthma and after bronchial provocation. Am Rev Respir Dis 1989; 139:806–817.
22. Huang J, Olivenstein R, Taha R, et al. Enhanced proteoglycan deposition in the airway wall of atopic asthmatics. Am J Respir Crit Care Med 1999; 160:725–729.
23. Mautino G, Capony F, Bousquet J, et al. Balance in asthma between matrix metalloproteinases and their inhibitors. J Allergy Clin Immunol 1999; 104:530–533.
24. Braunstahl GJ, Fokkens WJ, Overbeek SE, et al. Mucosal and systemic inflammatory changes in allergic rhinitis and asthma: a comparison between upper and lower airways. Clin Exp Allergy 2003; 33:579–587.
25. Chu HW, Halliday JL, Martin RJ, et al. Collagen deposition in large airways may not differentiate severe asthma from milder forms of the disease. Am J Respir Crit Care Med 1998; 158:1936–1944.
26. Pepe C, Foley S, Shannon J, et al. Differences in airway remodeling between subjects with severe and moderate asthma. J Allergy Clin Immunol 2005; 116:544–549.
27. Bergeron C, Hauber HP, Gotfried M, et al. Evidence of remodeling in peripheral airways of patients with mild to moderate asthma: effect of hydrofluoroalkane-flunisolide. J Allergy Clin Immunol 2005; 116:983–989.

28. Sont JK, Willems LN, Bel EH, et al. Clinical control and histopathologic outcome of asthma when using airway hyper-responsiveness as an additional guide to long-term treatment. The AMPUL Study Group. Am J Respir Crit Care Med 1999; 159:1043–1051.
29. Morcillo EJ, Cortijo J. Mucus and MUC in asthma. Curr Opin Pulm Med 2006; 12:1–6.
30. de Marco R, Marcon A, Jarvis D, et al. Prognostic factors of asthma severity: a 9-year international prospective cohort study. J Allergy Clin Immunol 2006; 117:1249–1256.
31. Aikawa T, Shimura S, Sasaki H, et al. Marked goblet cell hyperplasia with mucus accumulation in the airways of patients who died of severe acute asthma attack. Chest 1992; 101:916–921.
32. Flora GS, Sharma AM, Sharma OP. Asthma mortality in a metropolitan county hospital, a 38-year study. Allergy Proc 1991; 12:169–179.
33. Carroll N, Carello S, Cooke C, et al. Airway structure and inflammatory cells in fatal attacks of asthma. Eur Respir J 1996; 9:709–715.
34. Hashimoto M, Tanaka H, Abe S. Quantitative analysis of bronchial wall vascularity in the medium and small airways of patients with asthma and COPD. Chest 2005; 127:965–972.
35. Chetta A, Zanini A, Foresi A, et al. Vascular endothelial growth factor up-regulation and bronchial wall remodelling in asthma. Clin Exp Allergy 2005; 35:1437–1442.
36. Woodruff PG, Dolganov GM, Ferrando RE, et al. Hyperplasia of smooth muscle in mild to moderate asthma without changes in cell size or gene expression. Am J Respir Crit Care Med 2004; 169:1001–1006.
37. Joubert P, Hamid Q. Role of airway smooth muscle in airway remodeling. J Allergy Clin Immunol 2005; 116:713–716.

Airflow limitation

38. Irvin CG, Cherniack RM. Pathophysiology and physiological assessment of the asthmatic patient. Semin Respir Med 1987; 8:201–215.
39. Orehek J, Beaupre A, Badier M, et al. Perception of airway tone by asthmatic patients. Bull Eur Physiopathol Respir 1982; 18:601–607.
40. Burrows B. Course and prognosis of patients with chronic airways obstruction. Chest 1980; 77:250–251.
41. Ferguson GT, Enright PL, Buist AS, et al. Office spirometry for lung health assessment in adults: a consensus statement from the National Lung Health Education Program. Chest 2000; 117:1146–1161.
42. Mead J, Turner JM, Macklem PT, et al. Significance of the relationship between lung recoil and maximum expiratory flow. J Appl Physiol 1967; 22:95–108.
43. Cockcroft DW, Berscheid BA. Volume adjustment of maximal midexpiratory flow. Importance of changes in total lung capacity. Chest 1980; 78:595–600.
44. American Thoracic Society. Lung function testing: selection of reference values and interpretative strategies. Am Rev Respir Dis 1991; 144:1202–1218.
45. Paggiaro PL, Moscato G, Giannini D, et al. Relationship between peak expiratory flow (PEF) and FEV1. Eur Respir J 1997; 24:39S–41S.
46. Goldin JG, McNitt-Gray MF, Sorenson SM, et al. Airway hyperreactivity: assessment with helical thin-section CT. Radiology 1998; 208:321–329.
47. Irvin CG. Lessons from structure-function studies in asthma: myths and truths about what we teach. J Appl Physiol 2006; 101:7–9.
48. Dixon AE, Irvin CG. Early intervention of therapy in asthma. Curr Opin Pulm Med 2005; 11:51–55.
49. Enright PL, Lebowitz MD, Cockroft DW. Physiologic measures: pulmonary function tests. Asthma outcome. Am J Respir Crit Care Med 1994; 149:S9–S18, discussion S19–S20.
50. Kraft M, Cairns CB, Ellison MS, et al. Improvements in distal lung function correlate with asthma symptoms after treatment with oral montelukast. Chest 2006; 130:1726–1732.
51. Smith HR, Irvin CG, Cherniack RM. The utility of spirometry in the diagnosis of reversible airways obstruction. Chest 1992; 101:1577–1581.
52. Virchow JC Jr, Holscher U, Virchow C Sr. Sputum ECP levels correlate with parameters of airflow obstruction. Am Rev Respir Dis 1992; 146:604–606.

Airway hyper-responsiveness

53. Crapo RO, Casaburi R, Coates AL, et al. Guidelines for methacholine and exercise challenge testing, 1999. This official statement of the American Thoracic Society was adopted by the ATS Board of Directors, July 1999. Am J Respir Crit Care Med 2000; 161:309–329.
54. Vathenen AS, Knox AJ, Wisniewski A, et al. Time course of change in bronchial reactivity with an inhaled corticosteroid in asthma. Am Rev Respir Dis 1991; 143:1317–1321.
55. Overbeek SE, Kerstjens HA, Bogaard JM, et al. Is delayed introduction of inhaled corticosteroids harmful in patients with obstructive airways disease (asthma and COPD)? The Dutch CNSLD Study Group. The Dutch Chronic Nonspecific Lung Disease Study Groups. Chest 1996; 110:35–41.
56. Selroos O, Pietinalho A, Lofroos AB, et al. Effect of early vs late intervention with inhaled corticosteroids in asthma. Chest 1995; 108:1228–1234.
57. O'Byrne PM, Dolovich M, Dirks R, et al. Lung epithelial permeability: relation to nonspecific airway responsiveness. J Appl Physiol 1984; 57:77–84.
58. Armour CL, Lazar NM, Schellenberg RR, et al. A comparison of in vivo and in vitro human airway reactivity to histamine. Am Rev Respir Dis 1984; 129:907–910.
59. Roberts JA, Raeburn D, Rodger IW, et al. Comparison of in vivo airway responsiveness and in vitro smooth muscle sensitivity to methacholine in man. Thorax 1984; 39:837–843.

Lung parenchyma

60. Kraft M, Djukanovic R, Wilson S, et al. Alveolar tissue inflammation in asthma. Am J Respir Crit Care Med 1996; 154:1505–1510.
61. Kaminsky DA, Irvin CG, Gurka DA, et al. Peripheral airways responsiveness to cool, dry air in normal and asthmatic individuals. Am J Respir Crit Care Med 1995; 152:1784–1790.

62. Kraft M, Pak J, Martin RJ, et al. Distal lung dysfunction at night in nocturnal asthma. Am J Respir Crit Care Med 2001; 163:1551–1556.
63. Tomioka S, Bates JH, Irvin CG. Airway and tissue mechanics in a murine model of asthma: alveolar capsule vs. forced oscillations. J Appl Physiol 2002; 93:263–270.
64. Gelb AF, Zamel N. Unsuspected pseudophysiologic emphysema in chronic persistent asthma. Am J Respir Crit Care Med 2000; 162:1778–1782.
65. Gold WM, Kaufman HS, Nadel JA. Elastic recoil of the lungs in chronic asthmatic patients before and after therapy. J Appl Physiol 1967; 23:433–438.
66. Martin RJ. Therapeutic significance of distal airway inflammation in asthma. J Allergy Clin Immunol 2002; 109:S447–S460.
67. Juniper EF, Price DB, Stampone PA, et al. Clinically important improvements in asthma-specific quality of life, but no difference in conventional clinical indexes in patients changed from conventional beclomethasone dipropionate to approximately half the dose of extrafine beclomethasone dipropionate. Chest 2002; 121:1824–1832.
68. Kraft M, Cairns CB, Ellison MC, et al. Improvements in distal lung function correlate with asthma symptoms after treatment with oral montelukast. Chest 2006; 130:1726–1732.
69. Macklem PT. A theoretical analysis of the effect of airway smooth muscle load on airway narrowing. Am J Respir Crit Care Med 1996; 153:83–89.
70. Skloot G, Permutt S, Togias A. Airway hyper-responsiveness in asthma: a problem of limited smooth muscle relaxation with inspiration. J Clin Invest 1995; 96:2393–2403.
71. Irvin CG, Pak J, Martin RJ. Airway-parenchyma uncoupling in nocturnal asthma. Am J Respir Crit Care Med 2000; 161:50–56.
72. Fredberg JJ. Frozen objects: small airways, big breaths, and asthma. J Allergy Clin Immunol 2000; 106:615–624.
73. Irvin CG, Dempsey JA. Role of H1 and H2 receptors in increased small airways resistance in the dog. Respir Physiol 1978; 35:161–176.
74. Wiggs BR, Bosken C, Pare PD, et al. A model of airway narrowing in asthma and in chronic obstructive pulmonary disease. Am Rev Respir Dis 1992; 145:1251–1258.

Airway closure

75. In'tVeen JC, Beekman AJ, Bel EH, et al. Recurrent exacerbations in severe asthma are associated with enhanced airway closure during stable episodes. Am J Respir Crit Care Med 2000; 161:1902–1906.
76. Kaminsky DA, Bates JH, Irvin CG. Effects of cool, dry air stimulation on peripheral lung mechanics in asthma. Am J Respir Crit Care Med 2000; 162:179–186.
77. King GG, Eberl S, Salome CM, et al. Differences in airway closure between normal and asthmatic subjects measured with single-photon emission computed tomography and technegas. Am J Respir Crit Care Med 1998; 158:1900–1906.
78. Bates JH, Schuessler TF, Dolman C, et al. Temporal dynamics of acute isovolume bronchoconstriction in the rat. J Appl Physiol 1997; 82:55–62.
79. Wagers SS, Norton RJ, Rinaldi LM, et al. Extravascular fibrin, plasminogen activator, plasminogen activator inhibitors, and airway hyper-responsiveness. J Clin Invest 2004; 114:104–111.
80. Altes TA, Powers PL, Knight-Scott J, et al. Hyperpolarized 3He MR lung ventilation imaging in asthmatics: preliminary findings. J Magn Reson Imaging 2001; 13:378–384.

PFT interpretation

81. Pellegrino R, Viegi G, Brusasco V, et al. Interpretative strategies for lung function tests. Eur Respir J 2005; 26:948–968.
82. Pennock BE, Cottrell JJ, Rogers RM. Pulmonary function testing. What is 'normal'? Arch Intern Med 1983; 143:2123–2127.
83. Irvin CG. Guide to the evaluation of pulmonary function. In: Hamid Q, Shannon J, Martin J, eds. Physiological basis of respiratory disease. Hamilton: Decker; 2005.
84. Miller MR, Hankinson J, Brusasco V, et al. Standardisation of spirometry. Eur Respir J 2005; 26:319–338.
85. Hankinson JL, Bang KM. Acceptability and reproducibility criteria of the American Thoracic Society as observed in a sample of the general population. Am Rev Respir Dis 1991; 143:516–521.
86. Hankinson JL, Odencrantz JR, Fedan KB. Spirometric reference values from a sample of the general U.S. population. Am J Respir Crit Care Med 1999; 159:179–187.
87. Eliasson O, Degraff AC Jr. The use of criteria for reversibility and obstruction to define patient groups for bronchodilator trials. Influence of clinical diagnosis, spirometric, and anthropometric variables. Am Rev Respir Dis 1985; 132:858–864.
88. Kaminsky DA, Wenzel SE, Carcano C, et al. Hyperpnea-induced changes in parenchymal lung mechanics in normal subjects and in asthmatics. Am J Respir Crit Care Med 1997; 155:1260–1266.
89. The Childhood Asthma Management Program Research Group. Long-term effects of budesonide or nedocromil in children with asthma. N Engl J Med 2000; 343:1054–1063.
90. Ray CS, Sue DY, Bray G, et al. Effects of obesity on respiratory function. Am Rev Respir Dis 1983; 128:501–506.
91. Macintyre N, Crapo RO, Viegi G, et al. Standardisation of the single-breath determination of carbon monoxide uptake in the lung. Eur Respir J 2005; 26:720–735.
92. Gelb AF, Gold WM, Wright RR, et al. Physiologic diagnosis of subclinical emphysema. Am Rev Respir Dis 1973; 107:50–63.
93. Eliasson AH, Phillips YY, Rajagopal KR, et al. Sensitivity and specificity of bronchial provocation testing. An evaluation of four techniques in exercise-induced bronchospasm. Chest 1992; 102:347–355.

Airway Mucus and the Mucociliary System

39

Paula J Busse and John V Fahy

CONTENTS

SUMMARY OF IMPORTANT CONCEPTS

>> Airway mucus is an important component of the innate immune system which protects airway epithelium; however, increased production and secretion in asthma may also increase morbidity and mortality of this chronic airway disease

>> Mucus is composed of approximately 90% water; the remaining 10% contains proteins, of which the large mucin glycoproteins (encoded by the mucin (*MUC*) genes) are the most abundant

>> The mucin gene, *MUC*5AC has significantly higher expression in patients with asthma compared with normal controls

>> There are several growth factors driving the production of mucus by goblet and submucosal cells, including Th2 and some Th1 cytokines, leukotrienes, histamine, elastases, and environmental stimuli

>> Although there are currently no specific treatments for mucus hypersecretion in asthma, oral and inhaled corticosteroids are likely the most effective approved therapy which may decrease or prevent this pathologic change in the asthmatic airway

INTRODUCTION

Airway mucus has multiple functions (Table 39.1) that include hydration and protection of the airway epithelium and entrapment of foreign substances for their removal. Airway mucus forms two layers. The 'sol' layer is a watery mixture in direct contact with the airway epithelial cells. The 'gel' layer is a more elastic layer sitting on top of the sol in direct contact with the inhaled air. Cilia on epithelial cells beat freely in the sol layer, constituting an 'escalator' that moves trapped material in the gel toward the pharynx, in a process termed mucociliary clearance (MCC).

Airway mucus is a complex mixture of water, proteins, carbohydrates, and lipids. The components of mucus principally responsible for its viscoelastic properties are the mucin glycoproteins (mucins). Plasma proteins also contribute to airway mucus through processes of transudation or exudation. The cellular sources of airway mucus include airway submucosal glands (serous and mucous cells), goblet cells, ciliated epithelial cells, Clara cells, and possibly type 2 alveolar cells.

Abnormalities in mucus production, composition, and mucus clearance are a feature of most chronic airway diseases, including asthma, bronchitis, bronchiectasis, bronchiolitis, and cystic fibrosis. Mucus hypersecretion and abnormal mucus clearance in these diseases result in shared clinical features such as productive cough and airway obstruction; some of the pathophysiologic mechanisms of mucus hypersecretion may also be shared. It is beyond the scope of this chapter to review the clinical features and pathophysiologic mechanisms of mucus hypersecretion and abnormal mucus clearance in every airway disease. Instead, a review is presented of the normal physiology of airway mucus production and mucus clearance, followed by a review of abnormalities of mucus production and clearance in asthma.

Table 39.1 Functions of respiratory mucus

Preserves the mucous membrane
Lubricates
Humidifies
Waterproofs
Insulates
Provides appropriate environment for ciliary action

Acts as a barrier
Entraps microorganisms, irritants, and cellular debris
Provides extracellular surface for immunoglobulin and enzyme actions
Neutralizes toxic gases

Transports trapped materials
Works in concert with cilia to move trapped materials to nasopharynx

Modified from Kaliner M, Marom Z, Patow C, Shelhamer J. Human respiratory mucus. J Allergy Clin Immunol 1984; 73:318–323.

Table 39.2 Principal constituents of airway mucus and their sources

Constituent	Source
1. Ions and water	Ciliated epithelial cells and submucosal gland cells
2. Mucin glycoproteins	Goblet cells, mucous cells in submucosal glands
3. Proteoglycans	Serous cells
4. Proteins and peptides	
Secretory IgA	Serous cells
Lactoferrin	Serous cells, neutrophils
Lysozyme	Serous cells, macrophages
Trefoil factor peptides	Goblet cells, submucosal gland cells
5. Antiproteases and antioxidants	
Secretory leukocyte proteinase inhibitor	Serous cells, Clara cells
α_1-Antitrypsin	Transudate, macrophages
α_2-Macroglobulin	Macrophages
Peroxidases	Serous cells
6. Lipids	Clara cells, type II alveolar cells, all cell membranes
7. Albumin, plasma proteins	Plasma transudate
8. Products of cell lysis	
DNA	All cells, especially inflammatory leukocytes
Actin	All cells, especially inflammatory leukocytes

Modified and expanded from Jeffery PK. The origins of secretions in the lower respiratory tract. Eur Respir J Suppl 1987; 153:34–42.

■ CONSTITUENTS OF AIRWAY MUCUS ■

Detailed analysis of normal airway mucus reveals that approximately 90% is water and the remaining 10% is composed of protein, carbohydrate, and lipid. The non-aqueous constituents may be in the sol phase or gel phase or both, depending on their solubility. The protein constituents of airway mucus include mucin glycoproteins, proteoglycans, and a variety of other proteins important in airway host defense (Table 39.2). Glycoproteins and proteoglycans are distinct molecules characterized by the carbohydrate constituents of their oligosaccharide chains (glycans), by the nature of the glycosidic bond between the initial saccharide and the protein backbone, and by the types of amino acids in the protein backbone.[1] For example, mucin glycoproteins are 50–90% carbohydrate by weight and have O-glycosidic linkages between N-acetylactosamine and serine and/or threonine in the protein backbone, which is rich in threonine, serine, glycine, and alanine. Proteoglycans are 80–95% carbohydrate by weight and have O-glycosidic linkages between xylose and serine in the protein backbone, which is rich in serine and glycine. Whereas glycan chains in mucins typically comprise <10 sugar residues, the glycans attached to proteoglycans are very large, containing as many as a hundred residues.[2]

MUCIN GLYCOPROTEINS (MUCINS)

Although the name mucin suggests a specific molecule, mucin is a generic term denoting a group of highly glycosylated proteins synthesized by epithelial cells. Mucin glycoproteins are large complex molecules consisting of a peptide backbone and numerous oligosaccharide side chains that represent the products of mucin genes and glycosyltransferase genes, respectively.[1] Mucin molecules are among the largest in nature – ranging in size from 2 to 20×10^5 Da.[1] Electron microscopy reveals them to be linear

flexible threads. These threads are composed of a polypeptide backbone onto which multiple oligosaccharide side chains are attached (Fig. 39.1). Mucin glycoproteins may be either secreted or membrane-tethered.

The biosynthesis of a mucin glycoprotein is complex and involves several steps. The mucin glycoproteins are encoded by mucin *(MUC)* genes, which are translated to the mucin glycoprotein backbone. This backbone, in most mucin glycoproteins, is characterized by several tandem repeating nucleotides, which make up the central domain in the mucin molecule (Fig. 39.1). The tandem repeats are usually encoded by a single central exon in the *MUC* gene, although these genes can be polymorphic and can produce different repeating segments. Each tandem repeats contains a proline and several serine and/or threonine residues, which are the sites of O-glycosylation. The number of tandem repeats generally determines the mucin size; greater numbers correlate with larger mucin mass and can affect mucin conformation. Flanking the central tandem repeats, at the amino and carboxyl termini, are unique sequences of peptides which are only sparsely glycosylated and which are therefore sensitive to protease degradation (so called 'naked regions'). The backbone is then post-translationally modified by glycosyltransferases, typically resulting

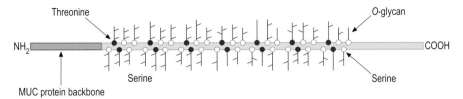

Fig. 39.1. Schematic drawing of a secretory mucin glycoprotein depicting a *MUC* protein backbone and its *O*-glycans. A *MUC* protein backbone typically consists of an NH$_2$-terminal domain (blue), one or more central domain(s) with a high number of tandem repeat (TR) domains (yellow), and a COOH-terminal domain (green). Numerous *O*-glycans are attached to threonine (●) or serine (○) residues in the TR domains. *O*-glycans exhibit size heterogeneity, which may reflect incomplete biosynthesis during elongation and termination of *O*-glycans or differences in substrate preferences of various GTs at specific serine or threonine sites. (Adapted from Rose MC, Voynow JA. Respiratory tract mucin genes and mucin glycoproteins in health and disease. Physiol Rev 2006; 86(1):245–278. Used with permissions.[1])

in the addition of several *O*-glycans. The mature, or glycosylated mucins are then either stored in granules ('secretory mucins') until specific stimuli produce their release, or remain attached to the cell membrane.

At least 20 human *MUC* genes have been identified and are numbered in chronological order of their description: *MUC*1–2, 3A, 3B, 4, *MUC*5AC, *MUC*5B, *MUC*6–9, and *MUC*11–13, and *MUC*15–20. The genes for *MUC*s 2, 5AC, 5B, and 6 are located on chromosome 11p15 and code for the major gel-forming secreted mucins. The genes for *MUC*s 1, 3, 4, 12, and 13 code for non-secreted transmembrane mucin molecules. All of these mucin genes, except *MUC*14, 15, 18, encode for mucin glycoproteins with tandem repeats in their backbone. The secretory mucins can be further classified as cysteine rich (e.g., *MUC*2, *MUC*5AC, *MUC*5B, *MUC*6) or cysteine poor (*MUC*7). Mucin gene expression may involve one or more of the MAP kinase pathways and activation of several transcription factors, including NF-κB, AP-1, and CREB.[1,3] However, the transcription factors involved may differ depending upon the initial 'trigger' of mucin gene expression.[4]

The first step in *O*-glycan synthesis is the transfer of GalNAc to Ser/Thr residues, by UDP-GalNAc:polypeptide α-GalNAc transferase (GalNAc transferase). A homologous family of UDP-GalNAc transferases initiate *O*-glycosylation, and three GalNAc transferase genes *(GALNT1, -T2, T3)* have been described.[5] A wide range of *O*-linked core structures is possible depending on the initial and subsequent substitutions on the GalNAc residue. For the terminal structures, alterations in Lewis type 1 (Le^a and Le^b) and type 2 (Le^x and Le^y) structures on mucin side chains have been described for gastric mucins.[6] The enzymes responsible for Lewis antigen synthesis are the fucosyltransferases, and 7 human 'FUT' genes have been cloned. Among them, *FUT1*, *FUT2*, and *FUT3* code for the enzymes that synthesize Lewis type 2 (Galβ1,4-GlcNAc) and type 1 (Galβ1–3-GlcNac) antigen precursors. In the stomach *FUT1* is exclusively detected with *MUC6*; *FUT2* is only detected when *MUC*5AC is present. Data for the glycosylation patterns of mucins in normal gastric epithelium show that it is dictated by the specific set of fucosyltransferases expressed by surface or gland cells, rather than by the apomucin peptide sequence.[7] Also, the development of intestinal metaplasia and gastric cancer is associated with the appearance of mucin glycosylation patterns that are absent in normal epithelium.[6] This suggests that goblet cell hyperplasia or submucosal gland hypertrophy in the airway in asthma may be accompanied by abnormal mucin glycosylation patterns. Little is known about this from clinical studies of airway disease, except for the observation that mucin-associated oligosaccharides in cystic fibrosis show increased sulfation.[8]

The polydiverse carbohydrate components of mucins bind surface adhesins or hemagglutinins on microorganisms and recognition sites on carbohydrates have been described for adhesins on *Mycoplasma pneumoniae*, *Streptococcus pneumoniae*, *Pseudomonas aeruginosa*, influenza virus, and *E. coli*.[9] Thus, mucin-associated carbohydrates may be an important host defense mechanism by presenting multiple potential sites for the attachment and clearance of microorganisms.[9] Another important function may be to bind with lysozyme, lactoferrin, or antiproteinases to protect these molecules and facilitate their role in host defense.

NON-MUCIN COMPONENTS OF MUCUS

In addition to mucins, airway mucus contains a variety of other proteins. These include proteoglycans, lactoferrin, lysozyme, secretory IgA, peroxidase, and antiproteases such as α$_1$-protease inhibitor (also known as α$_1$-antitrypsin), α$_2$-macroglobulin, secretory leukocyte proteinase inhibitor (also known as mucous proteinase inhibitor, bronchial inhibitor, or antileukoprotease), and trefoil factor peptides. The proteoglycans in serous cell granules include chondroitin sulfate and dermatan sulfate. The function of proteoglycans in airway mucus is unknown but their high anionic charge density is probably important. For example, ionic interactions between cationic proteins in the serous cell granule and proteoglycans may reduce the osmotic activity of the granule contents and thereby exclude water from the granule without the need for energy-dependent pumping mechanisms. In addition, because of their polyanionic charge, secreted proteoglycans in airway mucus provide a more readily hydrated network than that provided by mucins. The ratio of secreted proteoglycans and mucins may, therefore, determine the water content of mucus.

The other non-mucin components of airway mucus have important functions in airway host defense. Lysozyme is a bactericidal cationic protein that hydrolyzes components of bacterial cell walls. Lactoferrin is a cationic protein with high iron-binding capacity. One possible host defense function for lactoferrin is to reduce the growth of iron-dependent bacteria through iron-depravation; another is that lactoferrin prevents iron-catalyzed degradation of mucins. Secretory IgA is the major form of immunoglobulin present in airway mucus and has important antiviral and antibacterial functions. Peroxidases are a family of enzymes that catalyze the reduction of hydrogen peroxide to water by electron donors. In combination with hydrogen peroxide and either thiocyanate or halide ions, peroxidases are active against bacteria, viruses, fungi, and mycoplasma. The antiprotease activity of airway mucus is important in preventing protease-mediated epithelial injury[10] and mucus hypersecretion.[11] The lipids in mucus include free fatty acids, phospholipid, triglyceride, and cholesterol. The function of airway lipids is uncertain but may associate with mucins to change the rheology of airway mucus, alter the physical properties of periciliary fluid to facilitate effective ciliary beating, change the adhesiveness of airway mucus to the airway epithelium, or alter the surface activity of airway secretions to lessen the tendency of small airways collapse.

The trefoil factor family (TFF)-domain peptides (TFF1, TFF2, TFF3) is a group of mucin-associated peptides that were originally described in the gastrointestinal tract, but more recently have been found in the airways. In the former, the TFFs are localized to the mucus-producing cells[12] and have been linked with specific mucin-producing genes: TFF1 with $MUC5AC$, TFF2 with $MUC6$, and TFF3 with $MUC2$.[13] There, the TFFs function to increase mucus viscosity,[14] stimulate cell migration,[15] and protect against gastric injury.[16] In the airway mucosa (submucosal glands and goblet cells), TFF3 is present, but unlike in the intestine, pairs with $MUC5AC$.[17] TFF3 levels do not differ from normal in sputum from patients with asthma, cystic fibrosis, and chronic bronchitis.[17] $TFF2$ and to a lesser degree $TFF1$ gene expression, is increased in airway tissue from a murine model of asthma (and upregulated by cytokines IL-4 and IL-13), and in cultured airway epithelial cells from patients with asthma compared to control subjects.[18,19] However, the precise function of TFF domains and mucins in the respiratory epithelium and their role in asthma is not known, but most likely have similar functions to those seen in the gastrointestinal tract. TFF peptides promote cell migration in human bronchial epithelial cells,[20] and may be involved with airway remodeling, mucus viscosity, and mucus meta/hyperplasia.

■ CELLULAR REGULATION OF MUCOCILIARY CLEARANCE AND SECRETION ■

The principal cells in the airway that regulate mucus clearance and secretion include ciliated epithelial cells, goblet cells, and Clara cells in the airway surface epithelium, and serous cells and mucous cells in the submucosal glands (Fig. 39.2).

CILIATED AIRWAY EPITHELIAL CELLS

The cilia and microvilli located on the apical membranes of airway epithelial cells serve the important function of propelling airway secretions toward the mouth in the defense mechanism of mucociliary clearance. However, for normal mucociliary clearance to develop, the layer of fluid which bathes the cilia, termed the periciliary liquid layer (PCL), located between the apical membrane of the epithelial cells and the base of the overlying mucus, must be maintained at an optimal depth. Water movement into and out of the PCL is mediated by active ion transport in airway epithelial cells and probably plays a key role in regulating the depth of periciliary fluid in which the cilia beat. Increased Na^+ absorption decreases PCL and increases mucus obstruction in a mouse model of cystic fibrosis, but has not been studied in asthma.[21] Airway epithelial cells also regulate mucus secretion through expression of cytokines and other mediators.

GOBLET CELLS

Goblet cells take their name from the characteristic, but perhaps artifactual, goblet shape they exhibit in chemically fixed tissue. The normal airway goblet cells represent approximately 10% of the surface epithelial cells. At the basal part of the goblet cell is a nucleus surrounded by rough endoplasmic reticulum. The apical part of the cell is cup shaped and is filled with granules containing mucins and also a number of non-mucin components of mucus, including endoperoxidases, proteinase inhibitors, and lipids. The Golgi apparatus is between these two cell compartments. The mucin protein core is translated in the rough endoplasmic reticulum and is glycosylated in the Golgi apparatus before the mucin glycoproteins are packaged in mucin granules in the apical part of the cell (Fig. 39.2). Goblet cells are present at most airway levels but decrease in number peripherally, normally disappearing at the terminal bronchioles.

Goblet cell hyperplasia and metaplasia in the airway occurs in response to subacute or chronic stimuli and represent important mechanisms for mucus hypersecretion. Goblet cell hyperplasia involves cell division whereas goblet cell metaplasia involves differentiation of pre-existing epithelial cells into goblet cells, after stimuli encounter. Metaplasia is a more typical response in human peripheral airways or in the naive murine airway, both of which have few numbers of goblet cells. The mechanisms of metaplasia of normal airway epithelial cells to goblet cells are not entirely clear, but in a mouse model of asthma are regulated by EGFR and IL-13.[22] Increases in goblet cell number in the airway epithelium can occur quickly and are reversible when stimuli to secretion are removed or when treatment is instituted. For example, antiinflammatory agents such as indomethacin and corticosteroids attenuate the goblet cell hyperplasia associated with tobacco smoke and dexamethasone attenuates the goblet cell hyperplasia induced by neutrophil elastase or neutrophil lysates in animal models.[23,24]

The regulation of goblet cell secretion is poorly understood partly because experimental models in which secretory products and responses associated with goblet cells (and not with other secretory and non-secretory cell in the mucosa) are difficult to develop. It appears, however, that goblet cells in human airways do not have direct neuronal innervation. Rather, environmental stimuli (smoke, sulfur dioxide, chlorine, and ammonia) and inflammatory mediators with secretagogue activity seem to be the most important stimuli for mucin secretion from goblet cells.[25] For example, tachykinins, leukotrienes, histamine, neutrophil elastase, non-protease neutrophil products, and hypo-osmolar media all stimulate goblet cell secretion (Table 39.3). Goblet cells may not discharge all of their mucus when stimulated, since some studies have shown that stimulation leads to secretion of only 30% of the secretory granules.[26] This may be because loss of intracellular mucus to a critical level is a stimulus for goblet cells to enter the cell cycle.[25]

SUBMUCOSAL GLAND CELLS

The submucosal gland comprises a short ciliated duct that is a continuation of the surface epithelium, a non-ciliated collecting duct, and secretory tubules lined by mucous and serous cells. The products of serous cells must pass through tubules lined by mucous cells before reaching the collecting duct (Fig. 39.2). The body of these seromucous glands is located in the submucosa between the spiral bands of smooth muscle and the cartilaginous plates. They are not found in non-cartilaginous, membranous bronchioles. The mucus products of the mucous and serous cells

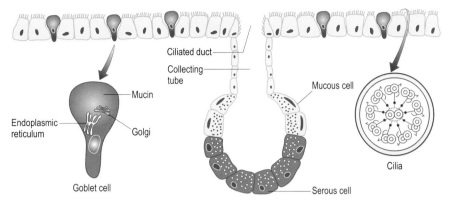

Fig. 39.2. Schematic representation of the airway epithelium showing goblet cells in the surface epithelium and mucous and serous cells in the submucosal gland. The basement membrane has been omitted for clarity of presentation. The submucosal gland comprises a short ciliated duct that is a continuation of the surface epithelium, a non-ciliated collecting duct, and secretory tubules lined by mucous and serous cells. The products of serous cells must pass through tubules lined by mucous cells before reaching the collecting duct. The schematic structure of the normal cilium shows an inner microtubule pair connected by radial spokes to nine outer microtubule doublets which are connected by nexin. The outer doublet each carry an outer and inner dynein arm. (Adapted from Basbaum C, Welsh MJ. Mucous secretion and ion transport in airways. In: Murray JF, Nadel JA, eds. Textbook of respiratory medicine, 2nd edn. Philadelphia: WB Saunders, 1994: pp 323–344; [37] Lundgren JD. J Allergy Clin Immunol 85:399–416; 1990; Elliasson J, Mosberg B, Camner P, et al. N Eng J Med 297; 1–6, 1997.)

are secreted into the lumen of the submucosal gland and are hydrated by water from the non-ciliated columnar epithelial cells in the gland duct.

Serous cells form crescentic caps, or demilunes, over the ends of the acini of the gland. In humans, serous cells exist in the surface epithelium before but not after birth. After birth, they are confined to the submucosal glands, where they comprise approximately 60% of the submucosal gland volume in healthy individuals. In the glands, the cells are pyramidal in shape and have small round nuclei in the basal region of the cell. Their supranuclear cytoplasm is rich in rough endoplasmic reticulum and Golgi apparatus. The apical portion of the cell contains numerous secretory granules. The granules of serous cells contain proteoglycans, lysozyme, lactoferrin, secretory IgA, peroxidase, antiproteases, and a variety of other proteins. Although serous cells themselves do not synthesize antibodies, they do synthesize the glycoprotein receptor (secretory component) that binds IgA released by plasma cells in the airway submucosal interstitium. This receptor, located on the basolateral surface of the serous cell, mediates the internalization and transport of IgA through the cell. 'Secretory IgA' (the term applied to the IgA-IgA receptor complex) is then secreted into the gland lumen and from there is transported to the airway lumen.

Mucous cells are the other cell type found in the acinar part of the submucosal gland. These are columnar cells whose nucleus is flattened against the base of the cell because the cell is packed with granules containing mucin. The free border of the cell is smooth and bulging. In response to injury such as sulfur dioxide or tobacco smoke, mucous cells are thought to form from serous cells by a process of serous cell transdifferentiation. Thus, in diseases such as chronic bronchitis, mucous cells rather than serous cells may be the predominant cell in the submucosal gland. This metaplastic response to injury can be expected to affect the type of mucus secreted by the submucosal gland.

Submucosal gland cells, unlike goblet cells, are neuronally innervated. Efferent cholinergic nerves originating in the vagi reach the trachea via the superior laryngeal nerves and the recurrent laryngeal nerves and cause mucus secretion when stimulated. Experimental studies in animal models suggest that the cholinergic nervous regulation of mucus secretion is mediated partly through pulmonary reflexes.[27] For example, stimulation of mechanoreceptors in the larynx, lung, and stomach as well as hypoxia, and chemical stimulation of cough receptors, bronchial C fibers, and pulmonary C fibers all reflexly increase glandular secretion via a cholinergic efferent pathway. It is not established, however, that all of these reflexes are present in humans. Postganglionic sympathetic nerves are also found in approximation with submucosal gland cells, at least in animals[28] and cause mucus secretion when stimulated.[29] Both sympathetic and parasympathetic ganglia contain cells that produce neuropeptides in addition to the classic neurotransmitters norepinephrine and acetylcholine. Candidate neurotransmitters for this non-adrenergic non-cholinergic (NANC) stimulation include neuropeptides such as substance P, neurokinin A, vasoactive intestinal peptide, and bradykinin. The Nκ-1 receptor mediates substance P- and neurokinin A-induced mucus secretion and β-adrenergic receptors mediate bradykinin-induced mucus secretion.

The relative contribution of goblet cells and submucosal gland cells to the mucin component of airway mucus is uncertain and is likely to vary by airway level and in health and disease. Reid estimated that the volume of glands in the airway mucosa was 40 times greater than the volume of goblet cells[30] but this calculation was based on several assumptions about the frequency and distribution of goblet cells and glands in the airway. Using quantitative morphometry to analyze mucins in the surface epithelium and submucosal glands of airways of macaque monkeys, Heidsiek et al[31] reported twice as much stainable stored mucins in the goblet cells in the epithelium of the tracheobronchial airway as in the submucosal glands. This suggests that in primates, goblet cells − not mucous cells − might be the principal source of airway mucins.

CLARA CELLS

These cells, also termed non-ciliated bronchial secretory cells, are most abundant in terminal bronchioles. They are columnar in shape and contain electron-dense granules. Clara cells synthesize and secrete Clara cell secretory protein (CCSP), of which the exact identity, function, and relationship to pulmonary surfactant is unknown. In the mouse, antigen challenge results in tracheobronchial Clara cells that retain their molecular and functional characteristics, but also develop the ability to secrete mucin.[32] Additionally, in healthy humans, goblet cells in the bronchiolar airways express CCSP,[33] suggesting that the Clara cell may be a precursor to goblet cells.

■ MUCIN PACKAGING AND DISCHARGE FROM AIRWAY SECRETORY CELLS ■

Mucins are oligomerized in the endoplasmic reticulum by disulfide bonding, an event that follows N-glycosylation, and then transferred to the Golgi in an energy-dependent step modulated by molecular chaperones.[34] In the Golgi there is further processing of mucins, including elongation of O-oligosaccharide side chains.[34] Mucin peptides may either then be secreted or remain membrane bound (e.g., $MUC1$), the former differing due to cysteine-rich domains at N and C termini.[1,35]

The packaging of the large secretory mucin molecules in the intracellular storage granules requires condensation – a process made difficult by the polyanionic nature of mucins. This is overcome by high concentrations of calcium in the granules which nullify the repulsive forces within the mucin molecule. Secretion of mucins from intracellular granules is induced by a variety of neural and humoral stimuli (Table 39.3).[25,36] However, for mucin granule exocytosis and secretion to occur, the granule matrix must first undergo decondensation. Activation of cell-surface receptors by signaling molecules (e.g., neurotransmitters) results in activation of signal transduction pathways and increases in intracellular calcium.[37] The outer surface of the granule fuses with the inner surface of the secretory cell to form a channel between the extracellular space and the granule. This channel provides a conduit for calcium to exit and extracellular water to enter the granule. The loss of calcium allows electrostatic repulsion to rapidly expand the mucin macromolecule, which is simultaneously hydrated with incoming water. To facilitate decondensation, the mucin granule lumen has been proposed to be organized into two phases: a mobile phase in which secretory proteins diffuse, and an immobile phase (matrix), in which proteins are immobilized by non-covalent pH-dependent interactions.[38] Recent studies also suggest that the myristoylated, alanine-rich C kinase substrate (MARCKS), along with chaperone proteins, cysteine string protein and heat shock protein 70, interacts with actin cytoskeleton and directs the mucin granules to the docking sites on the cell membrane.[39–41] The large hydrated macromolecule then erupts from the cell like a 'jack-in-the-box'.[34,36] Through this secretion mechanism, secreted mucin macromolecules are much greater in volume than the volume of stored mucins in the goblet cell granules.

■ MUCOCILIARY CLEARANCE ■

Airway mucus and the foreign material entrapped in it are normally removed from the tracheobronchial tree by a process known as mucociliary clearance (MCC). This process depends on the coordinated activity of ciliated airway epithelial cells. Rhythmic coordinated beating of cilia on ciliated cells propels mucus cephalad to clear a total daily volume of mucus of about 10 ml. The continuous motion of cilia results in continuous movement cephalad of lung secretions and the descriptive term 'mucus escalator' has been applied to this process.

The energy for ciliary bending is provided by adenosine triphosphate with the mechanism likely tied to its interaction with an intraciliary calcium-calmodulin complex. Temperature, pH, viscoelasticity, and volume of the overlying mucus all influence the activity of the ciliated cells. In addition, cholinergic and β-adrenergic stimulation increase ciliary activity markedly so that autonomic reflexes may be the most important defensive response to inhaled irritants.

The rhythmic synchronized beating of cilia on airway epithelial cells is facilitated by the specialized structure of the cilia (Fig. 39.2). The cilium is composed of a shaft anchored to the cell cytoplasm by a basal body from which rootlets extend into the apical part of the cell. The shaft of the cilium has longitudinal fibrils or axonemes, which are composed of nine outer pairs of microtubules (or doublets) and two central microtubules. The microtubules are composed of a contractile protein called tubulin. Dynein arms together with nexin arms join adjacent doublets. Radial spokes link with the central microtubules. The bending of the cilium is caused by an active sliding of the doublet microtubules. The dynein molecules undergo cyclical changes in shape as they engage with and disengage from the adjacent doublet. Fine claw-like projections have been observed on the apical but not the lateral aspect of the cilium tip (Fig. 39.3). These 'claws' may function to grip the overlying mucus and propel it toward the larynx.

The ciliary beat consists of an effective stroke and a recovery stroke. During the effective stroke, the cilium is extended and penetrates the mucus. The recovery stroke takes twice as long as the active stroke. The rhythmic beating of cilia, therefore, resembles repetitive cracking of a whip.

The effective clearance of mucus from the airway relies upon optimal rheologic properties of the mucus and normal functioning of cilia on epithelial cells. The optimal rheologic properties of mucus for maximum transport velocity along the mucociliary escalator are high elastic recoil and intermediate viscosity. The rheologic properties are altered when airway diseases such as asthma, bronchitis, or cystic fibrosis result in the secretion of 'pathologic' mucus (i.e., mucus that is abnormal in volume and/or composition). 'Primary ciliary dyskinesia', formerly known as the 'immotile cilia syndrome', describes a genetic disorder in the ultrastructure of the cilium and serves to emphasize the importance of normal ciliary function in the maintenance of upper and lower airway health. The inborn abnormalities of the ciliary cytoskeleton include lack of dynein arms and defective ciliary spokes and these abnormalities result in disruption of the ciliary motor so that, although the cilia may still move, they do not beat synchronously together and so do not function optimally. The airway consequences of this disorder include chronic rhinitis, sinusitis, otitis, bronchitis, and bronchiectasis. The non-airway manifestations include situs inversus, male sterility, and corneal abnormalities.

■ CLINICAL IMPORTANCE AND CELLULAR CHARACTERISTICS OF MUCUS HYPERSECRETION IN ASTHMA ■

Increased sputum production, typically with coughing, is a common symptom of asthma. Increased mucus production may contribute significantly to the morbidity related to this airway disease. A history of chronic mucus hypersecretion is associated with an accelerated loss

Table 39.3 Potential mediators of airway mucus secretion, goblet cell hyperplasia, MUC synthesis/gene expression, and plasma exudation in asthma

Stimulation	Secretion	Hyperplasia	MUC	Plasma exudation
Cytokines				
IL-1β	+	NP	NP	NP
IL-6	+	NP	Yes	NP
IL-9	NP	NP	Yes	NP
IL-13 (IL-4)	+	Yes	Yes	NP
TNF-α	++	Yes	Yes	NP
Gases				
Irritant gases (e.g., cigarette smoke)	++	Yes	Yes	+
Nitric oxide	−ve	NP	NP	+
Reactive oxygen species	0/+	NP	NP	+
Inflammatory mediators				
Bradykinin	+	NP	NP	++
Cysteinyl leukotrienes	++	NP	NP	++
Endothelin	0/+	NP	NP	+
Histamine	+	NP	NP	++
PAF	+	Yes[a]	Yes[a]	+++
Prostaglandins	0/+	NP	NP	0/+
Proteinases	+++	Yes[a]	NP	NP
Purine nucleotides	++	NP	NP	NP
Neural pathways				
Cholinergic nerves	++	NP	NP	0
Cholinoceptor agonists	++	Yes	NP	0
Nicotine	++	Yes	NP	++
Tachykininergic nerves	+	NP	NP	++
Substance P	++	NP	NP	+++
Neurokinin A	+	NP	NP	++
Miscellaneous				
EGF (+ TNF-α)	NP	Yes	Yes	NP
Sensitization followed by challenge	+	Yes	Yes	++

[a]Affect only observed with PAR and TNF-α in combination. +++, highly potent; ++, marked effect; +, lesser effect; 0, minimal effect; EGF, epidermal growth factor; NP, effect not published; PAF, platelet activating factor; TNF-α, tumour necrosis factor-α. (Adapted from Rogers.[43])

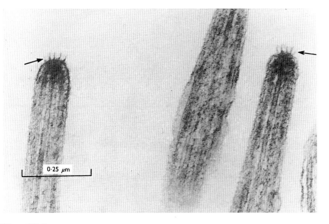

Fig. 39.3. An electron micrograph illustrating the claw-like projections (arrows) at the tip, but not on the lateral surface, of cilia on rat airway epithelial cells (×120 000). (From Jeffery PK, Reid L. New observations of rat airway epithelium: a quantitative and electron microscopic study. J Anat 1975; 120:295–320.)

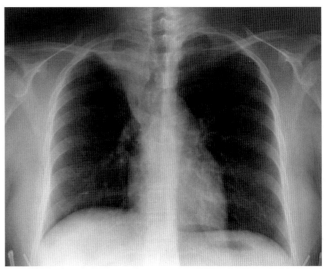

Fig. 39.4. Chest radiograph from a 20-year-old woman admitted to the intensive care unit for management of acute severe asthma. The chest radiograph shows collapse of the right upper lobe secondary to mucus impaction. The abnormality resolved completely within 24h of treatment with mechanical ventilation, corticosteroids, and bronchodilators.

of lung function in some asthmatic patients,[42] produces airway obstruction, and may increase airway hyperresponsiveness.[43] It has been long recognized that mucus plugging of the airways is an important pathologic feature of fatal asthma and is likely to be the principal cause of the asphyxiation leading to death in these patients.[44] It is only a small minority of asthma deaths that are not associated with mucus impaction of the airways.[45] Mucus hypersecretion can produce abnormalities of gas exchange, which can be further exacerbated by lobar or whole lung collapse secondary to mucus plugs in the large airways (Fig. 39.4). A history of recurrent episodes of lobar collapse, significant chronic mucus hypersecretion, and bronchiectasis should prompt consideration of a diagnosis of allergic bronchopulmonary aspergillosis (ABPA). Increased mucus production may produce increased airway hyperresponsiveness by reducing the airway luminal cross-sectional area or by changing the surface tension at the air–liquid interface. Additionally, it may prevent binding of inhaled medications needed to produce airway dilation and reduce hyperresponsiveness.

Mucociliary clearance may be abnormal in asthma and possibly contributes to increased airway obstruction by mucus, which cannot be properly removed. Assessment of the efficiency of mucociliary clearance in asthmatic subjects is performed by measuring the retention time of an inhaled radiolabeled aerosol. Asthmatic subjects, especially those with significant airway obstruction, demonstrate prolonged pulmonary retention of radioaerosol, indicating mucociliary dysfunction.[46] Using similar techniques, it has been documented that mucociliary clearance is severely impaired in asthmatic subjects requiring hospital admission for management of acute severe asthma,[47] which may improve after recovery from the exacerbation.

The sputum expectorated by asthmatic patients has long been recognized to have characteristically abnormal features. Abnormal bipyramidal crystals (Charcot–Leyden crystals) in asthmatic sputum were described by Leyden in 1872 (the constituents of these crystals were later determined to be eosinophil lysophospholipase). Corkscrew-shaped twists of inspissated mucus ('Curschmann's spirals') in asthmatic sputum were described by Curschmann in 1882, eosinophils were described

by Gollash in 1889, and multiple clumps of sloughed epithelial cells ('Creola bodies') were described later. More recent and more detailed cellular and biochemical analyses of asthmatic sputum have confirmed higher than normal percentages of eosinophils and have also shown higher than normal levels of eosinophil products such as eosinophil cationic protein and major basic protein.[48] The cytokine interleukin (IL-5), and the chemokines eotaxin and regulated on activation, normal T-cell expressed and secreted (RANTES) coordinate to direct migration of activated eosinophils to the airways.[49] Measuring sputum eosinophilia may become a useful clinical tool to predict onset of asthma exacerbations prior to symptoms, and to follow corticosteroid dosing during an exacerbation.[50]

Neutrophils are also an important cellular component of asthmatic mucus, constituting more than 75% of the sputum cells collected from the majority of asthmatic patients in one study.[51] Neutrophil percentages were significantly higher in the 50% of asthmatic subjects who reported that their asthma exacerbation was precipitated by a respiratory tract infection. Analysis of the sputum fluid phase revealed that many of the asthmatic sputum samples had free neutrophil elastase activity and that the levels of interleukin-8 and interleukin-6 were also very high. These findings may be linked together in a scheme where viral infection promotes IL-8 secretion by airway epithelial cells, IL-8 then mediates airway neutrophilia, and neutrophil elastase then mediates mucin glycoprotein hypersecretion. An independent role may also exist for IL-6 since recent in vitro experiments demonstrate that IL-6 is a mucin secretagogue.[52]

The consequences of the accumulation of inflammatory cells in airway mucus are at least two-fold. First, inflammatory cells secrete inflammatory mediators into the airway lumen – some of which (e.g. neutrophil elastase, chymase, eosinophil cationic protein, and LTD_4) function as mucus secretagogues (see below). Second, products of cell lysis (e.g., DNA and actin) have significant effects on the physical properties of sputum. For example, average DNA levels in CF sputum are very high (3–5 mg/ml) and contribute significantly to the viscoelastic properties of CF sputum[53] – findings which led to the development of recombinant human deoxyribonuclease I (DNase) as a therapeutic strategy for the treatment of CF-related airway disease. DNA levels in sputum from chronic stable asthmatics are low[54] but are much higher (0.5 mg/ml) when sputum is collected from asthmatic subjects experiencing an exacerbation.[51] The extent to which DNA in sputum from asthmatic subjects in exacerbation contributes to the abnormal viscoelastic properties of asthmatic sputum is unknown.

Actin is estimated to comprise 10% of total leukocyte protein and it forms long protease-resistant filaments that are highly viscoelastic. Actin levels in asthmatic sputum have not been reported but actin levels in CF sputum range from 0.5–5 mg/ml. Interestingly, human plasma gelsolin, a protein that severs actin filaments, rapidly decreases the viscosity of CF sputum samples in vitro and is more efficient in this regard than deoxyribonuclease I. Thus, gelsolin may have therapeutic potential as a mucolytic agent.

■ PATHOPHYSIOLOGY OF MUCUS HYPERSECRETION IN ASTHMA ■

The clinical and pathologic studies described above clearly show that the volume, composition, and clearance of airway secretions are abnormal in asthma. The pathophysiology of these changes in mucus and mucociliary clearance is unknown but clues have been obtained from detailed cellular and biochemical analysis of asthmatic sputum and from in vitro studies of mucociliary function. Taken together, the cellular and biochemical analyses of asthmatic sputum described above indicate a multifactorial etiology to mucus hypersecretion in asthma. These factors can be divided into those responsible for: (1) increased goblet cell numbers and gene expression of mucin glycoproteins, (2) mucin hypersecretion, (3) goblet cell degranulation, (4) increased bronchovascular permeability and leakage of plasma proteins, and (5) impaired mucociliary clearance.

INCREASED GOBLET CELL NUMBERS AND EXPRESSION OF MUCIN GENES

Goblet cell numbers are 2.5-fold higher than normal in the airway epithelium in subjects with asthma,[55] and store approximately three times higher than normal amounts of mucin (Fig. 39.5). Also, higher stored mucin levels in the epithelium are associated with lower secreted mucin in samples of induced sputum from patients with asthma, and vice versa. Because secreted mucin levels are higher in patients with lower FEV_1, it is possible that the pathogenesis of airway obstruction in more severe forms of asthma involves ongoing mucin hypersecretion from goblet cells. In addition, higher levels of stored mucins in goblet cells in patients with mild asthma suggest a mechanism for mucus formation and airway obstruction in these patients during acute exacerbations. Submucosal gland cells may also be hypertrophied in asthma, but this finding is less well established.

Measurement of different mucin gene transcripts in bronchial biopsies from asthmatic subjects and healthy controls show that the most frequently expressed mucin gene in the airways is $MUC5AC$,[55,56] which is localized to goblet cells regardless if the subject has asthma or is a normal control.[57]

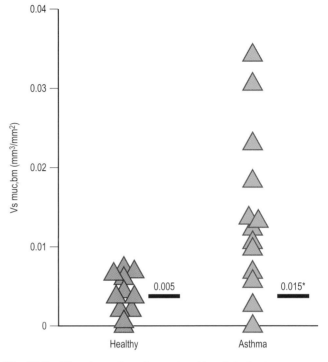

Fig. 39.5. The volume of stored mucin in goblet cells in the airway epithelium of 13 asthmatic and 12 healthy subjects. Measurements were made using methods of design based stereology and the data are presented as volume of mucin per surface area of basement membrane (Vs muc, bm). Solid bars indicate mean values. An asterisk (*) indicates that mucin volume in asthmatic subjects was significantly greater than in healthy subjects, p <0.05. (Reprinted from Ordoñez CL, Khashayar R, Wong HH, et al. American Journal of Respiratory and Critical Care Medicine 163:517–523, 2001. Official Journal of the American Thoracic Society. ©American Thoracic Society.[55])

However, $MUC5AC$ has significantly higher expression in patients with asthma (Fig. 39.6). Another gene which may be important in mucin production, and serve as a marker of mucus hyperproduction, is a member of the family of calcium-activated chloride channels in airway epithelial cells (hCLCA1 in humans and gob-5 in the mouse), although its role is not clearly defined. Initial studies suggested that they may function as an ion channel in mucus production, but more recent work has concluded that this is unlikely.[58] Lung tissue biopsies of patients with asthma demonstrate increased hCLCA1 expression compared to control subjects[56,59] which co-localizes with staining for goblet cells and $MUC5AC$.[56] Antigen sensitized and challenged mice developed increased gob-5 airway expression and mucus cell metaplasia, which was attenuated with either administration of an antisense gob-5 adenovirus, or in similarly treated gob-5 knockout mice.[60,61] However, not all studies have found gob-5 and hCLCA1 to be essential for mucus overproduction and $MUC5AC$ expression.[62,63]

Knowledge of the growth factors driving goblet cell hyperplasia or metaplasia in allergic airway diseases has advanced greatly due to experiments in animal models, immortalized lung cell lines, and cultured primary airway epithelial cells. For example, airway allergen challenge in sensitized animals causes marked goblet cell metaplasia (GCM) and increased mucin gene expression,[64] which are strongly driven by Th2

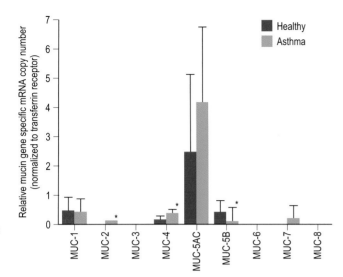

Fig. 39.6. Expression of nine mucin genes in homogenates of endobronchial biopsy specimens from eight healthy and 11 asthmatic subjects. Gene expression was measured by real-time reverse transcriptase–polymerase chain reaction (RT-PCR), and the expression of mucin genes is represented as the ratio of the copy number of mucin gene-specific messenger RNA (mRNA) to the copy number of the transferring receptor (a housekeeping gene). Data are presented as mean ± SD. An asterisk (*) indicates that mRNA expression in asthmatic subjects is significantly different from that in healthy subjects; p <0.005. (Reproduced from Ordoñez CL, Khashayar R, Wong HH, et al. American Journal of Respiratory and Critical Care Medicine 163:517–523, 2001. Official Journal of the American Thoracic Society. © American Thoracic Society.[55])

CD4+ T cells. Although several Th2-like cytokines (e.g., IL-4, IL-5, IL-9, IL-13, and more recently IL-17) induce mucus metaplasia and mucin gene expression in vivo and in vitro,[65–68] it appears that IL-13 and the IL-4Rα are critical, and may be necessary for mucus production by the other cytokines.[4] However, Th1 cytokines, including TNF-α and IL-1β, induce mucin gene expression in vitro[69–71] and gene expression and mucus metaplasia in vivo,[72] and Th1 cells enhanced mucus production if IFN-γ were blocked.[73] Additionally, increased expression of the growth factor thymic stromal lymphopoietin (TSLP), may be an initiating event in the inflammatory cascade producing mucus metaplasia. It induces expression of several Th2 cell chemokines, and dendritic cell production of cytokines IL-4, IL-5, IL-13, and TNF-α, and its overexpression in the airways of naive mice led to spontaneous airway mucus metaplasia, which was attenuated in antigen sensitized and challenged mice deficient for the TSLP receptor.[74]

The role of the eosinophil in mucus metaplasia is controversial. Some reports, using antigen sensitized and challenged IL-5-/- mice or antigen sensitized and challenged mice with a complete ablation of the eosinophil line, have demonstrated that the eosinophil is not important for mucus cell metaplasia.[75,76] In contrast, other studies using OVA-treated IL-5-/- mice with adoptive transfer of eosinophils, or OVA-treated mice congenitally deficient in eosinophils, show that this cell is necessary for, and may synergistically induce, mucus metaplasia with CD4+ T-cells.[77,78] The mechanism of eosinophil induction of mucus metaplasia may be through epidermal growth factor receptor (EGFR) activation (see below)[79] or release of proinflammatory cytokines.

It is well established that viral infections exacerbate asthma, and infected patients develop increased mucus secretions. Respiratory syncytial virus (RSV) is common in young children, whereas rhinovirus (RV) frequently affects children and adults. Infection with RSV in a murine system induces both gob-5 and MUC5AC expression, which may occur via an IL-17-dependent pathway or via the chemokine receptor CXCR2 induction.[80,81] Inoculation of normal volunteers and patients with asthma with RV16 increased MUC5AC expression in the airways.[82] The atypical bacteria, $M. pneumoniae$, shown to exacerbate asthma, upregulates MUC5AC expression.[83] Other stimuli which have been shown to induce goblet cell hyperplasia or metaplasia include cigarette smoke, sulfur dioxide, nitrogen dioxide, chlorine, adrenoceptor or cholinoceptor agonist drugs, and endotoxin.[24,84,85] In addition, neutrophil elastase and extracts from purified neutrophils cause goblet cell hyperplasia.[25]

The EGFR signaling cascade is an important common pathway for mucin gene translation activation for many of the above mentioned stimuli. Increased expression of the EGFR has been demonstrated in the airways of patients with asthma, which was noted in goblet cells.[86] Furthermore, selective inhibitors of EGFR tyrosine kinase inhibitors block IL-13-induced mucin gene expression in rat airways[87] and epithelial cell proliferation in cultured bronchial epithelial cells.[88] The critical ligand for the EGFR in these instances is TGF-α, released from neutrophils[87] or from the airway epithelium itself.[88] However, adenosine may also be an important ligand for the EGFR, at least for MUC2 expression.[89] A scheme for GCH in asthma is summarized in Figure 39.7.

Whether goblet cell hyperplasia is a transient or permanent change of the airways of asthmatics has not been definitively established. In murine models of asthma, without continual exposure to allergen or proinflammatory cytokines, in particular IL-13, the airway epithelium returns to near baseline structure without goblet cells.[90,91] Whether this occurs in humans with asthma after allergen avoidance has not been evaluated. The mechanisms governing resolution of goblet cell hyperplasia or metaplasia are poorly understood but appear to involve the BCL-2 family of apoptosis proteins.[92] Other proteins including BAX and BAK are proapoptotic. The role of these different protein families in mucus cells hyperplasia and metaplasia in allergic airway disease is just beginning to be investigated.

Overall, it is clear that the mechanisms of allergen-induced GCH are complex and CD4+ Th2 cells are critical; however, some Th1 cytokines and the eosinophil may also play important roles. However, much remains to be learned about the mechanisms of cytokine-induced goblet cell hyperplasia, the interaction of Th2 cytokines and the EGF receptor system, and the role of calcium-activated chloride channels in goblet cell differentiation.

MUCIN HYPERSECRETION

Higher than normal levels of mucin and lactoferrin in airway secretions indicate hypersecretion from goblet cells and submucosal gland cells. Fahy and colleagues found that mucin-like glycoprotein levels were higher in induced sputum from asthmatic subjects than from healthy subjects. The highest mucin levels were in the asthmatic subjects who gave a history of sputum production. Asthmatic subjects without a history of sputum production had mucin levels similar to those of healthy subjects.[54] However, little is known about the composition of secreted mucin gene products into the airways of asthmatics. Available data from

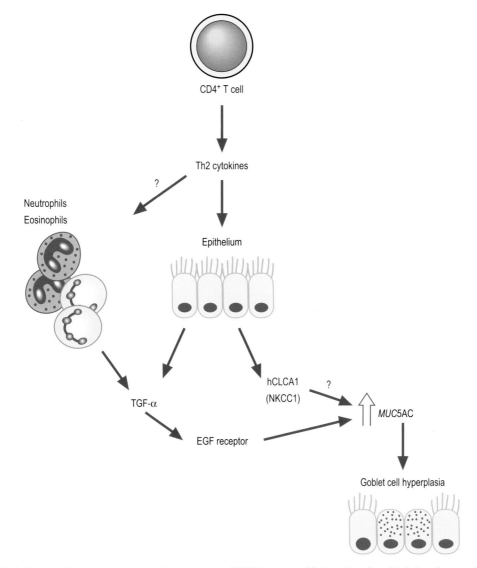

Fig. 39.7. Simplified schematic diagram showing possible mechanism of GCH in asthma. Th2 cytokines (e.g., IL-9, IL-13) secreted by CD4+ T cells cause increased $MUC5$AC gene expression, which may be a critical signal for goblet cell differentiation from basal cells or Clara cells. The effect of Th2 cytokines on $MUC5$AC in vivo may be mediated by a variety of other molecules, including the EGF receptor and its ligand TGF-α, and by ion channels such as the calcium-activated chloride channel (hCLCA1) or the sodium potassium chloride cotransporter (NKCC1). (From Fahy JV. Goblet cell and mucin gene abnormalities in asthma. Chest 2002; 122:320S–326S.)

healthy controls, and from patients with chronic bronchitis and cystic fibrosis show that $MUC5$AC and $MUC5$B are the principal secreted mucins in airway secretions,[55] and are increased in secretions from the airways of asthmatics compared with normal controls.[93]

Although hyperplasia/hypertrophy of mucus-secreting cells could account for increased mucin secretion, another mechanism is increased mucus secretagogue activity. Many inflammatory mediators secreted by cells such as mast cells, eosinophils, and neutrophils can stimulate secretion of mucin from goblet cells and submucosal gland cells (Table 39.3). Among the most potent mucin secretagogues are neutrophil elastase and

chymase. Neutrophil elastase activity increases in acute exacerbations of asthma and is detectable in sputum in this situation.[94] Mast cell chymase, eosinophil cationic protein, and leukotrienes C_4 and E_4 are likely to be important.[85,95,96] In addition, neuropeptides such as substance P vasoactive intestinal peptide and bradykinin cause mucin hypersecretion.[85,97] These peptides may be especially important when epithelial neutral endopeptidase activity is reduced. This occurs when the airway epithelium is sloughed as in asthma or damaged by injury such as viral infection. Neutral endopeptidase cleaves neuropeptides, thereby inactivating them.

GOBLET CELL DEGRANULATION

Goblet cell degranulation releases mucin glycoproteins. The mechanisms of goblet cell degranulation in vivo are separate from those of goblet cell hyperplasia or metaplasia. In rodents, goblet cell degranulation and mucus occlusion of the airways occurs following high-dose allergen challenge in sensitized animals.[98] The effect of allergen challenge on goblet cell degranulation in vivo in human subjects has been examined.[99] Eight allergic asthmatic subjects were challenged with aeroallergen aerosol using a whole lung challenge protocol. Although eosinophilic inflammation occurred as soon as 1 hour after challenge, there was no evidence of goblet cell degranulation in the airway biopsies or in lavage samples at either 1-h or 24-h time points after challenge (Fig. 39.8).[99] This suggests that the mechanisms of degranulation in human asthma are complex. Important inhibitory mechanisms must be in place in human asthma, which prevent degranulation of goblet cells even upon allergen exposure, except in specific clinical circumstances. An example of such a circumstance might be allergen exposure coincident with a viral infection of the airway. Other possible inflammatory mediators of allergen-induced goblet cell degranulation include chymase,[96] eosinophil cationic protein,[95] and neutrophil elastase.[11]

Extracellular nucleotide triphosphates such as ATP and UTP may have a role in goblet cell degranulation and in mechanisms of metaplasia. In the airways, both ATP and UTP are equally potent in causing mucin release from goblet cells, an effect that may be mediated by the G-protein-coupled receptor – P2Y2. The effects of extracellular ATP and UTP on goblet cell mucin production and mucin gene expression have been examined in more detail.[100] It was found that UTP is the only nucleotide that stimulates MUC5AC and MUC5B expression as well as mucin secretion in cultured human airway epithelial cells. Further, in mice, intratracheal instillation of UTP-saline causes similar effects. Preliminary studies with various inhibitors demonstrated that separate signaling pathways are involved in UTP regulation of mucin secretion and MUC expression.

Our knowledge of the mechanisms linking cell-surface stimulation with a mucin secretagogue and extracellular release of mucin granule contents is quite rudimentary, but recent advances have been made. Specifically, a role has been discovered for MARCKS protein (myristoylated alanine-rich C kinase substrate), whereby secretagogue-induced activation of protein kinase C phosphorylates MARCKS, causing translocation of MARCKS from the plasma membrane to the cytoplasm.[101] In the cytoplasm MARCKS is dephosphorylated, associates with both actin and myosin, and also interacts with mucin granule membranes. In this way, mucin granules are linked to the contractile cytoskeleton facilitating their movement to the cell periphery and subsequent exocytosis.

INCREASED BRONCHOVASCULAR PERMEABILITY

Higher than normal levels of plasma proteins in airway secretions indicate that bronchovascular permeability is abnormally increased in asthma. Increased bronchovascular permeability in asthma has a number of adverse consequences, including mucosal edema leading to airway narrowing and leakage of plasma proteins into the airway lumen. The mixing of plasma-derived proteins, plasma-derived inflammatory cells, excessive amounts of mucin glycoproteins, and sloughed airway epithelial cells results in abnormal mucus with abnormal viscoelastic properties. Coupled with reduced mucociliary clearance in asthma, a consequence of injury to cilia on airway epithelial cells, this 'pathologic' mucus proves difficult to expectorate and forms mucus 'plugs' that contribute significantly to airway obstruction in asthmatic patients. Interestingly, in acute asthma compared to CF-related lung disease, plasma-derived proteins contribute relatively more than mucin glycoproteins to luminal secretions.[102] Plasma proteins in airway mucus, especially albumin, may have important consequences for its physical properties. For example, the incubation of human serum albumin and pig gastric mucin results in a highly viscous solution.[103] Viscosity enhancement is proportional to the albumin concentration and is considerably greater than the additive or multiplicative viscosity values calculated for albumin or mucin solutions measured separately.

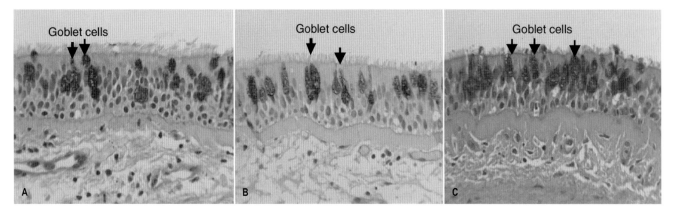

Fig. 39.8. Photomicrographs of 3-μm sections of bronchial biopsy specimens from an asthmatic subject before and after aerosolized allergen challenge. The stain is sequential Alcian blue periodic acid Schiff (AB/PAS). Representative biopsy sections are shown in the baseline state (A), 1 h after challenge (B), and 24 h after challenge (C). Allergen challenge did not result in a reduction in AB/PAS-stained mucins in the epithelial goblet cells; in fact, stained mucins tended to be increased in the epithelium 24 h after allergen challenge. (From Hays et al.[99])

ABNORMAL MUCOCILIARY CLEARANCE

The reduced clearance of airway mucus from the airways in asthma is multifactorial in etiology. Three of the more important mechanisms are abnormal viscoelastic properties of asthmatic mucus, cilioinhibitory effects of inflammatory mediators in asthmatic sputum, and disruption/destruction of the ciliated epithelial cell 'carpet'. First, as airway mucus in asthma is abnormal in volume and consistency, it leads to abnormal viscoelastic properties, abnormal interactions with cilia on epithelial cells, and delayed clearance. The ciliary beating frequency of bronchial mucosal explants was significantly decreased when the explants were incubated with sputum from asthmatic subjects.[104] This effect was greatest for sputum from asthmatic subjects experiencing an asthma exacerbation and was reversible, indicating that it was a functional (not a toxic) phenomenon. The mediators in the sputum responsible for this effect are unknown. Many inflammatory mediators in asthmatic sputum such as the leukotriene and prostaglandin products of arachidonic acid metabolism are ciliostimulatory so that the direct ciliary impairment of asthmatic sputum may be less important in impairing sputum clearance than its abnormal viscoelastic properties. Second, some inflammatory mediators found in the asthmatic airway decrease ciliary beat frequency directly; these include eosinophil major basic protein[105] and neutrophil elastase.[10] Finally, impairment of mucociliary clearance can also be expected as a consequence of reduced numbers of ciliated airway epithelial cells in the asthmatic airway. Reduction in ciliated epithelial cell numbers occurs because ciliated epithelial cells are exfoliated by mediators such as eosinophil granule proteins and because goblet cell and squamous cell numbers are increased as a result of metaplasia and hyperplasia in the airway epithelium. These cellular changes will result in a decrease in the normal complement of ciliated cells and a consequent decrease in the maximal efficiency of the mucociliary escalator.

■ TREATMENT OF MUCUS HYPERSECRETION IN ASTHMA ■

The goals of treatment for mucus hypersecretion in asthma should be to reduce mucus volume, normalize mucus composition, and improve mucus clearance. The effects of currently available antiasthma medications on mucus volume, mucus composition, or mucus clearance are largely unknown, however, because these outcomes are difficult to quantitate in clinical practice or in clinical research studies. Presently, the pharmacologic agents for mucus hypersecretion in asthma can be divided into established medications, including bronchodilators, antiinflammatory agents, mucolytic agents, and expectorants, and novel medications (Table 39.4).

ESTABLISHED MEDICATIONS

Bronchodilators

Beta agonists may potentially play important roles in the treatment of mucus hypersecretion independent of their bronchodilator activity: enhancing mucociliary clearance (MCC), and decreasing mucin secretion and goblet cell development. It is well established that β-agonists

Table 39.4 Pharmacotherapy of mucus hypersecretion in asthma

Bronchodilators
  β-Agonists
  Ipratropium bromide

Antiinflammatory agents
  Oral corticosteroids
  Inhaled corticosteroids
  Nedocromil sodium
  Drugs that interrupt the leukotriene pathway (Cys-LT$_1$ receptor antagonists)

Mucolytic agents
  N-acetylcysteine
  S-carboxymethylcysteine
  Bromhexine

Expectorants
  Guaifenesin
  Iodinated glycerol
  Potassium iodide
  Terpin hydrate

Novel therapies
  Recombinant human DNase
  Calcium-activated chloride channel (hCLCA1) inhibitor
  EGFR tyrosine kinase inhibitor
  p38MAPK inhibitor
  Anticytokine inhibitors (e.g., anti IL-13)
  Specific muscarinic (M$_3$) inhibitor
  Purine nucleotide receptor antagonist
  MARCKS inhibitors
  Alternative medications (e.g., herbal medications)

enhance mucociliary clearance in lung tissue cell culture and in patients without lung disease by increasing ciliary beat frequency.[106,107] However, the effect of β-agonists on MCC in patients with asthma is less consistent. Some studies show no effect of short-acting β-agonists on MCC (measured by radioaerosol clearance),[108,109] whereas others have demonstrated that these drugs, significantly improve MCC.[110,111] The use of long-acting β-agonists on MCC is even less well investigated, but most likely does not produce any significant improvement.[112,113] The effects of β-agonists on mucin secretion are also conflicting, with some studies demonstrating increased viscosity of the mucin secretion[29,114] and others finding no effect.[115,116] Treatment with both (R)- and (S)-enantiomers of albuterol reduced the numbers of airway goblet cells and airway mucus plugging in a mouse model of asthma, but has not been investigated in humans.[117] Finally, β-agonists may also have additional beneficial effects on mucus volume and composition by decreasing the plasma protein content of airway mucus by decreasing bronchovascular permeability.

The role of anticholinergic drugs such as ipratropium bromide, oxitropium bromide, or atropine in the treatment of mucus hypersecretion is uncertain because these drugs have multiple effects on mucus production and secretion, as well as the mucociliary apparatus;[118] some of these effects are beneficial whereas others are not. For example, since cholinergic stimuli are potent secretagogues for mucin and other products of goblet cells and submucosal gland cells (via muscarinic M_3 and M_1 receptor binding), anticholinergic drugs may decrease airway mucus levels. This effect might be beneficial in treating airway mucus hypersecretion as long as the reduction in secretion of mucus components does not render the residual mucus more difficult to clear by increasing its viscoelastic properties. Atropine decreases tracheal mucus secretion in dogs and changes some of the physical properties of residual mucus.[119] Ipratropium bromide, however, does not change the physical properties of sputum in patients with chronic bronchitis treatment and oxitropium bromide does not change the physical properties of sputum from patients with chronic bronchitis or asthma. These anticholinergic drugs, however, are non-selective for muscarinic receptor binding and will also bind the M_2 receptor which is autoinhibitory. Tiotropium bromide was recently approved for the use of COPD and is a long-acting anticholinergic with selectivity for the M_3 and M_1 receptors. Its use in asthma, especially to decrease mucus hypersecretion, has not been well studied, but may offer a potential benefit. In addition, since cholinergic stimuli increase ciliary beat frequency, anticholinergic drugs may decrease ciliary beat frequency and possibly decrease mucociliary clearance. This effect seems most marked for atropine, however; it does not occur with ipratropium bromide or oxitropium bromide. Finally, anticholinergic drugs are bronchodilators – an effect which will aid mucus clearance. Overall then, present data indicate that although atropine may have some deleterious effects on mucociliary clearance rate, mucus volume, and on the physical properties of mucus, ipratropium bromide or oxitropium bromide does not seem to share these deleterious effects and the bronchodilator effects of these agents are likely to aid mucus clearance.

Antiinflammatory agents

Although inhaled corticosteroids are the mainstay of asthma therapy, there are few studies investigating their role in the reduction of mucin expression and secretion, and their improvement of MCC. Most of these studies have demonstrated beneficial effects; however, there is some controversy. In vitro, dexamethasone decreased mRNA of mucin genes ($MUC2$ and $MUC5$),[120–122] protein expression[122] and mucus secretion[123,124] in several cell lines, including primary differentiated normal bronchial epithelial cells, but increased mucin gene expression in another study.[125] Furthermore, in primary rat tracheal surface epithelial cells, dexamethasone decreased $MUC5AC$ mRNA expression, but did not affect $MUC5AC$ protein levels or its stability.[122] In vivo studies have also demonstrated conflicting views on the effects of corticosteroids and mucus hyper/metaplasia. Dexamethasone pre-treatment of mice administered intratracheal IL-13 failed to suppress airway $MUC5AC$ expression or goblet cell numbers in one study,[126] but significantly decreased $MUC5AC$ airway expression in antigen sensitized and challenged mice in another.[127] There have been even fewer studies done in patients with asthma regarding the effects of steroid therapy on mucus hypersecretion; however, one study in stable asthmatics treated with inhaled budesonide resulted in decreased airway epithelial goblet cell numbers.[128] The benefits of corticosteroid treatment in decreasing mucin gene expression and secretion are most likely secondary to their antiinflammatory properties,

which include binding to two GRE sites in the $MUC5AC$ promoter.[121] The effect of corticosteroids on mucociliary clearance is difficult to study as MCC is usually impaired in patients with asthma which may or may not be reversible, and is probably best studied in steroid naive or newly diagnosed patients. However, administration of systemic, but not inhaled corticosteroids in a group of 13 patients with asthma, most of whom were previously taking inhaled corticosteroids, improved MCC.[129] Despite the controversies of corticosteroid treatment in mucus metaplasia, they represent important pharmacotherapy for the treatment of acute severe asthma exacerbations and for maintenance therapy in patients with persistent disease.

Leukotrienes are critical inflammatory mediators in asthma and in vivo work demonstrates that they induce mucus metaplasia[130] and produce mucociliary dysfunction.[131] Leukotriene receptor antagonists and selective 5-lipoxygenases inhibitors are useful adjunctive therapies for asthma. Inhibiting leukotriene receptor binding in a murine model of chronic asthma significantly decreased goblet cell metaplasia and mucus plugging of the airways.[132] Furthermore, pre-treatment with a leukotriene receptor antagonist prior to antigen challenge, but not after challenge, protected against the decrease in MCC in a sheep model of asthma.[133] A specific 5-lipoxygenaze inhibitor (Zileuton) prevents mucus cell degranulation, indicating that leukotrienes mediate this effect in this model.[130]

Finally, methylxanthines may also increase intracellular cyclic adenosine monophosphate levels, increasing ciliary beat frequency. Aminophylline acutely increases tracheal mucus velocity in dogs.[134]

Mucolytic agents

The use of the cysteine derivatives, N-acetylcysteine and S-carboxymethyl cysteine, has been advocated for the treatment of mucus hypersecretion for many decades. These agents break disulfide bonds that form bridges between mucin chains, and in vitro studies convincingly show that they have favorable effects on the viscoelastic properties of asthmatic sputum. In addition to these 'mucolytic' effects, N-acetylcysteine and S-carboxymethylcysteine have antioxidant effects which may have relevance for an effect on mucus hypersecretion. For example, N-acetylcysteine or S-carboxymethylcysteine administered concurrently during 2 weeks of cigarette smoke exposure, significantly inhibits the development of mucus hypersecretion in the rat.[135] The mechanism for this effect is probably a direct or indirect antioxidant effect. The direct antioxidant effect may be to increase intracellular stores of reduced glutathione or to block oxidant-induced depletion of glutathione. The indirect effect (relevant only for N-acetylcysteine) may be a direct oxygen scavenging effect. Despite these favorable in vitro and animal experiments with cysteine derivatives, the clinical experience with N-acetylcysteine in asthma has not been very favorable mainly because it causes bronchoconstriction when administered by aerosol.[136] Thus, the use of aerosolized or oral preparations of N-acetylcysteine or S-carboxymethylcysteine cannot be recommended.

Bromhexine is another oral agent classified as a mucolytic (although it does not break disulfide bonds) and it is one of the few mucolytic drugs whose therapeutic efficacy has been examined in a placebo-controlled trial in patients with acute severe asthma. Unfortunately, it proved no better than placebo in affecting outcomes that included rate of recovery, measures of oxygenation and ventilation, and measurements of peak flow.[137]

Expectorants

The term expectorant is derived from the Latin word *expectore,* which means 'from the chest'. Thus, drugs which allow patients to cough up sputum more easily are considered expectorants. Writing about expectorants in this chapter for the third edition of this textbook in 1983, Hirsch wrote: 'Of the areas in modern treatment, none remain more firmly attached to tradition than the use of bitter, sour, salty, and/or sweet medicaments in various preparations and at various temperatures as cough medicines. Each prescription of potassium iodide, ammonium chloride, terpin hydrate, guaifenesin, honey and lemon, or ethyl alcohol associated with antihistamines and cough depressants carries with it the fervent hope of the physician that the prescription will dislodge the phlegm and the cough will subside. It is my conviction that, although these drugs may have some therapeutic action in patients with acute bronchitis, the zeal with which the physician prescribes the drug is as therapeutic as the ingredients'.[138] Over 25 years later, the zeal with which expectorants are prescribed does not seem to have subsided despite the lack of any new body of research supporting their use.

Expectorants such as ammonium chloride and members of the terpin hydrate group may have some ciliostimulatory effects but there are no published reports of their efficacy in clinical trials. Some expectorants such as guaifenesin (glycerol guaiacolate) are emetics and are given in subemetic doses for the theoretic possibility that gastric irritation promotes an increase in mucus secretion by a cholinergic reflex mechanism. The clinical data to support the efficacy of guaifenesin in asthma is conflicting and, on balance, unimpressive.[139,140] The mechanism of action of the iodide salts expectorants (iodinated glycerol and potassium iodide) on the mucociliary system in unknown. They are thought to improve mucus expectoration by improving mucus hydration – perhaps through increased epithelial water secretion or serous cell secretion. In placebo-controlled trials, the administration of iodide salts results in improved symptoms in patients with airway disease, although lung function has not improved significantly. For example, iodinated glycerol treatment for 6 months in children with asthma resulted in improved asthma symptom scores but objective measures of pulmonary function did not change significantly and the treatment was associated with the development of palpable goiter in 15% of patients.[141] In addition, the administration of iodinated glycerol for 8 weeks in patients with COPD resulted in significant improvements in airway symptom scores but objective measures of pulmonary function, sputum volume, or mucus rheology were not measured.[142]

Miscellaneous pharmacologic agents

Sodium thiophene carboxylate decreases the viscosity and elasticity of pig mucin collected from a tracheal pouch but has no effect on pulmonary function or airway mucus rheology in patients with COPD and asthma.[143] Inhaled indomethacin has a significantly greater effect than inhaled placebo in reducing sputum volume in patients with bronchorrhea secondary to chronic bronchitis.[144] Two case reports have reported that erythromycin reduces sputum volume significantly in asthmatic patients with bronchorrhea.[145,146] This effect of erythromycin may be a mediated by directly downregulating *MUC*5AC mRNA and protein expression, rather than an indirect antibacterial effect.[147,148] Finally, a few studies have demonstrated that inhalation of hyperosmolar agents (e.g., hypertonic saline and mannitol) increases clearance of mucus in mild asthmatics. However, the data have not clearly demonstrated any

improvement in lung function from this treatment. Furthermore, the use of these agents may induce a significant fall in FEV_1 and should probably not be used in patients with moderate to severe asthma.[149]

Many of the medications used to decrease mucus hypersecretion in cystic fibrosis have not been studied in the treatment of asthma, but may be relevant. For example, aerosolized recombinant human DNase improves pulmonary function and reduces cystic fibrosis-related pulmonary exacerbations by liquefying DNA-rich CF sputum and enhancing mucus clearance. DNase has been used in patients with status asthmaticus in case reports.[150,151] In addition, aerosolized amiloride slows the loss of forced vital capacity and improves sputum viscosity and elasticity in patients with cystic fibrosis by blocking sodium channels in airway epithelial cells and increasing mucus hydration.[152] Finally, aerosolized uridine 5′-triphosphate (in combination with aerosolized amiloride) improves mucociliary clearance from the periphery of the lungs in patients with cystic fibrosis,[153] presumably by stimulating airway ciliary beat frequency.

Chest physical therapy

Chest physical therapy is probably most helpful in asthmatic patients with allergic bronchopulmonary aspergillosis since these patients have bronchiectasis. Chest physical therapy is usually not considered part of the regimen of management for acute severe asthma although a trial of chest physical therapy should be considered for patients with atelectasis secondary to mucus plugs. Bronchospasm and cough paroxysms are potential side effects of chest physical therapy in asthmatic subjects who are experiencing acute exacerbations.

Bronchoscopy

Bronchoscopy and bronchoalveolar lavage with saline or saline and *N*-acetylcysteine has been advocated as a treatment for acute severe asthma for over 30 years. No controlled trials of this therapy have been performed, however. The most recent uncontrolled series was in 19 asthmatic subjects refractory to at least 48–72 h of aggressive inpatient medical management.[154] A total of 51 bronchoscopies (1–6 per patient) were performed transnasally with local anesthesia. Mucus visualized in the large airways was removed by suction and mucus in smaller more peripheral airways was removed by lavage with a total of 50–300 ml of saline. Airway casts were recovered in the BAL in some instances (Fig. 39.9). Complications included three episodes of transient mild hypoxemia and four episodes of bronchospasm responsive to bronchodilator therapy. Mean FEV_1 values pre-bronchoscopy were 41% of predicted and increased to 60% of predicted within 96 h of bronchoscopy. Despite these encouraging uncontrolled data, the expense and potential dangers of bronchoscopy in acutely ill asthmatics require that a properly controlled randomized study be completed before BAL is recommended as a treatment for acute severe asthma refractory to usual therapeutic measures.

NOVEL TREATMENTS

The discovery that hCLCA1 – a calcium activated chloride channel – is upregulated in the airway epithelium and localizes to goblet cells in asthmatic subjects[56] provides a novel therapeutic target for decreasing airway goblet cell hyperplasia. An inhibitor of hCLCA1, niflumic acid,

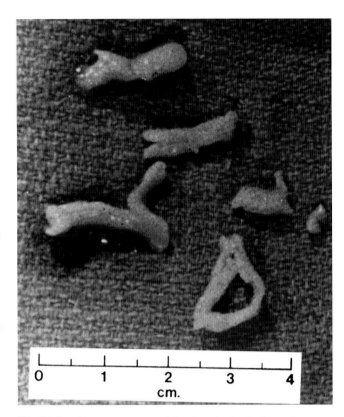

Fig. 39.9. Airway casts recovered from bronchoalveolar lavage from an asthmatic subject in acute exacerbation. (From Lang et al.[154])

decreases goblet cell hyperplasia and *MUC*5AC expression in cell culture and a murine model of asthma.[69,155] Currently, another inhibitor of hCLCA1, talniflumate, is in the early phases of clinical testing as a specific treatment for airway mucus hypersecretion.

It is also possible to target several arms of the inflammatory cascade leading to goblet cell hyperplasia. This may include administering inhibitors of EGFR tyrosine kinase (ZD1829, Iressa) or p38 MAPK activity, or antibodies against specific cytokines such as IL-13.[85] Selective phosophodiesterase-4 inhibitors have antiinflammatory properties and have decreased *MUC*5AC expression and goblet cell hyperplasia in an animal model and in human airway epithelial cell lines.[156] Alternative medications, such as a formulation of Traditional Chinese Medication for asthma decreased Th2 cytokine secretion with subsequent mucus cell metaplasia[157] and *MUC*5AC expression (PJ Busse, unpublished data) in a mouse model of allergic asthma.

Mucus hypersecretion may also be attenuated by preventing its release from secretory granules. The myristoylated, alanine-rich C kinase substrate (MARCKS) was demonstrated to be required for mucin secretion.[39] Inhibition of its action via pre-treating antigen-sensitized and challenged mice with a myristoylated N-terminal sequence (MANS) prevented mucin release from goblet cells[40] and decreased airway hyperresponsiveness.[158] Additionally, extracellular nucleotide triphosphates such as ATP and UTP release mucin from goblet cells, via binding to the P_{2Y2} receptors.[159] Therefore, P_{2Y2} receptor antagonists may be useful to prevent mucus hypersecretion in asthma, and are in clinical trials for CF.[160]

■ SUMMARY ■

Airway mucus is important for trapping inhaled foreign material, and the mucociliary escalator drives this material from the airways and to the mouth where it may be cleared. However, in chronic airway diseases such as asthma, the composition of airway mucus is altered. Specifically, there are increases in mucin levels, plasma protein levels, cell numbers, and products of cell lysis. These changes in mucus composition result in differences in viscosity and adhesiveness of mucus that render it more difficult to expectorate. These abnormalities, coupled with abnormalities in ciliary function, result in accumulation of mucus in the airways and airway obstruction. Consequently, mucus hypersecretion in asthma contributes significantly to the morbidity and mortality of the disease. The pathophysiology of mucus hypersecretion in asthma is probably closely linked to the pathophysiology of airway inflammation since important consequences of the abnormal cellular infiltration and vascular permeability that characterize asthma are higher than normal levels of cell-derived and plasma-derived mucus secretagogues in the airway as well as higher than normal levels of mediators that promote hyperplasia and metaplasia of goblet cells. Thus, it is not surprising that the most effective treatments for mucus hypersecretion in asthma are oral and inhaled corticosteroids. The role of mucolytics and expectorants in the treatment of mucus hypersecretion remains controversial. New therapeutic agents for mucus hypersecretion and mucus impaction are under development based on improved understanding of the mechanisms of mucus hypersecretion and on improved understanding of the contribution of mucus components such as mucins, albumin, DNA, and actin to the viscoelastic properties and rate of clearance of airway mucus.

References

Constituents of airway mucus

1. Rose MC, Voynow JA. Respiratory tract mucin genes and mucin glycoproteins in health and disease. Physiol Rev 2006; 86:245–278.
2. Taylor ME, Drickamer K. Introduction to glycobiology, 2nd edn. Oxford: Oxford University Press; 2003.
3. Voynow JA, Gendler SJ, Rose MC. Regulation of mucin genes in chronic inflammatory airway diseases. Am J Respir Cell Mol Biol 2006; 34:661–665.
4. Whittaker L, Niu N, Temann UA, et al. Interleukin-13 mediates a fundamental pathway for airway epithelial mucus induced by CD4 T cells and interleukin-9. Am J Respir Cell Mol Biol 2002; 27:593–602.
5. Bennett EP, Weghuis DO, Merkx G, et al. Genomic organization and chromosomal localization of three members of the UDP-N-acetylgalactosamine: polypeptide N-acetylgalactosaminyltransferase family. Glycobiology 1998; 8:547–555.
6. Lopez-Ferrer A, de Bolos C, Barranco C, et al. Role of fucosyltransferases in the association between apomucin and Lewis antigen expression in normal and malignant gastric epithelium. Gut 2000; 47:349–356.
7. de Bolos C, Guma M, Barranco C, et al. MUC6 expression in breast tissues and cultured cells: abnormal expression in tumors and regulation by steroid hormones. Int J Cancer 1998; 77:193–199.
8. Scanlin TF, Glick MC. Terminal glycosylation in cystic fibrosis. Biochim Biophys Acta 1999; 1455:241–253.
9. Lamblin G, Aubert JP, Perini JM, et al. Human respiratory mucins. Eur Respir J 1992; 5:247–256.
10. Tegner H, Ohlsson K, Toremalm NG, et al. Effect of human leukocyte enzymes on tracheal mucosa and its mucociliary activity. Rhinology 1979; 17:199–206.
11. Sommerhoff CP, Nadel JA, Basbaum CB, et al. Neutrophil elastase and cathepsin G stimulate secretion from cultured bovine airway gland serous cells. J Clin Invest 1990; 85:682–689.
12. Rasmussen TN, Raaberg L, Poulsen SS, et al. Immunohistochemical localization of pancreatic spasmolytic polypeptide (PSP) in the pig. Histochemistry 1992; 98:113–119.
13. Longman RJ, Douthwaite J, Sylvester PA, et al. Coordinated localisation of mucins and trefoil peptides in the ulcer associated cell lineage and the gastrointestinal mucosa. Gut 2000; 47:792–800.
14. Thim L, Madsen F, Poulsen SS. Effect of trefoil factors on the viscoelastic properties of mucus gels. Eur J Clin Invest 2002; 32:519–527.
15. Dignass A, Lynch-Devaney K, Kindon H, et al. Trefoil peptides promote epithelial migration through a transforming growth factor beta-independent pathway. J Clin Invest 1994; 94:376–383.

16. Babyatsky MW, deBeaumont M, Thim L, et al. Oral trefoil peptides protect against ethanol- and indomethacin-induced gastric injury in rats. Gastroenterology 1996; 110:489–497.
17. Wiede A, Jagla W, Welte T, et al. Localization of TFF3, a new mucus-associated peptide of the human respiratory tract. Am J Respir Crit Care Med 1999; 159:1330–1335.
18. Kuperman DA, Lewis CC, Woodruff PG, et al. Dissecting asthma using focused transgenic modeling and functional genomics. J Allergy Clin Immunol 2005; 116:305–311.
19. Nikolaidis NM, Zimmermann N, King NE, et al. Trefoil factor-2 is an allergen-induced gene regulated by Th2 cytokines and STAT6 in the lung. Am J Respir Cell Mol Biol 2003; 29:458–464.
20. Oertel M, Graness A, Thim L, et al. Trefoil factor family-peptides promote migration of human bronchial epithelial cells: synergistic effect with epidermal growth factor. Am J Respir Cell Mol Biol 2001; 25:418–424.

Cellular regulation of mucocillary clearance and secretion

21. Mall M, Grubb BR, Harkema JR, et al. Increased airway epithelial Na$^+$ absorption produces cystic fibrosis-like lung disease in mice. Nat Med 2004; 10:487–493.
22. Tyner JW, Kim EY, Ide K, et al. Blocking airway mucous cell metaplasia by inhibiting EGFR antiapoptosis and IL-13 transdifferentiation signals. J Clin Invest 2006; 116:309–321.
23. Lundgren JD, Kaliner M, Logun C, et al. Dexamethasone reduces rat tracheal goblet cell hyperplasia produced by human neutrophil products. Exp Lung Res 1988; 14:853–863.
24. Rogers DF, Jeffery PK. Inhibition of cigarette smoke-induced airway secretory cell hyperplasia by indomethacin, dexamethasone, prednisolone, or hydrocortisone in the rat. Exp Lung Res 1986; 10:285–298.
25. Rogers DF. Airway goblet cells: responsive and adaptable front-line defenders. Eur Respir J 1994; 7:1690–1706.
26. Tokuyama K, Kuo HP, Rohde JA, et al. Neural control of goblet cell secretion in guinea pig airways. Am J Physiol 1990; 259:L108–L115.
27. German VF, Ueki IF, Nadel JA. Micropipette measurement of airway submucosal gland secretion: laryngeal reflex. Am Rev Respir Dis 1980; 122:413–416.
28. Murlas C, Nadel JA, Basbaum CB. A morphometric analysis of the autonomic innervation of cat tracheal glands. J Auton Nerv Syst 1980; 2:23–37.
29. Gallagher JT, Kent PW, Passatore M, et al. The composition of tracheal mucus and the nervous control of its secretion in the cat. Proc R Soc Lond B Biol Sci 1975; 192:49–76.
30. Reid L. Measurement of the bronchial mucous gland layer: a diagnostic yardstick in chronic bronchitis. Thorax 1960; 15:132–141.
31. Heidsiek JG, Hyde DM, Plopper CG, et al. Quantitative histochemistry of mucosubstance in tracheal epithelium of the macaque monkey. J Histochem Cytochem 1987; 35:435–442.
32. Evans CM, Williams OW, Tuvim MJ, et al. Mucin is produced by Clara cells in the proximal airways of antigen-challenged mice. Am J Respir Cell Mol Biol 2004; 31:382–394.
33. Boers JE, Ambergen AW, Thunnissen FB. Number and proliferation of Clara cells in normal human airway epithelium. Am J Respir Crit Care Med 1999; 159:1585–1591.

Mucin packaging and discharge from airway secretory cells

34. Forstner G. Signal transduction, packaging and secretion of mucins. Annu Rev Physiol 1995; 57:585–605.
35. Hollingsworth MA, Swanson BJ. Mucins in cancer: protection and control of the cell surface. Nat Rev Cancer 2004; 4:45–60.
36. Rogers DF. The airway goblet cell. Int J Biochem Cell Biol 2003; 35:1–6.
37. Basbaum C, Welsh MJ. Mucous secretion and ion transport in airways. In: Murray JF, Nadel JA, eds. Textbook of respiratory medicine, 2nd edn. Philadelphia: WB Saunders; 1994 :323–344.
38. Perez-Vilar J. Mucin granule intraluminal organization. Am J Respir Cell Mol Biol 2007; 36:183–190.
39. Li Y, Martin LD, Spizz G, et al. MARCKS protein is a key molecule regulating mucin secretion by human airway epithelial cells in vitro. J Biol Chem 2001; 276:40982–40990.
40. Singer M, Martin LD, Vargaftig BB, et al. A MARCKS-related peptide blocks mucin hypersecretion in a mouse model of asthma. Nat Med 2004; 10:193–196.
41. Park J, Fang S, Adler KB. Regulation of airway mucin secretion by MARCKS protein involves the chaperones heat shock protein 70 and cysteine string protein. Proc Am Thorac Soc 2006; 3:493.

Clinical importance and cellular characteristics of mucus hypersecretion in asthma

42. Lange P, Parner J, Vestbo J, et al. A 15-year follow-up study of ventilatory function in adults with asthma. N Engl J Med 1998; 339:1194–1200.
43. Rogers DF. Airway mucus hypersecretion in asthma: an undervalued pathology? Curr Opin Pharmacol 2004; 4:241–250.
44. Dunhill M. The pathology of asthma with special reference to changes in the bronchial mucosa. J Clin Pathol 1960; 13:27–33.
45. Reid LM, O'Sullivan DD, Bhaskar KR. Pathophysiology of bronchial hypersecretion. Eur J Respir Dis Suppl 1987; 153:19–25.
46. O'Riordan TG, Zwang J, Smaldone GC. Mucociliary clearance in adult asthma. Am Rev Respir Dis 1992; 146:598–603.
47. Messina MS, O'Riordan TG, Smaldone GC. Changes in mucociliary clearance during acute exacerbations of asthma. Am Rev Respir Dis 1991; 143:993–997.
48. Fahy JV, Liu J, Wong H, et al. Cellular and biochemical analysis of induced sputum from asthmatic and from healthy subjects. Am Rev Respir Dis 1993; 147:1126–1131.
49. Gauvreau GM, Watson RM, O'Byrne PM. Kinetics of allergen-induced airway eosinophilic cytokine production and airway inflammation. Am J Respir Crit Care Med 1999; 160: 640–647.
50. Hargreave FE. Quantitative sputum cell counts as a marker of airway inflammation in clinical practice. Curr Opin Allergy Clin Immunol 2007; 7:102–106.
51. Fahy JV, Kim KW, Liu J, et al. Prominent neutrophilic inflammation in sputum from subjects with asthma exacerbation. J Allergy Clin Immunol 1995; 95:843–852.
52. Levine SJ LP, Logun C, Shelmaner JH. IL-6 induces respiratory mucous glycoprotein secretion and MUC-2 expression by human airway epithelial cells. Am J Resp Crit Care Med 1994; 149:A27.
53. Shak S, Capon DJ, Hellmiss R, et al. Recombinant human DNase I reduces the viscosity of cystic fibrosis sputum. Proc Natl Acad Sci U S A 1990; 87:9188–9192.
54. Fahy JV, Steiger DJ, Liu J, et al. Markers of mucus secretion and DNA levels in induced sputum from asthmatic and from healthy subjects. Am Rev Respir Dis 1993; 147:1132–1137.

Pathophysiology of mucus hypersecretion in asthma

55. Ordóñez CL, Khashayar R, Wong HH, et al. Mild and moderate asthma is associated with airway goblet cell hyperplasia and abnormalities in mucin gene expression. Am J Respir Crit Care Med 2001; 163:517–523.
56. Hoshino M, Morita S, Iwashita H, et al. Increased expression of the human Ca^{2+}-activated Cl$^-$ channel 1 (CaCC1) gene in the asthmatic airway. Am J Respir Crit Care Med 2002; 165:1132–1136.
57. Groneberg DA, Eynott PR, Lim S, et al. Expression of respiratory mucins in fatal status asthmaticus and mild asthma. Histopathology 2002; 40:367–373.
58. Erle DJ, Zhen G. The asthma channel? Stay tuned. Am J Respir Crit Care Med 2006; 173:1181–1182.
59. Toda M, Tulic MK, Levitt RC, et al. A calcium-activated chloride channel (HCLCA1) is strongly related to IL-9 expression and mucus production in bronchial epithelium of patients with asthma. J Allergy Clin Immunol 2002; 109:246–250.
60. Nakanishi A, Morita S, Iwashita H, et al. Role of gob-5 in mucus overproduction and airway hyperresponsiveness in asthma. Proc Natl Acad Sci U S A 2001; 98:5175–5180.
61. Long AJ, Sypek JP, Askew R, et al. Gob-5 contributes to goblet cell hyperplasia and modulates pulmonary tissue inflammation. Am J Respir Cell Mol Biol 2006; 35:357–365.
62. Robichaud A, Tuck SA, Kargman S, et al. Gob-5 is not essential for mucus overproduction in preclinical murine models of allergic asthma. Am J Respir Cell Mol Biol 2005; 33:303–314.
63. Thai P, Chen Y, Dolganov G, et al. Differential regulation of MUC5AC/Muc5ac and hCLCA-1/Gob-5 expression in airway epithelium. Am J Respir Cell Mol Biol 2005; 33:523–30.
64. Zuhdi Alimam M, Piazza FM, Selby DM, et al. Muc-5/5ac mucin messenger RNA and protein expression is a marker of goblet cell metaplasia in murine airways. Am J Respir Cell Mol Biol 2000; 22:253–260.
65. Temann UA, Prasad B, Gallup MW, et al. A novel role for murine IL-4 in vivo: induction of MUC5AC gene expression and mucin hypersecretion. Am J Respir Cell Mol Biol 1997; 16:471–478.
66. Reader JR, Hyde DM, Schelegle ES, et al. Interleukin-9 induces mucous cell metaplasia independent of inflammation. Am J Respir Cell Mol Biol 2003; 28:664–672.
67. Lee JJ, McGarry MP, Farmer SC, et al. Interleukin-5 expression in the lung epithelium of transgenic mice leads to pulmonary changes pathognomonic of asthma. J Exp Med 1997; 185:2143–2156.
68. Chen Y, Thai P, Zhao YH, et al. Stimulation of airway mucin gene expression by interleukin (IL)-17 through IL-6 paracrine/autocrine loop. J Biol Chem 2003; 278:17036 17043.
69. Hauber HP, Daigneault P, Frenkiel S, et al. Niflumic acid and MSI-2216 reduce TNF-alpha-induced mucin expression in human airway mucosa. J Allergy Clin Immunol 2005; 115:266–271.
70. Kim CH, Song KS, Koo JS, et al. IL-13 suppresses MUC5AC gene expression and mucin secretion in nasal epithelial cells. Acta Otolaryngol 2002; 122:638–643.
71. Song KS, Lee WJ, Chung KC, et al. Interleukin-1 beta and tumor necrosis factor-alpha induce MUC5AC overexpression through a mechanism involving ERK/p38 mitogen-activated protein kinases-MSK1-CREB activation in human airway epithelial cells. J Biol Chem 2003; 278:23243–23250.
72. Busse PJ, Zhang TF, Srivastava K, et al. Chronic exposure to TNF-alpha increases airway mucus gene expression in vivo. J Allergy Clin Immunol 2005; 116:1256–1263.
73. Cohn L, Homer RJ, Niu N, et al. T helper 1 cells and interferon gamma regulate allergic airway inflammation and mucus production. J Exp Med 1999; 190:1309–1318.
74. Zhou B, Comeau MR, De Smedt T, et al. Thymic stromal lymphopoietin as a key initiator of allergic airway inflammation in mice. Nat Immunol 2005; 6:1047–1053.
75. Humbles AA, Lloyd CM, McMillan SJ, et al. A critical role for eosinophils in allergic airways remodeling. Science 2004; 305:1776–1779.
76. Cohn L, Homer RJ, MacLeod H, et al. Th2-induced airway mucus production is dependent on IL-4Ralpha, but not on eosinophils. J Immunol 1999; 162:6178–6183.
77. Shen HH, Ochkur SI, McGarry MP, et al. A causative relationship exists between eosinophils and the development of allergic pulmonary pathologies in the mouse. J Immunol 2003; 170:3296–3305.
78. Lee JJ, Dimina D, Macias MP, et al. Defining a link with asthma in mice congenitally deficient in eosinophils. Science 2004; 305:1773–1776.
79. Burgel PR, Lazarus SC, Tam DC, et al. Human eosinophils induce mucin production in airway epithelial cells via epidermal growth factor receptor activation. J Immunol 2001; 167:5948–5954.
80. Miller AL, Strieter RM, Gruber AD, et al. CXCR2 regulates respiratory syncytial virus-induced airway hyperreactivity and mucus overproduction. J Immunol 2003; 170: 3348–3356.
81. Hashimoto K, Durbin JE, Zhou W, et al. Respiratory syncytial virus infection in the absence of STAT 1 results in airway dysfunction, airway mucus, and augmented IL-17 levels. J Allergy Clin Immunol 2005; 116:550–557.

82. Vrtis RF HE, Gern JE, Busse WW. MUC5AC gene expression in upper and lower airway samples following experimental rhinovirus (RV) 16 inoculation. J Allergy Clin Immunol 2005; 115:S142.
83. Chu HW, Rino JG, Wexler RB, et al. Mycoplasma pneumoniae infection increases airway collagen deposition in a murine model of allergic airway inflammation. Am J Physiol Lung Cell Mol Physiol 2005; 289:L125–L133.
84. Morcillo EJ, Cortijo J. Mucus and MUC in asthma. Curr Opin Pulm Med 2006; 12:1–6.
85. Rogers DF, Barnes PJ. Treatment of airway mucus hypersecretion. Ann Med 2006; 38: 116–125.
86. Takeyama K, Fahy JV, Nadel JA. Relationship of epidermal growth factor receptors to goblet cell production in human bronchi. Am J Respir Crit Care Med 2001; 163:511–516.
87. Shim JJ, Dabbagh K, Ueki IF, et al. IL-13 induces mucin production by stimulating epidermal growth factor receptors and by activating neutrophils. Am J Physiol Lung Cell Mol Physiol 2001; 280:L134–L140.
88. Booth BW, Adler KB, Bonner JC, et al. Interleukin-13 induces proliferation of human airway epithelial cells in vitro via a mechanism mediated by transforming growth factor-alpha. Am J Respir Cell Mol Biol 2001; 25:739–743.
89. McNamara N, Gallup M, Khong A, et al. Adenosine up-regulation of the mucin gene, MUC2, in asthma. FASEB J 2004; 18:1770–1772.
90. Shahzeidi S, Aujla PK, Nickola TJ, et al. Temporal analysis of goblet cells and mucin gene expression in murine models of allergic asthma. Exp Lung Res 2003; 29:549–565.
91. Kuperman DA, Huang X, Koth LL, et al. Direct effects of interleukin-13 on epithelial cells cause airway hyperreactivity and mucus overproduction in asthma. Nat Med 2002; 8: 885–889.
92. Shi ZO, Fischer MJ, De Sanctis GT, et al. IFN-gamma, but not Fas, mediates reduction of allergen-induced mucous cell metaplasia by inducing apoptosis. J Immunol 2002; 168: 4764–4771.
93. Kirkham S, Sheehan JK, Knight D, et al. Heterogeneity of airways mucus: variations in the amounts and glycoforms of the major oligomeric mucins MUC5AC and MUC5B. Biochem J 2002; 361:537–546.
94. Ordoñez CL, Shaughnessy TE, Matthay MA, et al. Increased neutrophil numbers and IL-8 levels in airway secretions in acute severe asthma: clinical and biologic significance. Am J Respir Crit Care Med 2000; 161:1185–1190.
95. Lundgren JD, Davey RT Jr, Lundgren B, et al. Eosinophil cationic protein stimulates and major basic protein inhibits airway mucus secretion. J Allergy Clin Immunol 1991; 87: 689–698.
96. Sommerhoff CP, Caughey GH, Finkbeiner WE, et al. Mast cell chymase. A potent secretagogue for airway gland serous cells. J Immunol 1989; 142:2450–2456.
97. Shimura S, Sasaki T, Ikeda K, et al. VIP augments cholinergic-induced glycoconjugate secretion in tracheal submucosal glands. J Appl Physiol 1988; 65:2537–2544.
98. Agusti C, Takeyama K, Cardell LO, et al. Goblet cell degranulation after antigen challenge in sensitized guinea pigs. Role of neutrophils. Am J Respir Crit Care Med 1998; 158:1253–1258.
99. Hays SR, Woodruff PG, Khashayar R, et al. Allergen challenge causes inflammation but not goblet cell degranulation in asthmatic subjects. J Allergy Clin Immunol 2001; 108:784–790.
100. Chen Y, Zhao YH, Wu R. Differential regulation of airway mucin gene expression and mucin secretion by extracellular nucleotide triphosphates. Am J Respir Cell Mol Biol 2001; 25:409–417.
101. Takashi S, Park J, Fang S, et al. A peptide against the N-terminus of myristoylated alanine-rich C kinase substrate inhibits degranulation of human leukocytes in vitro. Am J Respir Cell Mol Biol 2006; 34:647–652.
102. Widdicome J. Role of lipids in airway function. Eur J Resp Dis 1987; 71:197–204.
103. List SJ, Findlay BP, Forstner GG, et al. Enhancement of the viscosity of mucin by serum albumin. Biochem J 1978; 175:565–571.
104. Dulfano MJ, Luk CK. Sputum and ciliary inhibition in asthma. Thorax 1982; 37:646–651.
105. Hastie AT, Loegering DA, Gleich GJ, et al. The effect of purified human eosinophil major basic protein on mammalian ciliary activity. Am Rev Respir Dis 1987; 135:848–853.

Treatment of mucus hypersecretion in asthma

106. Houtmeyers E, Gosselink R, Gayan-Ramirez G, et al. Effects of drugs on mucus clearance. Eur Respir J 1999; 14:452–467.
107. Wanner A, Salathe M, O'Riordan TG. Mucociliary clearance in the airways. Am J Respir Crit Care Med 1996; 154:1868–1902.
108. Isawa T, Teshima T, Hirano T, et al. Does a beta 2-stimulator really facilitate mucociliary transport in the human lungs in vivo? A study with procaterol. Am Rev Respir Dis 1990; 141:715–720.
109. Bateman JR, Pavia D, Sheahan NF, et al. Effects of terbutaline sulphate aerosol on bronchodilator response and lung mucociliary clearance in patients with mild stable asthma. Br J Clin Pharmacol 1983; 15:695–700.
110. Mortensen J, Groth S, Lange P, et al. Effect of terbutaline on mucociliary clearance in asthmatic and healthy subjects after inhalation from a pressurised inhaler and a dry powder inhaler. Thorax 1991; 46:817–823.
111. Pavia D, Agnew JE, Sutton PP, et al. Effect of terbutaline administered from metered dose inhaler (2 mg) and subcutaneously (0.25 mg) on tracheobronchial clearance in mild asthma. Br J Dis Chest 1987; 81:361–370.
112. Hasani A, Toms N, O'Connor J, et al. Effect of salmeterol xinafoate on lung mucociliary clearance in patients with asthma. Respir Med 2003; 97:667–671.
113. Daviskas E, Anderson SD, Shaw J, et al. Mucociliary clearance in patients with chronic asthma: effects of beta agonists. Respirology 2005; 10:426–435.
114. Leikauf GD, Ueki IF, Nadel JA. Autonomic regulation of viscoelasticity of cat tracheal gland secretions. J Appl Physiol 1984; 56:426–430.
115. Shelhamer JH, Marom Z, Kaliner M. Immunologic and neuropharmacologic stimulation of mucous glycoprotein release from human airways in vitro. J Clin Invest 1980; 66:1400–1408.
116. Sturgess J, Reid L. An organ culture study of the effect of drugs on the secretory activity of the human bronchial submucosal gland. Clin Sci 1972; 43:533–543.
117. Henderson WR Jr., Banerjee ER, Chi EY. Differential effects of (S)- and (R)-enantiomers of albuterol in a mouse asthma model. J Allergy Clin Immunol 2005; 116:332–340.
118. Mann JS, George CF. Anticholinergic drugs in the treatment of airways disease. Br J Dis Chest 1985; 79:209–228.
119. King M, Cohen C, Viires N. Influence of vagal tone on rheology and transportability of canine tracheal mucus. Am Rev Respir Dis 1979; 120:1215–1219.
120. Kai H, Yoshitake K, Hisatsune A, et al. Dexamethasone suppresses mucus production and MUC-2 and MUC-5AC gene expression by NCI-H292 cells. Am J Physiol 1996; 271: L484–L488.
121. Chen Y, Nickola TJ, DiFronzo NL, et al. Dexamethasone-mediated repression of MUC5AC gene expression in human lung epithelial cells. Am J Respir Cell Mol Biol 2006; 34:338–347.
122. Lu W, Lillehoj EP, Kim KC. Effects of dexamethasone on Muc5ac mucin production by primary airway goblet cells. Am J Physiol Lung Cell Mol Physiol 2005; 288:L52–L60.
123. Shimura S, Sasaki T, Ikeda K, et al. Direct inhibitory action of glucocorticoid on glycoconjugate secretion from airway submucosal glands. Am Rev Respir Dis 1990; 141:1044–1049.
124. Marom Z, Shelhamer J, Alling D, et al. The effects of corticosteroids on mucous glycoprotein secretion from human airways in vitro. Am Rev Respir Dis 1984; 129:62–65.
125. Gollub EG, Waksman H, Goswami S, et al. Mucin genes are regulated by estrogen and dexamethasone. Biochem Biophys Res Commun 1995; 217:1006–1014.
126. Kibe A, Inoue H, Fukuyama S, et al. Differential regulation by glucocorticoid of interleukin-13-induced eosinophilia, hyperresponsiveness, and goblet cell hyperplasia in mouse airways. Am J Respir Crit Care Med 2003; 167:50–56.
127. Singer M, Lefort J, Vargaftig BB. Granulocyte depletion and dexamethasone differentially modulate airways hyperreactivity, inflammation, mucus accumulation, and secretion induced by rmIL-13 or antigen. Am J Respir Cell Mol Biol 2002; 26:74–84.
128. Laitinen LA, Heino M, Laitinen A, et al. Damage of the airway epithelium and bronchial reactivity in patients with asthma. Am Rev Respir Dis 1985; 131:599–606.
129. Shah RV, Amin M, Sangwan S, et al. Steroid effects on mucociliary clearance in outpatient asthma. J Aerosol Med 2006; 19:208–220.
130. Henderson WR Jr, Lewis DB, Albert RK, et al. The importance of leukotrienes in airway inflammation in a mouse model of asthma. J Exp Med 1996; 184:1483–1494.
131. Russi EW, Abraham WM, Chapman GA, et al. Effects of leukotriene D_4 on mucociliary and respiratory function in allergic and nonallergic sheep. J Appl Physiol 1985; 59:1416–1422.
132. Henderson WR Jr, Tang LO, Chu SJ, et al. A role for cysteinyl leukotrienes in airway remodeling in a mouse asthma model. Am J Respir Crit Care Med 2002; 165:108–116.
133. Sabater JR, Wanner A, Abraham WM. Montelukast prevents antigen-induced mucociliary dysfunction in sheep. Am J Respir Crit Care Med 2002; 166:1457–1460.
134. Serafini SM, Wanner A, Michaelson ED. Mucociliary transport in central and intermediate size airways: effect of aminophyllin. Bull Eur Physiopathol Respir 1976; 12:415–422.
135. Rogers DF, Turner NC, Marriott C, et al. Oral N-acetylcysteine or S-carboxymethylcysteine inhibit cigarette smoke-induced hypersecretion of mucus in rat larynx and trachea in situ. Eur Respir J 1989; 2:955–960.
136. Hirsch SR, Zastrow JE, Kory RC. Sputum liquefying agents: a comparative in vitro evaluation. J Lab Clin Med 1969; 74:346–353.
137. Rudolf M, Riordan JF, Grant BJ, et al. Bromhexine in severe asthma. Br J Dis Chest 1978; 72:307–312.
138. Hirsch SR. Airway mucus and the mucociliary system. In: Middleton E, ed. Allergy. Principles and Practice, Vol 1, 3 edn. St. Louis: Mosby, 1983.
139. Heilborn H, Pegelow K-O, Odeblad E. Effect of bromhexine and guaiphenesine on clinical state, ventilatory capacity and sputum viscosity in chronic asthma. Scand J Respir Dis 1976; 57:88–96.
140. Sisson JH, Yonkers AJ, Waldman RH. Effects of guaifenesin on nasal mucociliary clearance and ciliary beat frequency in healthy volunteers. Chest 1995; 107:747–751.
141. Falliers CJ, McCann WP, Chai H, et al. Controlled study of iodotherapy for childhood asthma. J Allergy 1966; 38:183–192.
142. Petty TL. The National Mucolytic Study. Results of a randomized, double-blind, placebo-controlled study of iodinated glycerol in chronic obstructive bronchitis. Chest 1990; 97:75–83.
143. Streit E, Medici TC. Sodium thiophene carboxylate does not facilitate expectoration. Eur Respir J 1991; 4:718–722.
144. Tamaoki J, Chiyotani A, Kobayashi K, et al. Effect of indomethacin on bronchorrhea in patients with chronic bronchitis, diffuse panbronchiolitis, or bronchiectasis. Am Rev Respir Dis 1992; 145:548–552.
145. Suez D, Szefler SJ. Excessive accumulation of mucus in children with asthma: a potential role for erythromycin? A case discussion. J Allergy Clin Immunol 1986; 77:330–334.
146. Marom ZM, Goswami SK. Respiratory mucus hypersecretion (bronchorrhea): a case discussion – possible mechanisms(s) and treatment. J Allergy Clin Immunol 1991; 87:1050–1055.
147. Shimizu T, Shimizu S, Hattori R, et al. In vivo and in vitro effects of macrolide antibiotics on mucus secretion in airway epithelial cells. Am J Respir Crit Care Med 2003; 168:581–587.
148. Imamura Y, Yanagihara K, Mizuta Y, et al. Azithromycin inhibits MUC5AC production induced by the Pseudomonas aeruginosa autoinducer N-(3-Oxododecanoyl) homoserine lactone in NCI-H292 cells. Antimicrob Agents Chemother 2004; 48:3457–3461.
149. Daviskas E, Anderson SD. Hyperosmolar agents and clearance of mucus in the diseased airway. J Aerosol Med 2006; 19:100–109.
150. Durward A, Forte V, Shemie SD. Resolution of mucus plugging and atelectasis after intratracheal rhDNase therapy in a mechanically ventilated child with refractory status asthmaticus. Crit Care Med 2000; 28:560–562.
151. Greally P. Human recombinant DNase for mucus plugging in status asthmaticus. Lancet 1995; 346:1423–1424.
152. Knowles MR, Church NL, Waltner WE, et al. A pilot study of aerosolized amiloride for the treatment of lung disease in cystic fibrosis. N Engl J Med 1990; 322:1189–1194.
153. Bennett WD, Olivier KN, Zeman KL, et al. Effect of uridine 5′-triphosphate plus amiloride on mucociliary clearance in adult cystic fibrosis. Am J Respir Crit Care Med 1996; 153: 1796–1801.

154. Lang DM, Simon RA, Mathison DA, et al. Safety and possible efficacy of fiberoptic bronchoscopy with lavage in the management of refractory asthma with mucous impaction. Ann Allergy 1991; 67:324–330.
155. Nakano T, Inoue H, Fukuyama S, et al. Niflumic acid suppresses interleukin-13-induced asthma phenotypes. Am J Respir Crit Care Med 2006; 173:1216–1221.
156. Mata M, Sarria B, Buenestado A, et al. Phosphodiesterase 4 inhibition decreases MUC5AC expression induced by epidermal growth factor in human airway epithelial cells. Thorax 2005; 60:144–152.
157. Li XM, Huang CK, Zhang TF, et al. The Chinese herbal medicine formula MSSM-002 suppresses allergic airway hyperreactivity and modulates TH1/TH2 responses in a murine model of allergic asthma. J Allergy Clin Immunol 2000; 106:660–668.
158. Agrawal A, Rengarajan S, Adler KB, et al. Inhibition of mucin secretion with MARCKS-related peptide improves airway obstruction in a mouse model of asthma. J Appl Physiol 2007; 102:399–405.
159. Kim KC, Park HR, Shin CY, et al. Nucleotide-induced mucin release from primary hamster tracheal surface epithelial cells involves the P2u purinoceptor. Eur Respir J 1996; 9:42–8.
160. Deterding RR, Lavange LM, Engels JM, et al. Phase 2 randomized safety and efficacy trial of nebulized denufosol tetrasodium in cystic fibrosis. Am J Respir Crit Care Med 2007; 176:362–9.

Aerosols and Aerosol Drug Delivery Systems

Myrna B Dolovich

40

SUMMARY OF IMPORTANT CONCEPTS

>> Deposition of aerosols in the lung depends on the combination of aerosol/inhaler technical factors, patient ventilatory factors and cooperation, and the nature of the airways/lung disease

>> Specific dose fractions within an aerosol as well as in vivo deposition measurements are important elements that provide a more accurate interpretation of clinical response

>> Some HFA propellant pMDIs provide a different quality and quantity of aerosolized medication, but with revised dosage regimens, a similar response is achieved to that obtained with the original CFC pMDIs

>> Physicians and healthcare workers need to understand how to use the aerosol inhalers that they are prescribing for their patients, and the features of each type of delivery system

>> More efficient inhaler devices with patient-friendly features are continually being designed and approved for human use

INTRODUCTION

Inhaled medications continue to be the most widely used form of therapy for treating respiratory disease in adults and children.[1–3] Over the last 30 years, developments in inhaler technology and design have led to improvements in the production of aerosols for therapy (Fig. 40.1).[4] Novel designs continue to be approved by the regulatory agencies and commercialized by manufacturers,[5] and numerous delivery systems are currently available for drugs administered in aerosol form. Devices range from hydrofluoroalkane (HFA) pressurized metered-dose inhalers (pMDIs) with and without attached spacer devices, dry powder inhalers (DPIs), and nebulizers for providing continuous or intermittent aerosols of liquid solutions or suspensions. Within these three categories are a variety of devices producing aerosols with somewhat similar characteristics but with a range of fine particle lung delivery efficiencies, the current indicator of lower respiratory tract deposition and anticipated clinical advantage. What distinguishes the different devices are the means used to produce and dispense the aerosols and the interface to the patient.

The inhaled route is the preferred route for administration of both bronchodilator and antiinflammatory drugs to patients with asthma and other respiratory diseases. Inhalation devices that deliver β_2-agonists, anticholinergics, and corticosteroids have become a mainstay in the management of asthma and chronic obstructive pulmonary disease (COPD).[6] Additionally, over the past several years, the benefit of using inhalation devices to deliver non-respiratory medications to the systemic circulation via the lung has been undertaken with success.[7]

Delivery of aerosolized medications to the lung is a challenge, a combination of several factors: the drug formulation properties, the delivery system characteristics, patient ventilatory technique and compliance and the nature of the lung disease.[8,9] The inhalation technique adopted by the patient (inspiratory flow rate, inspiratory volume, and breath-holding time) determines the dose of drug inhaled from the inhaler that deposits in the lung. Most importantly, the degree of airway narrowing, which varies with the type and severity of the lung disease, further influences the distribution of that dose within the lung and potentially, the response to the therapy.[10,11]

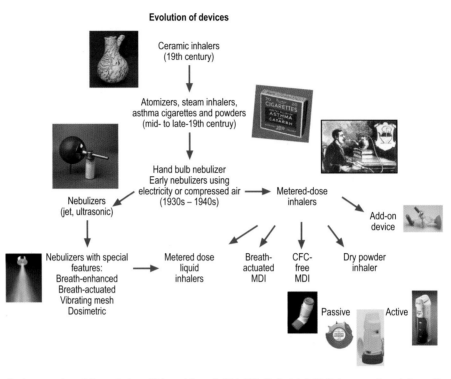

Fig. 40.1. Evolution of pulmonary drug delivery devices. (Adapted from Labiris NR, Dolovich MB. Pulmonary drug delivery. Part II: The role of inhalant delivery devices and drug formulations in therapeutic effectiveness of aerosolized medications. Br J Clin Pharmacol 2003; 56:600–612.[4])

In the last 10–15 years, major design changes have occurred in all three categories of drug delivery devices (pMDIs, DPIs, and nebulizers), giving the patient innovative inhalers with increased lung deposition along with improved control of aerosol production and inhalation flow rates.[5] The elimination of chlorofluorocarbon (CFC)-containing pMDIs has provided the impetus to develop alternative, non-propellant dependent aerosol delivery systems. Some elements that have been introduced into newer types of inhalers by device manufacturers are shown in Table 40.1. There are inhalers that provide low-velocity, fine aerosols to promote drug delivery to the more peripheral airways as well as incorporating features that limit the patient's breathing rate; all advantages for targeting drug to the lower rather than the upper respiratory tract. These key elements along with ease of use, portability and patient compliance monitors, such as dose counters and integrated electronic management systems to track treatments and treatment schedules, drive the current innovations in inhaler design.

Developments in device design have also been driven by the recognition that drugs to control pain and to treat a variety of systemic diseases, such as diabetes, can use the peripheral lung as part of the overall delivery system for these therapies.[12] Aerosols generated for these applications, of necessity, must be extra-fine to achieve high deposition in the peripheral lung for uptake by the systemic circulation to occur. A further interesting development is the nebulizing catheter that takes advantage of the bronchoscope channel to target treatment to specific sites within a lung lobe.[13]

■ DEFINITION AND TYPES OF AEROSOLS ■

An aerosol is a two-phase system defined as a dispersion or suspension of solid particles or liquid droplets in a gaseous medium (for example, air, oxygen, heliox). Other common two-phase systems are gels (liquid dispersed in a solid) and foams (gas dispersed in a liquid phase). Aerosols abound in nature, and our environment provides exposure to a wide variety of aerosols, both natural and man-made. Inhalation of pollen, bacteria, viruses, asbestos fibres, coal and mineral dusts, cigarette smoke, and house dust (to name just a few) can give rise to a variety of respiratory diseases. In medicine, aerosols are used for both diagnostic and therapeutic purposes. Diagnostic aerosols are used to confirm and monitor disease[14–17] and to categorize severity,[18,19] while therapeutic aerosols are employed to deliver active medication and agents in the treatment of lung, nasal and systemic diseases.[20–22] A list of the major advantages and disadvantages of using aerosol medications is given in Table 40.2.[13,23]

■ AEROSOLS FOR THERAPY ■

Therapeutic aerosols are produced by a variety of inhaler devices which are compared in terms of the proportion of available aerosol that would be likely to deposit in the lung. This variable, termed the fine particle or respirable fraction, is accepted as a good indicator of the ability of

Table 40.1 Trends in inhalation delivery system design

Breath-actuation (DPIs, pMDIs and high-tech nebulizers)
Inspiratory flow independence in delivered aerosol
Dose metering
Unit dose or multi-unit doses (capsules, blisters)
Dose counters; reservoir, multi-unit dose DPIs; pMDIs
Combination therapy
High delivery efficiency
Conservation of drug
Elimination of environmental contamination from drugs and discarded devices in landfills
Reduced volume of drug in device and reduced treatment time
Battery operated MDLIs
Miniaturization of device design
Smaller volume spacers/holding chambers; MDLIs
Metal or non-electrostatic spacers
Electronic monitoring including scheduling of treatments
Systemic delivery of drugs using extra-fine aerosols
Drug targeting

DPI, dry-powder inhaler; pMDI, pressurized metered dose inhaler

Table 40.2 Aerosol medications – advantages and disadvantages in respiratory disease

Advantages
Treatment of lungs directly
High drug concentrations in the airway
Reduced systemic adverse effects
Inhaled β_2-agonist bronchodilators produce a more rapid onset of action than oral delivery
Some drugs are only active with aerosol delivery
Aerosol drug delivery is painless and convenient

Disadvantages
Less than optimal technique decreases drug delivery and potentially reduces efficacy
The proliferation of inhalation devices has resulted in a confusing number of choices
Inhaler devices are less convenient than oral drug administration; greater time required for drug administration; some patients may find the device less portable

the inhaler to provide an aerosol that will successfully target the lower respiratory tract.[24] The devices currently available to patients for administering a variety of therapies have a range of delivery efficiencies, as high as 53% of the emitted dose for extra-fine solution pressurized aerosols. The amount of drug deposited in the lung impacts directly on the clinical response achieved and if sub-optimal, potentially on the level of compliance on the part of the patient in taking their medication.[25]

Interest in the delivery of drugs as inhaled therapy has increased over the past 30 years. Drugs such as insulin,[26,27] calcitonin,[28] vasodilators,[29,30] analgesics[31] and cyclosporine for lung transplant patients[32] have proven to be efficacious when administered topically as aerosols. A review of the literature discussing recent developments for gene therapies and vaccines delivered as aerosols have shown the lung to be an effective route for delivering these products systemically.[33] The advantage occurs for a variety of reasons, not the least being convenience, rapid absorption and in some instances, the sheer weight of drug that would need to be ingested by comparison to administration as an aerosol. New chemical entities and drugs used to treat other diseases such as diabetes are formulated initially in liquid form, usually aqueous-based solutions, thus favoring nebulization to produce an aerosol for therapy. The developments discussed below for both powder and liquid aerosol inhalers represent advances in the technology for generating respirable aerosols for therapy.

AEROSOL PROPERTIES AND THE RELATIONSHIP TO DRUG DELIVERY

The size range for environmental and occupational aerosols ranges from 0.001, termed ultrafine, to 1000 micrometers (μm) in diameter, termed supercoarse, while therapeutic and diagnostic aerosols targeted to the lower respiratory tract are composed of particles typically between 0.5 and 10 μm in diameter (fine to coarse distributions). The behavior of particles in this size range in air is described by Stokes' Law,[34–36] an equation which relates the viscous or frictional forces exerted against a spherical particle of density ρ, falling in still air under the force of gravity, to reach its final destination (e.g., airway wall) or:

$$F = 3\pi\eta vd$$

where:
F = friction or viscous force, dynes
η = viscosity of air, g/cm/s
v = particle velocity, cm/s
d = diameter of the particle, cm.

A particle falls in still air with velocity v until the viscous forces counter or are equal to the downward or gravitational forces (= mg or $(\pi/6)d^3\rho g$) on the particle. The particle reaches the terminal settling velocity (V_t) and maintains this velocity until it settles or deposits onto a surface. The terminal velocity, in cm/s, is given by:

$$V_t = \rho d^2/18\eta,$$

or, taking account of the viscosity of air:

$$V_t = 0.003\rho d^2$$

where:
ρ = particle density, g/cm^3
d = particle diameter, μm.

The rate at which inhaled particles or droplets deposit onto airway surfaces varies with their size. For example, the V_t of a 5 μm water droplet is 0.0740 cm/s, approximately 22 times greater than for a 1 μm water droplet but one-quarter that of a 10 μm water droplet. Ambient particulates with diameters 2.5 μm ($PM_{2.5}$) fall into the ultrafine or fine distribution categories. It is these particulates that can be troublesome to patients with asthma and COPD.

PARTICLE SIZE DISTRIBUTION

The size of an aerosol particle is the primary determinant of the site of lung deposition, distribution of the drug within the lung, and resulting deposition efficiency.[11,37–40] Particles or droplets comprising a therapeutic aerosol are heterodisperse with respect to physical diameter and are either spherical in shape if produced from a pure solution, or, if a suspension, will be a non-spherical core particle within a liquid carrier (saline) envelope. Size classification of the aerosol in terms of its aerodynamic behavior is performed using cascade impactors, multi-stage liquid impingers and optical systems, with chemical assay of the drug a major advantage of the impactor/impinger techniques.[41,42] While time-consuming and labor intensive compared with the laser techniques, the ability to quantify the amount of drug carried by aerosol particles of a specific size is useful for interpreting the resulting lung deposition patterns and clinical response to the inhaled drug dose.[43] Sizing data from light scattering instruments gives the median diameter of the aerosol, with the assumption that all particles in the aerosol being tested are spherical and of unit density. While this information predicts the site of deposition of aerosol in the lung, it says nothing of its drug content[44] and thus, what the patient could receive from the inhaler being tested. With all sizing measurements, the accuracy in measuring in vitro emitted doses is increased if the impactor/impinger flow rates used to sample the aerosol are matched to the conditions for optimal performance of the inhaler and the patient's IFR.

Using the data obtained from the sizing measurements, the distribution of particle diameters can be represented mathematically by a log-normal distribution, with the logarithm of the (aerodynamic) diameter plotted against frequency (of occurrence), expressed as particle number, surface area or mass (Fig. 40.2A).[24,45] This ideally results in a bell-shaped normal distribution curve,[46,47] but in practice, the curves are typically skewed or bimodal. When this same normal distribution data is replotted as a cumulative function on log probability graph paper, a 'straight' line is obtained (Fig. 40.2B).[24] The median diameter is read at the 50% point on the cumulative distribution curve, while the geometric standard deviation (GSD), a measure of the heterogeneity of the aerosol, is calculated as the ratio of median diameter to the diameter at one standard deviation from the median. Aerosols containing particles of uniform size, with a GSD of <1.2, are described as monodisperse.[48] While monodisperse aerosols do not occur naturally, they can be produced in the laboratory and have been used to measure lung deposition under a variety of conditions.[49,50] A change in the GSD from 1 to 2 will introduce less of an error than that due to an alteration in the subjects' breathing pattern.[48]

The prediction of deposition efficiency for a therapeutic aerosol has been based on its mass median aerodynamic diameter (MMAD). This parameter characterizes the aerosol in terms of mass (50% of the mass of the aerosol residing in particles less than the MMAD and 50% in particles greater than the MMAD). Characterizing aerosols in terms of mass enables an estimation of the dose of aerosolized medication delivered to the lung. Since the mass of a particle is proportional to the cube of its diameter, the majority of drug administered as an aerosol is contained in the larger droplets and these are fewer in number than those particles less than the MMAD. Conversely, the mass of drug in particles less than the MMAD is from a much greater number of particles, with each however, containing much less mass. More recently, predictions of deposition and therapeutic effect have been based on the percentage of the aerosol containing particles or droplets <5 μm in diameter as this is the size characteristic that can achieve deposition in the lower respiratory tract, specifically distal to the main stem bronchi and providing airways are patent and inspiratory flow rates are low.

AEROSOL DEPOSITION MECHANISMS

The deposition of particles onto surfaces in the lung mainly follow three physical principles: impaction – a function of particle inertia affecting particles greater than 5 μm, sedimentation due to gravitational forces acting on particles primarily between 0.5 and 5 μm, and diffusion resulting from Brownian motion affecting sub-micrometer particles in the low-flow regions of the lung (Fig. 40.3).[10,51–53] Factors affecting deposition of aerosols in the lung are listed in Table 40.3. Research into the use of drugs produced as nanoparticles, <1 μm median diameter is an expanding field with promise for high efficiency and targeted delivery to the specific sites within the lung.[54–56] Electrical charges carried by particles and, in the normal, patent lung, simple contact or interception of particles by airway walls are mechanisms considered less important and are usually ignored when determining lung deposition of medicinal aerosols. Electrostatic charge, however, not only enhances the deposition of environmental and occupational aerosols but also effects a reduction in the available aerosol from plastic spacer devices used to deliver pressurized metered doses of drugs. This is a direct result of the collection of the drug particles on the walls of the spacer due to charge effects between the drug and plastic.[57–59]

In addition to the influence of particle diameter on lung deposition, deposition by sedimentation or diffusion will be proportional to the residence time of the particle in the airway. The larger the particle, the more readily it will be influenced by gravity and removed from the air stream. Airflow directly influences impaction of particles onto airway walls. For example particles >5 μm inhaled at inspiratory flows comparable with taking a puff from an pMDI will impact in the oropharyngeal area, upper airways and at airway bifurcations.[60] Particles <5 μm tend to deposit by sedimentation and diffusion on successively smaller airways as both the mass of the aerosol particles and the air stream velocity decreases.[38,39] Thus, inhaling an aerosol at a low flow rate to minimize impaction[60,61] and by following the inhalation with a prolonged breath-hold allows greater time for sedimentation and diffusion to occur in the peripheral airways.[46,62]

In adults, particles >5 μm in diameter readily settle out of the air stream during normal tidal breathing, whereas particles between 0.1 and 1.0 μm likely remain suspended as the time required for these ultrafine particles to diffuse to an airway wall is typically greater than the time to complete the inspiratory phase of a normal breath.[36,63] Thus, these fine and ultrafine particles tend to be exhaled rather than deposited in the distal lung. Those that are retained in the lung may migrate from the lung surface to the interstitium, as has been demonstrated for insoluble, solid particles.[64] The implications from this research pertain to ambient and occupational exposures, such as road dust and toner particles, rather than to therapeutic aerosols.

It may be possible to target specific regions in the lung for therapy by selection of particle size[65–67] and inspiratory flow rate.[68] However,

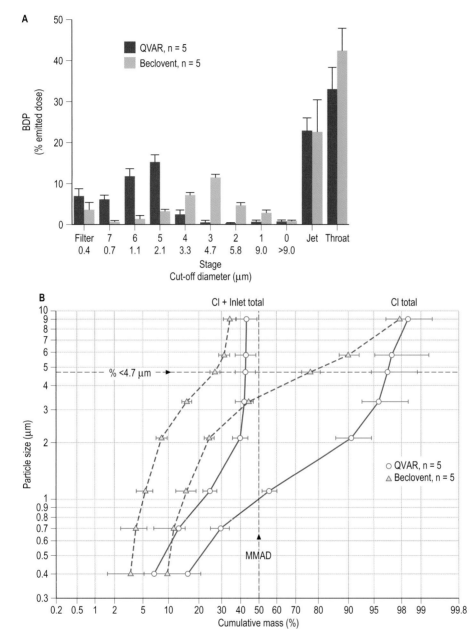

Fig. 40.2. (A) Histograms illustrating the percentage emitted dose (ED) that deposited on the individual cascade impactor (CI) stages, jet and throat (Inlet) for QVAR (3M Pharmaceuticals, USA) and Beclovent (A&H, USA). More of the HFA134a solution BDP aerosol deposited on the lower stages than from the CFC suspension BDP aerosol. (B) Cumulative mass distributions (derived from the histogram data for each drug) for HFA134a BDP pMDI aerosol QVAR, in comparison with the original CFC pMDI, Beclovent. Curves are shown for the emitted dose ex-actuator (CI+Inlet total) and the dose that is only deposited in the impactor (CI total). The mass median aerodynamic diameter (MMAD) of the aerosols deposited in the impactor is read from the CI curves at 50% of the cumulative mass and is 1.0 μm for QVAR (3M Pharmaceuticals, USA) and 3.3 μm for Beclovent. The fine particle fraction (% <4.7 μm) of the emitted dose is read from the CI+Inlet total curves. The HFA134a solution aerosol is a finer aerosol with significantly greater fine particle fraction compared with the CFC innovator suspension aerosol; 40% more drug is contained in the fine particle dose of QVAR compared with Beclovent forming the basis for the 2:1 dose substitution regimen.[24,45]

small particle therapeutic aerosols may also require a more concentrated formulation, longer treatment time or a greater number of doses to achieve the same clinical effect. Estimates of lung deposition fractions for stable, non-hygroscopic particles of varying aerodynamic size have been made using a variety of geometric models of the respiratory tract.[10,69–72] Above 5 µm, more particles deposit on airway surfaces and less in the peripheral lung, while for aerosols of <5 µm, the opposite occurs. Maximum deposition is obtained in the pulmonary region for particles ~3 µm in size, decreasing to only about 15% for 0.5 µm particles. At 0.5 µm, <5% will be deposited and retained in the lung, with maximal deposition in the 20th–21st generation of airway, at the level of the respiratory bronchioles. Particle size, airflow in the lung, and airway dimensions are the most influential factors in affecting the pattern of delivery of therapeutic aerosol to the lung. A reduction in airway calibre due to disease alters the air flow pattern in the lung and affects the distribution of inhaled aerosol, shifting deposition towards

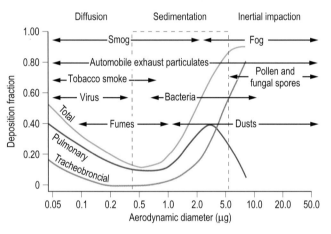

Fig. 40.3. Size-deposition relationships for stable particles of aerodynamic diameter 0.1 to 8 µm for the tracheobronchial (T-B) and pulmonary (P) compartments of the lung. Total curve represents the sum of T-B and P values. Deposition fractions are taken from calculations of Yu et al. (1979)[10] for mouth breathing at <0.25 L/s and account for intersubject variability in airway dimensions. Range of particle diameters over which diffusion, sedimentation, and inertial impaction are most important (as well as approximate size ranges of some commonly encountered aerosols) are shown. (Reproduced from Dolovich M, Newhouse M. Aerosols: generation, methods of administration and therapeutic applications in asthma. In: Middleton EJ, Reed C, Adkinson N, et al. Allergy: principles and practice, 4th edn. St Louis: Mosby; 1993:712–739.[53])

the central or proximal airways.[11,73,74] When conducting lung deposition studies, it is important to measure particle size and inspiratory flow rate for each subject. In a study of 10 healthy volunteers, the interaction of these two variables significantly influenced both the lung and oropharyngeal deposition from the same administered dose of radiolabeled albuterol sulfate powder, and even with small changes in either one of these factors.[75] Several attempts have also been made to correlate in vitro characteristics of administered aerosols with in vivo measurements of efficacy, with varying degrees of success.[50,76] Results from a study in asthmatic subjects inhaling dry powders of albuterol sulfate with different fine particle doses were unable to discriminate differences in FEV_1 response, even starting at a dose of 50 µg.[77] Many patients can achieve the plateau of the dose response curve inhaling low doses of albuterol and therefore, this outcome was not unexpected. This was also one of several reasons why a variety of settings and patient populations, clinical responses to the same bronchodilator drug inhaled from different devices failed to discriminate between device types.[78]

HYGROSCOPICITY

Therapeutic aerosols are often hygroscopic and may grow two- to three-fold in size when inhaled into the (humid) bronchial airways.[79,80] Similar growth may occur in ventilator circuits driven with humidified air.[81,82] In addition, characterization of aqueous aerosols under different conditions of relative humidity have been shown to be dependent on nebulizer design, with measurements of droplet size affected by the relative humidity of the ambient air entrained through conventional but not breath-enhanced (BE) nebulizers. This is likely because air drawn through BE designs becomes saturated prior to being drawn through the impactor or impinger.[83] Low ambient humidity causes droplet shrinkage prior to inhalation and possibly more distal distribution within the lung.

NOMENCLATURE FOR INDICATORS OF DRUG DELIVERY DEVICE PERFORMANCE

When assessing inhalers for regulatory approval and hence use with patients, the following information should be obtained: characterization of the delivery of aerosolized drug from the inhaler, measurement of lung deposition to estimate site of delivery of the drug within the respiratory tract, and clinical outcomes in response to the drug inhaled. Some or all of these measurements may be mandated by the regulatory

Table 40.3 Factors affecting deposition of aerosol in the lung

Physical	Particle diameter, particle shape, particle density, heterodisperse mass distribution of aerosol diameters, fine particle fraction of aerosol
Ventilatory	Inspiratory volume, inspiratory flow rate, breath-hold time, breathing rate, nose vs mouth breathing, ambient humidity, ambient temperature, requirement for facemask
Anatomic	Airway caliber, distortion due to disease, ventilation pattern
Patient related	Ability to use delivery system, compliance, response to therapy

agencies, and in particular when the drug and device (termed a combination product) are to be sold as a unit. (Aerosol drug delivery device design verification – Requirements and test methods. Draft International Standard ISO/DIS 20072© International Organization for Standardization, 2007; www.iso.org.) A number of guidance documents and standards have been published by various standards organizations and regulatory bodies worldwide which detail the requirements for obtaining measurements to determine acceptable performance of inhaler devices prior to approval for sale and use by patients.[84]

Variables used to describe the aerosol performance of inhaler devices in vitro are the emitted dose (ED), fine particle fraction (FPF), and fine particle dose (FPD). The ED is determined by collecting and quantifying unit doses released at the inhaler exit or mouthpiece: that is, the point at which the patient would be inhaling the drug aerosol. The ED is less than the unit drug dose specified on the package, termed the nominal dose or label claim (LC) (Fig. 40.4).[25] In the USA, the label claim is the emitted dose, while in Canada and Europe, the LC is the unit dose loaded into the inhaler.

The difference between the LC and ED reflects loss of drug on components within the inhaler, within add-on devices such as spacers or tubing placed between the mouthpiece and the drug reservoir or losses on the mouthpiece or actuator. The extent of these losses can be measured using chemical assays and can, in some systems, substantially reduce the nominal dose by up to 70%. This can occur, for example, when a spacer is used with a pMDI. It should be noted that pMDI mouthpiece actuator losses vary from 5% to 20%. The quantity of drug used to fill the inhaler reservoir, a term that applies to nebulizers, metered dose inhalers or dry powder inhalers is the maximum, but theoretical, amount of drug available for inhalation from the inhaler. Again, a portion of this total dose is unavailable for aerosolization and thus inhalation.

The term 'dead' volume is often applied to that portion of drug not nebulized from jet or ultrasonic nebulizers and often represents 20% or more of the total fill volume.[85] With pMDIs and DPIs, there is usually an 10–20% overfill in the amount of drug loaded into the bulk reservoir to guarantee that the total number of doses specified on the package are available to the patient. To normalize delivery performance between inhalers dispensing different formulations of the same drug, a change to the nominal unit dose can be made by the pharmaceutical company. This would occur during development as changes to an already marketed formulation would require, as a minimum, confirming bridging studies for re-approval. This circumvents inherent differences between systems without compromising treatment as patients are switched from one type of delivery system to another. Thus, while the dose of drug provided from one inhaler system may be greater or lesser than that from an alternative device, the clinical responses can still be the same.[78]

To obtain the fine particle fraction, the emitted dose of aerosol is fractionated according to particle or droplet diameters using impactors or other types of particle sizing systems. This sizing information provides estimates of that portion of the aerosol that is $<4.7\,\mu m$, termed the fine particle fraction, and that which is $>4.7\,\mu m$, termed the coarse particle fraction. The fine particle dose, also referred to as 'useful' aerosol, is that portion of the aerosol likely to be deposited within the lung and is obtained by multiplying the ED by the FPF:

$$FPD = FPF_{\%<4.7\mu m} \times ED, \mu g$$

The part of the inhaled dose that deposits in the oropharynx, larynx and on large airway surfaces can be estimated from the coarse particle fraction ($CPF_{\%>4.7\mu m}$) and dose and is the remainder of the ED:

$$CPD = ED - FPD, \mu g$$

In general, the percentage of particles with increasing likelihood for depositing in the distal lung increases as the FPF increases, also indicating that the aerosol has a smaller mass median aerodynamic diameter. While more drug is carried in larger droplets or particles, the probability of particles larger than $6\,\mu m$ depositing in the lower respiratory tract decreases with an increasing CPF. Submicronic droplets, $<1\,\mu m$ in diameter and present in increasing numbers in ethanolic pressurized steroid formulations such as HFA134a ciclesonide (Alvesco, Nycomed, USA) and HFA134a BDP (QVAR, TEVA Pharmaceuticals, USA) are retained less in the lung, but, due to their size and the vast number of submicron droplets in the aerosol, can penetrate into the pulmonary regions, even in the presence of airflow obstruction.[86,87] An extrafine particle fraction ($EFPF_{\%<1.0\,\mu m}$) and dose (EFPD) have been defined for those aerosols whose distributions contain a majority of particles $<1\,\mu m$ in diameter. Approximately 20% of these extrafine pMDI aerosols will be exhaled, as aerosols of this diameter behave as a gas and indeed, are widely used to measure lung ventilation in patients suspected of having a pulmonary embolism.[88] Of the dose of drug deposited in the lung, part is absorbed through the airway epithelium and lung parenchyma, part is cleared by mucociliary action, and part is retained in the lung. Each of these component doses contributes in part to the clinical efficacy as well as to any adverse effects experienced by the patient (Fig. 40.5).[25,89] Changes to the quality of the aerosol either through formulation changes, hardware changes or the use of baffles or spacers will be reflected in changes to the ED, FPF, CPF, FPD, and CPD.

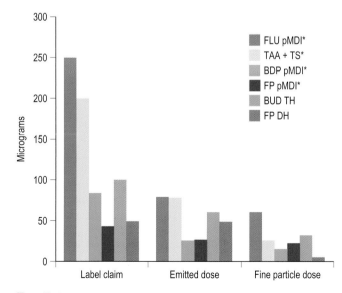

Fig. 40.4. Illustration showing the differences values for label claim (LC), emitted dose (ED), and fine particle dose (FPD) for six corticosteroid aerosols. The ED is less than the LC due to losses in the inhaler, while the FPD represents only that portion of the aerosol likely to achieve deposition in the lung. (Data plotted from Martin et al, 2002.[25])

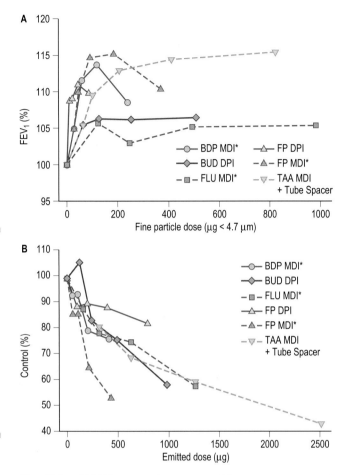

Table 40.4 Nebulizers – points to consider

Clinical benefit
Clinical setting (inpatient vs outpatient)
Ease of use
Patient compliance and competence
Assembly, cleaning, portability
Facemask vs mouthpiece
Rate of delivery of drug
Treatment time
Dose in single actuation vs nebulization over time
Frequency of treatments
Cost and convenience vs competition
Use with all drugs
Replacement parts, accessories
Reimbursement
Dose delivered
IFR-dependent
Breathing pattern required for optimal dosing
Breath-actuated, synchronization with actuation
Aerosol characteristics
Fine aerosol with sufficient respirable aerosol dose
Upper and lower respiratory tract deposition
Efficiency vs other aerosol systems
Side effects

IFR, inspiratory flow rate.

Fig. 40.5. (A) FEV_1 response (as percentage of the morning measurement) is shown for the corticosteroids used in the NIH/ACRN clinical trial,[25] plotted vs increasing fine particle dose, the portion of the inhaled dose likely to deposit in the lung and give rise to the response. (B) Measured cortisol levels (as percentage of baseline) plotted against increasing emitted (inhaled) doses for the corticosteroids used in the NIH/ACRN clinical trial. Suppression increased to varying degrees for these six steroid aerosols. Using ED, which includes the dose to the oropharynx, allows the response to be assessed at the actual microgram dose that caused the effect. The difference in cortisol levels for fluticasone propionate (FP) via the Diskhaler DPI compared to FP MDI inhaled from the spacer is the systemic absorption from the dose deposited in the oropharynx and the four-fold greater lung dose from the MDI. The oro-pharyngeal dose, which results in an increased total body dose, is typically greater from a DPI than when the drug is inhaled from a MDI used with a valved spacer.[89] *MDIs used with Optichamber™.

■ AEROSOL DRUG DELIVERY DEVICES ■

DELIVERY DEVICES PROVIDING AEROSOLS FOR THERAPY

Diagnostic and *therapeutic* aerosols are produced by mechanical, pneumatic or ultrasonic nebulizers, pMDIs, and dry powder inhaler devices. The pMDI, which creates therapeutic aerosols from pressurized solutions or suspensions, is the most widely used delivery system, followed by the DPI. In 1996, the signatories to the Montreal protocol, approximately 100 countries, agreed to eliminate pMDIs containing CFC propellants as delivery systems for respiratory medications. With this action, the development of new, CFC-free aerosol drug delivery systems was undertaken by the pharmaceutical industry.[90] This transition has severely limited the use of CFC propellants and the replacement formulations of these currently inhaled drugs, now containing hydrofluoroalkane (HFA) propellants are widely available, albeit at a higher cost to the patient.[91,92] As of 2008, CFC pMDI formulations will no longer be available in North America. Aerosolization of bronchodilators, steroid and anti-allergy medications via nebulizers as an alternative delivery system are still widely used despite the availability of proven alternatives.

Each class of delivery system has advantages and limitations,[78,93] many of which must be considered when selecting a device not only for ease of use by the adult or pediatric patient but primarily for the ability of the inhaler to provide the required therapeutic dose with minimal adverse effects.[78,94] Some factors to consider when selecting a nebulizer for liquid aerosols are given in Table 40.4. While choices in nebulizer systems are numerous, price, rather than performance, can often be the major determinant of use both for in-hospital and home therapy. In addition, economic considerations related to the development and approval of, in particular, new nebulizer technologies can play a decisive role in how and when the marketing of these developments to pharmacies, home care companies, hospitals, physicians and the public, where appropriate, occurs.[95] The costs associated with the purchase of an inhaler, filled with drug or without drug, such as a reusable nebulizer, can be an issue for many patients but will not be discussed in this chapter.

NEBULIZER DESIGNS FOR LIQUID FORMULATIONS

The most commonly used jet nebulizer is the constant output design with supplemental air drawn in across the top of the nebulizer, as necessitated by the patient's inspiratory volume. This pattern of airflow dilutes the aerosol produced within the nebulizer as it exits towards the patient. Aerosol is generated continuously, but with as much as 30–40% of the nominal dose trapped in the nebulizer, and >60% of the emitted dose wasted to atmosphere. This translates to <10% of the nebulizer contents being available to the patient. The advantage of these nebulizers is their low cost and the production of aerosol with little effort on the part of the patient.

Nebulizing liquid formulations: optimizing delivery

To reduce the waste of drug aerosolized during the expiratory phase of the breathing cycle, a thumb-control in the compressed air line allows the patient to divert gas flow from the atmosphere to the nebulizer during inspiration, allowing the patient to synchronize 'inhalation with actuation'. Patients with good hand/breath coordination receive similar amounts of aerosol per breath, but the time to aerosolize the reservoir contents or nominal dose are lengthened up to four-fold, with substantially greater dose of drug delivered to the lung. Unfortunately, many patients have difficulty coordinating the thumb-control with their inspiratory efforts during the course of therapy. The breath-actuated nebulizer was designed to circumvent this problem.[96,97] These nebulizers may also have the additional design feature that 'vents' supplemental air through the nebulizer across the Venturi emitting more aerosol from the nebulizer and providing an increased output of drug.[90,98] As inspiration ends, the flow through the nebulizer is reduced to the jet flow output, decreasing drug output and subsequent wastage during exhalation.[99] Dosimeters, used primarily in the pulmonary function lab, sense inspiration and pulse airflow to the jet orifice, transforming a standard nebulizer into a breath-actuated system.

Jet and ultrasonic nebulizers: principles of operation

Conventional pneumatic or jet nebulizers use compressed air or oxygen to break up a thin film or jet of fluid into droplets suitable for inhalation.[85,100] The nebulizer bowl is filled with drug in aqueous solution or suspension. Compressed air or oxygen is applied to the jet inlet and, travelling at a high velocity, exits through a narrow orifice, creating an area of low pressure at the outlet of the adjacent liquid feed tube, causing fluid from the reservoir to be drawn up (Venturi effect) and out of the tube where the liquid is then shattered into droplets of various sizes. These droplets are then carried by the air stream towards a wall or baffle within the nebulizer. The larger droplets impact on the walls or baffles positioned above this area and are returned to the fluid reservoir, while the finer droplets are carried out of the nebulizer to the patient by the flow of air. Impaction of particles >3 μm are the major form of loss of drug on the interior surfaces of the nebulizer, the connecting T-piece mounted on top of the nebulizer, or any mouthpiece, mask or tubing that may provide the interface for the nebulizer to the patient.

A multiplicity of factors and design features, such as the amount of jet air flow, valving to limit air flow during the expiratory phase of the breathing cycle, additional reservoirs that collect aerosol generated during expiration to be added to the aerosol inhaled with the subsequent inspiration, internal baffles to reduce the particle size of the aerosol cloud, diluent volume, the use of preservatives in the formulation, can all influence drug delivery to patients from nebulizers.

Some nebulizers are designed with a secondary air vent,[101] which allows additional room air to be entrained during inspiration. These nebulizers are classified as 'breath-enhanced' devices. If the nebulizer is operated with the vent open, auxiliary air flowing through the vent allows more of the aerosol cloud to be swept out of the nebulizer with each breath, thereby increasing the amount of useful aerosol for inhalation, albeit at a lower concentration due to the dilution effect.[102] During treatment, air may also be entrained through a T-piece or facemask, supplementing the jet air flow rate to meet the inspiratory flow requirement requirements of the patient. Overall, there will be an increase in the total drug delivered to the patient per unit time from nebulizers with additional air-entrainment. While higher plasma levels of albuterol following treatment with the Ventstream compared with a conventional constant flow nebulizer have been measured, indicating greater deposition of drug in the lung, somewhat greater systemic side effects from the higher administered dose were also noted.[101] Thus, while increasing the output may be convenient for patients, as treatment times may be shorter, adverse events may occur from bronchodilator therapy in particular.[103]

The MMAD of jet nebulizers used for therapy should be between 2 and 4 μm. The particle size is reduced by baffles within the nebulizer, one-way valves placed between the nebulizer and the mouthpiece or increasing the length of tubing between the nebulizer and the patient. These reductions in particle size come at the cost of reducing the rate of aerosol output to the patient. If one-way valves, mouthpieces or tubing are used in systems where precise doses are to be inhaled, such as in challenge testing with allergen and methacholine aerosols, the conditions should be fixed and the system calibrated with these added pieces in place.

Because of the high flow of gas through a jet nebulizer, solvent evaporates, resulting in a decrease in the temperature of the reservoir solution and a progressive increase in the concentration of drug in the reservoir and in the aerosol droplets produced.[104] The higher the flow driving the nebulizer, the greater the rate at which the solution undergoes increased concentration. As solvent evaporates from aerosol droplets, residual, dry (drug) particles are formed with diameters given by the following expression:[47,105]

$$D_p = (C/\rho_p)^{1/3}D$$

where:
D_p = diameter of dry particle (sphere), μm
C = solute concentration, g/mL of solution
ρ_p = density of dry particle, g/cc
D = diameter of droplet, μm.

This relationship shows that, as the concentration of the drug (solute) increases, the size of the residual (dry) particle will increase and more drug is thus potentially available for inhalation. However, while the droplets may contain more drug, the droplet diameter changes only marginally and hence the site of deposition of the drug in the lung remains essentially the same.[105] The aerodynamic diameter of a particle or droplet can be calculated by multiplying the physical diameter of the particle or droplet by the square root of its density, as shown in the formula above. The densities of most inhalant drugs are similar to water, but ambient particles have densities >1.

The rate at which the solution concentrates is affected by the volume of fluid placed in the reservoir. The larger volume of liquid cools more slowly, and the increase in the concentration of the drug will be less marked for the same operating time. A reservoir fill volume of 3–5 mL, compared with the 2 mL unit dose nebules, results in a greater total amount of drug aerosolized and delivered to the patient, albeit for a longer treatment time.[106]

The driving pressure or the flow rate of compressed air applied to the jet affects aerosol output and particle size from jet nebulizers. The higher the pressure or flow rate, the greater the output over time in terms of total solution aerosolized and the smaller the particle size.[107,108] The rate of nebulization, expressed as the loss of solution volume (usually <0.15 mL/min with pneumatic nebulizers), is due to drug leaving the nebulizer as aerosol (2/3), with one-third of the volume leaving as water vapor. The proportion of these two components varies with nebulizer design.[109] Therefore, to accurately gauge the dose provided to the patient, the amount of drug released from the nebulizer during the actual operating conditions should be measured.[78,110]

The greater the interior surface area within a nebulizer, the greater the volume of drug solution lost on the nebulizer walls. The time required to deliver the medication varies with the airflow rate used to drive the nebulizer, with typical treatment times varying between 5 and 15 min.[111] At the end of nebulization, when no further aerosol is produced, approximately 0.5–1.5 mL of concentrated solution is left in the nebulizer reservoir. This is referred to as 'dead volume', representing drug that is unavailable to the patient.[112] The greater the volume of residual drug remaining in the nebulizer after therapy, the lesser will be the amount of drug available to the patient. There are a number of jet nebulizers used for providing aerosols of bronchodilator, steroid, anti-allergy and antimicrobial drug solutions. Performance characteristics of these nebulizers vary somewhat in terms of the particle size of the aerosol produced as well as the mass of drug available for inhalation over a standard treatment time.[111] The differences, which may also be formulation dependent, can have substantial implications for patient management and should be known by the physician prior to selecting a delivery system for patients.[94,113–115]

Some nebulizer systems include an external reservoir for the aerosol to improve delivery efficiency. The reservoir is filled with aerosol produced during the expiratory phase, which is then inhaled with the next breath taken through the nebulizer. Reservoirs may also reduce particle size due to impaction of droplets on the interior walls, such as is seen with a valved spacer used with a pMDI. Adding a reservoir to nebulizers in ventilator circuits has been shown to increase aerosol drug output available to the patient.[116,117]

Thus, several factors influence the quantity and quality of drug aerosolized via conventional or continuous production nebulizers. In addition to variables mentioned above, the patient interface, particularly the design and fit of a facemask if used for young children and elderly patients, can change the amount of drug inhaled by the patient.[118,119] Drug dose prescribed along with treatment times required for complete nebulization need to be considered to provide sufficient therapy in a convenient manner.

Ultrasonic nebulizers

Ultrasonic nebulizers incorporate a piezoelectric crystal, vibrated at a high frequency with sufficient intensity to create standing waves on the surface of the liquid overlying the crystal. Droplets are formed which remain within the nebulizer until they are swept out by a fan or the patient's inspiratory breath. The diameter of the droplets (D) produced is inversely proportional to the oscillator frequency (f) applied to the crystal and expressed as:

$$D = \alpha \, (8\pi\gamma/\rho f^2)^\lambda$$

where:
D = average droplet diameter
α = constant
λ = wavelength of surface wave
γ = surface tension of liquid
ρ = density of liquid
f = oscillator frequency.

As the frequency increases, the median size of the droplets will decrease, with most current ultrasonic nebulizers operating at frequencies >1 megahertz (MHz), producing aerosols with MMADs ranging between 2 and 12 μm, with an output that is ≥2–3 fold more than most jet nebulizers.[100]

With ultrasonic nebulizers, heat is produced as the nebulizer solution is sonicated and the temperature can rise 10–15°C over a 10 min treatment which may adversely affect heat-sensitive formulations, such as proteins.[120] As with jet nebulizers, the drug becomes concentrated in the reservoir; however, only small decreases in particle size occur over the time required for complete nebulization.[108]

ADDITIVES IN NEBULIZER SOLUTIONS

In addition to the active ingredient, therapeutic nebulizer solutions may contain excipients such as buffers and preservatives (metabisulfite, benzalkonium chloride and ethylenediaminetetraacetic acid (EDTA)) that can produce, on inhalation, asthma-like symptoms, such as bronchoconstriction and cough, sometimes accompanied by a marked reduction in FEV_1.[121] The availability of unit-dose, preservative-free packaging for nebulizer formulations can eliminate these unpleasant side effects.[114] The effects observed from excipient inhalation are similar to what may occur on inhalation of either hypo- and hyperosmolar solutions,[122] the latter used for sputum induction in the investigation of inflammatory events in the lung. In this situation, cough is necessary for expectoration of the sputum sample that results from the inhalation of hypertonic saline aerosol.[123]

NEW-GENERATION NEBULIZERS: METERED-DOSE LIQUID INHALERS

The convenience of the portable pMDI, providing a unit dose of therapy in 1–2 actuations, has been recognized as the drug delivery system that the majority of patients and physicians favor for inhalant therapy.[90] Several new nebulizer systems can be categorized as metered-dose liquid inhalers (MDLIs) incorporating some of the pMDI features into their design (Table 40.5). Designs range from breath-enhanced nebulizers that entrain air through the nebulizer during inspiration[101,124] to breath-actuated nebulizers that reduce or eliminate aerosol generation during the patient's expiratory phase,[125] vibrating mesh or plate systems that produce aerosols through multiple holes or apertures[126] and systems that extrude or force liquid through precision-made nozzles.[127] Generation of low-velocity (soft mist) aerosol, improved particle characteristics for enhanced lower lung deposition, augmented aerosol output and systems that minimize residual volume of medication left in the nebulizer have substantially improved aerosol device efficiency and hence increased drug output to patients.[128] Along with their improved performance, some 'smart' nebulizers can also monitor patient compliance and management of the patient's treatment schedule.[129]

The newer designs are more efficient in providing aerosolized therapy, with pulmonary deposition improved from the old standard of approximately 10% to >60% of the nominal dose. In some cases, these device improvements may be accompanied by greater systemic side effects, unless the delivered dose is reduced. The key is to target effective doses to the lungs without adverse effects.[130]

Breath-actuated nebulizer

Breath-actuated nebulizers generate aerosol only during inspiration, eliminating wastage of aerosol during exhalation, increasing delivered dose ≥3-fold over continuous and breath-enhanced nebulizers. AeroEclipse™ (Trudell Medical International, London ON, Canada) (Fig. 40.6) is an example of a breath-actuated jet nebulizer. A unique, spring-loaded, one-way valve design draws the jet to the capillary tube during inspiration and causes nebulization to cease when the patient inspiratory flow reduces below threshold, or the patient exhales into the

device. Expiratory pressure on the valve at the initiation of exhalation moves the nebulizer baffle away from its position directly above the jet orifice, reducing the pressure in this area and stopping the aerosolization of the fluid. Thus drug wastage and contamination of the environment during the expiratory phase of the breathing cycle are almost completely eliminated.

The performance of the AeroEclipse under continuous, rather than intermittent, airflow conditions, has been compared to several other small-volume nebulizers. Using budesonide suspension as the test drug, the results showed a slightly better performance of the Aero-Eclipse compared to the Pari LC Star for the rate of delivery of budesonide, duration of nebulization, and the amount of budesonide delivered onto a filter. Further data from in vitro simulation experiments using an adult breathing pattern showed that while the AeroEclipse provided double the amount of aerosolized albuterol on the inhalation (lung) test filter, nebulization time was 70% longer than the comparator systems.[125] In vitro data from Leung et al[131] also using albuterol as the test drug but simulated breathing patterns representative of CF patients, confirmed reduced drug wastage and decreased environmental contamination during nebulization, but not the efficiency of delivery for the AeroEclipse. Thus, one has to weigh the advantages of recommending a potentially more efficient system in terms of drug output against prolonged treatment times. Alternatively, provided the required clinical response is obtained, the time to treat can be shortened because of the increased efficiency of delivery.

Adaptive aerosol delivery

The I-Neb (Respironics, USA), the third-generation design of the Halo-lite™ (Medic-Aid, UK) (Fig. 40.6) is a breath-actuated 'Smart' vibrating mesh nebulizer designed to control the inhaled dose to the patient. This is accomplished by monitoring the breathing pattern, specifically pressure

Table 40.5 New nebulizer technologies

Category	Device name	Manufacturer
Vibrating aperture	AeroNeb Go	Aerogen, USA
Vibrating mesh	MicroAir NE-U03, NE-U22	Omron, USA
	Touchspray	ODEM, UK
	e-Flow	Pari,GE
	I-Neb AAD System	Respironics, USA
Extrusion through nozzles	AERx	Aradigm,USA
	Respimat	Boehringer-Ingelheim,GE
Breath-actuated	AeroEclipse	TrudellMedical, CA
	Circulaire	WestMed, USA
Breath-enhanced	Ventstream Pro	Respironics, USA
	Pari LCD	Pari, GE
'Smart' nebulizers		
Control of dose during inhalation	I-Neb AAD System	Respironics, USA
Control of inhalation rate, volume	Akita system	InAMed, Munich, GE

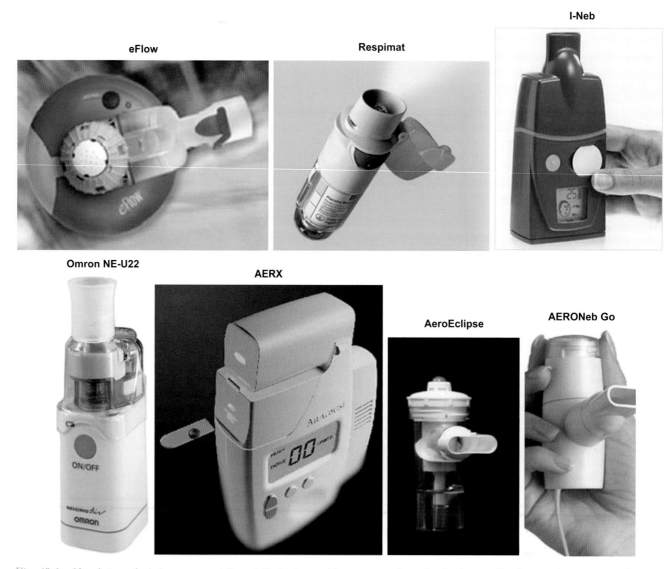

Fig. 40.6. New designs of nebulizers commercially available for therapy. All incorporate advanced technologies and/or features which are more efficient in producing and providing aerosol.

changes at the mouth and inspiratory time over consecutive tidal breaths of the patient.[132] Drug is then aerosolized over 50% of the inspiratory maneuver during the 4th and subsequent breaths until the pre-established total microgram dose to be inhaled by the patient has been aerosolized. The system then provides an audible signal indicating that the treatment should be stopped. Built-in electronics monitor patient treatment schedules and delivered doses with the intention to improve compliance with therapy. A radiolabeled lung deposition study using the Halolite in nine

normal and ten asthmatic subjects indicated that 60% of the emitted or delivered dose deposited in the lungs (coefficient of variation (CV) of 17%), with an oropharyngeal dose of approximately 40%.[90] The deposition measured is approximately 6 times greater than that from conventional jet nebulizers and similar to other new nebulizer technologies.

In a comparison, published by Leung, of the Halolite with other nebulizers, this nebulizer provided the most consistent and accurate output of the required dose for treatment. [131]

AERx™

The AERx™ (Aradigm Corp, USA) (Fig. 40.6) utilizes drug solution in a unit-dose, sterile, preservative-free blister pack containing 25–50 µL of fluid. The drug is extruded under pressure through a nozzle consisting of a number of small, precision-drilled holes to produce a fine, respirable spray on inhalation.[127,133] The aerosolization nozzle is a part of the disposable blister and not reused. The dose from a single blister is metered in approximately 1.5 s. The emitted dose is upwards of 70% of the dose loaded into the blister over an inspiratory flow rate range of 30–85 Lpm. The AERx™ is currently being tested with a number of drugs in liquid form to be used for topical and systemic therapy. Data have been published on its use with insulin and morphine. Using the current design, the in vitro (mean ± SD) emitted dose was shown to be 78 ± 3% of the dose of morphine sulphate loaded into the blister and, in patients with asthma, lung deposition has now been shown to be 75–80% of the loaded dose.[129,134] The AERx has built-in electronic monitoring capabilities, which measure the patient's IFR during dosing, and triggers the dispensing of the dose at the appropriate IFR for optimal delivery. The dosage administered is logged, providing a record of treatments and indication of patient compliance with therapy.

AeroNeb Go™

The AeroNeb Go™ (AeroGen Inc, USA) (Fig. 40.6) delivery device is a battery-operated, breath-actuated, liquid inhaler utilizing vibrating orifice technology to produce a fine aerosol.[126] The nebulizer consists of a dome-shaped plate containing approximately 1000 tapered apertures. The plate vibrates at ultrasonic frequencies, drawing (or pumping) the liquid through the apertures where it is broken up into fine droplets. The exit velocity of the aerosol is low, <10 m/s, and the particle size can be ≥2 µm (MMAD), varying with aperture size. Drug is packaged in miniature containers, ranging from 75 to 1200 µL, and the unit-dose is dispensed onto the dome when the patient pushes a button. Lung deposition in normals was measured using radiolabeled albuterol and found to be 70% of the nominal dose. This system is used with albuterol and has been tested with insulin, tobramycin, and ipratropium.

Respimat™

The Respimat™ soft-mist inhaler (Boehringer-Ingelheim, Germany) (Fig. 40.6) uses mechanical energy to create an aerosol from liquid solutions, producing a low-velocity spray (10 mm/s) and delivering of a unit-dose of drug in a single actuation. A detailed review of this device was published recently.[127] To operate, patients place the Respimat in the mouth and press the button to release the drug spray. The Respimat, as with the pMDI, requires hand–breath coordination on the part of the patient. The particle size of the aerosol released varies from 2.2 to 5.5 µm MMD (mass median diameter, depending on the formulation being aerosolized),[135] with oropharyngeal doses between 26 and 54%.

Deposition studies in normal volunteers using radiolabeled drug solutions in the Respimat have demonstrated mean delivery efficiencies to the lower respiratory tract of between 31% and 45% of the emitted dose.[136–138] Clinically, this device may provide an alternative,

easy-to-use, portable, multidose drug delivery system for a variety of medications.[139–142]

PRESSURIZED AEROSOLS: METERED DOSE INHALERS

Whether used alone, or in conjunction with a spacer or valved holding chamber, pressurized aerosols, metered-dose inhalers (pMDIs), are the most commonly used aerosol delivery devices in the world. pMDIs are portable, compact, and relatively easy to use. Two key advantages of propellant-based inhalers are that the aerosol is generated and a uniform dose of drug released from the inhaler within a fraction of a second following actuation and that the doses provided are reproducible throughout the canister life.[143,144] One of the major developments in recent years has been the introduction of and transition to hydrofluoroalkane (HFA) replacement propellant formulations for the CFC pMDIs,[145] as mandated by the Montreal Protocol. The criteria for these replacement formulations were that they were to: (1) use the same route for delivery of the drug, that is, the inhaled route; (2) be used for the same indication; (3) have the same safety and side-effect profile and (4) provide approximately the same level of convenience in terms of use and maintenance for the patient.

There have been three different strategies for reformulating and repackaging CFC pMDIs, namely (1) maintaining the same type of formulation: a suspension CFC pMDI to a suspension HFA pMDI; (2) changing the formulation: a suspension CFC pMDI to a solution HFA pMDI, and (3) a change in formulation + interface: a suspension CFC pMDI to a solution HFA pMDI + redesign to provide an integral actuator/spacer for the pMDI. Some examples of inhalers within the first category are salbutamol, fluticasone, salmeterol, within the second category beclomethasone dipropionate, ciclesonide, triamcinolone, and for the third category, flunisolide.

Substitution of HFA propellants for CFCs in pMDIs markedly reduces but does not totally eliminate concerns regarding environmental issues. While the Ozone Depleting Potential (ODP) for HFA134a is 0, it does have some global warming potential (GWP < 1). In time, this remaining concern may be eliminated as newer, more portable, propellant-free inhalers become more widely available.

Formulation properties

pMDIs contain drug as micronized powder, either dissolved or suspended in one of two HFA liquid propellants, namely HFA 134a or HFA 227. The former is the substitute for the high vapor pressure CFC-12, while the latter, HFA-227, is the replacement for CFC-11, the propellant that is liquid at room temperature and acted to reduce the vapor pressure in the CFC pMDI. The selection of the appropriate replacement HFA propellant was not a simple task. The choice was primarily based on compatibility with the drug and any additional excipients required during formulation. HFA134a has been the main replacement propellant for many of the transitioned inhalers. It is medically safe, is non-toxic to animals and humans, is devoid of pharmacologic activity and can be co-solved with corticosteroids to produce a solution formulation. One of the drawbacks of this propellant is that it is not compatible with the surfactants that were used in the CFC inhalers, namely oleic acid, lecithin, and sorbitan trioleate. This presented a challenge to the pharmaceutical industry and meant a revised approach to reformulating the existing drugs used to treat asthma and COPD to accommodate this incompatibility. It also provided an opportunity to redesign and improve the MDI hardware and componentry to provide better performance.[146]

Unlike the CFC pMDIs, only some HFA formulations contain excipients such as surfactants (oily, viscous, non-volatile substances that are used to keep the drug suspended in the propellant and to lubricate the valve mechanism).[147,148] Propellants comprise 60–80% of the spray from a pMDI on a per weight basis. The droplets created on firing a pMDI contain drug in an envelope of propellant and surfactant (if present). When the propellant completely evaporates, the residual dry drug particles are inhaled. When evaporation is incomplete, as is usually the case, liquid propellant or propellant vapor is inhaled along with drug and any excipients. One of the main differences in the HFA products immediately noticed by users was that the spray appeared to be softer (Fig. 40.7),[149] the product of a combination of formulation changes and valve and actuator redesign. In addition; the typical sound on firing was different as was the taste of the aerosol. All of these changes are related to the formulation ingredients and physicochemical properties of the propellant and discussed in detail in the literature.[150–152] When ethanol is used as a co-solvent for the drug in the HFA pMDI, the rate of evaporation of the propellants is decreased, resulting in a coarser spray.[153] Some products have concentrations of alcohol up to 37% (w/w) and may cause irritation on inhalation. Because of compatibility issues between surfactants used to formulate corticosteroid CFC pMDIs and HFA propellants, several CFC corticosteroid pMDI suspensions required reformulation to solution pressurized aerosols.[154] This resulted in the availability of finer corticosteroid aerosols, with an increased fine particle fraction.[150] The total lung dose as well as the dose delivered to the lung periphery has been shown to be approximately 3–5-fold greater compared with the CFC formulations,[148,155,156] necessitating a halving of the prescribed HFA134a BDP dose to reproduce the same clinical efficacy and side-effect profile as for CFC pMDI BDP. In contrast, Airomir, the albuterol sulfate HFA134a pMDI is a suspension formulation, containing a low concentration of alcohol and with aerosol characteristics and dose per actuation comparable with the existing CFC albuterol pMDI. This formulation provides similar clinical effects to the original CFC pMDI, Ventolin.[157,158]

The MMAD and pMDI spray pattern are influenced by the vapor pressure of the HFA propellant ambient temperature,[34,159,160] as well as the design of the valve stem and actuator orifices.[161–164] The vapor pressures of CFC pMDI formulations ranged from 275 to 575 kPa, resulting in heterodisperse aerosols with MMADs of approximately 3–6 μm.[165] HFA134a can produce sprays with similar characteristics. However, when the drug is dissolved in ethanol and co-solved with the propellant, the formulation becomes a solution rather than a suspension and the resulting aerosol becomes one with finer particle-size characteristics and MMADs in the 1 μm range. As with the CFC pMDIs, increasing the concentration of drug in the formulation can result in a coarser aerosol.[161,166]

In vitro studies with the new HFA134a formulations remeasured the amount of drug delivered ex-actuator and also from several spacer devices to determine how comparable the available doses and particle size distribution measurements were to the CFC pMDIs.[167] With Airomir, the emitted dose ex-actuator was reduced compared with Ventolin due to increased losses on the actuator but the fine particle doses tended to be similar when tested through the three spacers used in pediatrics (Fig. 40.8).[168] For an HFA134a pMDI used with the standard actuator mouthpiece,

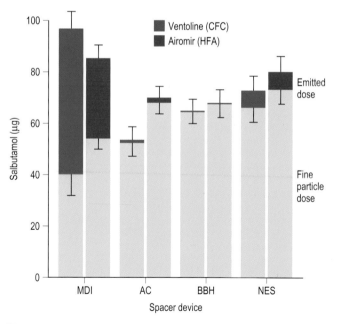

Fig. 40.8. Emitted dose (ED) and fine particle dose (FPD) from HFA 134a-salbutamol (Airomir™, 3M Pharmaceuticals, UK) measured from the pMDI (pressurized metered-dose inhalers) alone and with 3 spacers of different volumes and materials of manufacture – the Aerochamber™ (AC) (plastic, 145 mL), Babyhaler™ (BBH) (plastic, 350 mL), and Nebuchamber™ (NES) (metal, 280 mL) – in comparison to measurements with CFC-salbutamol (Ventoline™ GlaxoWellcome, France). ED for Airomir™ was significantly less than that for Ventolin due to losses on the actuator mouthpiece ($p<0.05$), but the Airomir™ FPD was greater. With all the spacers, EDs and FPDs for Airomir™ were either the same as ($p>0.05$) or greater ($p<0.05$) than those measured with Ventoline™.[168]

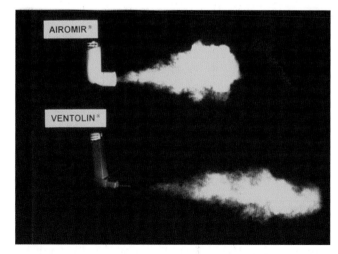

Fig. 40.7. High-speed photograph of the plume geometry of the albuterol aerosol emitted from (*Top*) HFA134a albuterol (Airomir, 3M Pharmaceuticals, MN) and (*Bottom*) CFC-albuterol (Ventolin, GlaxoSmithKline, USA).[149]

loss of drug in the valve stem housing and on the mouthpiece can amount to 10–15% of the nominal dose, somewhat greater than from CFC formulations; this loss is reflected in the label claim in some countries.

Changes in the dimensions of the actuator orifice or the placement of baffles within the actuator to reduce the spray forward velocity can also result in a finer spray due to impaction on the baffle.[162] This latter feature was incorporated into a redesigned pMDI actuator mouthpiece, producing a breath-actuated pMDI, the Gentlehaler. The baffle also effectively reduced the forward velocity of the drug spray, both of benefit to the patient taking their pMDI medication. In vivo studies comparing delivery with this new actuator to that from the original standard actuator, demonstrated a reduction in oropharyngeal deposition by approximately 50%; whole lung deposition was unchanged and a similar bronchodilator response measured.[169] However, extrapulmonary effects were greater from the aerosol produced by the new actuator, suggesting that it was the resulting changes to the aerosol cloud that gave rise to the observed enhanced absorption from the lung. A number of designs for breath-actuated pMDIs along with other novel designs for delivering pressurized aerosols have recently been described by Newman.[170] While the majority of these devices are not yet available in North America, once approved by the regulatory agencies, they may provide devices that ensure reliable drug delivery for pMDIs. However, while the coordination issue may be solved by these devices, oropharyngeal doses may still be high. Whether the patient could 'trigger' the actuation of the MDI with a spacer or holding chamber attached would need to be investigated.

With solution HFA pMDIs, the diameter of the actuator orifice is typically smaller, and the aerosol predictably finer.[90,171] When flunisolide CFC transitioned to an HFA solution product, Forest Laboratories redesigned the interface to the patient, extending the actuator mouthpiece to become a small open-tube spacer.[172] This actuator helped reduce the emitted dose to the same amount as from the CFC inhaler. However, patients still needed to coordinate actuation with inhalation as the redesign did not include a valve to allow the aerosol to be contained in the spacer.[173]

The volume of the formulation and the amount of drug released per actuation of the pMDI is a function of the physical size of the metering chamber, which ranges from 30 to 100 µL. pMDIs with larger metering chambers, used mainly to accommodate greater amounts of drug required to be released per actuation, cause a decrease in the rate of propellant evaporation due to the increased amount of propellent also released, further resulting in a greater loss of drug on the actuator mouthpiece.[147]

The liquid stream released from the canister metering chamber is atomized instantly as the propellant 'flashes' or vaporizes. This process continues as the stream of liquid is released from the metering chamber, taking approximately 20 ms to completely evaporate the propellant.[174,175] The liquid spray ejects from the CFC pMDI at about 15 m/s, depending on the formulation and rapidly decelerates to <7 m/s within 0.1 s as the spray cloud forms and moves away from actuator orifice.[176] This high velocity jet causes approximately 80% of the dose to impact in the oro- and hypopharynx when the canister is fired from inside the mouth. This may result in irritation and other side effects, especially with use of steroid aerosols.[53] Holding the canister outside the wide open mouth (at two fingers width) provides a space for the particles to decelerate while evaporating, enhancing the capacity to entrain the aerosol into the inspiratory airstream, and reducing the amount of propellant inhaled. Use of the open mouth technique, with a low inspiratory flow rate, can result in a doubling of the dose delivered to the lower respiratory tract in adults from approximately 7% to 14%.[177]

With CFC inhalers, the initial dose actuated from a new pMDI canister contains less active substance than subsequent actuations.[178] This 'loss of dose' from a pMDI appears to occur in formulations that tend to cream, i.e., where the drug particles rise to the top of the canister over time.[143] A reduction in emitted dose with the first actuation commonly occurs with a CFC pMDI following storage, particularly with the valve pointed in the downward position. 'Loss of prime' is related to valve design and occurs when propellant leaks out of the metering chamber during periods of non-use, for some drugs as short as 4 h, resulting in reduced pressure and hence less drug released with the next actuation. 'Tail-off' is the variability in the amount of drug dispensed towards the end of the life of the canister, resulting in swings from normal to virtually no dose emitted from one breath to the next. Improved designs of metering valves developed for use with HFA propellants have rectified these problems.[144] However, until all pMDIs are manufactured with these new valves, recommendations have been made that a single dose be wasted before the next dose is inhaled if the pMDI has not been used for even a period of 4–6 h. Given the cost of these medications, this suggestion is not seen to be a practical one for many patients, particularly those switched to HFA pMDIs. The data supporting the original claims of varying drug quantities emitted from the metering valve when left unused were obtained with CFC suspension formulations. Measurements need to be obtained with both solution and suspension HFA pMDIs to determine if the original findings still apply.

pMDI aerosol from spacers

Spacer devices and valved holding chambers (S/HC) have been developed for use with pMDIs in response to difficulties adult and pediatric patients encounter when taking their pMDI medication. The most common problems are related to timing or hand–breath coordination; that is, being able to coordinate actuating the pMDI and inhaling the spray at the same time.[179,180] The use of a S/HC device can overcome this problem, assuring delivery of the drug to the lung.

Three basic concepts for spacer devices include the open tube design, the reservoir or valved holding chamber design,[181,182] and the reverse-flow design in which the MDI, placed close to the mouth, is fired in the direction away from the patient (Fig. 40.9).[183,184] Approximately 12 different devices, based on these three concepts, and with volumes ranging from 15–750 mL, have been developed over the last 30 years. Factors to be considered when selecting a spacer are given in Table 40.6.

Modification of the particle size distribution of the aerosol dispensed and drug available at the device exit depend on a number of design factors.[185] The addition of a one-way valve to convert an open tube into a reservoir for the aerosol, the incorporation of the actuator for the MDI into the design, the shape of the device, flow of air through the device, edge effects, facemasks and manufacturing materials all affect aerosol characteristics and drug yield. The inhalation valve, which is used to contain the aerosol and reduce oropharyngeal deposition (as a baffle), must be able to withstand the initial pressure from the pMDI on firing, but have a sufficiently low resistance to open readily on inhalation, particularly when the device is used by children and infants. Exhalation valves in a facemask attached to a spacer device must also provide low resistance.[168,186] Issues of spacer volume, tidal volume, frequency of breathing and dead space between the spacer and mouth, are of particular concern when using these devices in children as differences of 2–3-fold in drug available at the mouth have been measured among spacers used for infants. Thus,

pMDI spacer designs

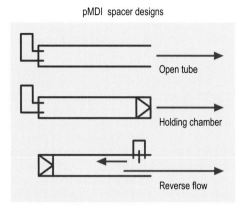

Open tube

Holding chamber

Reverse flow

Fig. 40.9. Schematic illustrating three current designs of spacer devices: (1) open-tube; (2) holding chamber with a one-way valve placed between the chamber and the mouthpiece, allowing the aerosol to be contained in the chamber after firing the pMDI; and (3) the reverse-flow design. This latter device contains a built-in actuator orifice for the pMDI. The one-way valve in the distal wall remains closed during actuation of the pMDI, opening to allow air entry on inhalation.[184]

clinicians should determine the delivery efficiencies of spacer devices prior to use in the target population. Recently, facemask design has received attention as it has been recognized that losses incurred with poor design can affect treatment, particularly in children.[187] Research is also needed to address facemask design for the elderly patient.[118,119,188]

The primary function of spacers is to eliminate the need to coordinate actuation of the pMDI with inhalation of the aerosol. Many patients, particularly children[189] and also the elderly, have difficulty performing this maneuver successfully, especially when short of breath.[190] Coordination is still required with all three types of spacer design, as even a 2 s delay between firing and inhaling the discharged spray will result in a substantial loss of drug and a reduced lung delivery. While drug loss due to sedimentation occurs during the interval between actuation and inhalation with valved holding chambers, the reduction in suspended dose is not as great as with the open tube spacers. The decrease in drug output from plastic spacers is largely due to the presence of electrostatic charge on the plastic.[58,59] Use of a metal spacer or spacer manufactured from a non-electrostatic plastic, or washing the plastic spacer periodically with de-ionizing detergent,[191] can overcome the loss of fine particle drug mass due to electrostatic charge.[192]

The coarse fraction of the aerosol is retained in the spacer through impaction on walls and on an inhalation valve, if present. With the retention of the larger droplets in the holding chamber, the 'cold Freon' effect, which causes many children to stop inhaling when using the pMDI alone, is reduced, as is the unpleasant taste associated with some of the drug aerosols. As the temperature of the HFA sprays is above freezing, this may no longer be as critical an issue when prescribing pMDIs for pediatric patients. Despite differences in design, all spacers reduce the initial forward velocity of the pMDI droplets, which occurs with partial evaporation of propellant in the time the aerosol traverses the length of the spacer, reducing non-respirable particles exiting the device.[193] The same drug used with different S/HC devices may only demonstrate small differences in MMAD, GSD and fine particle

Table 40.6 Spacer/holding chambers – points to consider
Design
Open tube vs valved holding chamber vs reverse-flow
Spacer volume
Materials of manufacture
Plastic vs metal, non-electrostatic material
Electrostatic charge
Clear vs opaque
Ability to clean
Valves
Placement
Design
Center cut vs flap vs duck-bill
Rubber vs plastic
Integrated expiratory valve
Resistance
Tidal volume/spacer volume ratio
Drug concentration within spacer due to differences in adult-pediatric-neonate tidal volumes
Requirement for multiple breaths to inhale drug dispensed into spacer/holding chamber
Inhalation technique
Coordination required for open tube spacer
Can delay up to 1 s for holding chamber
Tidal breathing through holding chamber (pediatric and neonatal) vs single breath
Facemask
Dead space
Expiratory valve resistance
Fit to face
Drug loss in spacer
Electrostatic charge
Delay between actuation and inhalation
Multiple breath inhalation protocol

fractions.[194] However, the quantity of aerosolized drug available at the spacer exit varies and is dependent on spacer volume and design, as well as formulation factors.[195,196]

Holding chambers produce a finer, slower-moving, more 'respirable' aerosol with less impaction of drug in the oropharyngeal area than simple spacers or the pMDI alone. Deposition following inhalation of a radiolabeled pMDI solution aerosol from the Aerochamber® compared with that from the same pMDI, inhaled using the open-mouth technique, showed a 10–17-fold decrease in the amount of radioactivity deposited in the oropharyngeal/laryngeal area in both normal and COPD subjects, while maintaining a similar lung dose.[182] Numerous other studies have demonstrated that the addition of a S/HC to the pMDI will reduce the oropharyngeal dose; the percentage decrease varies with the S/HC and drug pMDI aerosol tested.[173,197–199] The advantage of reduced oropharyngeal deposition is fewer side effects from steroid aerosols, demonstrated in a number of published clinical trials.[200,201]

The mass median aerodynamic diameter of the pMDI aerosol exiting a spacer is decreased by approximately 25% while the fraction containing particles <5 µm in diameter is increased.[185] With valved holding chambers, this fraction can be augmented by further evaporation of propellant in the finite time between actuation and inhalation; the increase in this fraction appears to depend on the pMDI formulation; the more concentrated the drug, the higher the fine particle fraction of aerosol exiting the device *relative* to the original pMDI aerosol.[193,202]

There are a variety of factors, both device and patient related, that contribute to poor aerosol delivery to both pediatric and adult patients. For example, multiple actuations or sprays from one or more drugs placed into a holding chamber, cause both the total dose and respirable dose of drug available for inhalation to be reduced. The extent of these losses may vary for different drugs and spacer designs.[57,203] A review of the issues contributing to poor aerosol delivery from holding chambers was recently published by Mitchell and Nagel.[204] Teaching patients proper inhaler technique, not only for pMDIs but also for spacer/holding chambers, is a subject of much discussion and often much frustration for healthcare workers and patients.[205–207] This issue is addressed on many levels, but it is clear that healthcare workers, including physicians, need to be familiar with device technology and proper technique to be able to teach patients how to correctly take their inhaled medication.[78,208,209]

There has been little data in the literature regarding the performance of spacers or holding chambers with generic CFC and HFA134a pMDI formulations. Significantly lower values were measured for the respirable fractions of generics of BDP compared with the innovator product when used with a large volume spacer,[210] while in another study, differences in emitted dose were noted for generic albuterol CFC pMDIs, but not HFA 134a Airomir when tested with both plastic and metal devices.[168] The observations may be drug-spacer specific. Information should be made available to ensure that the patient is benefiting from the particular generic drug/spacer combination selected to provide the therapy.

DRUGS IN POWDER FORM: DRY POWDER INHALERS

Aerosols of dry powder are created by directing air through an aliquot of loose powder. As dry powder inhalers are breath-actuated, the need to synchronize inhalation with actuation is eliminated. However, the dispersion of the powder into respirable particles is dependent upon the creation of turbulent flow in the powder container, or in the inhaler, which, in turn, is a function of both the ability of the patient to inhale the powder with a sufficiently high inspiratory flow rate and the design of the powder device. Factors to consider when selecting a DPI are given in Table 40.7.[208] Other considerations influence drug delivery and efficiency and these are discussed in detail in several reviews.[8,78,211,212] A number of dry powder inhaler (DPI) devices are commercially available in North America and many more in Europe;

some dispense individual doses of drug from punctured gelatin capsules such as the Aerolizer (Novartis Pharmaceuticals, USA) and HandiHaler (Boehringer Ingelheim, GER) and others from a tape system, containing multiple, sealed, single doses (Diskus™, Glaxo, UK). The Turbuhaler™ (Astra Draco, Sweden) is an example of a multi-dose reservoir powder system, preloaded with a quantity of pure drug sufficient for dispensing 200 doses of terbutaline sulfate, budesonide, formoterol, or formoterol/budesonide. The design and performance characteristics of various DPIs are discussed in a number of dedicated reviews.[213–215]

Most powder dispensing systems require the use of a carrier substance mixed into the drug to enable the drug powder to more readily flow out of the device. The carriers used are sugars, lactose or glucose and the size and surface characteristics of the particles used in a powder blend have been shown to affect how the formulation 'flows' out of its device.[216] Reactions to lactose and/or glucose appear to be fewer than to the surfactants and propellants used in pressurized MDIs, even though the amount of these substances is substantially greater than the drug and can represent 98% or more of the weight per inhaled dose in some blends. The particle size of the dry powder particles is of the order of 1–2 µm, but the size of the lactose or glucose particles can range from approximately 20–65 µm. Thus, most of the carrier deposits in the oropharynx. Using a drug with a carrier substance in a DPI originally designed to meter only pure drug has been shown to provide twice the clinical effect to the equivalent dose given as a pMDI aerosol.[164] Thus, using a more efficient delivery system may provide an opportunity to reduce the total body dose by decreasing the nominal dose.[217] Performance of DPIs can also be affected by the materials used in production and manufacturing and a multiplicity of factors related to design.[218]

DPIs: DESIGN, PROPERTIES, AND PERFORMANCE

DPI devices provide a drug as either single capsules, in a bulk reservoir or as multi-unit dose devices. These multi-unit dose systems can take the form of blisters, blister tape, capsules or multi-chambered cassettes. Most of the systems are designed to hold the drug powder in bulk in a reservoir. The Diskus (GlaxoSmithKline, USA) has an innovative multi-unit dose system for drug storage, storing 30–60 individual doses of drug in a coiled tape (Diskus), providing the patient the convenience of a month's supply of drug in one inhaler. DPIs supplying insulin powder

Table 40.7 DPIs – points to consider

Specific resistance of the device
Inspiratory flow rate required for optimal delivery
Emitted dose/nominal dose ratio (drug loss in device)
Reproducibility of the emitted dose
Lung deposition and regional distribution
Oropharyngeal deposition
Dose storage (capsules, reservoir, blisters)
Dose counter

DPI, dry-powder inhaler

use blisters[219] dispensed into a holding chamber, or capsules containing insulin powder.[220]

The specific resistance of a DPI device is determined by its geometry and governs the maximal inspiratory flow rate that can be drawn through the device. High resistance decreases the ability to draw air through the inhaler,[221] but use at the optimal IFR for the inhaler helps to produce a finer aerosol. The range of specific resistance values for current designs is approximately 0.02–$0.2 \, cmH_2O/L/s^{1/2}$.[222] Lung deposition varies between inhalers and is lower for DPIs with lower specific resistances.

Passive or patient-driven DPIs rely on the patient inspiratory effort to dispense the dose with resulting differences in lung delivery and, clinical response. Active or powered DPI devices are independent of patient effort. In some active DPI designs, such as the Inhale Powder Delivery System (PDS) (Inhale Therapeutics, USA)[219] a storage chamber is required to contain the powder cloud created on the release of the drug from the dosing blister, a design concept similar to the Aerochamber™ VHC (TMI, Int'l,Canada) used with pMDIs.

Optimal performance for an individual DPI design may occur at a specific inspiratory flow rate, different than for other inhaler devices.[223] The quality of the powder cloud leaving the DPI is influenced by flow rate, seen in the wide variability in the fine particle fraction of drug powders from existing DPIs, ranging from 10% to 60% of the nominal dose; this variability results in marked differences in lung deposition between the different devices and response.[193, 224] A concern for patients with compromised lung function is that they may not be able to inhale through high-resistance DPIs using the optimal inspiratory flow rate for the inhaler to obtain the maximum dose of drug from the device.[225] Despite the high resistance of the HandiHaler, patients with COPD, with FEV_1s below 27% predicted, were able to inhale through this device at the minimum target of 30 Lpm, particularly following training in proper technique.[226] An advantage of high-resistance devices is the potential for increasing delivery of drug to the lower respiratory tract.[227] This may though depend upon whether the powder is inhaled as a bolus or a cloud of suspended particles.

It has also recently been recognized that a truer comparison of emitted doses and aerosol particle size distributions between DPI devices should not be made at a universal flow rate, but at the flow rate indicated by the manufacturer of the device to produce optimal performance.[223,228] A comparison of measuring techniques was undertaken in an attempt to develop a standard methodology for in vitro testing of DPIs. The result, after several years of testing and discussions, are rigorous international standards for inhaler testing that manufacturer's implement prior to approval.

Ambient humidity can markedly affect drug powders delivered from DPIs.[229,230] The emitted dose will decrease in a humid environment, likely due to powder clumping and growth resulting from the added moisture.[231,232] Multiple unit dose DPIs, in which the powder is sealed until use, should minimize these effects.[233,234] The high peak inspiratory flow rates (>60 Lpm) required to dispense the drug powder from most current DPI designs result in a pharyngeal dose comparable with that received from a pMDI without an add-on device. The dose delivered to the respiratory tract from the Turbuhaler used at 60 Lpm has been measured in adults with lung disease and shown to be similar to that from a pMDI: 17% to the lungs and approximately 75% to the oropharynx.[235] If inhalation is not performed at the optimal inspiratory flow rate for a particular device, delivery to the lung will be reduced, as the

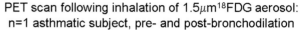

PET scan following inhalation of $1.5 \mu m$ [18]FDG aerosol: n=1 asthmatic subject, pre- and post-bronchodilation

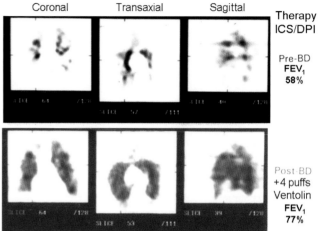

Fig. 40.10. PET scans (one example per plane) showing marked improvement in ventilation post-bronchodilator in an asthmatic subject. Deposition of [18]FDG aerosol (1.5 μm VMD) was poor pre-Ventolin.[239] [18]FDG, ^{18}F-labeled 2-deoxy-2-fluoro-D-glucose.

dose of drug dispensed is decreased and the particle size of the powder aerosol increased.

Lung deposition with radiolabeled powders

Lung deposition from various DPIs has been measured in a number of studies in adults and children[236,237] using the inhalation of radiolabeled drug powders and γ imaging or pharmacokinetic methods. The deposition studies have been performed with only a few drugs, mostly in normal subjects and at the manufacturer's suggested inspiratory flow rate for optimal performance. Deposition values vary three-fold between these DPIs, from 16 to 37% of the emitted dose. In general, these are much lower than the values for the new-generation liquid nebulizers and inhalers described above. Oropharyngeal doses are about 60% for all DPIs. Imaging can also demonstrate the effects of aerosol treatment.[238] One such example, shown in Figure 40.10,[239] demonstrates the change in distribution of ventilation post bronchodilator in a severe asthmatic subject.

Despite the above issues, DPIs, in general, are convenient and easy to use. Newer designs are being developed, providing more reproducible dosing, independent of inspiratory flow rate and aerosols with higher fine particle fractions. It remains to be seen if the dry powder inhaler can compete with the pressurized pMDI or the small-volume nebulizer for delivering the novel formulations being developed for inhalant therapy.[219,220,240,241]

■ INHALER SELECTION FOR THERAPY ■

There are a myriad of drug delivery devices used for taking the various aerosol therapies available. This wide range of devices, each with a different set of instructions for operation, can be confusing for both the physician and patient when trying to select an appropriate delivery system for the drug prescribed. The use of both solution inhalers and DPIs has broadened from systems for the delivery of traditional respiratory medications to treat asthma, COPD, and restrictive lung diseases to the delivery of inhaled proteins, peptides, and analgesics. Ultimately, the patient must be able to use the device easily, maintain it and derive clinical benefit from the drug delivered from the system.

The following is taken from the ACCP/ACACI Guidelines on device selection[78] and is a summary of the discussions that should be initiated with the patient and questions that should be asked by the physician or healthcare worker when selecting an inhaler for his/her patient. Whichever device is chosen, proper patient education on its use is critical and assessment of inhalation technique should be part of subsequent office visits. Physicians, respiratory therapists, and nurses caring for patients with respiratory diseases should be familiar with issues related to performance and correct use of aerosol delivery devices. They and their patients must recognize that if one system does not work, an alternative must be tried.

Aerosol device selection: nine questions to be asked by the prescribing physician or other healthcare worker when deciding which device to use:

1. What devices are available for the drug prescribed?
2. Given the patient's age and the clinical setting, what device will they be able to use properly?
3. Which drug/device combination is reimbursed?
4. Which are the most cost-effective devices?
5. Can all types of inhaled drugs for that patient be delivered with the same device type?
7. Which device is most convenient for patient or medical staff to use, considering administration time, cleaning of the device, and portability.
8. How durable is the device?
9. Does the patient or clinician have a specific preference?

■ SUMMARY ■

Medications delivered as pressurized aerosols using metered-dose inhalers (pMDIs), dry powders from dry powder inhalers (DPIs), and liquid aerosols from a variety of nebulizer systems remain the drug delivery options for treating asthma and other respiratory diseases by inhalation. New developments, both in formulation design and inhaler strategies, allow the use of the inhaled route for the treatment of systemic diseases such as diabetes. A current area of intense research is nanomedicine and the production of nanoparticle drugs that hold the potential for targeting very peripheral areas of the lung. It is important that physicians and other healthcare workers understand the basics of aerosol medicine and the implications of aerosol characteristics, such as particle size and emitted dose, and why attention to inhalation technique is key to successful aerosol delivery to the lung. This knowledge should be shared with patients where appropriate, allowing them to understand the importance of using proper inhaler technique and to recognize and attempt to remedy the situation when a particular device is not providing them with optimal benefit. It is important that patients comply in taking their medications and key to this is an understanding of how inhalers work.

If the lung is viewed as a black box with conventional clinical measures used as a guide to determining outcomes of a successful therapy, it can be quickly seen that if enough drug is given, responses using different inhalers can be the same. It is necessary to move beyond this paradigm and begin to consider how to target specific sites in the lung, delivering the minimum amount of therapy to provide the best possible response without side effects. This likely will require new and possibly more complex technologies for aerosol delivery systems, coupled with specific types of formulations for achieving these outcomes.

References

Introduction

1. Global Strategy for Asthma Management and Prevention, Global Initiative for Asthma (GINA) 2006. Online. Available: http://www.ginasthma.org
2. Global Strategy for the Diagnosis, Management and Prevention of COPD, Global Initiative for Chronic Obstructive Lung Disease (GOLD) 2006. Online. Available: http://www.goldcopd.org. http://www.goldcopd.org
3. Becker A, Berube D, Chad Z, et al. Canadian Pediatric Asthma Consensus Guidelines, 2003 (updated to December 2004): Introduction. CMAJ 2005; 173:S12–S14.
4. Labiris NR, Dolovich MB. Pulmonary drug delivery. Part II: The role of inhalant delivery devices and drug formulations in therapeutic effectiveness of aerosolized medications. Br J Clin Pharmacol 2003; 56:600–612.
5. Hess DR. Liquid nebulization: emerging technologies conference summary. Respir Care 2002; 47:1471–1476.
6. Dhand R. Aerosol therapy for asthma. Curr Opin Pulm Med 2000; 6:59–70.
7. Gonda I. Systemic delivery of drugs to humans via inhalation. J Aerosol Med 2006; 19:47–53.
8. Dolovich MB, MacIntyre NR, Anderson PJ, et al. Consensus statement: aerosols and delivery devices. American Association for Respiratory Care. Respir Care 2000; 45:589–596.
9. Scheuch G, Kohlhaeufl MJ, Brand P, et al. Clinical perspectives on pulmonary systemic and macromolecular delivery. Adv Drug Deliv Rev 2006; 58:996–1008.
10. Yu CP, Nicolaides P, Soong TT. Effect of random airway sizes on aerosol deposition. Am Ind Hyg Assoc J 1979; 40:999–1005.
11. Dolovich MB. Influence of inspiratory flow rate, particle size, and airway caliber on aerosolized drug delivery to the lung. Respir Care 2000; 45:597–608.
12. Patton JS, Byron PR. Inhaling medicines: delivering drugs to the body through the lungs. Nat Rev Drug Discov 2007; 6:67–74.
13. Waldrep JC, Selting KA, Reinero C, et al. Could inhaled chemotherapy be targeted to a specific lung lobe? J Aerosol Med 2007; 20:175, P036.

Definition and types of aerosols

14. Hargreave FE. Quantitative sputum cell counts as a marker of airway inflammation in clinical practice. Curr Opin Allergy Clin Immunol 2007; 7:102–106.
15. Anderson PJ, Dolovich MB. Aerosols as diagnostic tools. J Aerosol Med 1994; 7:77–88.
16. Dolovich M, Cockcroft D, Coates G. Aerosols in diagnosis: ventilation, airway penetrance, airway reactivity, epithelial permeability and mucociliary transport. In: Moren F, Dolovich M, Newhouse M, et al. eds. Aerosols in medicine: principles, diagnosis and therapy, 2nd edn. Amsterdam: Elsevier; 1993:195–234.
17. Kips JC, Inman MD, Jayaram L, et al. The use of induced sputum in clinical trials. Eur Respir J Suppl 2002; 37:47s–50s.
18. Leblanc M, Leveillee F, Turcotte E. Prospective evaluation of the negative predictive value of V/Q SPECT using 99mTc-Technegas. Nucl Med Commun 2007; 28:667–672.
19. D'silva L, Cook RJ, Allen CJ, Hargreave FE, Parameswaran K. Changing pattern of sputum cell counts during successive exacerbations of airway disease. Respir Med 2007; 101:2217–2220.
20. O'Byrne PM, Barnes PJ, Rodriguez-Roisin R, et al. Low dose inhaled budesonide and formoterol in mild persistent asthma: the OPTIMA randomized trial. Am J Respir Crit Care Med 2001; 164:1392–1397.
21. O'Byrne PM, Parameswaran K. Pharmacological management of mild or moderate persistent asthma. Lancet 2006; 368:794–803.
22. Hollander PA, Blonde L, Rowe R, et al. Efficacy and safety of inhaled insulin (Exubera) compared with subcutaneous insulin therapy in patients with type 2 diabetes: results of a 6-month, randomized, comparative trial. Diabetes Care 2004; 27:2356–2362.
23. Ellis AK, Keith PK. Nonallergic rhinitis with eosinophilia syndrome and related disorders. Clin Allergy Immunol 2007; 19:87–100.

Aerosols for therapy

24. Dolovich M. Aerosol delivery devices and airways/lung deposition. In: Schleimer R, O'Byrne P, Szefler SJ, et al, eds. Inhaled steroids in asthma: optimizing effects in the airways, New York: Marcel Dekker, 2002:169–211.
25. Martin RJ, Szefler SJ, Chinchilli VM, et al. Systemic effect comparisons of six inhaled corticosteroid preparations. Am J Respir Crit Care Med 2002; 165:1377–1383.
26. Laube BL, Georgopoulos A, Adams GK III. Preliminary study of the efficacy of insulin aerosol delivered by oral inhalation in diabetic patients (published erratum appears in JAMA 1993; 270:324). JAMA 1993; 269:2106–2109.

PHYSIOLOGY

27. Mudaliar S, Henry RR. Inhaled insulin in patients with asthma and chronic obstructive pulmonary disease. Diabetes Technol Ther 2007; 9:S83.

28. Yamamoto H, Kuno Y, Sugimoto S, et al. and Surface-modified PLGA nanosphere with chitosan improved pulmonary delivery of calcitonin by mucoadhesion and opening of the intercellular tight junctions. J Control Release 2005; 102:373–381.

29. Olschewski H, Simonneau G, Galie N, et al. and the Aerosolized Iloprost Randomized Study Group. Inhaled iloprost for severe pulmonary hypertension. N Engl J Med 2002; 347:322–329.

30. Yokoe K, Satoh K, Yamamoto Y, et al. Usefulness of 99mTc-Technegas and 133Xe dynamic SPECT in ventilatory impairment. Nucl Med Commun 2006; 27:887–892.

31. Hung OR, Whynot SC, Varvel JR, et al. Pharmacokinetics of inhaled liposome-encapsulated fentanyl. Anesthesiology 1995; 83:277–284.

32. Iacono AT, Johnson BA, Grgurich WF, et al. A randomized trial of inhaled cyclosporine in lung-transplant recipients. N Engl J Med 2006; 354:141–150.

33. Laube BL. The expanding role of aerosols in systemic drug delivery, gene therapy, and vaccination. Respir Care 2005; 50:1161–1176.

34. Hinds WC. Aerosol technology: properties, behavior, and measurement of airborne particles. New York: John Wiley & Sons; 1982.

35. Swift DL. Aerosol characterization and generation. In: Moren F, Dolovich MB, Newhouse MT, et al., eds. Aerosols in medicine: principles, diagnosis and therapy, 2nd revised edn. Amsterdam: Elsevier; 1993:64–81.

36. Brain JD, Valberg PA. Deposition of aerosol in the respiratory tract. Am Rev Respir Dis 1979; 120:1325–1373.

37. Lippmann M, Yeates DB, Albert RE. Deposition, retention, and clearance of inhaled particles. Br J Ind Med 1980; 37:337–362.

38. Yu CP, Diu CK. Total and regional deposition of inhaled aerosols in humans. J Aerosol Sci 1983; 14:599–609.

39. Heyder J. Deposition of inhaled particles in the human respiratory tract and consequences for regional targeting in respiratory drug delivery. Proc Am Thorac Soc 2004; 1:315–320.

40. Dolovich M, Ryan G, Newhouse MT. Aerosol penetration into the lung; influence on airway responses. Chest 1981; 80:834–836.

41. Willeke V, Baron PA. Aerosol measurement: principles, techniques and applications. New York: Van Nostrand Reinhold; 1993.

42. Mitchell JP, Nagel MW. Cascade impactors for the size characterization of aerosols from medical inhalers: their uses and limitations. J Aerosol Med 2003; 16:341–377.

43. Schmekel B, Hedenstrom H, Kampe M, et al. The bronchial response, but not the pulmonary response to inhaled methacholine is dependent on the aerosol deposition pattern. Chest 1994; 106:1781–1787.

44. Dahlback M. Behavior of nebulizing solutions and suspensions. J Aerosol Med 1994; 7:S13–S18.

45. Dolovich M, Rhem R. In vitro comparison of 2 strengths of Beclazone, a beclomethasone dipropionate (BDP) HFA 134 pMDI, with CFC Beclovent and Becloforte. Am J Resp Crit Care Med 2000; 161:A33.

46. Morrow PE. Conference on the scientific basis of respiratory therapy. Aerosol therapy. Aerosol characterization and deposition. Am Rev Respir Dis 1974; 110:88–99.

47. Dennis R. Handbook on aerosols. Tid-26608 National Technical Information Service US Department of Commerce; 1976.

48. Morrow PE. An evaluation of the physical properties of monodisperse and heterodisperse aerosols used in the assessment of bronchial function. Chest 1981; 80:809–813.

49. Biddiscombe MF, Usmani OS, Barnes PJ. A system for the production and delivery of monodisperse salbutamol aerosols to the lungs. Int J Pharma 2003; 254:243–253.

50. Usmani OS, Biddiscombe MF, Barnes PJ. Regional lung deposition and bronchodilator response as a function of beta2-agonist particle size. Am J Respir Crit Care Med 2005; 172:1497–1504.

Aerosol deposition mechanisms

51. Morrow PE. Physics of airborne particles and their deposition in the lung. Ann N Y Acad Sci 1980; 353:71–80.

52. Gonda I. Aerosols for delivery of therapeutic and diagnostic agents to the respiratory tract. Crit Rev Ther Drug Carrier Syst 1990; 6:273–313.

53. Dolovich M, Newhouse M. Aerosols: generation, methods of administration and therapeutic applications in asthma. In: Middleton EJ, Reed C, Adkinson N, et al., eds. Allergy: principles and practice, 4th edn. St Louis: Mosby; 1993:712–739.

54. Satoh K, Takahashi K, Kobayashi T, et al. The usefulness of 99mTc-Technegas scintigraphy for diagnosing pulmonary impairment caused by pulmonary emphysema. Acta Med Okayama 1998; 52:97–103.

55. Reilly RM. Carbon nanotubes: potential benefits and risks of nanotechnology in nuclear medicine. J Nucl Med 2007; 48:1039–1042.

56. Chan VS. Nanomedicine: an unresolved regulatory issue. Regul Toxicol Pharmacol 2006; 46:218–224.

57. O'Callaghan C, Lynch J, Cant M, et al. Improvement in sodium cromoglycate delivery from a spacer device by use of an antistatic lining, immediate inhalation, and avoiding multiple actuations of drug. Thorax 1993; 48:603–606.

58. Rau JL, Coppolo DP, Nagel MW, et al. The importance of nonelectrostatic materials in holding chambers for delivery of hydrofluoroalkane albuterol. Respir Care 2006; 51:503–510.

59. Mitchell JP, Coppolo DP, Nagel MW. Electrostatics and inhaled medications: influence on delivery via pressurized metered-dose inhalers and add-on devices. Respir Care 2007; 52:283–300.

60. Dolovich M, Ruffin RE, Roberts R, et al. Optimal delivery of aerosols from metered dose inhalers. Chest 1981; 80:911–915.

61. Anderson M, Philipson K, Svartengren M, et al. Human deposition and clearance of 6-micron particles inhaled with an extremely low flow rate. Exp Lung Res 1995; 21:187–195.

62. Newman SP, Pavia D, Garland N, et al. Effects of various inhalation modes on the deposition of radioactive pressurized aerosols. Eur J Respir Dis Suppl 1982; 119:57–65.

63. Hatch T, Gross P. Pulmonary deposition and retention of inhaled aerosols. New York: Academic Press, 1964.

64. Semmler-Behnke M, Takenaka S, Fertsch S, et al. Efficient elimination of inhaled nanoparticles from the alveolar region: evidence for interstitial uptake and subsequent reentrainment onto airways epithelium. Environ Health Perspect 2007; 115:728–733.

65. Rees PJ, Clark TJ, Moren F. The importance of particle size in response to inhaled bronchodilators. Eur J Respir Dis Suppl 1982; 119:73–78.

66. Zanen P, Go LT, Lammers JW. Optimal particle size for beta 2 agonist and anticholinergic aerosols in patients with severe airflow obstruction [see comments]. Thorax 1996; 51:977–980.

67. Usmani OS, Biddiscombe MF, Nightingale JA, et al. Effects of bronchodilator particle size in asthmatic patients using monodisperse aerosols. J Appl Physiol 2003; 95:2106–2112.

68. Ruffin RE, Dolovich MB, Wolff RK, et al. The effects of preferential deposition of histamine in the human airway. Am Rev Respir Dis 1978; 117:485–492.

69. Martonen TB, Schroeter JD, Hwang D, et al. Human lung morphology models for particle deposition studies. Inhal Toxicol 2000; 12(Suppl 4):109–121.

70. Martonen TB, Zhang Z, Yu G, et al. Three-dimensional computer modeling of the human upper respiratory tract. Cell Biochem Biophys 2001; 35:255–261.

71. Gerrity TR, Lee PS, Hass FJ, et al. Calculated deposition of inhaled particles in the airway generations of normal subjects. J Appl Physiol 1979; 47:867–873.

72. Gonda I. A semi-empirical model of aerosol deposition in the human respiratory tract for mouth inhalation. J Pharm Pharmacol 1981; 33:692–696.

73. Gerrity T. Pathophysiological and disease constraints on aerosol delivery. In: Byron PR, ed. Respiratory drug delivery. Boca Raton: CRC Press, 1990:1–38.

74. Martonen TB, Musante CJ, Segal RA, et al. Lung models: strengths and limitations. Respir Care 2000; 45:712–736.

75. Dolovich M, Rhem R. Small differences in inspiratory flow rate (IFR) and aerosol particle size can influence upper and lower respiratory tract deposition. J Aerosol Med 1997; 10:238.

76. Silkstone VL, Dennis JH, Pieron CA, et al. An investigation of in vitro/in vivo correlations for salbutamol nebulized by eight systems. J Aerosol Med 2002; 15:251–259.

77. Weda M, Zanen P, de Boer AH, et al. Equivalence testing of salbutamol dry powder inhalers: in vitro impaction results versus in vivo efficacy. Int J Pharm 2002; 249:247–255.

78. Dolovich MB, Ahrens RC, Hess DR, et al. Device selection and outcomes of aerosol therapy: Evidence-based guidelines: American College of Chest Physicians/American College of Asthma, Allergy, and Immunology. Chest 2005; 127:335–371.

79. Ferron GA. Aerosol properties and lung deposition. Eur Respir J 1994; 7:1392–1394.

80. Swift DL. Aerosols and humidity therapy. Generation and respiratory deposition of therapeutic aerosols. Am Rev Respir Dis 1980; 122:71–77.

81. Fuller HD, Dolovich M, Chambers C. Aerosol delivery during mechanical ventilation: a predictive in-vitro lung model. J Aerosol Med 1992; 5:251–259.

82. Mitchell JP, Nagel MW, Wiersema KJ, et al. The delivery of chlorofluorocarbon-propelled versus hydrofluoroalkane-propelled beclomethasone dipropionate aerosol to the mechanically ventilated patient: a laboratory study. Respir Care 2003; 48:1025–1032.

83. Nerbrink O, Pagels J, Pieron C, et al. Effect of humidity on constant output and breath enhanced nebulizer designs when tested in the EN 13544–1 EC Standard. Aerosol Sci Technol 2003; 37:282–292.

Nomenclature for indicators of drug delivery device performance

84. Canadian Standards Association. Spacers and holding chambers for use with metered-dose inhalers, Report Z264.1–02. 2002; Mississauga, ON: CSA.

85. Hess DR. Nebulizers: principles and performance. Respir Care 2000; 45:609–622.

86. Gerrity TR, Garrard CS, Yeates DB. Theoretic analysis of sites of aerosol deposition in the human lung. Chest 1981; 80:898–901.

87. Goldin JG, Tashkin DP, Kleerup EC, et al. Comparative effects of hydrofluoroalkane and chlorofluorocarbon beclomethasone dipropionate inhalation on small airways: assessment with functional helical thin-section computed tomography. J Allergy Clin Immunol 1999; 104:S258–S267.

88. Coates G, Dolovich M, Koehler D, et al. Ventilation scanning with technetium labeled aerosols. DTPA or sulfur colloid? Clin Nucl Med 1985; 10:835–838.

89. Parameswaran K, Leigh R, O'Byrne PM, et al. Clinical models to compare the safety and efficacy of inhaled corticosteroids in patients with asthma. Can Respir J 2003; 10:27–34.

Aerosol drug delivery devices

90. Dolovich M. New propellant-free technologies under investigation. J Aerosol Med 1999; 1:S9–S17.

91. Hendeles L, Colice GL, Meyer RJ. Withdrawal of albuterol inhalers containing chlorofluorocarbon propellants. N Engl J Med 2007; 356:1344–1351.

92. Gross NJ, Meyer RJ, Hendeles L, et al. Albuterol inhalers. N Engl J Med 2007; 356:2749.

93. De Benedictis FM, Selvaggio D. Use of inhaler devices in pediatric asthma. Paediatr Drugs 2003; 5:629–638.

94. Pedersen S. Inhalers and nebulizers: which to choose and why. Respir Med 1996; 90:69–77.

95. Dunne PJ. Economic aspects of introducing new nebulizer technology. Respir Care 2002; 47:1321–1331.

96. Nikander K, Turpeinen M, Wollmer P. Evaluation of pulsed and breath-synchronized nebulization of budesonide as a means of reducing nebulizer wastage of drug. Pediatr Pulmonol 2000; 29:120–126.

97. Mitchell JP, Nagel MW, Bates SL, et al. An in vitro study to investigate the use of a breath-actuated, small-volume, pneumatic nebulizer for the delivery of methacholine chloride bronchoprovocation agent. Respir Care 2003; 48:46–51.

98. Nikander K, Agertoft L, Pedersen S. Breath-synchronized nebulization diminishes the impact of patient-device interfaces (face mask or mouthpiece) on the inhaled mass of nebulized budesonide. J Asthma 2000; 37:451–459.
99. Nikander K, Bisgaard H. Impact of constant and breath-synchronized nebulization on inhaled mass of nebulized budesonide in infants and children. Pediatr Pulmonol 1999; 28:187–193.
100. Rau JL. Design principles of liquid nebulization devices currently in use. Respir Care 2002; 47:1257–1275.
101. Newnham DM, Lipworth BJ. Nebuliser performance, pharmacokinetics, airways and systemic effects of salbutamol given via a novel nebuliser delivery system ('Ventstream'). Thorax 1994; 49:762–770.
102. Mercer TT, Goddard RF, Flores RL. Effect of auxiliary air flow on the output characteristics of compressed-air nebulizers. Ann Allergy 1969; 27:211–217.
103. Newnham DM. Asthma medications and their potential adverse effects in the elderly: recommendations for prescribing. Drug Saf 2001; 24:1065–1080.
104. Phipps PR, Gonda I. Droplets produced by medical nebulizers. Some factors affecting their size and solute concentration. Chest 1990; 97:1327–1332.
105. Mercer TT, Tillery MI, Chow HY. Operating characteristics of some compressed-air nebulizers. Am Ind Hyg Assoc J 1968; 29:66–78.
106. Clay MM, Pavia D, Newman SP, et al. Assessment of jet nebulisers for lung aerosol therapy. Lancet 1983; 2:592–594.
107. Ryan G, Dolovich MB, Obminski G, et al. Standardization of inhalation provocation tests: influence of nebulizer output, particle size, and method of inhalation. J Allergy Clin Immunol 1981; 67:156–161.
108. Dolovich MB. Assessing nebulizer performance. Respir Care 2002; 47:1290–1301.
109. Mercer TT. Production and characterization of aerosols. Arch Intern Med 1973; 131:39–50.
110. Dennis JH, Stenton SC, Beach JR, et al. Jet and ultrasonic nebuliser output: use of a new method for direct measurement of aerosol output. Thorax 1990; 45:728–732.
111. Hess D, Fisher D, Williams P, et al. Medication nebulizer performance. Effects of diluent volume, nebulizer flow, and nebulizer brand [see comments]. Chest 1996; 110:498–505.
112. Clay MM, Pavia D, Newman SP, et al. Factors influencing the size distribution of aerosols from jet nebulisers. Thorax 1983; 38:755–759.
113. Alvine GF, Rodgers P, Fitzsimmons KM, et al. Disposable jet nebulizers. How reliable are they? Chest 1992; 101:316–319.
114. O'Riordan TG. Formulations and nebulizer performance. Respir Care 2002; 47:1305–1312.
115. Katz SL, Adatia I, Louca E, et al. Nebulized therapies for childhood pulmonary hypertension: an in vitro model. Pediatr Pulmonol 2006; 41:666–673.
116. Harvey CJ, O'Doherty MJ, Page CJ, et al. Effect of a spacer on pulmonary aerosol deposition from a jet nebuliser during mechanical ventilation. Thorax 1995; 50:50–53.
117. Coates AL, Fink J, Chantrel G, et al. In vivo justification of a physiological inspiratory: expiratory ratio to predict deposition of a novel valved spacer for liquid aerosol. Proc Am Thorac Soc 2006; 173:A84.
118. Nikander K, Berg E, Smaldone GC. Jet nebulizers versus pressurized metered dose inhalers with valved holding chambers: effects of the facemask on aerosol delivery. J Aerosol Med 2007; 20:S46–S58.
119. Smaldone GC, Sangwan S, Shah A. Facemask design, facial deposition, and delivered dose of nebulized aerosols. J Aerosol Med 2007; 20:S66–S77.
120. Oberdorster G, Utell MJ, Morrow PE, et al. Bronchial and alveolar absorption of inhaled 99mTc-DTPA. Am Rev Respir Dis 1986; 134:944–950.
121. Beasley R, Fishwick D, Miles JF, et al. Preservatives in nebulizer solutions: risks without benefit. Pharmacotherapy 1998; 18:130–139.
122. Phipps PR, Gonda I, Anderson SD, et al. Regional deposition of saline aerosols of different tonicities in normal and asthmatic subjects. Eur Respir J 1994; 7:1474–1482.
123. Hargreave FE. Quantitative sputum cell counts as a marker of airway inflammation in clinical practice. Curr Opin Allergy Clin Immunol 2007; 7:102–106.
124. Devadason SG, Everard ML, Linto JM, et al. Comparison of drug delivery from conventional versus 'Venturi' nebulizers. Eur Respir J 1997; 10:2479–2483.
125. Rau JL, Ari A, Restrepo RD. Performance comparison of nebulizer designs: constant-output, breath-enhanced, and dosimetric. Respir Care 2004; 49:174–179.
126. Dhand R. Nebulizers that use a vibrating mesh or plate with multiple apertures to generate aerosol. Respir Care 2002; 47:1406–1416.
127. Geller DE. New liquid aerosol generation devices: systems that force pressurized liquids through nozzles. Respir Care 2002; 47:1392–1404.
128. Ehtezazi T, Southern KW, Allanson D, et al. Suitability of the upper airway models obtained from MRI studies in simulating drug lung deposition from inhalers. Pharm Res 2005; 22:166–170.
129. Smaldone GC. Smart nebulizers. Respir Care 2002; 47:1434–1441.
130. Chou KJ, Cunningham SJ, Crain EF. Metered-dose inhalers with spacers vs nebulizers for pediatric asthma. Arch Pediatr Adolesc Med 1995; 149:201–205.
131. Leung K, Louca E, Coates AL. Comparison of breath-enhanced to breath-actuated nebulizers for rate, consistency, and efficiency. Chest 2004; 126:1619–1627.
132. Denyer J, Nikander K, Smith NJ. Adaptive Aerosol Delivery (AAD) technology. Expert Opin Drug Deliv 2004; 1:165–176.
133. Schuster J, Rubsamen R, Lloyd P, et al. The AERX aerosol delivery system. Pharm Res 1997; 14:354–357.
134. Sangwan S, Agosti JM, Bauer LA, et al. Aerosolized protein delivery in asthma: gamma camera analysis of regional deposition and perfusion. J Aerosol Med 2001; 14:185–195.
135. Zierenberg B. Optimizing the in vitro performance of Respimat. J Aerosol Med 1999; 1:S19–S24.
136. Newman SP, Steed KP, Reader SJ, et al. Efficient delivery to the lungs of flunisolide aerosol from a new portable hand-held multidose nebulizer. J Pharm Sci 1996; 85:960–964.
137. Newman SP, Brown J, Steed KP, et al. Lung deposition of fenoterol and flunisolide delivered using a novel device for inhaled medicines: comparison of RESPIMAT with conventional metered-dose inhalers with and without spacer devices. Chest 1998; 113:957–963.
138. Newman SP. Use of gamma scintigraphy to evaluate the performance of new inhalers. J Aerosol Med 1999; 1:S25–S31.
139. Iacono P, Velicitat P, Guemas E, et al. Improved delivery of ipratropium bromide using Respimat (a new soft mist inhaler) compared with a conventional metered dose inhaler: cumulative dose response study in patients with COPD. Respir Med 2000; 94:490–495.
140. Goldberg J, Freund E, Beckers B, et al. Improved delivery of fenoterol plus ipratropium bromide using Respimat compared with a conventional metered dose inhaler. Eur Respir J 2001; 17:225–232.
141. Ram FS, Brocklebank DM, Muers M, et al. Pressurised metered-dose inhalers versus all other hand-held inhalers devices to deliver bronchodilators for chronic obstructive pulmonary disease. Cochrane Database Syst Rev 2002; (1): CD002170.
142. Hodder R, Pavia D, Dewberry H, et al. Low incidence of paradoxical bronchoconstriction in asthma and COPD patients during chronic use of Respimat soft mist inhaler. Respir Med 2005; 99:1087–1095.
143. Schultz RK. Drug delivery characteristics of metered-dose inhalers. J Allergy Clin Immunol 1995; 96:284–287.
144. Cummings RH. Pressurized metered dose inhalers: chlorofluorocarbon to hydrofluoroalkane transition – valve performance. J Allergy Clin Immunol 1999; 104:s230–s235.
145. Noakes T. Medical aerosol propellants. J Fluorine Chem 2002; 118:35–45.
146. Nithyanandan P, Hoag S, Dalby R. The analysis and prediction of functional robustness of inhaler devices. J Aerosol Med 2007; 20:19–37.
147. Moren F. Aerosol dosage forms and formulation. In: Moren F. Dolovich MB, Newhouse MT, et al. eds Aerosols in medicine: principles, diagnosis and therapy, 2nd edn. Amsterdam: Elsevier; 1993:321–350.
148. Leach CL. The CFC to HFA transition and its impact on pulmonary drug development. Respir Care 2005; 50:1201–1208.
149. Dolovich M, Leach C. Drug delivery devices and propellants. In: Busse W, Holgate S, eds. Asthma and rhinitis, 2nd edn. Oxford: Blackwell Science; 2000:1719–1731.
150. Dolovich M. New delivery systems and propellants. Can Respir J 1999; 6:290–295.
151. Smyth HDC. The influence of formulation variables on the performance of alternative propellant-driven metered dose inhalers. Adv Drug Del Rev 2003; 55:807–828.
152. Smyth HD, Leach CL. Alternative propellant aerosol delivery systems. Crit Rev Ther Drug Carrier Syst 2005; 22:493–534.
153. Stein S, Myrdal P. The relative influence of atomization and evaporation on metered dose inhaler drug delivery efficiency. Aerosol Sci Technol 2006; 40:335–347.
154. Leach C. Effect of formulation parameters on hydrofluoroalkane-beclomethasone dipropionate drug deposition in humans. J Allergy Clin Immunol 1999; 104:S250–S252.
155. Dolovich MB, Rhem R, Gerrard L, et al. Lung deposition of coarse CFC vs fine HFA pMDI aerosols of beclomethasone dipropionate (BDP) in asthma. Am J Respir Crit Care Med 2000; 161:A62.
156. Vanden Burgt JA, Busse WW, Martin RJ, et al. Efficacy and safety overview of a new inhaled corticosteroid, QVAR (hydrofluoroalkane-beclomethasone extrafine inhalation aerosol), in asthma. J Allergy Clin Immunol 2000; 106:1209–1226.
157. Dockhorn R, Vanden Burgt JA, Ekholm BP, et al. Clinical equivalence of a novel non-chlorofluorocarbon-containing salbutamol sulfate metered-dose inhaler and a conventional chlorofluorocarbon inhaler in patients with asthma. J Allergy Clin Immunol 1995; 96: 50–56.
158. Kleerup EC, Tashkin DP, Cline AC, et al. Cumulative dose-response study of non-CFC propellant HFA 134a salbutamol sulfate metered-dose inhaler in patients with asthma. Chest 1996; 109:702–707.
159. Leach CL. Approaches and challenges to use freon propellant replacements. Aerosol Sci Technol 1995; 22:328–334.
160. Dolovich M, Leach C. Drug delivery devices and propellants. In: Busse WW, Holgate ST, eds. Asthma and rhinitis, 2nd edn. Oxford: Blackwell Science; 2000:1719–1731.
161. Porush I, Thiel CG, Young JG. Pressurized pharmaceutical aerosols for inhalation therapy. I. Physical testing methods. J Am Pharm Assoc Am Pharm Assoc 1960; 49:70–72.
162. Sanders P. Handbook of aerosol technology. NewYork: Van Nostrand Reinhold. 1979.
163. Polli GP, Grim WM, Bacher FA, et al. Influence of formulation on aerosol particle size. J Pharm Sci 1969; 58:484–486.
164. Niven RW, Kacmarek RM, Brain JD, et al. Small bore nozzle extensions to improve the delivery efficiency of drugs from metered dose inhalers: laboratory evaluation. Am Rev Respir Dis 1993; 147:1590–1594.
165. Kim CS, Trujillo D, Sackner MA. Size aspects of metered-dose inhaler aerosols. Am Rev Respir Dis 1985; 132:137–142.
166. Dolovich M. Measurement of particle size characteristics of metered dose inhaler (MDI) aerosols. J Aerosol Med 1991; 4:251–263.
167. Barry PW, O'Callaghan C. In vitro comparison of the amount of salbutamol available for inhalation from different formulations used with different spacer devices. Eur Respir J 1997; 10:1345–1348.
168. Dubus JC, Rhem R, Dolovich M. Delivery of HFA and CFC salbutamol from spacer devices used in infancy. Int J Pharm 2001; 222:101–108.
169. Newman SP, Clarke SW. Bronchodilator delivery from Gentlehaler, a new low-velocity pressurized aerosol inhaler[see comments]. Chest 1993; 103:1442–1446.
170. Newman SP. Principles of metered-dose inhaler design. Respir Care 2005; 50:1177–1190.
171. Leach CL. Enhanced drug delivery through reformulating MDIs with HFA propellants-drug deposition and its clinical effect on preclinical programs. In: Dalby RN, Byron PR, Farr SJ, eds. Respiratory drug delivery. Buffalo Grove, IL: Interpharm Press; 1996: V:133–144.
172. Morén F. Drug deposition of pressurized inhalation aerosols I. Influence of actuator tube design. Int J Pharm 1978; 1:205–212.
173. Richards J, Hirst P, Pitcairn G, et al. Deposition and pharmacokinetics of flunisolide delivered from pressurized inhalers containing non-CFC and CFC propellants. J Aerosol Med 2001; 14:197–208.
174. Wiener M. How to formulate aerosols to obtain the desired spray pattern. Soc Cos Chem 1958; 9:289–297.
175. Clark AR. MDIs: physics of aerosol formation. J Aerosol Med 1996; 1:S19–S26.
176. Dhand R, Malik SK, Balakrishnan M, et al. High speed photographic analysis of aerosols produced by metered dose inhalers. J Pharm Pharmacol 1988; 40:429–430.

177. Dolovich M, Ruffin RE, Roberts R, et al. Optimal delivery of aerosols from metered dose inhalers. Chest 1981; 80:911–915.

178. Cyr TD, Graham SJ, Li KY, et al. Low first-spray drug content in albuterol metered-dose inhalers. Pharm Res 1991; 8:658–660.

179. De Blaquiere P, Christensen DB, Carter WB, et al. Use and misuse of metered-dose inhalers by patients with chronic lung disease. A controlled, randomized trial of two instruction methods. Am Rev Respir Dis 1998; 140:910–916.

180. Crompton GK, Barnes PJ, Broeders M, et al. The need to improve inhalation technique in Europe: a report from the Aerosol Drug Management Improvement Team. Resp Med 2006; 100:1479–1494.

181. Moren F. Drug deposition of pressurized inhalation aerosols. Eur J Respir Dis Suppl 1982; 119:51–55.

182. Dolovich M, Ruffin R, Corr D, et al. Clinical evaluation of a simple demand inhalation MDI aerosol delivery device. Chest 1983; 84:36–41.

183. Sackner MA, Kim CS. Recent advances in the management of obstructive airways disease. Auxiliary MDI aerosol delivery systems. Chest 1985; 88:161S–170S.

184. Dolovich M. Inhalation technique and inhalation devices. In: Pauwels R, P. O'Byrne, eds. Beta2-agonists in asthma treatment. New York: Marcel Dekker; 1997:229–255.

185. Dolovich M. Lung dose, distribution, and clinical response to therapeutic aerosols. Aerosol Sci Technol 1993; 18:230–240.

186. Sennhauser FH, Sly PD. Pressure flow characteristics of the valve in spacer devices. Arch Dis Child 1989; 64:1305–1307.

187. Shah SA, Berlinski AB, Rubin BK. Force-dependent static dead space of face masks used with holding chambers. Respir Care 2006; 51:140–144.

188. Smaldone GC, Berg E, Nikander K. Variation in pediatric aerosol delivery: importance of facemask. J Aerosol Med 2005; 18:354–363.

189. O'Callaghan C. Delivery systems: the science. Pediatr Pulmonol 1997; 15:51–54.

190. Fink JB, Rubin BK. Problems with inhaler use: a call for improved clinician and patient education. Respir Care 2005; 50:1360–1374.

191. Wildhaber JH, Devadason SG, Eber E, et al. Effect of electrostatic charge, flow, delay and multiple actuations on the in vitro delivery of salbutamol from different small volume spacers for infants. Thorax 1996; 51:985–988.

192. Lauricella A, Dolovich M. The effects of inhalation delay and spacer pretreatment on HFA-pMDI delivery from several small volume valved holding chambers. J Aerosol Med 2007; 20:202.

193. Dolovich M. Characterization of medical aerosols: physical and clinical requirements for new inhalers. Aerosol Sci Technol 1995; 22:392–399.

194. Wilkes W, Fink J, Dhand R. Selecting an accessory device with a metered-dose inhaler: variable influence of accessory devices on fine particle dose, throat deposition, and drug delivery with asynchronous actuation from a metered-dose inhaler. J Aerosol Med 2001; 14:351–360.

195. Kim CS, Eldridge MA, Sackner MA. Oropharyngeal deposition and delivery aspects of metered-dose inhaler aerosols. Am Rev Respir Dis 1987; 135:157–164.

196. Ahrens RC. Inhaled drugs for treatment of asthma: nothing is ever as simple as it seems. Ann Allergy Asthma Immunol 1996; 77:260–262.

197. Thorsson L, Edsbacker S. Lung deposition of budesonide from a pressurized metered-dose inhaler attached to a spacer. Eur Respir J 1998; 12:1340–1345.

198. Newman SP. A comparison of lung deposition patterns between different asthma inhalers. J Aerosol Med 1995; 8:S21–S27.

199. Roller CM, Zhang G, Troedson RG, et al. Spacer inhalation technique and deposition of extrafine aerosol in asthmatic children. Eur Respir J 2007; 29:299–306.

200. Salzman GA, Pyszczynski DR. Oropharyngeal candidiasis in patients treated with beclomethasone dipropionate delivered by metered-dose inhaler alone and with Aerochamber. J Allergy Clin Immunol 1988; 81:424–428.

201. Meeran K, Burrin JM, Noonan KA, et al. A large volume spacer significantly reduces the effect of inhaled steroids on bone formation. Postgrad Med J 1995; 71:156–159.

202. Dolovich MB. Aerosol delivery devices and airways/lung deposition. In: Schleimer R, O'Byrne P, Szefler S, et al., eds. Inhaled steroids in asthma: optimizing effects in the airways, New York: Marcel Dekker; 2002:169–211.

203. Barry PW, O'Callaghan C. Multiple actuations of salbutamol MDI into a spacer device reduce the amount of drug recovered in the respirable range. Eur Respir J 1994; 7:1707–1709.

204. Mitchell JP, Nagel MW. Valved holding chambers (VHCs) for use with pressurised metered-dose inhalers (pMDIs): a review of causes of inconsistent medication delivery. Prim Care Respir J 2007; 16:207–214.

205. Melani AS, Zanchetta D, Barbato N, et al. Inhalation technique and variables associated with misuse of conventional metered-dose inhalers and newer dry powder inhalers in experienced adults. Ann Allergy Asthma Immunol 2004; 93:439–446.

206. Everard ML. Role of inhaler competence and contrivance in 'difficult asthma'. Paediatr Respir Rev 2003; 4:135–142.

207. Everard ML. Aerosol therapy: regimen and device compliance in daily practice. Paediatr Respir Rev 2006; 7:S80–S82.

208. Dolovich MB. In my opinion – interview with the expert. Pediatr Asthma Allergy Immunol 2004; 17:292–300.

209. Burkhart PV, Rayens MK, Bowman RK. An evaluation of children's metered-dose inhaler technique for asthma medications. Nurs Clin North Am 2005; 40:167–182.

210. Kenyon CJ, Thorsson L, Borgstrom L, et al. The effects of static charge in spacer devices on glucocorticosteroid aerosol deposition in asthmatic patients. Eur Respir J 1998; 11:606–610.

211. Ahrens RC. The role of the MDI and DPI in pediatric patients: 'Children are not just miniature adults'. Respir Care 2005; 50:1323–1328.

212. Selroos O, Borgstrom L, Ingelf J. Performance of Turbuhaler® in patients with acute airway obstruction and COPD, and in children with asthma: understanding the clinical importance of adequate peak inspiratory flow, high lung deposition, and low in vivo dose variability. Treat Respir Med 2006; 5:305–315.

213. Selroos O, Pietinalho A, Riska H. Delivery devices for inhaled asthma medication. Clin Immunother 1996; 6:273–299.

214. Newman SP, Busse WW. Evolution of dry powder inhaler design, formulation, and performance. Respir Med 2002; 96:293–304.

215. Atkins PJ. Dry powder inhalers: an overview. Respir Care 2005; 50:1304–1312.

216. Ganderton D. The generation of respirable clouds from coarse powder aggregates. J Biopharm Sci 1992; 3:101–105.

217. Lofdahl CG, Andersson L, Bondesson E, et al. Differences in bronchodilating potency of salbutamol in Turbuhaler as compared with a pressurized metered-dose inhaler formulation in patients with reversible airway obstruction. Eur Respir J 1997; 10:2474–2478.

218. Tobyn M, Staniforth JN, Morton D, et al. Active and intelligent inhaler device development. Int J Pharm 2004; 277:31–37.

219. Harper NJ, Gray S, Groot JD, et al. The design and performance of the Exubera pulmonary insulin delivery system. Diabet Technol Ther 2007; 9: S1–16.

220. Richardson PC, Boss AH. Technosphere insulin technology. Diabet Technol Ther 2007; 9:S–65.

221. Clark AR, Hollingworth AM. The relationship between powder inhaler resistance and peak inspiratory conditions in healthy volunteers – implications for in vitro testing. J Aerosol Med 1993; 6:99–110.

222. Frijlink HW, de Boer AH. Dry powder inhalers for pulmonary drug delivery. Expert Opin Drug Delivery 2004; 1:67–86.

223. Hindle M, Byron P. Dose emissions from marketed dry powder inhalers. Int J Pharm 1995; 116:169–177.

224. Nielsen KG, Auk IL, Bojsen K, et al. Clinical effect of Diskus dry-powder inhaler at low and high inspiratory flow-rates in asthmatic children. Eur Respir J 1998; 11:350–354.

225. Olsson B, Asking L. Critical aspects of the function of inspiratory flow driven inhalers. J Aerosol Med 1994; 7:S43–S47.

226. Al Showair RA, Tarsin WY, Assi KH, et al. Can all patients with COPD use the correct inhalation flow with all inhalers and does training help? Respir Med 2007; 101:2395–2401.

227. Svartengren K, Lindestad P, Svartengren M, et al. Added external resistance reduces oropharyngeal deposition and increases lung deposition of aerosol particles in asthmatics. Am J Respir Crit Care Med 1995; 152:32–37.

228. Richards R, Saunders M. Need for a comparative performance standard for dry powder inhalers. Thorax 1993; 48:1186–1187.

229. Hickey AJ, Martonen TB. Behavior of hygroscopic pharmaceutical aerosols and the influence of hydrophobic additives. Pharm Res 1993; 10:1–7.

230. Meakin BJ, Cainey J, Woodcock PM. Effect of exposure to humidity on terbutaline delivery from turbuhaler dry power inhalation devices. Eur Respir J 1993; 6:760–761.

231. Pitcairn G, Lunghetti G, Ventura P, et al. A comparison of the lung deposition of salbutamol inhaled from a new dry powder inhaler, at two inhaled flow rates. Int J Pharmaceut 1994; 102:11–18.

232. Telko MJ, Hickey AJ. Dry powder inhaler formulation. Respir Care 2005; 50:1209–1227.

233. Fuller R. The Diskus: a new multi-dose powder device – efficacy and comparison with Turbuhaler. J Aerosol Med 1995; 2:S11–7:S11–S17.

234. Sam T. Optimising the therapeutic trinity of active ingredient, delivery system and functional packaging. J Controlled Rel 2003; 87:153–157.

235. Newman S, Moren F, Trofast E, et al. Terbutaline sulphate Turbuhaler: effect of inhaled flow rate on drug deposition and efficacy. Int J Pharm 1991; 74:209–213.

236. Everard ML, Dolovich M. In vivo measurements of lung dose. In: Bisgaard H, O'Callaghan C, Smaldone GC, eds. Drug delivery to the lung. New York: Marcel Dekker; 2001:173–209.

237. Lahelma S, Kirjavainen M, Kela M, et al. Equivalent lung deposition of budesonide in vivo: a comparison of dry powder inhalers using a pharmacokinetic method. Br J Clin Pharmacol 2005; 59:167–173.

238. Dolovich M, Labiris R. Imaging drug delivery and drug responses in the lung. Proc Am Thorac Soc 2004; 1:329–337.

239. Dolovich M, Nahmias C, Coates G. Unleashing the PET: 3D imaging of the lung. In: Byron PR, Dalby R, Farr SJ, eds. Respiratory drug delivery, 7th edn. Raleigh, NC: Serentec, 2000:215–230.

240. Ganderton D, Lewis D, Davies R, et al. Modulite: a means of designing the aerosols generated by pressurized metered dose inhalers. Respir Med 2002; 96:S3–S8.

241. Ganderton D, Lewis D, Davies R, et al. The formulation and evaluation of a CFC-free budesonide pressurised metered dose inhaler. Respir Med 2003; 97:S4–S9.

Anatomy and Physiology of the Nose and Control of Nasal Airflow

Ronald Eccles

41

CONTENTS

- Functions of the nose 701
- Embryology and anatomy of the nose 702
- Nasal airflow 706

SUMMARY OF IMPORTANT CONCEPTS

>> The nose should be considered not as a single airway but as two separate nasal passages, each with its own blood supply and nervous pathways

>> The nasal airflow is usually asymmetrical due to the 'nasal cycle' of alternating congestion and decongestion of nasal venous sinuses

>> Nasal airway resistance is regulated at the level of the nasal valve, which is a dynamic valve controlled by swelling of the inferior turbinate

>> Nasal sensation of airflow is mediated by trigeminal nerves that are sensitive to the cooling action of inspired air

>> Any medicine or agent with an effect on blood vessels is likely to influence nasal airway resistance, such as histamine and sympathomimetics

FUNCTIONS OF THE NOSE

The nose is situated at the entrance of the airway and acts as an air conditioner and a chemosensor. The 10 000–20 000 L of air we breathe in each day is composed of a mixture of gases and suspended particulate matter. The nose acts as a very efficient filter and gas scrubber, and much of the suspended particulate matter and soluble gases such as sulfur dioxide are deposited there. The nasal epithelium is in direct contact with the external air and is exposed to a continuous threat of irritation, infection, and allergy, because the inspired air often contains air pollutants such as ozone, various pathogenic viruses, bacteria, fungal spores, and allergens derived from pollens, house dust mites, and animal dander.

The nose defends the lower airways from the harmful effects of the inspired air by acting as an efficient air conditioner. The nose warms, filters, and humidifies the inspired air so that clean air that is fully saturated with water vapor at a temperature of 37°C is delivered to the lungs.

FILTRATION

The nose acts as a very efficient filter of suspended particulate matter, and most suspended matter is either deposited in the nose or breathed in and out without respiratory deposition.[1] The filtration mechanism of the nose is firstly related to a sudden change in the direction of nasal airflow as the air stream passes upward through the nasal vestibule and then turns through 90 degrees to enter the nasal cavity. The sudden change in the direction of nasal airflow tends to spin suspended matter out of the main air stream and onto the surface of the nasal epithelium. Secondly, there is an acceleration of the airflow as it passes through the nasal valve region, which is the narrowest part of the nose, and then a deceleration of airflow as the air stream enters the nasal cavity. The changes in direction and velocity of the air stream occur over the same area of the nose, at the level of the anterior end of the inferior turbinate, and the slowing of the airflow at this point deposits particulate matter onto the nasal epithelium.

Much of the work of breathing is related to nasal filtration, because the nasal valve area forms the narrowest cross-sectional area of the whole airway and presents a considerable resistance to nasal airflow. Nasal airway resistance contributes up to two-thirds of the total airway resistance, and the work cost required from the respiratory muscles to move the airflow through the nasal valve area is the price that is paid for filtration of the inspired air.

Although nasal airflow may be laminar at very low levels of flow, for the greater part of the respiratory cycle, especially during inspiration, the flow is turbulent. The twisting course of nasal airflow, with changes in both velocity and direction, ensures that nasal airflow is mainly turbulent, and this is important for proper conditioning and mixing of the inspired air. If nasal airflow were mainly laminar, then only the portion of air directly in contact with the nasal epithelium would be conditioned by exchange of heat and water.

The tendency for a particle suspended in the air stream to be deposited in the nose is determined by factors such as its physical size, shape, density, and hygroscopicity. The physical size, shape, and density of a particle can be quantified as its aerodynamic equivalent diameter (AED). Particles with an AED larger than 180 μm are virtually non-inspirable. During nose breathing the majority of particles larger than 15 μm AED are deposited in the upper respiratory tract, but with mouth breathing some of these penetrate into the trachea. Particles with AEDs higher than 2.5 μm are primarily deposited in the trachea and bronchi, whereas those with lower AEDs penetrate into the gas exchange region of the lungs.[1]

HUMIDIFICATION OF INSPIRED AIR

Despite the fact that the upper airways condition the inspired air by increasing its humidity, so that air reaching the lungs is saturated with water, we often feel uncomfortable when the humidity of the air around us is high. This may be partly related to feeling 'hot and sticky,' but it may also be related to the fact that we often have a sensation of 'nasal stuffiness' when breathing air of high humidity, because the inspiratory nasal airflow does not provide the same cooling sensation of breathing.

The capacity of the upper airways to humidify the inspired air is very great, and no drying of the nasal epithelium is seen after prolonged exposure to dry air. The inhaled air rapidly reaches saturation with water vapor as it passes through the nose and upper airways, so that by the level of the trachea it is completely saturated. This saturation of the inhaled air is achieved despite a wide range of ambient air temperature and humidity. The water required for the humidification of the inhaled air is provided mainly by nasal glandular secretions, although it is unknown whether there are any control mechanisms linking the water requirement for air conditioning and the rate of glandular secretion.

The humidification of inspired air may also influence the filtration of particulate matter from the inspired air, because hydration of hygroscopic particulate matter may cause the particles to swell and thereby increase their AED.

Water is lost from the surface of the nasal epithelium during inspiration as it contributes to the humidification of the inspired air. The nasal epithelium is cooled as it gives up heat both for warming the inspired air and for evaporation of water. During expiration, warm and fully saturated air passes through the cooler nasal airway, and some water may be reclaimed from the expired air by condensation onto the cooler nasal epithelium. In cold weather this condensed water may drip from the nose.

HEAT EXCHANGE

In most environments, the temperature of the air we breathe is well below body temperature, and therefore the airway is always exposed to a degree of heat loss and cooling. Even in a temperate climate such as that of London (United Kingdom), air temperature extremes can vary seasonally from –13°C to +34°C.

The nasal epithelium contains a complex network of blood vessels with a relatively high blood flow. These blood vessels act as a heat exchanger so that, over a wide range of ambient temperatures, the temperature of the inspired air is brought close to body temperature by the time it leaves the nose. In extremely cold climates, there may be further warming of the inspired air along the trachea, so that the air temperature is close to 37°C by the time the air reaches the lungs.[2] Under usual laboratory conditions, the temperature of the nasal epithelium is approximately 30°C immediately after inspiration and rises to 32°C immediately after expiration, with the temperature of the expired air being close to 32°C.

■ EMBRYOLOGY AND ANATOMY OF THE NOSE ■

EMBRYOLOGY

The external nose and nasal airway are recent developments in the evolution of the respiratory system. Our ancestors developed in a watery environment, and chemoreception in the aqueous medium was well developed at an early stage of evolution. The evolution of the nose is recapitulated in the embryo. The growth of a nasal airway is preceded by the formation of an olfactory placode from ectoderm in the 5-mm embryo.[3] The olfactory placode sinks to form a nasal sac, connected by the external nares to the exterior. The nasal sac is the primitive nasal airway, which is at first separated from the nasopharynx by an oronasal membrane. Persistence of the oronasal membrane leads to the congenital malformation of choanal atresia.

The nasal cavity is divided into two halves by the nasal septum, which grows to separate the nasal cavity in the 19-mm embryo. At the same time as the nasal septum is developing, the maxillary processes grow from each side and fuse in the midline to form the palate. Failure of the maxillary processes to fuse causes a cleft palate.

The three bony shelves – nasal turbinates or conchae – that project from the lateral wall of the nasal cavity develop as outgrowths from the lateral wall between the 7th and 12th weeks of embryonic growth.

The paranasal sinuses develop in the embryo as outgrowths from the nasal cavity. The ethmoidal, sphenoidal, maxillary, and frontal sinuses are rudimentary at birth and slowly grow in size so that they are well developed by the seventh or eighth year of childhood, with further slow growth until puberty.

ANATOMY

The anatomy of the nose is depicted in Figure 41.1 and as a coronal computed tomographic scan in Figure 41.2. Two separate airways begin at the nostrils (anterior nares) and are divided by the nasal septum until the posterior nares, where the airways unite and join the nasopharynx. The external nose is formed from bone and cartilage and surrounds the nasal vestibule, which is lined with stratified squamous epithelium and hair. The nasal vestibules are trumpet-shaped orifices; each narrows from approximately 90 mm² at the nostril to a slit of 30 mm² that separates the nasal vestibule from the main nasal cavity.[1]

The narrowest point of the nasal airway is at the junction between the nasal vestibule and the main nasal cavity, just anterior to the tip of the inferior turbinate. This area is often called the nasal valve or internal ostium, and it is the narrowest point of the whole airway from nostril to alveoli, if one considers the total cross-sectional area at each level of the airway. At the junction of the nasal valve and the main nasal cavity, the airway abruptly expands to about 130 mm², and at this point the airflow bends through almost 90 degrees. The main airflow is directed around the inferior turbinate, with the major airflow traveling close to the floor of the nasal cavity, between the inferior turbinate and the nasal septum. With normal nasal breathing, relatively little airflow is directed upward toward the middle and superior turbinates, although sniffing is believed to direct more air toward the olfactory region in the upper part of the nasal cavity.

A coronal section through the nasal cavities, as illustrated in Figures 41.1 and 41.2, shows that the turbinates occupy much of the nasal cavity. The nasal airway is surrounded by the paranasal sinuses, which consist of the maxillary, frontal, sphenoidal, and ethmoidal sinuses. The anatomy of the paranasal sinuses is variable, especially in the ethmoidal region, where many cells join to form the sinuses. The paranasal sinuses communicate with the nasal cavity via small ostia of 2–6 mm in diameter, and this restricted access means that there is only a very slow exchange of air between the sinuses and the nasal cavity. The function of the nasal sinuses has been the source of much speculation.[4] From their position, wrapped around the nasal airway, the paranasal sinuses may act as air insulators and protect the brain from cooling with inspiration of cold air. A novel role for the paranasal sinuses may be as the source of the gas nitric oxide, which is found in high concentrations in the nasal airway.[5]

Nasal epithelium

The epithelium of the nasal airway comes into direct contact with the inspired air. The physical, chemical, and biologic characteristics of the air have great potential for causing damage and infection. The epithelium of the nose is directly exposed to the external environment; it acts as an air conditioner and as the first line of defense against toxic and infectious agents in the inspired air.

The nose is lined by three distinct types of epithelium: a stratified squamous epithelium in the nasal vestibule and nasopharynx, a pseudostratified ciliated columnar epithelium in the main respiratory area of the nasal cavity, and a specialized olfactory epithelium with ciliated receptor cells in the olfactory area.

The anterior portion of the nose forms the nasal vestibule, which is lined with a stratified squamous epithelium similar to that of the facial skin, almost as though a portion of the facial skin had been turned inward to form the vestibule. At the entrance to the nares, the skin is covered with short, stiff hairs that are extremely sensitive to certain kinds of mechanical stimuli that cause itching, tickling, and sneezing. The stiff nasal hairs are not stimulated by deformation resulting from forced inspiration or expiration. The stratified squamous epithelium lining the nasal vestibule has sensory properties similar to that of facial skin. The

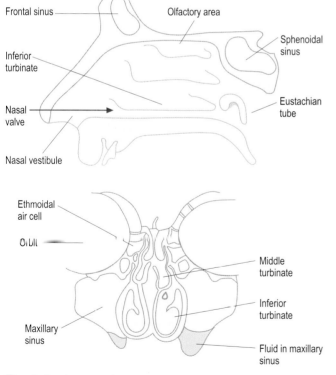

Fig. 41.1. Anatomy of the nasal cavity with a view of the lateral wall (top) and a coronal section through the middle of the nasal cavity (bottom). The coronal section is based on the computed tomographic scan illustrated in Figure 41.2. A fluid level in the maxillary sinuses is a common finding in patients who have acute rhinitis associated with a viral infection or allergy and does not necessarily indicate sinusitis.

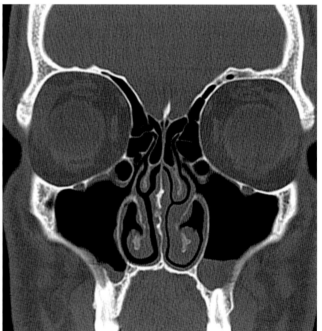

Fig. 41.2. A 2-mm-thick coronal computed tomographic scan of the nose in a patient who is lying prone with the neck extended, simulating erect posture. The scan is shown in diagrammatic form in Figure 41.1. The superior turbinate is not apparent in this scan, and the middle turbinate shows signs of pneumatization with large air spaces. Fluid levels are apparent in the maxillary sinuses. Note the asymmetry in size and degree of congestion of the nasal turbinates caused by the nasal cycle. (Courtesy Rhian Rhys, consultant radiologist at the Royal Glamorgan Hospital, Llantrisant, Wales, UK.)

thermoreceptors that are responsible for the cool sensation on inspiration may be situated in this region.[6]

The nasal valve area is strategically placed at the entrance of the nasal cavity, and the inspired air velocity is maximal at this point. Any cooling or mechanical stimulus from the inspired air would be greatest at this point, and the valve area may be of major importance as far as the sensation of nasal airflow is concerned.

Just past the nasal valve area, the skin gradually changes into a ciliated respiratory epithelium. At the junction between the squamous epithelium of the nasal vestibule and the respiratory epithelium of the nasal cavity lies a 1.5-mm-wide strip covering a region of capillary loops that are unusually wide and long, with dermal papillae.[3] In this transitional area, sometimes referred to as Kiesselbach's plexus, even mild trauma is a common source of nasal bleeding, particularly in childhood. The long capillary loops in this area may act as a source of plasma transudation and prevent drying of the transitional region between the keratinized skin of the nasal vestibule and the ciliated respiratory epithelium. Alternatively, the dermal papillae may act as sensitive mechanoreceptors or thermoreceptors that detect nasal airflow.

The inspiratory airflow is a source of trauma to the nasal epithelium, and this trauma stimulates the formation of a squamous epithelium in the anterior areas of the nose that are directly exposed to unconditioned air. The anterior edge of the inferior turbinate has a squamous epithelium, and, with increasing age, the surface area of squamous epithelium in the anterior part of the nose increases at the expense of the respiratory epithelium of the nasal cavity.

The typical respiratory epithelium is a pseudostratified ciliated columnar type, resting on a continuous basement membrane.[7] The epithelial cell types of the respiratory nasal epithelium are basal cells, goblet cells, and ciliated and non-ciliated columnar cells. The Clara cells, serous cells, and brush cells found in the tracheobronchial epithelium are not found in the human nose. The ratio of columnar cells to goblet cells is approximately 5:1, and there is a significant increase in the density of goblet cells in the anterior–posterior direction through the nasal cavity. The density of goblet cells in the respiratory epithelium is decreased by airflow trauma and increased by infection.[8] The goblet cells are not innervated by the autonomic nervous system, and local factors, such as inflammatory mediators or changes in osmolarity, may control the release of mucus precursors from the goblet cells.

The movements of cilia on the columnar cells propel the blanket of mucus that covers the nasal epithelium. The majority of columnar cells are covered with cilia 4–6 μm long, and there are about 100 cilia per cell. Each columnar cell is covered by 300–400 microvilli with a maximum length of 2 μm. Microvilli are not precursors for cilia, and they do not move. The microvilli may aid transport of fluid and electrolytes between the cells and nasal fluid.[1]

Nasal fluid and mucociliary clearance

Nasal fluid is a mixture of elements derived from glands, goblet cells, capillary plasma transudate, and cell debris. The relative contributions of these different elements to the blanket of mucus overlying the nasal epithelium are not well understood.

Nasal fluid acts as an interface between the air we breathe and the delicate epithelium of the nasal cavity. The respiratory epithelium continuously clears secretions through the beating action of cilia, and this is an important respiratory defense mechanism.

Nasal fluid is a mixture of elements derived from four sources in the respiratory area of the nasal cavity:[9]

1. Seromucous glands within the nasal epithelium
2. Goblet cells distributed along the surface of the nasal epithelium
3. Exudation of plasma from capillaries and veins within the nasal epithelium
4. Secretions and cell debris from leukocytes and epithelial cells.

Lacrimal gland secretions (via the nasolacrimal duct) and secretions from the specialized Bowman's glands of the olfactory epithelium also contribute to nasal secretions.

The glands found deep within the lamina propria of the nasal epithelium are of the compound alveolar type, and both mucous and serous glands may be present in one alveolus. The secretions from these glands flow onto the surface of the epithelium via large ducts. Some of the anterior nasal glands have long ducts that open in the anterior portion of the nose and produce a serous secretion. Secretions from these anterior nasal glands may be drawn out into a fine spray during inspiration, and this may contribute to the humidification of the inspired air.[10] The seromucous glands within the nasal epithelium have a parasympathetic cholinergic innervation, and electrical stimulation of these nerve fibers causes a watery nasal secretion.[11]

Goblet cells are distributed throughout the surface of the respiratory epithelium, and they release mucus directly onto the surface of the ciliated epithelium. The mucous blanket, composed of the secretions of goblet cells and mucous glands in the lamina propria, forms a protective layer overlying the delicate nasal epithelium and prevents the escape of water. There is some evidence that goblet cell secretion is influenced by neuropeptides such as substance P and neurokinin A via tachykinin receptors.[12] Nasal fluid is important in respiratory defense, because immunoglobulins such as immunoglobulin A (IgA) are secreted from the nasal glands and act as a first line of defense against infection. Antioxidants such as uric acid, glutathione, and vitamin C are found in nasal fluid; they may protect the nasal epithelium against the oxidizing action of air pollutants such as ozone and against the oxidative damage caused by peroxides released by leukocytes during periods of nasal inflammation.[13,14]

Plasma exudation directly from surface capillaries and small veins makes a contribution to nasal fluid, especially during nasal inflammation associated with infectious or allergic rhinitis. It has been proposed that exudation of plasma and plasma-derived mediators is a major respiratory defense mechanism.[15] In rhinitis, an outpouring of plasma from the subepithelial microcirculation provides mediators and substrates for the inflammatory response and immunoglobulins to defend against infection.

On the surface of the respiratory epithelium, the nasal fluid is found in two layers: a watery periciliary fluid in which the cilia beat freely, and an overlying layer of viscous, sticky mucus that is propelled by ciliary action. This mucus does not form a continuous blanket overlying the epithelium but rather consists of a discontinuous sheet or patches.[1]

The direction of mucociliary clearance in the nose is mainly toward the nasopharynx, where cleared mucus is swallowed. There is, however, some anterior clearance toward the nasal vestibule. The anterior clearance of material deposited in the anterior part of the nose ensures that deposited material is cleared forward toward the nares rather than being spread over the whole posterior part of the nasal epithelium.

Nasal mucociliary clearance can be measured in humans by placing a particle of saccharin on the anterior end of the inferior turbinate and timing the onset of a sweet taste when the saccharin reaches the pharynx and is swallowed. The rate of mucociliary clearance as measured by saccharin transport or other methods has a wide normal range, reported as 1–20 mm/min or as a clearance time of 7–11 minutes.[1,16] It is not clear why there should be such a large range of transport times for mucociliary clearance in normal healthy subjects, but this may be related to variation in the previous history of upper respiratory tract infections, which is not always documented in studies on mucociliary clearance.

Nasal blood vessels

The anatomy of the nasal blood vessels is complex but, to simplify matters, the vasculature can be discussed in terms of resistance and capacitance vessels. The resistance vessels are mainly small arteries, arterioles, and arteriovenous anastomoses. Blood flow to the nasal epithelium is regulated by constriction and dilation of these vessels.[17] The resistance vessels have a dense adrenergic innervation from the sympathetic nervous system. Stimulation of sympathetic nerves to the nose causes a marked vasoconstriction and reduction in blood flow. Under normal conditions, nasal blood flow is probably controlled by local mediators, because there is very little resting sympathetic vasoconstrictor tone to the resistance vessels, and sympathetic nerve section or blockade causes only a slight increase in nasal blood flow.[18]

Nasal blood flow is increased with nasal inflammation caused by infective rhinitis, but it is not clear how blood flow changes with allergic rhinitis. Nasal challenge with allergen in subjects with allergic rhinitis has been shown to cause both decreases and increases in nasal blood flow.[19,20]

A special feature of the vasculature of the nasal epithelium is that it contains large venous sinuses, which are especially well developed over the inferior and middle turbinates and the nasal septum. The venous sinuses are also referred to as capacitance vessels or venous erectile tissue. The venous erectile tissue of the nasal epithelium is well developed at the anterior end of the inferior turbinate, and swelling of the erectile tissue in this region controls nasal airway resistance. The venous erectile tissue has a dense adrenergic innervation, and congestion and constriction of the erectile tissue is regulated via the sympathetic nerve supply to the nose.[21]

The subepithelial capillaries and veins of the nasal epithelium are unusual in that they are fenestrated, and the large fenestrated areas of the endothelium face toward the respiratory epithelium.[22] Some capillaries penetrate the basement membrane and lie between the cells of the epithelium. The permeability of the capillaries is very high, and some endothelial cells are wide open, similar to the capillaries of the liver sinusoids, allowing free passage of large particles from the circulation.[23] The high permeability of nasal capillaries may also explain why drugs administered intranasally readily enter the bloodstream.

Nerve supply and nasal reflexes

The nose is ideally situated at the entrance to the respiratory tract to sample the inspired airflow and to detect chemical and physical irritants that could damage the airway. The sensory innervation of the nose is supplied mainly by the olfactory and trigeminal nerves. The olfactory nerves enter the nose through the cribriform plate and form a distinct olfactory area. Most of the sensory nerves to the nasal epithelium and nasal vestibule are supplied by two branches of the trigeminal nerve, the ophthalmic and maxillary nerves.[1]

The olfactory area acts as a long-distance chemoreceptor, sampling the odorants contained in the inspired air and giving us our appreciation of foods, perfumes, and other substances. The trigeminal nerves provide the sensations of touch, pain, hot, cold, and itch, as well as the sensation of nasal airflow, which is perceived as a cool sensation on inspiration. This sensation not only reassures us that breathing is taking place but also may influence the pattern of respiration and the activity of upper airway accessory respiratory muscles.[24] The trigeminal nerves also detect chemicals, such as ammonia and sulfur dioxide, and a range of organic substances, such as menthol, acetone, and pyridine.[25]

Chemical or physical stimuli to the nasal epithelium may initiate potent respiratory and cardiovascular reflexes via stimulation of trigeminal nerves, resulting in expiration with apnea, closure of the larynx, and bradycardia. Mild stimuli result in sneezing and nasal hypersecretion. These reflex responses protect the lower airways from inhalation of physical and chemical irritants. Sneezing may be initiated by a number of factors, such as mechanical stimulation of the nasal epithelium, cooling of the skin, bright light in the eyes, irritation of the scalp near the frontal hairline, challenge with allergen extract, and psychogenic causes.[1]

The trigeminal nerves in the nasal epithelium initiate the sneezing and hypersecretion associated with upper respiratory tract infection and allergy. They may also be responsible for neurogenic inflammation associated with nasal infection and allergy, because various inflammatory mediators (e.g., substance P, neurokinin A, calcitonin gene-related peptide) have been found in these nerves.[26]

The nasal epithelium is innervated by both sympathetic and parasympathetic nerve fibers, with the parasympathetic fibers supplying nasal glands and the sympathetic fibers controlling nasal blood flow and the filling of venous erectile tissue. The parasympathetic nerve supply to the nose originates in the salivatory nuclei of the brainstem and follows the greater superficial petrosal nerve and the nerve of the pterygoid canal (Vidian nerve). The parasympathetic fibers relay in the sphenopalatine ganglion, and postganglionic nerves reach the nasal glands via branches of the posterior nasal nerve. Electrical stimulation of parasympathetic nerves causes a profuse watery nasal secretion, and section of the nerve of the pterygoid canal, which contains parasympathetic fibers, has been used successfully for the treatment of rhinitis.[27] The parasympathetic nerves in the nasal epithelium release acetylcholine as their primary neurotransmitter and they also release vasoactive intestinal polypeptide, which is a potent vasodilator.

The activity of the sympathetic nerves to the nose can be influenced by electrical stimulation of areas of the hypothalamus and brainstem. Electrical stimulation of areas of the hypothalamus in the anesthetized cat causes a pronounced nasal vasoconstriction,[28] whereas stimulation of areas of the brainstem causes reciprocal changes in sympathetic tone to nasal blood vessels.[29] The preganglionic sympathetic nerve fibers originate in the thoracolumbar region of the spinal cord, relay in the superior cervical ganglion, and are distributed to the nasal blood vessels via the nerve of the pterygoid canal and branches of the trigeminal nerve. Electrical stimulation of the sympathetic nerves causes a pronounced nasal vasoconstriction and a reduction in nasal blood flow, accompanied by decongestion of venous erectile tissue and a subsequent decrease in nasal airway resistance. Norepinephrine is the primary neurotransmitter in the sympathetic nerves supplying the nasal blood vessels, and the vasoconstriction caused by norepinephrine is supplemented by the release of neuropeptide Y, which is also a potent vasoconstrictor.[30]

■ NASAL AIRFLOW ■

INFLUENCE OF NASAL BLOOD VESSELS ON NASAL AIRFLOW

The role of the nasal venous sinuses in the control of nasal airflow is now well recognized, and their ability to swell and completely obstruct the nasal passage has been reported.[31] A network of nasal venous sinuses is found throughout the epithelium of the nose, but they are particularly well developed at the tip of the inferior turbinate and on the nearby anterior end of the nasal septum. The location of nasal venous sinuses at the anterior tip of the inferior turbinate and nasal septum is critical for the control of nasal airflow, and this area of the nose is often referred to as the 'nasal valve.'

NASAL VALVE AND CONTROL OF NASAL AIRFLOW

The narrowest point of the nasal passage determines the nasal resistance to airflow; this is the area referred to as the nasal valve.[32] However, there is some dispute in the literature as to whether the nasal valve lies in the nasal vestibule or more posteriorly, within the bony cavum of the nose. The anatomic and physiologic evidence indicates that the nasal valve occurs at the entrance of the piriform aperture, with the major site of nasal resistance being just anterior to the tip of the inferior turbinate.

The nasal airway resistance can be thought of as consisting of three components: the nasal vestibule, the nasal valve, and the turbinated nasal passage. These three components are illustrated diagrammatically in Figure 41.3. The compliant nasal vestibule is stiffened by cartilage to which facial muscles such as the alae nasi muscles attach. During inspiration these muscles contract and splint the vestibule to prevent collapse.

The change in airway resistance along the nasal passage can be determined by passing a pressure-sensing cannula carefully along the passage and determining the relationships between pressure and flow during quiet breathing. Using this technique, researchers have demonstrated that the major site of nasal resistance lies at the anterior end of the inferior turbinate, within the first few millimeters of the bony nasal cavity.[32]

The nasal valve is a dynamic valve, not a fixed anatomic narrowing of the airway. The nasal airway resistance is determined by swelling and constriction of the venous sinuses of the inferior turbinate and nasal septum, which can cause complete obstruction of the nasal passage. The significance of the erectile properties of the inferior turbinate was discussed by Haight and Cole,[32] who found that the anterior end of the turbinate could advance by as much as 5 mm after application of histamine.

The anterior site of the major component of nasal resistance, at the level of the tip of the inferior turbinate, has important surgical implications. For example, treatments such as diathermy that aim to reduce the swelling of the inferior turbinate will have major effects on nasal resistance, whereas minor corrective surgery such as trimming of septal spurs posterior to the nasal valve region will have little effect on nasal resistance.

The turbinated region of the nasal passage has a relatively large cross-sectional area compared with the nasal valve area. In the normal nose, the turbinated area contributes minimally to the resistance of a nasal passage.

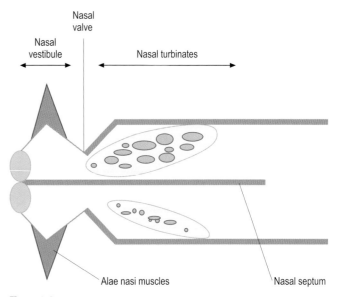

Fig. 41.3. Diagram of the nose. The compliant wall of the nasal vestibule is supported by the alae nasi muscles. The nasal valve is at the level of the anterior tip of the inferior turbinate. The degree of congestion of the tip of the inferior turbinate determines the dynamic cross-sectional area of the nasal valve and therefore the nasal airway resistance. The diagram illustrates the normal asymmetry of nasal congestion, with one side of the nose congested as a result of dilation of the venous sinuses in the inferior nasal turbinate and the other side open and decongested (i.e., venous sinuses constricted).

AUTONOMIC CONTROL OF NASAL AIRFLOW

In general, the autonomic innervation of the nose can be considered in terms of parasympathetic control of nasal secretion and sympathetic control of nasal airflow. Parasympathetic nerve stimulation causes a watery nasal secretion that is rapidly cleared from the nasal passages without any effect on nasal resistance. However, the thick, viscous mucus and plasma exudate associated with upper respiratory tract infection can influence nasal resistance by temporarily blocking the narrowed airway, and this can complicate the measurement of nasal resistance. Sympathetic nerve stimulation causes a pronounced vasoconstriction and shrinkage of the nasal venous sinuses, which have a dense adrenergic innervation.[33]

Although it is generally accepted that the nasal venous sinuses are involved in the regulation of airflow, and that the filling of these sinuses is controlled by the sympathetic nerves, the mechanism regulating the swelling of the veins is poorly understood. Cauna and Cauna[34] described throttle or cushion veins that may control the filling of the venous sinuses, but there is no information on how the autonomic nerves might control these throttle veins. The close apposition of arteries and veins in the bony canals of the turbinates may also be significant, because arterial dilation would cause compression of the venous plexus, draining the erectile venous sinuses, and this would lead to swelling of the venous sinuses.[33] The idea that dilation of arteries contained in the bony canals of the turbinates causes both an increased filling of the venous sinuses and a restriction of outflow from the venous sinuses is a reasonable hypothesis to explain the nasal congestion associated with a reduction in sympathetic tone.

Under normal conditions, there is a continuous sympathetic vasoconstrictor tone to the nasal venous sinuses, and section or local anesthesia of the cervical sympathetic nerves that supply the nasal epithelium causes Horner's syndrome, with ipsilateral nasal congestion and an increase in nasal resistance to air flow.[33]

NORMAL NASAL AIRFLOW

Rhinomanometry, which consists of the measurement of nasal pressure and airflow during breathing, is generally accepted as the standard technique of measuring nasal airway resistance and assessing the patency of the nose.[35] Acoustic rhinometry uses a reflected sound signal to measure the cross-sectional area and volume of the nasal passage. Acoustic rhinometry gives an anatomic description of a nasal passage, whereas rhinomanometry gives a functional measure of the pressure/flow relationships during the respiratory cycle. Reviews on the techniques of rhinomanometry, acoustic rhinometry, and other objective measures of nasal function are available, and the practical and theoretic aspects of these measurements will not be discussed here.[35]

In subjects free from signs of nasal disease, mean total resistance has been reported to be approximately $0.23\,Pa/cm^3/s$, with a range from 0.15 to $0.39\,Pa/cm^3/s$.[33] As a routine screening procedure, a total nasal resistance to airflow of $0.3\,Pa/cm^3/s$ may be considered as an upper limit of the normal range.

Nasal resistance is at a maximum in the infant, approximately $1.2\,Pa/cm^3/s$; declines to the adult value by 16 to 18 years of age; and then shows only a slow decline with increasing age. In a study on healthy volunteers, Vig and Zajac[36] reported that resistance declined with increasing age, from $0.6\,Pa/cm^3/s$ at age 5 to 12 years, to $0.29\,Pa/cm^3/s$ at 13 to 19 years and $0.22\,Pa/cm^3/s$ after 20 years of age, in male subjects. The relationship between age and nasal resistance was similar in female subjects, but in general nasal resistance was lower than in male subjects.[36]

Unlike other respiratory parameters (e.g., vital capacity), there is no established correlation in the adult between total nasal resistance and sex or height, although several authors claim to have shown a weak correlation with height and a negative correlation with age.[33] The lack of correlation between total nasal resistance and height may be related to the instability of nasal resistance that results from spontaneous congestion and decongestion of nasal venous sinuses. If the nose is decongested by exercise or by application of a topical decongestant, then any physiologic variation in resistance is eliminated, and one can investigate the anatomic factors that influence resistance. Studies by Broms[37] have provided a table of predictive values for height and nasal resistance in the decongested nose that is useful for assessing the extent of any deviation from normality in patients with nasal skeletal stenosis.

Total nasal resistance gives an overall measure of nasal function, but it is a very crude measure because it provides no information about the separate nasal passages. It is not very informative to quote the mean of unilateral resistance measured over several hours, because there will be a large standard deviation due to the instability of unilateral resistance. The range of unilateral nasal airway resistance in a group of healthy volunteers when recorded over a 6–8-hour period was shown to vary from 0.36 to $1.36\,Pa/cm^3/s$ in one study[38] and from 0.28 to $0.63\,Pa/cm^3/s$ in another.[39] This indicates that an almost four-fold change in unilateral resistance is often associated with spontaneous congestion and decongestion of the nasal venous sinuses.

One way to overcome the dilemma of spontaneous changes in unilateral nasal resistance is to decongest the nose before assessment. This technique is of use to the surgeon, who is interested in assessing the extent of any nasal anatomic problem.[37] However, decongestion of the nose cannot be used to stabilize nasal resistance when studying nasal physiology, because it is the spontaneous changes in unilateral resistance that are of interest to the physiologist. One solution is to quantify the extremes of unilateral resistance, or the amplitude of the unilateral changes in resistance, and study a period of several hours. This approach has been used to determine the unilateral changes in resistance in health, common cold, and allergic rhinitis;[33] to assess the effects of oral decongestants;[40] and to assess the efficacy of nasal surgery.[41] The disadvantage of unilateral nasal measurements is that, in order to assess the amplitude of changes in unilateral nasal resistance, it is necessary to make hourly measurements over several hours. The advantage of unilateral measurements is that they give a comprehensive assessment of the dynamic nose rather than the crude snapshot that is provided by a single measure of total resistance.

NASAL CYCLE

The term nasal cycle describes the spontaneous and often reciprocal changes in unilateral nasal airflow that are associated with congestion and decongestion of the nasal venous sinuses.[33] An example of the changes in nasal airflow associated with the nasal cycle is illustrated in Figure 41.4.

Spontaneous changes in unilateral congestion and decongestion of nasal venous sinuses were first described in the scientific literature over

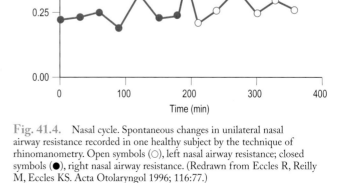

Fig. 41.4. Nasal cycle. Spontaneous changes in unilateral nasal airway resistance recorded in one healthy subject by the technique of rhinomanometry. Open symbols (○), left nasal airway resistance; closed symbols (●), right nasal airway resistance. (Redrawn from Eccles R, Reilly M, Eccles KS. Acta Otolaryngol 1996; 116:77.)

100 years ago, but these nasal responses have been known to the ancient Hindus, from as early as the Vedic period.[33] Heetderks in 1927[42] found that in 80% of 60 healthy volunteers there was a definite cycle of reaction, and this statement has been used many times in the literature to support the idea that 80% of the population exhibit a so-called nasal cycle.

In a study by Flanagan and Eccles[39] involving 52 healthy volunteers, unilateral nasal airflow was measured every hour over an 8-hour period. A wide range of patterns of airflow was observed, with some volunteers exhibiting regular spontaneous and reciprocal changes in unilateral airflow and others exhibiting irregular changes in airflow. The authors defined a nasal cycle in terms of numeric parameters of correlation and distribution of nasal airflow between the nasal passages and concluded that only 21% (11/52) of the volunteers exhibited airflow patterns that could be defined as a nasal cycle.

When present, the reciprocal changes in nasal airflow have been reported to occur over a time course of 0.5 to 3.0 hours.[39] The spontaneous, often reciprocal changes in nasal airflow are caused by congestion and decongestion of nasal venous sinuses under the influence of the sympathetic nervous system. Section or local anesthesia of the cervical sympathetic nerves that supply one side of the nose and face causes ipsilateral nasal congestion and abolition of the spontaneous changes in nasal airflow.[33]

Spontaneous congestion and decongestion of nasal blood vessels still occurs in the laryngectomized patient, in the absence of any nasal airflow.[43] The spontaneous changes in nasal airflow that are associated with the nasal cycle may be related to oscillations in the activity of autonomic control centers in the central nervous system (discussed later).

CENTRAL CONTROL OF NASAL AIRFLOW

The idea that the spontaneous changes in nasal airflow associated with the nasal cycle may be controlled from some center in the brain was first put forward by Stoksted in 1953,[44] who speculated that the nasal cycle was 'regulated by a central sympathetic centre possibly situated in the hypothalamus.' Studies on anesthetized animals demonstrate that pronounced nasal vasoconstriction and a reduction in nasal airway resistance may be induced on electric stimulation of areas of the hypothalamus but this may indicate control of a defense reaction rather than control of the nasal cycle.[28]

Reciprocal nasal vasomotor responses, with ipsilateral vasoconstriction and contralateral vasodilation, have been initiated on electric stimulation of areas of the brainstem in the anesthetized cat.[29] These reciprocal nasal vasomotor responses may be related to central control of the nasal cycle,[45] as illustrated in Figure 41.5.

EFFECT OF CHANGES IN POSTURE ON NASAL AIRFLOW

The changes in nasal airflow associated with changes in posture may be explained by two separate mechanisms: an increase in central venous pressure on moving from erect to supine, and a reflex change in nasal vasomotor activity on adoption of the lateral recumbent position. The postural changes in nasal airflow can be demonstrated in healthy volunteers, and they are often exaggerated in patients with rhinitis where they may cause unilateral or total nasal obstruction.[33]

The increase in venous pressure associated with a change from sitting to supine causes an increased filling of the nasal venous sinuses and an increase in nasal resistance to airflow. This passive hydrostatic effect of increased venous pressure is superimposed on any asymmetry of the nasal venous sinuses associated with the nasal cycle. The side of the nose with the greatest level of congestion in general exhibits the greatest increase in congestion and may become completely obstructed. Obstruction may alternate from one side of the nose to the other when the lateral recumbent position is adopted, so that the nasal passage on the down side congests and one on the up side decongests. This is not a passive effect of any further change in venous pressure but a reflex change in vasomotor activity associated with a pressure stimulus to one side of the body.

The reciprocal changes in nasal airflow observed on adoption of the lateral recumbent position are caused by pressure on the axilla and hip regions; these body surfaces have been shown to be the most sensitive regions to elicit the nasal response.[46] Local anesthesia to the skin surface of the axilla does not abolish the response, but intercostal nerve block does abolish the nasal response to axillary pressure.[46]

The reciprocal changes in nasal airflow associated with the lateral recumbent position may have a functional significance, because the reflex ensures that the upper nasal passage has the dominant airflow. In persons

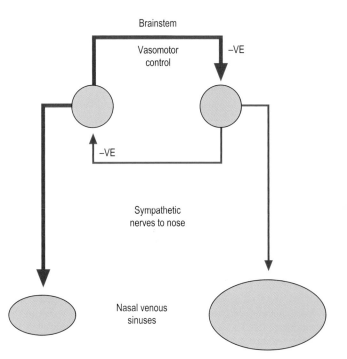

Fig. 41.5. Model illustrating the sympathetic nervous control of nasal venous sinuses. Vasomotor control is proposed to reside in two half-centers in the brainstem. The half-centers have reciprocal connections so that the dominance of activity oscillates over a period of hours, with only one center having dominance at any one time. The sympathetic vasoconstrictor tone exerted by the right and left cervical sympathetic nerves that supply the two halves of the nose is normally asymmetric. The asymmetric sympathetic tone causes decongestion of the venous sinuses on one side of the nose and congestion on the other side. The spontaneous changes in nasal congestion over a period of hours are often referred to as the nasal cycle. –VE, inhibition of neuronal activity.

with a marked asymmetry in nasal airflow associated with the nasal cycle, it would seem to be a functional advantage to decongest the upper nasal passage on adoption of the lateral recumbent position, because the dependent nasal passage could be obstructed by physical contact with the ground or other surface.

EFFECT OF EXERCISE ON NASAL AIRFLOW

Exercise causes a generalized increase in sympathetic nervous activity, with an increase in heart rate, bronchodilation, and a decrease in nasal resistance to airflow. The first study of the effect of exercise on nasal resistance was conducted by Richerson and Seebohm,[47] who demonstrated that when patients with allergic rhinitis performed strenuous exercise there was a marked reduction in nasal airway resistance. They also established that the reduction in nasal airway resistance was caused by an increase in sympathetic vasoconstrictor tone to the nasal venous sinuses, because the response was reduced by topical application of phentolamine or by local anesthesia of the stellate ganglion.[47]

The nasal decongestant response to exercise has been subsequently confirmed in healthy volunteers and in patients with asthma and rhinitis, and the response is reported to have some functional significance because it reduces the work of breathing by lowering nasal resistance to airflow.[33] However, exercise is normally accompanied by a switch to mouth breathing at a work rate of about 105 watts,[48] and may only be important for low to moderate work rates, when a significant proportion of the tidal volume passes through the nose.

EFFECT OF HYPERVENTILATION AND RE-BREATHING ON NASAL AIRFLOW

The partial pressure of carbon dioxide in arterial blood is the major factor that influences ventilation via peripheral and central chemoreceptors. The pressure can be lowered by hyperventilation and increased by breath-holding or asphyxia. These changes in the partial pressure of carbon dioxide are accompanied by changes in the drive to breathe and by changes in nasal airway resistance.

Tatum[49] studied anesthetized dogs and rabbits and demonstrated that partial asphyxia caused a nasal vasoconstrictor response, whereas hyperventilation caused nasal vasodilation. The nasal vasoconstrictor response to partial asphyxia was abolished on section of the cervical sympathetic nerves, whereas the vasodilator response to hyperventilation was unaffected. Furthermore, re-breathing from a bag or prolonged breath-holding in humans caused a decrease in nasal airway resistance, whereas hyperventilation caused an increase in nasal airway resistance.[50] This experimental work[49] has been repeated in both animals and humans, and the results confirm Tatum's conclusions that changes in blood carbon dioxide levels influence nasal airway resistance via the sympathetic nerve supply to nasal blood vessels.

The nasal vasoconstrictor response to an elevation in blood carbon dioxide can be explained by a reflex increase in sympathetic nervous activity mediated by peripheral and central chemoreceptors. The reduction in nasal airway resistance associated with asphyxia and re-breathing has some functional significance, because the increase in nasal patency facilitates ventilation. The nasal vasodilator response to a decrease in blood carbon dioxide is more difficult to explain, because it is unaffected by section of the sympathetic nerves[49] and may be mediated by parasympathetic pathways.[51]

ENDOCRINE INFLUENCE ON NASAL AIRFLOW

The development and activity of the nasal epithelium are influenced by many hormones, but epinephrine secreted from the adrenal medulla has the most obvious and acute effects. Epinephrine is released in response to stressful stimuli such as pain or asphyxia, and it causes a pronounced nasal vasoconstriction and a reduction in nasal airway resistance. The nasal blood vessels are extremely sensitive to circulating epinephrine, up to four times as sensitive as the heart.[52]

Considerable clinical and experimental evidence indicates that the male and female sex hormones have an influence on the nose. Nasal obstruction and hypersecretion are often associated with puberty, menstruation, and pregnancy.[53]

CEREBRAL EFFECTS OF NASAL AIRFLOW

Yoga breathing exercises often involve unilateral nasal airflow and are believed to alter mood and cerebral activity. Supporting evidence from the scientific and clinical literature suggests that airflow through the nose can influence cerebral activity. Deep nasal breathing has been found to have an activating effect on electroencephalographic (EEG) activity in humans to such an extent that it can trigger epileptic abnormalities in susceptible persons.[54] This arousal effect of nasal airflow is not caused by any change in blood gases with hyperventilation, because hyperventilation and passive airflow through the nose have similar effects, and the activating effect of nasal airflow is suppressed by local anesthesia of the nasal epithelium. Other human experiments have demonstrated that forced breathing through one nostril produces a relative increase in the amplitude of the EEG tracing in the contralateral hemisphere.[55] Any effects of nasal airflow on cerebral activity are likely to be mediated via nasal trigeminal nerves, although some influence of the olfactory nerves cannot be excluded.

SENSATION OF NASAL AIRFLOW

The cool sensation of nasal airflow we feel with each inspiration is mediated by cold receptors in the nose that are supplied by branches of the trigeminal nerves.[56] The sensation of nasal airflow is mainly related to a cool sensation in the nose rather than sensations from the respiratory muscles or lungs, and blockade of the trigeminal nerves supplying the nose or local anesthesia of the nasal epithelium causes a sensation of nasal obstruction.[57]

The sensation of nasal airflow is increased by intranasal application of menthol or inhalation of menthol, providing a false sensation of decongestion and improved airflow.[56] Oral administration of menthol by means of a lozenge causes a similar sensation of nasal coolness and increased nasal airflow.[58] The effects of ingestion of a menthol lozenge on the subjective sensation of nasal airflow and on total nasal airway resistance are illustrated in Figure 41.6. Menthol is believed to influence the activity of cold receptors by altering the conductance of calcium ions across the nerve cell membrane.[56] Menthol may have a specific pharmacologic effect on cold receptors, because L-menthol has cooling properties whereas D-menthol has little cooling activity.[59] In addition, by manipulating the chemical structure of menthol analogues, it is possible to produce cooling compounds that are more potent than menthol.[60]

Menthol is widely used as an ingredient of common cold medications, candy, chewing gum, cigarettes, and snuff; the popularity of menthol-containing products may be related to the pleasant and satisfying effect of menthol on the drive to breathe.[61]

PHARMACOLOGY OF NASAL AIRFLOW

Almost any substance that has an effect on vascular smooth muscle will have some influence on nasal airflow by causing changes in the activity of the smooth muscle of nasal venous sinuses. Similarly, any substance that influences the activity of sympathetic noradrenergic nerve endings is likely to influence nasal airflow by altering the sympathetic vasoconstrictor tone to nasal venous sinuses. Only the pharmacology relevant to effects on nasal airflow is discussed here.

Sympathomimetics and sympatholytics

The nasal blood vessels are extremely sensitive to sympathomimetic medications that mimic the vasoconstrictor effects of norepinephrine and epinephrine. These sympathomimetic medications cause decongestion of nasal venous sinuses and a decrease in nasal resistance to airflow. Nasal decongestant medications are sympathomimetics that act on α_1- and α_2-receptors on nasal venous sinuses. There is some evidence that α_1-receptors are the major receptor type on the smooth muscle of nasal venous sinuses. The pharmacology of sympathomimetics and nasal decongestants was reviewed in 1999.[21] Repeated application of topical sympathomimetics can cause a rebound vasodilation and nasal congestion that may be related to tissue hypoxia cause by pronounced vasoconstriction. Rhinitis medicamentosa can occur after prolonged abuse of topical nasal decongestants and this condition may be related more to chronic exposure to the preservatives used in topical nasal decongestants than to the vasoconstriction itself.[62]

Histamine and H$_1$ antihistamines

Histamine is a potent vasodilator mediator that is associated with the inflammatory allergic response. It has effects on nasal sensory nerves and blood vessels, causing sneezing, itching, runny nose, and nasal congestion.[63] The vasodilator actions of histamine influence nasal airflow by causing congestion of the nasal venous sinuses. Histamine challenge is often used as an experimental method to elicit nasal congestion and other symptoms of nasal allergy.[64]

The effects of histamine on the human nose are mediated by both H$_1$ and H$_2$ receptors. Both of these receptor types are involved in the dilation of venous sinuses, whereas only the H$_1$ receptors are involved in sneezing, itching, and hypersecretion.[65] The involvement of both H$_1$ and H$_2$ receptors in nasal congestion may explain why H$_1$ antihistamines are relatively ineffective in treating the nasal congestion associated with nasal allergy and histamine challenge.[65]

Bradykinin

The kallikrein enzyme that is responsible for the generation of bradykinin was first shown to be present in the nose in cat nasal secretions.[66] Bradykinin is a potent vasodilator mediator associated with the inflammatory response to acute upper respiratory tract infection. It has effects on both nasal blood vessels and nasal sensory nerves, causing nasal congestion, nasal irritation, and runny nose.[67] Although there has been considerable research to discover a bradykinin antagonist that could be useful in the treatment of symptoms associated with acute upper respiratory tract infection, at present no such agent is available. If a suitable bradykinin antagonist could be discovered, then it would be useful

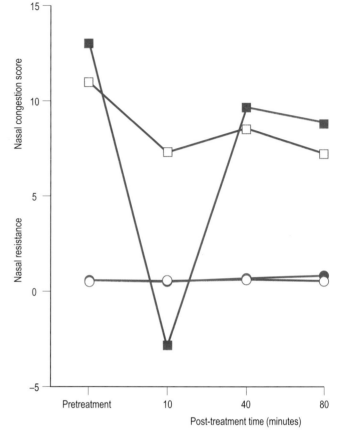

Fig. 41.6. The effects of ingestion of an 11 mg L-menthol lozenge on subjective sensation of nasal congestion and on nasal resistance to airflow in human volunteers with a common cold. The subjective sensation of nasal congestion was significantly reduced 10 minutes after ingestion of the lozenge, but nasal airway resistance as measured by rhinomanometry was unaffected. Shaded symbols represent mean values for the menthol-treated group; open symbols, mean values for the placebo-treated group. The congestion score represents change in score on a 100-mm visual analog scale. Nasal resistance is given in units of Pa cm^3 s. (Data from Eccles R, Jawad MS, Morris S. J Pharm Pharmacol 1990; 42:652.)

in the treatment of symptoms of the common cold, and would probably play a role similar to that of H$_1$ antihistamines in the treatment of allergic rhinitis.

Corticosteroids

Intranasal corticosteroids are widely used for the treatment of allergic rhinitis, but there have been very few studies of the effects of corticosteroids on nasal airflow. Unlike the H$_1$ antihistamines, which have a small effect on nasal congestion, intranasal corticosteroids are generally believed to provide relief of the symptom of nasal congestion associated with allergic rhinitis. Topical nasal steroid treatment has been shown to reduce the increase in nasal airway resistance that is associated with nasal challenge with grass pollen in allergic patients.[68]

Acknowledgment

Thanks to Rhian Rhys, consultant radiologist at the Royal Glamorgan Hospital, Llantrisant, Wales, UK, for providing the CT scan for Figure 41.2.

References

Functions of the nose

1. Proctor DF. The upper airway. In: Proctor DF, Andersen I, eds. The nose upper airway physiology and the atmospheric environment. Elsevier: Amsterdam; 1982:23.
2. Cole P. Modification of inspired air. In: Proctor DF, Andersen I, , eds. The nose upper airway physiology and the atmospheric environment. Amsterdam: Elsevier; 1982:351.

Embryology and anatomy of the nose

3. Langes J. Clinical anatomy of the nose, nasal cavity and paranasal sinuses. New York: Thieme Medical Publishers; 1989.
4. Blanton PL, Biggs NL. Eighteen hundred years of controversy: the paranasal sinuses. Am J Anat 1969; 124:135.
5. Proud D. Nitric oxide and the common cold. Curr Opin Allergy Clin Immunol 2005; 5:37.
6. Eccles R. Effects of menthol on nasal sensation of airflow. In: Green BG, ed. Chemical senses: 'irritation'. New York: Dekker; 1990:275.
7. Mygind N, Pedersen M, Nielsen M. Morphology of the upper airway epithelium. In: Proctor DF, Andersen I, eds. The nose, upper airways physiology and the atmospheric environment. Amsterdam: Elsevier; 1982:72.
8. Boyce J, Eccles R. Do chronic changes in nasal airflow have any physiological or pathological effect on the nose and paranasal sinuses? A systematic review. Clin Otolaryngol 2006; 31:15.
9. Eccles R. Nasal airflow of nasal secretion. Eur J Respir Dis 1983; 62:115.
10. Bojsen-Moller F. Glandulae nasales anteriores in the human nose. Ann Otol Rhinol Laryngol 1965; 74:363.
11. Eccles R, Wilson H. The parasympathetic secretory nerves of the nose of the cat. J Physiol 1973; 230:213.
12. Rogers DF. Motor control of airway goblet cells and glands. Respir Physiol 2001; 125:129.
13. Housley DG, Mudway I, Kelly FJ, et al. Depletion of urate in human nasal lavage following in-vitro ozone exposure. Int J Biochem Cell Biol 1995; 27:1153.
14. Mudway IS, Blomberg A, Frew AJ, et al. Antioxidant consumption and repletion kinetics in nasal lavage fluid following exposure of healthy human volunteers to ozone. Eur Respir J 1999; 13:1429.
15. Persson CGA, Erjefalt I, Alkner U, et al. Plasma exudation as a first line respiratory mucosal defence. Clin Exp Allergy 1991; 21:17.
16. Moriaty BG, Robson AM, Smallman LA, et al. Nasal mucociliary function: comparison of saccharin clearance with ciliary beat frequency. Rhinology 1991; 29:173.
17. Dawes JDK, Prichard MML. Studies of the vascular arrangements of the nose. J Anat 1953; 87:311.
18. Anggard A, Edwall L. The effects of sympathetic nerve stimulation on the tracer disappearance rate and local blood content in the nasal mucosa of the cat. Acta Otolaryngol 1974; 77:131.
19. Holmberg K, Bake B, Pipkorn U. Nasal mucosal blood flow after intranasal allergen challenge. J Allergy Clin Immunol 1988; 81:541.
20. Rangi SP, Serwonska MH, Lenahan GA, et al. Suppression by ingested eicosapentaenoic acid of the increases in nasal mucosal blood flow and eosinophilia of ryegrass-allergic reactions. J Allergy Clin Immunol 1990; 85:484.
21. Eccles R. Nasal airflow and decongestants. In: Naclerio RM, Durham SR, Mygind N, eds. Rhinitis mechanisms and management. New York: Marcel Dekker; 1999:291.
22. Grevers G. The role of fenestrated vessels for the secretory process in the nasal mucosa: a histological and transmission electron microscopic study in the rabbit. Laryngoscope 1993; 103:1255.
23. Watanabe K, Saito Y, Watanabe I, et al. Characteristics of capillary permeability in nasal mucosa. Ann Otol Rhinol Laryngol 1980; 89:377.
24. Davies AM, Eccles R. Electromyographic responses of a nasal muscle to stimulation of the nasal vestibule in the cat. J Physiol 1987; 391:25.
25. Doty R, Commetto-Muniz J. Trigeminal chemosensation. In: Doty R, ed. Handbook of olfaction and gustation, 2nd edn. New York: Marcel Dekker; 2003:981.
26. Woodhead CJ. Neuropeptides in nasal mucosa. Clin Otolaryngol 1994; 19:277.
27. Robinson SR, Wormald PJ. Endoscopic vidian neurectomy. Am J Rhinol 2006; 20:197.
28. Eccles R, Lee RL. The influence of the hypothalamus on the sympathetic innervation of the nasal vasculature of the cat. Acta Otolaryngol 1981; 91:127.
29. Bamford OS, Eccles R. The central reciprocal control of nasal vasomotor oscillations. Pflugers Arch 1982; 394:139.
30. Lacroix JS, Stjarne P, Anggard A, et al. Sympathetic vascular control of the pig nasal mucosa: (I) increased resistance and capacitance vessel responses upon stimulation with irregular bursts compared to continuous impulses. Acta Physiol Scand 1988; 132:83.

Nasal airflow

31. Davis SS, Eccles R. Nasal congestion: mechanisms, measurement and medications. Core information for the clinician. Clin Otolaryngol 2004; 29:659.
32. Haight JSJ, Cole P. Site and function of the nasal valve. Laryngoscope 1983; 93:49.
33. Eccles R. Nasal airflow in health and disease. Acta Otolaryngol 2000; 120:580.
34. Cauna N, Cauna D. The fine structure and innervation of the cushion veins of the human nasal respiratory mucosa. Anat Rec 1975; 181:1.
35. Nathan RA, Eccles R, Howarth PH, et al. Objective monitoring of nasal patency and nasal physiology in rhinitis. J Allergy Clin Immunol 2005; 115:S442.
36. Vig PS, Zajac DJ. Age and gender effects on nasal respiratory function in normal subjects. Cleft Palate-Craniofac 1993; 30:279.
37. Broms P. Rhinomanometry. III. Procedures and criteria for distinction between skeletal stenosis and mucosal swelling. Acta Otolaryngol 1982; 94:361.
38. Eccles R, Reilly M, Eccles KSJ. Changes in the amplitude of the nasal cycle associated with symptoms of acute upper respiratory tract infection. Acta Otolaryngol 1996; 116:77.
39. Flanagan P, Eccles R. Spontaneous changes of unilateral nasal airflow in man. A re-examination of the 'nasal cycle'. Acta Otolaryngol 1997; 117:590.
40. Jawad SSM, Eccles R. Effect of pseudoephedrine on nasal airflow in patients with nasal congestion associated with common cold. Rhinology 1998; 36:73.
41. Quine SM, Aitken PM, Eccles R. Effect of submucosal diathermy to the inferior turbinates on unilateral and total nasal airflow in patients with rhinitis. Acta Otolaryngol 1999; 119:911.
42. Heetderks DL. Observations on the reaction of normal nasal mucous membrane. Am J Med Sci 1927; 174:231.
43. Fisher EW, Liu M, Lung VJ. The nasal cycle after deprivation of airflow: a study of laryngectomy patients using acoustic rhinometry. Acta Otolaryngol 1994; 114:443.
44. Stoksted P. Rhinometric measurements for determination of the nasal cycle. Acta Otolaryngol 1953; (suppl) 109:159.
45. Eccles R. Sympathetic control of nasal erectile tissue. Eur J Respir Dis 1983; 64:150.
46. Haight JSJ, Cole P. Unilateral nasal resistance and asymmetrical body pressure. J Otolaryngol 1986; 16:1.
47. Richerson HB, Seebohm PM. Nasal airway response to exercise. J Allergy 1968; 41:269.
48. Niinma V, Cole P, Mintz Z, et al. The switching point from nasal to oronasal breathing. Respir Physiol 1980; 42:61.
49. Tatum AL. The effect of deficient and excessive pulmonary ventilation on nasal volume. Am J Physiol 1923; 65:229.
50. Dallimore NS, Eccles R. Changes in human nasal resistance associated with exercise, hyperventilation and rebreathing. Acta Otolaryngol 1977; 84:416.
51. Babatola FDO, Eccles R. Nasal vasomotor responses in man to breath holding and hyperventilation recorded by means of intranasal balloons. Rhinology 1986; 24:271.
52. Malcolmson KG. The vasomotor activities of the nasal mucous membrane. J Laryngol Otol 1959; 37:73.
53. Ellegard E, Karlsson G. Nasal congestion during the menstrual cycle. Clin Otolaryngol 1994; 19:400.
54. Servit Z, Kristof M, Strejckova A. Activating effect of nasal and oral hyperventilation on epileptic electrographic phenomena: reflex mechanisms of nasal origin. Epilepsia 1981; 22:321.
55. Werntz DA, Bickford RG, Shannahoff-Khalsa D. Selective hemispheric stimulation by unilateral forced nostril breathing. Human Neurobiol 1987; 6:165.
56. Eccles R. Menthol: effects on nasal sensation of airflow and the drive to breathe. Curr Allergy Asthma Rep 2003; 3:210.
57. Jones AS, Wight RG, Crosher R, et al. Nasal sensation of air-flow following blockade of the nasal trigeminal afferents. Clin Otolaryngol 1989; 14:285.
58. Eccles R, Jawad MS, Morris S. The effects of oral administration of (-)-menthol on nasal resistance to airflow and nasal sensation of airflow in subjects suffering from nasal congestion associated with the common cold. J Pharm Pharmacol 1990; 42:652.
59. Eccles R, Griffiths DH, Newton CG, et al. The effects of D and L isomers of menthol upon nasal sensation of airflow. J Laryngol Otol 1988; 102:506.
60. Eccles R. Menthol and related cooling compounds. J Pharm Pharmacol 1994; 46:618.
61. Eccles R. Role of cold receptors and menthol in thirst, the drive to breathe and arousal. Appetite 2000; 34:29.
62. Morris S, Eccles R, Jawad MSJ, et al. An evaluation of nasal response following different treatment regimes of oxymetazoline with reference to rebound congestion. Am J Rhinol 1997; 11:109.
63. Howarth PH. Mediators of nasal blockage in allergic rhinitis. Allergy 1997; 52:12.
64. Doyle WJ, Boehm S, Skoner DP. Physiological responses to intranasal dose-response challenges with histamine, methacholine, bradykinin, and prostaglandin in adult volunteers with and without nasal allergy. J Allergy Clin Immunol 1990; 86:924.
65. Shelton D, Eiser N. Histamine receptors in the human nose. Clin Otolaryngol 1994; 19:45.
66. Eccles R, Wilson H. A kallikrein-like substance in cat nasal secretion. Br J Pharmacol 1973; 49:712.
67. Proud D, Reynolds CJ, Lacapra S, et al. Nasal provocation with bradykinin induces symptoms of rhinitis and a sore throat. Am Rev Respir Dis 1988; 173:613.
68. Schmidt BMW, Timmer W, Georgens AC, et al. The new topical steroid ciclesonide is effective in the treatment of allergic rhinitis. J Clin Pharmacol 1999; 39:1062.

Index

Note: Page numbers followed by f indicate illustrations; t, tables; and b, boxed material.

INDEX

Airway remodeling *(Continued)*
 bronchial blood vessels, 929, 930f
 childhood asthma, 935, 1323
 epithelial basement membrane, 925–927
 epithelial cells, 379–380
  damage/desquamation, 924, 925f, 926f
  mesenchymal trophic dysfunction,
   912, 912f
 extracellular matrix, 638–639, 929–930
 functional impact, 912–913
 glucocorticoid therapy response, 913
 macrophages, 368–369
 mouse models, 439–440
 neutrophilic asthma, 291–292
Airway resistance measurement, 649, 653t
Airway smooth muscle, 399–408, 633–641
 asthma pathophysiology, 408, 639–640, 640f,
  641, 646
  airway narrowing, 633, 634, 636–637
  airway remodeling, 927–929, 929f, 930f
  hypertrophy/hyperplasia, 401–402, 464, 894,
   897–898, 927, 928, 934
  inflammatory changes, 463–464, 464f, 485,
   485f, 488f
 cell adhesion molecule expression, 405–406
 contractile units, 634, 636f
  plasticity, 634, 635, 928–929
 contraction
  airway hyperresponsiveness, 400, 400f
  cytokseletal element modulation, 637–638
  G protein-coupled receptor-associated
   calcium responses, 400–401
  length adaptation, 634–636
  length–force relationship, 635, 636f
  molecular basis, 400
  receptor signaling modulation, 401
  RhoA/Rho kinase regulation, 401
 cytokine/chemokine production, 405
  therapeutic targets, 406–407
 extracellular matrix interactions, 402,
  407–408, 634
  inflammation-related changes, 637, 640
  mechanical coupling, 636
 immunomodulatory protein expression, 406
 lung growth/development regulation, 399
 mast cell product responses, 932–933
 muscarinic receptors, 1603, 1604, 1605f
 parasympathetic nervous regulation, 1603
 peristalsis, 399
 proliferation regulation, 401–402
  antiasthma agent effects, 404–405
  cell cycle, 403
  extracellular signal-regulated kinase
   pathway, 404
  phosphatidylinositol 3-kinase
   pathway, 403–404
  signal transduction mechanisms, 403f
 protease-activated receptors, 428
 theophylline effects, 1508–1509, 1509f
 ultrastructure, 634, 635f
Airway–lung parenchyma mechanical coupling,
 636–637, 653, 654f
Akathisia, 1537
Akt signaling, 136, 266
 FcεRI, 239, 241
Albumin allergens, 586, 590

Albuterol (salbutamol), 406, 671, 691, 692, 1337,
 1356, 1635
 absorption, 1464, 1489
 aerosol delivery, 684, 1492
 asthma exacerbations management, 1371
 β$_2$-adrenoreceptor desensitization, 1495
 clinical pharmacology, 1462, 1486, 1487f, 1488
 enantiomer proinflammatory properties,
  1495–1486
 pharmacogenomics, 67, 68t, 1468, 1636–1637,
  1636f
 regular use (Beta Agonist Study; BAGS), 1496
 use in pregnancy, 1435
Alder (Betulaceae) pollen, 55, 522
Algal allergens, 535–536
Allergen avoidance, 557, 784, 1700
 allergic rhinitis, 984
 asthma, 749, 1333, 1355–1356, 1355t
  occupational, 950, 1355–1356, 1447
  prevention studies, 1339
 in pregnancy, 1427
 see also Environmental control; Food
  elimination therapy
Allergen exposure chambers, nasal provocation
 testing, 1284–1285
Allergen extracts, 557–567, 1251
 allergen content, 1666, 1666t
 bronchial challenge testing, 1302
 CBER regulation, 563–564, 565, 566–567
 diagnostic, 557
 immunotherapy *see* Immunotherapy
 insect venoms, 1008
 labeling, 561, 563, 564
 manufacture, 561–563
  aqueous/glycerinated, 561–562, 562f
  named-patient products, 563
 nasal provocation testing, 1283
 quality control, 564
  performance documentation, 1251, 1251f
  reference preparations, 562, 564
 skin test responses, 1272
 source materials, 558–561
  foods, 560–561
  fungi, 558
  mammals, 559–560
  pollen, 558, 559t
 stability, 563
 standardization, 557–558
  Europe, 567
  lot release limits, 566–567
  relative potency (RP), 564–565, 566
  skin tests, 1277
  specific allergen content, 565
  standardized tests, 565–567
  United States, 563–567
 see also Allergen vaccines
Allergen sensitization
 asthma, 901–902
  mouse models, 438
  in utero, 900
 dendritic cells, 350
 endotoxin exposure, 123
 isotype switching pathways, 123–124, 124f
Allergen vaccines, 557, 564
 clinical uses, 557
 currently licensed in USA, 561t

Allergen vaccines *(Continued)*
 house-dust mite allergens, 559
 national potency standards/reference
  preparations, 562, 564
Allergen-immunostimulatory complexes
 (AIC), 1671
Allergens, 4, 540, 569–607, 1250–1251
 allergic conjunctivitis, 1120
 allergic contact dermatitis, 1106, 1106t
 assay methods, 1261–1262
 asthma *see* Asthma
 atopic dermatitis, 1087–1088, 1091
 autoallergens, 595, 597, 599t
 exposure routes, 570
 food, 590–591, 1143–1147, 1144t
  cross-reactive, 1145t
  labeling, 1170
 immunogenicity
  biochemical activities, 599, 603t
  protease activity, 603
 immunotherapy *see* Immunotherapy
 indoor *see* Indoor allergens
 innate immune response, 30
 insect bites/stings, 591–592
 nomenclature, 570, 1251
 occupational *see* Occupational allergens;
  Occupational asthma
 outdoor *see* Outdoor allergens
 particle size, 539
 pathogen-derived, 595, 597, 598–599t
 proteases, 602
  apoptosis induction, 605–606
  desmosome effects, 605
  immune responses, 606–607
  inflammatory mediator effects, 606
  intermediate junction cleavage, 605
  tight junction cleavage, 603, 605f
  transepithelial delivery, 602–603
 sources, 570
 structure, 570, 597, 600–601t, 602f
Allergic bronchopulmonary aspergillosis, 364,
 365, 533, 576, 666, 967–968, 1360, 1399
 clinical features, 968
 complicating asthma, 290
 diagnosis, 968
 eosinophilia, 863, 870
 epidemiology, 967
 IgE levels, 849
 natural history, 968
 proteases in pathogenesis, 432
 skin tests, 1277
 treatment, 968
Allergic conjunctivitis, seasonal/perennial,
 1119–1122, 1120t, 1121t
 allergens, 1120
 clinical features, 1120–1121, 1121f
 diagnosis, 1122
 pathophysiology, 1121–1122
 treatment, 1128
  antihistamines, 1534
  cromolyn sodium, 1595
Allergic contact dermatitis, 1086–1087, 1106
 allergens, 1106, 1106t
  latex, 1022
  workplace exposure, 509
 clinical features, 1106

Index

Index

Index

Index

Index

INDEX

Index

Dendritic cells *(Continued)*
allergic inflammation, 457
allergic rhinitis, 352, 981–982
antigen presentation, 25, 27, 342–344, 906
cutaneous immune response, 623
inhaled allergens, 602–603
antigen processing, 272, 342–343, 344
antigen uptake, 342
apoptosis/survival regulation, 418
asthma, 350–351, 351f, 894, 906, 933
mouse models, 449
atopic dermatitis, 352
B cell interactions, 346
chemokine expression, 185–186t
cytokine production, 166, 167, 168, 172
dermis, 618, 622
epithelial cell interactions, 384
epithelial network formation, 344
FcεRI expression, 81, 331, 352, 474
omalizumab response, 1680
glucocorticoid responses, 1562
heterogeneity, 26, 27, 341–342
histamine
production, 1521
responses, 1522, 1523f, 1524f
HIV infection, 833
immune complex interactions, 790
indoleamine 2,3-dioxygenase expression, 307
lacotbacilli interactions, 1099
markers, 342
maturation, 26, 27, 272, 346
migration, 344, 345f
chemokines, 191, 344, 344t
to lymph nodes, 191, 344, 346
monocyte/macrophage interactions, 360
morphology, 342, 342f
myeloid, 25–26, 342, 344, 347, 352, 457, 982
subtypes, 26, 27
natural killer, 342
origins, 4, 342, 343f
pattern recognition receptors, 27
plasmatoid, 168, 331, 342, 344, 351, 457, 982
regulatory T cell interactions, 346, 348
in lung, 349–350
T cell activation, 27, 29t, 272, 346, 347f
terminology, 341–342
Th1/Th2 cell differentiation influence, 273–274, 346–349, 349f, 906
therapeutic targeting, 352–353
tolerance induction, 349
see also Langerhans cells
Dense bodies, 634
Dense deposit disease, 100
Depression, 1333, 1475
Der f 1, 543, 1262
protease-activated receptor 2 activation, 426
Der f 2, 543
Der p 1, 540, 542–543, 544, 546, 1262
airborne allergen, 548
airway Th2 cell differentiation response, 274
dendritic cell activation, 342, 349
inflammatory mediator induction, 606
protease activity, 349, 543, 546, 597
protease-activated receptor 2 activation, 426
recombinant allergen, 546
sequence data, 546
Der p *(Continued)*
structure, 597, 601t, 602f
tight junctional protein cleavage, 375, 603, 605f
Der p 2, 543, 544, 546
Dermal–epidermal junction, 615f, 617
Dermatitis herpetiformis, 1154
Dermatographism, 1070, 1072, 1536
Dermatomyositis, 1413
Dermatophagoides farinae, 30, 541, 544f, 583, 1261, 1262
allergens
extracts, 545, 558–559
quantitative measurement, 1262
structure, 601t
Dermatophagoides pteronyssinus, 30, 541, 583, 1261
allergens, 540
atopic dermatitis immunotherapy, 1098
extracts, 544, 545, 558–559
inflammatory mediator induction, 606
protease acitivity, 603
quantitative measurement, 1262
structure, 601t
Dermicidin, 21, 620
Dermis, 614f, 617–618
Desensitization
β_2-adrenoreceptor by β_2-agonists, 1495
IgE receptor downregulation, 246–250
Desensitization therapy
aspirin-induced asthma, 1237
complications, 1221
drug allergy, 1220–1221, 1221b
Desloratadine, 337, 985, 1533, 1534, 1535, 1536
adverse effects, 1540
clinical pharmacology, 1525, 1527, 1529
Desmocollins, 375, 605
Desmogleins, 375, 605
Desmoplakins, 375, 605
Desmosomes (macula adherens), 374, 374f, 604f
epidermis, 613
protease allergen effects, 605
respiratory epithelium, 374, 375
Detergent enzymes, 585
Detoxification therapy, 1698
Deuteromycete allergens (fungi imperfecti), 526, 527–528, 529, 531
Developmental cell movements, role of chemokines, 191–192
Dexamethasone, 672, 1550
Diabetes, asthma comorbidity, 1362
Diacyl glycerol (DAG), cell signaling, 136, 245
FcεRI, 241, 242
Diagnostic allergens, 557
Diagnostic tests
inappropriate, 1695–1697
unproven methods, 1692–1695
Dialysis patients, eosinophilia, 875
Dicer endonuclease, 55
Diclofenac allergy, 1239
Diesel exhaust particle exposure, 501, 504, 776, 1399
asthma associations, 1353
IgE levels, 854
nasal provocation testing, 1286, 1287
oxidative stress, 503, 504f
Diet diaries, 1157
Dietary factors
allergic disease, 774–775
asthma, 738–740, 738t, 1347
atopic dermatitis, 759
during pregnancy/breast-feeding, 774
Dietary protein-induced enteropathy, 1152
Dietary therapy, 1700
Diffuse cutaneous mastocytosis, 1053, 1055, 1055f, 1056f, 1058
Diffusing capacity of carbon monoxide (DLCO), 657
DiGeorge syndrome, 804, 818–819, 826, 1414, 1417, 1419
Diisocyanate-induced asthma, 939, 941, 942, 943, 952
bronchial challenge testing, 1305
genetic factors, 947
Diphenhydramine, 1045, 1072, 1073, 1079, 1161, 1525, 1537
adverse effects, 985, 1537, 1542
Diphenylhydantoin, 862
Diphtheria vaccine reactions, 1193
Disseminated intravascular coagulation, 95, 1033, 1038
Distribution, drug, 1463, 1463f, 1464–1464
antihistamines, 1525
DNA
denaturation, 46
genetic recombination, 43–44
methylation, 55, 56, 274
repair, 41
replication, 41–42, 41f
structure, 37–38, 38f
see also Recombinant DNA technology
DNA array technology, 53–54, 54f
DNA binding-site selection assay, 45
DNA footprinting, 45
DNA hybridization assays, 47
DNA polymerase, 41, 42
DNA probes, 45
gene isolation, 51–52
nucleic acid hybridization, 47
quantitative real-time polymerase chain reaction, 47
DNA sequencing, 45–46
DNA topoisomerases, 42
DNA vaccines, 1650, 1650f
asthma studies, 1650
DNA-based therapies, 1649–1653
Dock *(Rumex)* pollen, 513, 521
Dog allergens, 545, 559, 560, 582t, 1261
aerodynamic properties, 548, 1448, 1448t
allergic rhinitis, 973
asthma, 749, 1352
clinical relevance, 541
environmental control, 551, 1333, 1449–1450, 1449t, 1453
quantitative measurement, 1262
sensitization, 547
Dok proteins, 184, 248, 249
Domestic mites, 541
see also House-dust mites
Dopamine, 1275
Dose–outcome relationship, 1460f
Dose–response curves, 1461, 1461f, 1462
pathophysiologic variability, 1468

Dosimeters, 687
Doxepin, 1097
Doxycycline, 998
DP_1/DP_2 see Prostaglandin D_2 receptors
DPP10, asthma associations, 55, 62
Drug additives *see* Additives, food/drug
Drug allergy, 1205–1223, 1215t, 1635
  acute treatment, 1220
  anaphylaxis, 1028, 1046, 1047, 1440
    prevention, 1041–1042
  angioedema, 1066
  classification, 1206t
  contact dermatitis, 1106, 1211
  definition, 1205
  diagnosis, 1216–1219, 1216b, 1217f, 1220
    drug provocation testing, 1219
    history, 1217–1218
    skin testing, 1218–1219, 1218t
    in vitro evaluations, 1219
  drug interactions, 1469–1470
  eosinophilia, 861–862, 861t
  eosinophilic lung disease, 869
  epidemiology, 1206
  genetic factors, 1210, 1211t, 1214
  HIV-infected patients, 840–842, 841t
  immune mechanisms, 1206–1210, 1207t
    danger hypothesis, 1211
    drug immunogenicity determinants,
      1210–1211, 1210b
    hapten-carrier complexes, 1206–1207, 1207f
    metabolic intermediate reactivity, 1207
    T cell activation (*p–i* concept), 1208–1210,
      1209f
  immunopathology, 1212–1213, 1212t
  lupus-like syndrome, 1213
  non-allergic hypersensitivity (pseudoallery)
    differentiation, 1216, 1216t
  pharmacotherapy management, 1220–1222
    alternative medication, 1220
    potentially cross-reactive medication, 1220
    readministration of offending drug, 1222
    readministration of offending drug/
      desensitization, 1220–1221, 1221b
  photocontact dermatitis, 1105
  in pregnancy, 1440, 1442
  prophylaxis, 1041–1042, 1222–1223, 1222b
  pseuodanaphylaxis, 1040
  reevaluation, 1222–1223
  rhinitis, 978, 978t
  risk factors, 1213–1215, 1214t
  skin tests, 1277
  specificity of immune response, 1211–1212,
    1211f
  urticaria, 1066
Drug efficacy, 1461
Drug interactions, 1469–1470, 1470t
Drug intolerance, definition, 1205
Drug potency, 1461
Drug rash with eosinophilia and systemic
  symptoms (DRESS), 862
  HIV-infected patients, 840
Drug reactions
  delayed, 1205
  idiosyncratic, 1205, 1215, 1635
  immediate, 1205
  immunologic *see* Drug allergy

Drug reactions *(Continued)*
  non-allergic hypersensitivity (pseudoallergic),
    1215–1216, 1215t
    allergy differentiation, 1216, 1216t
  type A, 1205, 1206, 1206t
  type B, 1205, 1206, 1206t
Drug-induced autoimmune hemolytic
  anemia, 15
Dry powder inhalers, 679, 680, 686, 695–696,
  695t, 1356, 1463
  β_2-agonist delivery, 1491t, 1492
  bronchial challenge testing, 1299
  delivery performance, 685, 695–696
  glucocorticoids delivery, 1553
  lung deposition assessment, 696, 696f
  oral/pharyngeal drug deposition, 1464, 1553
Dry powder mannitol, bronchial challenge
  testing, 1299
DTP vaccine adverse reactions, 1197
Duchenne's muscular dystrophy, 50
Durham Sampler, 510
Dust extract allergen measurement, 1262
Dutch Chronic Nonspecific Lung Disease
  (CNSLD) study, 1581
Dysmorphic features, primary immunodeficiency
  disorders, 1414, 1416
Dyspnea, airway afferent innervation, 228
Dystonia, 1537

E

E-cadherin, 317, 375, 605
E-selectin, 150, 160, 161, 162, 167
  leukocyte adhesion/transmigration, 158, 284,
    285, 389, 619
  ligands, 151
E-selectin ligand-1 (ESL-1), 151
Early phase responses
  allergic rhinitis, 980
  asthma, 14, 901–902
  bronchial challenge testing, 1301, 1302f,
    1303–1304
  nasal provocation testing, 1282
Ebastine, 1525, 1537
Echimyopodid mite allergens, 584, 584t
Eczema *see* Atopic dermatitis
Eczema herpeticum (Kaposi's varicelliform
  eruption), 1097
Edible oil additives, 1185
Efalizumab, 154
Effector memory cells, 276
Efferocytosis, 26, 29–30, 30f, 287–288, 418–419
Efficacy, drug, 1461
Egg allergy, 560, 759, 779, 1140, 1151, 1152,
  1156, 1162
  allergens, 590, 1144–1145, 1144t
    occupational exposure, 585, 588t
    structure, 601t
  atopic dermatitis, 1093
  oral challenge tests, 1314
  vaccine adverse reactions, 1192, 1195, 1196
Egg content of vaccines, 1193b
Egg lecithin, 1183
Eicosanoids, 136, 203
  formation, 204–206, 205f
Elafin, 380, 381, 382, 614

Elastase, 390, 391
  extracellular matrix degradation, 637
  protease-activated receptor activation, 426, 428
Elastin, airway remodeling, 638–639
Electrodermal testing, 1694–1695
Electronic medication monitors, 1479
Electrophoretic mobility-shift assay, 45
Elemental diets, 885, 887
ELEX (systematic evolution of ligands by
  exponential enrichment) technology, 1248
Elimination diets
  eosinophilic gastritis/gastroenteritis, 887
  food hypersensitivity
    diagnosis, 1157, 1159
    management, 1159, 1161
  unconventional treatment programs, 1700
Elimination, drug, 1463, 1463f, 1465–1466
  antihistamines, 1525
  chromones, 1593
  clearance, 1466–1467, 1466f
  glucocorticoids, 1550, 1552
  half-life, 1467, 1467f
Elm (Ulmaceae) pollen, 515, 515f
Embryonic stem cells, 53, 259–260, 260f, 261
  cell-based therapy, 260
  self-renewal versus differentiation, 265–266
Emedastine, 1127, 1541
Emitted dose (ED), 685, 685f
Emollients, atopic dermatitis management, 1094
ENA-78 (CXCL5), 286, 390
  epithelial cell production, 377
  mast cell production, 323
Endoplasmic reticulum, signaling mechanisms,
  130, 243
Endothelial cells, 150, 152, 155, 387–397, 791
  chemokines, 182, 186, 187–188t, 190, 190f
    lymphocyte positioning in lymph nodes, 191
  endogenous antioxidants, 394
  hematopoietic stem cell vascular niche
    function, 265
  hemostastic activity, 388
  histamine receptors, 1521
  injury during acute inflammation, 390–395
    oxidant-induced, 392–394
    protective factors, 394
    reversible/irreversible, 391–392
  leukocyte adhesion/transmigration, 153,
    157–158, 157f, 158f, 190, 190f, 284, 285,
    297–298, 298f, 330, 389–390, 390f, 395,
    397, 791
    glucocorticoid effects, 1463
  lymphatic vessels, 619
  nitric oxide, 389, 394, 395f
  permeability barrier function, 389
  protease-activated receptors, 428
  pulmonary vasculature, 387–388, 388f
  repair mechanisms, 394–395
  skin vasculature, 619
  vascular tone regulation, 389
Endothelial progenitor cells, 395
Endothelins, 376, 402
  vascular tone regulation, 389
Endotoxin (lipopolysaccharide) exposure, 20, 27,
  123, 125, 363, 976
  airway response to inhalation, 357
    effects of atopy, 363

Index

Eotaxins, 181, 462, 485
basophil activation, 335
epithelial cell production, 377
EP_1 to EP_4 see Prostaglandin E_2 receptors
Ephedrine, 1485, 1486, 1487f
Epicoccum, 528, 529, 533, 534f, 558
Epidemiology, 4, 715–716
allergic rhinitis, 756–757, 758f, 975–976
asthma see Asthma; Exercise-induced asthma;
Occupational asthma
atopic dermatitis, 757, 759, 1083–1084
food allergy, 759–760
nasal polyps, 992
sinusitis, 999
study methods, 716, 717–718
Epidermal barrier, 613, 1087
Epidermal cells, 611, 613–617, 613t
Epidermal differentiation complex (EDC), 614
Epidermis, 611, 613–617, 614f
constitutive innate immunity, 620
cornified cell envelope, 613–614
stratum corneum lipid barrier, 613
Epidermolysis bullosa, 628
Epigenetic preprogramming, stem cell development, 262–263
Epigenetics, 55–56
Epinastine, 1129, 1541
Epinephrine
anaphylaxis management, 1042–1043
insect sting reactions, 1010
outpatient administration, 1042, 1045
physician administration, 1042, 1044
sublingual, 1045
autoinjectors, 1010, 1011, 1042, 1161, 1181, 1440
practical issues, 1042, 1047
mastocytosis, hypotension management, 1060
pharmacology, 1485, 1486, 1487f, 1488
safety in pregnancy, 1440–1441
sulfite adverse reactions, 1181
Episcleritis, 1132t, 1133–1134
Epithelial barriers to infection, 4, 26
Epithelial cells, 373–384
anatomy, 373–374, 374f
antimicrobial products, 20, 377, 382–384, 383f
cell–cell adhesion, 374–376
chemokines expression, 187–188t, 377, 378t
dendritic cell interactions, 384
immunoregulation, 384
inflammatory mediators production, 376–379
cytokines, 377–379, 378t
lipids, 376
peptides, 376–377
innate immune response, 25, 26, 381–384
leukocyte interactions, 379
neutrophil interactions, 285
pattern recognition receptors, 381
protease inhibitor production, 380–381
viral receptors, 381, 381t
see also Airway epithelial cells; Ciliated epithelium; Respiratory epithelium
Epstein–Barr virus, 10, 851, 1412, 1417
Equ c 1, 560

ERK pathway
airway smooth muscle mitogen signaling, 403, 404
basophil/mast cell signaling, 252, 253f
mite protease allergen activation, 606
muscarinic M2 receptor signaling, 1604
stem cells self-renewal regulation, 266
ERKs (extracellular signal-regulated kinases), 132, 138, 141, 144, 184
Erythema size, allergen extract standardization, 564
Erythromycin, 673
antihistamine interactions, 1525, 1527
theophylline interactions, 1469, 1510
use in pregnancy, 1433, 1438
Erythropoietin, 262
Eternacept, 641, 906, 1131, 1654
Ethnic/racial factors, asthma, 1320
epidemiology, 720, 720f, 1322
mortality (United States), 734, 735f
variability in therapy response, 1635
Euphorbiaceae, occupational aeroallergens, 586, 588–589t
Euroglyphus maynei, 541, 583
European allergen extracts
named-patient products, 563
quality control/reference preparations, 562–563, 567
standardization, 567
European Community Respiratory Health Survey (ECHRS), 717, 721, 743, 775, 894, 976
Exercise, 775
nasal airflow effects, 709
Exercise-induced anaphylaxis, 1071
food-associated, 1156
Exercise-induced asthma, 464, 1349, 1353, 1361, 1385–1392
anticholinergic agent effects, 1611
bronchial reactivity, 904–905, 905f, 1390
clinical features, 1389–1390, 1389f
diagnosis, 1385, 1390–1391, 1391b
exercise challenge testing, 1298–1299
late reactions, 1390
leukotriene modulator effects, 1623
pathogenesis, 1386–1389
airway cooling/rewarming, 1386–1387, 1387f, 1388f
airway drying, 1387, 1388f
hyperpnea, 1386, 1387
immediate hypersensitivity mediators, 1388–1389
respiratory heat exchange, 1386
prevalence, 1385–1386
refractory period, 1390
therapy/prevention, 1356, 1361, 1391–1392, 1392t
Exons, 39, 43
Expectorants, mucus hypersecretion management, 673
Experimental allergic encephalitis, 169
Experimental diagnostic/therapeutic methods, 1691
Extracellular matrix
airway remodeling, 638–639, 929–930
airway smooth muscle interactions, 407–408, 634, 637

Extracellular matrix *(Continued)*
inflammation-related changes, 637, 640
mechanical coupling, 636
mitogenesis, 402
airways, 637–638
asthma
subepithelial basement membrane, 897
therapeutic targets, 640–641
collagen, 638
elastic fibers, 637–638
leukocyte adhesion, 159–160
proteins, 375
respiratory epithelium basal cell binding, 375
skin, 617–618
Extrafine particle fraction (EFPF), 685
Eye, 1117–1135
allergic disease, 1119–1130, 1120t, 1121t
conjunctival provocation testing, 1126, 1127t
topical drug preparations, 1127, 1128t, 1129t
treatment principles, 1126–1128
anatomy, 1117–1119, 1118f
aspirin hypersensitivity symptoms, 1232
contact dermatoconjunctivitis, 1130–1131
immunologic disease, 1131–1134, 1132t
Eyelid anatomy, 1118

F

Fab (antigen-binding) fragments, 76, 77, 78f
Factor VIIa, 424, 425
Factor Xa, 424
Factor B, 10, 22, 92
deficiency, 103, 109
Factor D (adipsin), 10, 89, 92
deficiency, 103
Factor H, 92, 96
activator/non-activator surface binding, 92
antibodies, 101
deficiency, 106, 107, 109, 1413
Factor I, 96
deficiency, 106–107, 109, 1073
Fagales pollen, 515–516, 571–572
Familial cold urticaria, 167, 1073
Familial hemophagocytic lymphohistiocytosis syndromes, 1408t
Family history, 4
Family studies, gene–environment interactions, 735
Famotidine, 1053, 1060
Farm animals
allergens, 559, 560
sensitization, 123, 124
exposure-related allergic disease risk, 771–772, 783
Farming environment protective effect, 123, 125, 363, 500, 551, 741, 771, 783, 784, 976, 1339
Fas receptors, 27, 417, 418
Fas/Fas-ligand interaction, 625, 833
Fatty acids, dietary (*n*-3/*n*-6), 775
asthma studies, 739, 1347
atopic dermatitis, 1099
Fc domains, 81
Fc receptors, 8, 75t, 81
signal transduction, 145
Fc region, 76, 77, 78f, 79
FcαRI, 81

FcεRI, 81, 235, 473–474, 980, 1680
  aggregation reaction, 236–237
  expression, 331
    dendritic cells, 352
    eosinophils, 9, 298
    Langerhans cells, 615
    mast cells, 9, 318–319
    omalizumab response, 1680–1681
  loss from cell surface, 246–247
  monomeric IgE signaling, 236, 238
  signal termination/self-regulation, 237,
      246–248, 248f
    co-receptors, 249–250
    dok proteins, 248–249
    phosphatases, 247–248
    receptor-specific kinases, 246
    ubiquitinylation, 250
  signaling, 236, 237–255
    actin cytoskeleton/polymerization, 246
    adaptor proteins, 237, 241, 246, 248–249,
        249t
    calcium ions, 241, 242–245, 244f
    early stages, 237–239, 242f, 250–251
    feedback augmentation, 251
    modeling techniques, 250
    modulation, 237–238
    second messengers, 241, 242, 245
    therapeutic targets, 255–256
  signaling proteins, 242f
    domain structure, 239, 250
    phosphatidylinositol 3-kinase, 240–241
    phospholipase A2, 245–246
    phospholipase C, 240, 241–242
    phospholipase D, 245–246
    protein kinase C, 245, 246
    role of lipid rafts, 239, 240
    Src-family kinases, 239–240
    Syk kinase, 240, 250, 251
    Tec-family kinases, 242
  structure, 237, 331
FcεRIβ gene
  airway hyperresponsiveness
      associations, 910
  asthma association studies, 64, 737, 898
FcεRII, 7, 81, 365, 366, 474, 980, 1680
FCER1B see FcεRIβ gene
FcγRI, 81, 789
FcγRII, 81, 249, 250, 331, 789, 790
  monoclonal antibody (IDEC-152)
      therapy, 982
FcγRIII, 81, 319, 789, 790
Fel d 1, 540, 545, 546, 548, 560, 1262,
    1670, 1671
  allergen extracts
    preparations, 559
    standardization, 564, 565
Fel d 2 (cat albumin), 545
Fel d 3 (cystatin), 545
Fel d 4 (lipocalin), 545
Fenoterol, 734, 1356, 1488
  asthma deaths, 1497
  pharmacogenomics, 67
  pharmacology, 1486, 1487f, 1488
Fetal distress, anaphylaxis in pregnancy, 1439,
    1440
Fetal oxygenation determinants, 1424

FEV$_1$ (forced expiratory volume in 1 second),
    648, 649, 656, 1348
  acute asthma exacerbations, 1337, 1368
  bronchial challenge test response, 1296
  children, 646, 1326
  exercise-induced asthma, 1385, 1390
  long-term decline, 911
  post-bronchodilator therapy, 651, 652
  in pregnancy, 1424, 1435
  see also Lung function tests
FEV$_1$/FVC, 648, 649, 656
  children, 1326
Fexofenadine, 143, 985, 1053, 1060, 1078, 1273,
    1533, 1534, 1535, 1536
  adverse effects, 1540
  pharmacology, 1525, 1529
Fibroblast growth factors (FGFs), 267, 399
  stem cells self-renewal regulation, 265, 266
Fibroblasts, 618
  chemokines expression, 187–188t
Fibronectin
  airway remodeling, 638, 897, 926
  dermis, 617, 618
  eosinophil binding, 297, 298
  integrin interactions, 638
  leukocyte adhesion, 159
Ficolin, 622
Filaggrin, 613
  gene mutations, 1087
Filtration samplers, 511
Fine particle fraction (FPF), 685, 685f
FIP1L1-PDGFRA fusion gene
  eosinophilic leukemia, 867
  hypereosinophilic syndromes, 864, 865, 883,
      884
  mast cell-related disorders, 1052, 1060, 1061
First pass metabolism, 1462, 1464
Fish allergy, 560, 1151, 1152, 1161, 1162, 1184
  allergens, 590, 592t, 1144t, 1146
  atopic dermatitis, 1093
FLAP (5-lipoxygenase activating protein), 212,
    213, 299, 322, 368, 1620
Flavors, 1170, 1183
  protein hydrolysates, 1182, 1183
Flea bite allergic reactions, 1015
  salivary allergens, 592, 597t
Fletcher factor deficiency, 1064
Floristic zones (North America), 522, 523f, 524t
Flow cytometry, 1263, 1263f
Flow–volume loops, 648, 649f, 650f
  childhood asthma, 1326
Fluid therapy, anaphylaxis, 1045–1046
Flunisolide, 146, 691, 1331
  clinical pharmacology, 1553, 1577, 1578t
Fluorescence in situ hybridization (FISH), 48
Flushing, 1039, 1053
  anaphylaxis, 1033, 1035
Fluticasone, 146, 691, 885, 886, 1094, 1095, 1328,
    1331
  adverse effects, 1587, 1588
  clinical pharmacology, 1464, 1553, 1577, 1578t,
      1580, 1581, 1582, 1583, 1625
    montelukast comparison in children,
        1579–1580, 1580f
  salmeterol combined treatment, 1378
  use in pregnancy, 987

fMLP (f-Met-Leu-Phe), 241, 251
  basophil activation, 243, 244, 332, 335, 336
  leukocyte chemotaxis, 285, 390
Focal adhesion kinase, 637
Focal adhesions, 152, 637
Food additives see Additives, food/drug
Food adverse reactions
  definition, 1140
  non-allergic, 1140t
  see also Food hypersensitivity
Food allergens, 426, 590–591, 1143–1147, 1144t
  allergen extract sources, 560–561
  childhood sensitization, 779, 780, 780f, 1327
  cross-reactivity, 1145t
    syndromes, 591, 595t
  food labeling, 1170
Food aversions, 1140
Food challenge see Oral food challenge testing
Food elimination therapy
  dietary protein-induced enteropathy, 1152
  eosinophilic esophagitis, 885, 1151
  food protein-induced colitis, 1152
Food hypersensitivity, 31, 879, 880, 1139–1163,
    1309
  allergic rhinitis, 1163
  anaphylaxis, 1028, 1046, 1047, 1147, 1156, 1161
  angioedema, 1066
  arthritis, 1156
  asthma, 1155–1156, 1163, 1327
  atopic dermatitis, 1087, 1093, 1163
  atopy association, 1140, 1163
  chemokines, 196–197, 197f
  clinical features, 977, 1147, 1148–1156
  cutaneous symptoms, 1066, 1147, 1152–1154,
      1153t
  definitions, 1140
  diagnosis, 759, 1157–1159, 1696, 1697
    practical aspects, 1159, 1160f
    skin tests, 1277
  see also Oral food challenge testing
  differential diagnosis, 1157t
  eosinophilic esophagitis, 884
  epidemiology, 759–760, 1140–1141
  gastrointestinal symptoms, 1147, 1148,
      1149–1150t
  historical aspects, 1139–1140
  history-taking, 1157
  IgE-mediated responses, 196, 1147–1148
  management
    cromolyn sodium, 1599
    elimination diet, 1159, 1161
    emergency treatment plan, 1161
    immunotherapy, 1162
    medication, 1161–1162
    omalizumab, 1684–1685, 1685t
  mortality, 759
  natural history, 1161, 1162–1163
  non-IgE-mediated, 1148
  pathogenic mechanisms, 1147–1148, 1148t
  patient education, 1161
  prevention, 1163
  respiratory symptoms, 1147, 1154–1156, 1155t
  rhinitis, 977
  risk factors, 760
  urticaria, 1066
Food immune complex assay (FICA), 1696–1697

Food intolerance
  definition, 1140
  see also Food hypersensitivity
Food labeling, 1169–1170
  flavors, 1183
  protein hydrolysates, 1182
  sulfite residues, 1181
Food Labeling and Consumer Protection Act,
  1169–1170
Food protein-induced enterocolitis syndrome,
  1151–1152, 1312
Food toxic contamination, 1140
Food-associated exercise-induced anaphylaxis,
  1156
Food-induced contact dermatitis, 1154
Food-induced pulmonary siderosis (Heiner's
  syndrome), 1156
Foreign bodies
  aspiration, acute cough, 1396
  recurrent infection associations, 1411
Formoterol, 406, 1356, 1357, 1462, 1464
  budesonide combined therapy, 1357, 1378,
    1488, 1498
  childhood asthma, 1331–1332
  pharmacology, 1487f, 1489
  safety, 1332, 1497
Foxp3, 13, 467, 981
  gene mutations, 809, 1086, 1413
  regulatory T cell differentiation regulation, 175,
    175t, 625
FP (prostaglandin $F_{2\alpha}$ receptor), 210, 211t
Fractalkine, 181, 377
Fruit allergy, 1152, 1155
Fruit-derived allergens, 1147
  ingested, 591, 594t
  occupational aeroallergens, 587t
  structure, 600t
Fucosyltransferase genes, mucins biosynthesis,
  661
Fuel combustion emissions, 743
  asthma epidemiology, 748–749, 1353
  indoor air quality determinants, 498, 499
Fungal allergens, 576, 578–581, 579–581t
  air-borne, 522, 525–535
  allergic rhinitis, 976
  asthma, 525, 749
    immunotherapy, 1658–1659
  atopic dermatitis, 1087
  childhood sensitization, 1327
  environmental control, 551, 1333
  exposure assessment, 525, 531–532
  extract sources, 558
  indoor, 531, 551, 558, 749, 1261, 1262
  occupational, 587t
  outdoor, 558
  protease-activated receptor activation, 426
  seasonal variations, 529–530
  structure, 600t
  see also Fungal spores
Fungal infection, 1086, 1399, 1426
  immunodeficiency disorders, 1411, 1412
  sinusitis, 995–996, 996f
Fungal spores, 509, 576
  assay methods, 1261, 1262
  collection, 1261
  culture methods, 512

Fungal spores *(Continued)*
  development, 525
  dry-/wet-weather, 528, 530f
  microscopic examination, 511–512, 531
  sample analysis, 511
  sampling devices, 510–511, 510t, 531
  structure, 525, 525f
Fungi, 570
  allergenic phyla, 526–531
  common airborne genera, 532–535
  functional anatomy, 525
  growth conditions, 528–531, 558
  nomenclature, 525, 526
  prevalence/habitat, 529t
  taxonomy, 525–526
Furnishings, environmental control measures,
  1448, 1450
Fusarium, 526, 528, 533, 534f, 535, 558
FVC (forced vital capacity), 648, 656
  see also FEV$_1$/FVC
Fyn kinase, FcεRI signaling, 237, 239, 240

G

G protein-coupled receptors, 134, 134f, 135f, 141,
  183, 206, 208, 210, 235, 236
  agonist drug actions, 1461
  airway smooth muscle signaling, 400–401,
    403
  allergen responses, 143–144
  chemokine signaling, 181, 182–183, 189, 190
  FcεRI signaling, 241, 242
  leukocyte adhesion to endothelium, 158
  protease-activated, 423, 424, 425
G protein-related receptor for asthma (GPRA)
  gene, 910, 1324
G proteins
  FcεRI signaling, 240, 246
  intracellular signaling, 134–135, 134f,
    135f
  low-molecular weight, 135, 136–138
Galactosyltransferase genes, mucins biosynthesis,
  660, 661
Galectins, 156, 156f, 298
Gap junctions, 375–376, 613
Gastroesophageal reflux disease, 885, 885t, 1151,
  1411, 1435
  asthma comorbidity, 1328, 1360
  cough, 1400, 1401
  diagnosis, 1400t
  eosinophil accumulation, 879, 880
  treatment, 1403, 1435
Gastrointestinal disorders
  anaphylaxis, 1033, 1035
  aspirin hypersensitivity, 1232
  food hypersensitivity, 1149–1150t
    IgE-mediated, 1147, 1148,
      1150–1151
    immediate gastrointestinal allergic reaction,
      1151
    mixed IgE/non-IgE-mediated, 1151
    non-IgE-mediated, 1151–1152
  mastocytosis, 1055–1056, 1056f, 1060
  primary immunodeficiency disorders,
    1412–1413, 1413t
  see also Eosinophilic gastrointestinal disorders

Gastrointestinal mucosal barrier, 1141–1142, 1141t
  antigen penetration, 1142
  oral tolerance induction, 1142–1143
Gastrointestinal tract
  antigen handling, 1141–1143
  eosinophils, 880–881, 882t
  microflora, 21, 31
    atopy/allergic disease, 773, 774, 781, 784
    oral tolerance induction, 1142–1143
  normal antibody response to foods, 1143
  pattern recognition receptors, 26
  protease-activated receptors, 432
GATA-3, 127, 277, 467, 488–489, 489f, 981, 997
  Th2 cell differentiation regulation, 173,
    274–275, 276, 488
Gelatin, 1184
  protein hydrolysates manufacture, 1182
  vaccine additive, 1184, 1192b
    reactions, 1171, 1191–1192, 1194, 1196
Gell and Coombs classification, 13, 625
Gene cloning, 48–51
  gene libraries, 48, 51
  vectors, 49–51
Gene expression, 42–43, 52
  profiling, 444–445, 884
Gene libraries, 48, 51
Gene therapy, 812, 813
Gene–environment interactions, 65–67, 898, 899,
  899f
Genes, 37–38
  functional studies, 53
  isolation technology, 51–52
  mapping, 52–53
  transcription, 38–39
Genetic association studies
  asthma, 61–63, 63t, 69–70, 69f, 70f, 444, 718,
    737f
  linkage disequilibrium, 61, 61f
  pharmacogenomics, 1635, 1640
  replication of findings, 64, 69
  type I error (false-positive result), 63–64, 69
Genetic code, 40, 40t
Genetic engineering, 37–57
  see also Recombinant DNA technology
Genetic factors, 4, 59–70, 606
  air pollutant-related oxidative stress, 504
  airway hyperresponsiveness, 910
  aspirin hypersensitivity, 1229, 1230, 1236, 1238
  asthma, 277, 715, 718, 735, 737, 737f, 898–899,
    1323–1324, 1346
  atopic dermatitis, 1084
  drug hypersensitivity reactions, 1210, 1211t,
    1214
    HIV-infected patients, 840
  IgE responses, 126–127, 126t
  occupational asthma, 944
  see also Candidate gene studies;
    Pharmacogenomics
Genetic recombination, 43–44
Genomics, 53–55
German Infant Nutritional Intervention (GINI),
  784
Giardia lamblia infection, 1412, 1413
Gingivitis, 1411, 1412, 1417
Glafenine, 1239, 1240
Glaucoma, glucocorticoid-related, 1588, 1635

Index

Index

Immunoglobulin gene superfamily, 76, 82–84, 154
  cell adhesion molecules, 149, 154–156, 155f
  therapeutic targeting, 156
Immunoglobulin M (IgM), 79f, 80, 91, 276
  B cells, 6, 7
  immune complex biological activity, 788
  membrane-bound, 6, 80
  primary immune response, 74
Immunoglobulin-like domains, 76
Immunoglobulin-like transcripts see LIRs
  (leukocyte inhibitory receptors)
Immunoglobulins, 4, 73–86
  allotypes, 79
  antigen binding, 73, 77–78
    affinity, 78, 1249
    avidity, 78–79, 1250
    sites, 76, 77
  classification, 86b
  cleavage fragments, 77, 78f
  diversity generation, 7, 82–84, 86b, 276
  effector functions, 80, 80t
  Fab (antigen-binding) fragments, 76, 77, 78f
  Fc portion, 76
  idiotypes, 76, 77
  isotype switching see Isotype switching
  isotypes, 79–81, 79f, 80t
  membrane-bound, 73, 74
  primary immune response, 74, 76f, 80
  secondary immune response, 74, 76, 76f
    affinity maturation, 84
  secreted, 73
  structure, 76–79, 77f, 78f
    carbohydrate content, 76
  therapeutic applications, 84–86, 85t, 86f
  total serum levels, 1695
  variable regions, 76, 77
  see also Antibodies
Immunologic synapse, 76, 346, 348f
Immunometric assays, 1254f, 1255
Immunomodulators, 1643–1655
  asthma, 1359
  Wegener's granulomatosis, 961–962
Immunophenotyping, 1262
  flow cytometry, 1263, 1263f
  monoclonal antibody panel specificities, 1264t
Immunostimulatory DNA therapy (CpG DNA),
  1650–1651
  asthma/allergy studies, 1651
  immune response, 1650–1651, 1651t
Immunostimulatory sequences (ISS), 364
Immunotherapy, 557, 1657–1674
  adherence, 1669
  adverse reactions, 1012, 1029, 1668–1669, 1670
  allergen doses, 1660–1661, 1660t
  allergen extracts, 1665–1668
    allergen content, 1666, 1666t
    cross-reactivity, 1665, 1665b
    labeling of treatment vials, 1667, 1668f
    modified, 1669–1670, 1670b
    prescription, 1665–1666, 1667t
    recombinant technology, 1670–1671
    storage/handling, 1667–1668
  allergic rhinitis, 982, 986, 1658, 1669
    asthma development prevention, 1661
    nasal glucocorticoids comparison, 1661

Immunotherapy (Continued)
  asthma, 1359, 1658, 1659f, 1669
    childhood, 1333
    guideline recommendations, 1665
  atopic dermatitis, 1098, 1658
  B cell responses, 1663
  basophil responses, 1663
  clinical efficacy, 1658–1661
    atopy progression prevention, 1661
    persistence of improvement, 1668
    singel versus multiple allergens, 1659
  cytokine responses, 1663–1664
  duration, 1668
  food hypersensitivity, 1162
  historical development, 1657
  immunologic response, 1662–1664, 1662b
    clinical outcome correlations, 1664
    end-organ inflammation, 1662–1663
    end-organ sensitivity, 1662
    immunoglobulins (IgE/IgG), 1663
  immunologic specificity, 1660
  insect venom see Insect venom allergy,
    immunotherapy
  intranasal/intrabronchial administration, 1673
  latex allergy, 1023
  monitoring
    nasal provocation testing, 1282
    skin tests, 1278
  omalizumab combined therapy, 1673,
    1684–1685
  oral administration, 1672
  oral allergy syndrome, 1661
  patient selection, 1664–1665
  in pregnancy, 1427, 1669
  pretreatment, 1669
  skin test response effects, 1275
  sublingual/swallow (SLIT), 982, 1162,
    1672–1673
  T cell responses, 13, 1663–1664
  treatment schedule, 1666, 1667b, 1668
    modification, 1671
Impulse oscillometry, 1327
Inab phenotype (decay accelerating factor
  deficiency), 107
Inappropriate therapy, 1699–1700
Incidence rate, 716
Indacaterol, 1486, 1487f, 1489
Indoleamine 2,3-dioxygenase, 307, 349
Indomethacin, 505, 673
Indoor allergens, 498–499, 509, 539–552, 776
  airborne, 547–549
  assays, 1261–1262
  asthma associations, 748–748, 1327, 1352,
    1355
  atopy relationship, 782–783, 782f
  childhood sensitization, 546–547, 779, 780,
    780f, 1327
  clinical relevance, 541, 541t, 542f
  endotoxin, 548–549
  environmental control see Environmental control
  historical background, 539–541
  house-dust mite see House-dust mite
  immune response, 551–552, 552t
  sequence data, 546
  sources, 541–546
  T cell responses, 546

Inducible co-stimulator (ICOS), 118, 272
  deficiency, 822
Infantile colic, 1151
Infection susceptibility see Recurrent infections
Inflammation
  anaphylaxis pathophysiology, 1032–1033,
    1034–1035
  cardinal signs, 456, 465
  complement system activation, 92, 93,
    95, 95f
  histamine mediation, 1521–1522
  regulation, 467, 468f
  skin, 620, 622–623
Inflammatory bowel disease, 175, 196, 432, 879,
  886, 887, 1143
Inflammatory dendritic epidermal cells (IDEC),
  352, 623
Inflammatory mediators
  allergic inflammation, 459–462, 460f
  mast cell products, 26
  neurotransmission effects, 465, 465f
  protease allergen induction, 606
Infliximab, 641, 967, 1654
Influenza, 383, 1321, 1396
  asthma exacerbation, 291, 1353
  vaccination
    adverse reactions, 1193, 1195
    asthma patients, 1360, 1381
    during pregnancy, 1425, 1433
    egg allergic recipients, 1192
Inhalers, 679, 680, 680f, 685, 686–696
  β_2-agonist delivery, 1490, 1491t
  costs, 686–687
  delivery efficiency, 680–681
  design trends, 680, 681t
  indicators of performance, 684–685, 685f,
    686f
  selection, 696–697
  types, 686–687
  see also Dry powder inhalers; Metered-dose
    inhalers; Nebulizers
Inhibitor of apoptosis (IAP) family, 413, 415,
  415f
Initiation factors (IFs), 41
Innate immune response, 4, 19–32
  adaptive immune response linkage, 27, 29f, 363,
    384, 623
  allergen induction, 30
  allergy pathogenesis, 32
  cellular responses
    infiltrative, 26–27
    resident cells, 25–26, 25f, 357
  complement activation, 92–93
  epithelial cells, 381–384
  genetic defects, 819–821, 1410t
    laboratory evaluation, 1418–1419,
      1418t
  glucocorticoid effects, 1562–1563
  homeostasis, 27, 29–30
  microbial pattern recognition, 20
  mouse models, 449–450
  neutrophil recruitement, 286, 286f
  neutrophilic asthma pathogenesis, 289,
    290f, 291
  protease-activated pathways, 424
  skin, 620–623, 621f

Index

Levocetirizine, 784, 985, 1273, 1533, 1534, 1536, 1537
  adverse effects, 1540, 1541
  pharmacology, 1525, 1529
LFA-1 (CD11a/CD18), 190, 191, 276, 285, 316–317
Lichen sclerosis, 617
Ligand-induced receptor internalization, 141
Ligand–receptor interactions, 131
Ligase 4 deficiency, 812, 813–814
Light chain, 76
  complementarity-determining regions (CDRs), 82
  constant region, 76
  types/subtypes, 79–80
  variable region, 76, 77
  V(D)J gene rearrangements, 82–84
Linkage analysis, asthma, 718, 737
Linkage disequilibrium, 61, 61f
Lipid bodies, 300
Lipid mediators, 203–218
  allergic inflammation, 460
  antiinflammatory activities, 468
Lipid rafts, 237, 240, 246
  FcεRI signaling, 239, 240
Lipid transfer protein allergens, 571, 572, 574
  foods, 1144t
Lipocalin-prostaglandin D2 synthase, 206
Lipocalins, 21, 560, 583
Lipodystrophy, 100
Lipoid pneumonia, 1401
Lipoid proteinosis, 617
Lipopolysaccharide, 166
  see also Endotoxin
Lipopolysaccharide-binding protein, 20, 23, 291
Lipoxin A, 376
Lipoxins, 136, 299
  aspirin hypersensitivity, 1231–1232, 1233f
5-Lipoxygenase, 299, 322, 368, 376
  gene (ALOX5) polymorphism, 1468, 1620
    aspirin hypersensitivity association, 1230
    pharmacogenomics, 899, 1626, 1638, 1639f
5-Lipoxygenase inhibitors, 213, 1620, 1621
  asthma, 1358, 1623–1625, 1627
    childhood, 1625
    guidelines, 1629
    inhaled glucocorticoids comparison, 1626
    theophylline comparison, 1626–1627
  dose, 1626, 1628, 1628t
  pharmacogenomics, 1635t, 1638–1639
15-Lipoxygenase, 299–300, 376
Lipoxygenase pathway, 212–216, 213f, 332, 1620
LIRs (leukocyte inhibitory receptors), 145, 235, 250, 332, 336
Literacy, adherence influence, 1477
Lobar collapse, 666, 666f
Local anaestheic agent reactions, 1216, 1442
Locust tree pollen, 518
Lodoxamide, 1127, 1129
Lofgren's syndrome, 965, 966
Loratadine, 143, 1060, 1078, 1273, 1533, 1534, 1535, 1536
  adverse effects, 1540
  levels in breast milk, 1433

Loratadine (Continued)
  pharmacology, 1525, 1527, 1529
  use in pregnancy, 987, 1428, 1439, 1441
Loricrin, 614
Löffler's syndrome, 869
Low birth weight
  asthma association, 742, 776, 777, 1347
  maternal asthma association, 1433, 1438
Low-molecular weight G proteins, 135, 136–138, 139f, 143
Lung, 645–657
  acute inflammatory injury, 390
  development, 399, 645–646
  function
    childhood asthma prediction, 754–755
    IgE level associations, 849–850
  growth, 399, 645, 646
Lung function tests
  asthma, 1350
    children, 1326–1327
    infants, 1327
  interpretation, 653–657, 656t
Lung volumes, 651f, 656
  measurement, 648–649
    childhood asthma, 1326–1327
Lupus nephritis, 797, 797f
Lupus-like illness
  complement deficiencies, 1413
  drug-induced, 1213
Lymph nodes, 191
  dendritic cells
    B cell interactions, 346
    migration, 344, 346
    T cell interactions, 346, 347f, 348f
  leukocyte trafficking
    during inflammation, 191, 193f
    role of chemokines, 191, 192f, 193t
  lymphocyte positioning, 191
  T cell differentiation, 191
Lymphatic vessels, 619
Lymphocyte function assays, 1696
Lymphocytes, 271–280
  laboratory assays, 1262–1264
    enumeration, 1262–1263
    functional evaluation (proliferation tests), 1263–1264
    subset counts, 1695–1696
  muscarinic receptors, 1605
Lymphoid stem cells, 4
Lymphokines, allergic inflammation, 460–461
Lymphotoxin-α gene (LTA), asthma association, 64
Lymphotoxins, 166, 173, 181, 273
Lyn kinase, 138, 144, 297, 403
  FcεRI signaling, 237, 239, 240, 250, 251
Lysoglycero-phospholipid metabolism, 203–204
Lysophosphatidic acid, 203–204, 245
Lysosomal hydrolases, 402
Lysosphingolipids, 217
Lysozyme, 21, 373, 382, 620, 661, 663

M

M cells, 1141
M13 phagemid vector, 50
Ma Huang, 1485

Mac-1 (CD11b/CD18), 191, 285
Macrolide antibiotics
  nasal polyposis, 998
  neutrophilic asthma, 292–293, 292f
Macrophages, 4, 8, 11, 355–369, 1521, 1620
  airway remodeling, 368–369
  allergic inflammation, 457
  antigen processing/presentation, 30, 272, 357, 359
  antigen-dependent activation, 364
  antiinflammatory role, 27, 29, 30f
  asthma, 356, 933
  chemokine expression, 182, 185–186t
  co-stimulatory molecule expression, 359
  cytokine production, 166, 166f
  dendritic cell interactions, 360
  dermis, 618, 622
  development, 355
  effector mechanisms, 356t
  efferocytosis, 26, 29, 30f, 418–419
  food hypersensitivity, 1147
  glucocorticoid responses, 1562
  gut-associated lymphoid tissue (GALT), 1141
  heterogeneity, 364
  innate immune response, 25, 26, 357
  lung see Alveolar macrophages; Pulmonary interstitial macrophages
  MHC Class II molecule expression, 357
  surface receptors, 24, 25, 355, 356t, 357, 1605
    pattern recognition receptors, 24–25, 357, 360t
  T cell activation, 359–360, 362f
Macrophagic myofasciitis, 1200
Macula adherens see Desmosomes
Macular degeneration, 107
MAdCAM-1, leukocyte trafficking, 151, 158, 190, 316, 330
MAFA (mast cell function associated antigen), 250
Magnesium sulfate, 1337, 1375t, 1438
Major basic protein, 14, 295, 296, 296f, 300, 304, 332, 391, 462, 475, 666, 881, 981
  airway cytotoxicity, 300, 376
Major basic protein, 2, 881
Malaria, 198
Malassezia, 527, 576, 578, 620
  allergens, 581t
Manchester Allergy and Asthma Study (MAAS), 784, 1455
Mannitol, dry powder, 1299
Mannose-binding lectin, 22, 26, 29, 381
  complement activation, 9, 93
  deficiency, 93, 102–103
MAP kinase signaling, 74, 137, 138, 141, 144, 184, 252, 262, 298, 357, 425, 1519, 1604
  apoptosis, 415, 416
  gene transcription, 138
  low molecular weight G protein regulation, 138, 139f
  mite allergen activation, 606
Maple (Aceraceae) pollen, 517
MASP1, 93
MASP2, 93
  deficiency, 103

Index

Index

Mucus *(Continued)*
  gel/sol layers, 659
  mediators of secretion, 665t
  mucociliary clearance, 664
  parasympathetic regulation of production, 227, 1603
Mucus hypersecretion, 277, 659, 664, 666–667
  asthma, 442, 465, 465f, 646
  bronchoscopy and bronchoalveolar lavage, 673, 674f
  chest physical therapy, 673
  chronic obstructive pulmonary disease, 922, 924, 927
  glucocorticoid responses, 1565
  goblet cell
    degranulation, 670, 670f
    hyperplasia, 667–668, 667f, 669f
  inflammatory changes, 465, 465f, 666
  mediators, 665t
  mucin gene expression, 667–668, 668f
  mucin hypersecretion, 668–669
  pharmacotherapy, 671–674, 671t
    new agents, 673–674
Mucus plugging, 646, 653, 666, 670, 894, 927, 933
  anaphylactic death, 1031
  asthma, 924
Mugwort *(Artemisia vulgaris)* pollen, 520, 520f, 522
  oral allergy syndrome, 1150
Mulberry (Moraceae) pollen, 516, 516f
MULTICASE, 941
Multiple drug allergy syndrome, 1214
Multiple food and chemical sensitivities, 1701–1704, 1705
Multiple sclerosis, 175, 325
  hepatitis B vaccination, relapse activation, 1199–1200
  natalizumab treatment, 154, 162
Munchausen stridor, 1039, 1040
Mupirocin, 1097
Mus m 1, 560, 1262
Muscarinic M1 receptors, 1604, 1605, 1606
Muscarinic M2 receptors, 1604, 1606, 1608
  parasympathetic nerves
    acetylcholine release inhibition, 1606
    asthma pathophysiology, 1606–1607, 1607f
Muscarinic M3 receptors, 1604, 1605, 1608
  selective antagonists, 1608
Muscarinic receptors
  agonists, G protein-coupled receptor interactions, 1461
  airway, 1604–1607, 1605f
    epithelium, 1604
    glands, 1604
    inflammatory cells, 1605, 1605f
    smooth muscle, 1603, 1604
  antagonists *see* Anticholinergic agents
  subtypes, 1604
Mycelia sterilia, 527–528
Mycetoma, 995
Mycobacteria, 773, 783, 1411, 1412, 1425
  toll-like receptor recognition, 357
  vaccines, 1653–1654
Mycobacterium avium intracellulare, 1412
Mycobacterium leprae, 273

Mycobacterium tuberculosis, 21, 357
Mycobacterium vaccae vaccines, 1653, 1654
Mycophenolate mofetil, 1099
Mycoplasm infection, 223, 668, 773, 1329, 1398, 1418, 1438
  asthma associations, 900, 901, 1353
  cough, 1396
  pattern recognition receptors, 24
Mycotoxins, 532
MyD88 signaling pathway, 23, 24, 286, 357
Myeloglycans, 151
Myeloid stem cells, 4, 8
Myosin, airway smooth muscle, 400, 634
Myosin light chain kinase, 132
Myrmecia (Australian jack jumper ant), 1008

N

NADPH oxidase, 26, 392
  eosinophil respiratory burst, 304, 305f
Nanoparticle technology, 682
NAP-2 (CLCL7), 286, 390
Naphazoline, 1127
Naproxen allergy, 1239
Nasal airflow, 702–703, 704, 706–710, 983, 1288
  cerebral effects, 709
  control, 706–707, 706f, 708
  endocrine influences, 709
  hyperventilation effects, 709
  nasal cycle, 707–708, 707f
  nasal provocation test endpoints, 1288
  normal flow, 707
  paranasal sinuses ventilation, 999
  pharmacology, 710
  posture-related changes, 708–709
  sensation, 709
Nasal airway resistance, 706, 707, 709
  measurement, 707
  nasal provocation test outcome measures, 1288–1289
Nasal anatomy, 701–711, 974–975
Nasal biopsy, 984, 1292
Nasal blood vessels, 705, 974
Nasal cavity, 702–703, 703f
Nasal congestion, 710, 973
  aspirin hypersensitivity, 1232
  food hypersensitivity, 1147
  see also Nasal airflow
Nasal cycle, 707–708, 707f
Nasal eosinophilia, 860–861
Nasal epithelium, 701, 702, 703–704, 974
  allergen exposure responses
    chemokine expression, 485, 486f, 487f
    IgE expression, 124–125, 474–475, 474f, 475f
    Th2 cytokines production, 477–478, 479f
  eosinophils, 475–476, 477f
  goblet cells, 704, 974
  imprints, 1292
  mucociliary clearance, 704–705, 974
  sensitivity following immunotherapy, 1662
  seromucous glands, 704, 1289
  sources of nasal fluid, 704
  vasculature, 705, 974
Nasal filtration, 701–702

Nasal fluid, 704, 705
  collection, 1281
  nasal provocation test response, 1289–1291
Nasal innervation, 975, 980
Nasal lavage
  cellular contents collection, 1292
  nasal secretions collection, 1290–1291, 1291f
Nasal polyps, 991–998
  aspirin sensitivity-related, 978, 991, 992, 993–995, 1233, 1237
  atopy association, 995
  classification, 992–993, 993b
  clinical features, 992
  cystic fibrosis comorbidity, 995, 995f
  diagnosis, 992, 992f
  differential diagnosis, 996
  eosinophilia, 861
  eosinophils, 996, 997, 997f
  epidemiology, 992
  fungal infection association, 995–996, 996f
  histopathology, 996–997, 997f
  imaging, 992, 993f, 994t
  physical examination, 983
  in pregnancy, 1439
  protease/protease-activated receptor interactions, 431–432
  rhinitis comorbidity, 984
  staging, 993, 994t
  Staphylococcus aureus enterotoxins, 998
  T helper 2 (Th2) cells, 997–998
  treatment, 998, 1237
Nasal provocation testing, 1281–1292
  adenosine, 1287
  air pollutants, 1286–1287
  allergen exposure chambers, 1284–1285
  allergic rhinitis diagnosis, 1282–1283
  capsaicin, 1286
  cellular response evaluation, 1291–1292
  early phase response, 1282
  histamine, 1287
  immunotherapy monitoring, 1282
  irritant stimuli, 1286–1287
  late phase response, 1282
  local delivery systems, 1283–1284, 1284f
  methacholine, 1287
  nasal patency measurements, 1288–1289
    acoustic rhinometry, 1289
    active rhinomanometry, 1288–1289, 1288f
    nasal peak flow, 1288
  nasal secretions evaluation, 1289
    collection methods, 1290–1291, 1291f
    composition/biomarkers, 1289, 1290t
    quantification, 1289
  nasal symptom endpoints, 1287–1288, 1288f
  neuropeptides, 1287
  patient selection, 1283
  pharmacologic studies, 1282
  physical stimuli, 1286
  precautions, 1283
  prior medication discontinuation, 1283, 1283t
  repeated allergen provocations, 1285
  unilateral, 1284f, 1285–1286, 1285f
Nasal pyogenic granuloma gravidarum, 987
Nasal reflexes, 705
Nasal scrapings/brushings, 1292
Nasal swabs/smears, 984, 1000, 1292

Nasal valve, 702, 704, 706, 706f, 974
Nasal venous sinuses, 705, 706
  pharmacology, 710
  spontaneous congestion/decongestion
    (nasal cycle), 707, 708
  sympathetic innervation, 706, 707, 708, 708f
Nasal vestibule, 703, 706, 706f, 974
Natalizumab, 154, 162
National ambient air quality standards (NAAQS),
    496–497, 497t
National Cooperative Inner-City Asthma Study
    (NCICAS), 1480
National Health Interview Survey (NHIS), 718,
    719–720, 1320
National Health and Nutrition Examination
    Survey (NHANES), 718, 739, 740, 743,
    750, 894
Natural antibodies, 790
Natural killer (NK) cells, 9, 26–27, 28f, 168, 191, 1426
  allergic contact dermatitis, 1113
  assay methods, 1262
  asthma, 278, 279, 894
  cytokine/chemokine production, 27, 168, 169
  origins, 4
Natural killer dendritic cells, 342
Natural killer T cells, 173, 191
  allergic contact dermatitis, 1112
  asthma, 448, 458
  cytokines production, 169, 173, 278
Nebulizer solution adverse reactions, 688, 1185
Nebulizers, 679, 680, 684, 686, 686t, 1356,
    1463
  adaptive aerosol delivery, 689–691
  β_2-agonist delivery, 1334, 1337, 1371, 1491t,
    1492, 1494
  breath-actuated, 687, 689
  bronchial challenge testing applications, 1299
  budesonide suspension for young children,
    1582–1583
  cromolyn sodium delivery, 1593, 1597
  delivery performance, 685
  designs for liquid formulations, 687–688
  inhalation with actuation, 687
  metered-dose liquid inhalers, 688–689
  new technologies, 689t, 690f
Nebulizing catheters, 680
Nedocromil sodium, 505, 985, 1127, 1129, 1391
  adverse effects, 1599
  allergic eye disease, 1598
  antiinflammatory effects, 1596
  asthma, 1359
    adults, 1597
    children, 1331, 1332, 1597–1598
    cromolyn sodium comparison, 1598
    dose, 1598
  mechanism of action, 125, 1596
  pharmacology, 1464, 1465, 1591, 1592,
    1593–1594, 1595
  structure, 1592f
Neisseria infection, 101, 103, 104, 106, 109, 1412
Neomycin sensitivity, 1106, 1131
  vaccine adverse reactions, 1196
Neonatal aspiration syndrome, 1401
Neoplastic disease, IgE levels, 853–854
Nephelometry, 1253, 1255, 1260, 1418
Nephritic factor, 100

Nerve growth factor, 231, 262, 302, 335, 466
  biological activities, 171
Nervous system–immune system interactions, 223
Nettle (Urtica) pollen, 520, 521f
Neurogenic inflammation, 223, 227, 433, 466,
    466f, 975, 1519–1520
Neurological diseases, eosinophilia, 872, 872t
Neuromuscular blocking drug allergy, 1206, 1218,
    1219
Neuropeptide Y, 227, 705
Neuropeptides, nasal provocation testing, 1287
Neurotransmission, inflammatory mediators, 465,
    465f
Neurotrophins, 466, 480, 480f, 481f, 482f
Neutralization, 80
Neutralization therapy, 1697
Neutrophil elastase, 26, 286–287, 288, 290, 668
Neutrophilic asthma, 288–293, 291b
  definition, 288, 289f
  pathogenesis, 289–290, 290f
  smoking influence, 292
  treatment, 292–293, 292f, 293b
  triggers, 291, 291b
Neutrophils, 9, 14, 91, 95, 96, 283–293, 1426
  allergic inflammation, 458
  apoptosis, 287, 288, 417
    cell clearance, 26, 29, 287–288
    associated tissue damage, 283, 390–391
  asthma, 666, 908, 923–924
    see also Neutrophilic asthma
  cell adhesion molecules, 152, 153t, 285
  chemoattractants, 22, 92, 182, 186, 285, 377,
    390, 1622
  chemokine expression, 185–186t
  cytokine synthesis, 288
  defensins, 287
  drug allergy (type IVd hypersensitivity), 1213
  FcγRII–immune complex interactions, 789
  food hypersensitivity, 1147
  genetic defects, 1409t
  glucocorticoid responses, 1559
  granules, 283, 284, 390–391
    contents, 20, 21, 26, 283, 284f, 424
  innate immune response, 26
  mediators, 284f, 286–287, 1521, 1620
  migration, 283–286, 284f, 1522
    endothelial cell interactions, 284–285,
      389–390, 390f, 397
    epithelial cell interactions, 285
  muscarinic receptors, 1605
  origins, 4, 283, 284
  pattern recognition receptors, 26, 286
  proteases, 286–287
    protease-activated receptor activation, 424
  reactive oxygen species (ROS) generation, 287,
    390, 391
    endothelial cell damage, 392–393, 392f
  skin inflammatory response, 623
Nevirapine hypersensitivity, 12, 840, 862
Nickel, 1106, 1131
Nicotinamide adenine dinucleotide (phosphate)
    reduced:quinone oxidoreducatse (NQO1)
    polymorphism, 504
Niflumic acid, 673
Nimesulide, 1234, 1236
Ninhydrin protein assays, 566

Nitrate/nitrite additives, 1183
Nitric oxide
  airway smooth muscle effects, 227, 406
  allergic inflammation, 462
  anaphylaxis, 1035
  antimicrobial activity, 384
  endothelial cell functions, 389, 394, 395f
  epithelial cell production, 384
  exercise-induced asthma, 1389
  exhaled
    asthma diagnosis, 1323, 1350
    occupational asthma, 949, 950
    omalizumab response, 1681
    rhinitis diagnosis, 983
  nasal airway, 703
  parasympathetic neurotransmission, 227, 228, 231
  vascular tone regulation, 389
Nitric oxide synthase, 1035
  airway smooth muscle expression, 406
  asthma, 367, 445, 912
    genetic association studies, 899
  endothelial cells production, 389, 394
  epithelial cell expression, 384, 912
Nitrogen dioxide, 498, 499, 749
  asthma epidemiology, 743, 748
  biological effects of exposure, 502
Nitrogen oxides, 495, 496, 1353, 1355
  sources, 498
Nociceptors, airway, 225–226, 227, 229
  cough reflex, 228
NODs, 24, 357, 622
Nodule, eosinophilia, rheumatism, dermatitis
    and swelling (NERDS), 867
Nominal dose (label claim), 685, 685f
Non-allergic rhinitis with eosinophilia syndrome
    (NARES), 861, 978, 986
Non-nucleoside reverse transcriptase inhibitors
    (NNRTIs), hypersensitivity reactions, 840
Non-steroidal antiinflammatory drugs
  allergic eye disease, 1128, 1128t
  aspirin sensitive nasal polyposis/rhinosinusitis,
    994
  asthma improvement, 1237
  eosinophilia stimulation, 862
  hypersensitivity, 1206, 1227–1240, 1353
    avoidance measures, 1356
    classification, 1228
    cross-reactivity, 1229, 1233–1234, 1234t
    diagnosis, 1219
    tolerated drugs, 1234, 1234t
    see also Aspirin-induced asthma
  mode of action, 204
  non-allergic (pseudoallergic) hypersensitivity,
    1215
  non-allergic rhinitis, 978
  urticaria/angioedema, 1066
Nordic skin test, 567
Norepinephrine neurotransmission, 226, 705
Northern blotting, 47
Nose
  anatomy, 702–705, 703f
  blood vessels, 705, 974
  embryology, 702
  functions, 701–702, 974
  innervation, 705, 974–975
  physical examination, 983

Index

Notch signaling, stem cell self-renewal, 265, 267
Nuclear factor of activated T cells (NF-AT), 253, 275, 337
    calcineurin inhibitor effects, 1646–1647
Nuclear factor-κB essential modulator (NEMO) deficiency, 804, 807, 1412, 1416, 1417
Nuclear factor-κB genes, pharmacogenomics, 1639
Nuclear factor-κB signaling pathway, 140, 140f
    allergic inflammation, 467, 488
    asthma, 367, 912
    cytokine production, 253, 275
    dendritic cell survival, 418
    endothelial cells, 392
    isotype switching to IgE synthesis, 119
    mite allergen activation, 606
    T cell activation, 272
    theophylline inhibition, 1506–1507
    therapeutic targeting, 146
    toll-like receptors, 23, 24, 286, 357
Nucleic acid hybridization, 46–48, 52
Nucleoside/nucleotide receptors, 144
Nucleotides, 37
Nucleus
    cell signaling, 130
    receptors, 130, 131
Nucleus tractus solitarius, 224, 229, 230, 231f
Nurses' Health Study, 739, 740
Nutrient supplements, 1699–1700

O

Oak (Fagaceae) pollen, 515–516, 516f
Obesity, 775, 1381–1382
    asthma comorbidity, 740, 740f, 1347, 1360, 1381
Occludin, 375, 603
Occupational allergens, 509, 545, 559, 570, 585–586, 587–590t, 742
    high-molecular weight, 939, 940t
    low-molecular weight, 939, 940t, 941, 977
    prediction of activity, 941, 950
    see also Occupational asthma
Occupational asthma, 585, 903–904, 939–953, 1352
    airway pathology, 942–943, 943f
    allergen avoidance, 950, 1355–1356, 1447
    allergens, 742, 1352–1353
        food/drug additives, 1171, 1177, 1184
        high-molecular weight, 939, 940t, 951–952
        low-molecular weight, 939, 940t, 952–953
        Permissible Exposure Limits, 944, 950
        prediction of activity, 941, 950
        sensitization potency, 941
        structure, 940–941
    atopy associations, 944
    clinical investigation, 947–950, 948f
        history, 948–949
        immunological tests, 949
        inhalation challenge tests, 949, 1300, 1305, 1306
        non-invasive airway inflammation detection, 949–950

Occupational asthma (Continued)
        serial non-specific bronchial hyper-responsiveness measurements, 949
        serial peak expiratory flow measurements, 949
    definition, 742, 939–940
    epidemiology, 943–944, 945–946t
    exposure-related risk, 944
    genetic factors, 944, 947
    medicolegal aspects, 950
    natural history, 947, 947f
    pathogenesis, 940–941
        immunological, 941, 942
        non-immunological, 941–942
        role of adjuvant exposure, 942
    pre-empolyment surveillance, 951
    prevention, 950–951
    rhinoconjunctivitis association, 944, 948
    risk factors, 742–743, 944
    social impact, 950
Occupational contact dermatitis, 1105, 1154
Occupational exposure-related cough, 1399–1400
Occupational rhinitis, 973, 977
Ocular cicatricial pemphigoid, 1131, 1132t
Odorant sampling, 705, 974
Okasaki fragments, 42
Older sibling effects, 711, 770, 776, 976
Olfactory area, 705
Olfactory mucosa, 705, 974
Olfactory nerve, 705, 974
Olfactory tests, rhinitis diagnosis, 984
Olive (Oleaceae) pollen, 517, 571
Olopatadine, 1127, 1128, 1129, 1525, 1541
Omalizumab, 457, 986, 1079, 1099, 1679–1687
    allergic rhinitis, 1684, 1684t
    asthma, 1333, 1359, 1361, 1682–1684, 1684t
    atopic dermatitis, 1685
    dose, 1248, 1686, 1686t
    food allergy, 1684–1685, 1685t
    IgE complex formation, 1679–1680, 1681f
    immunotherapy combination, 1673, 1684–1685
    mechanisms of actions, 1680–1682, 1682f, 1683t
    safety, 1686–1687
    structure, 1679, 1681f
Omenn syndrome, 147, 804, 875
Oomycete allergens, 528
Opsonins/opsonization, 9, 15, 22, 23, 80
    complement system functions, 90, 91, 93, 96
    skin inflammatory response, 622, 623
Optic nerve, 1119
Orai1 (CRACM1), 243, 814
Oral allergy syndrome, 571, 591, 977, 1150–1151
    allergens, 426, 1150
    immunotherapy, 1661
Oral contraception, 776, 777
Oral drug formulations, 1463, 1464
Oral food challenge testing, 1140, 1158–1159, 1309–1316
    data collection, 1312, 1313f
    dosing strategies, 1313–1314, 1314t
    indications, 1309–1310, 1310f
    methods, 1310–1314, 1311t
    reactions, 1314, 1315t

Oral food challenge testing (Continued)
        treatment, 1315–1316
    research applications, 1310
    risk reduction, 1314–1316t
    risk–benefit considerations, 1310, 1312
Oral tolerance induction, 1142–1143
Orbicularis oculi, 1118
Orbicules (Ubisch bodies), 571
Orbital anatomy, 1117
Organochlorides, 776
ORMDL3, asthma associations, 70, 70f
Osteoblastic stem cell niche, 265, 266f, 267
Osteoporosis
    glucocorticoid-related, 1553, 1554, 1585–1586, 1587–1588, 1635
        prophylaxis, 1357, 1359
    mastocytosis, 1056, 1060
    treatment, 1586
Otitis media, 984, 1411, 1417, 1535
Outdoor air pollutants see Air pollutants
Outdoor allergens, 509–536
    algae, 535–536
    analytic methods, 511–512, 512t
    assay methods, 1261
    childhood sensitization, 779, 780, 780f
    determinants of clinical significance, 509–510
    fungi see Fungal allergens
    particle size, 509–510
    pollen see Pollen
    sampling devices, 510–511, 510t
    sources, 509, 570
    see also Aeroallergens
Ovalbumin, 438, 439
Oxidative stress, 462
    particulate air pollutant exposure, 503–504, 504f
Oxitropium bromide, 671, 672, 1604
Oxygen therapy, 1371, 1435
Oxymetazoline, 978, 1439
Oxytocin allergy, 1442
Ozone, 495, 496, 506, 701, 776, 942, 1353
    asthma epidemiology, 743, 748
    biological effects of exposure, 502–503
    nasal provocation testing, 1286
    sources, 498, 498f

P

P-particles, 571
P-selectin, 150, 160, 162
    leukocyte adhesion/transmigration, 158, 284, 285, 389, 619
    ligands, 151
P-selectin glycoprotein ligand-1 (PSGL-1; CD162), 151
Pachycondyla (Asian ant), 1008
Pancreatic supplement enzymes, 585
Papain, 1184
Papular urticaria, 1067
Parabens, 1182–1183
Paragonimus, 869
Parainfluenza virus, 740, 1321, 1347, 1396
Parallel-line bioassay, 564, 565f
Paranasal sinuses, 703, 703f, 975, 999
    development, 702
Paraphenylenediamine (PPD), 1107

Index

INDEX

Phospholipase C, 136, 183, 401, 415
  FcεRI signaling, 239, 240, 241–242
  muscarinic M3 receptor signaling, 1604
  protease-activated receptor signaling, 425
Phospholipase C family, 241
Phospholipase D, 136, 141
  FcεRI signaling, 239, 245–246
  histamine H1 receptor signaling, 1519
Phospholipases, signal transduction, 136
Phospholipids, cell signaling, 133, 136, 137f
Phosphoprotein phosphatases, 132
Phosphorylation events
  FcεRI signaling, 239
  gene transcription regulation, 138, 139f,
    140–141, 140f
  intracellular signaling, 132, 132f, 184
    cyclic AMP, 135–136
Photochemical smog, 498
Photocontact dermatitis, 1105, 1106–1107
Photodermatitis, drug hypersensitivity in
    HIV-infected patients, 840
Pigweed pollen, 518–519
Pimecrolimus, 1645–1647
  atopic dermatitis, 1648
Pirbuterol, 1356, 1371, 1486, 1487f
Pityrosporum ovale, 853, 1086, 1087, 1088
Plague vaccine, 1199
Plakoglobin, 375, 605
Plakophilin, 1, 375
Plant pathogenesis-related proteins, 575,
    578t
Plantain (Plantago) pollen, 512, 513, 520–521,
    521f
Plaque proteins, 375
Plasma cells, 74, 76
Plasma membrane, 130
  microdomains, 130
    signaling mechanisms, 141, 142f
  receptors, 130, 131
Plasmid vectors, 48–49
  eukaryote (shuttle vectors), 50
Plasmids, 48
Platelet-activating factor (PAF), 14, 389, 390,
    460, 1033
  eosinophil production/responses, 299, 300,
    457–458
Platelet-activating factor acetylhydrolase, 204,
    204t
Platelet-activating factor receptor (PAFR), 298,
    332
Platelet-derived growth factor (PDGF), 389, 402,
    404, 408
Platelet-endothalial cell adhesion molecule-1
    (PECAM-1), 155–156, 285
Platelets, 150, 424, 459, 1520, 1521
  aspirin hypersensitivity, 1229
Plectomycete allergens, 526
Plesthysmography, 1326
  aiway resistance measurement, 649–650, 653f
  lung volume measurement, 648, 649
  specific conductance measurement, 649, 650,
    653f
Pleural eosinophilia, 871
Plodia interpunctella (Indian meal moth) allergens,
    585, 586t
Pneumococcal vaccine, 1194, 1425, 1433

Pneumocystis carinii, 1412
Pneumonia, 1397, 1411
Poaceae, occupational aeroallergens, 586,
    589–590t
Pogonomyrmex (harvester ant), 1008
Poison ivy/poison oak, 15, 1106
Polio vaccine, oral, 1191
Polistes, 1005, 1006
  venom, 592, 1008
    immunotherapy, 1012
    skin tests, 1010
Pollen, 509, 510, 551, 570–575
  allergens, 342, 512–522
    content variation, 558, 560t
    extracts, 558, 559t, 1665, 1665b
    pathogenesis-related proteins, 575, 578t
    protease-activated receptor activation, 426
    structure, 597, 600t
    submicronic particles, 570–571
  allergic conjunctivitis, 1120
  allergic rhinitis, 973, 976
  challenge tests, 1284–1285, 1301
  childhood sensitization, 780, 1327
  collection methods, 558, 1261
  cross-reactivity syndromes, 591, 595t, 1150
  exposure outside North America, 522
  immunotherapy, 1657, 1658, 1665, 1665b
  microscopic examination, 511–512
  morphology, 512–513
  North American floristic zones, 522, 523f, 524t
  particle size, 570
  plants of regional importance, 521–522
  proteins, 572, 574–575, 577t
  proteomics, 572
  sample analysis, 511
  sampling devices, 510–511, 510t
  storage, 558
  see also Grass pollen; Tree pollen; Weed pollen
    and specific species
Pollen tube growth, 571, 574
Poly-A tail, 39, 43
Polyclonal antibodies, 84
Polymerase chain reaction, 47–48, 48f, 52
Poplar (Populus) pollen, 512, 518, 518f
Positional cloning, asthma-related genes, 61, 62,
    63t, 444
Postinfectious cough, 1395, 1397–1398
Postprandial syndromes (restaurant syndromes),
    1039
Poststreptococcal glomerulonephritis, 797
Potassium ion channels, mast cells, 244
Potency, drug, 1461
Pranlukast, 143, 144, 215, 1231, 1236
  pharmacology, 1621, 1623, 1625
Prausnitz-Küstner (P-K) reaction, 845, 1139, 1179
Pre-B cells, 6, 74, 82, 192
Precipitin reaction, 1252, 1252f, 1261
Prednisolone, 1337, 1549
Prednisone, 866, 966, 968, 969, 1010, 1078, 1337,
    1549
  acute asthma
    adults, 1575–1576
    children, 1576
Pregnancy, 1423–1442
  allergen avoidance, 1427
  anaphylaxis, 1439–1441

Pregnancy (Continued)
  differential diagnosis, 1440
  prevention, 1440
  treatment, 1440–1441
  angioedema, 1441
  asthma, 1362, 1423, 1433–1438
    acute management, 1435–1436, 1437f
    adverse perinatal outcome associations, 1433,
      1434t
    chronic management, 1435, 1436b
    effects of pregnancy on symptoms,
      1433–1435
    effects on pregnancy outcome, 1433
    fetal hypoxia, 1424
    fetal monitoring, 1438
    labor/delivery management, 1438
    medication safety, 1428, 1429–1432t, 1438,
      1543
  atopic dermatitis, 1441–1442
  drug allergy, 1442
  fetal oxygenation determinants, 1424
  immunization responses, 1425
  immunotherapy, 1427, 1669
  non-infectious ear symptoms, 1439
  pharmacologic therapy, 1427–1433
    teratogenesis, 1427–1428
  pruritic conditions, 1441, 1442
  psychologic management, 1426–1427
  respiratory physiologic changes, 1423–1424
  response to infection, 1425–1426
  rhinitis, 986–987, 987f, 1438–1439
  serum immunoglobulin levels, 1424–1425
  sinusitis, 1438, 1439
  urticaria, 1441
Premature birth
  asthma associations, 742, 744–747t, 777
  pulmonary sequelae, 742
Pressure urticaria, 1071–1072
Pressurized metered-dose inhalers
  see Metered-dose inhalers
Prevalence/prevalence rate, 715, 716
Prevention of Early Asthma in Kids (PEAK),
    755, 1579
Prevention and Incidence of Asthma and Mite
    Allergy (PIAMA), 748, 784, 1454–1455
Primaquine-sensitive anemia, 1216
Primary Prevention of Asthma in Children
    (PREVASC) study, 1454
Pro-B cells, 82, 192
Probiotics, 784, 1099, 1143
Profilins, 574, 590, 591, 1147
Progesterone-in-oil allergy, 1442
Progesterone-related anaphylaxis, 1040
Progressive multifocal leukoencephalitis, 162
Promethazine, 1537
Promoter, 38
  transcription complex interaction, 42
Properidin, 10, 89, 92, 96
  deficiency, 101, 103, 109, 825
Propylene glycol, 1185
Propyphenazone, 1240
Prostaglandin D2, 204, 205, 206–208, 460, 980,
    1064
  allergic inflammation, 207–208
  dendritic cell migration, 346
  mast cell/basophil release, 236, 311, 322

Recurrent infections *(Continued)*
  screening laboratory tests, 1418–1420
  sites of infection, 1411
Recurrent laryngeal nerves, 224
Reflex bronchospasm, 227, 228
  central neuronal changes, 230
Reflex pathways, airway, 228–229, 229f
  allergy-related up-regulation, 228, 228f
Regulators of G protein signaling (RGS)
      proteins, 189
Regulatory T cells, 13, 14t, 169, 175, 175t, 273,
      981
  allergic contact dermatitis, 1113
  asthma, 279–280, 448–449, 459, 478, 907
  atopic dermatitis, 1089
  cutaneous immune response modulation, 625
  cytokine production, 172t
  cytokines involved in differentiation, 174t
  dendritic cell interactions, 346, 348, 349–350
  food allergen tolerance induction, 1142
  glucocorticoid responses, 1561–1562
  immunotherapy responses, 1664
  indoleamine 2,3-dioxygenase expression, 307
  nasal polyposis, 997
Rel, 119, 140
Remote practice, 1705
Renal disease, eosinophilia, 874–875
Replicon, 50
Reslizumab, 997
Respimat, 691
Respiratory cycle, mechanoreceptor activity, 225,
      226f
Respiratory epithelium, 373–374, 374f
  airway remodeling, 912, 912f
  asthma
    basement membrane thickening, 925–927,
        928f
    damage/desquamation, 376, 462–463,
        894–895, 896f, 897f, 909, 924, 925f,
        926f, 941
    fibrosis, 463
    irritant-induced, 941
    submucosal gland enlargement, 927
  barrier function, 380–381
  basal cell extracellular matrix binding, 375
  ciliated cells, 373
  desmosomes, 374, 375
  gap junctions, 375–376
  goblet cells, 373
  hemidesmosomes, 375
  intermediate junctions, 374, 375
  leukocyte transmigration, 379
  mucociliary clearance, 380–381
  nasal cavity, 704
  tight junctions, 374–375, 374f, 375f
  see also Airway epithelial cells; Epithelial cells
Respiratory food hypersensitivity reactions, 1147,
      1154–1156, 1155t
Respiratory irritants, asthma associations, 1353,
      1355
Respiratory syncytial virus, 383, 851, 1275, 1396,
      1398
  asthma
    exacerbation, 291
    risk associations, 740, 741, 773, 900, 902f,
        1321, 1347

Respiratory syncytial virus *(Continued)*
    secondary prevention, 1339
  montelukast treatment, 1625
  mucin gene expression induction, 668
Restriction endonucleases, 44, 45t, 48, 49
  cleavage sites, 44, 46f
Restriction fragment length polymorphism
      (RFLP), 52–53
Restriction maps, 44
Reticular dysgenesis, 823
Retina, 1119
Retroviral vectors, 50, 51
Rett syndrome, 56
Revatropate, 1608
Rheumatoid arthritis, 15, 93, 103, 325
  therapeutic targets, 146, 156
Rhinitis, 973
  allergic *see* Allergic rhinitis
  anticholinergic agents, 1614
  atrophic, 978–979, 979f
  comorbidity, 984
  diagnosis, 982–984
  differential diagnosis, 983t
  drug-induced, 978, 978t
  food/drug additive reactions, 1179, 1181, 1182
  history-taking, 982, 983t
  idiopathic, 978
  imaging, 984, 984f
  inflammatory, 977–978
  investigation, 983
  mucociliary clearance assessment, 983
  nasal hyperresponsiveness, 975
  non-allergic, 977–979
    causes, 977t
    treatment, 985f
  non-inflammatory, 978–979
  olfactory tests, 984
  physical examination, 983
  in pregnancy, 986–987, 1438–1439
  rhinosinusitis comorbidity, 999
  socioeconomic impact, 979
Rhinitis medicamentosa, 710, 978, 985, 1438,
      1439
Rhinomanometry, nasal patency evaluation, 707,
      983, 1288–1289
  anterior, 1289
  posterior, 1288, 1288f
Rhinosinusitis, 431–432, 998–1002
  acute, 998, 999
  allergic fungal, 996
  anatomical considerations, 999
  aspirin hypersensitivity, 1232, 1236–1237
  asthma comorbidity, 999–1000, 1360
  chronic, 991, 998–1002
    definition, 999
    diagnosis, 1000, 1001f
    differential diagnosis, 1000, 1000b
    imaging, 1000, 1000f
    pathophysiology, 1000–1001, 1001f, 1002f
    symptoms, 999, 999b
  classification, 999
  clinical features, 999, 1396, 1398
  complications, 1001
  microbiology, 1000
  prevalence, 999
  treatment, 1001–1002

Rhinovirus, 740, 741, 851, 1535
  asthma
    aspirin-induced, 1229
    exacerbation, 291, 1353
    risk associations, 900, 901, 902, 903, 1321
  mucin gene expression induction, 668
Rhizopus, 526, 528, 531, 535, 558, 996
Rho, 135, 136, 143, 184
  airway smooth muscle signaling, 401, 404
  cytoskeleton regulation, 246
  protease-activated receptor signaling, 425
Rhodosporidium, 527
Ribosomal RNA (rRNA), 38, 40
Ribosomes, 38, 39, 40, 41
Rice allergy, 1151
Rifampicin, 862
Rituximab, 798, 962
RNA, 38, 39t
  post-transcriptional processing, 43
  primary transcripts, 39
  splicing, 39, 43, 73, 84
RNA hybridization assays, 47
RNA interference/silencing, 55, 56f
RNA polymerase, 38, 39, 42
RNA-induced silencing complex (RISC), 55
Rodent allergens, 545, 547, 548, 559, 560, 1261
  environmental control, 1333
  quantitative measurement, 1262
Rofecoxib, 994, 1234
Roflumilast, 1513
Rolipram, 407
RORγt, Th17 lymphocyte differentiation
      regulation, 175, 275
Rotavirus vaccine, 1191
Rotorod samplers, 510, 511, 531, 1261
Rupatadine, 1524, 1525
Russian thistle *(Salsola kali)* pollen, 519, 522
RWJ-56110, 433

S

S-protein, 98
Saccharomyces, 526, 535
Sagebrush *(Artemisia tridentata)* pollen, 520, 520f
Salbutamol *see* Albuterol
Salicylsulfapyridine, 862
Salmeterol, 337, 406, 407, 691, 1357, 1391, 1635
  β₂-adrenoreceptor desensitization, 1495
  childhood asthma, 1331, 1332
  fluticasone combined treatment, 1378
  inhaled glucocorticoid reduction study,
      1496–1497
  masking of airway inflammation, 1498–1499
  monotherapy, 1496, 1498
  pharmacogenomics, 67, 68t, 1637, 1637f
  pharmacology, 1461, 1462, 1464, 1486, 1487f,
      1489
  safety, 1332, 1358, 1497
  theophylline comparisons, 1498
Salmeterol +/- Inhaled glucocorticoids (SLIC),
      1496–1497
Salmeterol or glucocorticoids Study (SOCS),
      1496
Salmeterol Multi-center Asthma trial (SMART),
      1358
Saltbush *(Atriplex)* pollen, 519, 519f

Index

Index

Thrombin, protease-activated receptor activation, 424, 426, 428
Thrombocytopenia, 15
Thrombopoietin, 262
Thrombospondin, 617
Thromboxane A_2, 204, 211–212, 402
  role in allergic inflammation, 212
Thromboxane A_2 receptor (TP), 211–212, 211t
Thromboxane B_2, 211
Thromboxane synthase, 211
Thromboxanes, 136
  eosinophil production, 299, 300
Thymic stromal lymphopoietin, 384, 450, 906
  asthma/inflammation pathogenesis, 350, 461, 461f
  dendritic cell activation, 384
  Th2 cell differentiation induction, 173, 174
Thymoma-related immunodeficiency, 823
Thymus, T cell maturation, 4, 5, 6, 13
Thymus-dependent antigen B cell activation, 74
Thymus-independent antigen B cell activation, 74
Thyrotropin receptor, autoantibody reactions, 15–16
Tight junctions (zonula occludens), 374–375, 374f, 375f, 603
  allergen protease cleavage, 603, 605t
  epidermis, 613
  proteins, 375
  structure, 603, 604f
  viral receptor components, 381
TIM-1, asthma associations, 444
TIMs (T-cell immunoglobulin and mucin-containing molecules), 444, 774
Tiotropium bromide, 672, 1359, 1402, 1612, 1613, 1614
  pharmacology, 1608, 1611
Tissue inhibitor of metalloproteinase 1 (TIMP-1), 287, 290, 369, 380, 640
TLR1, 24, 26, 286, 332
TLR2, 20, 25, 26, 123, 125, 286, 332, 336
  activation pathway, 24
  epithelial cell expression, 381
  neutrophilic asthma, 289
  pathogen recognition, 357
  peptidoglycan/lipoprotein ligands, 24
  stimulation-mediated vitamin D metabolism, 21
TLR3, 24
  activation pathway, 24
  epithelial cell respiratory virus responses, 381, 382f
TLR4, 20, 23–24, 25, 26, 123, 125, 166, 286, 332, 336
  activation pathway, 24
  endotoxin (lipopolysaccharide) interactions, 20, 21f, 23, 31, 291, 357, 359f
  enhancer proteins, 23
  epithelial cell expression, 381
  genetic polymorphism, 357, 363
  Gram-negative bacteria recognition, 357
  neutrophilic asthma, 289, 291
TLR5, 24, 381
TLR6, 24, 26, 286, 332
TLR7, 24, 26, 168, 344

TLR8, 24
TLR9, 24, 26, 32, 125, 168, 332, 336, 344, 357, 364, 552, 1651
TLRs (toll-like receptors), 20, 23–24, 24t, 125, 166, 286, 357
  activation/signaling pathway, 24, 145, 357, 361f
  airway epithelial cells, 26
  allergen ligands, 30
  associated detection-enhancing proteins, 20
  basophils, 332, 336
  dendritic cells, 26, 27, 344, 348, 418
  epithelial cells, 381
  ligand exposure
    allergy, 30–31, 144–145
    epidemiological studies, 31–32
  macrophages, 357, 360t
  mast cells, 26, 324
  natural killer cells, 26
  neutrophils, 286
  skin, 622
Tobacco smoke exposure, 750, 854, 1399, 1557
  asthma associations, 65, 749–750, 754, 755–756, 776, 783, 1340, 1347, 1353, 1379, 1410
    active smoking, 749, 755–756, 944
    childhood exposure, 65–66
    intrauterine exposure, 65, 750
    neutrophilic asthma, 292
    occupational asthma, 944
    passive smoking, 65–66, 750, 783
  atopy associations, 783, 1410
  biomarkers, 750
  childhood infection risk associations, 1410
  environmental control, 506, 1333
  genetic factor interactions, 1640
  IgE levels, 854
  indoor air quality, 498–499
    biological effects, 502, 504
  nasal provocation testing, 1286
  oxidative stress, 503
  in pregnancy, 504, 645, 750, 783, 1427
    transient early wheezing in infant, 1320–1321
  secondhand smoke, 750, 854
  smoking cessation programs, 1356, 1379
Tolerance
  drug, 1468–1469
  immune, 3, 13, 349
Toll-like receptors see TLRs
Topoisomerases, 42
Total lung capacity (TLC), 648, 649, 1424
Tourette's syndrome, 1401
Toxic oil syndrome, 873
Toxic shock, 167
Toxocara, 863, 1067
Toxoplasma gondii, 774
TP (thromboxane A_2 receptor), 211–212, 211t
Tr1 lymphocytes, 175, 175t, 176
Traditional Chinese herbal therapy, 1099
Traffic exposure, asthma associations, 500
Traffic-Related Air Pollution and Childhood Asthma (TRAPCA), 748
TRAIL, 27, 625
TRAIL receptors, 416, 417

Tranexamic acid, 1074, 1441
Transcortin, 1550
Transcription, 38–39
  complex assembly, 42, 43f
  gene expression regulation, 42–43, 43f
  histone modification, 141
  protein phosphorylation in regulation, 138, 140–141
Transcription factors, 42, 43f, 130
  allergic inflammation pathogenesis, 466–467, 467f, 488–490, 489f
  glucocorticoid receptor interactions, 1555, 1556–1557
  phosphorylation, 136, 138
  therapeutic targets, 146
Transfer RNA (tRNA), 38, 40, 41
Transferrin receptor (CD71), 81
Transforming growth factor α, 379
Transforming growth factor β, 13, 84, 171–172, 175, 176, 265
  airway remodeling/subepithelial fibrosis, 291, 292, 379, 638, 912, 913
  biological activities, 29, 171–172
Transgenic mice
  asthma models, 443
  gene function studies, 53
Transient early wheezing, 1319, 1320–1321
Transient hypogammaglobulinemia of infancy, 823
Transient neonatal immunodeficiency, 116
Transient receptor potential vanilloid 1 (TRPV1), 1395
  airway nociceptor signaling regulation, 226
Translation, 40–41
Transplant rejection, 875
Travel, asthma management, 1362–1363
Tree nut allergy, 560, 759, 1141, 1151, 1152, 1161, 1162
  allergens, 590, 593t, 1146
  anaphylaxis, 1047, 1156
Tree pollen, 513–518, 522, 551, 570, 976
  allergens, 571–572, 575t
    extract sources, 558, 559t
  genera/species, 514t
  proteomics, 574
Trefoil factor peptides, 444, 661, 662
  mucin gene interactions, 662
Tregs see Regulatory T cells
Tri r 2, 546
Triamcinolone, 146, 691, 1331
  clinical pharmacology, 1553, 1577, 1578t
  Salmeterol or glucocorticoids Study (SOCS), 1496
Triatoma (kissing bug) allergens/allergic reactions, 592, 597t, 853, 1015
Triazolam, 862
Trichoderma, 526, 528, 535
Trichophyton, 526, 546, 576, 853, 1086, 1087
  allergens, 580t
Trichuris trichiura, 853
Trigeminal nerve, nasal innervation, 705, 974, 975
Trimethoprim–sulfamethoxazole, 962, 1439
  desensitization therapy, 1221
  hypersensitivity reactions, 840, 842
Troleandomycin, 1552

Trombicula (chiggers), 853
Tropical house mite species, 541
Tropical pulmonary eosinophilia, 849, 869–870
Trp channels, mast cells, 244–245
Trypsin, protease-activated receptor activation,
424, 424f, 426, 431
gastrointestinal disease, 432
Tryptase (mast cell tryptase), 332, 402, 456
allergic rhinitis, 980
anaphylaxis, 323, 432, 1031, 1032, 1033, 1035,
1036, 1041
endothelial permeability effects, 389
mast cell production, 312, 313, 320, 321, 618
mastocytosis, 1053, 1059
protease-activated receptor activation, 423, 426,
428, 431
skin disease, 432
serum level measurement, 1041, 1260
Tuberculosis, 1398–1399, 1425
Tumor necrosis factor receptor superfamily, 116
Tumor necrosis factor receptors, 166, 417, 1108
gene mutations, 1413
Tumor necrosis factor-α, 166–167, 273, 302, 401
biological activation, 166–167
cell adhesion molecule expression stimulation,
160
gene *(TNF)*, asthma associations, 64, 737, 899
mast cell production, 26, 322–323
Tumor necrosis factor-α converting enzyme
(TACE), 166
Tumor necrosis factor-α inhibitors, 167, 1654
asthma, 641
Tumor-associated eosinophilia, 867
Turbinates, 702, 703, 706, 706f, 974
Twin studies
airway hyperresponsiveness, 910
asthma, 61, 735, 737
Typhoid vaccine adverse reactions, 1197
Tyrophagus, 583, 584
Tyrosine kinases, 74, 138
gene transcription regulation, 138

U

Ubiquitinylation, signal transduction, 141
FcεRI signaling, 250
Ulcerative colitis, 872
Ultrasonic nebulizers, 688
Unconventional therapies, 1700–1705, 1706t
Undifferentiated somatoform anaphylaxis, 1039,
1040
Unproven methods, 1691
diagnostic tests, 1692–1695
treatments, 1697–1699
Upper airway cough syndrome, 1396, 1402
Uracil-DNA glycosylase deficiency, 818
Ureaplasma urealyticum infection, 1412, 1418
Urticaceae pollen, 512, 520, 521f, 571
Urticaria, 625, 1063–1079
acute, 1535–1536
anaphylaxis, 1033, 1035, 1036
antihistamines, 1535–1536
aquagenic, 1073
aspirin hypersensitivity, 1228, 1237–1239,
1238f, 1239f
genetic factors, 1238

Urticaria *(Continued)*
causes, 1065–1067
cholinergic, 1070–1071
chronic, 1536, 1536f
autoimmune, 1077
idiopathic, 1040, 1075–1077, 1076f, 1077f
treatment, 1078
clinical features, 1063, 1238, 1238f
cold, 1067–1070, 1068f
familial, 1073
contact, 1106
drug hypersensitivity, 1206, 1212, 1212t
HIV-infected patients, 840
evaluation, 1067, 1068t
food hypersensitivity, 1147, 1152–1153
food/drug additive reactions, 1171, 1175, 1176,
1181, 1182, 1183, 1184
challenge studies, 1171–1173
sulfites, 1179
heat, 1070–1071, 1071f
hereditary forms, 1073–1075
mediator pathways, 1063–1065, 1064t
physical, 1067–1073
in pregnancy, 1441
pressure-induced, 1071–1072
protease-activated receptor activation, 433
solar, 1072–1073
vaccine reactions, 1193, 1194
vasculitis association, 1078
Urticaria pigmentosa (cutaneous mastocytosis),
323, 1053, 1054f, 1055, 1058, 1067
Urushiol, 1106
Uvea, 1119
Uveitis, 1132t, 1134

V

V (variable region) gene rearrangements
immunoglobuin heavy/light chains, 7, 276
T cell receptor, 5
Vaccination
atopic/allergic disease association studies, 774,
783, 1199
biological agents used as weapons, 1198–1199
during pregnancy, 1425, 1433
immunocompromised recipients, 1200
impact on infectious diseases, 1189, 1190t
interval following immunoglobulin-containing
products, 1200, 1201t
risk–benefit considerations, 1190–1191
theoretical evolution of programs, 1190,
1190f
Vaccine Adverse Event Reporting System
(VAERS), 1189, 1191
Vaccine adverse reactions, 1189–1201
anaphylaxis, 1191
egg allergic recipients, 1192
evaluation approach, 1195–1196, 1195f
gelatin additive reactions, 1191–1192, 1194
IgE-mediated, 1191–1196
immunodeficiency disorders association, 1414,
1414t
latex-allergic recipients, 1192–1193
monitoring, 1191
non-IgE-mediated, 1196–1198
rarity, 1189

Vaccine adverse reactions *(Continued)*
to specific vaccines, 1193–1196
yeast protein sensitivity, 1193
Vaccine egg content, 1193b
Vaccine gelatin content, 1192b
Vaccine Safety Datalink (VSD), 1191
Vaccine-associated paralytic poliomyelitis,
1191
Vaccinia immunoglobulin, 1199
Vaccinia vaccination, 1198–1199
Vacuum collection, pollen, 558
Vagotomy, asthma treatment, 1610–1611
Vagus nerve, 229, 1605, 1606
airway hyperresponsiveness, 1603, 1611
airway innervation, 224, 225
asthma involvement, 1610–1611
cough regulation, 228, 1395, 1396
reflex bronchoconstriction, 1610
Valved holding chambers, 693, 694–695, 1490,
1491t, 1492
VAMPs, 252, 306
Variable number tandem repeats (VNTRs;
microsatellites), 1634
Varicella
immune response in pregnancy, 1425
vaccine reactions, 1194, 1197
to gelatin additive, 1191
Vascular changes, airway inflammation, 464, 464f,
646
glucocorticoid effects, 1564
Vascular endothelial growth factor (VEGF), 379,
389, 395
airway remodeling, 292
glucocorticoid effects, 1564
Vascular stem cell niche, 265, 267
Vascular tone regulation, 389
Vasculitis, 795–796, 796f
Churg-Strauss syndrome, 963
complement component deficiencies, 1413
cutaneous necrotizing eosinophilic, 868, 874
eosinophilia, 873–874
eosinophilic colitis, 887
gastric eosinophil infiltration, 886
urticaria association, 1078
Wegener's granulomatosis, 958
Vasculogenesis, 395
Vasoactive intestinal peptide (VIP), 226, 227, 231,
466, 705, 930
Vasoconstrictors, allergic eye disease, 1127, 1128t
Vasopressin, 1045
VCAM-1 (vascular cell adhesion molecule-1),
155, 160, 161, 162, 167, 170, 267, 397, 405,
931
leukocyte adhesion/barrier transmigration, 158,
190, 297, 298, 330, 389, 619
mast cell trafficking, 316
V(D)J gene rearrangements, 82–84, 83f, 276
Vegetable allergy, 1152, 1155
allergens, 591, 1147
Velocardial facial syndrome, 1414
Vernal keratoconjunctivitis, 1120t, 1121t,
1124–1125, 1124f
diagnosis, 1126
treatment, 1130
Vertigo, 1537
Very low birth weight, asthma associations, 742